Ebola
Scientific Abstracts

This collection includes the abstracts of articles published on the topic of Ebola Virus.

1. J Biomol Struct Dyn. 2015 Mar;33(3):461-470. Epub 2014 Nov 26.

Ebola virus envelope glycoprotein derived peptide in human Furin-bound state: computational studies.

Omotuyi IO(1).

Author information: (1)a Department of Pharmacology and Therapeutic Innovation , Graduate School of Biomedical Science, Nagasaki University , Nagasaki , Japan.

Ebola virus (EboV) is currently ravaging West Africa with estimated case fatality rate of 52%. Currently, no drug treatment is available and immunoglobulin therapy is still at the rudimentary stage. For anti-EboV drug development, druggable viral and host protein targets, including human Furin are under intense investigation. Here, molecular dynamics simulation was performed on Apo-Furin, meta-guanidinomethyl-Phac-RVR-Amba-bound, and two EboV glycoprotein (GP) 494-TGGRRTRREA-503/Furin complexes (Accurate and one amino acid shift alignment). The results of the simulation established ligand-induced desolvation of Furin active site and structural compactness. Accurately aligned EboV-GP peptide exhibited a tighter binding mode with Furin and showed 1.5- and 3.0-fold MMPBSA binding free energy estimate compared with the displaced peptide and inhibitor, respectively. The difference in free energy was traced to the difference in contribution of threonine residues of the peptides. Furthermore, Furin subsites I conferred substrate specificity and ligand binding accuracy. Accurately aligned peptide trapped active site His194 side chain into gauche (-) (+60(o)) χ1-dihedral compared with gauche+ (-60(o)) in other biosystems while Asp153 is trapped in gauche+ (-60(o)) in ligand bound not Apo state. Ramachandran plot showed that the scissile Arg8 of the accurately aligned peptide showed β conformation distribution as apposed to 310R, αL, and 310L. Finally, the active site proximal Na(+) binding is dependent on substrate peptide occupancy of the active site but detaches in the absence of a ligand. In conclusion, Furin might represent candidate drug target for Ebola virus disease treatment via therapeutic target of the active site and Na(+) binding pocket.

PMID: 25347780 [PubMed - as supplied by publisher]

2. Int J Cardiol. 2015 Jan 20;179:325. doi: 10.1016/j.ijcard.2014.11.092. Epub 2014 Nov 11.

Ebola therapy: Developing new drugs or repurposing old ones?

Lentini G(1), Habtemariam S(2).

Author information: (1)Dipartimento di Farmacia-Scienze del Farmaco, Università degli Studi di Bari Aldo Moro, via E. Orabona 4, 70126 Bari, Italy. Electronic address: giovanni.lentini@uniba.it. (2)Pharmacognosy Research Laboratories, Medway School of Science, University of Greenwich, Chatham-Maritime, Kent ME4 4TB, UK.

PMID: 25464477 [PubMed - in process]

3. Proc Biol Sci. 2015 Jan 7;282(1798). pii: 20142124.

Ecological dynamics of emerging bat virus spillover.

Plowright RK(1), Eby P(2), Hudson PJ(3), Smith IL(4), Westcott D(5), Bryden WL(6), Middleton D(4), Reid PA(7), McFarlane RA(8), Martin G(9), Tabor GM(10), Skerratt LF(9), Anderson DL(6), Crameri G(4), Quammen D(11), Jordan D(12), Freeman P(12), Wang LF(13), Epstein JH(14), Marsh GA(4), Kung NY(15), McCallum H(16).

Author information: (1)Department of Microbiology and Immunology, Montana State University, Bozeman, MT 59717, USA Center for Infectious Disease Dynamics, Pennsylvania State University, State College, PA, USA raina.plowright@montana.edu. (2)School of Biological, Earth and Environmental Sciences, University of New South Wales, Sydney, New South Wales 2052, Australia. (3)Center for Infectious Disease Dynamics, Pennsylvania State University, State College, PA, USA. (4)New and Emerging Zoonotic Diseases, CSIRO, Australian Animal Health Laboratory, East Geelong, Victoria 3220, Australia. (5)CSIRO Ecosystem Sciences and Tropical Environment and Sustainability Sciences, James Cook University, Atherton, Queensland 4883, Australia. (6)Equine Research Unit, School of Agriculture and Food Sciences, University of Queensland, Gatton, Queensland 4343, Australia. (7)Equine Veterinary Surgeon, Brisbane, Queensland 4034, Australia. (8)National Centre for Epidemiology and Population Health, Australian National University, Canberra 0200, Australia. (9)School of Public Health, Tropical Medicine and Rehabilitation Sciences, James Cook University, Townsville, Queensland 4811, Australia. (10)Center for Large Landscape Conservation, Bozeman, MT 59771, USA. (11)414 South Third Avenue, Bozeman, MT 59715, USA. (12)New South Wales Department of Primary Industries, 1423 Bruxner Highway, Wollongbar, New South Wales 2477, Australia. (13)New and Emerging Zoonotic Diseases, CSIRO, Australian Animal Health Laboratory, East Geelong, Victoria 3220, Australia Program in Emerging Infectious Diseases, Duke-NUS Graduate Medical School, Singapore 169857. (14)EcoHealth Alliance, New York, NY 10001, USA. (15)Animal Biosecurity and Welfare Program, Biosecurity Queensland, Department of Agriculture, Fisheries and Forestry, Brisbane, Queensland 4001, Australia. (16)Griffith School of Environment, Griffith University, Brisbane 4111, Australia.

Viruses that originate in bats may be the most notorious emerging zoonoses that spill over from wildlife into domestic animals and humans. Understanding how these infections filter through ecological systems to cause disease in humans is of profound importance to public health. Transmission of viruses from bats to humans requires a hierarchy of enabling conditions that connect the distribution of reservoir hosts, viral infection within these hosts, and exposure and susceptibility of recipient hosts. For many emerging bat viruses, spillover also requires viral shedding from bats, and survival of the virus in the environment. Focusing on Hendra virus, but also addressing Nipah virus, Ebola virus, Marburg virus and coronaviruses, we delineate this cross-species spillover dynamic from the within-host processes that drive virus excretion to land-use changes that increase interaction among species. We describe how land-use changes may affect co-occurrence and contact between bats and recipient hosts. Two hypotheses may explain temporal and spatial pulses of virus shedding in bat populations: episodic shedding from persistently infected bats or transient epidemics that occur as virus is transmitted among bat populations. Management of livestock also may affect the probability of exposure and disease. Interventions to decrease the probability of virus spillover can be implemented at multiple levels from targeting the reservoir host to managing recipient host exposure and susceptibility.

PMCID: PMC4262174 [Available on 2015/1/7] PMID: 25392474 [PubMed - as supplied by publisher]
4. Acta Obstet Gynecol Scand. 2015 Jan;94(1):5-7. doi: 10.1111/aogs.12540.

Enhancing access to emergency obstetric care through surgical task shifting in Sierra Leone: confrontation with Ebola during recovery from civil war.

Milland M(1), Bolkan HA.

Author information: (1)Department of Obstetrics, Rigshospitalet, Copenhagen University Hospital, Copenhagen, Denmark; CapaCare, Department of Surgery, St. Olavs Hospital, Trondheim.
PMID: 25522776 [PubMed - in process]
5. Am J Clin Pathol. 2015 Jan;143(1):4-5. doi: 10.1309/AJCP26MIFUIETBPL.

Safety considerations in the laboratory testing of specimens suspected or known to contain ebola virus.

Iwen PC(1), Smith PW(2), Hewlett AL(2), Kratochvil CJ(3), Lisco SJ(4), Sullivan JN(4), Gibbs SG(5), Lowe JJ(5), Fey PD(6), Herrera VL(7), Sambol AR(7), Wisecarver JL(6), Hinrichs SH(6).

Author information: (1)From the Department of Pathology and Microbiology, College of Medicine, University of Nebraska Medical Center, Omaha; Nebraska Public Health Laboratory, Omaha; (2)Department of Internal Medicine, Division of Infectious Diseases, University of Nebraska Medical Center, Omaha; (3)Department of Psychiatry, College of Medicine, University of Nebraska Medical Center, Omaha; (4)Department of Anesthesiology, Division of Critical Care, University of Nebraska Medical Center, Omaha; and. (5)Department of Environmental, Agricultural, and Occupational Health, College of Public Health, University of Nebraska Medical Center, Omaha. (6)From the Department of Pathology and Microbiology, College of Medicine, University of Nebraska Medical Center, Omaha; (7)Nebraska Public Health Laboratory, Omaha;
PMID: 25511134 [PubMed - in process]
6. Am J Public Health. 2015 Jan;105(1):6-8.

The Moral Challenge of Ebola.

Rothstein MA(1).

Author information: (1)Mark A. Rothstein is with the Institute for Bioethics, Health Policy and Law, University of Louisville School of Medicine, Louisville, KY. He is also a Department Editor for the American Journal of Public Health.
PMID: 25354202 [PubMed - as supplied by publisher]
7. Ann Emerg Med. 2015 Jan;65(1):101-108. doi: 10.1016/j.annemergmed.2014.10.009. Epub 2014 Oct 23.

Ebola Virus Outbreak 2014: Clinical Review for Emergency Physicians.

Meyers L(1), Frawley T(2), Goss S(2), Kang C(2).

Author information: (1)Madigan Army Medical Center, Department of Emergency Medicine, Fort Lewis, WA. Electronic address: linda.y.meyers.mil@mail.mil. (2)Madigan Army Medical Center, Department of Emergency Medicine, Fort Lewis, WA.

The 2014 Ebola outbreak in West Africa is the largest in history. Ebola viral disease is a severe and fatal illness characterized by a nonspecific viral syndrome followed by fulminant septic shock and coagulopathy. Despite ongoing efforts directed at experimental treatments and vaccine development, current medical management of Ebola viral disease is largely limited to supportive therapy, thus making early case identification and immediate implementation of appropriate control measures critical. Because a case of Ebola viral disease was confirmed in the United States on September 30, 2014, emergency medicine providers should be knowledgeable about it for a number of reasons: we are being called on to answer questions about Ebola and allay public fears, we are likely to be first to encounter an infected patient, and there are increasing numbers of US emergency physicians working in Africa who risk coming in direct contact with the disease. This article seeks to provide emergency physicians with the essential and up-to-date information required to identify, evaluate, and manage Ebola viral disease and to join global efforts to contain the current outbreak.

PMID: 25455908 [PubMed - as supplied by publisher]
8. Intensive Care Med. 2015 Jan;41(1):118-9. doi: 10.1007/s00134-014-3562-7. Epub 2014 Nov 28.

Preparing an ICU room to welcome a critically ill patient with Ebola virus disease.

Pasquier P(1), Ficko C, Mérens A, Dubost C.

Author information: (1)Intensive Care Unit, Bégin Military Teaching Hospital, Saint-Mandé, France, pasquier9606@me.com.
PMID: 25431367 [PubMed - in process]
9. Intensive Care Med. 2015 Jan;41(1):111-4. doi: 10.1007/s00134-014-3568-1. Epub 2014 Nov 27.

Ebola care and research protocols.

Perner A(1), Fowler RA, Bellomo R, Roberts I.

Author information: (1)Department of Intensive Care, Rigshospitalet, University of Copenhagen, Copenhagen, Denmark, anders.perner@rh.regionh.dk.
PMID: 25427868 [PubMed - in process]
10. Intensive Care Med. 2015 Jan;41(1):115-7. doi: 10.1007/s00134-014-3529-8. Epub 2014 Nov 11.

Treatment of Ebola virus disease.

Yazdanpanah Y(1), Arribas JR, Malvy D.

Author information: (1)Service de Maladies Infectieuses et tropicales, Hôpital Bichat Claude Bernard, Paris, France, yazdan.yazdanpanah@bch.aphp.fr.

PMID: 25385474 [PubMed - in process]

11. J Clin Microbiol. 2015 Jan;53(1):4-8. Epub 2014 Nov 12.

Ebola Virus: a Clear and Present Danger.

Burd EM(1).

Author information: (1)Department of Pathology and Laboratory Medicine and Department of Medicine, Division of Infectious Diseases, Emory University School of Medicine, Atlanta, Georgia eburd@emory.edu.

An epidemic of Ebola virus disease is occurring in Western Africa on a scale not seen before, particularly in the countries of Guinea, Liberia, and Sierra Leone. The continued spread is facilitated by insufficient medical facilities, poor sanitation, travel, and unsafe burial practices. Several patients diagnosed with Ebola virus disease in Africa have been evacuated to the United States for treatment, and several other patients have been diagnosed in the United States. It is important for laboratories to be aware of available tests, especially those granted emergency use authorization, as hospitals prepare protocols for the diagnosis and management of high-risk patients.

PMID: 25392362 [PubMed - as supplied by publisher]

12. J Med Ethics. 2015 Jan;41(1):107-10. doi: 10.1136/medethics-2014-102304.

Ebola: what it tells us about medical ethics.

Dawson AJ.

Good medical ethics needs to look more to the resources of public health ethics and use more societal, population or community values and perspectives, rather than defaulting to the individualistic values that currently dominate discussion. In this paper I argue that we can use the recent response to Ebola as an example of a major failure of the global community in three ways. First, the focus has been on the treatment of individuals rather than seeing that the priority ought to be public health measures. Second, the advisory committee on experimental interventions set up by the WHO has focused on ethical issues related to individuals and their guidance has been unclear. Third, the Ebola issue can be seen as a symptom of a massive failure of the global community to take sufficient notice of global injustice.

PMID: 25516949 [PubMed - in process]

13. J Med Ethics. 2015 Jan;41(1):103-6. doi: 10.1136/medethics-2014-102356.

Good medical ethics, justice and provincial globalism.

Ruger JP.

The summer 2014 Ebola virus outbreak in Western Africa illustrates global health's striking inequalities. Globalisation has also increased pandemics, and disparate health system conditions mean that where one falls ill or is injured in the world can mean the difference between quality care, substandard care or no care at all, between full recovery, permanent ill effects and death. Yet attention to the normative underpinnings of global health justice and distribution remains, despite some important exceptions, inadequate in medical ethics, bioethics and political philosophy. We need a theoretical foundation on which to build a more just world. Provincial globalism (PG), grounded in capability theory, offers a foundation; it provides the components of a global health justice framework that can guide implementation. Under PG, all persons possess certain health entitlements. Global health justice requires progressively securing this health capabilities threshold for every person.

PMID: 25516948 [PubMed - in process]

14. J Pathol. 2015 Jan;235(2):149-52. doi: 10.1002/path.4476.

Viruses and disease: emerging concepts for prevention, diagnosis and treatment.

Herrington C(1), Coates P, Duprex W.

Author information: (1)Medical Research Institute, University of Dundee Medical School, Ninewells Hospital, Dundee, UK.

Viruses cause a wide range of human diseases, ranging from acute self-resolving conditions to acute fatal diseases. Effects that arise long after the primary infection can also increase the propensity for chronic conditions or lead to the development of cancer. Recent advances in the fields of virology and pathology have been fundamental in improving our understanding of viral pathogenesis, in providing improved vaccination strategies and in developing newer, more effective treatments for patients worldwide. The reviews assembled here focus on the interface between virology and pathology and encompass aspects of both the clinical pathology of viral disease and the underlying disease mechanisms. Articles on emerging diseases caused by Ebola virus, Marburg virus, coronaviruses such as SARS and MERS, Nipah virus and noroviruses are followed by reviews of enteroviruses, HIV infection, measles, mumps, human respiratory syncytial virus (RSV), influenza, cytomegalovirus (CMV) and varicella zoster virus (VZV). The issue concludes with a series of articles reviewing the relationship between viruses and cancer, including the role played by Epstein-Barr virus (EBV) in the pathogenesis of lymphoma and carcinoma; how human papillomaviruses (HPVs) are involved in the development of skin cancer; the involvement of hepatitis B virus infection in hepatocellular carcinoma; and the mechanisms by which Kaposi's sarcoma-associated herpesvirus (KSHV) leads to Kaposi's sarcoma. We hope that this collection of articles will be of interest to a wide range of scientists and clinicians at a time when there is a renaissance in the appreciation of the power of pathology as virologists dissect the processes of disease. Copyright © 2014 Pathological Society of Great Britain and Ireland. Published by John Wiley & Sons, Ltd.

PMID: 25366544 [PubMed - in process]

15. J Pathol. 2015 Jan;235(2):153-74. doi: 10.1002/path.4456.

Tissue and cellular tropism, pathology and pathogenesis of Ebola and Marburg viruses.

Martines RB(1), Ng DL, Greer PW, Rollin PE, Zaki SR.

Author information: (1)Infectious Diseases Pathology Branch, Division of High Consequence Pathogens and Pathology, Centers for Disease Control and Prevention, Atlanta, GA, USA.

Ebola viruses and Marburg viruses include some of the most virulent and fatal pathogens known to humans. These viruses cause severe haemorrhagic fevers, with case fatality rates in the range 25-90%. The diagnosis of filovirus using formalin-fixed tissues from fatal cases poses a significant challenge. The most characteristic histopathological findings are seen in the liver; however, the findings overlap with many other viral and non-viral haemorrhagic diseases. The need to distinguish filovirus infections from other haemorrhagic fevers, particularly in areas with multiple endemic viral haemorrhagic agents, is of paramount importance. In this review we discuss the current state of knowledge of filovirus infections and their pathogenesis, including histopathological findings, epidemiology, modes of transmission and filovirus entry and spread within host organisms. The pathogenesis of filovirus infections is complex and involves activation of the mononuclear phagocytic system, with release of pro-inflammatory cytokines, chemokines and growth factors, endothelial dysfunction, alterations of the innate and adaptive immune systems, direct organ and endothelial damage from unrestricted viral replication late in infection, and coagulopathy. Although our understanding of the pathogenesis of filovirus infections has rapidly increased in the past few years, many questions remain unanswered. Copyright © 2014 Pathological Society of Great Britain and Ireland. Published by John Wiley & Sons, Ltd.

PMID: 25297522 [PubMed - in process]

16. J Transcult Nurs. 2015 Jan;26(1):6-7. doi: 10.1177/1043659614561680.

Thoughts on transcultural nursing and ebola.

Gray J(1).

Author information: (1)The University of Texas at Arlington, TX, USA jgray@uta.edu.

PMID: 25505166 [PubMed - in process]

17. J Virol. 2015 Jan 1;89(1):844-56. doi: 10.1128/JVI.02697-14. Epub 2014 Oct 29.

Simian Hemorrhagic Fever Virus Cell Entry Is Dependent on CD163 and Uses a Clathrin-Mediated Endocytosis-Like Pathway.

Caì Y(1), Postnikova EN(1), Bernbaum JG(1), Yú SQ(1), Mazur S(1), Deiuliis NM(1), Radoshitzky SR(2), Lackemeyer MG(1), McCluskey A(3), Robinson PJ(4), Haucke V(5), Wahl-Jensen V(1), Bailey AL(6), Lauck M(6), Friedrich TC(6), O'Connor DH(6), Goldberg TL(6), Jahrling PB(1), Kuhn JH(7).

Author information: (1)Integrated Research Facility at Fort Detrick, National Institute of Allergy and Infectious Diseases, National Institutes of Health, Fort Detrick, Frederick, Maryland, USA. (2)United States Army Medical Research Institute of Infectious Diseases, Fort Detrick, Frederick, Maryland, USA. (3)Department of Chemistry, Centre for Chemical Biology, School of Environmental and Life Sciences, University of Newcastle, Callaghan, New South Wales, Australia. (4)Cell Signaling Unit, Children's Medical Research Institute, The University of Sydney, Sydney, New South Wales, Australia. (5)Leibniz Institut für Molekulare Pharmakologie, Berlin, Germany. (6)Wisconsin National Primate Research Center, Madison, Wisconsin, USA. (7)Integrated Research Facility at Fort Detrick, National Institute of Allergy and Infectious Diseases, National Institutes of Health, Fort Detrick, Frederick, Maryland, USA kuhnjens@mail.nih.gov.

Simian hemorrhagic fever virus (SHFV) causes a severe and almost uniformly fatal viral hemorrhagic fever in Asian macaques but is thought to be nonpathogenic for humans. To date, the SHFV life cycle is almost completely uncharacterized on the molecular level. Here, we describe the first steps of the SHFV life cycle. Our experiments indicate that SHFV enters target cells by low-pH-dependent endocytosis. Dynamin inhibitors, chlorpromazine, methyl-β-cyclodextrin, chloroquine, and concanamycin A dramatically reduced SHFV entry efficiency, whereas the macropinocytosis inhibitors EIPA, blebbistatin, and wortmannin and the caveolin-mediated endocytosis inhibitors nystatin and filipin III had no effect. Furthermore, overexpression and knockout study and electron microscopy results indicate that SHFV entry occurs by a dynamin-dependent clathrin-mediated endocytosis-like pathway. Experiments utilizing latrunculin B, cytochalasin B, and cytochalasin D indicate that SHFV does not hijack the actin polymerization pathway. Treatment of target cells with proteases (proteinase K, papain, α-chymotrypsin, and trypsin) abrogated entry, indicating that the SHFV cell surface receptor is a protein. Phospholipases A2 and D had no effect on SHFV entry. Finally, treatment of cells with antibodies targeting CD163, a cell surface molecule identified as an entry factor for the SHFV-related porcine reproductive and respiratory syndrome virus, diminished SHFV replication, identifying CD163 as an important SHFV entry component.IMPORTANCE: Simian hemorrhagic fever virus (SHFV) causes highly lethal disease in Asian macaques resembling human illness caused by Ebola or Lassa virus. However, little is known about SHFV's ecology and molecular biology and the mechanism by which it causes disease. The results of this study shed light on how SHFV enters its target cells. Using electron microscopy and inhibitors for various cellular pathways, we demonstrate that SHFV invades cells by low-pH-dependent, actin-independent endocytosis, likely with the help of a cellular surface protein.

PMID: 25355889 [PubMed - in process]

18. Nat Rev Microbiol. 2015 Jan;13(1):3. doi: 10.1038/nrmicro3412. Epub 2014 Dec 8.

Viral pathogenesis: Ebola virus' shed GP activates immune cells.

Nunes-Alves C.

PMID: 25488766 [PubMed - in process]

19. Oral Dis. 2015 Jan;21(1):1-6. doi: 10.1111/odi.12298.

Viral haemorrhagic fevers with emphasis on Ebola virus disease and oro-dental healthcare.

Samaranayake L, Scully C, Nair RG, Petti S.

PMID: 25399654 [PubMed - in process]

20. Vaccine. 2015 Jan 1;33(1):73-5. doi: 10.1016/j.vaccine.2014.09.035. Epub 2014 Oct 8

The Brighton Collaboration Viral Vector Vaccines Safety Working Group (V3SWG).

Chen RT(1), Carbery B(2), Mac L(3), Berns KI(4), Chapman L(3), Condit RC(4), Excler JL(5), Gurwith M(6), Hendry M(3), Khan AS(7), Khuri-Bulos N(8), Klug B(9), Robertson JS(10), Seligman SJ(11), Sheets R(12), Williamson AL(13); V3SWG.

Author information: (1)DHAP, NCHHSTP, Centers for Disease Control and Prevention, 1600 Clifton Road, Atlanta, GA 30333, USA. Electronic address: brightoncollaborationv3swg@gmail.com. (2)DHAP, NCHHSTP, Centers for Disease Control and Prevention, 1600 Clifton Road, Atlanta, GA 30333, USA; Division of Infectious Diseases, Beth Israel Deaconess Medical Center, Boston, MA 02215, USA. (3)DHAP, NCHHSTP, Centers for Disease Control and Prevention, 1600 Clifton Road, Atlanta, GA 30333, USA. (4)Department of Molecular Genetics and Microbiology, University of Florida College of Medicine, P.O. Box 100266, Gainesville, FL 32610, USA. (5)International AIDS Vaccine Initiative, New York, NY, USA; U.S. Military HIV Research Program (MHRP), Bethesda, MD 20817, USA. (6)PaxVax, San Diego, CA 92121, USA. (7)Laboratory of Retroviruses, Division of Viral Products, Center for Biologics Evaluation and Research, US Food and Drug Administration, Bethesda, MD 20892, USA. (8)Division of Infectious Disease, Jordan University Hospital, Amman, Jordan. (9)Paul-Ehrlich-Institut, 63225 Langen, Germany. (10)Independent Adviser (formerly of National Institute for Biological Standards and Control, Potters Bar, ENG 3QG, UK). (11)Department of Microbiology and Immunology, New York Medical College, Valhalla, NY 10595, USA. (12)Division of AIDS, National Institute of Allergy and Infectious Diseases, U.S. National Institutes of Health, Bethesda, MD 20892, USA. (13)Institute of Infectious Disease and Molecular Medicine, University of Cape Town and National Health Laboratory Service, Cape Town, South Africa.

Recombinant viral vectors provide an effective means for heterologous antigen expression in vivo and thus represent promising platforms for developing novel vaccines against human pathogens from Ebola to tuberculosis. An increasing number of candidate viral vector vaccines are entering human clinical trials. The Brighton Collaboration Viral Vector Vaccines Safety Working Group (V3SWG) was formed to improve our ability to anticipate potential safety issues and meaningfully assess or interpret safety data, thereby facilitating greater public acceptance when licensed.

Published by Elsevier Ltd.

PMID: 25305565 [PubMed - in process]

21. JAMA. 2014 Dec 22. doi: 10.1001/jama.2014.17934. [Epub ahead of print]

The 2014 Ebola Outbreak and Mental Health: Current Status and Recommended Response.

Shultz JM(1), Baingana F(2), Neria Y(3).

Author information: (1)Center for Disaster and Extreme Event Preparedness, University of Miami Miller School of Medicine, Miami, Florida. (2)Makerere University School of Public Health, Kampala, Uganda. (3)New York State Psychiatric Institute, Departments of Psychiatry and Epidemiology, Columbia University Medical Center, New York, New York.

PMID: 25532102 [PubMed - as supplied by publisher]

22. Viral Immunol. 2014 Dec 22. [Epub ahead of print]

Multiple Circulating Infections Can Mimic the Early Stages of Viral Hemorrhagic Fevers and Possible Human Exposure to Filoviruses in Sierra Leone Prior to the 2014 Outbreak.

Boisen ML(1), Schieffelin JS, Goba A, Dottamasathien D, Jones AB, Shaffer JG, Hastie KM, Hartnett JN, Momoh M, Fullah M, Gabiki M, Safa S, Zandonatti M, Fusco M, Bornholdt Z, Abelson D, Gire SK, Andersen KG, Tariyal R, Stremlau M, Cross RW, Geisbert JB, Pitts KR, Geisbert TW, Kulakoski P, Wilson RB, Henderson L, Sabeti PC, Grant DS, Garry RF, Saphire EO, Branco LM, Khan SH.

Author information: (1)I Corgenix Medical Corporation, Inc. , Broomfield, Colorado.

Abstract Lassa fever (LF) is a severe viral hemorrhagic fever caused by Lassa virus (LASV). The LF program at the Kenema Government Hospital (KGH) in Eastern Sierra Leone currently provides diagnostic services and clinical care for more than 500 suspected LF cases per year. Nearly two-thirds of suspected LF patients presenting to the LF Ward test negative for either LASV antigen or anti-LASV immunoglobulin M (IgM), and therefore are considered to have a non-Lassa febrile illness (NLFI). The NLFI patients in this study were generally severely ill, which accounts for their high case fatality rate of 36%. The current studies were aimed at determining possible causes of severe febrile illnesses in non-LF cases presenting to the KGH, including possible involvement of filoviruses. A seroprevalence survey employing commercial enzyme-linked immunosorbent assay tests revealed significant IgM and IgG reactivity against dengue virus, chikungunya virus, West Nile virus (WNV), Leptospira, and typhus. A polymerase chain reaction-based survey using sera from subjects with acute LF, evidence of prior LASV exposure, or NLFI revealed widespread infection with Plasmodium falciparum malaria in febrile patients. WNV RNA was detected in a subset of patients, and a 419 nt amplicon specific to filoviral L segment RNA was detected at low levels in a single patient. However, 22% of the patients presenting at the KGH between 2011 and 2014 who were included in this survey registered anti-Ebola virus (EBOV) IgG or IgM, suggesting prior exposure to this agent. The 2014 Ebola virus disease (EVD) outbreak is already the deadliest and most widely dispersed outbreak of its kind on record. Serological evidence reported here for possible human exposure to filoviruses in Sierra Leone prior to the current EVD outbreak supports genetic analysis that EBOV may have been present in West Africa for some time prior to the 2014 outbreak.

PMID: 25531344 [PubMed - as supplied by publisher]

23. Biol Chem. 2014 Dec 19. pii: /j/bchm.just-accepted/hsz-2014-0273/hsz-2014-0273.xml. doi: 10.1515/hsz-2014-0273. [Epub ahead of print]

Sphingolipids in viral infection.

Schneider-Schaulies J, Schneider-Schaulies S.

Abstract Viruses exploit membranes and their components such as sphingolipids in all steps of their life cycle including attachment and membrane fusion, intracellular transport, replication, protein sorting and budding. Examples for sphingolipid-dependent virus entry are found for human immunodeficiency virus (HIV), which besides its protein receptors also interacts with glycosphingolipids (GSLs), or rhinovirus, which promotes the formation of ceramide-enriched platforms and endocytosis, or measles virus (MV), which induces the surface expression of its own receptor CD150 via activation of sphingomyelinases (SMases). While SMase activation was implicated in Ebola virus (EBOV) attachment, the virus utilizes the cholesterol transporter Niemann-Pick C protein 1 (NPC1) as 'intracellular' entry receptor after uptake into endosomes. Differential activities of SMases also affect the intracellular milieu required for virus replication. Sindbis virus (SINV), for example, replicates better in cells lacking acid SMase (ASMase). Defined lipid compositions of viral assembly and budding sites influence virus release and infectivity, as found for hepatitis C virus (HCV) or HIV. And finally, viruses manipulate cellular signalling and the sphingolipid metabolism to their advantage, as for example influenza A virus (IAV), which activates sphingosine kinase 1 and the transcription factor NF-κB.

PMID: 25525752 [PubMed - as supplied by publisher]

24. Br Dent J. 2014 Dec 19;217(12):685. doi: 10.1038/sj.bdj.2014.1120.

Editorial - Rationality and coordination for Ebola outbreak in west Africa and Commentary - Ebola: no time to waste.

[No authors listed]

See http://ebola.thelancet.com/ for The Lancet Ebola Resource Centre.

PMID: 25525013 [PubMed - in process]

25. Br Dent J. 2014 Dec 19;217(12):661. doi: 10.1038/sj.bdj.2014.1108.

Infection control: Ebola aware; Ebola beware; Ebola healthcare.

Scully C, Samaranayake L, Petti S, Nair RG.

PMID: 25525000 [PubMed - in process]

26. MMWR Morb Mortal Wkly Rep. 2014 Dec 19;63(50):1207-9.

Reintegration of ebola survivors into their communities - firestone district, liberia, 2014.

Arwady MA, Garcia EL, Wollor B, Mabande LG, Reaves EJ, Montgomery JM.

The current Ebola virus disease (Ebola) epidemic in West Africa is unprecedented in size and duration. Since the outbreak was recognized in March 2014, the World Health Organization (WHO) has reported 17,145 cases with 6,070 deaths, primarily in Guinea, Liberia, and Sierra Leone. Combined data show a case-fatality rate of approximately 70% in patients with a recorded outcome; a 30% survival rate means that thousands of patients have survived Ebola. An important component of a comprehensive Ebola response is the reintegration of Ebola survivors into their communities.

PMID: 25522091 [PubMed - in process]

27. MMWR Morb Mortal Wkly Rep. 2014 Dec 19;63(50):1205-6.

Support services for survivors of ebola virus disease - sierra leone, 2014.

Lee-Kwan SH, DeLuca N, Adams M, Dalling M, Drevlow E, Gassama G, Davies T.

As of December 6, 2014, Sierra Leone reported 6,317 laboratory-confirmed cases of Ebola virus disease (Ebola), the highest number of reported cases in the current West Africa epidemic. The Sierra Leone Ministry of Health and Sanitation reported that as of December 6, 2014, there were 1,181 persons who had survived and were discharged. Survivors from previous Ebola outbreaks have reported major barriers to resuming normal lives after release from treatment, such as emotional distress, health issues, loss of possessions, and difficulty regaining their livelihoods. In August 2014, a knowledge, attitude, and practice survey regarding the Ebola outbreak in Sierra Leone, administered by a consortium of partners that included the Ministry of Health and Sanitation, UNICEF, CDC, and a local nongovernmental organization, Focus 1000, found that 96% of the general population respondents reported some discriminatory attitude towards persons with suspected or known Ebola. Access to increased psychosocial support, provision of goods, and family and community reunification programs might reduce these barriers. Survivors also have unique potential to contribute to the Ebola response, particularly because survivors might have some immunity to the same virus strain. In previous outbreaks, survivors served as burial team members, contact tracers, and community educators promoting messages that seeking treatment improves the chances for survival and that persons who survived Ebola can help their communities. As caregivers in Ebola treatment units, survivors have encouraged patients to stay hydrated and eat and inspired them to believe that they, too, can survive. Survivors regaining livelihood through participation in the response might offset the stigma associated with Ebola.

PMID: 25522090 [PubMed - in process]

28. MMWR Morb Mortal Wkly Rep. 2014 Dec 19;63(50):1202-4.

Challenges in responding to the ebola epidemic - four rural counties, liberia, august-november 2014.

Summers A, Nyenswah TG, Montgomery JM, Neatherlin J, Tappero JW, T N, M F, M M.

The first cases of Ebola virus disease (Ebola) in West Africa were identified in Guinea on March 22, 2014. On March 30, the first Liberian case was identified in Foya Town, Lofa County, near the Guinean border. Because the majority of early cases occurred in Lofa and Montserrado counties, resources were

concentrated in these counties during the first several months of the response, and these counties have seen signs of successful disease control. By October 2014, the epidemic had reached all 15 counties of Liberia. During August 27-September 10, 2014, CDC in collaboration with the Liberian Ministry of Health and Social Welfare assessed county Ebola response plans in four rural counties (Grand Cape Mount, Grand Bassa, Rivercess, and Sinoe, to identify county-specific challenges in executing their Ebola response plans, and to provide recommendations and training to enhance control efforts. Assessments were conducted through interviews with county health teams and health care providers and visits to health care facilities. At the time of assessment, county health teams reported lacking adequate training in core Ebola response strategies and reported facing many challenges because of poor transportation and communication networks. Development of communication and transportation network strategies for communities with limited access to roads and limited means of communication in addition to adequate training in Ebola response strategies is critical for successful management of Ebola in remote areas.
PMID: 25522089 [PubMed - in process]

29. MMWR Morb Mortal Wkly Rep. 2014 Dec 19;63(50):1199-1201.

Update: Ebola Virus Disease Epidemic - West Africa, December 2014.

Incident Management System Ebola Epidemiology Team, CDC; Guinea Interministerial Committee for Response Against the Ebola Virus; World Health Organization; CDC Guinea Response Team; Liberia Ministry of Health and Social Welfare; CDC Liberia Response Team; Sierra Leone Ministry of Health and Sanitation; CDC Sierra Leone Response Team; Viral Special Pathogens Branch, National Center for Emerging and Zoonotic Infectious Diseases, CDC.

CDC is assisting ministries of health and working with other organizations to end the ongoing epidemic of Ebola virus disease (Ebola) in West Africa. The updated data in this report were compiled from situation reports from the Guinea Interministerial Committee for Response Against the Ebola Virus, the World Health Organization, the Liberia Ministry of Health and Social Welfare, and the Sierra Leone Ministry of Health and Sanitation. Total case counts include all suspected, probable, and confirmed cases, which are defined similarly by each country. These data reflect reported cases, which make up an unknown proportion of all cases, and reporting delays that vary from country to country.
PMID: 25522088 [PubMed - as supplied by publisher]

30. Virology. 2014 Dec 19;476C:85-91. doi: 10.1016/j.virol.2014.12.002. [Epub ahead of print]

Recombinant Marburg viruses containing mutations in the IID region of VP35 prevent inhibition of Host immune responses.

Albariño CG(1), Wiggleton Guerrero L(1), Spengler JR(1), Uebelhoer LS(1), Chakrabarti AK(1), Nichol ST(1), Towner JS(2).

Author information: (1)Centers for Disease Control and Prevention, Atlanta, USA. (2)Centers for Disease Control and Prevention, Atlanta, USA. Electronic address: jit8@cdc.gov.

Previous in vitro studies have demonstrated that Ebola and Marburg virus (EBOV and MARV) VP35 antagonize the host cell immune response. Moreover, specific mutations in the IFN inhibitory domain (IID) of EBOV and MARV VP35 that abrogate their interaction with virus-derived dsRNA, lack the ability to inhibit the host immune response. To investigate the role of MARV VP35 in the context of infectious virus, we used our reverse genetics system to generate two recombinant MARVs carrying specific mutations in the IID region of VP35. Our data show that wild-type and mutant viruses grow to similar titers in interferon deficient cells, but exhibit attenuated growth in interferon-competent cells. Furthermore, in contrast to wild-type virus, both MARV mutants were unable to inhibit expression of various antiviral genes. The MARV VP35 mutants exhibit similar phenotypes to those previously described for EBOV, suggesting the existence of a shared immune-modulatory strategy between filoviruses.

Published by Elsevier Inc.
PMID: 25531184 [PubMed - as supplied by publisher]

31. Am J Obstet Gynecol. 2014 Dec 18. pii: S0002-9378(14)02485-5. doi: 10.1016/j.ajog.2014.12.026. [Epub ahead of print]

Physicians' Obligations to Patients Infected with Ebola: Echoes of AIDS.

Minkoff H(1), Ecker J(2).

Author information: (1)Department of Obstetrics and Gynecology at Maimonides Medical Center, SUNY Downstate. Electronic address: hminkoff@maimonidesmed.org. (2)Department of Obstetrics and Gynecology, Massachusetts General Hospital, Harvard Medical School.

Physicians across the United States are engaged in training in the identification, isolation and initial care of patients with Ebola. Some will be asked to do more. The issue this viewpoint will address is the moral obligation of physicians to participate in these activities. In order to do so the implicit contract between society and its physicians will be considered, as will many of the arguments that are redolent of those that were litigated 30 years ago when AIDS was raising public fears to similar levels, and some physicians were publically proclaiming their unwillingness to render care to those individuals. We will build the case that if steps are taken to reduce risks-optimal personal protective equipment (PPE) and training-- to what is essentially the lowest possible level then rendering care should be seen as obligatory. If not, as in the AIDS era there will be an unfair distribution of risk, with those who take their obligations seriously having to go beyond their fair measure of exposure. It would also potentially undermine patients' faith in the altruism of physicians and thereby degrade the esteem in which our profession is held and the trust that underpins the therapeutic relationship. Finally there is an implicit contract with society. Society gives tremendously to us; we encumber a debt from all society does and offers, a debt for which recompense is rarely sought. The mosaic of moral, historical and professional imperatives to render care to the infected all echoes the word's of medicine's moral leaders in the AIDS epidemic. Arnold Relman perhaps put it most succinctly, "the risk of contracting the patient's disease is one of the risks that is inherent in the profession of medicine. Physicians who are not willing to accept that risk....ought not be in the practice of medicine."

Copyright © 2014 Elsevier Inc. All rights reserved.
PMID: 25530596 [PubMed - as supplied by publisher]

32. Evid Based Med. 2014 Dec 18. pii: ebmed-2014-110127. doi: 10.1136/ebmed-2014-110127. [Epub ahead of print]

The unprecedented scale of the West African Ebola virus disease outbreak is due to environmental and sociological factors, not special attributes of the currently circulating strain of the virus.

Gatherer D(1).

Author information: (1)Division of Biomedical & Life Sciences, Faculty of Health & Medicine, Lancaster University, Lancaster, UK.

PMID: 25525042 [PubMed - as supplied by publisher]
33. Genome Announc. 2014 Dec 18;2(6). pii: e01331-14. doi: 10.1128/genomeA.01331-14.

Complete genome sequences of three ebola virus isolates from the 2014 outbreak in west Africa.

Hoenen T(1), Groseth A(2), Feldmann F(3), Marzi A(2), Ebihara H(2), Kobinger G(4), Günther S(5), Feldmann H(6).

Author information: (1)Laboratory of Virology, Division of Intramural Research, National Institute of Allergy and Infectious Diseases, National Institutes of Health, Hamilton, Montana, USA thomas.hoenen@nih.gov feldmannh@niaid.nih.gov. (2)Laboratory of Virology, Division of Intramural Research, National Institute of Allergy and Infectious Diseases, National Institutes of Health, Hamilton, Montana, USA. (3)Rocky Mountain Veterinary Branch, Division of Intramural Research, National Institute of Allergy and Infectious Diseases, National Institutes of Health, Hamilton, Montana, USA. (4)Special Pathogens Program, Public Health Agency of Canada, Winnipeg, Manitoba, Canada. (5)Bernard Nocht Institute for Tropical Medicine, Hamburg, Germany. (6)Laboratory of Virology, Division of Intramural Research, National Institute of Allergy and Infectious Diseases, National Institutes of Health, Hamilton, Montana, USA Rocky Mountain Veterinary Branch, Division of Intramural Research, National Institute of Allergy and Infectious Diseases, National Institutes of Health, Hamilton, Montana, USA Special Pathogens Program, Public Health Agency of Canada, Winnipeg, Manitoba, Canada Bernard Nocht Institute for Tropical Medicine, Hamburg, Germany thomas.hoenen@nih.gov feldmannh@niaid.nih.gov.

Here, we report the complete genome sequences, including the genome termini, of three Ebola virus isolates (species Zaire ebolavirus) originating from Guinea that are now being widely used in laboratories in North America for research regarding West African Ebola viruses.

PMID: 25523781 [PubMed]
34. N Engl J Med. 2014 Dec 18;371(25):2350-1. doi: 10.1056/NEJMp1414145. Epub 2014 Dec 3.

Evaluating Ebola therapies--the case for RCTs.

Cox E(1), Borio L, Temple R.

Author information: (1)From the Center for Drug Evaluation and Research (E.C., R.T.) and the Office of the Commissioner (L.B.), Food and Drug Administration, Silver Spring, MD.

PMID: 25470568 [PubMed - in process]
35. N Engl J Med. 2014 Dec 18;371(25):2439-40. doi: 10.1056/NEJMc1412662. Epub 2014 Nov 19.

The first case of Ebola virus disease acquired outside Africa.

Parra JM(1), Salmerón OJ, Velasco M.

Author information: (1)Hospital Universitario Fundación Alcorcón, Madrid, Spain mvelasco@fhalcorcon.es.

PMID: 25409262 [PubMed - in process]
36. N Engl J Med. 2014 Dec 18;371(25):2430-2. doi: 10.1056/NEJMe1412744. Epub 2014 Nov 12.

Out of Africa--caring for patients with Ebola.

Rubin EJ, Baden LR.

Comment on N Engl J Med. 2014 Dec 18;371(25):2402-9. N Engl J Med. 2014 Dec 18;371(25):2394-401.

PMID: 25390461 [PubMed - in process]
37. N Engl J Med. 2014 Dec 18;371(25):2402-9. doi: 10.1056/NEJMoa1409838. Epub 2014 Nov 12.

Clinical care of two patients with Ebola virus disease in the United States.

Lyon GM(1), Mehta AK, Varkey JB, Brantly K, Plyler L, McElroy AK, Kraft CS, Towner JS, Spiropoulou C, Ströher U, Uyeki TM, Ribner BS; Emory Serious Communicable Diseases Unit.

Collaborators: Bell S, Ash T, Barnes C, Calhoun J, Chapman L, Daye T, Durr H, Evans S, Gentry J, Ginnane J, Grant S, Haynes C, Hickey P, Hill C, Hillis D, Johnson C, Loomis J, Mamora J, Mitchell L, Morgan J, Owen J, Piazza S, Shirley K, Siddens J, Slabach J, Tirador E, Todd D, Vanairsdale S, Adebayo L, Bowker K, Clark B, Hines N, Kugbila L, Lalor M, Morfaw P, Osakwe N, Silas C, Brammer N, Buchanan J, Burd E, Cardella J, Eaves B, Evans C, Hill C, Hostetler K, Jenkins K, Lindsey M, Magee J, Powers R, Ritchie J, Ryan E, Adams A, Allen MB, Bachman R, Bornstein W, Cantrell D, Cosper P, Feistritzer N, Fox J, Gartland B, Goodman J, Grant S, Howard-Crow D, Horowitz I, Pugh D, Ritenour C, Golston G, Kaufman S, Olinger P, Olinger S, Rengarajan K, Thomaston S, Beck E, Desroches P, Hall C, Walker C, Bryant C, Hackman B, Howard R, Jones M, Broughton J, Frisle B, Jackson R, Lewis J, Brown-Haithco R, Gartin ML, Geralds-Washington E, James-Jones R, Miller D, Stark D, McGee G, Jones P, Scott-Harris L, Cain J, Davis R, Johnson T, Pickett T, Shaw A, Truesdale T, Blum J, Klopman M, Hill L, Matkins R, Meechan C, Meechan P, Schwock K, Schuck J, Sevransky J, Stack K, Wolf F, Zivot J, Walker S, Bray B, Isakov A, Shartar S, Christenbury J, Dollard V, De Gennaro M, Korschun H, Seideman N, Emamifar A, Kuban T, Pack J, Rogers S.

Author information: (1)From the Departments of Medicine (G.M.L., A.K. Mehta, J.B.V., C.S.K., B.S.R.), Pathology (C.S.K.), and Pediatrics (A.K. McElroy), Division of Infectious Diseases, Emory University School of Medicine, and the Centers for Disease Control and Prevention (A.K. McElroy, J.S.T., C.S., U.S., T.M.U.) - both in Atlanta; and Samaritan's Purse, Boone, NC (K.B., L.P.).

Comment in N Engl J Med. 2014 Dec 18;371(25):2430-2.

West Africa is currently experiencing the largest outbreak of Ebola virus disease (EVD) in history. Two patients with EVD were transferred from Liberia to our hospital in the United States for ongoing care. Malaria had also been diagnosed in one patient, who was treated for it early in the course of EVD. The two patients had substantial intravascular volume depletion and marked electrolyte abnormalities. We undertook aggressive supportive measures of hydration (typically, 3 to 5 liters of intravenous fluids per day early in the course of care) and electrolyte correction. As the patients' condition improved clinically, there was a concomitant decline in the amount of virus detected in plasma.
PMID: 25390460 [PubMed - in process]

38. N Engl J Med. 2014 Dec 18;371(25):2348-9. doi: 10.1056/NEJMp1413425. Epub 2014 Nov 5.

Panic, paranoia, and public health--the AIDS epidemic's lessons for Ebola.

Gonsalves G(1), Staley P.

Author information: (1)Mr. Gonsalves is the codirector of the Yale Global Health Justice Partnership, Yale Law School and Yale School of Public Health, New Haven, CT, and an AIDS activist; Mr. Staley is a longtime AIDS activist.
PMID: 25372947 [PubMed - in process]

39. N Engl J Med. 2014 Dec 18;371(25):2394-401. doi: 10.1056/NEJMoa1411677. Epub 2014 Oct 22.

A case of severe Ebola virus infection complicated by gram-negative septicemia.

Kreuels B(1), Wichmann D, Emmerich P, Schmidt-Chanasit J, de Heer G, Kluge S, Sow A, Renné T, Günther S, Lohse AW, Addo MM, Schmiedel S.

Author information: (1)From the Division of Tropical Medicine, First Department of Medicine (B.K., A.W.L., M.M.A., S.S.), Department of Intensive Care Medicine (D.W., G.H., S.K.), Institute for Clinical Chemistry and Laboratory Medicine (T.R.), and Infectious Disease Unit for Outpatient Care (S.S.), University Medical Center Hamburg-Eppendorf, the German Center for Infection Research, Hamburg-Borstel-Lübeck (B.K., J.S.-C., S.G., A.W.L., M.M.A., S.S.), the Research Group for Infectious Disease Epidemiology, Bernhard Nocht Institute for Tropical Medicine (B.K.), and the Bernhard Nocht Institute for Tropical Medicine, World Health Organization Collaborating Center for Arbovirus and Hemorrhagic Fever Reference and Research (P.E., J.S.-C., S.G.) - all in Hamburg, Germany; Arboviruses and Hemorrhagic Fever Viruses Unit, Pasteur Institute, and Public Health and Development Institute, Cheikh Anta Diop University - both in Dakar, Senegal (A.S.); Bordeaux Public Health Institute, INSERM Unité 897, Bordeaux University, Bordeaux, France (A.S); the Department of Molecular Medicine and Surgery, Karolinska Institutet, Stockholm (T.R.); and the Infectious Diseases Unit, Massachusetts General Hospital, Boston (M.M.A.).

Comment in N Engl J Med. 2014 Dec 18;371(25):2430-2.

Ebola virus disease (EVD) developed in a patient who contracted the disease in Sierra Leone and was airlifted to an isolation facility in Hamburg, Germany, for treatment. During the course of the illness, he had numerous complications, including septicemia, respiratory failure, and encephalopathy. Intensive supportive treatment consisting of high-volume fluid resuscitation (approximately 10 liters per day in the first 72 hours), broad-spectrum antibiotic therapy, and ventilatory support resulted in full recovery without the use of experimental therapies. Discharge was delayed owing to the detection of viral RNA in urine (day 30) and sweat (at the last assessment on day 40) by means of polymerase-chain-reaction (PCR) assay, but the last positive culture was identified in plasma on day 14 and in urine on day 26. This case shows the challenges in the management of EVD and suggests that even severe EVD can be treated effectively with routine intensive care.
PMID: 25337633 [PubMed - in process]

40. Trop Doct. 2014 Dec 18. pii: 0049475514564269. [Epub ahead of print]

Ebola virus disease: the 'Black Swan' in West Africa.

Brown C(1), Arkell P(2), Rokadiya S(2).

Author information: (1)King's Centre for Global Health, Denmark Hill, London colinstewartbrown@gmail.com. (2)King's Centre for Global Health, Denmark Hill, London.
PMID: 25527679 [PubMed - as supplied by publisher]

41. Am J Epidemiol. 2014 Dec 17. pii: kwu354. [Epub ahead of print]

Ebola: The Natural and Human History of a Deadly Virus.

Levin-Sparenberg E(1), Gicquelais R(1), Blanco N(1), Ismail MD(1), Lee KH(1), Foxman B(1).

Author information: (1)University of Michigan, School of Public Health, Ann Arbor, MI.
PMID: 25520259 [PubMed - as supplied by publisher]

42. BJOG. 2014 Dec 17. doi: 10.1111/1471-0528.13232. [Epub ahead of print]

Obstetrics in the time of Ebola: challenges and dilemmas in providing lifesaving care during a deadly epidemic.

Black B(1).

Author information: (1)Médecins Sans Frontières, London, UK.
PMID: 25515060 [PubMed - as supplied by publisher]

43. JAMA. 2014 Dec 17;312(23):2495-6. doi: 10.1001/jama.2014.15497.

Ebola virus disease and the need for new personal protective equipment.

Edmond MB(1), Diekema DJ(1), Perencevich EN(2).

Author information: (1)Department of Internal Medicine, University of Iowa Carver College of Medicine, Iowa City. (2)Department of Internal Medicine, University of Iowa Carver College of Medicine, Iowa City2Iowa City VA Health System, Iowa City.
PMID: 25350321 [PubMed - in process]

44. JAMA. 2014 Dec 17;312(23):2499-500. doi: 10.1001/jama.2014.15064.

Ebola in the United States: EHRs as a public health tool at the point of care.

Mandl KD(1).

Author information: (1)Children's Hospital Informatics Program, Boston Children's Hospital, Boston, Massachusetts2Center for Biomedical Informatics, Harvard Medical School, Boston, Massachusetts.

PMID: 25329170 [PubMed - in process]

45. JAMA. 2014 Dec 17;312(23):2497-8. doi: 10.1001/jama.2014.15041.

Is the United States prepared for Ebola?

Gostin LO(1), Hodge JG Jr(2), Burris S(3).

Author information: (1)O'Neill Institute for National and Global Health Law, Georgetown University Law Center, Washington, DC. (2)Sandra Day O'Connor College of Law, Arizona State University, Tempe. (3)Public Health Law Research Program, Beasley School of Law, Temple University, Philadelphia, Pennsylvania.

PMID: 25325877 [PubMed - in process]

46. Lancet. 2014 Dec 17. pii: S0140-6736(14)62388-6. doi: 10.1016/S0140-6736(14)62388-6. [Epub ahead of print]

Sierra Leone doctors call for better Ebola care for colleagues.

Shuchman M.

PMID: 25530440 [PubMed - as supplied by publisher]

47. N Engl J Med. 2014 Dec 17. [Epub ahead of print]

License to Serve - U.S. Trainees and the Ebola Epidemic.

Rosenbaum L(1).

Author information: (1)Dr. Rosenbaum is a national correspondent for the Journal.

Before medical school, Sara L., now a fourth-year resident, worked for 6 years as a microbiologist at the Centers for Disease Control and Prevention. While there, she focused on hemorrhagic fevers, and she went to West Africa several times to assist in outbreaks. Indeed, until recently, Sara was one of only a few hundred people in the United States who was trained to work in a biosafety level 4 spacesuit laboratory, which requires the same personal protective equipment (PPE) needed for working with Ebola. As the current Ebola epidemic exploded, and after careful deliberation, Sara sought and secured a position . . .

PMID: 25517575 [PubMed - as supplied by publisher]

48. Nature. 2014 Dec 17;516(7531):323-5. doi: 10.1038/516323a.

Infectious disease: Mobilizing Ebola survivors to curb the epidemic.

Epstein JM(1), Sauer LM(2), Chelen J(3), Hatna E(3), Parker J(3), Rothman RE(4), Rubinson L(5).

Author information: (1)Center for Advanced Modeling, and director for systems science of the Johns Hopkins Systems Institute, Johns Hopkins University, Baltimore, Maryland, USA. J.M.E. is also external professor at the Santa Fe Institute, Santa Fe, New Mexico, USA. (2)Department of Emergency Medicine, Johns Hopkins School of Medicine, Baltimore, Maryland, USA. (3)Johns Hopkins Center for Advanced Modeling, Baltimore, Maryland, USA. (4)Department of Emergency Medicine, Johns Hopkins University School of Medicine, Baltimore, Maryland, USA. (5)R Adams Cowley Shock Trauma Center, University of Maryland School of Medicine, Baltimore, Maryland, USA.

PMID: 25519116 [PubMed - in process]

49. Nature. 2014 Dec 17;516(7531):295-6. doi: 10.1038/516295a.

Ebola threatens a way of life.

Hayden EC.

PMID: 25519108 [PubMed - in process]

50. Pediatr Infect Dis J. 2014 Dec 17. [Epub ahead of print]

Ebola in children: Epidemiology, clinical features, diagnosis and outcomes.

Olupot-Olupot P.

Ebola virus disease (EVD) is caused by a highly contagious and pathogenic threadlike RNA virus of the Filoviridae family. The index human case is usually a zoonosis that launches human-to-human transmission interface with varying levels of sustainability of the epidemic depending on the level of public health preparedness of the affected country and the Ebola virus strain. The disease affects all age groups in the population.Clinical diagnosis is challenging in index cases especially in the early stages of the disease when the presenting features are usually non-specific and only similar to a flu-like illness. However, in the agonal stages, haemorrhage frequently occurs in a high proportion of cases. The diagnostic gold standard is by detecting the antigen using Reverse Transcription - PCR (RT - PCR).Mortality rates in the last 28 outbreaks since 1976 have ranged from 30% to 100% in different settings among adults, but lower mortality rates have been documented in children. This review aims to describe Ebola virus infection, clinical presentation, diagnosis and outcomes in children.

PMID: 25522340 [PubMed - as supplied by publisher]

51. Microbes Infect. 2014 Dec 16. pii: S1286-4579(14)00312-8. doi: 10.1016/j.micinf.2014.12.004. [Epub ahead of print]

Development of vaccines for prevention of Ebola virus infection.

Ye L(1), Yang C(2).

Author information: (1)Department of Microbiology and Immunology, Emory University School of Medicine, Atlanta, GA, United States of America. (2)Department of Microbiology and Immunology, Emory University School of Medicine, Atlanta, GA, United States of America. Electronic address: chyang@emory.edu.

Ebola virus infection causes severe hemorrhagic fevers with high fatality rates up to 90% in humans, for which no effective treatment is currently available. The ongoing Ebola outbreak in West Africa that has caused over 14,000 human infections and over 5000 deaths underscores its serious threat to the public health. While licensed vaccines against Ebola virus infection are still not available, a number of vaccine approaches have been developed and shown to protect against lethal Ebola virus infection in animal models. This review aims to summarize the advancement of different strategies for Ebola vaccine development with a focus on the discussion of their protective efficacies and possible limitations. In addition, the development of animal models for efficacy evaluation of Ebola vaccines and the mechanism of immune protection against Ebola virus infection are also discussed.

PMID: 25526819 [PubMed - as supplied by publisher]

52. Reprod Sci. 2014 Dec 16. pii: 1933719114563733. [Epub ahead of print]

Male Ebola Survivors: Do Not Forget to Use a Condom!

Cardona-Maya WD(1), Hernandez PA(2), Henao DE(3).

Author information: (1)Grupo Reproducción, Estrategia de Sostenibilidad 2014-2015, Universidad de Antioquia, Medellin, Colombia. (2)Grupo de Inmunovirología, Estrategia de Sostenibilidad 2014-2015, Universidad de Antioquia, Medellin, Colombia. (3)Observatorio EcoRegional de Salud Pública, Departamento de Medicina Comunitaria, Universidad Tecnológica de Pereira, Pereira, Colombia d.henao@utp.edu.co.

PMID: 25515607 [PubMed - as supplied by publisher]

53. Sci China Life Sci. 2014 Dec 16. [Epub ahead of print]

A new chapter for China's public health security-aids offered to Africa to combat Ebola.

Zhang B(1), Gao GF.

Author information: (1)Chinese Center for Disease Control and Prevention, Beijing, 102206, China.

PMID: 25514849 [PubMed - as supplied by publisher]

54. Viral Immunol. 2014 Dec 16. [Epub ahead of print]

Characterization of Clinical and Immunological Parameters During Ebola Virus Infection of Rhesus Macaques.

Martins K(1), Cooper C, Warren T, Wells J, Bell T, Raymond J, Stuthman K, Benko J, Garza N, van Tongeren S, Donnelly G, Retterer C, Dong L, Bavari S.

Author information: (1)1 Department of Molecular and Translational Sciences, United States Army Medical Research Institute of Infectious Diseases (USAMRIID), Frederick, Maryland.

Abstract The rhesus macaque serves as an animal model for Ebola virus (EBOV) infection. A thorough understanding of EBOV infection in this species would aid in further development of filovirus therapeutics and vaccines. In this study, pathological and immunological data from EBOV-infected rhesus macaques are presented. Changes in blood chemistries, hematology, coagulation, and immune parameters during infection, which were consistently observed in the animals, are presented. In an animal that survived challenge, a delay was observed in the detection of viral RNA and inflammatory cytokines and chemokines which may have contributed to survival. Collectively, these data add to the body of knowledge regarding EBOV pathogenesis in rhesus macaques and emphasize the reproducibility of the rhesus macaque challenge model.

PMID: 25514385 [PubMed - as supplied by publisher]

55. Viral Immunol. 2014 Dec 16. [Epub ahead of print]

Cross-Protection Conferred by Filovirus Virus-Like Particles Containing Trimeric Hybrid Glycoprotein.

Martins K(1), Carra JH, Cooper CL, Kwilas SA, Robinson CG, Shurtleff AC, Schokman RD, Kuehl KA, Wells JB, Steffens JT, van Tongeren SA, Hooper JW, Bavari S.

Author information: (1)1 Department of Molecular and Translational Sciences, United States Army Medical Research Institute of Infectious Diseases (USAMRIID), Frederick, Maryland.

Abstract Filoviruses are causative agents of hemorrhagic fever, and to date no effective vaccine or therapeutic has been approved to combat infection. Filovirus glycoprotein (GP) is the critical immunogenic component of filovirus vaccines, eliciting high levels of antibody after successful vaccination. Previous work has shown that protection against both Ebola virus (EBOV) and Marburg virus (MARV) can be achieved by vaccinating with a mixture of virus-like particles (VLPs) expressing either EBOV GP or MARV GP. In this study, the potential for eliciting effective immune responses against EBOV, Sudan virus, and MARV with a single GP construct was tested. Trimeric hybrid GPs were produced that expressed the sequence of Marburg GP2 in conjunction with a hybrid GP1 composed EBOV and Sudan virus GP sequences. VLPs expressing these constructs, along with EBOV VP40, provided comparable protection against MARV challenge, resulting in 75 or 100% protection. Protection from EBOV challenge differed depending upon the hybrid used, however, with one conferring 75% protection and one conferring no protection. By comparing the overall antibody titers and the neutralizing antibody titers specific for each virus, it is shown that higher antibody responses were elicited by the C terminal region of GP1 than by the N terminal region, and this correlated with protection. These data collectively suggest that GP2 and the C terminal region of GP1 are highly immunogenic, and they advance progress toward the development of a pan-filovirus vaccine.

PMID: 25514232 [PubMed - as supplied by publisher]

56. Am J Transplant. 2014 Dec 15. doi: 10.1111/ajt.13093. [Epub ahead of print]

Ebola Virus Disease: Implications for Solid Organ Transplantation.

Kaul DR(1), Mehta AK, Wolfe CR, Blumberg E, Green M.

Author information: (1)Department of Internal Medicine, Division of Infectious Diseases, University of Michigan Medical School, Ann Arbor, MI.

PMID: 25510898 [PubMed - as supplied by publisher]

57. Am J Trop Med Hyg. 2014 Dec 15. pii: 14-0746. [Epub ahead of print]

Being Ready to Treat Ebola Virus Disease Patients.

Brett-Major DM(1), Jacob ST(2), Jacquerioz FA(2), Risi GF(2), Fischer WA 2nd(2), Kato Y(2), Houlihan CF(2), Crozier I(2), Bosa HK(2), Lawler JV(2), Adachi T(2), Hurley SK(2), Berry LE(2), Carlson JC(2), Button TC(2), McClellan SL(2), Shea BJ(2), Kuniyoshi GG(2), Ferri M(2), Murthy SG(2), Petrosillo N(2), Lamontagne F(2), Porembka DT(2), Schieffelin J(2), Rubinson L(2), O'Dempsey T(2), Donovan SM(2), Bausch DG(2), Fowler RA(2), Fletcher TE(2).

Author information: (1)Naval Medical Research Center, Silver Spring, Maryland; Uniformed Services University, Bethesda, Maryland; University of Washington, Seattle, Washington; Tulane University Health Sciences Center, New Orleans, Louisiana; Infectious Disease Specialists, PC, Missoula, Montana; Division of Pulmonary and Critical Care Medicine, The University of North Carolina at Chapel Hill, North Carolina; Division of Preparedness and Emerging Infections, Disease Control and Prevention Center, National Center for Global Health and Medicine, Tokyo, Japan; Clinical Research Department, London School of Hygiene and Tropical Medicine, London, United Kingdom; Infectious Diseases Institute, College of Health Sciences, Makerere University, Kampala, Uganda; Uganda Peoples Defence Forces, Kampala, Uganda; Naval Medical Research Center- Frederick, Fort Detrick, Maryland; Austere Environment Consortium for Enhanced Sepsis Outcomes (ACESO), Fort Detrick, Maryland; Toshima Hospital, Tokyo, Japan; Providence St. Patrick Hospital, Missoula, Montana; Department of Infectious Diseases, Nottingham University Hospitals, National Health Service Trust, Nottingham, United Kingdom; Truman Medical Centers, Kansas City, Missouri; Toronto, Ontario, Canada; The Queen's Medical Center, Honolulu, Hawaii; Department of Community Health Sciences, University of Calgary, Calgary, Alberta, Canada; University of British Columbia, Vancouver, British Columbia, Canada; National Institute for Infectious Diseases, Lazzaro Spallanzani, Rome, Italy; Centre de Recherche, Clinique Centre Hospitalier Universitaire de Sherbrooke, Sherbrooke, Quebec, Canada; Department of Medicine, Sanford School of Medicine, University of South Dakota, Sioux Falls, South Dakota; Avera McKenna Medical Center, Sioux Falls, South Dakota; Critical Care Receiving Unit, University of Maryland Shock Trauma Center, Baltimore, Maryland; Liverpool School of Tropical Medicine, Liverpool, United Kingdom; Division Infectious Diseases, Olive View UCLA Medical Center, David Geffen School of Medicine at UCLA, Los Angeles, California; U.S. Naval Medical Research Unit No. 6 (NAMRU-6), Lima, Peru; University of Toronto, Toronto, Ontario, Canada David.Brett-Major@usuhs.edu. (2)Naval Medical Research Center, Silver Spring, Maryland; Uniformed Services University, Bethesda, Maryland; University of Washington, Seattle, Washington; Tulane University Health Sciences Center, New Orleans, Louisiana; Infectious Disease Specialists, PC, Missoula, Montana; Division of Pulmonary and Critical Care Medicine, The University of North Carolina at Chapel Hill, North Carolina; Division of Preparedness and Emerging Infections, Disease Control and Prevention Center, National Center for Global Health and Medicine, Tokyo, Japan; Clinical Research Department, London School of Hygiene and Tropical Medicine, London, United Kingdom; Infectious Diseases Institute, College of Health Sciences, Makerere University, Kampala, Uganda; Uganda Peoples Defence Forces, Kampala, Uganda; Naval Medical Research Center- Frederick, Fort Detrick, Maryland; Austere Environment Consortium for Enhanced Sepsis Outcomes (ACESO), Fort Detrick, Maryland; Toshima Hospital, Tokyo, Japan; Providence St. Patrick Hospital, Missoula, Montana; Department of Infectious Diseases, Nottingham University Hospitals, National Health Service Trust, Nottingham, United Kingdom; Truman Medical Centers, Kansas City, Missouri; Toronto, Ontario, Canada; The Queen's Medical Center, Honolulu, Hawaii; Department of Community Health Sciences, University of Calgary, Calgary, Alberta, Canada; University of British Columbia, Vancouver, British Columbia, Canada; National Institute for Infectious Diseases, Lazzaro Spallanzani, Rome, Italy; Centre de Recherche, Clinique Centre Hospitalier Universitaire de Sherbrooke, Sherbrooke, Quebec, Canada; Department of Medicine, Sanford School of Medicine, University of South Dakota, Sioux Falls, South Dakota; Avera McKenna Medical Center, Sioux Falls, South Dakota; Critical Care Receiving Unit, University of Maryland Shock Trauma Center, Baltimore, Maryland; Liverpool School of Tropical Medicine, Liverpool, United Kingdom; Division Infectious Diseases, Olive View UCLA Medical Center, David Geffen School of Medicine at UCLA, Los Angeles, California; U.S. Naval Medical Research Unit No. 6 (NAMRU-6), Lima, Peru; University of Toronto, Toronto, Ontario, Canada.

As the outbreak of Ebola virus disease (EVD) in West Africa continues, clinical preparedness is needed in countries at risk for EVD (e.g., United States) and more fully equipped and supported clinical teams in those countries with the epidemic spread of EVD in Africa. Clinical staff must approach the patient with a very deliberate focus on providing effective care while assuring personal safety. To do this, both individual health care providers and health systems must improve EVD care. Although formal guidance toward these goals exists from the World Health Organization, Medecin Sans Frontières, the Centers for Disease Control and Prevention, and other groups, some of the most critical lessons come from personal experience. In this narrative, clinicians deployed by the World Health Organization into a wide range of clinical settings in West Africa distill key, practical considerations for working safely and effectively with patients with EVD.

PMID: 25510724 [PubMed - as supplied by publisher]
58. Am J Trop Med Hyg. 2014 Dec 15. pii: 14-0753. [Epub ahead of print]

Out of (West) Africa-Who Lost in the End?

Olliaro P(1), Lasry E(2), Tiffany A(2).

Author information: (1)UNICEF/UNDP/World Bank/WHO Special Programme for Research and Training in Tropical Diseases (TDR), Geneva, Switzerland; Centre for Tropical Medicine, Nuffield Department of Medicine, University of Oxford, Churchill Hospital, Oxford, United Kingdom; Médecins Sans Frontières (MSF)/Doctors Without Borders, New York, New York; Epicentre and Médecins Sans Frontières (MSF) Switzerland, Geneva, Switzerland olliarop@who.int. (2)UNICEF/UNDP/World Bank/WHO Special Programme for Research and Training in Tropical Diseases (TDR), Geneva, Switzerland; Centre for Tropical Medicine, Nuffield Department of Medicine, University of Oxford, Churchill Hospital, Oxford, United Kingdom; Médecins Sans Frontières (MSF)/Doctors Without Borders, New York, New York; Epicentre and Médecins Sans Frontières (MSF) Switzerland, Geneva, Switzerland.

On October 29, 2014, 4 days before the annual meeting of the American Society of Tropical Medicine and Hygiene (ASTMH) to be held in New Orleans, LA, meeting registrants received an e-mail letter from the Louisiana Department of Health and Hospitals stating "we have requested that any individuals that will be traveling to Louisiana following a trip to the West African countries of Guinea, Liberia, and Sierra Leone or have had contact with an Ebola-infected individual remain in a self-quarantine for the 21 days following their relevant travel history...we see no use in you traveling to New Orleans to simply be confined to your room." This communication made it clear that those recently in countries experiencing the 2014 Ebola epidemic would not be able to participate in the meeting. The ASTMH sent their own communication stating that the Society did not agree with the State's policy, but had no choice but to abide. However inconvenient and upsetting this decision might have been, what really matters transcends the mere disturbance of long-planned schedules. More broadly, we lost on five levels.

© The American Society of Tropical Medicine and Hygiene.

PMID: 25510720 [PubMed - as supplied by publisher]

59. Am J Trop Med Hyg. 2014 Dec 15. pii: 14-0769. [Epub ahead of print]

From Clinician to Suspect Case: My Experience After a Needle Stick in an Ebola Treatment Unit in Sierra Leone.

Rubinson L(1).

Author information: (1)R. Adams Cowley Shock Trauma Center, University of Maryland School of Medicine, Baltimore, Maryland lrubinson@umm.edu.

From clinician to suspect case: My experience after a needle stick in an ebola treatment unit in Sierra Leone.

© The American Society of Tropical Medicine and Hygiene.

PMID: 25510717 [PubMed - as supplied by publisher]

60. BMJ. 2014 Dec 15;349:g7668. doi: 10.1136/bmj.g7668.

West African countries plan to strengthen health systems after Ebola.

Gulland A(1).

Author information: (1)London.

PMID: 25512385 [PubMed - in process]

61. Clin Infect Dis. 2014 Dec 15. pii: ciu1131. [Epub ahead of print]

Epidemiological and viral genomic sequence analysis of the 2014 Ebola outbreak reveals clustered transmission.

Scarpino SV(1), Iamarino A(2), Wells C(3), Yamin D(3), Ndeffo-Mbah M(3), Wenzel NS(4), Fox SJ(5), Nyenswah T(6), Altice FL(7), Galvani AP(8), Meyers LA(9), Townsend JP(10).

Author information: (1)Santa Fe Institute, Santa Fe, NM 87501, USA. (2)Department of Biostatistics, Yale School of Public Health, 135 College St, New Haven, CT 06510, USA Department of Microbiology, Biomedical Sciences Institute, University of São Paulo, São Paulo, Brazil. (3)Center for Infectious Disease Modeling, Yale School of Public Health, New Haven, CT 06510, USA Department of Epidemiology of Microbial Diseases, Yale School of Public Health, New Haven, CT, USA. (4)Center for Infectious Disease Modeling, Yale School of Public Health, New Haven, CT 06510, USA. (5)Department of Integrative Biology, University of Texas at Austin, Austin, TX 78712, USA. (6)Ministry of Health and Social Welfare, Monrovia, Liberia. (7)Department of Epidemiology of Microbial Diseases, Yale School of Public Health, New Haven, CT, USA Section of Infectious Diseases, Yale University School of Medicine, New Haven, CT, USA. (8)Center for Infectious Disease Modeling, Yale School of Public Health, New Haven, CT 06510, USA Department of Epidemiology of Microbial Diseases, Yale School of Public Health, New Haven, CT, USA Program in Computational Biology and Bioinformatics, Yale University, New Haven, CT 06520 Department of Ecology and Evolutionary Biology, Yale University, New Haven, CT 06520. (9)Santa Fe Institute, Santa Fe, NM 87501, USA Department of Integrative Biology, University of Texas at Austin, Austin, TX 78712, USA. (10)Department of Biostatistics, Yale School of Public Health, 135 College St, New Haven, CT 06510, USA Program in Computational Biology and Bioinformatics, Yale University, New Haven, CT 06520 Department of Ecology and Evolutionary Biology, Yale University, New Haven, CT 06520 Jeffrey.Townsend@yale.edu.

Using Ebolavirus genomic and epidemiological data, we conduct the first joint analysis where both data types are used to fit dynamic transmission models for an ongoing outbreak. Our results indicate that transmission is clustered, highlighting a potential bias in medical demand forecasts, and provide the first empirical estimate of underreporting.

© The Author 2014. Published by Oxford University Press on behalf of the Infectious Diseases Society of America. All rights reserved. For Permissions, please e-mail: journals.permissions@oup.com.

PMID: 25516185 [PubMed - as supplied by publisher]

62. Clin Infect Dis. 2014 Dec 15. pii: ciu978. [Epub ahead of print]

Traffic Control Bundling Is Essential for Protecting Healthcare Workers and Controlling the 2014 Ebola Epidemic.

Yen M(1), Schwartz J(2), Hsueh P(3), Chiu AW(4), Armstrong D(5).

Author information: (1)Section of Infectious Diseases, Taipei City Hospital, Department of Medicine, National Yang-Ming University School of Medicine, Taipei, Taiwan. (2)Department of Political Science, State University of New York, New Paltz. (3)Department of Laboratory Medicine and Internal Medicine, National Taiwan University Hospital, National Taiwan University College of Medicine. (4)Department of Surgery, Taipei City Hospital, Department of Health, Taipei City Government and National Yang-Ming University School of Medicine, Taiwan. (5)Memorial Sloan Kettering Cancer Center, New York, New York.

PMID: 25512433 [PubMed - as supplied by publisher]

63. CMAJ. 2014 Dec 15. pii: cmaj.109-4961. [Epub ahead of print]

Ebola-free in Africa's most populous nation.

Walji M(1).

Author information: (1)CMAJ.

PMID: 25512655 [PubMed - as supplied by publisher]

64. Int J Cardiol. 2014 Dec 15;177(2):524-6. doi: 10.1016/j.ijcard.2014.08.114. Epub 2014 Aug 26.

Ebola: Is there a hope from treatment with cardiovascular drugs?

Patanè S(1).

Author information: (1)Cardiologia Ospedale San Vincenzo - Taormina (Me) Azienda Sanitaria Provinciale di Messina, Contrada Sirina, 98039 Taormina (Messina), Italy. Electronic address: patane-@libero.it.

PMID: 25205490 [PubMed - in process]

65. J Virol. 2014 Dec 15;88(24):14458-66. doi: 10.1128/JVI.02267-14. Epub 2014 Oct 8.

Putative domain-domain interactions in the vesicular stomatitis virus L polymerase protein appendage region.

Ruedas JB(1), Perrault J(2).

Author information: (1)Department of Biology and Center for Microbial Sciences, San Diego State University, San Diego, California, USA. (2)Department of Biology and Center for Microbial Sciences, San Diego State University, San Diego, California, USA jperrault@mail.sdsu.edu.

The multidomain polymerase protein (L) of nonsegmented negative-strand (NNS) RNA viruses catalyzes transcription and replication of the virus genome. The N-terminal half of the protein forms a ring-like polymerase structure, while the C-terminal half encoding viral mRNA transcript modifications consists of a flexible appendage with three distinct globular domains. To gain insight into putative transient interactions between L domains during viral RNA synthesis, we exchanged each of the four distinct regions encompassing the appendage region of vesicular stomatitis virus (VSV) Indiana serotype L protein with their counterparts from VSV New Jersey and analyzed effects on virus polymerase activity in a minigenome system. The methyltransferase domain exchange yielded a fully active polymerase protein, which functioned as well as wild-type L in the context of a recombinant virus. Exchange of the downstream C-terminal nonconserved region abolished activity, but coexchanging it with the methyltransferase domain generated a polymerase favoring replicase over transcriptase activity, providing strong evidence of interaction between these two regions. Exchange of the capping enzyme domain or the adjacent nonconserved region thought to function as an "unstructured" linker also abrogated polymerase activity even when either domain was coexchanged with other appendage domains. Further probing of the putative linker segment using in-frame enhanced green fluorescent protein (EGFP) insertions similarly abrogated activity. We discuss the implications of these findings with regard to L protein appendage domain structure and putative domain-domain interactions required for polymerase function.IMPORTANCE: NNS viruses include many well-known human pathogens (e.g., rabies, measles, and Ebola viruses), as well as emerging viral threats (e.g., Nipah and Hendra viruses). These viruses all encode a large L polymerase protein similarly organized into multiple domains that work in concert to enable virus genome transcription and replication. But how the unique L protein carries out the multiplicity of individual steps in these two distinct processes is poorly understood. Using two different approaches, i.e., exchanging individual domains in the C-terminal appendage region of the protein between two closely related VSV serotypes and inserting unrelated protein domains, we shed light on requirements for domain-domain interactions and domain contiguity in polymerase function. These findings further our understanding of the conformational dynamics of NNS L polymerase proteins, which play an essential role in the pathogenic properties of these viruses and represent attractive targets for the development of antiviral measures.

PMCID: PMC4249160 [Available on 2015/6/1] PMID: 25297996 [PubMed - in process]

66. J Virol. 2014 Dec 15;88(24):14440-50. doi: 10.1128/JVI.02069-14. Epub 2014 Oct 8.

The VP40 Protein of Marburg Virus Exhibits Impaired Budding and Increased Sensitivity to Human Tetherin following Mouse Adaptation.

Feagins AR(1), Basler CF(2).

Author information: (1)Icahn School of Medicine at Mount Sinai, Department of Microbiology, New York, New York, USA. (2)Icahn School of Medicine at Mount Sinai, Department of Microbiology, New York, New York, USA chris.basler@mssm.edu.

The Marburg virus VP40 protein is a viral matrix protein that spontaneously buds from cells. It also functions as an interferon (IFN) signaling antagonist by targeting Janus kinase 1 (JAK1). A previous study demonstrated that the VP40 protein of the Ravn strain of Marburg virus (Ravn virus [RAVV]) failed to block IFN signaling in mouse cells, whereas the mouse-adapted RAVV (maRAVV) VP40 acquired the ability to inhibit IFN responses in mouse cells. The increased IFN antagonist function of maRAVV VP40 mapped to residues 57 and 165, which were mutated during the mouse adaptation process. In the present study, we demonstrate that maRAVV VP40 lost the capacity to efficiently bud from human cell lines, despite the fact that both parental and maRAVV VP40s bud efficiently from mouse cell lines. The impaired budding in human cells corresponds with the appearance of protrusions on the surface of maRAVV VP40-expressing Huh7 cells and with an increased sensitivity of maRAVV VP40 to restriction by human tetherin but not mouse tetherin. However, transfer of the human tetherin cytoplasmic tail to mouse tetherin restored restriction of maRAVV VP40. Residues 57 and 165 were demonstrated to contribute to the failure of maRAVV VP40 to bud from human cells, and residue 57 was demonstrated to alter VP40 oligomerization, as assessed by coprecipitation assay, and to determine sensitivity to human tetherin. This suggests that RAVV VP40 acquired, during adaptation to mice, changes in its oligomerization potential that enhanced IFN antagonist function. However, this new capacity impaired RAVV VP40 budding from human cells.IMPORTANCE: Filoviruses, which include Marburg viruses and Ebola viruses, are zoonotic pathogens that cause severe disease in humans and nonhuman primates but do not cause similar disease in wild-type laboratory strains of mice unless first adapted to these animals. Although mouse adaptation has been used as a method to develop small animal models of pathogenesis, the molecular determinants associated with filovirus mouse adaptation are poorly understood. Our study demonstrates how genetic changes that accrued during mouse adaptation of the Ravn strain of Marburg virus have impacted the budding function of the viral VP40 matrix protein. Strikingly, we find impairment of mouse-adapted VP40 budding function in human but not mouse cell lines, and we correlate the impairment with an increased sensitivity of VP40 to restriction by human but not mouse tetherin and with changes in VP40 oligomerization. These data suggest that there are functional costs associated with filovirus adaptation to new hosts and implicate tetherin as a filovirus host restriction factor.

PMCID: PMC4249122 [Available on 2015/6/1] PMID: 25297995 [PubMed - in process]

67. Antiviral Res. 2014 Dec 13;114C:53-56. doi: 10.1016/j.antiviral.2014.12.005. [Epub ahead of print]

Could pharmacological curtailment of the RhoA/Rho-kinase pathway reverse the endothelial barrier dysfunction associated with Ebola virus infection?

Eisa-Beygi S(1), Wen X(2).

Author information: (1)Program in Development and Stem Cell Biology, The Hospital for Sick Children, Toronto, ON, Canada. Electronic address: shahram.eisa.beygi@utoronto.ca. (2)Keenan Research Centre for Biomedical Science and the Li Ka Shing Knowledge Institute of St. Michael's Hospital, Canada; Institute of Medical Science, University of Toronto, Toronto, Ontario, Canada.

Activation of the RhoA/Rho-kinase (ROCK) pathway induces endothelial barrier dysfunction and increased vascular permeability, which is a hallmark of various life-threatening vascular pathologies. Therapeutic approaches aimed at inhibiting the RhoA/ROCK pathway have proven effective in the attenuation of vascular leakage observed in animal models of endotoxin-induced lung injury/sepsis, edema, autoimmune disorders, and stroke. These findings suggest that treatments targeting the ROCK pathway might be of benefit in the management of the Ebola virus disease (EVD), which is characterized by severe vascular leak, likely involving pro-inflammatory cytokines, such as tumor necrosis factor-alpha, released from virus-infected macrophages. In this paper, we review evidence from in vivo and in vitro models of vascular leakage, suggesting that the RhoA/ROCK pathway is an important therapeutic target for the reversal of the vascular permeability defects associated with EVD. Future studies should explore the efficacy of pharmacological inhibition of RhoA/ROCK pathway on reversing the endothelial barrier dysfunction in animal models of EVD and other hemorrhagic fever virus infections as part of an adjunctive therapy. Such experimental studies should focus, in particular, on the small molecule fasudil (HA-1077), a derivative of isoquinoline, which is a safe and clinically approved inhibitor of ROCK, making it an excellent candidate in this context.

PMID: 25512227 [PubMed - as supplied by publisher]

68. Lancet. 2014 Dec 13;384(9960):2105. doi: 10.1016/S0140-6736(14)62364-3.

Ebola in Africa: beyond epidemics, reproductive health in crisis.

Delamou A(1), Hammonds RM(2), Caluwaerts S(3), Utz B(4), Delvaux T(4).

Author information: (1)Centre de Formation et Recherche en Santé Rurale, Maferinyah, Guinea; Department of Public Health, Institute of Tropical Medicine, Antwerp, Belgium; Woman and Child Health Research Centre, Institute of Tropical Medicine, Antwerp, Belgium. Electronic address: alexdelamou@yahoo.fr. (2)Department of Public Health, Institute of Tropical Medicine, Antwerp, Belgium. (3)Department of Clinical Sciences, Institute of Tropical Medicine, Antwerp, Belgium; Woman and Child Health Research Centre, Institute of Tropical Medicine, Antwerp, Belgium; Médecins sans Frontières Operational Centre, Brussels, Belgium. (4)Department of Public Health, Institute of Tropical Medicine, Antwerp, Belgium; Woman and Child Health Research Centre, Institute of Tropical Medicine, Antwerp, Belgium.

PMID: 25497191 [PubMed - in process]

69. Lancet. 2014 Dec 13;384(9960):2105-6. doi: 10.1016/S0140-6736(14)62250-9. Epub 2014 Dec 2.

Provision of care for Ebola.

Jacobs M(1), Beadsworth M(2), Schmid M(3), Tunbridge A(4).

Author information: (1)Department of Infectious Diseases, Royal Free London NHS Foundation Trust, London NW3 2QG, UK. Electronic address: michael.jacobs@ucl.ac.uk. (2)Tropical and Infectious Disease Unit, Royal Liverpool University Hospital, Liverpool, UK. (3)Infection & Tropical Medicine, Royal Victoria Infirmary, Newcastle upon Tyne, UK. (4)Department of Infection and Tropical Medicine, Royal Hallamshire Hospital, Glossop Road, Sheffield, UK.

PMID: 25479694 [PubMed - in process]

70. Lancet. 2014 Dec 13;384(9960):2091-3. doi: 10.1016/S0140-6736(14)61412-4. Epub 2014 Sep 19.

Ebola and human rights in West Africa.

Eba PM(1).

Author information: (1)UNAIDS, Geneva, 1211 Geneva 27, Switzerland. Electronic address: ebap@unaids.org.

PMID: 25245179 [PubMed - in process]

71. Nurse Pract. 2014 Dec 13;39(12):7. doi: 10.1097/01.NPR.0000456399.15780.34.

Ebola: The power of nursing overcomes fear.

[No authors listed]

PMID: 25539741 [PubMed - in process]

72. Vet Rec. 2014 Dec 13;175(23):575. doi: 10.1136/vr.g7592.

Assessing the risk to people from pets exposed to Ebola virus.

[No authors listed]

PMID: 25501514 [PubMed - in process]

73. Virulence. 2014 Dec 13:0. [Epub ahead of print]

Quantifying the epidemic spread of Ebola virus (EBOV) in Sierra Leone using phylodynamics.

Alizon S(1), Lion S, Murall CL, Abbate JL.

Author information: (1)a CNRS , Montpellier , France.

Measuring epidemic parameters early in an outbreak is essential to inform control efforts. Using the viral genome sequence and collection date from 74 infections in the 2014 Ebola virus outbreak in Sierra Leone, we estimate key epidemiological parameters such as infectious period duration (approximately 71 hours) and date of the first case in Sierra Leone (approximately April 25(th)). We also estimate the effective reproduction number, Re, (approximately 1.26), which is the number of secondary infections effectively caused by an infected individual and accounts for public health control measures. This study illustrates that phylodynamics methods, applied during the initial phase of an outbreak on fewer and more easily attainable data, can yield similar estimates to count-based epidemiological studies.

PMID: 25495064 [PubMed - as supplied by publisher]

74. Am J Physiol Lung Cell Mol Physiol. 2014 Dec 12:ajplung.00354.2014. doi: 10.1152/ajplung.00354.2014. [Epub ahead of print]

Ebola: History, treatment and lessons from a new emerging pathogen.

Harrod KS(1).

Author information: (1)University of Alabama-Birmingham kharrod@uab.edu.

No abstract.

PMID: 25502503 [PubMed - as supplied by publisher]

75. Biochem Biophys Res Commun. 2014 Dec 12;455(3-4):223-8. doi: 10.1016/j.bbrc.2014.10.144. Epub 2014 Nov 4.

A polymorphism of the TIM-1 IgV domain: Implications for the susceptibility to filovirus infection.

Kuroda M(1), Fujikura D(2), Noyori O(1), Kajihara M(1), Maruyama J(1), Miyamoto H(1), Yoshida R(1), Takada A(3).

Author information: (1)Division of Global Epidemiology, Hokkaido University Research Center for Zoonosis Control, Sapporo 001-0020, Japan. (2)Division of Infection and Immunity, Hokkaido University Research Center for Zoonosis Control, Sapporo 001-0020, Japan. (3)Division of Global Epidemiology, Hokkaido University Research Center for Zoonosis Control, Sapporo 001-0020, Japan; Global Institution for Collaborative Research and Education, Hokkaido University, Sapporo 001-0020, Japan; School of Veterinary Medicine, The University of Zambia, P.O. Box 32379, Lusaka, Zambia. Electronic address: atakada@czc.hokudai.ac.jp.

Filoviruses, including Ebola and Marburg viruses, cause severe hemorrhagic fever in humans and nonhuman primates with mortality rates of up to 90%. Human T-cell immunoglobulin and mucin domain 1 (TIM-1) is one of the host proteins that have been shown to promote filovirus entry into cells. In this study, we cloned TIM-1 genes from three different African green monkey kidney cell lines (Vero E6, COS-1, and BSC-1) and found that TIM-1 of Vero E6 had a 23-amino acid deletion and 6 amino acid substitutions compared with those of COS-1 and BSC-1. Interestingly, Vero E6 TIM-1 had a greater ability to promote the infectivity of vesicular stomatitis viruses pseudotyped with filovirus glycoproteins than COS-1-derived TIM-1. We further found that the increased ability of Vero E6 TIM-1 to promote virus infectivity was most likely due to a single amino acid difference between these TIM-1s. These results suggest that a polymorphism of the TIM-1 molecules is one of the factors that influence cell susceptibility to filovirus infection, providing a new insight into the molecular basis for the filovirus host range.

PMID: 25449273 [PubMed - in process]

76. Curr Opin Infect Dis. 2014 Dec 12. [Epub ahead of print]

Ebola virus as a sexually transmitted infection.

Rogstad KE(1), Tunbridge A.

Author information: (1)aHIV and Sexual Health, Sheffield Teaching Hospitals NHS Foundation Trust and Undergraduate Dean, University of Sheffield School of Medicine bInfectious Diseases, Sheffield Teaching Hospitals NHS Foundation Trust, Department of Infectious Diseases and Tropical Medicine, Royal Hallamshire Hospital, Sheffield, UK.

PURPOSE OF REVIEW: The ongoing Ebola virus epidemic in West Africa is a major global health challenge. The main mode of transmission is through contact with bodily fluids and skin of those infected or who have died. This review was undertaken to consider the evidence for transmission by contact with bodily fluids occurring through sexual activity. RECENT FINDINGS: No cases in the previous 20 outbreaks or the current outbreak in West Africa have been shown to be sexually transmitted, although other types of viral haemorrhagic fever have had sexual transmission implicated. Ebola virus is found in sites and fluids associated with sexual activity but this occurs at different stages of the disease. Persistence in the convalescent period occurs in rectum, vagina and semen, with persistence in semen being longest of up to at least 101 days. Recommendations based on this data are that those recovering from Ebola virus disease should abstain from all sexual intercourse, or if this is not possible, use condoms, for 3 months after the onset of symptoms. SUMMARY: There is theoretical plausibility for sexual transmission of Ebola virus but there has been no evidence of this occurring. Further research is needed to consider if sexual activity contributes to the epidemic in order to inform individuals with regard to avoiding acquisition or transmission by those recovering from Ebola virus disease.

PMID: 25501666 [PubMed - as supplied by publisher]

77. MMWR Morb Mortal Wkly Rep. 2014 Dec 12;63(49):1175-9.

Clinical Inquiries Regarding Ebola Virus Disease Received by CDC - United States, July 9-November 15, 2014.

Karwowski MP, Meites E, Fullerton KE, Ströher U, Lowe L, Rayfield M, Blau DM, Knust B, Gindler J, Beneden CV, Bialek SR, Mead P, Oster AM.

Since early 2014, there have been more than 6,000 reported deaths from Ebola virus disease (Ebola), mostly in Guinea, Liberia, and Sierra Leone. On July 9, 2014, CDC activated its Emergency Operations Center for the Ebola outbreak response and formalized the consultation service it had been providing to assist state and local public health officials and health care providers evaluate persons in the United States thought to be at risk for Ebola. During July 9-November 15, CDC responded to clinical inquiries from public health officials and health care providers from 49 states and the District of Columbia regarding 650 persons thought to be at risk. Among these, 118 (18%) had initial signs or symptoms consistent with Ebola and epidemiologic risk factors placing them at risk for infection, thereby meeting the definition of persons under investigation (PUIs). Testing was not always performed for PUIs because alternative diagnoses were made or symptoms resolved. In total, 61 (9%) persons were tested for Ebola virus, and four, all of whom met PUI criteria, had laboratory-confirmed Ebola. Overall, 490 (75%) inquiries concerned persons who had neither traveled to an Ebola-affected country nor had contact with an Ebola patient. Appropriate medical evaluation and treatment for other conditions were noted in some instances to have been delayed while a person was undergoing evaluation for Ebola. Evaluating and managing persons who might have Ebola is one component of the overall approach to domestic surveillance, the goal of which is to rapidly identify and isolate Ebola patients so that they receive appropriate medical care and secondary transmission is prevented. Health care providers should remain vigilant and consult their local and state health departments and CDC when assessing ill travelers from Ebola-affected countries. Most of these persons do not have Ebola; prompt diagnostic assessments, laboratory testing, and provision of appropriate care for other conditions are essential for appropriate patient care and reflect hospital preparedness.

PMID: 25503923 [PubMed - in process]

78. MMWR Morb Mortal Wkly Rep. 2014 Dec 12;63(49):1172-4.

Rapid assessment of ebola infection prevention and control needs - six districts, sierra leone, october 2014.

Pathmanathan I, O'Connor KA, Adams ML, Rao CY, Kilmarx PH, Park BJ, Mermin J, Kargbo B, Wurie AH, Clarke KR.

As of October 31, 2014, the Sierra Leone Ministry of Health and Sanitation had reported 3,854 laboratory-confirmed cases of Ebola virus disease (Ebola) since the outbreak began in May 2014; 199 (5.2%) of these cases were among health care workers. Ebola infection prevention and control (IPC) measures are essential to interrupt Ebola virus transmission and protect the health workforce, a population that is disproportionately affected by Ebola because of its increased risk of exposure yet is essential to patient care required for outbreak control and maintenance of the country's health system at large. To rapidly identify existing IPC resources and high priority outbreak response needs, an assessment by CDC Ebola Response Team members was conducted in six of the 14 districts in Sierra Leone, consisting of health facility observations and structured interviews with key informants in facilities and government district health management offices. Health system gaps were identified in all six districts, including shortages or absence of trained health care staff, personal protective equipment (PPE), safe patient transport, and standardized IPC protocols. Based on rapid assessment findings and key stakeholder input, priority IPC actions were recommended. Progress has since been made in developing standard operating procedures, increasing laboratory and Ebola treatment capacity and training the health workforce. However, further system strengthening is needed. In particular, a successful Ebola outbreak response in Sierra Leone will require an increase in coordinated and comprehensive district-level IPC support to prevent ongoing Ebola virus transmission.

PMID: 25503922 [PubMed - in process]

79. MMWR Morb Mortal Wkly Rep. 2014 Dec 12;63(49):1168-71.

Ebola virus disease in health care workers - sierra leone, 2014.

Kilmarx PH, Clarke KR, Dietz PM, Hamel MJ, Husain F, McFadden JD, Park BJ, Sugerman DE, Bresee JS, Mermin J, McAuley J, Jambai A.

Health care workers (HCWs) are at increased risk for infection in outbreaks of Ebola virus disease (Ebola). To characterize Ebola in HCWs in Sierra Leone and guide prevention efforts, surveillance data from the national Viral Hemorrhagic Fever database were analyzed. In addition, site visits and interviews with HCWs and health facility administrators were conducted. As of October 31, 2014, a total of 199 (5.2%) of the total of 3,854 laboratory-confirmed Ebola cases reported from Sierra Leone were in HCWs, representing a much higher estimated cumulative incidence of confirmed Ebola in HCWs than in non-HCWs, based on national data on the number of HCW. The peak number of confirmed Ebola cases in HCWs was reported in August (65 cases), and the highest number and percentage of confirmed Ebola cases in HCWs was in Kenema District (65 cases, 12.9% of cases in Kenema), mostly from Kenema General Hospital. Confirmed Ebola cases in HCWs continued to be reported through October and were from 12 of 14 districts in Sierra Leone. A broad range of challenges were reported in implementing infection prevention and control measures. In response, the Ministry of Health and Sanitation and partners are developing standard operating procedures for multiple aspects of infection prevention, including patient isolation and safe burials; recruiting and training staff in infection prevention and control; procuring needed commodities and equipment, including personal protective equipment and vehicles for safe transport of Ebola patients and corpses; renovating and constructing Ebola care facilities designed to reduce risk for nosocomial transmission; monitoring and evaluating infection prevention and control practices; and investigating new cases of Ebola in HCWs as sentinel public health events to identify and address ongoing prevention failures.

PMID: 25503921 [PubMed - in process]

80. MMWR Morb Mortal Wkly Rep. 2014 Dec 12;63(49):1163-7.

Airport exit and entry screening for ebola - august-november 10, 2014.

Brown CM, Aranas AE, Benenson GA, Brunette G, Cetron M, Chen TH, Cohen NJ, Diaz P, Haber Y, Hale CR, Holton K, Kohl K, Le AW, Palumbo GJ, Pearson K, Phares CR, Alvarado-Ramy F, Roohi S, Rotz LD, Tappero J, Washburn FM, Watkins J, Pesik N.

In response to the largest recognized Ebola virus disease epidemic now occurring in West Africa, the governments of affected countries, CDC, the World Health Organization (WHO), and other international organizations have collaborated to implement strategies to control spread of the virus. One strategy recommended by WHO calls for countries with Ebola transmission to screen all persons exiting the country for "unexplained febrile illness consistent with potential Ebola infection." Exit screening at points of departure is intended to reduce the likelihood of international spread of the virus. To initiate this strategy, CDC, WHO, and other global partners were invited by the ministries of health of Guinea, Liberia, and Sierra Leone to assist them in developing and implementing exit screening procedures. Since the program began in August 2014, an estimated 80,000 travelers, of whom approximately 12,000 were en route to the United

States, have departed by air from the three countries with Ebola transmission. Procedures were implemented to deny boarding to ill travelers and persons who reported a high risk for exposure to Ebola; no international air traveler from these countries has been reported as symptomatic with Ebola during travel since these procedures were implemented.

PMID: 25503920 [PubMed - in process]

81. Ann Emerg Med. 2014 Dec 11. pii: S0196-0644(14)01571-6. doi: 10.1016/j.annemergmed.2014.12.003. [Epub ahead of print]

Health Care Worker Quarantine for Ebola: To Eradicate the Virus or Alleviate Fear?

Koenig KL(1).

Author information: (1)Center for Disaster Medical Sciences, University of California at Irvine, Orange, CA. Electronic address: kkoenig@uci.edu.

PMID: 25499243 [PubMed - as supplied by publisher]

82. Clin Infect Dis. 2014 Dec 11. pii: ciu981. [Epub ahead of print]

Sexual and mother-to-child transmission of Ebola virus in the post-convalescent period.

Sonnenberg P(1), Field N(1).

Author information: (1)Research Department of Infection and Population Health, University College of London.

PMID: 25501984 [PubMed - as supplied by publisher]

83. Euro Surveill. 2014 Dec 11;19(49). pii: 20983.

Management of pregnant women infected with Ebola virus in a treatment centre in Guinea, June 2014.

Baggi F(1), Taybi A, Kurth A, Van Herp M, Di Caro A, Wolfel R, Gunther S, Decroo T, Declerck H, Jonckheere S.

Author information: (1)Medecins Sans Frontieres - Operational Centre Brussels, Gueckedou, Guinea.

PMID: 25523968 [PubMed - in process]

84. Int J Clin Pract. 2014 Dec 11. doi: 10.1111/ijcp.12593. [Epub ahead of print]

What is Ebola?

Stein RA(1).

Author information: (1)Department of Biochemistry and Molecular Pharmacology, New York University School of Medicine, New York, NY, USA.

On 23 March 2014, the World Health Organization first announced a new Ebola virus outbreak that started in December 2013 in the eastern part of the Republic of Guinea. Human infections shortly emerged in Liberia, Sierra Leone, and Nigeria. On 30 September 2014, the Centers for Disease Control and Prevention confirmed through laboratory testing the first Ebola virus infection diagnosed in the USA, in a patient who travelled from West Africa to Texas. On 6 October 2014, the first human infection occurring outside of Africa was reported, in a Spanish nurse who treated two priests, both of whom died, and on 23 October 2014, the first human infection was reported in New York City. To date, the 2014 Ebola virus outbreak is the longest, largest, and most persistent one since 1976, when the virus was first identified in humans, and the number of human cases exceeded, as of mid-September 2014, the cumulative number of infections from all the previous outbreaks. The early clinical presentation overlaps with other infectious diseases, opening differential diagnosis difficulties. Understanding the transmission routes and identifying the natural reservoir of the virus are additional challenges in studying Ebola hemorrhagic fever outbreaks. Ebola virus is as much a public health challenge for developing countries as it is for the developed world, and previous outbreaks underscored that the relative contribution of the risk factors may differ among outbreaks. The implementation of effective preparedness plans is contingent on integrating teachings from previous Ebola virus outbreaks with those from the current outbreak and with lessons provided by other infectious diseases, along with developing a multifaceted inter-disciplinary and cross-disciplinary framework that should be established and shaped by biomedical as well as sociopolitical sciences.

© 2014 John Wiley & Sons Ltd.

PMID: 25496121 [PubMed - as supplied by publisher]

85. Intensive Care Med. 2014 Dec 11. [Epub ahead of print]

Isolation in patients with Ebola virus disease.

Wichmann D(1), Schmiedel S, Kluge S.

Author information: (1)Department of Intensive Care Medicine, University Medical Center Hamburg-Eppendorf, Martinistr. 52, 20246, Hamburg, Germany, d.wichmann@uke.de.

PMID: 25502094 [PubMed - as supplied by publisher]

86. J Public Health Policy. 2014 Dec 11. doi: 10.1057/jphp.2014.51. [Epub ahead of print]

Lessons from the public health response to Ebola.

Robbins A Co-Editor, Berkelman R Member Jphp Editorial Board.

PMID: 25501973 [PubMed - as supplied by publisher]

87. Microbes Infect. 2014 Dec 11. pii: S1286-4579(14)00311-6. doi: 10.1016/j.micinf.2014.11.012. [Epub ahead of print]

Development of therapeutics for treatment of Ebola virus infection.

Li H(1), Ying T(1), Yu F(1), Lu L(2), Jiang S(3).

Author information: (1)Key Lab of Medical Molecular Virology of MOE/MOH, Shanghai Medical College, Fudan University, 130 Dong An Rd., Xuhui District, Shanghai 200032, China. (2)Key Lab of Medical Molecular Virology of MOE/MOH, Shanghai Medical College, Fudan University, 130 Dong An Rd., Xuhui District, Shanghai 200032, China. Electronic address: lul@fudan.edu.cn. (3)Key Lab of Medical Molecular Virology of MOE/MOH, Shanghai Medical College, Fudan University, 130

Dong An Rd., Xuhui District, Shanghai 200032, China; Lindsley F. Kimball Research Institute, New York Blood Center, New York, NY 10065, USA. Electronic address: shibojiang@fudan.edu.cn.

Ebola virus infection can cause Ebola virus disease (EVD). Patients usually show severe symptoms, and the fatality rate can reach up to 90%. No licensed medicine is available. In this review, development of therapeutics for treatment of Ebola virus infection and EVD will be discussed.

PMID: 25498866 [PubMed - as supplied by publisher]

88. N Engl J Med. 2014 Dec 11;371(24):2249-51. doi: 10.1056/NEJMp1412166. Epub 2014 Oct 7.

Ebola vaccine--an urgent international priority.

Kanapathipillai R(1), Henao Restrepo AM, Fast P, Wood D, Dye C, Kieny MP, Moorthy V.

Author information: (1)Dr. Kanapathipillai is an editorial fellow at the Journal. Other authors are from the World Health Organization, Geneva.

PMID: 25289888 [PubMed - in process]

89. BMJ. 2014 Dec 10;349:g7608. doi: 10.1136/bmj.g7608.

US provides immunity from legal claims related to three Ebola vaccines.

McCarthy M(1).

Author information: (1)Seattle.

PMID: 25499701 [PubMed - in process]

90. BMJ. 2014 Dec 10;349:g7518. doi: 10.1136/bmj.g7518.

Ebola virus vaccine trials: the ethical mandate for a therapeutic safety net.

Bellan SE(1), Pulliam JR(2), Dushoff J(3), Meyers LA(4).

Author information: (1)Center for Computational Biology and Bioinformatics, The University of Texas at Austin, Austin, TX 78712, USA steve.bellan@gmail.com. (2)Department of Biology and Emerging Pathogens Institute, University of Florida, Gainesville, FL, USA. (3)Department of Biology and Institute of Infectious Disease Research, McMaster University, Hamilton, ON, Canada. (4)Department of Integrative Biology, The University of Texas at Austin, Austin, TX, USA.

PMID: 25498325 [PubMed - in process]

91. BMJ. 2014 Dec 10;349:g7348. doi: 10.1136/bmj.g7348.

Ebola virus disease.

Beeching NJ(1), Fenech M(2), Houlihan CF(3).

Author information: (1)Liverpool School of Tropical Medicine, Royal Liverpool University Hospital, Liverpool, UK Royal Liverpool University Hospital, Liverpool, UK nicholas.beeching@rlbuht.nhs.uk. (2)Royal Liverpool University Hospital, Liverpool, UK. (3)London School of Hygiene and Tropical Medicine, London, UK.

PMID: 25497512 [PubMed - as supplied by publisher]

92. Nurs Stand. 2014 Dec 10;29(15):32. doi: 10.7748/ns.29.15.32.s37.

Reddit: Tracking the 2014 Ebola Outbreak across the World.

Arthur M(1).

Author information: (1)Living in London.

Reddit is a source for what's new and popular on the web. Users provide all the content and decide, through voting, what is good, interesting and informative.

PMID: 25492780 [PubMed - in process]

93. Nurs Stand. 2014 Dec 10;29(15):11. doi: 10.7748/ns.29.15.11.s12.

Clinicians told to stay alert to Ebola, despite low risk in UK.

[No authors listed]

England's chief nurse has urged nurses to remain vigilant to the threat of the Ebola virus.

PMID: 25492753 [PubMed - in process]

94. Viral Immunol. 2014 Dec 10. [Epub ahead of print]

VSVΔG/EBOV GP-Induced Innate Protection Enhances Natural Killer Cell Activity to Increase Survival in a Lethal Mouse Adapted Ebola Virus Infection.

Williams KJ(1), Qiu X, Fernando L, Jones SM, Alimonti JB.

Author information: (1)1 Department of Medical Microbiology and Immunology, University of Alberta , Edmonton, Canada .

Abstract Members of the species Zaire ebolavirus cause severe hemorrhagic fever with up to a 90% mortality rate in humans. The VSVΔG/EBOV GP vaccine has provided 100% protection in the mouse, guinea pig, and nonhuman primate (NHP) models, and has also been utilized as a post-exposure therapeutic to protect mice, guinea pigs, and NHPs from a lethal challenge of Ebola virus (EBOV). EBOV infection causes rapid mortality in human and animal models, with death occurring as early as 6 days after infection, suggesting a vital role for the innate immune system to control the infection before cells of the adaptive immune system can assume control. Natural killer (NK) cells are the predominant cell of the innate immune response, which has been shown to expand with VSVΔG/EBOV GP treatment. In the current study, an in vivo mouse model of the VSVΔG/EBOV GP post-exposure treatment was used for a mouse adapted (MA)-EBOV infection, to determine the putative VSVΔG/EBOV GP-induced protective mechanism of NK cells. NK depletion studies demonstrated that mice with NK cells survive longer in a MA-EBOV infection, which is further enhanced with VSVΔG/EBOV GP treatment. NK cell mediated cytotoxicity and IFN-γ secretion was significantly higher with VSVΔG/EBOV GP treatment. Cell mediated cytotoxicity assays and perforin knockout mice experiments suggest that there are

perforin-dependent and -independent mechanisms involved. Together, these data suggest that NK cells play an important role in VSVΔG/EBOV GP-induced protection of EBOV by increasing NK cytotoxicity, and IFN-γ secretion.
PMID: 25494457 [PubMed - as supplied by publisher]
95. Viral Immunol. 2014 Dec 10. [Epub ahead of print]

Ebola Virus Infection Induces Irregular Dendritic Cell Gene Expression.

Melanson VR(1), Kalina WV, Williams P.
Author information: (1)1 Entomology Department, Walter Reed Army Institute of Research , Silver Spring, Maryland.

Abstract Filoviruses subvert the human immune system in part by infecting and replicating in dendritic cells (DCs). Using gene arrays, a phenotypic profile of filovirus infection in human monocyte-derived DCs was assessed. Monocytes from human donors were cultured in GM-CSF and IL-4 and were infected with Ebola virus Kikwit variant for up to 48 h. Extracted DC RNA was analyzed on SuperArray's Dendritic and Antigen Presenting Cell Oligo GEArray and compared to uninfected controls. Infected DCs exhibited increased expression of cytokine, chemokine, antiviral, and anti-apoptotic genes not seen in uninfected controls. Significant increases of intracellular antiviral and MHC I and II genes were also noted in EBOV-infected DCs. However, infected DCs failed to show any significant difference in co-stimulatory T-cell gene expression from uninfected DCs. Moreover, several chemokine genes were activated, but there was sparse expression of chemokine receptors that enabled activated DCs to home to lymph nodes. Overall, statistically significant expression of several intracellular antiviral genes was noted, which may limit viral load but fails to stop replication. EBOV gene expression profiling is of vital importance in understanding pathogenesis and devising novel therapeutic treatments such as small-molecule inhibitors.
PMID: 25493356 [PubMed - as supplied by publisher]
96. CMAJ. 2014 Dec 9;186(18):E669. doi: 10.1503/cmaj.109-4934. Epub 2014 Nov 3.

Call for Ebola medics falls on deaf ears: MSF.

Vogel L(1).
Author information: (1)CMAJ.
PMID: 25367423 [PubMed - in process]
97. Int J Epidemiol. 2014 Dec 9. pii: dyu233. [Epub ahead of print]

To hasten Ebola containment, mobilize survivors.

Stein ZA(1), Tocco JU(2), Mantell JE(3), Smith RA(3).
Author information: (1)HIV Center for Clinical and Behavioral Studies, Division of Gender, Sexuality and Health, New York State Psychiatric Institute and Columbia University, New York, NY, USA HIV Center for Clinical and Behavioral Studies, Division of Gender, Sexuality and Health, New York State Psychiatric Institute and Columbia University, New York, NY, USA. (2)HIV Center for Clinical and Behavioral Studies, Division of Gender, Sexuality and Health, New York State Psychiatric Institute and Columbia University, New York, NY, USA jt2830@columbia.edu. (3)HIV Center for Clinical and Behavioral Studies, Division of Gender, Sexuality and Health, New York State Psychiatric Institute and Columbia University, New York, NY, USA.
PMID: 25492949 [PubMed - as supplied by publisher]
98. J Community Health. 2014 Dec 9. [Epub ahead of print]

Ebola Therapy and Health Equity.

Nusbaum NJ(1).
Author information: (1)VA Central Western Massachusetts Healthcare System, Leeds, MA, 01053, USA, NusbN@aol.com.

Current care for Ebola patients in resource poor countries is hampered by a lack of resources to isolate patients and their close contacts. The current Ebola epidemic offers the opportunity to harvest convalescent serum to help contain this and future outbreaks. A systemic and just process to accomplish this goal can incorporate procedures to improve care for current Ebola patients and their close contacts.
PMID: 25488847 [PubMed - as supplied by publisher]
99. Med Clin (Barc). 2014 Dec 9;143(11):495-7. doi: 10.1016/j.medcli.2014.10.002. Epub 2014 Oct 25.

[The African tragedy of Ebola].

[Article in Spanish]
Reina J(1).
Author information: (1)Unidad de Virología, Servicio de Microbiología, Hospital Universitario Son Espases, Palma de Mallorca, Spain. Electronic address: jorge.reina@ssib.es.
PMID: 25458517 [PubMed - in process]
100. Med Clin (Barc). 2014 Dec 9;143(11):492-4. doi: 10.1016/j.medcli.2014.10.001. Epub 2014 Oct 23.

[Ebola ad portas].

[Article in Spanish]
Trilla A(1).
Author information: (1)Centro de Investigación en Salud Internacional de Barcelona (CRESIB), Hospital Clínic, Universidad de Barcelona, Barcelona, España. Electronic address: atrilla@clinic.cat.
PMID: 25458516 [PubMed - in process]
101. Nature. 2014 Dec 9;516(7530):154-5. doi: 10.1038/516154a.

Ebola experts seek to expand testing.

Butler D.

PMID: 25503213 [PubMed - in process]

102. BMJ. 2014 Dec 8;349:g7559. doi: 10.1136/bmj.g7559.

Quarantining health workers returning from Ebola affected countries is "bad science," says public health adviser.

Gulland A(1).

Author information: (1)Venice.

PMID: 25486942 [PubMed - in process]

103. J Am Med Dir Assoc. 2014 Dec 6. pii: S1525-8610(14)00755-5. doi: 10.1016/j.jamda.2014.11.008. [Epub ahead of print]

Borrowing From Geriatrics to Treat Ebola in Africa.

Hassid EJ(1).

Author information: (1)California Pacific Medical Center, San Francisco, California.

PMID: 25492640 [PubMed - as supplied by publisher]

104. Lancet. 2014 Dec 6;384(9959):2023. doi: 10.1016/S0140-6736(14)62330-8.

Ebola, International Health Regulations, and global safety.

Kimball AM(1), Heymann D(2).

Author information: (1)Department of Epidemiology, University of Washington, Seattle, WA 98195, USA. Electronic address: amkimball@gmail.com. (2)Chatham House, London, UK.

Comment on Lancet. 2014 Oct 11;384(9951):1321.

PMID: 25483162 [PubMed - in process]

105. Lancet. 2014 Dec 6;384(9959):2022. doi: 10.1016/S0140-6736(14)62329-1.

Ebola control: the Cuban approach.

Ebrahim S(1), Squires N(2), Díaz MB(3), di Fabio JL(3), Reed G(4), Bourne PG(5), Keck W(6), Chalkidou K(7).

Author information: (1)London School of Hygiene & Tropical Medicine, London, UK. (2)Public Health England, London, UK. (3)Pan American Health Organisation, La Habana, Cuba. (4)Medical Education Cooperation with Cuba, Oakland, CA, USA. (5)Medical Education Cooperation with Cuba, Oakland, CA, USA; Green Templeton College, Oxford, UK. (6)Medical Education Cooperation with Cuba, Oakland, CA, USA; Northeast Ohio Medical University, Rootstown, OH, USA. (7)National Institute for Health and Care Excellence International, London, UK. Electronic address: kalipso.chalkidou@gmail.com.

PMID: 25483161 [PubMed - indexed for MEDLINE]

106. Lancet. 2014 Dec 6;384(9959):2001-2. doi: 10.1016/S0140-6736(14)62316-3.

Ebola virus disease: clinical care and patient-centred research.

Roberts I(1), Perner A(2).

Author information: (1)Clinical Trials Unit, London School of Hygiene & Tropical Medicine, London WC1E 7HT, UK. Electronic address: ian.roberts@lshtm.ac.uk. (2)Department of Intensive Care, Rigshospitalet, University of Copenhagen, Denmark.

PMID: 25483156 [PubMed - indexed for MEDLINE]

107. Lancet. 2014 Dec 6;384(9959):2023-4. doi: 10.1016/S0140-6736(14)62226-1. Epub 2014 Nov 19.

Ebola: should we consider influenza vaccination?

Matheron S(1), Baize S(2), Lerat I(3), Houhou N(4), Yazdanpanah Y(3).

Author information: (1)Infectious and Tropical Diseases Department, Hôpital Bichat-Claude-Bernard, Assistance Publique-Hôpitaux de Paris, 75018 Paris, France; Université Paris Diderot, Paris 7, Paris, France; Unité mixte de recherche 1137 (Infection, Antimicrobiens, Modélisation, Evolution), Institut national de la santé et de la recherche médicale, Paris, France. Electronic address: sophie.matheron@bch.aphp.fr. (2)National Reference Center for Viral Hemorrhagic Fevers, Unité de Biologie des Infections Virales Emergentes, Institut Pasteur-Centre International de Recherche en Infectiologie, Lyon, France. (3)Infectious and Tropical Diseases Department, Hôpital Bichat-Claude-Bernard, Assistance Publique-Hôpitaux de Paris, 75018 Paris, France; Université Paris Diderot, Paris 7, Paris, France; Unité mixte de recherche 1137 (Infection, Antimicrobiens, Modélisation, Evolution), Institut national de la santé et de la recherche médicale, Paris, France. (4)Virology Department, Hôpital Bichat-Claude-Bernard, Assistance Publique-Hôpitaux de Paris, 75018 Paris, France.

PMID: 25467571 [PubMed - indexed for MEDLINE]

108. BMJ. 2014 Dec 5;349:g7503. doi: 10.1136/bmj.g7503.

Obama calls on Congress to fund $6.2bn emergency Ebola initiative.

McCarthy M(1).

Author information: (1)Seattle.

PMID: 25497740 [PubMed - in process]

109. Cell Stress Chaperones. 2014 Dec 5. [Epub ahead of print]

The transition from a rural to an urban environment alters expression of the human Ebola virus receptor Neiman-Pick C1: implications for the current epidemic in West Africa.

Bickler SW(1), Lizardo RE, De Maio A.

Author information: (1)Center for Investigations of Health and Education Disparities, University of California San Diego, 9500 Gilman Drive, #0739, La Jolla, CA, 92093-0739, USA, sbickler@ucsd.edu.
PMID: 25477151 [PubMed - as supplied by publisher]
110. Ann N Y Acad Sci. 2014 Dec 4. doi: 10.1111/nyas.12601. [Epub ahead of print]

One Medicine One Science: a framework for exploring challenges at the intersection of animals, humans, and the environment.

Travis DA(1), Srirama Rao P, Cardona C, Steer CJ, Kennedy S, Sreevatsan S, Murtaugh MP.

Author information: (1)Department of Veterinary Population Medicine, College of Veterinary Medicine, University of Minnesota, St. Paul, Minnesota.
Characterizing the health consequences of interactions among animals, humans, and the environment in the face of climatic change, environmental disturbance, and expanding human populations is a critical global challenge in today's world. Exchange of interdisciplinary knowledge in basic and applied sciences and medicine that includes scientists, health professionals, key sponsors, and policy experts revealed that relevant case studies of monkeypox, influenza A, tuberculosis, and HIV can be used to guide strategies for anticipating and responding to new disease threats such as the Ebola and Chickungunya viruses, as well as to improve programs to control existing zoonotic diseases, including tuberculosis. The problem of safely feeding the world while preserving the environment and avoiding issues such as antibiotic resistance in animals and humans requires cooperative scientific problem solving. Food poisoning outbreaks resulting from Salmonella growing in vegetables have demonstrated the need for knowledge of pathogen evolution and adaptation in developing appropriate countermeasures for prevention and policy development. Similarly, pesticide use for efficient crop production must take into consideration bee population declines that threaten the availability of the two-thirds of human foods that are dependent on pollination. This report presents and weighs the objective merits of competing health priorities and identifies gaps in knowledge that threaten health security, to promote discussion of major public policy implications such that they may be decided with at least an underlying platform of facts.
PMID: 25476836 [PubMed - as supplied by publisher]
111. Biochem Pharmacol. 2014 Dec 4. pii: S0006-2952(14)00689-3. doi: 10.1016/j.bcp.2014.11.008. [Epub ahead of print]

Ebola virus (EBOV) infection: Therapeutic strategies.

De Clercq E(1).

Author information: (1)Rega Institute for Medical Research, KU Leuven, Minderbroedersstraat 10, B-3000 Leuven, Belgium. Electronic address: erik.declercq@rega.kuleuven.be.
Within less than a year after its epidemic started (in December 2013) in Guinea, Ebola virus (EBOV), a member of the filoviridae, has spread over a number of West-African countries (Guinea, Sierra Leone and Liberia) and gained allures that have been unprecedented except by human immunodeficiency virus (HIV). Although EBOV is highly contagious and transmitted by direct contact with body fluids, it could be counteracted by the adequate chemoprophylactic and -therapeutic interventions: vaccines, antibodies, siRNAs (small interfering RNAs), interferons and chemical substances, i.e. neplanocin A derivatives (i.e. 3-deazaneplanocin A), BCX4430, favipiravir (T-705), endoplasmic reticulum (ER) α-glucosidase inhibitors and a variety of compounds that have been found to inhibit EBOV infection blocking viral entry or by a mode of action that still has to be resolved. Much has to be learned from the mechanism of action of the compounds active against VSV (vesicular stomatitis virus), a virus belonging to the rhabdoviridae, that in its mode of replication could be exemplary for the replication of filoviridae.
PMID: 25481298 [PubMed - as supplied by publisher]
112. Euro Surveill. 2014 Dec 4;19(48). pii: 20980.

Preparedness for admission of patients with suspected Ebola virus disease in European hospitals: a survey, August-September 2014.

de Jong M(1), Reusken C, Horby P, Koopmans M, Bonten M, Chiche J, Giaquinto C, Welte T, Leus F, Schotsman J, Goossens H; PREPARE consortium and affiliated clinical networks.

Author information: (1)Department of Medical Microbiology, Academic Medical Center, Amsterdam, the Netherlands.
PMID: 25496571 [PubMed - in process]
113. J Hosp Med. 2014 Dec 4. doi: 10.1002/jhm.2298. [Epub ahead of print]

The role of hospitalists in the Ebola response in the United States and abroad.

Waters A(1), Wu E, Shamasunder S, Le P.

Author information: (1)Division of Hospital Medicine, University of California San Francisco, San Francisco, California.
PMID: 25471530 [PubMed - as supplied by publisher]
114. J Perinat Med. 2014 Dec 4. pii: /j/jpme.ahead-of-print/jpm-2014-0334/jpm-2014-0334.xml. doi: 10.1515/jpm-2014-0334. [Epub ahead of print]

Ebola viral infection in pregnancy: a plea for specific clinical recommendations.

Santolaya JL, Santolaya-Forgas J.

PMID: 25473800 [PubMed - as supplied by publisher]
115. Nat Med. 2014 Dec 4;20(12):1359. doi: 10.1038/nm1214-1359.

University travel bans and quarantines may impede Ebola response.

Willyard C.

PMID: 25473907 [PubMed - in process]

116. Nat Med. 2014 Dec 4;20(12):1356-7. doi: 10.1038/nm1214-1356.

Advances in marmoset and mouse models buoy Ebola research.

Willyard C.

PMID: 25473905 [PubMed - in process]

117. Nature. 2014 Dec 4;516(7529):15-6. doi: 10.1038/516015a.

Positive results spur race for Ebola vaccine.

Callaway E.

PMID: 25471858 [PubMed - in process]

118. Virus Res. 2014 Dec 4. pii: S0168-1702(14)00503-6. doi: 10.1016/j.virusres.2014.11.028. [Epub ahead of print]

Controlled viral glycoprotein expression as a safety feature in a bivalent rabies-ebola vaccine.

Papaneri A(1), Bernbaum J(1), Blaney JE(1), Jahrling PB(1), Schnell M(1), Johnson RF(2).

Author information: (1)NIH/NIAID, Ft. Detrick, MD, USA. (2)NIH/NIAID, Ft. Detrick, MD, USA. Electronic address: johnsonreed@mail.nih.gov.

Using a recombinant rabies (RABV) vaccine platform, we have developed several safe and effective vaccines. Most recently, we have developed a RABV-based ebolavirus (EBOV) vaccine that is efficacious in nonhuman primates. One safety feature of this vaccine is the utilization of a live but replication-deficient RABV construct. In this construct, the RABV glycoprotein (G) has been deleted from the genome, requiring G trans complementation in order for new infectious viruses to be released from the initial infected cell. Here we analyze this safety feature of the bivalent RABV-based EBOV vaccine comprised of the G-deleted RABV backbone expressing EBOV glycoprotein (GP). We found that, while the level of RABV genome in infected cells is equivalent regardless of G supplementation, the production of infectious virus is indeed restricted by the lack of G, and most importantly, that the presence of EBOV GP does not substitute for G. These findings further support the safety profile of this replication-deficient RABV-EBOV bivalent vaccine.

PMID: 25481284 [PubMed - as supplied by publisher]

119. BMJ. 2014 Dec 3;349:g7402. doi: 10.1136/bmj.g7402.

The west African Ebola disaster has stretched us to near breaking point: MSF's volunteer doctors need your support.

Godlee F.

PMID: 25477504 [PubMed - in process]

120. Int J Infect Dis. 2014 Dec 3;30C:85-86. doi: 10.1016/j.ijid.2014.12.002. [Epub ahead of print]

Guidelines for treatment of patients with Ebola Virus Diseases are urgently needed.

Petersen E(1), Maiga B(2).

Author information: (1)Editor-in-Chief, International Journal of Infectious Diseases, Professor of Tropical Medicine, Department of Infectious Diseases and Clinical Microbiology, Aarhus University Hospital, Aarhus, Denmark. (2)Faculty of Medicine and Odonto-Stomatology, University of Sciences, Techniques and, Technology of Bamako (USTTB) of Bamako, Mali.

PMID: 25481049 [PubMed - as supplied by publisher]

121. J Virol. 2014 Dec 3. pii: JVI.02752-14. [Epub ahead of print]

GB virus C co-infections in West African Ebola patients.

Lauck M(1), Bailey AL(1), Andersen KG(2), Goldberg TL(3), Sabeti PC(2), O'Connor DH(4).

Author information: (1)Department of Pathology and Laboratory Medicine, University of Wisconsin-Madison, Madison, Wisconsin, USA Wisconsin National Primate Research Center, Madison, Wisconsin, USA. (2)The Broad Institute of MIT and Harvard, Cambridge, Massachusetts, USA Center for Systems Biology, Department of Organismic and Evolutionary Biology, Harvard University, Cambridge, Massachusetts, USA. (3)Wisconsin National Primate Research Center, Madison, Wisconsin, USA Department of Pathobiological Sciences, University of Wisconsin-Madison. (4)Department of Pathology and Laboratory Medicine, University of Wisconsin-Madison, Madison, Wisconsin, USA Wisconsin National Primate Research Center, Madison, Wisconsin, USA doconnor@primate.wisc.edu.

In 49 patients with known Ebolavirus (EBOV) outcomes during the ongoing outbreak in Sierra Leone, 13 were co-infected with the immunomodulatory pegivirus GB virus C (GBV-C). 53% of these GBV-C+ patients survived; in contrast, only 22% of GBV-C(-) patients survived. Both survival and GBV-C status were associated with age, with older patients having lower survival rates and intermediate-age patients (21-45 years) having the highest rate of GBV-C infection. Understanding the separate and combined effects of GBV-C and age on EBOV survival could lead to new treatment and prevention strategies, perhaps through age-related pathways of immune activation.

PMID: 25473056 [PubMed - as supplied by publisher]

122. Kidney Int. 2014 Dec 3. doi: 10.1038/ki.2014.375. [Epub ahead of print]

Minimizing risks associated with renal replacement therapy in patients with Ebola virus disease.

Wolf T(1), Ross MJ(2), Davenport A(3).

Author information: (1)Facharzt für Innere Medizin und Infektiologie, Universitätsklinikum Frankfurt, Medizinische Klinik II, Infektiologie, Frankfurt, Germany. (2)Division of Nephrology, Icahn School of Medicine at Mount Sinai, New York, New York, USA. (3)UCL Centre for Nephrology, Royal Free Hospital, University College London Medical School, London, UK.

PMID: 25469847 [PubMed - as supplied by publisher]

123. Virol J. 2014 Dec 3;11(1):205. [Epub ahead of print]

Plant-based vaccines against viruses.

Rybicki EP.

Plant-made or ¿biofarmed¿ viral vaccines are some of the earliest products of the technology of plant molecular farming, and remain some of the brightest prospects for the success of this field. Proofs of principle and of efficacy exist for many candidate viral veterinary vaccines; the use of plant-made viral antigens and of monoclonal antibodies for therapy of animal and even human viral disease is also well established. This review explores some of the more prominent recent advances in the biofarming of viral vaccines and therapies, including the recent use of ZMapp for Ebolavirus infection, and explores some possible future applications of the technology.

PMCID: PMC4264547 PMID: 25465382 [PubMed - as supplied by publisher]

124. Ann Intern Med. 2014 Dec 2;161(11):829-30. doi: 10.7326/M14-2084.

Safe management of patients with serious communicable diseases: recent experience with ebola virus.

Isakov A, Jamison A, Miles W, Ribner B.

PMID: 25244492 [PubMed - in process]

125. Ann Intern Med. 2014 Dec 2;161(11):831-2. doi: 10.7326/M14-2141.

Preparing for critical care services to patients with ebola.

Decker BK, Sevransky JE, Barrett K, Davey RT, Chertow DS.

PMID: 25244048 [PubMed - in process]

126. BMJ. 2014 Dec 2;349:g7424. doi: 10.1136/bmj.g7424.

WHO warns over complacency as targets on Ebola are met.

Gulland A(1).

Author information: (1)London.

PMID: 25468873 [PubMed - in process]

127. Int J Palliat Nurs. 2014 Dec 2;20(12):575.

Palliative nursing and the Ebola crisis.

[No authors listed]

PMID: 25526285 [PubMed - as supplied by publisher]

128. MBio. 2014 Dec 2;5(6):e02145. doi: 10.1128/mBio.02145-14.

Genomics and proteomics of mycobacteriophage patience, an accidental tourist in the Mycobacterium neighborhood.

Pope WH(1), Jacobs-Sera D(1), Russell DA(1), Rubin DH(2), Kajee A(3), Msibi ZN(4), Larsen MH(5), Jacobs WR Jr(6), Lawrence JG(1), Hendrix RW(1), Hatfull GF(7).

Author information: (1)Department of Biological Sciences, University of Pittsburgh, Pittsburgh, Pennsylvania, USA. (2)Harvard College, Cambridge, Massachusetts, USA. (3)University of KwaZulu-Natal, School of Laboratory Medicine, College of Health Sciences, Inkosi Albert Luthuli Hospital, Durban, South Africa. (4)Department of Infection Prevention and Control, University of KwaZulu-Natal, Durban, South Africa. (5)Department of Medicine, Albert Einstein College of Medicine, Bronx, New York, USA. (6)Howard Hughes Medical Institute, Department of Microbiology and Immunology, Albert Einstein College of Medicine, Bronx, New York, USA. (7)Department of Biological Sciences, University of Pittsburgh, Pittsburgh, Pennsylvania, USA gfh@pitt.edu.

Newly emerging human viruses such as Ebola virus, severe acute respiratory syndrome (SARS) virus, and HIV likely originate within an extant population of viruses in nonhuman hosts and acquire the ability to infect and cause disease in humans. Although several mechanisms preventing viral infection of particular hosts have been described, the mechanisms and constraints on viral host expansion are ill defined. We describe here mycobacteriophage Patience, a newly isolated phage recovered using Mycobacterium smegmatis mc(2)155 as a host. Patience has genomic features distinct from its M. smegmatis host, including a much lower GC content (50.3% versus 67.4%) and an abundance of codons that are rarely used in M. smegmatis. Nonetheless, it propagates well in M. smegmatis, and we demonstrate the use of mass spectrometry to show expression of over 75% of the predicted proteins, to identify new genes, to refine the genome annotation, and to estimate protein abundance. We propose that Patience evolved primarily among lower-GC hosts and that the disparities between its genomic profile and that of M. smegmatis presented only a minimal barrier to host expansion. Rapid adaptions to its new host include recent acquisition of higher-GC genes, expression of out-of-frame proteins within predicted genes, and codon selection among highly expressed genes toward the translational apparatus of its new host.IMPORTANCE: The mycobacteriophage Patience genome has a notably lower GC content (50.3%) than its Mycobacterium smegmatis host (67.4%) and has markedly different codon usage biases. The viral genome has an abundance of codons that are rare in the host and are decoded by wobble tRNA pairing, although the phage grows well and expression of most of the genes is detected by mass spectrometry. Patience thus has the genomic profile of a virus that evolved primarily in one type of host genetic landscape (moderate-GC bacteria) but has found its way into a distinctly different high-GC environment. Although Patience genes are ill matched to the host expression apparatus, this is of little functional consequence and has not evidently imposed a barrier to migration across the microbial landscape. Interestingly, comparison of expression levels and codon usage profiles reveals evidence of codon selection as the genome evolves and adapts to its new environment.

Copyright © 2014 Pope et al.

PMID: 25467442 [PubMed - in process]

129. Proc Natl Acad Sci U S A. 2014 Dec 2;111(48):17182-7. doi: 10.1073/pnas.1414164111. Epub 2014 Nov 17.

Structures of protective antibodies reveal sites of vulnerability on Ebola virus.

Murin CD(1), Fusco ML(2), Bornholdt ZA(2), Qiu X(3), Olinger GG(4), Zeitlin L(5), Kobinger GP(6), Ward AB(7), Saphire EO(8).
Author information: (1)Department of Integrative Structural and Computational Biology, Department of Immunology and Microbial Science, and. (2)Department of Immunology and Microbial Science, and. (3)National Microbiology Laboratory, Public Health Agency of Canada, Winnipeg, MB, Canada R3E 3R2; (4)National Institute of Allergy and Infectious Diseases/Integrated Research Facility, National Institutes of Health, Frederick, MD 21702; (5)Mapp Biopharmaceutical, San Diego, CA 92121; (6)National Microbiology Laboratory, Public Health Agency of Canada, Winnipeg, MB, Canada R3E 3R2; Department of Medical Microbiology, University of Manitoba, Winnipeg, MB, Canada R3E 0J9; and Department of Immunology, University of Manitoba, Winnipeg, MB, Canada R3E 0T5. (7)Department of Integrative Structural and Computational Biology, abward@scripps.edu erica@scripps.edu. (8)Department of Immunology and Microbial Science, and The Skaggs Institute for Chemical Biology, The Scripps Research Institute, La Jolla, CA 92037; abward@scripps.edu erica@scripps.edu.

Ebola virus (EBOV) and related filoviruses cause severe hemorrhagic fever, with up to 90% lethality, and no treatments are approved for human use. Multiple recent outbreaks of EBOV and the likelihood of future human exposure highlight the need for pre- and postexposure treatments. Monoclonal antibody (mAb) cocktails are particularly attractive candidates due to their proven postexposure efficacy in nonhuman primate models of EBOV infection. Two candidate cocktails, MB-003 and ZMAb, have been extensively evaluated in both in vitro and in vivo studies. Recently, these two therapeutics have been combined into a new cocktail named ZMapp, which showed increased efficacy and has been given compassionately to some human patients. Epitope information and mechanism of action are currently unknown for most of the component mAbs. Here we provide single-particle EM reconstructions of every mAb in the ZMapp cocktail, as well as additional antibodies from MB-003 and ZMAb. Our results illuminate key and recurring sites of vulnerability on the EBOV glycoprotein and provide a structural rationale for the efficacy of ZMapp. Interestingly, two of its components recognize overlapping epitopes and compete with each other for binding. Going forward, this work now provides a basis for strategic selection of next-generation antibody cocktails against Ebola and related viruses and a model for predicting the impact of ZMapp on potential escape mutations in ongoing or future Ebola outbreaks.

PMCID: PMC4260551 [Available on 2015/6/2] PMID: 25404321 [PubMed - in process]

130. Am J Health Syst Pharm. 2014 Dec 1;71(23):2000-6. doi: 10.2146/news140080.

Pharmacists' investigational drug services aid Ebola response.

Traynor K.

PMID: 25404587 [PubMed - in process]

131. Am J Infect Control. 2014 Dec;42(12):1256-7. doi: 10.1016/j.ajic.2014.10.006. Epub 2014 Nov 25.

Nebraska Biocontainment Unit perspective on disposal of Ebola medical waste.

Lowe JJ(1), Gibbs SG(2), Schwedhelm SS(3), Nguyen J(4), Smith PW(5).
Author information: (1)Department of Environmental, Agricultural & Occupational Health, University of Nebraska Medical Center College of Public Health, Omaha, NE; Nebraska Biocontainment Unit, The Nebraska Medical Center, Omaha, NE. Electronic address: jjlowe@unmc.edu. (2)Department of Environmental, Agricultural & Occupational Health, University of Nebraska Medical Center College of Public Health, Omaha, NE; Nebraska Biocontainment Unit, The Nebraska Medical Center, Omaha, NE. (3)Nebraska Biocontainment Unit, The Nebraska Medical Center, Omaha, NE; The Nebraska Medical Center, Omaha, NE. (4)The Nebraska Medical Center, Omaha, NE. (5)Nebraska Biocontainment Unit, The Nebraska Medical Center, Omaha, NE; Division of Infectious Diseases, Department of Internal Medicine, University of Nebraska Medical Center, Omaha, NE.

PMID: 25465251 [PubMed - in process]

132. Am J Nurs. 2014 Dec;114(12):14-15.

Caring for Patients with Ebola.

Wallis L.

Nurses at Emory University Hospital shine.

PMID: 25423377 [PubMed - as supplied by publisher]

133. Am J Nurs. 2014 Dec;114(12):7.

Our Ebola Wake-Up Call.

Kennedy MS(1).
Author information: (1)AJN Editor-in-Chief E-mail: shawn.kennedy@wolterskluwer.com.

What have we learned from this crisis?

PMID: 25423370 [PubMed - as supplied by publisher]

134. Am J Trop Med Hyg. 2014 Dec 1. pii: 14-0719. [Epub ahead of print]

Rethinking the Discharge Policy for Ebola Convalescents in an Accelerating Epidemic.

O'Dempsey T(1), Khan SH(1), Bausch DG(2).
Author information: (1)Liverpool School of Tropical Medicine, Liverpool, United Kingdom; Kenema Government Hospital, Ministry of Health and Sanitation, Sierra Leone; Tulane University Health Sciences Center, New Orleans, Louisiana; U.S. Naval Medical Research Unit No. 6, Lima, Peru. (2)Liverpool School of Tropical Medicine, Liverpool, United Kingdom; Kenema Government Hospital, Ministry of Health and Sanitation, Sierra Leone; Tulane University Health Sciences Center, New Orleans, Louisiana; U.S. Naval Medical Research Unit No. 6, Lima, Peru dbausch@tulane.edu.

The outbreak of Ebola virus disease (EVD) in West Africa has outstripped available resources. Novel strategies are desperately needed to streamline operations. The present norm of requiring negative results on polymerase chain reaction for EVD convalescent patients to be discharged is not evidence-based and often results in asymptomatic patients competing for beds in dangerously crowded Ebola Treatment Units, posing risks to ward staff and patients and the community if infected persons are turned away. We summarize the relevant data and call for a change in discharge criteria for convalescent patients that can safely help reduce the strain on resources and direct energies where they are most needed. In the longer term, research is needed to assess the true infectivity of EVD convalescent patients to establish evidence-based criteria and guidelines for discharge.

©The American Society of Tropical Medicine and Hygiene.

PMID: 25448238 [PubMed - as supplied by publisher]

135. Antiviral Res. 2014 Dec;112:1-7. doi: 10.1016/j.antiviral.2014.09.012. Epub 2014 Oct 5.

The cyanobacterial lectin scytovirin displays potent in vitro and in vivo activity against Zaire Ebola virus.

Garrison AR(1), Giomarelli BG(2), Lear-Rooney CM(1), Saucedo CJ(3), Yellayi S(4), Krumpe LR(3), Rose M(2), Paragas J(1), Bray M(5), Olinger GG Jr(1), McMahon JB(2), Huggins J(1), O'Keefe BR(6).

Author information: (1)Department of Viral Therapeutics, Virology Division, United States Army Medical Research Institute of Infectious Disease, Ft. Detrick, Frederick, MD 21702, United States. (2)Molecular Targets Laboratory, Center for Cancer Research, National Cancer Institute, National Institutes of Health, Frederick National Laboratory for Cancer Research, Frederick, MD 21702, United States. (3)Molecular Targets Laboratory, Center for Cancer Research, National Cancer Institute, National Institutes of Health, Frederick National Laboratory for Cancer Research, Frederick, MD 21702, United States; Basic Science Program, Leidos Biomedical Research Inc., Frederick National Laboratory for Cancer Research, Frederick, MD 21702, United States. (4)Office of the Chief Scientist, Integrated Research Facility, Division of Clinical Research, National Institute of Allergy and Infectious Diseases, Frederick, MD 2170, United States. (5)Department of Viral Therapeutics, Virology Division, United States Army Medical Research Institute of Infectious Disease, Ft. Detrick, Frederick, MD 21702, United States; Division of Clinical Research, National Institute of Allergy and Infectious Disease, National Institutes of Health, Bethesda, MD 20892, United States. (6)Molecular Targets Laboratory, Center for Cancer Research, National Cancer Institute, National Institutes of Health, Frederick National Laboratory for Cancer Research, Frederick, MD 21702, United States. Electronic address: okeefeba@mail.nih.gov.

The cyanobacterial lectin scytovirin (SVN) binds with high affinity to mannose-rich oligosaccharides on the envelope glycoprotein (GP) of a number of viruses, blocking entry into target cells. In this study, we assessed the ability of SVN to bind to the envelope GP of Zaire Ebola virus (ZEBOV) and inhibit its replication. SVN interacted specifically with the protein's mucin-rich domain. In cell culture, it inhibited ZEBOV replication with a 50% virus-inhibitory concentration (EC50) of 50nM, and was also active against the Angola strain of the related Marburg virus (MARV), with a similar EC50. Injected subcutaneously in mice, SVN reached a peak plasma level of 100nm in 45min, but was cleared within 4h. When ZEBOV-infected mice were given 30mg/kg/day of SVN by subcutaneous injection every 6h, beginning the day before virus challenge, 9 of 10 animals survived the infection, while all infected, untreated mice died. When treatment was begun one hour or one day after challenge, 70-90% of mice survived. Quantitation of infectious virus and viral RNA in samples of serum, liver and spleen collected on days 2 and 5 postinfection showed a trend toward lower titers in treated than control mice, with a significant decrease in liver titers on day 2. Our findings provide further evidence of the potential of natural lectins as therapeutic agents for viral infections.

Published by Elsevier B.V.

PMCID: PMC4258435 [Available on 2015/12/1] PMID: 25265598 [PubMed - in process]

136. Biomedica. 2014 Dec;34(4):503-5. doi: 10.1590/S0120-41572014000400001.

[Ebola hemorrhagic fever and the threat it poses to health systems].

[Article in Spanish]

De la Hoz F(1).

Author information: (1)Instituto Nacional de Salud, Bogotá, D.C, Colombia.

PMID: 25504237 [PubMed - in process]

137. Br J Gen Pract. 2014 Dec;64(629):636. doi: 10.3399/bjgp14X682909.

GPs and the Ebola patient: working safely in primary care.

Stockley SN(1), Rafi I(2), Baker M(2).

Author information: (1)Eaglescliffe, Stockton-On-Tees, North East England. (2)Royal College of General Practitioners, London.

PMCID: PMC4240134 PMID: 25452526 [PubMed - in process]

138. Can J Surg. 2014 Dec;57(6):366-367.

[La chirurgie chez le patient atteint de la maladie à virus Ebola.]

[Article in French]

McAlister V(1).

Author information: (1)Co-rédacteur, Journal canadien de chirurgie.

PMCID: PMC4245264 PMID: 25421076 [PubMed - as supplied by publisher]

139. Can J Surg. 2014 Dec;57(6):364-5. doi: 10.1503/cjs.015514.

Surgery in patients with Ebola virus disease.

McAlister V(1).

Author information: (1)Coeditor, Canadian Journal of Surgery.

PMCID: PMC4245263 PMID: 25354163 [PubMed - in process]

140. Cleve Clin J Med. 2014 Dec;81(12):729-35. doi: 10.3949/ccjm.81gr.14007.

Ebola virus: Questions, answers, and more questions.

Brizendine KD(1).

Author information: (1)Department of Infectious Disease, Cleveland Clinic.

Ebola virus causes a hemorrhagic fever with a high case-fatality rate. Treatment remains supportive although a variety of specific treatments are still in the early stages of investigation. This report reviews the clinical virology of Ebola virus, the reported proposed treatments, and the current outbreak.

PMID: 25452350 [PubMed - in process]

141. Cleve Clin J Med. 2014 Dec;81(12):708. doi: 10.3949/ccjm.81b.12014.

Ebola-lessons still to be learned.

Mandell BF.

PMID: 25452343 [PubMed - in process]

142. Clin Chem Lab Med. 2014 Dec 1;52(12):1681-4. doi: 10.1515/cclm-2014-0960.

Laboratory preparedness to face infectious outbreaks. Ebola and beyond.

Lippi G, Mattiuzzi C, Plebani M.

PMID: 25324450 [PubMed - in process]

143. Clin Vaccine Immunol. 2014 Dec;21(12):1605-12. doi: 10.1128/CVI.00484-14. Epub 2014 Sep 17.

Determination of specific antibody responses to the six species of ebola and marburg viruses by multiplexed protein microarrays.

Kamata T(1), Natesan M(1), Warfield K(2), Aman MJ(2), Ulrich RG(3).

Author information: (1)United States Army Medical Research Institute for Infectious Diseases, Frederick, Maryland, USA. (2)Integrated BioTherapeutics, Inc., Gaithersburg, Maryland, USA. (3)United States Army Medical Research Institute for Infectious Diseases, Frederick, Maryland, USA rulrich@bhsai.org.

Infectious hemorrhagic fevers caused by the Marburg and Ebola filoviruses result in human mortality rates of up to 90%, and there are no effective vaccines or therapeutics available for clinical use. The highly infectious and lethal nature of these viruses highlights the need for reliable and sensitive diagnostic methods. We assembled a protein microarray displaying nucleoprotein (NP), virion protein 40 (VP40), and glycoprotein (GP) antigens from isolates representing the six species of filoviruses for use as a surveillance and diagnostic platform. Using the microarrays, we examined serum antibody responses of rhesus macaques vaccinated with trivalent (GP, NP, and VP40) virus-like particles (VLP) prior to infection with the Marburg virus (MARV) (i.e., Marburg marburgvirus) or the Zaire virus (ZEBOV) (i.e., Zaire ebolavirus). The microarray-based assay detected a significant increase in antigen-specific IgG resulting from immunization, while a greater level of antibody responses resulted from challenge of the vaccinated animals with ZEBOV or MARV. Further, while antibody cross-reactivities were observed among NPs and VP40s of Ebola viruses, antibody recognition of GPs was very specific. The performance of mucin-like domain fragments of GP (GP mucin) expressed in Escherichia coli was compared to that of GP ectodomains produced in eukaryotic cells. Based on results with ZEBOV and MARV proteins, antibody recognition of GP mucins that were deficient in posttranslational modifications was comparable to that of the eukaryotic cell-expressed GP ectodomains in assay performance. We conclude that the described protein microarray may translate into a sensitive assay for diagnosis and serological surveillance of infections caused by multiple species of filoviruses.

PMCID: PMC4248775 [Available on 2015/6/1] PMID: 25230936 [PubMed - in process]

144. Dev World Bioeth. 2014 Dec;14(3):ii-iii. doi: 10.1111/dewb.12073.

Bioethics and the ebola outbreak in West Africa.

Schuklenk U.

PMID: 25359688 [PubMed - in process]

145. Dtsch Med Wochenschr. 2014 Dec;139(49):2510-2. doi: 10.1055/s-0034-1387472. Epub 2014 Nov 25.

[Ebola virus disease].

[Article in German]

Grünewald T(1).

Author information: (1)Behandlungszentrum Leipzig des Ständigen Arbeitskreises der Kompetenz- und Behandlungszentren für hochkontagiöse und lebensbedrohliche Erkrankungen (STAKOB), Klinik für Infektiologie/Tropenmedizin und Nephrologie, Zentrum für Innere Medizin, Klinikum St. Georg Leipzig.

The current Ebola outbreak in Western Africa differs from previous ones due to its extent. Serious shortcomings in the on-site management in Africa are obvious. In addition to the situation in the countries affected media and medical interests also focus on detection and management of imported cases in Germany. From the experience with such patients already treated in Germany the existing medical concepts have been updated and expanded. This overview addresses not only the latest clinical knowledge and epidemiological developments but also outlines the key measures as well as the practical procedure when there is a suspected case.

PMID: 25423458 [PubMed - in process]

146. ED Manag. 2014 Dec;26(12):138-41.

Hospitals prepare plans, drill staff to ensure that potential Ebola patients are identified, isolated, and managed safely.

[No authors listed]

Hospitals around the country have stepped up their efforts to train staff and implement procedures to ensure the safe identification and management of any patients with signs of Ebola virus disease (EVD). Ronald Reagan UCLA Medical Center in Los Angeles, CA, held an "Ebola preparedness exercise" to give staff an opportunity to walk through the hospital's protocol for handling a simulated patient with EVD. The University of Alabama at Birmingham (UAB) Medical Center has held similar exercises, and is now holding twice-weekly meetings of its leadership team to make sure that all new developments in the Ebola outbreak are communicated. UCLA Medical Center has prepared PPE kits based on the practices developed at Emory University Hospital, which has thus far had the most experience in this country in caring for patients with EVD. The UCLA Health System has adjusted its medical record system so that a red flag is placed on the electronic medical record [EMR] of any patient who has recently traveled to a high-risk area. UAB Medical Center has incorporated what had been a paper-and-pencil screening tool for EVD into its electronic medical record. Training on PPE as well as EVD screening is being provided to first-responders and 911 call center dispatchers in the UAB system.

PMID: 25522495 [PubMed - in process]

147. ED Manag. 2014 Dec;26(12):136-8.

State, local authorities in the driver's seat for much of the Ebola response.

[No authors listed]

PMID: 25522494 [PubMed - in process]

148. ED Manag. 2014 Dec;26(12):133-6.

With strengthened guidelines for health care workers, the CDC ups its game against the deadly Ebola virus.

[No authors listed]

Informed by the cases of two nurses who contracted Ebola virus disease (EVD) while caring for a patient with the disease in Dallas, TX, the Centers for Disease Control and Prevention (CDC) in Atlanta, GA, has unveiled strengthened guidance for health care workers. Further, nursing organizations are pledging to work together to identify gaps and make system-level improvements to protect both patients and caregivers. The CDC's new recommendations emphasize rigorous training for health care workers in how to put on and take off personal protective equipment (PPE), and they state that this activity should always be carefully supervised by a monitor. The guidance also states that health care workers should use either an N-95' respirator mask or a powered air purifying respirator (PAPR) when they are providing care to a patient with Ebola. Experts stress that the new guidance does not change the fundamental issue that Ebola is transmitted through contact with infectious substances from patients. Nursing organizations are pledging to work together to identify problems and improve safety for both caregivers and patients.

PMID: 25522493 [PubMed - in process]

149. Emerg Nurse. 2014 Dec;22(8):26-32. doi: 10.7748/en.22.8.26.e1383.

Assessing and treating fever in returned travellers.

Poulter K(1).

Author information: (1)Local Care Direct, Wharfedale Hospital, Otley, West Yorkshire, University of Leeds.

As population mobility and global interconnectedness increase, and more people travel to tropical regions, the risk of importing infectious diseases has become higher than ever before. This risk has been highlighted by the recent outbreak in West Africa of the Ebola virus, isolated cases of which have been reported in Europe and the United States. Many infectious diseases are associated with similar generic symptoms, and assessing febrile illness in patients who have recently travelled can be difficult for primary and urgent care practitioners. This article explains how to assess the risk of specific travel-related conditions in such patients and to recognise when urgent actions, such as malaria testing, are required.

PMID: 25466755 [PubMed - in process]

150. Epidemics. 2014 Dec;9:70-8. doi: 10.1016/j.epidem.2014.09.003. Epub 2014 Oct 6.

Potential for large outbreaks of Ebola virus disease.

Camacho A(1), Kucharski AJ(2), Funk S(3), Breman J(4), Piot P(5), Edmunds WJ(3).

Author information: (1)Centre for the Mathematical Modelling of Infectious Diseases, Department of Infectious Disease Epidemiology, London School of Hygiene and Tropical Medicine, London, United Kingdom. Electronic address: anton.camacho@lshtm.ac.uk. (2)Centre for the Mathematical Modelling of Infectious Diseases, Department of Infectious Disease Epidemiology, London School of Hygiene and Tropical Medicine, London, United Kingdom. Electronic address: adam.kucharski@lshtm.ac.uk. (3)Centre for the Mathematical Modelling of Infectious Diseases, Department of Infectious Disease Epidemiology, London School of Hygiene and Tropical Medicine, London, United Kingdom. (4)Fogarty International Center, National Institutes of Health, United States. (5)London School of Hygiene and Tropical Medicine, London, United Kingdom.

Outbreaks of Ebola virus can cause substantial morbidity and mortality in affected regions. The largest outbreak of Ebola to date is currently underway in West Africa, with 3944 cases reported as of 5th September 2014. To develop a better understanding of Ebola transmission dynamics, we revisited data from the first known Ebola outbreak, which occurred in 1976 in Zaire (now Democratic Republic of Congo). By fitting a mathematical model to time series stratified by disease onset, outcome and source of infection, we were able to estimate several epidemiological quantities that have previously proved challenging to measure, including the contribution of hospital and community infection to transmission. We found evidence that transmission decreased considerably before the closure of the hospital, suggesting that the decline of the outbreak was most likely the result of changes in host behaviour. Our analysis suggests that the person-to-person reproduction number was 1.34 (95% CI: 0.92-2.11) in the early part of the outbreak. Using stochastic simulations we demonstrate that the same epidemiological conditions that were present in 1976 could have generated a large outbreak purely by chance. At the same time, the relatively high person-to-person basic reproduction number suggests that Ebola would have been difficult to control through hospital-based infection control measures alone.

PMCID: PMC4255970 PMID: 25480136 [PubMed - in process]
151. Eur J Phys Rehabil Med. 2014 Dec;50(6):601-8.

Current research funding methods dumb down health care and rehabilitation for disabled people and aging population: a call for a change.

Negrini S(1), Padua L, Kiekens C, Michail X, Boldrini P.

Author information: (1)Department of Clinical and Experimental Sciences University of Brescia, Brescia, Italy - stefano.negrini@unibs.it.

Health care systems in Western societies are faced with two major challenges: aging populations and the growing burden of chronic conditions. This translates into more persons with disabilities and the need for more Physical and Rehabilitation Medicine (PRM) services. We raise the point of how these emerging needs are faced by the actual research funding. We briefly present the results of an analysis we made about research funding by the Italian National Health Service as an interesting case study, since it relates to Italy (the financer) and the United States, where National Institutes of Health (NIH) reviewers were identified according to their classification of research topics. The topics of potentially greatest interest for aging Western societies, like chronicity, disability and rehabilitation, were among those least often funded and considered in the traditional method of financing research projects. These results could be based on those PRM peculiarities that make the specialty different from all other classical biomedical specialties, namely the bio-psycho-social approach and its specific research methodologies. Moreover, PRM researchers are spread among the different topics as usually classified, and it is probable that PRM projects are judged by non-PRM reviewers. There are at least two possible ways in which research can be better placed to meet the emerging needs of Western societies (chronicity, disability and consequently also rehabilitation). One is to create specific keywords on these topics so as to improve the match between researchers and reviewers; the second is to allocate specific funds to research in these areas. In fact, the not coherence between emerging needs and research priorities have already been periodically addressed in the past with specific "political" and/or "social" initiatives, when researchers were forced to respond to new emergencies: some historical examples include cancer or HIV and viral diseases or the recent Ebola outbreak.
PMID: 25521703 [PubMed - in process]

152. Germs. 2014 Dec 1;4(4):97-9. doi: 10.11599/germs.2014.1063. eCollection 2014.

Utility of contact tracing in reducing the magnitude of Ebola disease.

Shrivastava SR(1), Shrivastava PS(1), Ramasamy J(2).

Author information: (1)MD, Assistant Professor, Department of Community Medicine, Shri Sathya Sai Medical College & Research Institute, Kancheepuram, India. (2)MD, Professor & Head, Department of Community Medicine, Shri Sathya Sai Medical College & Research Institute, Kancheepuram, India.
PMCID: PMC4258401 PMID: 25505743 [PubMed]

153. Hosp Peer Rev. 2014 Dec;39(12):140-1.

Ebola fears remain high, despite new guidelines.

[No authors listed]
PMID: 25513698 [PubMed - in process]

154. Int J Health Policy Manag. 2014 Nov 1;3(7):417-8. doi: 10.15171/ijhpm.2014.117. eCollection 2014.

Preventing the emergence of Ebola disease in unaffected countries: necessity of preparedness.

RamBihariLal Shrivastava S(1), Shrivastava PS(1), Ramasamy J(1).

Author information: (1)Department of Community Medicine, Shri Sathya Sai Medical College and Research Institute, Kancheepuram, TamilNadu, India.
PMCID: PMC4258895 PMID: 25489601 [PubMed]

155. Int J Nurs Stud. 2014 Dec;51(12):1694-5. doi: 10.1016/j.ijnurstu.2014.10.004. Epub 2014 Oct 12.

Response to Martin-Moreno et al. (2014) Surgical mask or no mask for health workers not a defensible position for Ebola.

MacIntyre CR(1), Chughtai AA(2), Seale H(3), Richards GA(4), Davidson PM(5).

Author information: (1)School of Public Health and Community Medicine, Faculty of Medicine, University of New South Wales, Sydney, Australia. Electronic address: r.macintyre@unsw.edu.au. (2)School of Public Health and Community Medicine, Faculty of Medicine, University of New South Wales, Sydney, Australia. Electronic address: abrar.chughtai@unsw.edu.au. (3)School of Public Health and Community Medicine, Faculty of Medicine, University of New South Wales, Sydney, Australia. Electronic address: h.seale@unsw.edu.au. (4)University of the Witwatersrand Johannesburg, South Africa; Critical Care Charlotte Maxeke Johannesburg Academic Hospital, Johannesburg, South Africa. Electronic address: Guy.Richards@wits.ac.za. (5)Johns Hopkins University, Baltimore, USA; University of Technology, Sydney, Australia. Electronic address: pdavidson@jhu.edu.
PMID: 25457271 [PubMed - in process]

156. Int J Nurs Stud. 2014 Dec;51(12):1693. doi: 10.1016/j.ijnurstu.2014.10.005. Epub 2014 Oct 13.

Response to "MacIntyre et al., 2014: Respiratory protection for healthcare workers treating Ebola virus disease (EVD): are facemasks sufficient to meet occupational health and safety obligations?".

Martin-Moreno JM(1), Llinás G(2), Martínez-Hernández J(3).

Author information: (1)University of Valencia Medical School, Valencia, Spain; University Clinical Hospital, Valencia, Spain. Electronic address: dr.martinmoreno@gmail.com. (2)University of Valencia Medical School, Valencia, Spain. (3)Hospital La Paz-Carlos III, Madrid, Spain.
PMID: 25457270 [PubMed - in process]

157. Int Nurs Rev. 2014 Dec;61(4):443-4. doi: 10.1111/inr.12149.

Ebola: a global challenge for nurses and other health workers.

[No authors listed]

PMID: 25411069 [PubMed - in process]
158. Intensive Care Med. 2014 Dec;40(12):1936-9. doi: 10.1007/s00134-014-3515-1. Epub 2014 Nov 1.

Understanding organ dysfunction in Ebola virus disease.

Fletcher TE(1), Fowler RA, Beeching NJ.

Author information: (1)WellcomeTraining Fellow and Lecturer, Liverpool School of Tropical Medicine, Pembroke Place, Liverpool, L3 5QA, UK, tomfletcher@doctors.org.uk.

PMID: 25366120 [PubMed - in process]
159. J Autoimmun. 2014 Dec;55C:1-9. doi: 10.1016/j.jaut.2014.09.001. Epub 2014 Sep 26.

Clinical features and pathobiology of Ebolavirus infection.

Ansari AA(1).

Author information: (1)Department of Pathology & Laboratory Medicine, Emory University School of Medicine, Atlanta, GA 30322, USA. Electronic address: pathaaa@emory.edu.

There has clearly been a deluge of international press coverage of the recent outbreak of Ebolavirus in Africa and is partly related to the "fear factor" that comes across when one is confronted with the fact that once infected, not only is the speed of death in a majority of cases rapid but also the images of the cause of death such as bleeding from various orifices gruesome and frightening. The fact that it leads to infection and death of health care providers (10% during the current epidemic) and the visualization of protective gear worn by these individuals to contain such infection adds to this "fear factor". Finally, there is a clear perceived notion that such an agent can be utilized as a bioterrorism agent that adds to the apprehension. Thus, in efforts to gain an objective view of the growing threat Ebolavirus poses to the general public, it is important to provide some basic understanding for the lethality of Ebolavirus infection that is highlighted in Fig. 1. This virus infection first appears to disable the immune system (the very system needed to fight the infection) and subsequently disables the vascular system that leads to blood leakage (hemorrhage), hypotension, drop in blood pressure, followed by shock and death. The virus appears to sequentially infect dendritic cells disabling the interferon system (one of the major host anti-viral immune systems) then macrophages (that trigger the formation of blood clots, release of inflammatory proteins and nitric oxide damaging the lining of blood vessels leading to blood leakage) and finally endothelial cells that contribute to blood leakage. The virus also affects organs such as the liver (that dysregulates the formation of coagulation proteins), the adrenal gland (that destroys the ability of the patient to synthesize steroids and leads to circulation failure and disabling of regulators of blood pressure) and the gastro-intestinal tract (leading to diarrhea). The ability of the virus to disable such major mechanisms in the body facilitates the ability of the virus to replicate in an uncontrolled fashion leading to the rapidity by which the virus can cause lethality. Various laboratories have been working on defining such mechanisms utilizing in vitro culture systems, a variety of animal models including inbred strains of normal and select gene knock out mice, guinea pigs and nonhuman primates that have led to a better understanding of the potential mechanisms involved. There have also been some major advances made in the identification of therapies from the very simple (major supportive type of therapy), to the identification of a number of highly effective chemotherapeutic agents, a variety of highly effective preventive (demonstrating 100% effectiveness in nonhuman primate models) recombinant formulations (adenovirus based, VSV-based, rabies virus based), therapeutic candidate vaccines (cocktail of monoclonal antibodies such as ZMAPP) and alternate approaches (RNAi-based such as TKM-Ebola and antisense based such as AVI-7537) that show great promise and at an unprecedented rate of discovery that speaks well for the scientific research community at large.

PMID: 25260583 [PubMed - as supplied by publisher]
160. J Bioeth Inq. 2014 Dec;11(4):413-4. doi: 10.1007/s11673-014-9581-9. Epub 2014 Dec 12

Ebola, ethics, and the question of culture.

Komesaroff P(1), Kerridge I.

Author information: (1)Centre for Ethics in Medicine and Society, Monash University Faculty of Medicine, Nursing and theHealth Sciences, Melbourne, Australia, paul.komesaroff@monash.edu.

PMID: 25501565 [PubMed - in process]
161. J Bioeth Inq. 2014 Dec;11(4):415-6. doi: 10.1007/s11673-014-9590-8. Epub 2014 Nov 25

Using the ebola outbreak as an opportunity to educate on vaccine utility.

Brown B(1).

Author information: (1)Program in Public Health, Department of Population Health & Disease Prevention, University of California, Irvine, 653 E. Peltason Drive, 2024 AIRB, Irvine, CA, 92697-3957, USA, Brandon.brown@uci.edu.

PMID: 25421820 [PubMed - in process]
162. J Bioeth Inq. 2014 Dec;11(4):405-11. doi: 10.1007/s11673-014-9589-1. Epub 2014 Nov 23.

Art, (in)visibility, and ebola : "what are the consequences of a digitally-created society in the psyche of the global community?".

Rich LE(1), Ashby MA, Shaw DM.

Author information: (1)Department of Health Sciences (Public Health), Armstrong State University, 11935 Abercorn Street, University Hall 154F, Savannah, GA, 31419, USA, leigh.rich@armstrong.edu.

PMID: 25417004 [PubMed - in process]

163. J Bioeth Inq. 2014 Dec;11(4):441-4. doi: 10.1007/s11673-014-9588-2. Epub 2014 Nov 13

Disease, communication, and the ethics of (in) visibility.

Pietrzak-Franger MM(1), Holmes MS.

Author information: (1)Department of English and American Studies, University of Hamburg, Von-Melle-Park 6, 20146, Hamburg, Germany.

As the recent Ebola outbreak demonstrates, visibility is central to the shaping of political, medical, and socioeconomic decisions. The symposium in this issue of the Journal of Bioethical Inquiry explores the uneasy relationship between the necessity of making diseases visible, the mechanisms of legal and visual censorship, and the overall ethics of viewing and spectatorship, including the effects of media visibility on the perception of particular "marked" bodies. Scholarship across the disciplines of communication, anthropology, gender studies, and visual studies, as well as a photographer's visual essay and memorial reflection, throw light on various strategies of visualization and (de)legitimation and link these to broader socioeconomic concerns. Questions of the ethics of spectatorship, such as how to evoke empathy in the representation of individuals' suffering without perpetuating social and economic inequalities, are explored in individual, (trans-)national, and global contexts, demonstrating how disease (in)visibility intersects with a complex nexus of health, sexuality, and global/national politics. A sensible management of visibility-an "ecology of the visible"-can be productive of more viable ways of individual and collective engagement with those who suffer.

PMID: 25391918 [PubMed - in process]

164. J Bioeth Inq. 2014 Dec;11(4):417-20. doi: 10.1007/s11673-014-9587-3. Epub 2014 Nov 12.

Ethical challenges posed by the ebola virus epidemic in west Africa.

Omonzejele PF(1).

Author information: (1)Department of Philosophy, University of Benin, Benin-City, Nigeria, pfomonzejele@yahoo.com.

This paper examines how people in West Africa are reacting to the Ebola virus disease, an epidemic presently prevalent in the region. Certain lifestyle changes are suggested. Additionally, the heart of the paper focuses on the request by governments to be allowed access to experimental drugs, such as Zmapp and TKM-Ebola, for their infected populations. The author argues that granting such a request would circumvent research ethics procedures, which could potentially constitute significant risk to users of the drugs. The Pfizer Kano meningitis trial of 1996 is cited as an example to buttress how unapproved drugs could prove fatal.

PMID: 25387576 [PubMed - in process]

165. J Bioeth Inq. 2014 Dec;11(4):421-3. doi: 10.1007/s11673-014-9580-x. Epub 2014 Oct 8

Ebola virus in west Africa: waiting for the owl of minerva.

Upshur RE(1).

Author information: (1)Department of Family and Community Medicine and Dalla Lana School of Public Health, Division of Clinical Public Health, University of Toronto, Toronto, ON, Canada, ross.upshur@gmail.com.

The evolving Ebola epidemic in West Africa is unprecedented in its size and scope, requiring the rapid mobilization of resources. It is too early to determine all of the ethical challenges associated with the outbreak, but these should be monitored closely. Two issues that can be discussed are (1) the decision to implement and evaluate unregistered agents to determine therapeutic or prophylactic safety and efficacy and (2) the justification behind this decision. In this paper, I argue that it is not compassionate use that justifies this decision and suggest three lines of reasoning to support the decision.

PMID: 25294651 [PubMed - in process]

166. J Health Commun. 2014 Dec;19(12):1327-9. doi: 10.1080/10810730.2014.989098.

Twenty Years Later: Ebola, AIDS, BSE and NCDs-What Have We Learned?

Ratzan SC.

PMID: 25491578 [PubMed - in process]

167. J Perianesth Nurs. 2014 Dec;29(6):526-8. doi: 10.1016/j.jopan.2014.10.001. Epub 2014 Nov 20.

Ebola-a crisis.

Odom-Forren J.

PMID: 25458636 [PubMed - in process]

168. J Public Health (Oxf). 2014 Dec;36(4):525-6. doi: 10.1093/pubmed/fdu094.

The international Ebola response: heroes and bystanders in the chronicle of an epidemic foretold.

Martin-Moreno JM(1).

Author information: (1)Department of Preventive Medicine and Public Health and INCLIVA Research Institute, University of Valencia, Valencia 46010, Spain Department of Epidemiology, Johns Hopkins Bloomberg School of Public Health, Baltimore, MD 21205, USA.

PMID: 25431471 [PubMed - in process]

169. J R Soc Med. 2014 Dec;107(12):463. doi: 10.1177/0141076814562296.

Ebola and the wisdom of Haygarth.

Abbasi K(1).

Author information: (1)Editor, JRSM.

PMID: 25504600 [PubMed - in process]

170. J Vasc Nurs. 2014 Dec;32(4):157. doi: 10.1016/j.jvn.2014.09.002. Epub 2014 Nov 15

Ebola virus disease.

Thomson L(1).

Author information: (1)Department of Vascular Surgery, Health Sciences Centre, Winnipeg, Manitoba, Canada. Electronic address: lthomson@sbgh.mb.ca.

PMID: 25455323 [PubMed - in process]

171. J Virol. 2014 Dec 1;88(23):13626-37. doi: 10.1128/JVI.02234-14. Epub 2014 Sep 10.

The HERV-K Human Endogenous Retrovirus Envelope Protein Antagonizes Tetherin Antiviral Activity.

Lemaître C(1), Harper F(2), Pierron G(2), Heidmann T(3), Dewannieux M(3).

Author information: (1)CNRS, UMR 8122, Institut Gustave Roussy, Villejuif, France Université Paris-Sud, Orsay, France Université Paris Denis Diderot, Sorbonne Paris-Cité, Paris, France. (2)CNRS, UMR 8122, Institut Gustave Roussy, Villejuif, France Université Paris-Sud, Orsay, France. (3)CNRS, UMR 8122, Institut Gustave Roussy, Villejuif, France Université Paris-Sud, Orsay, France heidmann@igr.fr marie.dewannieux@igr.fr.

Endogenous retroviruses are the remnants of past retroviral infections that are scattered within mammalian genomes. In humans, most of these elements are old degenerate sequences that have lost their coding properties. The HERV-K(HML2) family is an exception: it recently amplified in the human genome and corresponds to the most active proviruses, with some intact open reading frames and the potential to encode viral particles. Here, using a reconstructed consensus element, we show that HERV-K(HML2) proviruses are able to inhibit Tetherin, a cellular restriction factor that is active against most enveloped viruses and acts by keeping the viral particles attached to the cell surface. More precisely, we identify the Envelope protein (Env) as the viral effector active against Tetherin. Through immunoprecipitation experiments, we show that the recognition of Tetherin is mediated by the surface subunit of Env. Similar to Ebola glycoprotein, HERV-K(HML2) Env does not mediate Tetherin degradation or cell surface removal; therefore, it uses a yet-undescribed mechanism to inactivate Tetherin. We also assessed all natural complete alleles of endogenous HERV-K(HML2) Env described to date for their ability to inhibit Tetherin and found that two of them (out of six) can block Tetherin restriction. However, due to their recent amplification, HERV-K(HML2) elements are extremely polymorphic in the human population, and it is likely that individuals will not all possess the same anti-Tetherin potential. Because of Tetherin's role as a restriction factor capable of inducing innate immune responses, this could have functional consequences for individual responses to infection.IMPORTANCE: Tetherin, a cellular protein initially characterized for its role against HIV-1, has been proven to counteract numerous enveloped viruses. It blocks the release of viral particles from producer cells, keeping them tethered to the cell surface. Several viruses have developed strategies to inhibit Tetherin activity, allowing them to efficiently infect and replicate in their host. Here, we show that human HERV-K(HML2) elements, the remnants of an ancient retroviral infection, possess an anti-Tetherin activity which is mediated by the envelope protein. It is likely that this activity was an important factor that contributed to the recent, human-specific amplification of this family of elements. Also, due to their recent amplification, HERV-K(HML2) elements are highly polymorphic in the human population. Since Tetherin is a mediator of innate immunity, interindividual variations among HERV-K(HML2) Env genes may result in differences in immune responses to infection.

PMCID: PMC4248984 [Available on 2015/6/1] PMID: 25210194 [PubMed - in process]

172. JAMA Pediatr. 2014 Dec 1;168(12):1087-8. doi: 10.1001/jamapediatrics.2014.2835.

Ebola virus disease and children: what pediatric health care professionals need to know.

Peacock G(1), Uyeki TM(1), Rasmussen SA(1).

Author information: (1)Centers for Disease Control and Prevention, Atlanta, Georgia.

PMID: 25325785 [PubMed - in process]

173. Lancet Glob Health. 2014 Dec;2(12):e686. doi: 10.1016/S2214-109X(14)70341-9. Epub 2014 Oct 30.

Hyperimmune serum from healthy vaccinated individuals for Ebola virus disease?

Almansa R(1), Eiros JM(1), Fedson D(2), Bermejo-Martin JF(3).

Author information: (1)Hospital Clínico Universitario de Valladolid, SACYL/IECSYL, 47005 Valladolid, Spain. (2)Sergy Haut, France. (3)Hospital Clínico Universitario de Valladolid, SACYL/IECSYL, 47005 Valladolid, Spain. Electronic address: jfbermejo@saludcastillayleon.es.

PMID: 25433619 [PubMed - in process]

174. Lancet Glob Health. 2014 Dec;2(12):e685. doi: 10.1016/S2214-109X(14)70339-0. Epub 2014 Oct 30.

Ebola in urban slums: the elephant in the room.

Snyder RE(1), Marlow MA(2), Riley LW(3).

Author information: (1)Division of Epidemiology, University of California-Berkeley, Berkeley, CA 94720, USA. (2)Division of Epidemiology, University of California-Berkeley, Berkeley, CA 94720, USA; Division of Infectious Diseases and Vaccinology, University of California-Berkeley, Berkeley, CA 94720, USA. (3)Division of Infectious Diseases and Vaccinology, University of California-Berkeley, Berkeley, CA 94720, USA. Electronic address: lwriley@berkeley.edu.

PMID: 25433618 [PubMed - in process]

175. Lancet Infect Dis. 2014 Dec;14(12):1189-95. doi: 10.1016/S1473-3099(14)70995-8. Epub 2014 Oct 23.

Dynamics and control of Ebola virus transmission in Montserrado, Liberia: a mathematical modelling analysis.

Lewnard JA(1), Ndeffo Mbah ML(1), Alfaro-Murillo JA(1), Altice FL(2), Bawo L(3), Nyenswah TG(3), Galvani AP(4).

Author information: (1)Department of Epidemiology of Microbial Diseases, Yale School of Public Health, New Haven, CT, USA; Center for Infectious Disease Modeling and Analysis, Yale School of Public Health, New Haven, CT, USA. (2)Department of Epidemiology of Microbial Diseases, Yale School of Public Health, New Haven, CT, USA; Infectious Diseases Section, Yale University School of Medicine, New Haven, CT, USA. (3)Ministry of Health and Social Welfare, Monrovia, Liberia.

(4)Department of Epidemiology of Microbial Diseases, Yale School of Public Health, New Haven, CT, USA; Center for Infectious Disease Modeling and Analysis, Yale School of Public Health, New Haven, CT, USA. Electronic address: alison.galvani@yale.edu.

BACKGROUND: A substantial scale-up in public health response is needed to control the unprecedented Ebola virus disease (EVD) epidemic in west Africa. Current international commitments seek to expand intervention capacity in three areas: new EVD treatment centres, case ascertainment through contact tracing, and household protective kit allocation. We aimed to assess how these interventions could be applied individually and in combination to avert future EVD cases and deaths. METHODS: We developed a transmission model of Ebola virus that we fitted to reported EVD cases and deaths in Montserrado County, Liberia. We used this model to assess the effectiveness of expanding EVD treatment centres, increasing case ascertainment, and allocating protective kits for controlling the outbreak in Montserrado. We varied the efficacy of protective kits from 10% to 50%. We compared intervention initiation on Oct 15, 2014, Oct 31, 2014, and Nov 15, 2014. The status quo intervention was defined in terms of case ascertainment and capacity of EVD treatment centres on Sept 23, 2014, and all behaviour and contact patterns relevant to transmission as they were occurring at that time. The primary outcome measure was the expected number of cases averted by Dec 15, 2014. FINDINGS: We estimated the basic reproductive number for EVD in Montserrado to be 2·49 (95% CI 2·38-2·60). We expect that allocating 4800 additional beds at EVD treatment centres and increasing case ascertainment five-fold in November, 2014, can avert 77 312 (95% CI 68 400-85 870) cases of EVD relative to the status quo by Dec 15, 2014. Complementing these measures with protective kit allocation raises the expectation as high as 97 940 (90 096-105 606) EVD cases. If deployed by Oct 15, 2014, equivalent interventions would have been expected to avert 137 432 (129 736-145 874) cases of EVD. If delayed to Nov 15, 2014, we expect the interventions will at best avert 53 957 (46 963-60 490) EVD cases. INTERPRETATION: The number of beds at EVD treatment centres needed to effectively control EVD in Montserrado substantially exceeds the 1700 pledged by the USA to west Africa. Accelerated case ascertainment is needed to maximise effectiveness of expanding the capacity of EVD treatment centres. Distributing protective kits can further augment prevention of EVD, but it is not an adequate stand-alone measure for controlling the outbreak. Our findings highlight the rapidly closing window of opportunity for controlling the outbreak and averting a catastrophic toll of EVD cases and deaths. FUNDING: US National Institutes of Health.

PMID: 25455986 [PubMed - in process]
176. Lancet Infect Dis. 2014 Dec;14(12):1164-5. doi: 10.1016/S1473-3099(14)70851-5. Epub 2014 Oct 23.

Ebola: no time to waste.

Fisman D(1), Tuite AR(2).
Author information: (1)Dalla Lana School of Public Health, University of Toronto, Toronto, ON, Canada M5T 3M7. Electronic address: david.fisman@utoronto.ca. (2)Dalla Lana School of Public Health, University of Toronto, Toronto, ON, Canada M5T 3M7.

PMID: 25455968 [PubMed - in process]
177. Lancet Infect Dis. 2014 Dec;14(12):1163. doi: 10.1016/S1473-3099(14)71020-5. Epub 2014 Nov 10.

Rationality and coordination for Ebola outbreak in west Africa.

The Lancet Infectious Diseases.

PMID: 25455967 [PubMed - in process]
178. Mayo Clin Proc. 2014 Dec;89(12):1710-1717. doi: 10.1016/j.mayocp.2014.10.010. Epub 2014 Oct 30.

What Clinicians Should Know About the 2014 Ebola Outbreak.

Tosh PK(1), Sampathkumar P(2).
Author information: (1)Division of Infectious Diseases, Mayo Clinic, Rochester, MN. (2)Division of Infectious Diseases, Mayo Clinic, Rochester, MN. Electronic address: sampathkumar.priya@mayo.edu.

The ongoing Ebola outbreak that began in Guinea in February 2014 has spread to Liberia, Sierra Leone, Nigeria, Senegal, Spain, and the United States and has become the largest Ebola outbreak in recorded history. It is important for frontline medical providers to understand key aspects of Ebola virus disease (EVD) to quickly recognize an imported case, provide appropriate medical care, and prevent transmission. Furthermore, an understanding of the clinical presentation, clinical course, transmission, and prevention of EVD can help reduce anxiety about the disease and allow health care providers to calmly and confidently provide medical care to patients suspected of having EVD.

PMID: 25467644 [PubMed - as supplied by publisher]
179. Mayo Clin Proc. 2014 Dec;89(12):1596-8. doi: 10.1016/j.mayocp.2014.10.006. Epub 2014 Nov 6.

Ebola virus: exposing the inadequacies of public health in liberia.

Butler YS(1).
Author information: (1)Division of Obstetrics, Department of Obstetrics and Gynecology, Mayo Clinic, Rochester, MN. Electronic address: butler.yvonne@mayo.edu.

PMID: 25467643 [PubMed - in process]
180. Med Mal Infect. 2014 Dec;44(11-12):491-4. doi: 10.1016/j.medmal.2014.09.009. Epub 2014 Oct 23.

Ebola outbreak in Conakry, Guinea: Epidemiological, clinical, and outcome features.

Barry M(1), Traoré FA(2), Sako FB(3), Kpamy DO(1), Bah EI(1), Poncin M(4), Keita S(5), Cisse M(6), Touré A(7).
Author information: (1)Service des maladies infectieuses et tropicales, hôpital national Donka, CHU de Conakry, Quartier Cameroun, Conakry, Guinea. (2)Service des maladies infectieuses et tropicales, hôpital national Donka, CHU de Conakry, Quartier Cameroun, Conakry, Guinea; Chaire de dermatologie et maladies

infectieuses, département de médecine, université de Conakry, Conakry, Guinea. Electronic address: fatraore01@gmail.com. (3)Service des maladies infectieuses et tropicales, hôpital national Donka, CHU de Conakry, Quartier Cameroun, Conakry, Guinea; Chaire de dermatologie et maladies infectieuses, département de médecine, université de Conakry, Conakry, Guinea. (4)Coordonateur projet MSF urgence Ebola, hôpital Donka, Conakry, Guinea. (5)Division de la prévention et de la lutte contre la maladie, ministère de la Santé, Guinea. (6)Chaire de dermatologie et maladies infectieuses, département de médecine, université de Conakry, Conakry, Guinea. (7)Chaire de santé publique, département de pharmacie, université de Conakry, Conakry, Guinea.

OBJECTIVES: The authors studied the epidemiological, clinical, and outcome features of the Ebola virus disease in patients hospitalized at the Ebola treatment center (ETC) in Conakry to identify clinical factors associated with death. MATERIALS AND METHODS: A prospective study was conducted from March 25 to August 20, 2014. The diagnosis of Ebola virus infection was made on real-time PCR. RESULTS: Ninety patients, with a positive test result, were hospitalized. Their mean age was 34.12 ± 14.29 years and 63% were male patients. Most worked in the informal sector (38%) and in the medical and paramedical staff (physicians 12%, nurses 6%, and laboratory technicians 1%). Most patients lived in the Conakry suburbs (74%) and in Boffa (11%). The main clinical signs were physical asthenia (80%) and fever (72%). Hemorrhagic signs were observed in 26% of patients. The comparison of clinical manifestations showed that hiccups (P=0.04), respiratory distress (P=0.04), and hemorrhagic symptoms (P=0.01) were more frequent among patients who died. Malaria (72%) and diabetes (2%) were the most frequent co-morbidities. The crude case fatality rate was 44% [95% confidence interval (33-54%)]. The average hospital stay was 7.96 ± 5.81 days. CONCLUSION: The first Ebola outbreak in Conakry was characterized by the young age of patients, discrete hemorrhagic signs related to lethality. Its control relies on a strict use of preventive measures.

PMID: 25391486 [PubMed - in process]

181. Microb Pathog. 2014 Dec;77:136-41. doi: 10.1016/j.micpath.2014.09.002. Epub 2014 Sep 18.

Arthropods as a source of new RNA viruses.

Bichaud L(1), de Lamballerie X(2), Alkan C(3), Izri A(4), Gould EA(5), Charrel RN(6).

Author information: (1)Aix Marseille Université, IRD French Institute of Research for Development, EHESP French School of Public Health, EPV UMR_D 190 "Emergence des Pathologies Virales", 13385 Marseille, France; IHU Méditerranée Infection, APHM Public Hospitals of Marseille 13385 Marseille, France. Electronic address: laurencebichaud@gmail.com. (2)Aix Marseille Université, IRD French Institute of Research for Development, EHESP French School of Public Health, EPV UMR_D 190 Emergence des Pathologies Virales, 13385 Marseille, France; IHU Méditerranée Infection, APHM Public Hospitals of Marseille 13385 Marseille, France. Electronic address: xavier.de-lamballerie@univ-amu.fr. (3)Aix Marseille Université, IRD French Institute of Research for Development, EHESP French School of Public Health, EPV UMR_D 190 "Emergence des Pathologies Virales", 13385 Marseille, France; IHU Méditerranée Infection, APHM Public Hospitals of Marseille 13385 Marseille, France. Electronic address: cgdmalkan@gmail.com. (4)Aix Marseille Université, IRD French Institute of Research for Development, EHESP French School of Public Health, EPV UMR_D 190 "Emergence des Pathologies Virales", 13385 Marseille, France; IHU Méditerranée Infection, APHM Public Hospitals of Marseille 13385 Marseille, France. Electronic address: arezki.izri@avc.aphp.fr. (5)Aix Marseille Université, IRD French Institute of Research for Development, EHESP French School of Public Health, EPV UMR_D 190 "Emergence des Pathologies Virales", 13385 Marseille, France; IHU Méditerranée Infection, APHM Public Hospitals of Marseille 13385 Marseille, France. Electronic address: eag@ceh.ac.uk. (6)Aix Marseille Université, IRD French Institute of Research for Development, EHESP French School of Public Health, EPV UMR_D 190 "Emergence des Pathologies Virales", 13385 Marseille, France; IHU Méditerranée Infection, APHM Public Hospitals of Marseille 13385 Marseille, France. Electronic address: remi.charrel@univ-amu.fr.

The discovery and development of methods for isolation, characterisation and taxonomy of viruses represents an important milestone in the study, treatment and control of virus diseases during the 20th century. Indeed, by the late-1950s, it was becoming common belief that most human and veterinary pathogenic viruses had been discovered. However, at that time, knowledge of the impact of improved commercial transportation, urbanisation and deforestation, on disease emergence, was in its infancy. From the late 1960s onwards viruses, such as hepatitis virus (A, B and C) hantavirus, HIV, Marburg virus, Ebola virus and many others began to emerge and it became apparent that the world was changing, at least in terms of virus epidemiology, largely due to the influence of anthropological activities. Subsequently, with the improvement of molecular biotechnologies, for amplification of viral RNA, genome sequencing and proteomic analysis the arsenal of available tools for virus discovery and genetic characterization opened up new and exciting possibilities for virological discovery. Many recently identified but "unclassified" viruses are now being allocated to existing genera or families based on whole genome sequencing, bioinformatic and phylogenetic analysis. New species, genera and families are also being created following the guidelines of the International Committee for the Taxonomy of Viruses. Many of these newly discovered viruses are vectored by arthropods (arboviruses) and possess an RNA genome. This brief review will focus largely on the discovery of new arthropod-borne viruses.

PMID: 25239874 [PubMed - in process]

182. Milbank Q. 2014 Dec;92(4):662-6. doi: 10.1111/1468-0009.12089.

Ethical allocation of drugs and vaccines in the west african ebola epidemic.

Gostin LO.

PMID: 25492601 [PubMed - in process]

183. Milbank Q. 2014 Dec;92(4):633-9. doi: 10.1111/1468-0009.12084.

Ebola Fever and global health responsibilities.

Markel H.

PMID: 25492594 [PubMed - in process]

184. Nat Rev Genet. 2014 Dec;15(12):781. doi: 10.1038/nrg3865. Epub 2014 Nov 11.

Model organisms: Host determinants of Ebola virus pathogenicity.

Burgess DJ.

PMID: 25385126 [PubMed - in process]

185. Pediatr Dev Pathol. 2014 Dec 1. [Epub ahead of print]

Ebolavirus Hemorrhagic Fever (EHF) and the Obstetric Patient.

Pinar H(1), Goldenberg RL.

Author information: (1)a Women and Infants Hospital, Division of Perinatal and Pediatric Pathology.

PMID: 25437511 [PubMed - as supplied by publisher]

186. PLoS Comput Biol. 2014 Dec 11;10(12):e1004004. doi: 10.1371/journal.pcbi.1004004. eCollection 2014.

Vesicular Stomatitis Virus Polymerase's Strong Affinity to Its Template Suggests Exotic Transcription Models.

Tang X(1), Bendjennat M(1), Saffarian S(2).

Author information: (1)Department of Physics and Astronomy, University of Utah, Salt Lake City, Utah, United States of America. (2)Department of Physics and Astronomy, University of Utah, Salt Lake City, Utah, United States of America; Center for Cell and Genome Science, University of Utah, Salt Lake City, Utah, United States of America; Department of Biology, University of Utah, Salt Lake City, Utah, United States of America.

Vesicular stomatitis virus (VSV) is the prototype for negative sense non segmented (NNS) RNA viruses which include potent human and animal pathogens such as Rabies, Ebola and measles. The polymerases of NNS RNA viruses only initiate transcription at or near the 3' end of their genome template. We measured the dissociation constant of VSV polymerases from their whole genome template to be 20 pM. Given this low dissociation constant, initiation and sustainability of transcription becomes nontrivial. To explore possible mechanisms, we simulated the first hour of transcription using Monte Carlo methods and show that a one-time initial dissociation of all polymerases during entry is not sufficient to sustain transcription. We further show that efficient transcription requires a sliding mechanism for non-transcribing polymerases and can be realized with different polymerase-polymerase interactions and distinct template topologies. In conclusion, we highlight a model in which collisions between transcribing and sliding non-transcribing polymerases result in release of the non-transcribing polymerases allowing for redistribution of polymerases between separate templates during transcription and suggest specific experiments to further test these mechanisms.

PMCID: PMC4263359 PMID: 25501005 [PubMed - in process]

187. Prehosp Disaster Med. 2014 Dec;29(6):553-4. doi: 10.1017/S1049023X14001307.

Ebola: Who is Responsible for the Political Failures?

[No authors listed]

PMID: 25515002 [PubMed - in process]

188. Simul Healthc. 2014 Dec;9(6):337-8. doi: 10.1097/SIH.0000000000000068.

Simulation as a critical resource in the response to ebola virus disease.

Gaba DM(1).

Author information: (1)From the Department of Anesthesiology, Perioperative, and Pain Medicine, Stanford University School of Medicine, Stanford, CA.

PMID: 25503528 [PubMed - in process]

189. Surg Infect (Larchmt). 2014 Dec;15(6):671. doi: 10.1089/sur.2014.9985.

Surgical infection society statement on ebola hemorrhagic Fever.

[No authors listed]

PMID: 25313927 [PubMed - in process]

190. Trans R Soc Trop Med Hyg. 2014 Dec;108(12):741-2. doi: 10.1093/trstmh/tru177.

Ebola: controlling the nightmare.

Carson GL(1), Dunning J(2), Longuere KS(2), Brooks WA(2).

Author information: (1)International Severe Acute Respiratory and Emerging Infection Consortium (ISARIC) Coordinating Centre, University of Oxford, Centre for Tropical Medicine, NDM Research Building, Old Road Campus, Roosevelt Drive, Oxford, OX3 7FZ, UK gail.carson@ndm.ox.ac.uk. (2)International Severe Acute Respiratory and Emerging Infection Consortium (ISARIC) Coordinating Centre, University of Oxford, Centre for Tropical Medicine, NDM Research Building, Old Road Campus, Roosevelt Drive, Oxford, OX3 7FZ, UK.

PMID: 25398779 [PubMed - in process]

191. Transfusion. 2014 Dec;54(12):3247-51. doi: 10.1111/trf.12913. Epub 2014 Nov 18.

Ebola virus disease, transmission risk to laboratory personnel, and pretransfusion testing.

Katz LM(1), Tobian AA.

Author information: (1)America's Blood Centers, Washington, DC; Internal Medicine, Infectious Diseases, Carver College of Medicine, University of Iowa, Iowa City, IA.

As Ebola virus has infected thousands of individuals in West Africa, there is growing concern about the appropriate response of hospitals in developed nations caring for patients and handling laboratory specimens for patients suspected of Ebola virus disease (EVD). Guidelines for caring for EVD patients are proliferating rapidly from national and state public health authorities, professional societies, and individual hospitals. It is no surprise that they differ from one another, and some very conservative recommendations call for suspension of routine laboratory testing, including pretransfusion testing. EVD is transmitted by direct contact with blood, secretions, organs, and other body fluids and not by airborne routes. Based on experimental and observational data, the US Centers for Disease Control and Prevention (CDC) recommends that clinicians follow contact and droplet precautions. Laboratory personnel are required to follow the blood-borne pathogen standard, especially the use of appropriate barriers consisting of gloves, gown, goggles, mask to cover nose and mouth, and plexiglass shield, where splashes of potentially infectious materials may be generated. Their recommendations are permissive of clinically appropriate laboratory testing, including pretransfusion testing, using barrier isolation precautions. Most individuals with suspected EVD will have a fever of another etiology, such as Plasmodium falciparum malaria. We believe that forgoing all routine pretransfusion laboratory testing may result in a greater increase in poor clinical outcomes than any diminution in the risks to laboratory personnel will justify. It is imperative for all laboratory directors, working with institutional infection control and safety personnel, to evaluate their hospital policies for potentially infectious patients and provide a safe environment for their patients and employees.

© 2014 AABB.

PMID: 25403825 [PubMed - in process]

192. Yale J Biol Med. 2014 Dec 12;87(4):473-479. eCollection 2014.

Reducing Outbreaks: Using International Governmental Risk Pools to Fund Research and Development of Infectious Disease Medicines and Vaccines.

Erfe JM(1).

Author information: (1)Yale School of Medicine, New Haven, Connecticut.

The deadliest Ebola outbreak the world has ever seen is currently ravaging West Africa, despite the concerted efforts of the World Health Organization and many national governments. The current picture is troubling, but not altogether unexpected. Ebola was initially identified in 1976, and since that time, few drugs have been developed to combat it. The same is true for myriad other dangerous infectious diseases to which the world is currently susceptible. One proposal that might prevent outbreaks of this scale and magnitude from recurring would be to have the World Health Organization (WHO) and its technical partners assess which of its member states are at high risk for a disease, either directly or indirectly, and facilitate the creation of international governmental risk pools of those member states. Risk pools would offer open-indexed grant contracts to fund vaccine and drug development for a particular disease, and pharmaceutical companies could browse the index to apply for these grants. If the risk-pool states and a particular company sign a contract, a mutually agreed upon amount of the vaccine or drug would be produced at a below-market purchase price for those states. In return, the company would keep any patents or intellectual property rights for the developed vaccines or drugs. Risk-pool countries that did not use their vaccine or drug could resell that supply on secondary markets to other countries outside of the risk pool. This arrangement will increase the supply of tested drug and vaccine candidates available for combatting unexpected outbreaks of any previously discovered major infectious disease in the future.

PMCID: PMC4257034 PMID: 25506281 [PubMed - as supplied by publisher]

193. Retrovirology. 2014 Nov 30;11(1):110. [Epub ahead of print]

How will the ebola crisis impact the HIV epidemic?

Wainberg MA, Lever AM.

No abstract.

PMCID: PMC4260236 PMID: 25472763 [PubMed - as supplied by publisher]

194. BMC Biol. 2014 Nov 29;12:100. doi: 10.1186/s12915-014-0100-6.

Vaccines, emerging viruses, and how to avoid disaster.

Rappuoli R(1).

Author information: (1)Novartis Vaccines, Siena 53100, Italy. rino.rappuoli@novartis.com.

Rino Rappuoli is a graduate of Siena University, where he also earned his PhD before moving to the Sclavo Research Center, the Italian vaccine institute, also in Siena. He then spent two years in the USA, mostly at Harvard with John Murphy and Alwin Pappenheimer working on a new diphtheria vaccine based on a non-toxic mutant of diphtheria toxin which has since become the basis for conjugate vaccines against haemophilus, meningococcus, and pneumococcal infections, before returning to the Sclavo Research Center where he developed an acellular vaccine based on a mutant pertussis toxin. With many achievements in vaccine development to his credit, he is now Global Head of Vaccines Research and Development for Novartis Vaccines in Siena, and has most recently pioneered reverse vaccinology, in which the genome of the pathogen is screened for candidate antigenic and immunogenic vaccine components. We spoke to him about the potential for outbreaks of the kind we are now seeing with Ebolavirus in West Africa, and what can be done to prevent them.

PMCID: PMC4247664 PMID: 25432510 [PubMed - in process]

195. Lancet. 2014 Nov 29;384(9958):e61.

Is Canada patent deal obstructing Ebola vaccine development?

Attaran A, Nickerson JW.

PMID: 25513416 [PubMed - in process]

196. Lancet. 2014 Nov 29;384(9958):e61.

Is Canada patent deal obstructing Ebola vaccine development?

Attaran A, Nickerson JW.

PMID: 25467593 [PubMed - in process]

197. Microbes Infect. 2014 Nov 29. pii: S1286-4579(14)00303-7. doi: 10.1016/j.micinf.2014.11.007. [Epub ahead of print]

Ebola virus disease: A highly fatal and panic-generating infectious disease reemerging in West Africa.

To KK(1), Chan JF(1), Tsang AK(2), Cheng VC(2), Yuen KY(3).

Author information: (1)State Key Laboratory for Emerging Infectious Diseases, The University of Hong Kong, Hong Kong, China; Carol Yu Centre for Infection, The University of Hong Kong, Hong Kong, China; Research Centre of Infection and Immunology, The University of Hong Kong, Hong Kong, China; Department of Microbiology, The University of Hong Kong, Hong Kong, China. (2)Department of Microbiology, The University of Hong Kong, Hong Kong, China. (3)State Key Laboratory for Emerging Infectious Diseases, The University of Hong Kong, Hong Kong, China; Carol Yu Centre for Infection, The University of Hong Kong, Hong Kong, China; Research Centre of Infection and Immunology, The University of Hong Kong, Hong Kong, China; Department of Microbiology, The University of Hong Kong, Hong Kong, China. Electronic address: kyyuen@hku.hk.

Ebolavirus can cause a highly fatal and panic-generating human disease which may jump from bats to other mammals and human. High viral loads in body fluids allow efficient transmission by contact. Lack of effective antivirals, vaccines and public health infrastructures in parts of Africa allow the disease to spread unchecked.

PMID: 25456100 [PubMed - as supplied by publisher]

198. J Biol Chem. 2014 Nov 28;289(48):33590-7. doi: 10.1074/jbc.M114.586396. Epub 2014 Oct 14.

The Ebola Virus Matrix Protein VP40 Selectively Induces Vesiculation from Phosphatidylserine-enriched Membranes.

Soni SP(1), Stahelin RV(2).

Author information: (1)From the Department of Biochemistry and Molecular Biology, Indiana University School of Medicine, South Bend, Indiana 46617 and. (2)From the Department of Biochemistry and Molecular Biology, Indiana University School of Medicine, South Bend, Indiana 46617 and the Department of Chemistry and Biochemistry and the Eck Institute for Global Health, University of Notre Dame, Notre Dame, Indiana 46556 rstaheli@iu.edu.

Ebola virus is from the Filoviridae family of viruses and is one of the most virulent pathogens known with ~60% clinical fatality. The Ebola virus negative sense RNA genome encodes seven proteins including viral matrix protein 40 (VP40), which is the most abundant protein found in the virions. Within infected cells VP40 localizes at the inner leaflet of the plasma membrane (PM), binds lipids, and regulates formation of new virus particles. Expression of VP40 in mammalian cells is sufficient to form virus-like particles that are nearly indistinguishable from the authentic virions. However, how VP40 interacts with the PM and forms virus-like particles is for the most part unknown. To investigate VP40 lipid specificity in a model of viral egress we employed giant unilamellar vesicles with different lipid compositions. The results demonstrate VP40 selectively induces vesiculation from membranes containing phosphatidylserine (PS) at concentrations of PS that are representative of the PM inner leaflet content. The formation of intraluminal vesicles was not significantly detected in the presence of other important PM lipids including cholesterol and polyvalent phosphoinositides, further demonstrating PS selectivity. Taken together, these studies suggest that PM phosphatidylserine may be an important component of Ebola virus budding and that VP40 may be able to mediate PM scission.

PMCID: PMC4246110 [Available on 2015/11/28] PMID: 25315776 [PubMed - in process]

199. Science. 2014 Nov 28;346(6213):1039-40. doi: 10.1126/science.346.6213.1039.

Infectious diseases. A new phase in the Ebola war.

Kupferschmidt K.

PMID: 25430746 [PubMed - indexed for MEDLINE]

200. BMJ. 2014 Nov 27;349:g7328. doi: 10.1136/bmj.g7328.

India's health ministry inspects airports for Ebola preparedness.

Bagcchi S(1).

Author information: (1)Kolkata.

PMID: 25430549 [PubMed - in process]

201. BMJ. 2014 Nov 27;349:g7198. doi: 10.1136/bmj.g7198.

Doctors trial amiodarone for Ebola in Sierra Leone.

Turone F(1).

Author information: (1)Milan.

PMID: 25429872 [PubMed - in process]

202. Br J Nurs. 2014 Nov 27;23(21):1104. doi: 10.12968/bjon.2014.23.21.1104.

Soluble chlorine disinfectants for Ebola.

Barton A(1).

Author information: (1)Consultant, GV Health.

PMID: 25426522 [PubMed - in process]

203. Int J Nurs Stud. 2014 Nov 27. pii: S0020-7489(14)00303-4. doi: 10.1016/j.ijnurstu.2014.11.009. [Epub ahead of print]

Nurses as scapegoats in Ebola virus disease response.

Menzel NN(1).

Author information: (1)Associate Professor, School of Nursing, University of Nevada, Las Vegas, 4505 S. Maryland Parkway, Box 453018, Las Vegas, NV 89154-3018, United States. Electronic address: Nancy.menzel@unlv.edu.

PMID: 25498741 [PubMed - as supplied by publisher]
204. J Public Health Policy. 2014 Nov 27. doi: 10.1057/jphp.2014.50. [Epub ahead of print]

Ebola: The haves and the have-nots.

Palomo AM(1).

Author information: (1)Center for Advanced Studies, Molecular Pathogenesis, Avenida IPN 2508, Mexico City (D.F.) 01030, Mexico. E-mail: amartine@cinvestav.mx.

The Ebola epidemic exemplifies the importance of social determinants of health: poverty and illiteracy, among others.Journal of Public Health Policy advance online publication, 27 November 2014; doi:10.1057/jphp.2014.50.

PMID: 25428190 [PubMed - as supplied by publisher]
205. Lancet Infect Dis. 2014 Nov 27. pii: S1473-3099(14)71047-3. doi: 10.1016/S1473-3099(14)71047-3. [Epub ahead of print]

Dose regimen of favipiravir for Ebola virus disease.

Mentré F(1), Taburet AM(2), Guedj J(3), Anglaret X(4), Keïta S(5), de Lamballerie X(6), Malvy D(4).

Author information: (1)INSERM, IAME, UMR 1137, F-75018 Paris, France; Université Paris Diderot, Sorbonne Paris Cité, Paris, France. Electronic address: france.mentre@inserm.fr. (2)Assistance-Publique Hôpitaux de Paris, Hôpital Bicêtre, Université Paris-Sud, Kremin Bicêtre, France; Assistance-Publique Hôpitaux de Paris, Hôpital Bicêtre, Université Paris-Sud, Kremin Bicêtre, France; INSERM U1012, Kremlin Bicêtre, France; DHU Hepatinov, Kremlin Bicêtre, France. (3)INSERM, IAME, UMR 1137, F-75018 Paris, France; Université Paris Diderot, Sorbonne Paris Cité, Paris, France. (4)UMR 897, INSERM, Bordeaux, France. (5)Ministry of Health, Conakry, Guinea. (6)UMR_D 190, Aix-Marseille Université, Institut de Recherche pour le Développement, Marseille, France.

PMID: 25435054 [PubMed - as supplied by publisher]
206. N Engl J Med. 2014 Nov 27;371(22):2054-7. doi: 10.1056/NEJMp1413084. Epub 2014 Nov 5.

Ebola virus disease in West Africa--clinical manifestations and management.

Chertow DS(1), Kleine C, Edwards JK, Scaini R, Giuliani R, Sprecher A.

Author information: (1)From the Liberia Mission, Médecins sans Frontières, Brussels (D.S.C., C.K., J.K.E., R.S., R.G., A.S.); the Critical Care Medicine Department, Clinical Center, National Institutes of Health, Bethesda, MD (D.S.C.); and the Department of Infectious Diseases and Tropical Medicine, J.W. Goethe-University Hospital, Frankfurt, Germany (C.K.).

PMID: 25372854 [PubMed - indexed for MEDLINE]
207. N Engl J Med. 2014 Nov 27;371(22):2092-100. doi: 10.1056/NEJMoa1411680. Epub 2014 Oct 29.

Clinical illness and outcomes in patients with Ebola in Sierra Leone.

Schieffelin JS(1), Shaffer JG, Goba A, Gbakie M, Gire SK, Colubri A, Sealfon RS, Kanneh L, Moigboi A, Momoh M, Fullah M, Moses LM, Brown BL, Andersen KG, Winnicki S, Schaffner SF, Park DJ, Yozwiak NL, Jiang PP, Kargbo D, Jalloh S, Fonnie M, Sinnah V, French I, Kovoma A, Kamara FK, Tucker V, Konuwa E, Sellu J, Mustapha I, Foday M, Yillah M, Kanneh F, Saffa S, Massally JL, Boisen ML, Branco LM, Vandi MA, Grant DS, Happi C, Gevao SM, Fletcher TE, Fowler RA, Bausch DG, Sabeti PC, Khan SH, Garry RF; KGH Lassa Fever Program; Viral Hemorrhagic Fever Consortium; WHO Clinical Response Team.

Collaborators: Adachi T, Bhdella N, Bausch D, Brett-Major D, Crozier I, Donovan S, Ferri M, Fletcher T, Fowler R, Houlihan C, Hurley K, Jacob S, O'Dempsey SM, Porembka D, Risi G, Rubinson L, Schieffelin J, Abu J, Allieu A, Bangura J, Dukullay B, Fomgbeh M, Kamara B, Kamara F, Kainesie G, Kallon M, Kallon T, Kargbo K, Karbgo D, Koninga J, Konneh V, Koroma V, Lungay V, Massaquoi E, Moseray J, Musa J, Robert W, Samai S, Sannoh P, Sesay J, Shaw S, Sow M, Wilson RB, Kulakosky PC, Simpson K, Charbonnet M, Butts M, Burchfield L, Gladden A, Hlastava A, Hueklom S, Karlsson E, Phelan E, Tariyal R, Matranga C, Shlyakhter I, Tareila A, Tewhey R, Vitti J, Simpson D, Simpson D, Saphire EO, Hastie K, Oldstone MB, de la Torre JC, Sullivan B, Hutto S, Gaither C, Tubre' S, Gale TV, Hoffmann A, Melnik LI, Yenni RB, Haislip AM, Li S, Geisbert TW, Geisbert J, Cross R, Mire CE, Fish W, Folarin O, Adomeh D, Adun O, Agbukor J, Airende M, Akpede GO, Aire C, Akhaine I, Asogun D, Ayepada J, Ekaete T, Ehikhametalor S, Eromon PE, Ifeh V, Ighenegbale G, Ighodalo YO, Muoebonam E, Odia I, Okokhere PO, Olokor T, Omomoh E, Omoniwa O, Oyakhilome J, Uyigue E.

Author information: (1)The authors' affiliations are listed in the Appendix.

BACKGROUND: Limited clinical and laboratory data are available on patients with Ebola virus disease (EVD). The Kenema Government Hospital in Sierra Leone, which had an existing infrastructure for research regarding viral hemorrhagic fever, has received and cared for patients with EVD since the beginning of the outbreak in Sierra Leone in May 2014. METHODS: We reviewed available epidemiologic, clinical, and laboratory records of patients in whom EVD was diagnosed between May 25 and June 18, 2014. We used quantitative reverse-transcriptase-polymerase-chain-reaction assays to assess the load of Ebola virus (EBOV, Zaire species) in a subgroup of patients. RESULTS: Of 106 patients in whom EVD was diagnosed, 87 had a known outcome, and 44 had detailed clinical information available. The incubation period was estimated to be 6 to 12 days, and the case fatality rate was 74%. Common findings at presentation included fever (in 89% of the patients), headache (in 80%), weakness (in 66%), dizziness (in 60%), diarrhea (in 51%), abdominal pain (in 40%), and vomiting (in 34%). Clinical and laboratory factors at presentation that were associated with a fatal outcome included fever, weakness, dizziness, diarrhea, and elevated levels of blood urea nitrogen, aspartate aminotransferase, and creatinine. Exploratory analyses indicated that patients under the age of 21 years had a lower case fatality rate than those over the age of 45 years (57% vs. 94%, P=0.03), and patients presenting with fewer than 100,000 EBOV copies per milliliter had a lower case fatality rate than those with 10 million EBOV copies per milliliter or more (33% vs. 94%, P=0.003). Bleeding occurred in only 1 patient. CONCLUSIONS: The incubation period and case fatality rate among patients with EVD in Sierra Leone are similar to those observed elsewhere in the 2014 outbreak and in previous outbreaks. Although bleeding was an infrequent finding, diarrhea and other gastrointestinal manifestations were common. (Funded by the National Institutes of Health and others.).

PMID: 25353969 [PubMed - indexed for MEDLINE]
208. N Engl J Med. 2014 Nov 27;371(22):2083-91. doi: 10.1056/NEJMoa1411099. Epub 2014 Oct 15.

Ebola virus disease in the Democratic Republic of Congo.

Maganga GD(1), Kapetshi J, Berthet N, Kebela Ilunga B, Kabange F, Mbala Kingebeni P, Mondonge V, Muyembe JJ, Bertherat E, Briand S, Cabore J, Epelboin A, Formenty P, Kobinger G, González-Angulo L, Labouba I, Manuguerra JC, Okwo-Bele JM, Dye C, Leroy EM.

Author information: (1)From the Centre International de Recherches Médicales de Franceville, World Health Organization (WHO) Collaborating Center, Franceville, Gabon (G.D.M., N.B., I.L., E.M.L.); Ministry of Health (B.K.I., F.K.), Institut National de Recherche Biomédicale (J.K., P.M.K., J.-J.T.M.), and the WHO (V.M., J.C.), Kinshasa, Democratic Republic of Congo; Centre National de la Recherche Scientifique, Unité Epidémiologie et Physiopathologie des Virus Oncogènes (CNRS UMR3569) (N.B.), Eco-anthropologie et Ethnobiologie, UMR 7206 CNRS-MNHN (A.E.), and Institut Pasteur, Unité de Recherche et d'Expertise Environnement et Risques Infectieux, Cellule d'Intervention Biologique d'Urgence (J.-C.M.), Paris, and Institut de Recherche pour le Développement, Unité Maladies Infectieuses et Vecteurs Ecologie, Genetique, Evolution et Controle IRD 224-CNRS 5290-UMI-UM2, Montpellier (E.M.L.) - all in France; Public Health Agency of Canada, Winnipeg (G.K.); and the WHO, Geneva (E.B., S.B., P.F., L.G.-A., J.-M.O.-B., C.D.).

BACKGROUND: The seventh reported outbreak of Ebola virus disease (EVD) in the equatorial African country of the Democratic Republic of Congo (DRC) began on July 26, 2014, as another large EVD epidemic continued to spread in West Africa. Simultaneous reports of EVD in equatorial and West Africa raised the question of whether the two outbreaks were linked. METHODS: We obtained data from patients in the DRC, using the standard World Health Organization clinical-investigation form for viral hemorrhagic fevers. Patients were classified as having suspected, probable, or confirmed EVD or a non-EVD illness. Blood samples were obtained for polymerase-chain-reaction-based diagnosis, viral isolation, sequencing, and phylogenetic analysis. RESULTS: The outbreak began in Inkanamongo village in the vicinity of Boende town in Équateur province and has been confined to that province. A total of 69 suspected, probable, or confirmed cases were reported between July 26 and October 7, 2014, including 8 cases among health care workers, with 49 deaths. As of October 7, there have been approximately six generations of cases of EVD since the outbreak began. The reported weekly case incidence peaked in the weeks of August 17 and 24 and has since fallen sharply. Genome sequencing revealed Ebola virus (EBOV, Zaire species) as the cause of this outbreak. A coding-complete genome sequence of EBOV that was isolated during this outbreak showed 99.2% identity with the most closely related variant from the 1995 outbreak in Kikwit in the DRC and 96.8% identity to EBOV variants that are currently circulating in West Africa. CONCLUSIONS: The current EVD outbreak in the DRC has clinical and epidemiologic characteristics that are similar to those of previous EVD outbreaks in equatorial Africa. The causal agent is a local EBOV variant, and this outbreak has a zoonotic origin different from that in the 2014 epidemic in West Africa. (Funded by the Centre International de Recherches Médicales de Franceville and others.).

PMID: 25317743 [PubMed - indexed for MEDLINE]
209. Nature. 2014 Nov 27;515(7528):492. doi: 10.1038/515492a.

Ebola: models do more than forecast.

Rivers C(1).

Author information: (1)Virginia Bioinformatics Institute, Virginia Tech, Blacksburg, USA.

Comment on Nature. 2014 Nov 6;515(7525):18.

PMID: 25428492 [PubMed - in process]
210. Nature. 2014 Nov 27;515(7528):492. doi: 10.1038/515492b.

Ebola: the power of behaviour change.

Funk S(1), Knight GM(1), Jansen VA(2).

Author information: (1)London School of Hygiene &Tropical Medicine, London, UK. (2)Royal Holloway University of London, Egham, Surrey, UK.

Comment on Nature. 2014 Nov 6;515(7525):18.

PMID: 25428491 [PubMed - in process]
211. Nature. 2014 Nov 27;515(7528):465-6. doi: 10.1038/515465b.

Ebola opportunity.

[No authors listed]

PMID: 25428460 [PubMed - in process]
212. Ann Pharmacother. 2014 Nov 26. pii: 1060028014561782. [Epub ahead of print]

Ebola Virus Disease: Roles and Considerations for Pharmacists.

Guarascio AJ(1), Faust AC(2), Sheperd L(2), O'Donnell LA(3).

Author information: (1)Mylan School of Pharmacy at Duquesne University, Pittsburgh, PA, USA guarascioa@duq.edu. (2)Texas Health Presbyterian Hospital, Dallas, TX, USA. (3)Mylan School of Pharmacy at Duquesne University, Pittsburgh, PA, USA.

Ebola virus disease (EVD) poses significant clinical care implications for pharmacists. Emergency preparedness efforts should be undertaken to ensure vital response to EVD. Pharmacists should consider factors such as enhanced use of resources for front-line EVD patient care along with procurement of investigational medications. Appropriate and timely preparation, distribution, and administration of treatment for patients with EVD in the setting of substantial critical illness as well as infection control measures are essential. Aggressive supportive care and early, goal-directed therapy are cornerstones of therapy, whereas investigational treatments for EVD will likely play a larger, more well-defined role as future clinical trials are conducted.

PMID: 25429092 [PubMed - as supplied by publisher]

213. N Engl J Med. 2014 Nov 26. [Epub ahead of print]

One Step Closer to an Ebola Virus Vaccine.

Bausch DG(1).

Author information: (1)From the Tulane University Health Sciences Center, New Orleans; and the U.S. Naval Medical Research Unit No. 6, Lima, Peru.

Despite cautious optimism from the apparent recent slowing of the spread of Ebola virus disease (EVD) in some parts of West Africa,(1) the remaining pockets of intense transmission and the recent incursion of the virus into Mali(2) remind us that the battle for control is still on. This is no time to be complacent. The scale of this outbreak, in which every few days about the same number of cases accrue as occurred during the entire 3-month outbreak in Gulu, Uganda, in 2000-2001 - previously the largest outbreak on record - has prompted us to pull out all the stops, . . .

PMID: 25426836 [PubMed - as supplied by publisher]

214. N Engl J Med. 2014 Nov 26. [Epub ahead of print]

Chimpanzee Adenovirus Vector Ebola Vaccine - Preliminary Report.

Ledgerwood JE(1), DeZure AD, Stanley DA, Novik L, Enama ME, Berkowitz NM, Hu Z, Joshi G, Ploquin A, Sitar S, Gordon IJ, Plummer SA, Holman LA, Hendel CS, Yamshchikov G, Roman F, Nicosia A, Colloca S, Cortese R, Bailer RT, Schwartz RM, Roederer M, Mascola JR, Koup RA, Sullivan NJ, Graham BS; the VRC 207 Study Team.

Author information: (1)From the Vaccine Research Center (J.E.L., A.D.D., D.A.S., L.N., M.E.E., N.M.B., A.P., S.S., I.J.G., S.A.P., L.A.H., C.S.H., G.Y., R.T.B., R.M.S., M.R., J.R.M., R.A.K., N.J.S., B.S.G.) and the Biostatistics Research Branch, Division of Clinical Research (Z.H., G.J.), National Institute of Allergy and Infectious Diseases, National Institutes of Health, Bethesda, MD; GlaxoSmithKline Vaccines, Rixensart, Belgium (F.R.); ReiThera, Rome (A.N., S.C.), and CEINGE and the Department of Molecular Medicine and Medical Biotechnology, University of Naples Federico II, Naples (A.N.) - both in Italy; and Keires, Basel, Switzerland (R.C.).

Background The unprecedented 2014 epidemic of Ebola virus disease (EVD) has prompted an international response to accelerate the availability of a preventive vaccine. A replication-defective recombinant chimpanzee adenovirus type 3-vectored ebolavirus vaccine (cAd3-EBO), encoding the glycoprotein from Zaire and Sudan species that offers protection in the nonhuman primate model, was rapidly advanced into phase 1 clinical evaluation. Methods We conducted a phase 1, dose-escalation, open-label trial of cAd3-EBO. Twenty healthy adults, in sequentially enrolled groups of 10 each, received vaccination intramuscularly in doses of $2\times10(10)$ particle units or $2\times10(11)$ particle units. Primary and secondary end points related to safety and immunogenicity were assessed throughout the first 4 weeks after vaccination. Results In this small study, no safety concerns were identified; however, transient fever developed within 1 day after vaccination in two participants who had received the $2\times10(11)$ particle-unit dose. Glycoprotein-specific antibodies were induced in all 20 participants; the titers were of greater magnitude in the group that received the $2\times10(11)$ particle-unit dose than in the group that received the $2\times10(10)$ particle-unit dose (geometric mean titer against the Zaire antigen, 2037 vs. 331; P=0.001). Glycoprotein-specific T-cell responses were more frequent among those who received the $2\times10(11)$ particle-unit dose than among those who received the $2\times10(10)$ particle-unit dose, with a CD4 response in 10 of 10 participants versus 3 of 10 participants (P=0.004) and a CD8 response in 7 of 10 participants versus 2 of 10 participants (P=0.07). Conclusions Reactogenicity and immune responses to cAd3-EBO vaccine were dose-dependent. At the $2\times10(11)$ particle-unit dose, glycoprotein Zaire-specific antibody responses were in the range reported to be associated with vaccine-induced protective immunity in challenge studies involving nonhuman primates. Clinical trials assessing cAd3-EBO are ongoing. (Funded by the Intramural Research Program of the National Institutes of Health; VRC 207 ClinicalTrials.gov number, NCT02231866 .).

PMID: 25426834 [PubMed - as supplied by publisher]

215. Nurs Stand. 2014 Nov 26;29(13):30. doi: 10.7748/ns.29.13.30.s35.

Ebola virus disease: clinical management and guidance.

Evans R(1).

Author information: (1)Nursing Standard.

As part of the UK government's response to the outbreak of Ebola in west Africa, Public Health England has launched a health protection resource on the Gov.UK website.

PMID: 25424098 [PubMed - in process]

216. Nurs Stand. 2014 Nov 26;29(13):11. doi: 10.7748/ns.29.13.11.s11.

More Sierra Leone volunteers fly out.

[No authors listed]

Another group of more than 30 NHS healthcare staff left for Sierra Leone last week to join the fight against Ebola. They are among more than 1,000 NHS staff who have volunteered to help.

PMID: 25424072 [PubMed - in process]

217. J Obstet Gynecol Neonatal Nurs. 2014 Nov 24. doi: 10.1111/1552-6909.12518. [Epub ahead of print]

Ebola: Caring for Pregnant and Postpartum Women and Newborns in the United States: AWHONN Practice Brief Number 3.

[No authors listed]

PMID: 25421426 [PubMed - as supplied by publisher]

218. Nat Genet. 2014 Nov 24;46(12):1257. doi: 10.1038/ng.3158.

Modeling Ebola hemorrhagic fever in mice.

Vogan K.

PMID: 25418746 [PubMed - in process]
219. Viruses. 2014 Nov 24;6(11):4760-99. doi: 10.3390/v6114760.

Nomenclature- and Database-Compatible Names for the Two Ebola Virus Variants that Emerged in Guinea and the Democratic Republic of the Congo in 2014.

Kuhn JH(1), Andersen KG(2), Baize S(3), Bào Y(4), Bavari S(5), Berthet N(6), Blinkova O(7), Brister JR(8), Clawson AN(9), Fair J(10), Gabriel M(11), Garry RF(12), Gire SK(13), Goba A(14), Gonzalez JP(15), Günther S(16), Happi CT(17), Jahrling PB(18), Kapetshi J(19), Kobinger G(20), Kugelman JR(21), Leroy EM(22), Maganga GD(23), Mbala PK(24), Moses LM(25), Muyembe-Tamfum JJ(26), N'Faly M(27), Nichol ST(28), Omilabu SA(29), Palacios G(30), Park DJ(31), Paweska JT(32), Radoshitzky SR(33), Rossi CA(34), Sabeti PC(35), Schieffelin JS(36), Schoepp RJ(37), Sealfon R(38), Swanepoel R(39), Towner JS(40), Wada J(41), Wauquier N(42), Yozwiak NL(43), Formenty P(44).

Author information: (1)Integrated Research Facility at Fort Detrick, National Institute of Allergy and Infectious Diseases, National Institutes of Health, Fort Detrick, Frederick, MD 21702, USA. kuhnjens@mail.nih.gov. (2)FAS Center for Systems Biology, Harvard University, Cambridge, MA 02138, USA. kandersen@oeb.harvard.edu. (3)Unité de Biologie des Infections Virales Emergentes, Institut Pasteur, Lyon, France. sylvain.baize@inserm.fr. (4)Information Engineering Branch, National Center for Biotechnology Information, National Library of Medicine, National Institutes of Health, Bethesda, MD 20894, USA. bao@ncbi.nlm.nih.gov. (5)United States Army Medical Research Institute of Infectious Diseases, Fort Detrick, Frederick, MD 21702, USA. sina.bavari.civ@mail.mil. (6)Centre International de Recherches Médicales de Franceville, B. P. 769, Franceville, Gabon. nicolas.berthet@pasteur.fr. (7)Information Engineering Branch, National Center for Biotechnology Information, National Library of Medicine, National Institutes of Health, Bethesda, MD 20894, USA. olga.blinkova@nih.gov. (8)Information Engineering Branch, National Center for Biotechnology Information, National Library of Medicine, National Institutes of Health, Bethesda, MD 20894, USA. jamesbr@ncbi.nlm.nih.gov. (9)Integrated Research Facility at Fort Detrick, National Institute of Allergy and Infectious Diseases, National Institutes of Health, Fort Detrick, Frederick, MD 21702, USA. anna@logosconsulting.us. (10)Fondation Mérieux, Washington, DC 20036, USA. joseph.fair@fondation-merieux.org. (11)Bernhard Nocht Institute for Tropical Medicine, World Health Organization (WHO) Collaborating Center for Arbovirus and Hemorrhagic Fever Reference and Research, and the German Center for Infection Research (DZIF), Partner Site Hamburg, 20259 Hamburg, Germany. gabriel@bni-hamburg.de. (12)Tulane University School of Medicine, New Orleans, LA 70112, USA. rfgarry@tulane.edu. (13)FAS Center for Systems Biology, Harvard University, Cambridge, MA 02138, USA. sgire@oeb.harvard.edu. (14)Integrated Research Facility at Fort Detrick, National Institute of Allergy and Infectious Diseases, National Institutes of Health, Fort Detrick, Frederick, MD 21702, USA. augstgoba@yahoo.com. (15)Integrated Research Facility at Fort Detrick, National Institute of Allergy and Infectious Diseases, National Institutes of Health, Fort Detrick, Frederick, MD 21702, USA. jpgonzalez@metabiota.com. (16)Bernhard Nocht Institute for Tropical Medicine, World Health Organization (WHO) Collaborating Center for Arbovirus and Hemorrhagic Fever Reference and Research, and the German Center for Infection Research (DZIF), Partner Site Hamburg, 20259 Hamburg, Germany. guenther@bni.uni-hamburg.de. (17)Integrated Research Facility at Fort Detrick, National Institute of Allergy and Infectious Diseases, National Institutes of Health, Fort Detrick, Frederick, MD 21702, USA. happic@run.edu.ng. (18)Integrated Research Facility at Fort Detrick, National Institute of Allergy and Infectious Diseases, National Institutes of Health, Fort Detrick, Frederick, MD 21702, USA. jahrlingp@niaid.nih.gov. (19)Integrated Research Facility at Fort Detrick, National Institute of Allergy and Infectious Diseases, National Institutes of Health, Fort Detrick, Frederick, MD 21702, USA. jimmy_kap@hotmail.com. (20)Integrated Research Facility at Fort Detrick, National Institute of Allergy and Infectious Diseases, National Institutes of Health, Fort Detrick, Frederick, MD 21702, USA. gary.kobinger@phac-aspc.gc.ca. (21)United States Army Medical Research Institute of Infectious Diseases, Fort Detrick, Frederick, MD 21702, USA. jeffrey.r.kugelman.mil@mail.mil. (22)Centre International de Recherches Médicales de Franceville, B. P. 769, Franceville, Gabon. eric.leroy@ird.fr. (23)Centre International de Recherches Médicales de Franceville, B. P. 769, Franceville, Gabon. gael_maganga@yahoo.fr. (24)Integrated Research Facility at Fort Detrick, National Institute of Allergy and Infectious Diseases, National Institutes of Health, Fort Detrick, Frederick, MD 21702, USA. mbalaplacide@gmail.com. (25)Tulane University School of Medicine, New Orleans, LA 70112, USA. lmoses2@tulane.edu. (26)Integrated Research Facility at Fort Detrick, National Institute of Allergy and Infectious Diseases, National Institutes of Health, Fort Detrick, Frederick, MD 21702, USA. muyembejj@gmail.com. (27)Integrated Research Facility at Fort Detrick, National Institute of Allergy and Infectious Diseases, National Institutes of Health, Fort Detrick, Frederick, MD 21702, USA. cmagassouba01@gmail.com. (28)Integrated Research Facility at Fort Detrick, National Institute of Allergy and Infectious Diseases, National Institutes of Health, Fort Detrick, Frederick, MD 21702, USA. stn1@cdc.gov. (29)Integrated Research Facility at Fort Detrick, National Institute of Allergy and Infectious Diseases, National Institutes of Health, Fort Detrick, Frederick, MD 21702, USA. omilabusa@yahoo.com. (30)United States Army Medical Research Institute of Infectious Diseases, Fort Detrick, Frederick, MD 21702, USA. gustavo.f.palacios.ctr@us.army.mil. (31)Integrated Research Facility at Fort Detrick, National Institute of Allergy and Infectious Diseases, National Institutes of Health, Fort Detrick, Frederick, MD 21702, USA. dpark@broadinstitute.org. (32)Integrated Research Facility at Fort Detrick, National Institute of Allergy and Infectious Diseases, National Institutes of Health, Fort Detrick, Frederick, MD 21702, USA. januszp@nicd.ac.za. (33)United States Army Medical Research Institute of Infectious Diseases, Fort Detrick, Frederick, MD 21702, USA. sheli.r.radoshitzky.ctr@mail.mil. (34)United States Army Medical Research Institute of Infectious Diseases, Fort Detrick, Frederick, MD 21702, USA. cynthia.a.rossi.civ@mail.mil. (35)FAS Center for Systems Biology, Harvard University, Cambridge, MA 02138, USA. pardis@broadinstitute.org. (36)Tulane University School of Medicine, New Orleans, LA 70112, USA. jschieff@tulane.edu. (37)United States Army Medical Research Institute of Infectious Diseases, Fort Detrick, Frederick, MD 21702, USA. randal.j.schoepp.civ@mail.mil. (38)FAS Center for Systems Biology, Harvard University, Cambridge, MA 02138, USA. sealfon@gmail.com. (39)FAS Center for Systems Biology, Harvard University, Cambridge, MA 02138, USA. bobswanepoel@gmail.com. (40)Integrated Research Facility at Fort Detrick, National Institute of Allergy and Infectious Diseases, National Institutes of Health, Fort Detrick, Frederick, MD 21702, USA. jit8@cdc.gov. (41)Integrated Research Facility at Fort Detrick, National Institute of Allergy and Infectious Diseases, National Institutes of Health, Fort Detrick, Frederick, MD 21702, USA. wadaj@niaid.nih.gov. (42)Integrated Research Facility at Fort Detrick, National Institute of Allergy and Infectious Diseases, National Institutes of

Health, Fort Detrick, Frederick, MD 21702, USA. nadia.wauquier@gmail.com. (43)FAS Center for Systems Biology, Harvard University, Cambridge, MA 02138, USA. nyozwiak@broadinstitute.org. (44)FAS Center for Systems Biology, Harvard University, Cambridge, MA 02138, USA. formentyp@who.int.

In 2014, Ebola virus (EBOV) was identified as the etiological agent of a large and still expanding outbreak of Ebola virus disease (EVD) in West Africa and a much more confined EVD outbreak in Middle Africa. Epidemiological and evolutionary analyses confirmed that all cases of both outbreaks are connected to a single introduction each of EBOV into human populations and that both outbreaks are not directly connected. Coding-complete genomic sequence analyses of isolates revealed that the two outbreaks were caused by two novel EBOV variants, and initial clinical observations suggest that neither of them should be considered strains. Here we present consensus decisions on naming for both variants (West Africa: "Makona", Middle Africa: "Lomela") and provide database-compatible full, shortened, and abbreviated names that are in line with recently established filovirus sub-species nomenclatures.

PMCID: PMC4246247 PMID: 25421896 [PubMed - in process]

220. Viruses. 2014 Nov 24;6(11):4666-82. doi: 10.3390/v6114666.

Euthanasia assessment in ebola virus infected nonhuman primates.

Warren TK(1), Trefry JC(2), Marko ST(3), Chance TB(4), Wells JB(5), Pratt WD(6), Johnson JC(7), Mucker EM(8), Norris SL(9), Chappell M(10), Dye JM(11), Honko AN(12).

Author information: (1)US Army Medical Research Institute for Infectious Diseases, 1425 Porter St., Fort Detrick, MD 21702, USA. travis.k.warren.ctr@mail.mil. (2)US Army Medical Research Institute for Infectious Diseases, 1425 Porter St., Fort Detrick, MD 21702, USA. john.c.trefry.ctr@mail.mil. (3)US Army Medical Research Institute for Infectious Diseases, 1425 Porter St., Fort Detrick, MD 21702, USA. shannon.t.marko.mil@mail.mil. (4)US Army Medical Research Institute for Infectious Diseases, 1425 Porter St., Fort Detrick, MD 21702, USA. taylor.b.chance.mil@mail.mil. (5)US Army Medical Research Institute for Infectious Diseases, 1425 Porter St., Fort Detrick, MD 21702, USA. jay.b.wells.ctr@mail.mil. (6)US Army Medical Research Institute for Infectious Diseases, 1425 Porter St., Fort Detrick, MD 21702, USA. william.d.pratt4.civ@mail.mil. (7)US Army Medical Research Institute for Infectious Diseases, 1425 Porter St., Fort Detrick, MD 21702, USA. joshua.johnson@nih.gov. (8)US Army Medical Research Institute for Infectious Diseases, 1425 Porter St., Fort Detrick, MD 21702, USA. eric.m.mucker.ctr@mail.mil. (9)US Army Medical Research Institute for Infectious Diseases, 1425 Porter St., Fort Detrick, MD 21702, USA. sarah.l.norris2.civ@mail.mil. (10)US Army Medical Research Institute for Infectious Diseases, 1425 Porter St., Fort Detrick, MD 21702, USA. mark.chappell@usuhs.edu. (11)US Army Medical Research Institute for Infectious Diseases, 1425 Porter St., Fort Detrick, MD 21702, USA. john.m.dye1.civ@mail.mil. (12)US Army Medical Research Institute for Infectious Diseases, 1425 Porter St., Fort Detrick, MD 21702, USA. anna.honko@nih.gov.

Multiple products are being developed for use against filoviral infections. Efficacy for these products will likely be demonstrated in nonhuman primate models of filoviral disease to satisfy licensure requirements under the Animal Rule, or to supplement human data. Typically, the endpoint for efficacy assessment will be survival following challenge; however, there exists no standardized approach for assessing the health or euthanasia criteria for filovirus-exposed nonhuman primates. Consideration of objective criteria is important to (a) ensure test subjects are euthanized without unnecessary distress; (b) enhance the likelihood that animals exhibiting mild or moderate signs of disease are not prematurely euthanized; (c) minimize the occurrence of spontaneous deaths and loss of end-stage samples; (d) enhance the reproducibility of experiments between different researchers; and (e) provide a defensible rationale for euthanasia decisions that withstands regulatory scrutiny. Historic records were compiled for 58 surviving and non-surviving monkeys exposed to Ebola virus at the US Army Medical Research Institute of Infectious Diseases. Clinical pathology parameters were statistically analyzed and those exhibiting predicative value for survival are reported. These findings may be useful for standardization of objective euthanasia assessments in rhesus monkeys exposed to Ebola virus and may serve as a useful approach for other standardization efforts.

PMCID: PMC4246243 PMID: 25421892 [PubMed - in process]

221. Genome Biol. 2014 Nov 22;15(11):540. [Epub ahead of print]

Elucidating variations in the nucleotide sequence of Ebola virus associated with increasing pathogenicity.

Dowall SD, Matthews DA, García-Dorival I, Taylor I, Kenny J, Hertz-Fowler C, Hall N, Corbin-Lickfett K, Empig C, Schlunegger K, Barr JN, Carroll MW, Hewson R, Hiscox JA.

BackgroundEbolaviruses causes a severe and often fatal hemorrhagic fever in humans, with some species such as Ebola virus having case fatality rates approaching 90%. Currently the worst Ebola virus outbreak since the disease was discovered is occurring in West Africa. Although thought to be a zoonotic infection, a concern is that with increasing numbers of humans being infected, Ebola virus variants could be selected which are better adapted for human-to-human transmission.ResultsTo investigate whether genetic changes in Ebola virus become established in response to adaptation in a different host, a guinea pig model of infection was used. In this experimental system, guinea pigs were infected with Ebola virus (EBOV), which initially did not cause disease. To simulate transmission to uninfected individuals, the virus was serially passaged five times in naive animals. As the virus was passaged, virulence increased and clinical effects were observed in the guinea pig. An RNAseq and consensus mapping approach was then used to evaluate potential nucleotide changes in the Ebola virus genome at each passage.ConclusionsUpon passage in the guinea pig model, EBOV become more virulent, RNA editing and also coding changes in key proteins become established. The data suggest that the initial evolutionary trajectory of EBOV in a new host can lead to a gain in virulence. Given the circumstances of the sustained transmission of EBOV in the current outbreak in West Africa, increases in virulence may be associated with prolonged and uncontrolled epidemics of EBOV.

PMID: 25416632 [PubMed - as supplied by publisher]

222. Lancet. 2014 Nov 22;384(9957):1833.

First trials for Ebola treatments announced.

Mohammadi D.

PMID: 25513402 [PubMed - in process]

223. Lancet. 2014 Nov 22;384(9957):1833.

First trials for Ebola treatments announced.

Mohammadi D.

PMID: 25478606 [PubMed - in process]

224. Lancet. 2014 Nov 22;384(9957):1844. doi: 10.1016/S0140-6736(14)62236-4. Epub 2014 Nov 21.

Compassionate use of experimental drugs in the Ebola outbreak - Authors' reply.

Rid A(1), Emanuel EJ(2).

Author information: (1)Department of Social Science, Health & Medicine, King's College London, London WC2R 2LS, UK. Electronic address: annette.rid@kcl.ac.uk. (2)Department of Medical Ethics & Health Policy, Perelman School of Medicine, University of Pennsylvania, Philadelphia, PA, USA.

Comment on Lancet. 2014 Nov 22;384(9957):1896-9. Lancet. 2014 Nov 22;384(9957):1843. Lancet. 2014 Nov 22;384(9957):1843-4.

PMID: 25457910 [PubMed - in process]

225. Lancet. 2014 Nov 22;384(9957):1843. doi: 10.1016/S0140-6736(14)61609-3. Epub 2014 Sep 25.

Priorities for Ebola virus disease response in west Africa.

Jacob ST(1), Crozier I(2), Schieffelin JS(3), Colebunders R(4).

Author information: (1)Department of Medicine, University of Washington, Seattle, WA 98109, USA. Electronic address: sjacob2@uw.edu. (2)Accordia Global Health Foundation, Washington, DC, USA. (3)Department of Tropical Medicine, Tulane University School of Public Health and Tropical Medicine, LA, USA. (4)Department of Clinical Sciences, Institute of Tropical Medicine, and Epidemiology and Social Medicine, University of Antwerp, Antwerp, Belgium.

Comment in Lancet. 2014 Nov 22;384(9957):1844.

Comment on Lancet. 2014 Nov 22;384(9957):1896-9.

PMID: 25262343 [PubMed - in process]

226. Lancet. 2014 Nov 22;384(9957):1843-4. doi: 10.1016/S0140-6736(14)61605-6. Epub 2014 Sep 11.

Compassionate use of experimental drugs in the Ebola outbreak.

Folayan M(1), Brown B(2), Yakubu A(3), Peterson K(4), Haire B(5).

Author information: (1)Obafemi Awolowo University, Ile-Ife, Nigeria. (2)Program in Public Health, University of California-Irvine, Irvine, CA 92697, USA. Electronic address: brandojb@uci.edu. (3)National Health Research Ethics Committee, Abuja, Nigeria. (4)Department of Anthropology, University of California-Irvine, Irvine, CA 92697, USA. (5)School of Public Health and Community Medicine, University of New South Wales, Sydney, NSW, Australia.

Comment in Lancet. 2014 Nov 22;384(9957):1844.

Comment on Lancet. 2014 Nov 22;384(9957):1896-9.

PMID: 25220192 [PubMed - in process]

227. Lancet. 2014 Nov 22;384(9957):1896-9. doi: 10.1016/S0140-6736(14)61315-5. Epub 2014 Aug 22.

Ethical considerations of experimental interventions in the Ebola outbreak.

Rid A(1), Emanuel EJ(2).

Author information: (1)Department of Social Science, Health & Medicine, King's College London, London, UK. Electronic address: annette.rid@kcl.ac.uk. (2)Department of Medical Ethics & Health Policy, Perelman School of Medicine, University of Pennsylvania, Philadelphia, PA, USA.

Comment in Lancet. 2014 Nov 22;384(9957):1843-4. Lancet. 2014 Nov 22;384(9957):1844. Lancet. 2014 Nov 22;384(9957):1843.

PMID: 25155413 [PubMed - in process]

228. MMWR Morb Mortal Wkly Rep. 2014 Nov 21;63(46):1089-91.

Response to importation of a case of ebola virus disease - ohio, october 2014.

McCarty CL, Basler C, Karwowski M, Erme M, Nixon G, Kippes C, Allan T, Parrilla T, DiOrio M, Fijter Sd, Stone ND, Yost DA, Lippold SA, Regan JJ, Honein MA, Knust B, Braden C.

On September 30, 2014, the Texas Department of State Health Services reported a case of Ebola virus disease (Ebola) diagnosed in Dallas, Texas, and confirmed by CDC, the first case of Ebola diagnosed in the United States. The patient (patient 1) had traveled from Liberia, a country which, along with Sierra Leone and Guinea, is currently experiencing the largest recorded Ebola outbreak. A nurse (patient 2) who provided hospital bedside care to patient 1 in Texas visited an emergency department (ED) with fever and was diagnosed with laboratory-confirmed Ebola on October 11, and a second nurse (patient 3) who also provided hospital bedside care visited an ED with fever and rash on October 14 and was diagnosed with laboratory-confirmed Ebola on October 15. Patient 3 visited Ohio during October 10-13, traveling by commercial airline between Dallas, Texas, and Cleveland, Ohio. Based on the medical history and clinical and laboratory findings on October 14, the date of illness onset was uncertain; therefore, CDC, in collaboration with state and local partners, included the period October 10-13 as being part of the potentially infectious period, out of an abundance of caution to ensure all potential contacts were monitored. On October 15, the Ohio Department of Health requested CDC assistance to identify and monitor contacts of patient 3, assess the risk for disease transmission, provide infection control recommendations, and assess and guide regional health care system preparedness. The description of this contact investigation and hospital assessment is provided to help other states in planning for similar events.

PMID: 25412070 [PubMed - in process]

229. MMWR Morb Mortal Wkly Rep. 2014 Nov 21;63(46):1087-8.

Ebola virus disease cluster in the United States - dallas county, Texas, 2014.

Chevalier MS, Chung W, Smith J, Weil LM, Hughes SM, Joyner SN, Hall E, Srinath D, Ritch J, Thathiah P, Threadgill H, Cervantes D, Lakey DL.

Since March 10, 2014, Guinea, Liberia, and Sierra Leone have experienced the largest known Ebola virus disease (Ebola) epidemic with approximately 13,000 persons infected as of October 28, 2014. Before September 25, 2014, only four patients with Ebola had been treated in the United States; all of these patients had been diagnosed in West Africa and medically evacuated to the United States for care.

PMID: 25412069 [PubMed - in process]

230. MMWR Morb Mortal Wkly Rep. 2014 Nov 21;63(46):1082-6.

Ebola epidemic - liberia, march-october 2014.

Nyenswah T, Fahnbulleh M, Massaquoi M, Nagbe T, Bawo L, Falla JD, Kohar H, Gasasira A, Nabeth P, Yett S, Gergonne B, Casey S, Espinosa B, McCoy A, Feldman H, Hensley L, Baily M, Fields B, Lo T, Lindblade K, Mott J, Boulanger L, Christie A, Wang S, Montgomery J, Mahoney F.

On March 21, 2014, the Guinea Ministry of Health reported the outbreak of an illness characterized by fever, severe diarrhea, vomiting and a high fatality rate (59%), leading to the first known epidemic of Ebola virus disease (Ebola) in West Africa and the largest and longest Ebola epidemic in history. As of November 2, Liberia had reported the largest number of cases (6,525) and deaths (2,697) among the three affected countries of West Africa with ongoing transmission (Guinea, Liberia, and Sierra Leone). The response strategy in Liberia has included management of the epidemic through an incident management system (IMS) in which the activities of all partners are coordinated. Within the IMS, key strategies for epidemic control include surveillance, case investigation, laboratory confirmation, contact tracing, safe transportation of persons with suspected Ebola, isolation, infection control within the health care system, community engagement, and safe burial. This report provides a brief overview of the progression of the epidemic in Liberia and summarizes the interventions implemented.

PMID: 25412068 [PubMed - in process]

231. MMWR Morb Mortal Wkly Rep. 2014 Nov 21;63(46):1077-81.

Ebola virus disease cases among health care workers not working in ebola treatment units - liberia, june-august, 2014.

Matanock A, Arwady MA, Ayscue P, Forrester JD, Gaddis B, Hunter JC, Monroe B, Pillai SK, Reed C, Schafer IJ, Massaquoi M, Dahn B, De Cock KM.

West Africa is experiencing the largest Ebola virus disease (Ebola) epidemic in recorded history. Health care workers (HCWs) are at increased risk for Ebola. In Liberia, as of August 14, 2014, a total of 810 cases of Ebola had been reported, including 10 clusters of Ebola cases among HCWs working in facilities that were not Ebola treatment units (non-ETUs). The Liberian Ministry of Health and Social Welfare and CDC investigated these clusters by reviewing surveillance data, interviewing county health officials, HCWs, and contact tracers, and visiting health care facilities. Ninety-seven cases of Ebola (12% of the estimated total) were identified among HCWs; 62 HCW cases (64%) were part of 10 distinct clusters in non-ETU health care facilities, primarily hospitals. Early recognition and diagnosis of Ebola in patients who were the likely source of introduction to the HCWs (i.e., source patients) was missed in four clusters. Inconsistent recognition and triage of cases of Ebola, overcrowding, limitations in layout of physical spaces, lack of training in the use of and adequate supply of personal protective equipment (PPE), and limited supervision to ensure consistent adherence to infection control practices all were observed. Improving infection control infrastructure in non-ETUs is essential for protecting HCWs. Since August, the Liberian Ministry of Health and Social Welfare with a consortium of partners have undertaken collaborative efforts to strengthen infection control infrastructure in non-ETU health facilities.

PMID: 25412067 [PubMed - in process]

232. MMWR Morb Mortal Wkly Rep. 2014 Nov 21;63(46):1072-6.

Evidence for declining numbers of ebola cases - montserrado county, liberia, june-october 2014.

Nyenswah TG, Westercamp M, Kamali AA, Qin J, Zielinski-Gutierrez E, Amegashie F, Fallah M, Gergonne B, Nugba-Ballah R, Singh G, Aberle-Grasse JM, Havers F, Montgomery JM, Bawo L, Wang SA, Rosenberg R.

The epidemic of Ebola virus disease (Ebola) in West Africa that began in March 2014 has caused approximately 13,200 suspected, probable, and confirmed cases, including approximately 6,500 in Liberia. About 50% of Liberia's reported cases have been in Montserrado County (population 1.5 million), the most populous county, which contains the capital city, Monrovia. To examine the course of the Ebola epidemic in Montserrado County, data on Ebola treatment unit (ETU) admissions, laboratory testing of patient blood samples, and collection of dead bodies were analyzed. Each of the three data sources indicated consistent declines of 53%-73% following a peak incidence in mid-September. The declines in ETU admissions, percentage of patients with reverse transcription-polymerase chain reaction (RT-PCR) test results positive for Ebola, and dead bodies are the first evidence of reduction in disease after implementation of multiple prevention and response measures. The possible contributions of these interventions to the decline is not yet fully understood or corroborated. A reduction in cases suggests some progress; however, eliminating Ebola transmission is the critical goal and will require greatly intensified efforts for complete, high-quality surveillance to direct and drive the rapid intervention, tracking, and response efforts that remain essential.

PMID: 25412066 [PubMed - in process]

233. MMWR Morb Mortal Wkly Rep. 2014 Nov 21;63(46):1067-71.

Evidence for a decrease in transmission of ebola virus - lofa county, liberia, june 8-november 1, 2014.

Sharma A, Heijenberg N, Peter C, Bolongei J, Reeder B, Alpha T, Sterk E, Robert H, Kurth A, Cannas A, Bocquin A, Strecker T, Logue C, Caro AD, Pottage T, Yue C, Stoecker K, Wölfel R, Gabriel M, Günther S, Damon I.

Lofa County has one of the highest cumulative incidences of Ebola virus disease (Ebola) in Liberia. Recent situation reports from the Liberian Ministry of Health and Social Welfare (MoHSW) have indicated a decrease in new cases of Ebola in Lofa County. In October 2014, the Liberian MoHSW requested the assistance of CDC to further characterize recent trends in Ebola in Lofa County. Data collected during June 8-November 1, 2014 from three sources were analyzed: 1) aggregate data for newly reported cases, 2) case-based data for persons admitted to the dedicated Ebola treatment unit (ETU) for the county, and 3) test results for community decedents evaluated for Ebola. Trends from all three sources suggest that transmission of Ebola virus decreased as early as August 17, 2014, following rapid scale-up of response activities in Lofa County after a resurgence of Ebola in early June 2014. The comprehensive response strategy developed with participation from the local population in Lofa County might serve as a model to implement in other affected areas to accelerate control of Ebola.

PMID: 25412065 [PubMed - in process]

234. MMWR Morb Mortal Wkly Rep. 2014 Nov 21;63(46):1064-6.

Update: ebola virus disease epidemic - west Africa, november 2014.

System Ebola Epidemiology Team IM.

CDC is assisting ministries of health and working with other organizations to end the ongoing epidemic of Ebola virus disease (Ebola) in West Africa. The updated data in this report were compiled from situation reports from the Guinea Interministerial Committee for Response Against the Ebola Virus and the World Health Organization, the Liberia Ministry of Health and Social Welfare, and the Sierra Leone Ministry of Health and Sanitation. Total case counts include all suspected, probable, and confirmed cases, which are defined similarly by each country. These data reflect reported cases, which make up an unknown proportion of all cases, and reporting delays that vary from country to country.

PMID: 25412064 [PubMed - in process]

235. Science. 2014 Nov 21;346(6212):991-5. doi: 10.1126/science.1260612. Epub 2014 Oct 30.

Strategies for containing Ebola in West Africa.

Pandey A(1), Atkins KE(2), Medlock J(3), Wenzel N(1), Townsend JP(4), Childs JE(5), Nyenswah TG(6), Ndeffo-Mbah ML(1), Galvani AP(7).

Author information: (1)Center for Infectious Disease Modeling and Analysis, Yale School of Public Health, New Haven, CT, USA. (2)Center for Infectious Disease Modeling and Analysis, Yale School of Public Health, New Haven, CT, USA. Department of Infectious Disease Epidemiology, London School of Hygiene and Tropical Medicine, London, UK. (3)Department of Biomedical Sciences, Oregon State University, Corvallis, OR, USA. (4)Department of Biostatistics, Yale School of Public Health, New Haven, CT, USA. (5)Department of Epidemiology of Microbial Diseases, Yale School of Public Health, New Haven, CT, USA. (6)Ministry of Health and Social Welfare, Monrovia, Liberia. (7)Center for Infectious Disease Modeling and Analysis, Yale School of Public Health, New Haven, CT, USA. Department of Epidemiology of Microbial Diseases, Yale School of Public Health, New Haven, CT, USA. alison.galvani@yale.edu.

The ongoing Ebola outbreak poses an alarming risk to the countries of West Africa and beyond. To assess the effectiveness of containment strategies, we developed a stochastic model of Ebola transmission between and within the general community, hospitals, and funerals, calibrated to incidence data from Liberia. We find that a combined approach of case isolation, contact-tracing with quarantine, and sanitary funeral practices must be implemented with utmost urgency in order to reverse the growth of the outbreak. As of 19 September, under status quo, our model predicts that the epidemic will continue to spread, generating a predicted 224 (134 to 358) daily cases by 1 December, 280 (184 to 441) by 15 December, and 348 (249 to 545) by 30 December.

Copyright © 2014, American Association for the Advancement of Science.

PMID: 25414312 [PubMed - indexed for MEDLINE]

236. Science. 2014 Nov 21;346(6212):911. doi: 10.1126/science.346.6212.911.

Saving lives without new drugs.

Cohen J.

PMID: 25414286 [PubMed - indexed for MEDLINE]

237. Science. 2014 Nov 21;346(6212):908-11. doi: 10.1126/science.346.6212.908.

A dose of reality.

Cohen J, Kupferschmidt K.

PMID: 25414285 [PubMed - indexed for MEDLINE]

238. Science. 2014 Nov 21;346(6212):987-91. doi: 10.1126/science.1259595. Epub 2014 Oct 30.

Host genetic diversity enables Ebola hemorrhagic fever pathogenesis and resistance.

Rasmussen AL(1), Okumura A(2), Ferris MT(3), Green R(1), Feldmann F(4), Kelly SM(1), Scott DP(4), Safronetz D(5), Haddock E(5), LaCasse R(4), Thomas MJ(1), Sova P(1), Carter VS(1), Weiss JM(1), Miller DR(3), Shaw GD(3), Korth MJ(1), Heise MT(6), Baric RS(7), de Villena FP(3), Feldmann H(5), Katze MG(8).

Author information: (1)Department of Microbiology, University of Washington, Seattle, WA, USA. (2)Department of Microbiology, University of Washington, Seattle, WA, USA. Laboratory of Virology, National Institute of Allergy and Infectious Diseases, National Institutes of Health, Rocky Mountain Laboratories, Hamilton, MT, USA. (3)Department of Genetics, University of North Carolina, Chapel Hill, NC, USA. (4)Rocky Mountain Veterinary Branch, National Institute of Allergy and Infectious Diseases, National Institutes of Health, Rocky Mountain Laboratories, Hamilton, MT, USA. (5)Laboratory of Virology, National Institute of Allergy and Infectious Diseases, National Institutes of Health, Rocky Mountain Laboratories, Hamilton, MT, USA. (6)Department of Genetics, University of North Carolina, Chapel Hill, NC, USA. Department of Microbiology and Immunology, University of North Carolina, Chapel Hill, NC, USA. (7)Department of Microbiology and Immunology, University of North Carolina, Chapel Hill, NC, USA. (8)Department of Microbiology, University of Washington, Seattle, WA, USA. Washington National Primate Research Center, Seattle, WA, USA. honey@uw.edu.

Existing mouse models of lethal Ebola virus infection do not reproduce hallmark symptoms of Ebola hemorrhagic fever, neither delayed blood coagulation and disseminated intravascular coagulation nor death from shock, thus restricting pathogenesis studies to nonhuman primates. Here we show that mice from the Collaborative Cross panel of recombinant inbred mice exhibit distinct disease phenotypes after mouse-adapted Ebola virus infection. Phenotypes range from complete resistance to lethal disease to severe hemorrhagic fever characterized by prolonged coagulation times and 100% mortality. Inflammatory signaling was associated with vascular permeability and endothelial activation, and resistance to lethal infection arose by induction of lymphocyte differentiation and cellular adhesion, probably mediated by the susceptibility allele Tek. These data indicate that genetic background determines susceptibility to Ebola hemorrhagic fever.

PMCID: PMC4241145 PMID: 25359852 [PubMed - indexed for MEDLINE]
239. Ann Pharmacother. 2014 Nov 20. pii: 1060028014561227. [Epub ahead of print]

Potential and Emerging Treatment Options for Ebola Virus Disease.

Bishop BM(1).

Author information: (1)St Rita's Medical Center, Lima, OH, USA Rudolph H. Raabe College of Pharmacy at Ohio Northern University, Ada, OH, USA bryan.bishop.2006@gmail.com.

OBJECTIVE: To describe the current Ebola virus epidemic and the potential options for treatment and prevention of Ebola virus disease. DATA SOURCES: A PubMed literature search (1976 through October 20, 2014) was conducted using the search term Ebola. STUDY SELECTION AND DATA EXTRACTION: Animal and human studies published in English were selected. Studies published within the past 5 years were the primary focus of this review. DATA SYNTHESIS: The current Ebola virus epidemic has primarily been contained in West Africa though it has subsequently spread to other areas, including the United States. The first patient in the United States infected with Ebola virus was diagnosed, treated, and expired in Texas. Two nurses caring for this patient also were diagnosed with Ebola virus and have been successfully treated. Treatment options for patients infected with Ebola virus are limited. Supportive therapy is centered on fluid resuscitation, electrolyte imbalance correction, treating complicating infections, and preventing complications of shock. Experimental therapies (ZMapp, brincidofovir, TKM-Ebola, and favipiravir) have been used during this current outbreak. Several medications such as amiodarone, chloroquine, and clomiphene may prevent the transmission of or treat Ebola virus. Different vaccine therapies are also in early-stage development. One of the vaccine strategies using recombinant vesicular stomatitis virus as a delivery vector has demonstrated efficacy when used for preexposure and postexposure prophylaxis. CONCLUSION: Ebola virus is highly virulent and fatal, and treatment options are limited. Several experimental and existing therapies may be options for preventing and treating Ebola virus disease.

PMID: 25414384 [PubMed - as supplied by publisher]
240. Genome Announc. 2014 Nov 20;2(6). pii: e01178-14. doi: 10.1128/genomeA.01178-14.

Reidentification of Ebola Virus E718 and ME as Ebola Virus/H.sapiens-tc/COD/1976/Yambuku-Ecran.

Kuhn JH(1), Lofts LL(2), Kugelman JR(2), Smither SJ(3), Lever MS(3), van der Groen G(4), Johnson KM(5), Radoshitzky SR(2), Bavari S(2), Jahrling PB(6), Towner JS(7), Nichol ST(7), Palacios G(2).

Author information: (1)Integrated Research Facility at Fort Detrick (IRF-Frederick), National Institute of Allergy and Infectious Diseases, National Institutes of Health, Fort Detrick, Frederick, Maryland, USA kuhnjens@mail.nih.gov. (2)United States Army Medical Research Institute of Infectious Diseases (USAMRIID), Fort Detrick, Frederick, Maryland, USA. (3)Biomedical Sciences Department, Dstl, Porton Down, Salisbury, Wiltshire, United Kingdom. (4)Prins Leopold Instituut voor Tropische Geneeskunde (ITG), Antwerp, Belgium. (5)Retired, Portland, Oregon, USA. (6)Integrated Research Facility at Fort Detrick (IRF-Frederick), National Institute of Allergy and Infectious Diseases, National Institutes of Health, Fort Detrick, Frederick, Maryland, USA. (7)Viral Special Pathogens Branch, Division of High-Consequence Pathogens Pathology, National Center for Emerging and Zoonotic Infectious Diseases, Centers for Disease Control and Prevention (CDC), Atlanta, Georgia, USA.

Ebola virus (EBOV) was discovered in 1976 around Yambuku, Zaire. A lack of nomenclature standards resulted in a variety of designations for each isolate, leading to confusion in the literature and databases. We sequenced the genome of isolate E718/ME/Ecran and unified the various designations under Ebola virus/H.sapiens-tc/COD/1976/Yambuku-Ecran.

PMCID: PMC4239354 PMID: 25414499 [PubMed]
241. J Am Acad Dermatol. 2014 Nov 20. pii: S0190-9622(14)02117-3. doi: 10.1016/j.jaad.2014.10.037. [Epub ahead of print]

Effect of recent Ebola outbreaks on estimating the global burden of diseases with skin manifestations.

Vaughan V(1), Boyers L(2), Karimkhani C(3), Dellavalle R(4).

Author information: (1)Medical College of Georgia, Augusta, Georgia. (2)Georgetown University School of Medicine, Washington, District of Columbia. (3)Columbia University College of Physicians and Surgeons, New York, New York. (4)Eastern Colorado Health Care System, Department of Veterans Affairs, Denver, Colorado; University of Colorado School of Medicine, Anschutz Medical Campus, Aurora, Colorado; Department of Epidemiology, Colorado School of Public Health, Aurora, Colorado. Electronic address: robert.dellavalle@ucdenver.edu.

PMID: 25464860 [PubMed - as supplied by publisher]
242. JAMA. 2014 Nov 20. doi: 10.1001/jama.2014.16572. [Epub ahead of print]

The President's National Security Agenda: Curtailing Ebola, Safeguarding the Future.

Gostin LO(1), Waxman HA(2), Foege W(3).

Author information: (1)O'Neill Institute for National and Global Health Law, Georgetown University, Washington, DC. (2)US House of Representatives, Washington, DC. (3)Emory University School of Public Health, Atlanta, Georgia.

PMID: 25412348 [PubMed - as supplied by publisher]

243. N Engl J Med. 2014 Nov 20;371(21):2029-30. doi: 10.1056/NEJMe1413139. Epub 2014 Oct 27.

Ebola and quarantine.

Drazen JM, Kanapathipillai R, Campion EW, Rubin EJ, Hammer SM, Morrissey S, Baden LR.

PMID: 25347231 [PubMed - indexed for MEDLINE]

244. Travel Med Infect Dis. 2014 Nov 20. pii: S1477-8939(14)00218-X. doi: 10.1016/j.tmaid.2014.11.004. [Epub ahead of print]

What makes people talk about Ebola on social media? A retrospective analysis of Twitter use.

Rodriguez-Morales AJ(1), Castañeda-Hernández DM(2), McGregor A(3).

Author information: (1)Research Group Public Health and Infection, Faculty of Health Sciences, Universidad Tecnológica de Pereira, Pereira, Risaralda, Colombia; Fundación Cenit Colombia, Pereira, Risaralda, Colombia; Fundación Universitaria del Área Andina, Seccional Pereira, Pereira, Risaralda, Colombia. Electronic address: arodriguezm@utp.edu.co. (2)Fundación Cenit Colombia, Pereira, Risaralda, Colombia; Fundación Universitaria del Área Andina, Seccional Pereira, Pereira, Risaralda, Colombia. (3)Rare and Imported Pathogens Laboratory, Public Health England, Porton, Salisbury, UK.

PMID: 25468077 [PubMed - as supplied by publisher]

245. Mass Thermography Screening for Infection and Prevention: A Review of the Clinical Effectiveness [Internet].

Ottawa (ON): Canadian Agency for Drugs and Technologies in Health; 2014 Nov. CADTH Rapid Response Reports.

Thermography involves the quantification of emitted radiation to measure temperature, and provides a quick non-invasive means to measure body temperature. Infrared thermography (IRT) can be implemented at international airports in order to detect febrile passengers and prevent the introduction and spread of infectious diseases to other countries. Border control strategies were enacted as a response to the emergence of Severe Acute Respiratory Syndrome (SARS) in 2003, which included the introduction of non-contact infrared thermal scanners at international airports and bus or railway stations for mass screening of individuals. IRT has also been used as a measure to detect and prevent influenza outbreaks and transmission of dengue fever across borders. IRT may be influenced by several confounding factors including age and outdoor temperature. In addition, results from studies looking at IRT as a tool to detect fever tend to have small positive predictive values due to the small prevalence of febrile passengers. However, advantages of using IRT include its ability to screen mass numbers of individuals and reduce close contacts with infected individuals. Recently, the 2014 Ebola epidemic in West Africa has renewed concerns of disease transmission across borders and increased vigilance to identify individuals entering the country who may harbour infection. The purpose of this review is to examine the effectiveness of screening for fever at border crossings to reduce the risk of infectious disease outbreaks.

PMID: 25520988 [PubMed]

246. BMJ. 2014 Nov 19;349:g6946. doi: 10.1136/bmj.g6946.

How Twitter may have helped Nigeria contain Ebola.

Carter M.

PMID: 25410185 [PubMed - in process]

247. Lancet Infect Dis. 2014 Nov 19. pii: S1473-3099(14)71033-3. doi: 10.1016/S1473-3099(14)71033-3. [Epub ahead of print]

Ebola virus in the semen of convalescent men.

Mackay IM(1), Arden KE(2).

Author information: (1)Sir Albert Sakzewski Virus Research Centre and Clinical Medical Virology Centre, Queensland Paediatric Infectious Diseases Laboratory, QLD 4029, Australia. Electronic address: ian.mackay@uq.edu.au. (2)Sir Albert Sakzewski Virus Research Centre and Clinical Medical Virology Centre, Queensland Paediatric Infectious Diseases Laboratory, QLD 4029, Australia.

PMID: 25467652 [PubMed - as supplied by publisher]

248. Lancet Infect Dis. 2014 Nov 19. pii: S1473-3099(14)71035-7. doi: 10.1016/S1473-3099(14)71035-7. [Epub ahead of print]

Ebola control: rapid diagnostic testing.

Dhillon RS(1), Srikrishna D(2), Garry RF(3), Chowell G(4).

Author information: (1)Brigham and Women's Hospital, Boston, MA 02115, USA; Earth Institute, Columbia University, New York, NY, USA. Electronic address: rsdhillon@partners.org. (2)Patient Knowhow, San Mateo, CA, USA. (3)Viral Hemorrhagic Fever Consortium and Tulane University, New Orleans, LA, USA. (4)Arizona State University, Tempe, AZ, USA.

PMID: 25467648 [PubMed - as supplied by publisher]

249. Nurs Stand. 2014 Nov 19;29(12):32. doi: 10.7748/ns.29.12.32.s37.

Disasters emergency committee.

Evans R(1).

Author information: (1)Nursing Standard.

The Disasters Emergency Committee (DEC) has launched an unprecedented public appeal in the UK to tackle the Ebola virus disease epidemic in west Africa.

PMID: 25408035 [PubMed - in process]

250. Nurs Stand. 2014 Nov 19;29(12):26-7. doi: 10.7748/ns.29.12.26.s29.

Inequality epidemic.

Wright S(1).

Author information: (1)Cumbria.

The Ebola virus in west Africa has infected more than 10,000 people, claiming almost 5,000 lives since the outbreak was reported in March.
PMID: 25408027 [PubMed - in process]
251. Nurs Stand. 2014 Nov 19;29(12):21. doi: 10.7748/ns.29.12.21.s25.

Ebola.
[No authors listed]
Essential facts Ebola virus disease is a severe viral haemorrhagic fever (VHF). It was first recognised in 1976, and since then there have been sporadic outbreaks in several African countries. There are five different strains, four of which have caused disease in humans. The current outbreak of the Zaire strain began in March 2014. It is the largest and most complicated ever seen, so far affecting five West African countries: Liberia, Sierra Leone, Guinea, Nigeria and Senegal. A small number of cases have occurred outside Africa, including one involving a nurse in Spain.
PMID: 25408023 [PubMed - in process]
252. Ann Intern Med. 2014 Nov 18;161(10):753-4. doi: 10.7326/M14-1953.

Protecting health care workers from ebola: personal protective equipment is critical but is not enough.
Fischer WA 2nd, Hynes NA, Perl TM.
PMID: 25155746 [PubMed - in process]
253. Ann Intern Med. 2014 Nov 18;161(10):751-2. doi: 10.7326/M14-1918.

Ebola Fever: reconciling planning with risk in u.s. Hospitals.
Klompas M, Diekema DJ, Fishman NO, Yokoe DS.
PMID: 25141883 [PubMed - in process]
254. Ann Intern Med. 2014 Nov 18;161(10):749-50. doi: 10.7326/M14-1904.

Ebola vaccination: if not now, when?
Galvani AP, Ndeffo-Mbah ML, Wenzel N, Childs JE.
PMID: 25141813 [PubMed - in process]
255. Ann Intern Med. 2014 Nov 18;161(10):744-5. doi: 10.7326/M14-1864.

Ebola, ethics, and public health: what next?
Kass N.
PMID: 25133473 [PubMed - in process]
256. Ann Intern Med. 2014 Nov 18;161(10):746-8. doi: 10.7326/M14-1880.

Ebola hemorrhagic Fever in 2014: the tale of an evolving epidemic.
Del Rio C, Mehta AK, Lyon GM 3rd, Guarner J.
PMID: 25133433 [PubMed - in process]
257. Ann Intern Med. 2014 Nov 18;161(10):742-3. doi: 10.7326/M14-1810.

Serotherapy for ebola: back to the future.
Podolsky SH.
PMID: 25110967 [PubMed - in process]
258. BMJ. 2014 Nov 18;349:g6837. doi: 10.1136/bmj.g6837.

We mustn't forget other essential health services during the Ebola crisis.
Nam SL(1), Blanchet K(2).
Author information: (1)Options Consultancy Services, Devon House, London E1W 1LB, UK s.nam@options.co.uk. (2)Public Health in Humanitarian Crises Group, London School of Hygiene and Tropical Medicine, London, UK.
PMID: 25406151 [PubMed - in process]
259. BMJ. 2014 Nov 18;349:g6942. doi: 10.1136/bmj.g6942.

Surgeon from Sierra Leone treated for Ebola in Nebraska dies.
McCarthy M(1).
Author information: (1)Seattle.
PMID: 25406131 [PubMed - in process]
260. Clin Infect Dis. 2014 Nov 18. pii: ciu921. [Epub ahead of print]

Estimates of Ebola Virus Case-Fatality Ratio in the 2014 West African Outbreak.
Focosi D(1), Maggi F(1).
Author information: (1)Division of Virology and Retrovirus Centre, Pisa University Hospital, Italy.
PMID: 25409472 [PubMed - as supplied by publisher]
261. CMAJ. 2014 Nov 18;186(17):E643-4. doi: 10.1503/cmaj.109-4919. Epub 2014 Oct 14.

WMA calls for urgent support to fight Ebola.
Shuchman M(1).
Author information: (1)Durban, South Africa.

PMCID: PMC4234729 [Available on 2015/11/18] PMID: 25316902 [PubMed - in process]
262. CMAJ. 2014 Nov 18;186(17):E642. doi: 10.1503/cmaj.109-4913. Epub 2014 Oct 6.

Physician pushes for improved Ebola care.

Shuchman M(1).
Author information: (1)Toronto, Ont.

PMCID: PMC4234728 [Available on 2015/11/18] PMID: 25288317 [PubMed - in process]
263. Genome Biol. 2014 Nov 18;15(11):519. [Epub ahead of print]

Enhanced methods for unbiased deep sequencing of Lassa and Ebola RNA viruses from clinical and biological samples.

Matranga CB, Andersen KG, Winnicki S, Busby M, Gladden AD, Tewhey R, Stremlau M, Berlin A, Gire SK, England E, Moses LM, Mikkelsen TS, Odia I, Ehiane PE, Folarin O, Goba A, Kahn S, Grant DS, Honko A, Hensley L, Happi C, Garry RF, Malboeuf CM, Birren BW, Gnirke A, Levin JZ, Sabeti PC.

We have developed a robust RNA sequencing method for generating complete de novo assemblies with intra-host variant calls of Lassa and Ebola virus genomes in clinical and biological samples. Our method uses targeted RNase H-based digestion to remove contaminating poly(rA) carrier and ribosomal RNA. This depletion step improves both the quality of data and quantity of informative reads in unbiased total RNA sequencing libraries. We have also developed a hybrid-selection protocol to further enrich the viral content of sequencing libraries. These protocols have enabled rapid deep sequencing of both Lassa and Ebola virus and are broadly applicable to other viral genomics studies.

PMCID: PMC4262991 PMID: 25403361 [PubMed - as supplied by publisher]
264. Radiology. 2014 Nov 18:142502. [Epub ahead of print]

Ebola Virus Disease: Radiology Preparedness.

Bluemke DA(1), Meltzer CC.
Author information: (1)From the Department of Radiology and Imaging Sciences, National Institutes of Health, 10 Center Dr, Room 1C355, Bethesda, MD 20892 (D.A.B.); and Departments of Radiology and Imaging Sciences, Psychiatry and Behavioral Sciences, and Neurology, Emory University School of Medicine, Atlanta, Ga (C.C.M.).

At present, there is a major emphasis on Ebola virus disease (EVD Ebola virus disease) preparedness training at medical facilities throughout the United States. Failure to have proper EVD Ebola virus disease procedures in place was cited as a major reason for infection of medical personnel in the United States. Medical imaging does not provide diagnosis of EVD Ebola virus disease , but patient assessment in the emergency department and treatment isolation care unit is likely to require imaging services. The purpose of this article is to present an overview of relevant aspects of EVD Ebola virus disease disease and preparedness relevant to the radiologic community. © RSNA, 2014.

PMID: 25405643 [PubMed - as supplied by publisher]
265. AJR Am J Roentgenol. 2014 Nov 17:1-5. [Epub ahead of print]

Radiographic Imaging for Patients With Contagious Infectious Diseases: How to Acquire Chest Radiographs of Patients Infected With the Ebola Virus.

Auffermann WF(1), Kraft CS, Vanairsdale S, Lyon GM 3rd, Tridandapani S.
Author information: (1)1 Department of Radiology and Imaging Sciences, Emory University School of Medicine, Atlanta, GA.

OBJECTIVE. Contagious infectious diseases add a new dimension to radiology and pose many unanswered questions. In particular, what is the safest way to image patients with contagious and potentially lethal infectious diseases? Here, we describe protocols used by Emory University to successfully acquire chest radiographs of patients with Ebola virus disease. CONCLUSION. Radiology departments need to develop new protocols for various modalities used in imaging patients with contagious and potentially lethal infectious diseases.

PMID: 25402496 [PubMed - as supplied by publisher]
266. Disaster Med Public Health Prep. 2014 Nov 17:1-5. [Epub ahead of print]

Ebola Virus Disease: Preparedness in Japan.

Ashino Y(1), Chagan-Yasutan H(1), Egawa S(2), Hattori T(1).
Author information: (1)1Division of Disaster-Related Infectious Disease,International Research Institute of Disaster Science (IRIDeS),Tohoku University,Sendai,Japan. (2)2Division of International Cooperation for Disaster Medicine,IRIDeS,Tohoku University,Sendai,Japan.

ABSTRACT The current outbreak of Ebola virus disease (EVD) is due to a lack of resources, untrained medical personnel, and the specific contact-mediated type of infection of this virus. In Japan's history, education and mass vaccination of the native Ainu people successfully eradicated epidemics of smallpox. Even though a zoonotic virus is hard to control, appropriate precautions and personal protection, as well as anti-symptomatic treatment, will control the outbreak of EVD. Ebola virus utilizes the antibody-dependent enhancement of infection to seed the cells of various organs. The pathogenesis of EVD is due to the cytokine storm of pro-inflammatory cytokines and the lack of antiviral interferon-$\alpha 2$. Matricellular proteins of galectin-9 and osteopontin might also be involved in the edema and abnormality of the coagulation system in EVD. Anti-fibrinolytic treatment will be effective. In the era of globalization, interviews of travelers with fever within 3 weeks of departure from the affected areas will be necessary. Not only the hospitals designated for specific biohazards but every hospital should be aware of the biology of biohazards and establish measures to protect both patients and the community. (Disaster Med Public Health Preparedness. 2014;0:1-5).

PMID: 25399765 [PubMed - as supplied by publisher]
267. Mod Healthc. 2014 Nov 17;44(46):39.

On the VA, Ebola trials and the SHOP exchanges.

Goozner M.

PMID: 25509539 [PubMed - in process]

268. Mod Healthc. 2014 Nov 17;44(46):12.

Immigration, Ebola will dominate lame-duck session in Congress.

Demko P.

PMID: 25509535 [PubMed - in process]

269. Lancet. 2014 Nov 15;384(9956):1740-1.

Ebola: epidemic echoes and the chronicle of a tragedy foretold.

Honigsbaum M.

PMID: 25513381 [PubMed - in process]

270. Lancet. 2014 Nov 15;384(9956):1740-1.

Ebola: epidemic echoes and the chronicle of a tragedy foretold.

Honigsbaum M.

PMID: 25473684 [PubMed - in process]

271. Lancet. 2014 Nov 15;384(9956):1743. doi: 10.1016/S0140-6736(14)61787-6. Epub 2014 Nov 3.

Ebola: fever definitions might delay detection in non-epidemic areas.

Dananché C(1), Bénet T(2), Vanhems P(3).

Author information: (1)Infection Control and Epidemiology Unit, Edouard Herriot Hospital, Hospices Civils de Lyon, Lyon 69437, France. (2)Infection Control and Epidemiology Unit, Edouard Herriot Hospital, Hospices Civils de Lyon, Lyon 69437, France; Epidemiology and Public Health Group, Centre National de la Recherche Scientifique, Unité Mixte de Recherche 5558, University of Lyon I, Lyon, France. (3)Infection Control and Epidemiology Unit, Edouard Herriot Hospital, Hospices Civils de Lyon, Lyon 69437, France; Epidemiology and Public Health Group, Centre National de la Recherche Scientifique, Unité Mixte de Recherche 5558, University of Lyon I, Lyon, France. Electronic address: philippe.vanhems@chu-lyon.fr.

PMID: 25455239 [PubMed - in process]

272. Vet Rec. 2014 Nov 15;175(19):471. doi: 10.1136/vr.g6767.

Health professionals in Europe urged to be prepared for Ebola virus.

[No authors listed]

PMID: 25395561 [PubMed - in process]

273. BMJ. 2014 Nov 14;349:g6827. doi: 10.1136/bmj.g6827.

Clinical trials of Ebola therapies to begin in December.

Gulland A(1).

Author information: (1)London.

PMID: 25398534 [PubMed - in process]

274. J Am Soc Nephrol. 2014 Nov 14. pii: ASN.2014111057. [Epub ahead of print]

Successful Delivery of RRT in Ebola Virus Disease.

Connor MJ Jr(1), Kraft C(2), Mehta AK(3), Varkey JB(3), Lyon GM(3), Crozier I(4), Ströher U(5), Ribner BS(3), Franch HA(6).

Author information: (1)Divisions of Pulmonary, Allergy, and Critical Care, Renal Medicine, and michael.connor@emory.edu hfranch@emory.edu. (2)Infectious Diseases, Department of Medicine, Emory University School of Medicine, Atlanta, Georgia; Department of Pathology and Laboratory Medicine, Emory University School of Medicine, Atlanta, Georgia; (3)Infectious Diseases, Department of Medicine, Emory University School of Medicine, Atlanta, Georgia; (4)Infectious Diseases Institute, Mulago Hospital Complex, Kampala, Uganda; (5)US Centers for Disease Control and Prevention, Atlanta, Georgia; and. (6)Renal Medicine, and Research Service, Atlanta Department of Veterans Affairs Medical Center, Decatur, Georgia michael.connor@emory.edu hfranch@emory.edu.

AKI has been observed in cases of Ebola virus disease. We describe the protocol for the first known successful delivery of RRT with subsequent renal recovery in a patient with Ebola virus disease treated at Emory University Hospital, in Atlanta, Georgia. Providing RRT in Ebola virus disease is complex and requires meticulous attention to safety for the patient, healthcare workers, and the community. We specifically describe measures to decrease the risk of transmission of Ebola virus disease and report pilot data demonstrating no detectable Ebola virus genetic material in the spent RRT effluent waste. This article also proposes clinical practice guidelines for acute RRT in Ebola virus disease.

Copyright © 2014 by the American Society of Nephrology.

PMID: 25398785 [PubMed - as supplied by publisher]

275. Mol Pharm. 2014 Nov 14. [Epub ahead of print]

A Single Dose Respiratory Recombinant Adenovirus-Based Vaccine Provides Long-Term Protection for Non-Human Primates from Lethal Ebola Infection.

Choi JH(1), Jonsson-Schmunk K, Qiu X, Shedlock DJ, Strong J, Xu JX, Michie KL, Audet J, Fernando L, Myers MJ, Weiner D, Bajrovic I, Tran LQ, Wong G, Bello A, Kobinger GP, Schafer SC, Croyle MA.

Author information: (1)Division of Pharmaceutics, College of Pharmacy, The University of Texas at Austin , Austin, Texas 78712, United States.

As the Ebola outbreak in West Africa continues and cases appear in the United States and other countries, the need for long-lasting vaccines to preserve global health is imminent. Here, we evaluate the long-term efficacy of a respiratory and sublingual (SL) adenovirus-based vaccine in non-human primates in two phases. In the first, a single respiratory dose of 1.4 × 10(9) infectious virus particles (ivp)/kg of Ad-CAGoptZGP induced strong Ebola glycoprotein (GP) specific CD8(+) and CD4(+) T cell responses and Ebola GP-specific antibodies in systemic and mucosal compartments and was partially (67%) protective from challenge 62 days after immunization. The same dose given by the SL route induced Ebola GP-specific CD8(+) T cell responses similar to that of intramuscular (IM) injection, however, the Ebola GP-specific antibody response was low. All primates succumbed to infection. Three primates were then given the vaccine in a formulation that improved the immune response to Ebola in rodents. Three primates were immunized with 2.0 × 10(10) ivp/kg of vaccine by the SL route. Diverse populations of polyfunctional Ebola GP-specific CD4(+) and CD8(+) T cells and significant anti-Ebola GP antibodies were present in samples collected 150 days after respiratory immunization. The formulated vaccine was fully protective against challenge 21 weeks after immunization. While diverse populations of Ebola GP-specific CD4(+) T cells were produced after SL immunization, antibodies were not neutralizing and the vaccine was unprotective. To our knowledge, this is the first time that durable protection from a single dose respiratory adenovirus-based Ebola vaccine has been demonstrated in primates.
PMID: 25363619 [PubMed - as supplied by publisher]
276. Nat Rev Microbiol. 2014 Nov 14;12(12):792. doi: 10.1038/nrmicro3392.

Ebola Crisis continues.

Kåhrström CT.
PMID: 25396719 [PubMed - in process]
277. Science. 2014 Nov 14;346(6211):791. doi: 10.1126/science.aaa2692.

Out of sight, out of mind.

Woolley M(1), Leshner AI(2).

Author information: (1)Mary Woolley is the president and chief executive officer of Research!America. mwoolley@researchamerica.org. (2)Alan I. Leshner is the chief executive officer of the American Association for the Advancement of Science and executive publisher of Science.

PMID: 25395507 [PubMed - indexed for MEDLINE]
278. Viral Immunol. 2014 Nov 14. [Epub ahead of print]

Immune Evasion in Ebolavirus Infections.

Audet J(1), Kobinger GP.

Author information: (1)1 Department of Medical Microbiology, University of Manitoba , Winnipeg, Manitoba, Canada .

Abstract Ebola virus (EBOV) infects humans as well as several animal species. It can lead to a highly lethal disease, with mortality rates approaching 90% in primates. Recent advances have deepened our understanding of how this virus is able to prevent the development of protective immune responses. The EBOV genome encodes eight proteins, four of which were shown to interact with the host in ways that counteract the immune response. The viral protein 35 (VP35) is capable of capping dsRNA and interacts with IRF7 to prevent detection of the virus by immune cells. The main role of the soluble glycoprotein (sGP) is still unclear, but it is capable of subverting the anti-GP1,2 antibody response. The GP1,2 protein has shown anti-tetherin activity and the ability to hide cell-surface proteins. Finally, VP24 interferes with the production of interferons (IFNs) and with IFN signaling in infected cells. Taken together, these data point to extensive adaptation of EBOV to evade the immune system of dead end hosts. While our understanding of the interactions between the human and viral proteins increases, details of those interactions in other hosts remain largely unclear and represent a gap in our knowledge.
PMID: 25396298 [PubMed - as supplied by publisher]
279. Virus Res. 2014 Nov 14;196C:87-93. doi: 10.1016/j.virusres.2014.11.005. [Epub ahead of print]

Genome-wide analysis of codon usage bias in Ebolavirus.

Cristina J(1), Moreno P(2), Moratorio G(3), Musto H(4).

Author information: (1)Laboratorio de Virología Molecular, Centro de Investigaciones Nucleares, Facultad de Ciencias, Universidad de la República, Iguá 4225, 11400 Montevideo, Uruguay. Electronic address: cristina@cin.edu.uy. (2)Laboratorio de Virología Molecular, Centro de Investigaciones Nucleares, Facultad de Ciencias, Universidad de la República, Iguá 4225, 11400 Montevideo, Uruguay. (3)Laboratorio de Virología Molecular, Centro de Investigaciones Nucleares, Facultad de Ciencias, Universidad de la República, Iguá 4225, 11400 Montevideo, Uruguay; Viral Populations and Pathogenesis Laboratory, Institut Pasteur, CNRS UMR 3569, Paris, France. (4)Laboratorio de Organización y Evolución del Genoma, Instituto de Biología, Facultad de Ciencias, Universidad de la República, Iguá 4225, 11400 Montevideo, Uruguay.

Ebola virus (EBOV) is a member of the family Filoviridae and its genome consists of a 19-kb, single-stranded, negative sense RNA. EBOV is subdivided into five distinct species with different pathogenicities, being Zaire ebolavirus (ZEBOV) the most lethal species. The interplay of codon usage among viruses and their hosts is expected to affect overall viral survival, fitness, evasion from host's immune system and evolution. In the present study, we performed comprehensive analyses of codon usage and composition of ZEBOV. Effective number of codons (ENC) indicates that the overall codon usage among ZEBOV strains is slightly biased. Different codon preferences in ZEBOV genes in relation to codon usage of human genes were found. Highly preferred codons are all A-ending triplets, which strongly suggests that mutational bias is a main force shaping codon usage in ZEBOV. Dinucleotide composition also plays a role in the overall pattern of ZEBOV codon usage. ZEBOV does not seem to use the most abundant tRNAs present in the human cells for most of their preferred codons.
PMID: 25445348 [PubMed - as supplied by publisher]
280. Am J Med. 2014 Nov 13. pii: S0002-9343(14)00981-4. doi: 10.1016/j.amjmed.2014.10.038. [Epub ahead of print]

Death by Caring: Ebola and Alcott's "Little Women"

Swanson J(1), Potyk D(2).

Author information: (1)Clinical Associate Professor of Medicine, University of Washington School of Medicine, Clinical Associate Professor Biomedical Sciences, Washington State University, Faculty, Providence Internal Medicine Residency Spokane. Electronic address: Judy.Swanson@providence.org. (2)Clinical Professor of Medicine, University of Washington School of Medicine, Assistant Program Director, Providence Internal Medicine Residency Spokane.

PMID: 25446300 [PubMed - as supplied by publisher]

281. Euro Surveill. 2014 Nov 13;19(45). pii: 20960.

The Innovative Medicines Initiative launches call on Ebola and other filoviral haemorrhagic fevers.

Eurosurveillance editorial team.

PMID: 25411693 [PubMed - in process]

282. J Infect Dev Ctries. 2014 Nov 13;8(11):1378-80. doi: 10.3855/jidc.6142.

The current Ebola outbreak: old and new contexts.

Bellizzi S(1).

Author information: (1)Via Verona 22, 07100 Sassari, Italy. saverio.bellizzi@gmail.com.

Within the ongoing Ebola outbreak in West Africa, separate scenarios reflect old contexts with well-known strategies to face the epidemic on one side and completely new and unprecedented situations requiring new approaches on the other side. While Senegal and Nigeria represent success stories on the implementation of appropriate standard public health measures for containment, Liberia, Sierra Leone, and Guinea require a major and innovative scale of actions to halt even more catastrophic consequences.

PMID: 25390049 [PubMed - in process]

283. Lancet. 2014 Nov 13. pii: S0140-6736(14)61894-8. doi: 10.1016/S0140-6736(14)61894-8. [Epub ahead of print]

Effectiveness of screening for Ebola at airports.

Read JM(1), Diggle PJ(2), Chirombo J(1), Solomon T(3), Baylis M(1).

Author information: (1)Institute of Infection and Global Health, University of Liverpool, Liverpool L69 7BE, UK; Health Protection Research Unit in Emerging and Zoonotic Infections, University of Liverpool, Liverpool, UK. (2)Institute of Infection and Global Health, University of Liverpool, Liverpool L69 7BE, UK; Division of Medicine, Lancaster University, Lancaster, UK; Health Protection Research Unit in Emerging and Zoonotic Infections, University of Liverpool, Liverpool, UK. (3)Institute of Infection and Global Health, University of Liverpool, Liverpool L69 7BE, UK; Walton Centre NHS Foundation Trust, Liverpool, UK; Health Protection Research Unit in Emerging and Zoonotic Infections, University of Liverpool, Liverpool, UK. Electronic address: tsolomon@liv.ac.uk.

PMID: 25467590 [PubMed - as supplied by publisher]

284. N Engl J Med. 2014 Nov 13. [Epub ahead of print]

Communicating Uncertainty - Ebola, Public Health, and the Scientific Process.

Rosenbaum L(1).

Author information: (1)Dr. Rosenbaum is a national correspondent for the Journal.

The levees of the Red River in Grand Forks, North Dakota, are built to withstand 51-ft water levels. In 1997, the National Weather Service predicted a flood, but despite a 35% margin of error for previous estimates, it emphasized that the river would crest at 49 ft at most. When the waters rose to 54 ft, wreaking havoc on the area, local inhabitants were shocked and angry. Why had forecasters projected such confidence in their prediction? According to Nate Silver, who describes the incident in The Signal and the Noise, "The forecasters later told researchers that they were afraid the . . .

PMID: 25394322 [PubMed - as supplied by publisher]

285. Nature. 2014 Nov 13;515(7526):192-4. doi: 10.1038/515192a.

Infectious disease: tough choices to reduce Ebola transmission.

Whitty CJ, Farrar J, Ferguson N, Edmunds WJ, Piot P, Leach M, Davies SC.

PMID: 25391946 [PubMed - indexed for MEDLINE]

286. Nature. 2014 Nov 13;515(7526):177-8. doi: 10.1038/515177a.

Ethical dilemma for Ebola drug trials.

Hayden EC.

PMID: 25391940 [PubMed - indexed for MEDLINE]

287. Travel Med Infect Dis. 2014 Nov 13;12(6PA):690-692. doi: 10.1016/j.tmaid.2014.10.019. [Epub ahead of print]

Ebola and travel, Personal Protective Equipment (PPE) - Useful web links and video clips.

Chiodini J(1).

Author information: (1)Travel Health Specialist Nurse, The Village Medical Centre, Bedfordshire, UK. Electronic address: janechiodini@btinternet.com.

PMID: 25468530 [PubMed - as supplied by publisher]

288. BMJ. 2014 Nov 12;349:g6777. doi: 10.1136/bmj.g6777.

NHS leaders remind frontline staff to be alert to Ebola infection.

Kmietowicz Z(1).

Author information: (1)The BMJ.

PMID: 25391842 [PubMed - in process]
289. BMJ. 2014 Nov 12;349:g6776. doi: 10.1136/bmj.g6776.

Time to think Ebola: a message from NHS England to frontline clinical staff.

Finn RP(1), Smith C(2), Ghafur S(2), Zarkali A(2), Adlington K(2), Winter B(2), Keogh BE(2).

Author information: (1)NHS England, Skipton House, London SE1 6LH, UK roisinfinn@nhs.net. (2)NHS England, Skipton House, London SE1 6LH, UK.
PMID: 25391841 [PubMed - in process]
290. BMJ. 2014 Nov 12;349:g6788. doi: 10.1136/bmj.g6788.

UK's plan to build community care centres for Ebola patients is questioned.

Gulland A(1).

Author information: (1)London.
PMID: 25391517 [PubMed - in process]
291. Daru. 2014 Nov 12;22(1):70. doi: 10.1186/s40199-014-0070-9.

Ebola hemorrhagic fever: current outbreak and progress in finding a cure.

Saeidnia S, Abdollahi M(1).

Author information: (1)Faculty of Pharmacy, and Pharmaceutical Sciences Research Center, Tehran University of Medical Sciences, Tehran 1417614411, Iran. Mohammad@TUMS.Ac.Ir.
PMCID: PMC4228070 PMID: 25392051 [PubMed - in process]
292. J Virol. 2014 Nov 12. pii: JVI.02836-14. [Epub ahead of print]

Ebola virus transmission in guinea pigs.

Wong G(1), Qiu X(2), Richardson JS(2), Cutts T(2), Collignon B(3), Gren J(2), Aviles J(4), Embury-Hyatt C(3), Kobinger GP(5).

Author information: (1)Special Pathogens Program, National Microbiology Laboratory, Public Health Agency of Canada, Winnipeg, MB, Canada Department of Medical Microbiology. (2)Special Pathogens Program, National Microbiology Laboratory, Public Health Agency of Canada, Winnipeg, MB, Canada. (3)National Centre for Foreign Animal Disease, Canadian Food Inspection Agency, Winnipeg, MB, Canada. (4)Special Pathogens Program, National Microbiology Laboratory, Public Health Agency of Canada, Winnipeg, MB, Canada Department of Immunology, University of Manitoba, Winnipeg, MB, Canada. (5)Special Pathogens Program, National Microbiology Laboratory, Public Health Agency of Canada, Winnipeg, MB, Canada Department of Medical Microbiology Department of Immunology, University of Manitoba, Winnipeg, MB, Canada Department of Pathology and Laboratory Medicine, University of Pennsylvania School of Medicine, Philadelphia, PA, USA gary.kobinger@phac-aspc.gc.ca.

Ebola virus (EBOV) transmission is currently poorly characterized and thought to occur primarily by direct contact with infectious material; however transmission from swine to nonhuman primates via the respiratory tract has been documented. To establish an EBOV transmission model for performing studies with statistical significance, groups of six guinea pigs (gps) were challenged intranasally (IN) or intraperitoneally (IP) with 10,000 x LD50 of gp-adapted EBOV, and naïve gps were then introduced as cage-mates for contact exposure at 1 day post-infection (dpi). Animals were monitored for survival and clinical signs of disease, and quantitated for virus shedding post-exposure. Changes in contact duration of naïve gps with infected animals were evaluated for impact on transmission efficiency. Transmission was more efficient from IN compared to IP-challenged gps, with 17% versus 83% of naïve gps surviving exposure, respectively. Virus shedding was detected beginning at 3 dpi from both IN- and IP-challenged animals. Contact duration positively correlated with transmission efficiency, and the abrogation of direct contact between infected and naïve animals through the erection of a steel mesh is effective at stopping virus spread, provided that infectious animal bedding was absent in the cages. Histopathological and immunohistochemical findings show that IN-infected gps display enhanced lung pathology and EBOV antigen in the trachea, which support increased virus transmission from these animals. The results suggest that IN-challenged gps are more infectious to naïve animals than their systemically-infected counterparts, and that transmission occurs through direct contact with infectious materials, including those transported through air movement over short distances.IMPORTANCE: Ebola is generally thought to be spread between humans though infectious bodily fluids. However, a study has shown that Ebola can be spread from pigs to monkeys without direct contact. Further studies have been hampered, because an economical animal model for Ebola transmission is not available. To address this, we established a transmission model in guinea pigs, and determined the mechanisms behind virus spread. The survival data, in addition to microscopic examination of lung and trachea sections, show that mucosal infection of guinea pigs is an efficient model for Ebola transmission. Virus spread is increased with longer contact times to an infected animal and is possible without direct contact between an infected and naïve host, but can be stopped if infectious materials were absent. These results warrant consideration for the development of future strategies against Ebola transmission, and a better understanding of the parameters involved with virus spread.
PMID: 25392221 [PubMed - as supplied by publisher]
293. J Virol. 2014 Nov 12. pii: JVI.01810-14. [Epub ahead of print]

Less is More: Ebola Surface Glycoprotein Expression Levels Regulate Virus Production and Infectivity.

Mohan GS(1), Ye L(1), Li W(1), Monteiro A(2), Lin X(1), Sapkota B(3), Pollack BP(4), Compans RW(5), Yang C(6).

Author information: (1)Department of Microbiology and Immunology, Emory University, Atlanta, Georgia, United States of America. (2)Department of Pathology, Emory University, Atlanta, Georgia, United States of America. (3)Department of Dermatology, Emory University, Atlanta, Georgia, United States of America. (4)Department of Veterans' Affairs, Atlanta VA Medical Center, Decatur Georgia, United States of America Department of Dermatology, Emory University,

Atlanta, Georgia, United States of America. (5)Department of Microbiology and Immunology, Emory University, Atlanta, Georgia, United States of America rcompan@emory.edu. (6)Department of Microbiology and Immunology, Emory University, Atlanta, Georgia, United States of America chyang@emory.edu.

The Ebola virus surface glycoprotein (GP1,2) mediates host cell attachment and fusion, and is the primary target for host neutralizing antibodies. Expression of GP1,2 at high levels disrupts normal cell physiology, and EBOV uses an RNA editing mechanism to regulate expression of the GP gene. In this study, we demonstrate that high levels of GP1,2 expression impair production and release of EBOV VLPs, as well as infectivity of GP1,2-pseudotyped viruses. We further show that this effect is mediated through two mechanisms. First, high levels of GP1,2 expression reduce synthesis of other proteins needed for virus assembly. Second, viruses containing high levels of GP1,2 are intrinsically less infectious, possibly due to impaired receptor binding or endosomal processing. Importantly, proteolysis can rescue the infectivity of high-GP1,2 containing viruses. Taken together, our findings indicate that GP1,2 expression levels have a profound effect on factors that contribute to virus fitness, and that RNA editing may be an important mechanism employed by EBOV to regulate GP1,2 expression in order to optimize virus production and infectivity.IMPORTANCE: The Ebola virus (EBOV), as well as other members of the Filoviridae family, causes severe hemorrhagic fever that is highly lethal with up to 90% mortality. The EBOV surface glycoprotein (GP1,2) plays important roles in virus infection and pathogenesis, and its expression is tightly regulated by an RNA editing mechanism during virus replication. Our study demonstrates that the level of GP1,2 expression profoundly affects virus particle production and release and uncovers a new mechanism by which Ebola virus infectivity is regulated by the level of GP1,2 expression. These findings extend our understanding of EBOV infection and replication in adaptation of host environments, which will aid the development of countermeasures against EBOV infection.

PMID: 25392212 [PubMed - as supplied by publisher]

294. JAMA. 2014 Nov 12;312(18):1859-60. doi: 10.1001/jama.2014.14387.

The Ebola outbreak, fragile health systems, and quality as a cure.

Boozary AS(1), Farmer PE(2), Jha AK(3).

Author information: (1)Department of Health Policy and Management, Harvard School of Public Health, Boston, Massachusetts. (2)Division of Global Health Equity, Brigham and Women's Hospital, Boston. (3)Department of Health Policy and Management, Harvard School of Public Health, Boston, Massachusetts3Division of General Internal Medicine, Brigham and Women's Hospital, Boston4Harvard Medical School, Boston.
PMID: 25285459 [PubMed - indexed for MEDLINE]

295. JAMA. 2014 Nov 12;312(18):1942. doi: 10.1001/jama.2014.13759.

JAMA patient page. Ebola virus disease.

Jin J.
PMID: 25285380 [PubMed - indexed for MEDLINE]

296. Nurs Stand. 2014 Nov 12;29(11):30. doi: 10.7748/ns.29.11.30.s36.

UN: Global Ebola Response.

Evans R(1).

Author information: (1)Nursing Standard.

The United Nations has been criticised for being slow to react to the latest Ebola outbreak in West Africa. But it is now making up for lost time with a concerted response to help the countries most affected.

PMID: 25388723 [PubMed - in process]

297. Travel Med Infect Dis. 2014 Nov 11;12(6PA):688-689. doi: 10.1016/j.tmaid.2014.11.002. [Epub ahead of print]

Ebola: A latent threat to Latin America. Are we ready?

Rodríguez-Morales AJ(1), Henao DE(2), Franco TB(3), Mayta-Tristán P(4), Alfaro-Toloza P(5), Paniz-Mondolfi AE(6).

Author information: (1)Public Health and Infection Group of Research, Faculty of Health Sciences, Universidad Tecnológica de Pereira, Pereira, Risaralda, Colombia. Electronic address: arodriguezm@utp.edu.co. (2)Public Health and Infection Group of Research, Faculty of Health Sciences, Universidad Tecnológica de Pereira, Pereira, Risaralda, Colombia. (3)Universidade Federal Fluminense, Rio de Janeiro, Brazil. (4)Universidad Peruana de Ciencias Aplicadas, Lima, Peru. (5)Asociación Chilena de Seguridad, Chillán, Chile. (6)Department of Pathology and Laboratory Medicine, Hospital Internacional Barquisimeto, Venezuela and the Laboratory of Biochemistry, Instituto de Biomedicina, Caracas, Venezuela.
PMID: 25468529 [PubMed - as supplied by publisher]

298. Mod Healthc. 2014 Nov 10;44(45):27.

In long term, much good can come from the tragedy of Ebola.

Moore S.
PMID: 25509518 [PubMed - in process]

299. Nat Med. 2014 Nov 10. doi: 10.1038/nm.3763. [Epub ahead of print]

University travel bans and quarantines may impede Ebola response.

Willyard C.
PMID: 25384084 [PubMed - as supplied by publisher]

300. Small. 2014 Nov 10. doi: 10.1002/smll.201402184. [Epub ahead of print]

Quantifying Lipid Contents in Enveloped Virus Particles with Plasmonic Nanoparticles.

Feizpour A(1), Yu X, Akiyama H, Miller CM, Edmans E, Gummuluru S, Reinhard BM.

Author information: (1)Department of Chemistry and the Photonics Center, Boston University, Boston, MA, 02215, USA.

Phosphatidylserine (PS) and monosialotetrahexosylganglioside (GMI) are examples of two host-derived lipids in the membrane of enveloped virus particles that are known to contribute to virus attachment, uptake, and ultimately dissemination. A quantitative characterization of their contribution to the functionality of the virus requires information about their relative concentrations in the viral membrane. Here, a gold nanoparticle (NP) binding assay for probing relative PS and GMI lipid concentrations in the outer leaflet of different HIV-1 and Ebola virus-like particles (VLPs) using sample sizes of less than $3 \times 10(6)$ particles is introduced. The assay evaluates both scattering intensity and resonance wavelength, and determines relative NP densities through plasmon coupling as a measure for the target lipid concentrations in the NP-labeled VLP membrane. A correlation of the optical observables with absolute lipid contents is achieved by calibration of the plasmon coupling-based methodology with unilamellar liposomes of known PS or GMI concentration. The performed studies reveal significant differences in the membrane of VLPs that assemble at different intracellular sites and pave the way to an optical quantification of lipid concentration in virus particles at physiological titers.

PMID: 25382201 [PubMed - as supplied by publisher]
301. Lancet. 2014 Nov 8;384(9955):1658-9.

International community ramps up Ebola vaccine effort.

Mohammadi D.

PMID: 25513370 [PubMed - in process]
302. Lancet. 2014 Nov 8;384(9955):1658-9.

International community ramps up Ebola vaccine effort.

Mohammadi D.

PMID: 25473675 [PubMed - in process]
303. Lancet. 2014 Nov 8;384(9955):1667. doi: 10.1016/S0140-6736(14)61735-9. Epub 2014 Oct 27.

Randomisation is essential in Ebola drug trials.

Shaw D(1).

Author information: (1)Institute for Biomedical Ethics, University of Basel, 4056 Basel, Switzerland. Electronic address: david.shaw@unibas.ch.

Comment on Lancet. 2014 Oct 18;384(9952):1423-4.

PMID: 25441188 [PubMed - in process]
304. Lancet. 2014 Nov 8;384(9955):1660. doi: 10.1016/S0140-6736(14)61738-4. Epub 2014 Nov 3.

Adrian Hill: accelerating the pace of Ebola vaccine research.

Mohammadi D.

PMID: 25441187 [PubMed - in process]
305. Lancet. 2014 Nov 8;384(9955):1641. doi: 10.1016/S0140-6736(14)62016-X. Epub 2014 Nov 7.

The medium and the message of Ebola.

[No authors listed]

PMID: 25441179 [PubMed - in process]
306. Vet Rec. 2014 Nov 8;175(18):441. doi: 10.1136/vr.g6615.

Spain explains reasons for euthanasia of Ebola nurse's dog.

[No authors listed]

PMID: 25377193 [PubMed - in process]
307. BMJ. 2014 Nov 7;349:g6704. doi: 10.1136/bmj.g6704.

UK built Ebola treatment centre opens in Sierra Leone.

Gulland A(1).

Author information: (1)London.

PMID: 25380747 [PubMed - in process]
308. BMJ. 2014 Nov 7;349:g6672. doi: 10.1136/bmj.g6672.

Ebola is causing moral distress among African healthcare workers.

Ulrich CM.

PMID: 25380700 [PubMed - in process]
309. BMJ. 2014 Nov 7;349:g6712. doi: 10.1136/bmj.g6712.

Response to Ebola in the US: misinformation, fear, and new opportunities.

Merino JG(1).

Author information: (1)The BMJ, USA jmerino@bmj.com.

PMID: 25380659 [PubMed - in process]
310. J Proteome Res. 2014 Nov 7;13(11):5120-35. doi: 10.1021/pr500556d. Epub 2014 Oct 23

Elucidation of the Ebola Virus VP24 Cellular Interactome and Disruption of Virus Biology through Targeted Inhibition of Host-Cell Protein Function.

García-Dorival I(1), Wu W, Dowall S, Armstrong S, Touzelet O, Wastling J, Barr JN, Matthews D, Carroll M, Hewson R, Hiscox JA.

Author information: (1)Department of Infection Biology, Institute of Infection and Global Health, University of Liverpool , Liverpool L3 5RF, United Kingdom.

Viral pathogenesis in the infected cell is a balance between antiviral responses and subversion of host-cell processes. Many viral proteins specifically interact with host-cell proteins to promote virus biology. Understanding these interactions can lead to knowledge gains about infection and provide potential targets for antiviral therapy. One such virus is Ebola, which has profound consequences for human health and causes viral hemorrhagic fever where case fatality rates can approach 90%. The Ebola virus VP24 protein plays a critical role in the evasion of the host immune response and is likely to interact with multiple cellular proteins. To map these interactions and better understand the potential functions of VP24, label-free quantitative proteomics was used to identify cellular proteins that had a high probability of forming the VP24 cellular interactome. Several known interactions were confirmed, thus placing confidence in the technique, but new interactions were also discovered including one with ATP1A1, which is involved in osmoregulation and cell signaling. Disrupting the activity of ATP1A1 in Ebola-virus-infected cells with a small molecule inhibitor resulted in a decrease in progeny virus, thus illustrating how quantitative proteomics can be used to identify potential therapeutic targets.

PMID: 25158218 [PubMed - in process]

311. MMWR Morb Mortal Wkly Rep. 2014 Nov 7;63(44):1010-2.

Establishment of a community care center for isolation and management of ebola patients - bomi county, liberia, october 2014.

Logan G, Vora NM, Nyensuah TG, Gasasira A, Mott J, Walke H, Mahoney F, Luce R, Flannery B.

As of October 29, 2014, a total of 6,454 Ebola virus disease (Ebola) cases had been reported in Liberia by the Liberian Ministry of Health and Social Welfare, with 2,609 deaths. Although the national strategy for combating the ongoing Ebola epidemic calls for construction of Ebola treatment units (ETUs) in all 15 counties of Liberia, only a limited number are operational, and most of these are within Montserrado County. ETUs are intended to improve medical care delivery to persons whose illnesses meet Ebola case definitions, while also allowing for the safe isolation of patients to break chains of transmission in the community. Until additional ETUs are constructed, the Ministry of Health and Social Welfare is supporting development of community care centers (CCCs) for isolation of patients who are awaiting Ebola diagnostic test results and for provision of basic care (e.g., oral rehydration salts solutions) to patients confirmed to have Ebola who are awaiting transfer to ETUs. CCCs often have less bed capacity than ETUs and are frequently placed in areas not served by ETUs; if built rapidly enough and in sufficient quantity, CCCs will allow Ebola-related health measures to reach a larger proportion of the population. Staffing requirements for CCCs are frequently lower than for ETUs because CCCs are often designed such that basic patient needs such as food are provided for by friends and family of patients rather than by CCC staff. (It is customary in Liberia for friends and family to provide food for hospitalized patients.) Creation of CCCs in Liberia has been led by county health officials and nongovernmental organizations, and this local, community-based approach is intended to destigmatize Ebola, to encourage persons with illness to seek care rather than remain at home, and to facilitate contact tracing of exposed family members. This report describes one Liberian county's approach to establishing a CCC.

PMID: 25375073 [PubMed - in process]

312. N Z Med J. 2014 Nov 7;127(1405):6-8.

Ebola, should we be concerned?

Jennings LC(1), Werno A.

Author information: (1)Microbiology Department, Canterbury Health Laboratories, Cnr Hagley Ave and Tuam St, Christchurch 8011, New Zealand. lance.jennings@cdhb.health.nz.

PMID: 25399035 [PubMed - in process]

313. Prehosp Emerg Care. 2014 Nov 7. [Epub ahead of print]

Considerations for Safe EMS Transport of Patients Infected with Ebola Virus.

Lowe JJ, Jelden KC, Schenarts PJ, Rupp LE, Hawes KJ, Tysor BM, Swansiger RG, Schwedhelm SS, Smith PW, Gibbs SG.

Abstract The Nebraska Biocontainment Unit through the Nebraska Medical Center in Omaha, Nebraska, recently received patients with confirmed Ebola virus from West Africa. The Nebraska Biocontainment Unit and Omaha Fire Department's emergency medical services (EMS) coordinated patient transportation from airport to the high-level isolation unit. Transportation of these highly infectious patients capitalized on over 8 years of meticulous planning and rigorous infection control training to ensure the safety of transport personnel as well as the community during transport. Although these transports occurred with advanced notice and after confirmed Ebola virus disease (EVD) diagnosis, approaches and key lessons acquired through this effort will advance the ability of any EMS provider to safely transport a confirmed or suspected patient with EVD. Three critical areas have been identified from our experience: ambulance preparation, appropriate selection and use of personal protective equipment, and environmental decontamination.

PMID: 25380073 [PubMed - as supplied by publisher]

314. Science. 2014 Nov 7;346(6210):684-5. doi: 10.1126/science.346.6210.684.

Infectious Diseases. Delays hinder Ebola genomics.

Vogel G.

PMID: 25378599 [PubMed - indexed for MEDLINE]

315. Can J Anaesth. 2014 Nov 6. [Epub ahead of print]

Ebola virus disease: an update for anesthesiologists and intensivists.

Funk DJ(1), Kumar A.

Author information: (1)Departments of Anesthesiology and Medicine, Section of Critical Care, Faculty of Medicine, University of Manitoba, 2nd Floor Harry Medovy House, 671 William Avenue, Winnipeg, MB, Canada, funk@cc.umanitoba.ca.

PURPOSE: Ebola virus disease (EVD) is a viral hemorrhagic fever that is highly transmissible and all too often rapidly fatal. Recent outbreaks in West Africa reveal that this infection has the potential to be transmitted worldwide. Anesthesiologists and intensivists, due to their training in the management of the critically ill, may be called upon to assist in the management of these patients. The focus of this brief review is on the epidemiology, pathogenesis, and management of patients with EVD. SOURCE: Review of the current literature. PRINCIPAL FINDINGS: Ebola virus disease causes severe diarrhea, electrolyte disturbances and other major end-organ dysfunction. Early aggressive resuscitation may reduce the mortality of this disease. There is presently no available vaccine nor cure, with experimental therapies having yielded limited success. Personal protective equipment (PPE) is necessary for all patient contact, and enhanced PPE is required for all aerosol-generating medical procedures. CONCLUSION: Anesthesiologists and intensivists may be called upon to manage patients with EVD. It is important that these clinicians have an appreciation for the epidemiology and pathogenesis of this disease and for the proper utilization of PPE when treating these patients.

PMID: 25373801 [PubMed - as supplied by publisher]

316. Can J Anaesth. 2014 Nov 6. [Epub ahead of print]

Ebola and the Journal's response to "the most severe acute health emergency seen in modern times"

Grocott HP(1).

Author information: (1)Departments of Anesthesia & Perioperative Medicine and Surgery, St. Boniface Hospital, University of Manitoba, CR3008-369 Tache Avenue, Winnipeg, MB, R2H 2A6, Canada, hgrocott@sbgh.mb.ca.

PMID: 25373800 [PubMed - as supplied by publisher]

317. Cell. 2014 Nov 6;159(4):940-54. doi: 10.1016/j.cell.2014.10.004. Epub 2014 Oct 23

Paper-based synthetic gene networks.

Pardee K(1), Green AA(1), Ferrante T(2), Cameron DE(3), DaleyKeyser A(2), Yin P(2), Collins JJ(4).

Author information: (1)Wyss Institute for Biological Inspired Engineering, Harvard University, Boston, MA 02115, USA; Department of Biomedical Engineering and Center of Synthetic Biology, Boston University, Boston, MA 02215, USA. (2)Wyss Institute for Biological Inspired Engineering, Harvard University, Boston, MA 02115, USA. (3)Department of Biomedical Engineering and Center of Synthetic Biology, Boston University, Boston, MA 02215, USA; Howard Hughes Medical Institute, Chevy Chase, MD 20815, USA. (4)Wyss Institute for Biological Inspired Engineering, Harvard University, Boston, MA 02115, USA; Department of Biomedical Engineering and Center of Synthetic Biology, Boston University, Boston, MA 02215, USA; Howard Hughes Medical Institute, Chevy Chase, MD 20815, USA. Electronic address: jcollins@bu.edu.

Synthetic gene networks have wide-ranging uses in reprogramming and rewiring organisms. To date, there has not been a way to harness the vast potential of these networks beyond the constraints of a laboratory or in vivo environment. Here, we present an in vitro paper-based platform that provides an alternate, versatile venue for synthetic biologists to operate and a much-needed medium for the safe deployment of engineered gene circuits beyond the lab. Commercially available cell-free systems are freeze dried onto paper, enabling the inexpensive, sterile, and abiotic distribution of synthetic-biology-based technologies for the clinic, global health, industry, research, and education. For field use, we create circuits with colorimetric outputs for detection by eye and fabricate a low-cost, electronic optical interface. We demonstrate this technology with small-molecule and RNA actuation of genetic switches, rapid prototyping of complex gene circuits, and programmable in vitro diagnostics, including glucose sensors and strain-specific Ebola virus sensors.

PMCID: PMC4243060 [Available on 2015/11/6] PMID: 25417167 [PubMed - in process]

318. N Engl J Med. 2014 Nov 6;371(19):1763-5. doi: 10.1056/NEJMp1411244. Epub 2014 Sep 17

Ebola in a stew of fear.

Mitman G(1).

Author information: (1)From the Departments of Medical History and Bioethics, History of Science, and History, and the Nelson Institute for Environmental Studies, University of Wisconsin-Madison.

PMID: 25229794 [PubMed - indexed for MEDLINE]

319. Nature. 2014 Nov 6;515(7525):18. doi: 10.1038/515018a.

Models overestimate Ebola cases.

Butler D.

Comment in Nature. 2014 Nov 27;515(7528):492. Nature. 2014 Nov 27;515(7528):492.

PMID: 25373654 [PubMed - indexed for MEDLINE]

320. Obstet Gynecol. 2014 Nov 6. [Epub ahead of print]

Ebola Virus Disease: Understanding the Facts, Putting Fears in Perspective, and Being Prepared.

Hill WC(1).

Author information: (1)Dr. Hill is with the Human Resources for Health Program Rwanda, http://hrhconsortium.moh.gov.rw, Department of Obstetrics and Gynecology Maternal-Fetal Medicine at the Duke University School of Medicine, Kigali, Rwanda; e-mail: dr.washingtonhill@gmail.com.

PMID: 25376638 [PubMed - as supplied by publisher]

321. Sci Rep. 2014 Nov 6;4:6881. doi: 10.1038/srep06881.

Molecular Characterization of the Monoclonal Antibodies Composing ZMAb: A Protective Cocktail Against Ebola Virus.

Audet J(1), Wong G(2), Wang H(3), Lu G(3), Gao GF(3), Kobinger G(4), Qiu X(2).

Author information: (1)Department of Medical Microbiology, Faculty of Medicine, University of Manitoba, Winnipeg, Canada, R3E 0J9. (2)Special Pathogens Program, Canadian Science Center for Human and Animal Health, Public Health Agency of Canada, Winnipeg, Canada, R3E 3R2. (3)CAS Key Laboratory of Pathogenic Microbiology and Immunology, Institute of Microbiology, Chinese Academy of Sciences, Beijing 100101, P.R. China. (4)1] Department of Medical Microbiology, Faculty of Medicine, University of Manitoba, Winnipeg, Canada, R3E 0J9 [2] Special Pathogens Program, Canadian Science Center for Human and Animal Health, Public Health Agency of Canada, Winnipeg, Canada, R3E 3R2 [3] Department of Immunology, Faculty of Medicine, University of Manitoba, Winnipeg, Canada, R3E 0J9 [4] Department of Pathology and Laboratory Medicine, University of Pennsylvania School of Medicine, Philadelphia, PA, USA.

Ebola virus (EBOV) causes severe viral hemorrhagic fever in humans and non-human primates, with a case fatality rate of up to 88% in human outbreaks. Over the past 3 years, monoclonal antibody (mAb) cocktails have demonstrated high efficacy as treatments against EBOV infection. One such cocktail is ZMAb, which consists of three mouse antibodies, 1H3, 2G4, and 4G7. Here, we present the epitope binding properties of mAbs 1H3, 2G4, and 4G7. We showed that these antibodies have different variable region sequences, suggesting that the individual mAbs are not clonally related. All three antibodies were found to neutralize EBOV variant Mayinga. Additionally, 2G4 and 4G7 were shown to cross-inhibit each other in vitro and select for an escape mutation at the same position on the EBOV glycoprotein (GP), at amino acid 508. 1H3 selects an escape mutant at amino acid 273 on EBOV GP. Surface plasmon resonance studies showed that all three antibodies have dissociation constants on the order of 10(-7). In combination with previous studies evaluating the binding sites of other protective antibodies, our results suggest that antibodies targeting the GP1-GP2 interface and the glycan cap are often selected as efficacious antibodies for post-exposure interventions against EBOV.

PMID: 25375093 [PubMed - in process]

322. BMJ. 2014 Nov 5;349:g6576. doi: 10.1136/bmj.g6576.

Is the United Nations catching up with Ebola at last?

Hawkes N, Arie S.

PMID: 25378433 [PubMed - in process]

323. N Engl J Med. 2014 Nov 5. [Epub ahead of print]

Clinical Presentation of Patients with Ebola Virus Disease in Conakry, Guinea.

Bah EI(1), Lamah MC, Fletcher T, Jacob ST, Brett-Major DM, Sall AA, Shindo N, Fischer WA, Lamontagne F, Saliou SM, Bausch DG, Moumié B, Jagatic T, Sprecher A, Lawler JV, Mayet T, Jacquerioz FA, Baggi MF, Vallenas C, Clement C, Mardel S, Faye O, Faye O, Soropogui B, Magassouba N, Koivogui L, Pinto R, Fowler RA.

Author information: (1)The authors' affiliations are listed in the Appendix.

Background In March 2014, the World Health Organization was notified of an outbreak of Zaire ebolavirus in a remote area of Guinea. The outbreak then spread to the capital, Conakry, and to neighboring countries and has subsequently become the largest epidemic of Ebola virus disease (EVD) to date. Methods From March 25 to April 26, 2014, we performed a study of all patients with laboratory-confirmed EVD in Conakry. Mortality was the primary outcome. Secondary outcomes included patient characteristics, complications, treatments, and comparisons between survivors and nonsurvivors. Results Of 80 patients who presented with symptoms, 37 had laboratory-confirmed EVD. Among confirmed cases, the median age was 38 years (interquartile range, 28 to 46), 24 patients (65%) were men, and 14 (38%) were health care workers; among the health care workers, nosocomial transmission was implicated in 12 patients (32%). Patients with confirmed EVD presented to the hospital a median of 5 days (interquartile range, 3 to 7) after the onset of symptoms, most commonly with fever (in 84% of the patients; mean temperature, 38.6°C), fatigue (in 65%), diarrhea (in 62%), and tachycardia (mean heart rate, >93 beats per minute). Of these patients, 28 (76%) were treated with intravenous fluids and 37 (100%) with antibiotics. Sixteen patients (43%) died, with a median time from symptom onset to death of 8 days (interquartile range, 7 to 11). Patients who were 40 years of age or older, as compared with those under the age of 40 years, had a relative risk of death of 3.49 (95% confidence interval, 1.42 to 8.59; P=0.007). Conclusions Patients with EVD presented with evidence of dehydration associated with vomiting and severe diarrhea. Despite attempts at volume repletion, antimicrobial therapy, and limited laboratory services, the rate of death was 43%.

PMID: 25372658 [PubMed - as supplied by publisher]

324. Nurs Stand. 2014 Nov 5;29(10):10. doi: 10.7748/ns.29.10.10.s9.

False alarms give hospital staff practice in managing Ebola care.

Osborne K.

Most London hospitals have dealt with at least one patent with suspected Ebola virus in the past month, a leading infection control nurse has claimed.

PMID: 25370224 [PubMed - in process]

325. BMJ. 2014 Nov 4;349:g6585. doi: 10.1136/bmj.g6585.

Advantages of airport screening for Ebola.

Cosford P(1).

Author information: (1)Public Health England, London SE1 8UG, UK paul.cosford@phe.gov.uk.

Comment on BMJ. 2014;349:g6202.

PMID: 25371224 [PubMed - in process]

326. BMJ. 2014 Nov 4;349:g6571. doi: 10.1136/bmj.g6571.

Airport screening for Ebola: current thermal scanning procedures are unreliable.

Kumana CR(1), Cheung BM(1), Chan LS(2).

Author information: (1)Department of Medicine, University of Hong Kong, Queen Mary Hospital, Hong Kong. (2)Department of Earth Sciences, University of Hong Kong, Hong Kong.
Comment on BMJ. 2014;349:g6202.
PMID: 25371221 [PubMed - in process]
327. CMAJ. 2014 Nov 4;186(16):1206. doi: 10.1503/cmaj.109-4910. Epub 2014 Oct 6.

Ebola research fueled by bioterrorism threat.

Strauss S(1).

Author information: (1)Toronto, Ont.
PMCID: PMC4216251 [Available on 2015/11/4] PMID: 25288318 [PubMed - in process]
328. CMAJ. 2014 Nov 4;186(16):1204. doi: 10.1503/cmaj.109-4906. Epub 2014 Sep 22.

Could interferon help treat Ebola?

Shuchman M(1).

Author information: (1)Toronto, Ont.
PMCID: PMC4216250 [Available on 2015/11/4] PMID: 25246419 [PubMed - in process]
329. MBio. 2014 Nov 4;5(6):e02011. doi: 10.1128/mBio.02011-14.

Deep sequencing identifies noncanonical editing of Ebola and Marburg virus RNAs in infected cells.

Shabman RS, Jabado OJ(1), Mire CE(2), Stockwell TB(3), Edwards M(4), Mahajan M(1), Geisbert TW(2), Basler CF(5).

Author information: (1)Institute for Genomics and Multiscale Biology, Icahn School of Medicine at Mount Sinai, New York, New York, USA. (2)Department of Microbiology and Immunology, Galveston National Laboratory, University of Texas Medical Branch, Galveston, Texas, USA. (3)Virology Group, J. Craig Venter Institute, Rockville, Maryland, USA. (4)Department of Microbiology, Icahn School of Medicine at Mount Sinai, New York, New York, USA. (5)Department of Microbiology, Icahn School of Medicine at Mount Sinai, New York, New York, USA chris.basler@mssm.edu.

Deep sequencing of RNAs produced by Zaire ebolavirus (EBOV) or the Angola strain of Marburgvirus (MARV-Ang) identified novel viral and cellular mechanisms that diversify the coding and noncoding sequences of viral mRNAs and genomic RNAs. We identified previously undescribed sites within the EBOV and MARV-Ang mRNAs where apparent cotranscriptional editing has resulted in the addition of non-template-encoded residues within the EBOV glycoprotein (GP) mRNA, the MARV-Ang nucleoprotein (NP) mRNA, and the MARV-Ang polymerase (L) mRNA, such that novel viral translation products could be produced. Further, we found that the well-characterized EBOV GP mRNA editing site is modified at a high frequency during viral genome RNA replication. Additionally, editing hot spots representing sites of apparent adenosine deaminase activity were found in the MARV-Ang NP 3'-untranslated region. These studies identify novel filovirus-host interactions and reveal production of a greater diversity of filoviral gene products than was previously appreciated.IMPORTANCE: This study identifies novel mechanisms that alter the protein coding capacities of Ebola and Marburg virus mRNAs. Therefore, filovirus gene expression is more complex and diverse than previously recognized. These observations suggest new directions in understanding the regulation of filovirus gene expression.

PMCID: PMC4222107 PMID: 25370495 [PubMed - in process]
330. Nurs Stand. 2014 Nov 4;29(9):13. doi: 10.7748/ns.29.9.13.s17.

Nurses close to Heathrow take part in Ebola simulation exercise.

[No authors listed]

Nursing staff and other healthcare professionals at Hillingdon Hospital near Heathrow airport have taken part in an Ebola containment and treatment simulation exercise.
PMID: 25351060 [PubMed - in process]
331. BMJ. 2014 Nov 3;349:g6542. doi: 10.1136/bmj.g6542.

WHO reports decline in number of new Ebola cases in Liberia.

Gulland A(1).

Author information: (1)London.
PMID: 25368391 [PubMed - in process]
332. BMJ. 2014 Nov 3;349:g6606. doi: 10.1136/bmj.g6606.

Maine judge refuses to quarantine nurse who cared for Ebola patients.

McCarthy M(1).

Author information: (1)Seattle.
PMID: 25368390 [PubMed - in process]
333. Mod Healthc. 2014 Nov 3;44(44):18.

Can transfusions aid Ebola fight?

Johnson SR.
PMID: 25509447 [PubMed - in process]
334. Mod Healthc. 2014 Nov 3;44(44):12.

Demand soars for Ebola supplies as cost and safety concerns rise.

Lee J.

PMID: 25509445 [PubMed - in process]

335. Mod Healthc. 2014 Nov 3;44(44):10.

Divisions surface between healthcare workers, public over Ebola quarantines.

Johnson SR.

PMID: 25509444 [PubMed - in process]

336. Am J Health Syst Pharm. 2014 Nov 1;71(21):1822-3, 1827. doi: 10.2146/news140073.

Ebola cases bring practical and clinical challenges.

Traynor K.

PMID: 25320125 [PubMed - in process]

337. Am J Ther. 2014 Nov-Dec;21(6):441. doi: 10.1097/MJT.0000000000000181.

The failing ebola policy.

Somberg JC(1).

Author information: (1)Editor.

PMID: 25373311 [PubMed - in process]

338. Ann Am Thorac Soc. 2014 Nov;11(9):1341-50. doi: 10.1513/AnnalsATS.201410-481PS.

Clinical presentation and management of severe ebola virus disease.

West TE(1), von Saint André-von Arnim A.

Author information: (1)1 Division of Pulmonary & Critical Care Medicine, Department of Medicine, and.

Clinicians caring for patients infected with Ebola virus must be familiar not only with screening and infection control measures but also with management of severe disease. By integrating experience from several Ebola epidemics with best practices for managing critical illness, this report focuses on the clinical presentation and management of severely ill infants, children, and adults with Ebola virus disease. Fever, fatigue, vomiting, diarrhea, and anorexia are the most common symptoms of the 2014 West African outbreak. Profound fluid losses from the gastrointestinal tract result in volume depletion, metabolic abnormalities (including hyponatremia, hypokalemia, and hypocalcemia), shock, and organ failure. Overt hemorrhage occurs infrequently. The case fatality rate in West Africa is at least 70%, and individuals with respiratory, neurological, or hemorrhagic symptoms have a higher risk of death. There is no proven antiviral agent to treat Ebola virus disease, although several experimental treatments may be considered. Even in the absence of antiviral therapies, intensive supportive care has the potential to markedly blunt the high case fatality rate reported to date. Optimal treatment requires conscientious correction of fluid and electrolyte losses. Additional management considerations include searching for coinfection or superinfection; treatment of shock (with intravenous fluids and vasoactive agents), acute kidney injury (with renal replacement therapy), and respiratory failure (with invasive mechanical ventilation); provision of nutrition support, pain and anxiety control, and psychosocial support; and the use of strategies to reduce complications of critical illness. Cardiopulmonary resuscitation may be appropriate in certain circumstances, but extracorporeal life support is not advised. Among other ethical issues, patients' medical needs must be carefully weighed against healthcare worker safety and infection control concerns. However, meticulous attention to the use of personal protective equipment and strict adherence to infection control protocols should permit the safe provision of intensive treatment to severely ill patients with Ebola virus disease.

PMID: 25369317 [PubMed - in process]

339. Antimicrob Agents Chemother. 2014 Nov;58(11):6639-47. doi: 10.1128/AAC.03442-14. Epub 2014 Aug 25.

Safety and pharmacokinetic profiles of phosphorodiamidate morpholino oligomers with activity against ebola virus and marburg virus: results of two single-ascending-dose studies.

Heald AE(1), Iversen PL(2), Saoud JB(3), Sazani P(3), Charleston JS(3), Axtelle T(3), Wong M(3), Smith WB(4), Vutikullird A(5), Kaye E(3).

Author information: (1)Sarepta Therapeutics, Inc., Cambridge, Massachusetts, USA healda@uw.edu. (2)Sarepta Therapeutics, Inc., Cambridge, Massachusetts, USA Oregon State University, Corvallis, Oregon, USA. (3)Sarepta Therapeutics, Inc., Cambridge, Massachusetts, USA. (4)New Orleans Center for Clinical Research-Knoxville, Knoxville, Tennessee, USA. (5)West Coast Clinical Trials, Cypress, California, USA.

Two identical single-ascending-dose studies evaluated the safety and pharmacokinetics (PK) of AVI-6002 and AVI-6003, two experimental combinations of phosphorodiamidate morpholino oligomers with positive charges (PMOplus) that target viral mRNA encoding Ebola virus and Marburg virus proteins, respectively. Both AVI-6002 and AVI-6003 were found to suppress disease in virus-infected nonhuman primates in previous studies. AVI-6002 (a combination of AVI-7537 and AVI-7539) or AVI-6003 (a combination of AVI-7287 and AVI-7288) were administered as sequential intravenous (i.v.) infusions of a 1:1 fixed dose ratio of the two subcomponents. In each study, 30 healthy male and female subjects between 18 and 50 years of age were enrolled in six-dose escalation cohorts of five subjects each and received a single i.v. infusion of active study drug (0.005, 0.05, 0.5, 1.5, 3, and 4.5 mg/kg per component) or placebo in a 4:1 ratio. Both AVI-6002 and AVI-6003 were safe and well tolerated at the doses studied. A maximum tolerated dose was not observed in either study. The four chemically similar PMOplus components exhibited generally similar PK profiles. The mean peak plasma concentration and area under the concentration-time curve values of the four components exhibited dose-proportional PK. The estimated plasma half-life of all four components was 2 to 5 h. The safety of the two combinations and the PK of the four components were similar, regardless of the target RNA sequence.

PMCID: PMC4249403 [Available on 2015/5/1] PMID: 25155593 [PubMed - in process]

340. Antiviral Res. 2014 Nov;111:33-5. doi: 10.1016/j.antiviral.2014.09.001. Epub 2014 Sep 6.

A tribute to Sheik Humarr Khan and all the healthcare workers in West Africa who have sacrificed in the fight against Ebola virus disease: Mae we hush.

Bausch DG(1), Bangura J(2), Garry RF(3), Goba A(4), Grant DS(4), Jacquerioz FA(3), McLellan SL(3), Jalloh S(4), Moses LM(3), Schieffelin JS(3).
Author information: (1)Tulane University Health Sciences Center, New Orleans, USA; U.S. Naval Medical Research Unit No. 6, Lima, Peru. Electronic address: dbausch@tulane.edu. (2)Kenema Government Hospital, Ministry of Health and Sanitation, Kenema, Sierra Leone. (3)Tulane University Health Sciences Center, New Orleans, USA. (4)Tulane University Health Sciences Center, New Orleans, USA; Kenema Government Hospital, Ministry of Health and Sanitation, Kenema, Sierra Leone.

The Kenema Government Hospital Lassa Fever Ward in Sierra Leone, directed since 2005 by Dr. Sheikh Humarr Khan, is the only medical unit in the world devoted exclusively to patient care and research of a viral hemorrhagic fever. When Ebola virus disease unexpectedly appeared in West Africa in late 2013 and eventually spread to Kenema, Khan and his fellow healthcare workers remained at their posts, providing care to patients with this devastating illness. Khan and the chief nurse, Mbalu Fonnie, became infected and died at the end of July, a fate that they have sadly shared with more than ten other healthcare workers in Kenema and hundreds across the region. This article pays tribute to Sheik Humarr Khan, Mbalu Fonnie and all the healthcare workers who have acquired Ebola virus disease while fighting the epidemic in West Africa. Besides the emotional losses, the death of so many skilled and experienced healthcare workers will severely impair health care and research in affected regions, which can only be restored through dedicated, long-term programs.

PMID: 25196533 [PubMed - in process]

341. Biomed Instrum Technol. 2014 Nov-Dec;48(6):425-9. doi: 10.2345/0899-8205-48.6.425.

Ebola virus poses new challenge to healthcare community.

Hollis E.

PMID: 25408978 [PubMed - in process]

342. Biosecur Bioterror. 2014 Nov-Dec;12(6):373. doi: 10.1089/bsp.2014.1031.

Re: optimization of interventions in ebola.

Wiwanitkit V.

PMID: 25470466 [PubMed - in process]

343. Biosecur Bioterror. 2014 Nov-Dec;12(6):306-9. doi: 10.1089/bsp.2014.1030.

Travel bans will increase the damage wrought by ebola.

Nuzzo JB, Cicero AJ, Waldhorn R, Inglesby TV.

PMID: 25397355 [PubMed - in process]

344. Biosecur Bioterror. 2014 Nov-Dec;12(6):301-5. doi: 10.1089/bsp.2014.1002.

Sociocultural dimensions of the ebola virus disease outbreak in liberia.

Ravi SJ(1), Gauldin EM.
Author information: (1)Sanjana J. Ravi, MPH, is an Analyst, UPMC Center for Health Security, Baltimore, Maryland. Eric M. Gauldin is a graduate student at Texas State University , San Marcos, Texas.

PMID: 25341052 [PubMed - in process]

345. Biosecur Bioterror. 2014 Nov-Dec;12(6):299-300. doi: 10.1089/bsp.2014.0925.

Optimization of interventions in ebola: differential contagion.

Adalja AA, Henderson DA.

PMCID: PMC4248254 [Available on 2015/12/1] PMID: 25265478 [PubMed - in process]

346. Cad Saude Publica. 2014 Nov;30(11):2256-2258.

Ethical issues in the management of patients with Ebola virus disease.

Cerbino Neto J.

PMID: 25493980 [PubMed - as supplied by publisher]

347. Clin Microbiol Infect. 2014 Nov;20(11):O794-5. doi: 10.1111/1469-0691.12792.

Coordinating the clinical management of imported human cases suspected of being infected with a highly pathogenic virus such as Ebola.

de Lamballerie X(1).
Author information: (1)Aix Marseille Université, IRD French Institute of Research for Development, EHESP French School of Public Health, EPV UMR_D 190 Emergence des Pathologies Virales, Marseille, France; IHU Méditerranée Infection, APHM Public Hospitals of Marseille, Marseille, France.

PMID: 25273076 [PubMed - in process]

348. Emerg Nurse. 2014 Nov;22(7):15. doi: 10.7748/en.22.7.15.s17.

Answering the call.

Brysiewicz P(1).
Author information: (1)The School of Nursing and Public Health, University of KwaZulu-Natal, Durban, South Africa.

EBOLA IS a highly dangerous infection and its management requires a great many resources. The recent outbreak of the virus has occurred in a rural area of west Africa with little medical infrastructure and technology, and few health facilities and professionals.

PMID: 25369960 [PubMed - in process]
349. Emerg Nurse. 2014 Nov;22(7):11. doi: 10.7748/en.22.7.11.s11.

Emergency nurses test NHS response to Ebola outbreak.

Dean E.

URGENT CARE staff should be aware that Ebola must be ruled out in all patients at their first point of contact in emergency departments (EDs), new guidance warns.

PMID: 25369954 [PubMed - in process]
350. Genet Test Mol Biomarkers. 2014 Nov;18(11):715-6. doi: 10.1089/gtmb.2014.1560. Epub 2014 Oct 23.

Ebola hemorrhagic fever: genetic biomarkers and vaccine development.

Oliphant E(1).

Author information: (1)Genetic Alliance , Washington, District of Columbia.

PMCID: PMC4216996 [Available on 2015/11/1] PMID: 25340986 [PubMed - in process]
351. IEEE Pulse. 2014 Nov-Dec;5(6):30-2. doi: 10.1109/MPUL.2014.2355302.

Nigeria in the Spotlight : This African country is faced with multiple challenges to delivering quality care. Health advisor Femi Olugbile offers his perspective on the current situation.

Fischer S.

As immediate past permanent secretary of the Lagos State Ministry of Health in Nigeria and former chief medical director of one of the country?s top medical centers, Lagos State University Teaching Hospital (LASUTH), Femi Olugbile has had a close view of his country?s health care progress over the years. Despite decades of economic booms and busts and sociopolitical turmoil, Nigeria?s health systems have grown, Olugbile says?but not enough. The average life expectancy is around 52 years. Ongoing problems with extremist groups like Boko Haram have hamstrung vaccination programs, and this year, the country experienced the first Ebola threat in its history.

PMID: 25415881 [PubMed - in process]
352. Int J Infect Dis. 2014 Nov;28:217-8. doi: 10.1016/j.ijid.2014.09.001. Epub 2014 Oct 18.

Are we ready for a global pandemic of Ebola virus?

Ross AG(1), Olveda RM(2), Yuesheng L(3).

Author information: (1)Department of Medical Sciences, Griffith Health Institute, Griffith University, Gold Coast Campus, Southport, Queensland, Australia. Electronic address: a.ross@griffith.edu.au. (2)Research Institute for Tropical Medicine, Department of Health, Manila, the Philippines. (3)Division of Infectious Diseases, QIMR Berghofer Medical Research Institute, Brisbane, Queensland, Australia.

We are not ready for a global pandemic of Ebola virus. The current West African epidemic should serve as a dire warning of things to come.

PMID: 25403915 [PubMed - in process]
353. Int J Nurs Stud. 2014 Nov;51(11):1421-6. doi: 10.1016/j.ijnurstu.2014.09.002. Epub 2014 Sep 8.

Respiratory protection for healthcare workers treating Ebola virus disease (EVD): are facemasks sufficient to meet occupational health and safety obligations?

MacIntyre CR(1), Chughtai AA(2), Seale H(2), Richards GA(3), Davidson PM(4).

Author information: (1)School of Public Health and Community Medicine, Faculty of Medicine, University of New South Wales, Australia. Electronic address: r.macintyre@unsw.edu.au. (2)School of Public Health and Community Medicine, Faculty of Medicine, University of New South Wales, Australia. (3)University of the Witwatersrand Johannesburg, South Africa; Critical Care Charlotte Maxeke Johannesburg Academic Hospital, Johannesburg, South Africa. (4)Johns Hopkins University, Baltimore, USA; University of Technology, Sydney, Australia.

PMID: 25218265 [PubMed - in process]
354. Intensive Care Med. 2014 Nov;40(11):1742-5. doi: 10.1007/s00134-014-3497-z. Epub 2014 Sep 25.

Ebola in West Africa: be aware and prepare.

Parkes-Ratanshi R(1), Ssekabira U, Crozier I.

Author information: (1)Infectious Diseases Institute, College of Health Sciences, Makerere University, P.O. Box 22418, Mulago Hospital Complex, Kampala, Uganda, rratanshi@idi.co.ug.

PMID: 25253023 [PubMed - in process]
355. Intensive Care Med. 2014 Nov;40(11):1738-41. doi: 10.1007/s00134-014-3473-7. Epub 2014 Sep 3.

Does this patient have Ebola virus disease?

Tattevin P(1), Durante-Mangoni E, Massaquoi M.

Author information: (1)Infectious Diseases and Intensive Care Unit, Pontchaillou University Hospital, INSERM U835, Université Rennes-1, Rennes, France, pierre.tattevin@chu-rennes.fr.

PMID: 25183574 [PubMed - in process]
356. J Am Pharm Assoc (2003). 2014 Nov 1;54(6):654-7. doi: 10.1331/JAPhA.2014.14541.

Progress toward vaccines for cholera, dengue, malaria, and Ebola.

Cunningham KC, Hayney MS.

PMID: 25379984 [PubMed - in process]

357. J Contin Educ Nurs. 2014 Nov;45(11):479-81. doi: 10.3928/00220124-20141027-12.

Care of patients with Ebola virus disease.

Feistritzer NR, Hill C, Vanairsdale S, Gentry J.

Caring for patients with Ebola virus disease requires strict biosafety protocols to eliminate exposure and ensure containment. Training and competency verification were critical to creation of a safe environment for nursing staff involved in the direct care of two patients with Ebola virus disease at Emory University Hospital.

Copyright 2014, SLACK Incorporated.

PMID: 25365183 [PubMed - in process]

358. J Contin Educ Nurs. 2014 Nov;45(11):475-6. doi: 10.3928/00220124-20141027-10.

Blame free-"Bah, humbug!" the need for responsible media about Ebola.

Yoder-Wise PS.

PMID: 25365181 [PubMed - in process]

359. J Health Commun. 2014 Nov;19(11):1213-5. doi: 10.1080/10810730.2014.977680.

Ebola crisis-communication chaos we can avoid.

Ratzan SC, Moritsugu KP.

PMID: 25356719 [PubMed - in process]

360. J Pineal Res. 2014 Nov;57(4):381-4. doi: 10.1111/jpi.12186. Epub 2014 Oct 14.

Ebola virus disease: potential use of melatonin as a treatment.

Tan DX(1), Korkmaz A, Reiter RJ, Manchester LC.

Author information: (1)Department of Cellular and Structural Biology, The University of Texas Health Science Center at San Antonio, San Antonio, TX, USA.

The purpose of this report is to emphasize the potential utility for the use of melatonin in the treatment of individuals who are infected with the Ebola virus. The pathological changes associated with an Ebola infection include, most notably, endothelial disruption, disseminated intravascular coagulation and multiple organ hemorrhage. Melatonin has been shown to target these alterations. Numerous similarities between Ebola virus infection and septic shock have been recognized for more than a decade. Moreover, melatonin has been successfully employed for the treatment of sepsis in many experimental and clinical studies. Based on these factors, as the number of treatments currently available is limited and the useable products are not abundant, the use of melatonin for the treatment of Ebola virus infection is encouraged. Additionally, melatonin has a high safety profile, is readily available and can be orally self-administered; thus, the use of melatonin is compatible with the large scale of this serious outbreak.

© 2014 John Wiley & Sons A/S. Published by John Wiley & Sons Ltd.

PMID: 25262626 [PubMed - in process]

361. J Virol. 2014 Nov;88(21):12703-14. doi: 10.1128/JVI.01643-14. Epub 2014 Aug 20.

Establishment and characterization of a lethal mouse model for the Angola strain of Marburg virus.

Qiu X(1), Wong G(2), Audet J(2), Cutts T(3), Niu Y(4), Booth S(4), Kobinger GP(5).

Author information: (1)Special Pathogens Program, National Microbiology Laboratory, Public Health Agency of Canada, Winnipeg, Manitoba, Canada xiangguo.qiu@phac-aspc.gc.ca gary.kobinger@phac-aspc.gc.ca. (2)Special Pathogens Program, National Microbiology Laboratory, Public Health Agency of Canada, Winnipeg, Manitoba, Canada Department of Medical Microbiology, University of Manitoba, Winnipeg, Manitoba, Canada. (3)Applied Biosafety and Research Program, JC Wilt Infectious Diseases Research Centre, Public Health Agency of Canada, Winnipeg, Manitoba, Canada. (4)Molecular PathoBiology, National Microbiology Laboratory, Public Health Agency of Canada, Winnipeg, Manitoba, Canada. (5)Special Pathogens Program, National Microbiology Laboratory, Public Health Agency of Canada, Winnipeg, Manitoba, Canada Department of Medical Microbiology, University of Manitoba, Winnipeg, Manitoba, Canada Department of Immunology, University of Manitoba, Winnipeg, Manitoba, Canada Department of Pathology and Laboratory Medicine, University of Pennsylvania School of Medicine, Philadelphia, Pennsylvania, USA xiangguo.qiu@phac-aspc.gc.ca gary.kobinger@phac-aspc.gc.ca.

Infections with Marburg virus (MARV) and Ebola virus (EBOV) cause severe hemorrhagic fever in humans and nonhuman primates (NHPs) with fatality rates up to 90%. A number of experimental vaccine and treatment platforms have previously been shown to be protective against EBOV infection. However, the rate of development for prophylactics and therapeutics against MARV has been lower in comparison, possibly because a small-animal model is not widely available. Here we report the development of a mouse model for studying the pathogenesis of MARV Angola (MARV/Ang), the most virulent strain of MARV. Infection with the wild-type virus does not cause disease in mice, but the adapted virus (MARV/Ang-MA) recovered from liver homogenates after 24 serial passages in severe combined immunodeficient (SCID) mice caused severe disease when administered intranasally (i.n.) or intraperitoneally (i.p.). The median lethal dose (LD50) was determined to be 0.015 50% TCID50 (tissue culture infective dose) of MARV/Ang-MA in SCID mice, and i.p. infection at a dose of 1,000× LD50 resulted in death between 6 and 8 days postinfection in SCID mice. Similar results were obtained with immunocompetent BALB/c and C57BL/6 mice challenged i.p. with 2,000× LD50 of MARV/Ang-MA. Virological and pathological analyses of MARV/Ang-MA-infected BALB/c mice revealed that the associated pathology was reminiscent of observations made in NHPs with MARV/Ang. MARV/Ang-MA-infected mice showed most of the clinical hallmarks observed with Marburg hemorrhagic fever, including lymphopenia, thrombocytopenia, marked liver damage, and uncontrolled viremia. Virus titers reached 10(8) TCID50/ml in the blood and between 10(6) and 10(10) TCID50/g tissue in the intestines, kidney, lungs, brain, spleen, and liver. This model provides an important tool to screen candidate vaccines and therapeutics against MARV infections.IMPORTANCE: The Angola strain of Marburg virus (MARV/Ang) was responsible for the largest outbreak ever documented for Marburg viruses. With a 90% fatality rate, it is similar to Ebola virus, which makes it one of the most lethal viruses known to humans. There are currently no approved interventions for Marburg virus, in part because a small-animal model that is vulnerable to MARV/Ang infection is not available to screen and test potential vaccines and therapeutics in a quick and economical manner. To address this need, we have adapted MARV/Ang so that it causes illness in mice resulting in death. The signs of disease in these mice are reminiscent of wild-type MARV/Ang infections in humans and nonhuman primates. We believe that this will be of help in accelerating the development of life-saving measures against Marburg virus infections.

PMCID: PMC4248893 [Available on 2015/5/1] PMID: 25142608 [PubMed - in process]
362. J Virol. 2014 Nov;88(21):12500-10. doi: 10.1128/JVI.02163-14. Epub 2014 Aug 20.

Molecular basis for ebolavirus VP35 suppression of human dendritic cell maturation.

Yen B(1), Mulder LC(2), Martinez O(3), Basler CF(4).

Author information: (1)Department of Microbiology, Icahn School of Medicine at Mount Sinai, New York, New York, USA. (2)Department of Microbiology, Icahn School of Medicine at Mount Sinai, New York, New York, USA Global Health and Emerging Pathogens Institute, Icahn School of Medicine at Mount Sinai, New York, New York, USA. (3)Department of Biology, Winona State University, Winona, Minnesota, USA. (4)Department of Microbiology, Icahn School of Medicine at Mount Sinai, New York, New York, USA chris.basler@mssm.edu.

Zaire ebolavirus (EBOV) VP35 is a double-stranded RNA (dsRNA)-binding protein that inhibits RIG-I signaling and alpha/beta interferon (IFN-α/β) responses by both dsRNA-binding-dependent and -independent mechanisms. VP35 also suppresses dendritic cell (DC) maturation. Here, we define the pathways and mechanisms through which VP35 impairs DC maturation. Wild-type VP35 (VP35-WT) and two well-characterized VP35 mutants (F239A and R322A) that independently ablate dsRNA binding and RIG-I inhibition were delivered to primary human monocyte-derived DCs (MDDCs) using a lentivirus-based expression system. VP35-WT suppressed not only IFN-α/β but also proinflammatory responses following stimulation of MDDCs with activators of RIG-I-like receptor (RLR) signaling, including RIG-I activators such as Sendai virus (SeV) or 5'-triphosphate RNA, or MDA5 activators such as encephalomyocarditis virus (EMCV) or poly(I · C). The F239A and R322A mutants exhibited greatly reduced suppression of IFN-α/β and proinflammatory cytokine production following treatment of DCs with RLR agonists. VP35-WT also blocked the upregulation of DC maturation markers and the stimulation of allogeneic T cell responses upon SeV infection, whereas the mutants did not. In contrast to the RLR activators, VP35-WT and the VP35 mutants impaired IFN-β production induced by Toll-like receptor 3 (TLR3) or TLR4 agonists but failed to inhibit proinflammatory cytokine production induced by TLR2, TLR3, or TLR4 agonists. Furthermore, VP35 did not prevent lipopolysaccharide (LPS)-induced upregulation of surface markers of MDDC maturation and did not prevent LPS-triggered allogeneic T cell stimulation. Therefore, VP35 is a general antagonist of DC responses to RLR activation. However, TLR agonists can circumvent many of the inhibitory effects of VP35. Therefore, it may be possible to counteract EBOV immune evasion by using treatments that bypass the VP35-imposed block to DC maturation.IMPORTANCE: The VP35 protein, which is an inhibitor of RIG-I signaling and alpha/beta interferon (IFN-α/β) responses, has been implicated as an EBOV-encoded factor that contributes to suppression of dendritic cell (DC) function. We used wild-type VP35 and previously characterized VP35 mutants to clarify VP35-DC interactions. Our data demonstrate that VP35 is a general inhibitor of RIG-I-like receptor (RLR) signaling that blocks not only RIG-I- but also MDA5-mediated induction of IFN-α/β responses. Furthermore, in DCs, VP35 also impairs the RLR-mediated induction of proinflammatory cytokine production, upregulation of costimulatory markers, and activation of T cells. These inhibitory activities require VP35 dsRNA-binding activity, an activity previously correlated to VP35 RIG-I inhibitory function. In contrast, while VP35 can inhibit IFN-α/β production induced by TLR3 or TLR4 agonists, this occurs in a dsRNA-independent fashion, and VP35 does not inhibit TLR-mediated expression of proinflammatory cytokines. These data suggest strategies to overcome VP35 inhibition of DC function.

PMCID: PMC4248944 [Available on 2015/5/1] PMID: 25142601 [PubMed - in process]
363. J Virol. 2014 Nov;88(21):12558-71. doi: 10.1128/JVI.01863-14. Epub 2014 Aug 20.

Analysis of the highly diverse gene borders in Ebola virus reveals a distinct mechanism of transcriptional regulation.

Brauburger K(1), Boehmann Y(2), Tsuda Y(3), Hoenen T(3), Olejnik J(4), Schümann M(2), Ebihara H(3), Mühlberger E(5).

Author information: (1)Department of Microbiology, Boston University School of Medicine, Boston, Massachusetts, USA National Emerging Infectious Diseases Laboratories, Boston University School of Medicine, Boston, Massachusetts, USA Department of Virology, Philipps University of Marburg, Marburg, Germany. (2)Department of Virology, Philipps University of Marburg, Marburg, Germany. (3)Laboratory of Virology, Division of Intramural Research, National Institute of Allergy and Infectious Diseases, National Institutes of Health, Hamilton, Montana, USA. (4)Department of Microbiology, Boston University School of Medicine, Boston, Massachusetts, USA National Emerging Infectious Diseases Laboratories, Boston University School of Medicine, Boston, Massachusetts, USA. (5)Department of Microbiology, Boston University School of Medicine, Boston, Massachusetts, USA National Emerging Infectious Diseases Laboratories, Boston University School of Medicine, Boston, Massachusetts, USA muehlber@bu.edu.

Ebola virus (EBOV) belongs to the group of nonsegmented negative-sense RNA viruses. The seven EBOV genes are separated by variable gene borders, including short (4- or 5-nucleotide) intergenic regions (IRs), a single long (144-nucleotide) IR, and gene overlaps, where the neighboring gene end and start signals share five conserved nucleotides. The unique structure of the gene overlaps and the presence of a single long IR are conserved among all filoviruses. Here, we sought to determine the impact of the EBOV gene borders during viral transcription. We show that readthrough mRNA synthesis occurs in EBOV-infected cells irrespective of the structure of the gene border, indicating that the gene overlaps do not promote recognition of the gene end signal. However, two consecutive gene end signals at the VP24 gene might improve termination at the VP24-L gene border, ensuring efficient L gene expression. We further demonstrate that the long IR is not essential for but regulates transcription reinitiation in a length-dependent but sequence-independent manner. Mutational analysis of bicistronic minigenomes and recombinant EBOVs showed no direct correlation between IR length and reinitiation rates but demonstrated that specific IR lengths not found naturally in filoviruses profoundly inhibit downstream gene expression. Intriguingly, although truncation of the 144-nucleotide-long IR to 5 nucleotides did not substantially affect EBOV transcription, it led to a significant reduction of viral growth.IMPORTANCE: Our current understanding of EBOV transcription regulation is limited due to the requirement for high-containment conditions to study this highly pathogenic virus. EBOV is thought to share many mechanistic features with well-analyzed prototype nonsegmented negative-sense RNA viruses. A single polymerase entry site at the 3' end of the genome determines that transcription of the genes is mainly controlled by gene order and cis-acting signals found at the gene borders. Here, we examined the regulatory role of the structurally unique EBOV gene borders during viral transcription. Our data suggest that transcriptional regulation in EBOV is highly complex and differs from that in prototype viruses and further the understanding of this most fundamental process in the filovirus replication cycle. Moreover, our results with recombinant EBOVs suggest a novel role of the long IR found in all filovirus genomes during the viral replication cycle.

PMCID: PMC4248908 [Available on 2015/5/1] PMID: 25142600 [PubMed - in process]
364. J Virol Methods. 2014 Nov;208:1-5. doi: 10.1016/j.jviromet.2014.07.023. Epub 2014 Jul 27.

A new approach to determining whole viral genomic sequences including termini using a single deep sequencing run.

Alfson KJ(1), Beadles MW(2), Griffiths A(3).

Author information: (1)Department of Virology and Immunology, Texas Biomedical Research Institute, PO Box 760549, San Antonio, TX 78245, USA; Department of Microbiology and Immunology, University of Texas Health Science Center at San Antonio, Mail Code 7758, 7703 Floyd Curl Drive, San Antonio, TX 78229, USA. (2)Department of Virology and Immunology, Texas Biomedical Research Institute, PO Box 760549, San Antonio, TX 78245, USA. (3)Department of Virology and Immunology, Texas Biomedical Research Institute, PO Box 760549, San Antonio, TX 78245, USA; Department of Microbiology and Immunology, University of Texas Health Science Center at San Antonio, Mail Code 7758, 7703 Floyd Curl Drive, San Antonio, TX 78229, USA. Electronic address: agriffiths@txbiomed.org.

Next-generation sequencing is now commonly used for a variety of applications in virology including virus discovery, investigation of quasispecies, viral evolution, metagenomics, and analyses of antiviral resistance. However, there are limitations with the current sample preparation methods used for deep sequencing of viral genomes, especially during de novo sequencing. For example, current methods are unable to capture the terminal sequences of viral genomes in an efficient and effective manner; data representing the 3' and 5' ends are typically insufficient. Methods such as Rapid Amplification of cDNA Ends address this issue but these methods can be time consuming, may require some prior knowledge of the viral sequence, and require multiple independent procedures. The current study outlines a sample preparation technique that overcomes some of these shortcomings. The method relied on random fragmentation with divalent cations and subsequent adapter ligation directly to RNA, rather than cDNA, to maximize the quality and quantity of terminal reads. The technique was tested on RNA samples from two different RNA viruses, Ebola virus and hepatitis C virus. This method permits rapid preparation of samples for deep sequencing while eliminating the use of sequence specific primers and captures the entire genome sequence, including the 5' and 3' ends. This could improve the efficiency of virus discovery projects where the terminal ends are unknown.

PMID: 25075935 [PubMed - in process]
365. Lancet Infect Dis. 2014 Nov;14(11):1045-6. doi: 10.1016/S1473-3099(14)70954-5. Epub 2014 Oct 1.

Ebola and compliance with infection prevention measures in Nigeria.

Yusuf I(1), Adam RU(2), Ahmad SA(3), Yee PL(3).

Author information: (1)Microbiology and Medical Laboratory Sciences, Bayero University, 3011, Kano, Nigeria. Electronic address: iyusuf.bio@buk.edu.ng. (2)Pathology Department, Sir Muhammad Sunusi Specialist Hospital Kano, Nigeria. (3)Faculty of Biotechnology and Biomolecular Sciences, Universiti Putra Malaysia, Selangor, Malaysia.

PMID: 25282666 [PubMed - in process]
366. Lancet Infect Dis. 2014 Nov;14(11):1034-5. doi: 10.1016/S1473-3099(14)70956-9. Epub 2014 Oct 1.

Ebola in west Africa: from disease outbreak to humanitarian crisis.

Piot P(1), Muyembe JJ(2), Edmunds WJ(3).

Author information: (1)London School of Hygiene & Tropical Medicine, Keppel Street, London, WC1E 7HT, UK. Electronic address: peter.piot@lshtm.ac.uk. (2)Institut National de Recherche Biomédicale, Kinshasa, Democratic Republic of the Congo. (3)London School of Hygiene & Tropical Medicine, Keppel Street, London, WC1E 7HT, UK.

PMID: 25282665 [PubMed - in process]
367. Lancet Infect Dis. 2014 Nov;14(11):1045. doi: 10.1016/S1473-3099(14)70924-7. Epub 2014 Sep 10.

Ebola in west Africa.

Trad MA(1), Fisher DA(2), Tambyah PA(2).

Author information: (1)National University Hospital, Singapore, Singapore. Electronic address: m.a.trad@hotmail.com. (2)National University Hospital, Singapore, Singapore.

PMID: 25218096 [PubMed - in process]
368. Neth J Med. 2014 Nov;72(9):442-8.

Ebola virus disease: a review on epidemiology, symptoms, treatment and pathogenesis.

Goeijenbier M(1), van Kampen JJ, Reusken CB, Koopmans MP, van Gorp EC.

Author information: (1)Department of Viroscience, Erasmus MC, Rotterdam, the Netherlands.

Currently, West Africa is facing the largest outbreak of Ebola virus disease (EVD) in history. The virus causing this outbreak, the Zaire Ebolavirus (EBOV), belongs to the genus Ebolavirus which together with the genus Marburgvirus forms the family of the Filoviridae. EBOV is one of the most virulent pathogens among the viral haemorrhagic fevers, and case fatality rates up to 90% have been reported. Mortality is the result of multi-organ failure and severe bleeding complications. By 18 September 2014, the WHO reported of 5335 cases (confirmed, suspected and probable) with 2622 deaths, resulting in a case fatality rate of around 50%. This review aims to provide an overview of EVD for clinicians, with the emphasis on pathogenesis, clinical manifestations, and treatment options.
PMID: 25387613 [PubMed - in process]

369. Nurs Child Young People. 2014 Nov;26(9):7. doi: 10.7748/ncyp.26.9.7.s7.

Call to support orphans of outbreak, as death toll rises.

[No authors listed]

INTERNATIONAL CHARITIES are rallying to provide food, shelter, health care and support for children orphaned by the outbreak of the Ebola virus.

PMID: 25369087 [PubMed - in process]

370. Nurs Child Young People. 2014 Nov;26(9):7. doi: 10.7748/ncyp.26.9.7.s6.

RCN publishes advice on identifying and managing children with Ebola.

Sprinks J.

NURSES SHOULD apply the same measures for identifying and caring for children with suspected Ebola virus as required for adult nursing care, according to the RCN.

PMID: 25369086 [PubMed - in process]

371. Nurs Child Young People. 2014 Nov;26(9):5. doi: 10.7748/ncyp.26.9.5.s1.

Effects of Ebola hit children most.

[No authors listed]

International charities working in West Africa are warning that children are bearing the brunt of the Ebola crisis.

PMID: 25369081 [PubMed - in process]

372. Nurs Outlook. 2014 Nov-Dec;62(6):379-81. doi: 10.1016/j.outlook.2014.09.002. Epub 2014 Sep 22.

Ebola: The new HIV?

Smith BA(1), DeMarco R(2).

Author information: (1)Michigan State University, College of Nursing, East Lansing, MI. Electronic address: Barbara.Smith@hc.msu.edu. (2)Department of Nursing, College of Nursing and Health Sciences, University of Massachusetts Boston, Boston, MA.

PMID: 25455707 [PubMed - in process]

373. Obstet Gynecol. 2014 Nov;124(5):1005-10. doi: 10.1097/AOG.0000000000000533.

What obstetrician-gynecologists should know about ebola: a perspective from the centers for disease control and prevention.

Jamieson DJ(1), Uyeki TM, Callaghan WM, Meaney-Delman D, Rasmussen SA.

Author information: (1)Division of Reproductive Health, National Center for Chronic Disease Prevention and Health Promotion, the Influenza Division, National Center for Immunization and Respiratory Diseases, the National Center for Emerging and Zoonotic Infectious Diseases, and the Office of Public Health Preparedness and Response, Centers for Disease Control and Prevention, Atlanta, Georgia.

West Africa is currently in the midst of the largest Ebola outbreak in history. Although there have been no Ebola virus disease cases identified in the United States, two U.S. health care workers with Ebola virus disease were medically evacuated from Liberia to the United States in early August 2014. The Centers for Disease Control and Prevention has been working closely with other U.S. government agencies and international and nongovernmental partners for several months to respond to this global crisis. Limited evidence suggests that pregnant women are at increased risk for severe illness and death when infected with Ebola virus, but there is no evidence to suggest that pregnant women are more susceptible to Ebola virus disease. In addition, pregnant women with Ebola virus disease appear to be at an increased risk for spontaneous abortion and pregnancy-associated hemorrhage. Neonates born to mothers with Ebola virus disease have not survived. Although it is very unlikely that obstetrician-gynecologists (ob-gyns) in the United States will diagnose or treat a patient with Ebola virus disease, it is important that all health care providers are prepared to evaluate and care for these patients. Specifically, U.S. health care providers, including ob-gyns, should ask patients about recent travel and should know the signs and symptoms of Ebola virus disease and what to do if assessing a patient with compatible illness. This article provides general background information on Ebola and specifically addresses what is known about Ebola virus disease in pregnancy and the implications for practicing ob-gyns in the United States.

PMID: 25203368 [PubMed - in process]

374. Pharmacotherapy. 2014 Nov;34(11):1115-7. doi: 10.1002/phar.1520.

Basic science and the ebola virus infection epidemic.

DeVane CL(1).

Author information: (1)Medical University of South Carolina, Charleston, South Carolina.

PMID: 25382095 [PubMed - in process]

375. PLoS Negl Trop Dis. 2014 Nov 13;8(11):e3257. doi: 10.1371/journal.pntd.0003257. eCollection 2014.

The Global One Health Paradigm: Challenges and Opportunities for Tackling Infectious Diseases at the Human, Animal, and Environment Interface in Low-Resource Settings.

Gebreyes WA(1), Dupouy-Camet J(2), Newport MJ(3), Oliveira CJ(4), Schlesinger LS(5), Saif YM(6), Kariuki S(7), Saif LJ(6), Saville W(1), Wittum T(1), Hoet A(1), Quessy S(8), Kazwala R(9), Tekola B(10), Shryock T(11), Bisesi M(12), Patchanee P(13), Boonmar S(14), King LJ(1).

Author information: (1)Global Health Programs, College of Veterinary Medicine, The Ohio State University and VPH-Biotec Global Consortium, Columbus, Ohio, United States of America. (2)Department of Parasitology, Hôspital Cochin, Paris Descartes University, Paris, France. (3)Centre for Global Health Research, Brighton and Sussex Medical School, Sussex, United Kingdom. (4)College of Agricultural Sciences, Federal University of Paraiba, Brazil (CCA/UFPB), Areia, Paraiba, Brazil. (5)Department of Microbial Infection and Immunity, Center for Microbial Interface Biology, The Ohio State University, Columbus, Ohio, United States of America. (6)Food Animal Health Research Program, The Ohio State University, Wooster, Ohio, United States of America. (7)Centre for Microbiology Research, Kenya Medical Research Institute (KEMRI), Nairobi, Kenya. (8)Department of Pathology and Microbiology University of Montreal, Saint-Hyacinthe, Québec, Canada. (9)Faculty of Veterinary Medicine, Sokoine University of Agriculture, Chuo Kikuu, Morogoro, Tanzania. (10)United Nations Food and Agriculture Organization (FAO), Rome, Italy. (11)Elanco Animal Health, Greenfield, Indiana, United States of America. (12)The Ohio State University College of Public Health, Columbus, Ohio, United States of America. (13)Chiang Mai University, Chiang Mai, Thailand. (14)Thailand MOPH-U.S. CDC Collaboration, Bangkok, Thailand.

Zoonotic infectious diseases have been an important concern to humankind for more than 10,000 years. Today, approximately 75% of newly emerging infectious diseases (EIDs) are zoonoses that result from various anthropogenic, genetic, ecologic, socioeconomic, and climatic factors. These interrelated driving forces make it difficult to predict and to prevent zoonotic EIDs. Although significant improvements in environmental and medical surveillance, clinical diagnostic methods, and medical practices have been achieved in the recent years, zoonotic EIDs remain a major global concern, and such threats are expanding, especially in less developed regions. The current Ebola epidemic in West Africa is an extreme stark reminder of the role animal reservoirs play in public health and reinforces the urgent need for globally operationalizing a One Health approach. The complex nature of zoonotic diseases and the limited resources in developing countries are a reminder that the need for implementation of Global One Health in low-resource settings is crucial. The Veterinary Public Health and Biotechnology (VPH-Biotec) Global Consortium launched the International Congress on Pathogens at the Human-Animal Interface (ICOPHAI) in order to address important challenges and needs for capacity building. The inaugural ICOPHAI (Addis Ababa, Ethiopia, 2011) and the second congress (Porto de Galinhas, Brazil, 2013) were unique opportunities to share and discuss issues related to zoonotic infectious diseases worldwide. In addition to strong scientific reports in eight thematic areas that necessitate One Health implementation, the congress identified four key capacity-building needs: (1) development of adequate science-based risk management policies, (2) skilled-personnel capacity building, (3) accredited veterinary and public health diagnostic laboratories with a shared database, and (4) improved use of existing natural resources and implementation. The aim of this review is to highlight advances in key zoonotic disease areas and the One Health capacity needs.

PMCID: PMC4230840 PMID: 25393303 [PubMed - as supplied by publisher]

376. PLoS Pathog. 2014 Nov 20;10(11):e1004509. doi: 10.1371/journal.ppat.1004509. eCollection 2014.

Shed GP of Ebola Virus Triggers Immune Activation and Increased Vascular Permeability.

Escudero-Pérez B(1), Volchkova VA(1), Dolnik O(1), Lawrence P(1), Volchkov VE(1).

Author information: (1)Molecular Basis of Viral Pathogenicity, CIRI, INSERM U1111- CNRS UMR5308, Université de Lyon, Université Claude Bernard Lyon 1, Ecole Normale Supérieure de Lyon, Lyon, France.

During Ebola virus (EBOV) infection a significant amount of surface glycoprotein GP is shed from infected cells in a soluble form due to cleavage by cellular metalloprotease TACE. Shed GP and non-structural secreted glycoprotein sGP, both expressed from the same GP gene, have been detected in the blood of human patients and experimentally infected animals. In this study we demonstrate that shed GP could play a particular role during EBOV infection. In effect it binds and activates non-infected dendritic cells and macrophages inducing the secretion of pro- and anti-inflammatory cytokines (TNFα, IL1β, IL6, IL8, IL12p40, and IL1-RA, IL10). Activation of these cells by shed GP correlates with the increase in surface expression of co-stimulatory molecules CD40, CD80, CD83 and CD86. Contrary to shed GP, secreted sGP activates neither DC nor macrophages while it could bind DCs. In this study, we show that shed GP activity is likely mediated through cellular toll-like receptor 4 (TLR4) and is dependent on GP glycosylation. Treatment of cells with anti-TLR4 antibody completely abolishes shed GP-induced activation of cells. We also demonstrate that shed GP activity is negated upon addition of mannose-binding sera lectin MBL, a molecule known to interact with sugar arrays present on the surface of different microorganisms. Furthermore, we highlight the ability of shed GP to affect endothelial cell function both directly and indirectly, demonstrating the interplay between shed GP, systemic cytokine release and increased vascular permeability. In conclusion, shed GP released from virus-infected cells could activate non-infected DCs and macrophages causing the massive release of pro- and anti-inflammatory cytokines and effect vascular permeability. These activities could be at the heart of the excessive and dysregulated inflammatory host reactions to infection and thus contribute to high virus pathogenicity.

PMCID: PMC4239094 PMID: 25412102 [PubMed - in process]

377. Postgrad Med J. 2014 Nov;90(1069):610-2. doi: 10.1136/postgradmedj-2014-133068.

Ebola virus disease: where are we now and where do we go?

Brown CS(1), Cropley IM(2).

Author information: (1)Royal Free London NHS Foundation Trust, London, UK King's Sierra Leone Partnership, London, UK. (2)Royal Free London NHS Foundation Trust, London, UK.

PMID: 25335794 [PubMed - in process]

378. Presse Med. 2014 Nov;43(11):1159-61. doi: 10.1016/j.lpm.2014.09.001. Epub 2014 Sep 26.

[Alert - epidemic due to the Ebola virus].

[Article in French]

Bricaire F(1).

Author information: (1)Groupe hospitalier Pitié-Salpêtrière, service des maladies infectieuses, 47, boulevard de l'Hôpital, 75013 Paris, France. Electronic address: francois.bricaire@psl.aphp.fr.

PMID: 25261916 [PubMed - in process]

379. Protein Sci. 2014 Nov;23(11):1519-27. doi: 10.1002/pro.2541. Epub 2014 Sep 4.

Conformational plasticity of the Ebola virus matrix protein.

Radzimanowski J(1), Effantin G, Weissenhorn W.

Author information: (1)University Grenoble Alpes, UVHCI, F-38000, Grenoble, France; CNRS, UVHCI, F-38000, Grenoble, France.

Filoviruses are the causative agents of a severe and often fatal hemorrhagic fever with repeated outbreaks in Africa. They are negative sense single stranded enveloped viruses that can cross species barriers from its natural host bats to primates including humans. The small size of the genome poses limits to viral adaption, which may be partially overcome by conformational plasticity. Here we review the different conformational states of the Ebola virus (EBOV) matrix protein VP40 that range from monomers, to dimers, hexamers, and RNA-bound octamers. This conformational plasticity that is required for the viral life cycle poses a unique opportunity for development of VP40 specific drugs. Furthermore, we compare the structure to homologous matrix protein structures from Paramyxoviruses and Bornaviruses and we predict that they do not only share the fold but also the conformational flexibility of EBOV VP40.

PMCID: PMC4241103 [Available on 2015/11/1] PMID: 25159197 [PubMed - in process]

380. Recenti Prog Med. 2014 Nov;105(11):405-6. doi: 10.1701/1680.18396.

[Ebola and the global governance of health].

[Article in Italian]

Dentico N.

The high state of anxiety about Ebola virus and its possible spread in the Western world has seemingly changed the route of the disease, for which effective vaccines and medicines do not exist. The rapid spread of the virus provides a paradigmatic narrative about the failure of today's governance for health, grounded on a series of global initiatives focussed on pathologies prioritized by the donors' community, at the detriment of health promotion and the strengthening of health systems in countries. The Ebola crisis also delivers a powerful account about the consequences of the de-potentiation of the World Health Organization (WHO), once the leading organization in public health policy-making. Today, the WHO is increasingly weak technically, politically and financially. While the virus remains out of control, the WHO's capacity to play a role in accompanying the development of the new essential vaccines and in brokering the conditions for accessibility and availability of the new medical tools remains to be questioned.

PMID: 25424232 [PubMed - in process]

381. Rev Med Virol. 2014 Nov;24(6):363-4. doi: 10.1002/rmv.1812. Epub 2014 Oct 15.

Ebola and ethics.

Griffiths PD.

PMID: 25318448 [PubMed - in process]

382. Virology. 2014 Nov;468-470:637-46. doi: 10.1016/j.virol.2014.08.019. Epub 2014 Oct 11.

Cell entry by a novel European filovirus requires host endosomal cysteine proteases and Niemann-Pick C1.

Ng M(1), Ndungo E(1), Jangra RK(1), Cai Y(2), Postnikova E(2), Radoshitzky SR(3), Dye JM(3), Ramírez de Arellano E(4), Negredo A(4), Palacios G(3), Kuhn JH(2), Chandran K(5).

Author information: (1)Department of Microbiology and Immunology, Albert Einstein College of Medicine, Bronx, NY 10461, United States. (2)Integrated Research Facility at Fort Detrick, National Institute for Allergy and Infectious Diseases, National Institutes of Health, Frederick, MD 21702, United States. (3)United States Army Medical Research Institute of Infectious Diseases, Fort Detrick, Frederick, MD 21702, United States. (4)National Center of Microbiology, Instituto de Salud Carlos III, 28220 Madrid, Spain. (5)Department of Microbiology and Immunology, Albert Einstein College of Medicine, Bronx, NY 10461, United States. Electronic address: kartik.chandran@einstein.yu.edu.

Lloviu virus (LLOV), a phylogenetically divergent filovirus, is the proposed etiologic agent of die-offs of Schreibers's long-fingered bats (Miniopterus schreibersii) in western Europe. Studies of LLOV remain limited because the infectious agent has not yet been isolated. Here, we generated a recombinant vesicular stomatitis virus expressing the LLOV spike glycoprotein (GP) and used it to show that LLOV GP resembles other filovirus GP proteins in structure and function. LLOV GP must be cleaved by endosomal cysteine proteases during entry, but is much more protease-sensitive than EBOV GP. The EBOV/MARV receptor, Niemann-Pick C1 (NPC1), is also required for LLOV entry, and its second luminal domain is recognized with high affinity by a cleaved form of LLOV GP, suggesting that receptor binding would not impose a barrier to LLOV infection of humans and non-human primates. The use of NPC1 as an intracellular entry receptor may be a universal property of filoviruses.

PMCID: PMC4252868 [Available on 2015/11/1] PMID: 25310500 [PubMed - in process]

383. West J Emerg Med. 2014 Nov;15(7):728-31. doi: 10.5811/westjem.2014.9.24011. Epub 2014 Sep 26.

Ebola virus disease: essential public health principles for clinicians.

Koenig KL(1), Majestic C(1), Burns MJ(2).
Author information: (1)University of California at Irvine, Center for Disaster Medical Sciences and Department of Emergency Medicine, Orange, California. (2)University of California at Irvine, Department of Emergency Medicine and Department of Medicine, Division of Infectious Diseases, Orange, California.
Ebola Virus Disease (EVD) has become a public health emergency of international concern. The World Health Organization and Centers for Disease Control and Prevention have developed guidance to educate and inform healthcare workers and travelers worldwide. Symptoms of EVD include abrupt onset of fever, myalgias, and headache in the early phase, followed by vomiting, diarrhea and possible progression to hemorrhagic rash, life-threatening bleeding, and multi-organ failure in the later phase. The disease is not transmitted via airborne spread like influenza, but rather from person-to-person, or animal to person, via direct contact with bodily fluids or blood. It is crucial that emergency physicians be educated on disease presentation and how to generate a timely and accurate differential diagnosis that includes exotic diseases in the appropriate patient population. A patient should be evaluated for EVD when both suggestive symptoms, including unexplained hemorrhage, AND risk factors within 3 weeks prior, such as travel to an endemic area, direct handling of animals from outbreak areas, or ingestion of fruit or other uncooked foods contaminated with bat feces containing the virus are present. There are experimental therapies for treatment of EVD virus; however the mainstay of therapy is supportive care. Emergency department personnel on the frontlines must be prepared to rapidly identify and isolate febrile travelers if indicated. All healthcare workers involved in care of EVD patients should wear personal protective equipment. Despite the intense media focus on EVD rather than other threats, emergency physicians must master and follow essential public health principles for management of all infectious diseases. This includes not only identification and treatment of individuals, but also protection of healthcare workers and prevention of spread, keeping in mind the possibility of other more common disease processes.

PMCID: PMC4251210 PMID: 25493109 [PubMed - in process]

384. West J Emerg Med. 2014 Nov;15(7):723-727. Epub 2014 Oct 10.

Emergency Medical Services Public Health Implications and Interim Guidance for the Ebola Virus in the United States.

McCoy CE(1), Lotfipour S(1), Chakravarthy B(1), Schultz C(1), Barton E(1).
Author information: (1)University of California, Irvine, Department of Emergency Medicine, Orange, California.

The 25th known outbreak of the Ebola Virus Disease (EVD) is now a global public health emergency and the World Health Organization (WHO) has declared the epidemic to be a Public Health Emergency of International Concern (PHEIC). Since the first cases of the West African epidemic were reported in March 2014, there has been an increase in infection rates of over 13,000% over a 6-month period. The Ebola virus has now arrived in the United States and public health professionals, doctors, hospitals, Emergency Medial Services Administrators, Medical Directors, and policy makers have been working with haste to develop strategies to prevent the disease from reaching epidemic proportions. Prehospital care providers (emergency medical technicians and paramedics) and medical first responders (including but not limited to firefighters and law enforcement) are the healthcare systems front lines when it comes to first medical contact with patients outside of the hospital setting. Risk of contracting Ebola can be particularly high in this population of first responders if the appropriate precautions are not implemented. This article provides a brief clinical overview of the Ebola Virus Disease and provides a comprehensive summary of the Center for Disease Control and Prevention's Interim Guidance for Emergency Medical Services (EMS) Systems and 9-1-1 Public Safety Answering Points (PSAPS) for Management of Patients with Known of Suspected Ebola Virus Disease in the United States.

PMCID: PMC4251209 PMID: 25493108 [PubMed - as supplied by publisher]

385. Workplace Health Saf. 2014 Nov;62(11):484. doi: 10.3928/21650799-20141014-02.

Ebola virus disease epidemic.

Phillips JA.

The Ebola virus disease epidemic now constitutes an international public health emergency. Occupational and environmental health nurses can collaborate with international colleagues to halt Ebola virus transmission within Africa, protect workers from exposures, and prevent another pandemic. [Workplace Health Saf 2014;62(11):484.].

Copyright 2014, SLACK Incorporated.

PMID: 25373029 [PubMed - in process]

386. BMJ. 2014 Oct 31;349:g6584. doi: 10.1136/bmj.g6584.

Louisiana tells Ebola doctors to stay away from tropical medicine conference.

McCarthy M(1).
Author information: (1)Seattle.

PMID: 25361732 [PubMed - indexed for MEDLINE]

387. MMWR Morb Mortal Wkly Rep. 2014 Oct 31;63(43):984.

Announcement: Interim U.S. guidance for monitoring and movement of persons with potential Ebola virus exposure.

Centers for Disease Control and Prevention (CDC).

PMID: 25518066 [PubMed - indexed for MEDLINE]

388. MMWR Morb Mortal Wkly Rep. 2014 Oct 31;63(43):978-81.

Update: Ebola virus disease outbreak--West Africa, October 2014.

Incident Management System Ebola Epidemiology Team, CDC; Guinea Interministerial Committee for Response Against the Ebola Virus; CDC Guinea Response Team; Liberia Ministry of Health and Social Welfare; CDC Liberia Response Team; Sierra Leone Ministry of Health and Sanitation; CDC Sierra Leone Response Team; Viral Special Pathogens Branch, National Center for Emerging and Zoonotic Infectious Diseases, CDC; Centers for Disease Control and Prevention (CDC).

CDC is assisting ministries of health and working with other organizations to control and end the ongoing outbreak of Ebola virus disease (Ebola) in West Africa. The updated data in this report were compiled from situation reports from the Guinea Interministerial Committee for Response Against the Ebola Virus and the World Health Organization, the Liberia Ministry of Health and Social Welfare, and the Sierra Leone Ministry of Health and Sanitation. Total case counts include all suspected, probable, and confirmed cases as defined by each country. These data reflect reported cases, which make up an unknown proportion of all actual cases and reporting delays that vary from country to country.

PMID: 25356606 [PubMed - indexed for MEDLINE]

389. Nat Rev Drug Discov. 2014 Oct 31;13(11):812. doi: 10.1038/nrd4466.

Infectious disease: Durable protection against Ebola virus.

Crunkhorn S.

PMID: 25359380 [PubMed - in process]

390. Science. 2014 Oct 31;346(6209):666. doi: 10.1126/science.346.6209.666.

On the ground in Sierra Leone.

Gao GF(1), Feng Y(1).

Author information: (1)George F. Gao is deputy director general of the Chinese Center for Disease Control and Prevention. Yong Feng is director of the Division of African Affairs in the Department of International Cooperation at China's National Health and Family Planning Commission.

PMID: 25359978 [PubMed - indexed for MEDLINE]

391. Science. 2014 Oct 31;346(6209):534. doi: 10.1126/science.346.6209.534.

Infectious diseases. The Ebola vaccine underdog.

Link C Jr, Cohen J.

PMID: 25359944 [PubMed - indexed for MEDLINE]

392. BMJ. 2014 Oct 30;349:g6555. doi: 10.1136/bmj.g6555.

US nurse says she will fight Ebola quarantine.

McCarthy M(1).

Author information: (1)Seattle.

PMID: 25360033 [PubMed - in process]

393. BMJ. 2014 Oct 30;349:g6543. doi: 10.1136/bmj.g6543.

Doctors and politicians must unite in public health messages on Ebola, says expert.

Kmietowicz Z(1).

Author information: (1)The BMJ.

PMID: 25358540 [PubMed - in process]

394. Int J Nurs Stud. 2014 Oct 30;52(1):491. doi: 10.1016/j.ijnurstu.2014.10.012. [Epub ahead of print]

Threat of Ebola infection may lead nurses to adopt self-protection behaviours.

Jackson C(1).

Author information: (1)Department of Postgraduate Research, Florence Nightingale Faculty of Nursing and Midwifery, King's College London, Room 1.21a, James Clerk Maxwell Building, Waterloo Campus, 57 Waterloo Road, London SE1 8WA, United Kingdom. Electronic address: carole.jackson@kcl.ac.uk.

PMID: 25468133 [PubMed - as supplied by publisher]

395. N Engl J Med. 2014 Oct 30;371(18):1663-6. doi: 10.1056/NEJMp1410540. Epub 2014 Sep 10.

Ebola then and now.

Breman JG(1), Johnson KM.

Author information: (1)From the Fogarty International Center, National Institutes of Health, Bethesda, MD (J.G.B.); and Portland, OR (K.M.J.).

PMID: 25207624 [PubMed - indexed for MEDLINE]

396. Nature. 2014 Oct 30;514(7524):554-7. doi: 10.1038/514554a.

The Ebola questions.

Check Hayden E.

PMID: 25355344 [PubMed - indexed for MEDLINE]

397. Nature. 2014 Oct 30;514(7524):537. doi: 10.1038/514537a.

Developed nations must not fear sending Ebola help.

Inglis T(1).

Author information: (1)University of Western Australia in Nedlands.

PMID: 25355324 [PubMed - indexed for MEDLINE]

398. Nature. 2014 Oct 30;514(7524):535-6. doi: 10.1038/514535b.

Call to action.

[No authors listed]

PMID: 25355322 [PubMed - indexed for MEDLINE]

399. Disaster Med Public Health Prep. 2014 Oct 29:1-2. [Epub ahead of print]

Identify, Isolate, Inform: A 3-pronged Approach to Management of Public Health Emergencies.

Koenig KL(1).

Author information: (1)Center for Disaster Medical Sciences,University of California at Irvine,Orange,California.

During an evolving public health emergency, a simple algorithm for initial patient identification and management is essential for providers on the front lines. This article recommends a 3-pronged system of Identify, Isolate, Inform to describe the actions necessary in the first few minutes of encountering a potential Ebola patient. Application of the "vital sign zero" triage concept of early recognition of potential threats coupled with this novel algorithm will optimize protection of health care workers and the public health while concurrently providing a safe method for individual patient care. (Disaster Med Public Health Preparedness. 2014;0:1-2).

PMID: 25351772 [PubMed - as supplied by publisher]

400. Disaster Med Public Health Prep. 2014 Oct 29:1-2. [Epub ahead of print]

Ebola Triage Screening and Public Health: The New "Vital Sign Zero"

Koenig KL(1).

Author information: (1)Center for Disaster Medical Sciences,University of California at Irvine,Orange,California.

During public health emergencies of international concern such as the 2014 Ebola event, health care leaders need to educate clinicians on the front lines to make uncomfortable, but real triage decisions that focus on optimization of population health outcomes over individual care. Health care workers must consider their own protection first before direct contact with potentially contagious patients. In an era of globalization and emerging infectious disease, routine triage including evaluation of the standard vital signs must shift to include public health considerations with immediate consequences. A new "vital sign zero" should be taken at the time of initial patient evaluation to assess for risk and exposure to potentially contagious infectious diseases.

PMID: 25351634 [PubMed - as supplied by publisher]

401. Travel Med Infect Dis. 2014 Oct 29;12(6PA):682-683. doi: 10.1016/j.tmaid.2014.10.014. [Epub ahead of print]

Ebola virus disease: An emerging zoonosis with importance for travel medicine.

Cardona-Ospina JA(1), Giselle-Badillo A(1), Calvache-Benavides CE(1), Rodriguez-Morales AJ(2).

Author information: (1)Public Health and Infection Research Group and Incubator, Faculty of Health Sciences, Universidad Tecnologica de Pereira, Pereira, Risaralda, Colombia. (2)Working Group on Zoonoses, International Society for Chemotherapy, Public Health and Infection Research Group, Faculty of Health Sciences, Universidad Tecnologica de Pereira, Pereira, Risaralda, Colombia. Electronic address: arodriguezm@utp.edu.co.

PMID: 25467087 [PubMed - as supplied by publisher]

402. Viral Immunol. 2014 Oct 29. [Epub ahead of print]

The Multiple Roles of sGP in Ebola Pathogenesis.

de La Vega MA(1), Wong G, Kobinger GP, Qiu X.

Author information: (1)1 Special Pathogens Program, National Microbiology Laboratory, Public Health Agency of Canada , Winnipeg, Manitoba, Canada .

Abstract Ebola causes severe hemorrhagic fever in humans and nonhuman primates, and there are currently no approved therapeutic countermeasures. The virulence of Ebola virus (EBOV) may be partially attributed to the secreted glycoprotein (sGP), which is the main product transcribed from its GP gene. sGP is secreted from infected cells and can be readily detected in the serum of EBOV-infected hosts. This review summarizes the multiple roles that sGP may play during infection and highlights the implications for the future design of vaccines and treatments.

PMID: 25354393 [PubMed - as supplied by publisher]

403. Ann Intern Med. 2014 Oct 28. doi: 10.7326/M14-2255. [Epub ahead of print]

Effect of Ebola Progression on Transmission and Control in Liberia.

Yamin D, Gertler S, Ndeffo-Mbah ML, Skrip LA, Fallah M, Nyenswah TG, Altice FL, Galvani AP.

Background: The Ebola outbreak that is sweeping across West Africa is the largest, most volatile, and deadliest Ebola epidemic ever recorded. Liberia is the most profoundly affected country, with more than 3500 infections and 2000 deaths recorded in the past 3 months. Objective: To evaluate the contribution of disease progression and case fatality to transmission and to examine the potential for targeted interventions to eliminate the disease. Design: Stochastic transmission model that integrates epidemiologic and clinical data on incidence and case fatality, daily viral load among survivors and nonsurvivors evaluated on the basis of the 2000-2001 outbreak in Uganda, and primary data on contacts of patients with Ebola in Liberia. Setting: Montserrado County Liberia, July to September 2014. Measurements: Ebola incidence and case fatality records from 2014 Liberian Ministry of Health and Social Welfare. Results: The average number of secondary infections generated throughout the entire infectious period of a single infected case, R0, was estimated as 1.73 (95% CI, 1.66 to 1.83). There was substantial stratification between survivors (R0Survivors), for whom the estimate was 0.66 (CI, 0.10 to 1.69) and nonsurvivors (the R0Nonsurvivors), for whom the estimate was 2.36 (CI, 1.72 to 2.80). The nonsurvivors had the highest risk for transmitting the virus later in the course of disease progression. Consequently, the isolation of 75% of infected individuals in critical condition within 4 days from symptom onset has a high chance of eliminating the disease. Limitations: Projections are based on the initial dynamics of the epidemic, which may change as the outbreak and interventions evolve. Conclusion: These results underscore the importance of isolating the most severely ill patients with Ebola within the first few days of their symptomatic phase. Primary Funding Source: National Institutes of Health.

PMID: 25347321 [PubMed - as supplied by publisher]

404. BMJ. 2014 Oct 28;349:g6499. doi: 10.1136/bmj.g6499.

CDC rejects mandatory quarantine for travelers arriving from Ebola stricken nations.

McCarthy M(1).

Author information: (1)Seattle.

PMID: 25352542 [PubMed - in process]

405. BMJ. 2014 Oct 28;349:g6497. doi: 10.1136/bmj.g6497.

EU appoints Ebola coordinator.

Watson R(1).

Author information: (1)Brussels.

PMID: 25351197 [PubMed - in process]

406. Nurs Stand. 2014 Oct 28;29(8):8. doi: 10.7748/ns.29.8.8.s4.

Clinicians deployed at more UK entry points as Ebola screening increases.

[No authors listed]

PMID: 25335584 [PubMed - in process]

407. Vet Pathol. 2014 Oct 28. pii: 0300985814556781. [Epub ahead of print]

Mission Critical: Mobilization of Essential Animal Models for Ebola, Nipah, and Machupo Virus Infections.

Zumbrun EE(1).

Author information: (1)Department of Pathology, Microbiology and Immunology, University of South Carolina School of Medicine, Columbia, SC, USA Elizabeth.Zumbrun@uscmed.sc.edu.

The reports for Ebola virus Zaire (EBOV), Nipah virus, and Machupo virus (MACV) pathogenesis, in this issue of Veterinary Pathology, are timely considering recent events, both nationally and internationally. EBOV, Nipah virus, and MACV cause highly lethal infections for which no Food and Drug Administration (FDA) licensed vaccines or therapies exist. Not only are there concerns that these agents could be used by those with malicious intent, but shifts in ecological distribution of viral reservoirs due to climate change or globalization could lead to more frequent infections within remote regions than previously seen as well as outbreaks in more populous areas. The current EBOV epidemic shows no sign of abating across 3 West African nations (as of October 2014), including densely populated areas, far outpacing infection rates of previous outbreaks. A limited number of cases have also arisen in the United States and Europe. With few treatment options for these deadly viruses, development of animal models reflective of human disease is paramount to combat these diseases. As an example of this potential, a new treatment compound, ZMapp, that had demonstrated efficacy against EBOV infection in nonhuman primates (NHPs) received an emergency compassionate use exception from the FDA for the treatment of 2 American medical workers infected with EBOV, and they are currently virus free and recovering.

© The Author(s) 2014.

PMID: 25352204 [PubMed - as supplied by publisher]

408. BMJ. 2014 Oct 27;349:g6469. doi: 10.1136/bmj.g6469.

Tough quarantine plans may hurt Ebola fight, Obama administration warns.

McCarthy M(1).

Author information: (1)Seattle.

PMID: 25348209 [PubMed - in process]

409. BMJ. 2014 Oct 27;349:g6468. doi: 10.1136/bmj.g6468.

US nurse who contracted Ebola leaves hospital.

McCarthy M(1).

Author information: (1)Seattle.

PMID: 25348101 [PubMed - in process]

410. Mod Healthc. 2014 Oct 27;44(43):29.

CDC demonstrates new Ebola protocols.

McKinney M.

PMID: 25509620 [PubMed - in process]

411. Mod Healthc. 2014 Oct 27;44(43):26.

Learning the lessons of Ebola as events continue to unfold.

Leavitt M.

PMID: 25509618 [PubMed - in process]

412. Mod Healthc. 2014 Oct 27;44(43):12.

Clumsy Ebola response tests country's faith in health leaders.

Johnson SR.

PMID: 25509614 [PubMed - in process]

413. Time. 2014 Oct 27;184(16):20-3.

The new Ebola protocols.

Von Drehle D.
PMID: 25509763 [PubMed - in process]
414. Travel Med Infect Dis. 2014 Oct 27;12(6PA):650-658. doi: 10.1016/j.tmaid.2014.10.015. [Epub ahead of print]

Risk of imported Ebola virus disease in China.

Chen T(1), Ka-Kit Leung R(2), Liu R(1), Chen F(1), Zhang X(1), Zhao J(1), Chen S(1).

Author information: (1)Changsha Center for Disease Control and Prevention, People's Republic of China. (2)Stanley Ho Centre for Emerging Infectious Diseases, Faculty of Medicine, The Chinese University of Hong Kong, Hong Kong Special Administrative Region. Electronic address: ross@cuhk.edu.hk.

BACKGROUND: More than 600,000 annual arrivals from Africa, 1.4 billion population and developing health care systems render China at non-negligible risk of imported Ebola virus disease (EVD). METHOD: According to the natural history of EVD, we constructed a deterministic SEIR model. Three published EVD outbreaks in Africa were enrolled to calculate the basic reproduction number (R0) of EVD. Scenarios representing unreported and reported (with n weeks delay) imported EVD in China were simulated to evaluate the effectiveness of interventions assumed to be implemented in different periods of the outbreaks. RESULTS: Based on previous Africa outbreak incidence datasets, our mathematical model predicted the basic reproduction number of EVD in the range of 1.53-3.54. Adopting EVD prevalence at 0.04-0.16% from the same datasets and estimated missing information and monitoring rates at 1-10%, a total of 6-194 imported cases were predicted. Be a single case left unidentified/unreported, total attack rate was predicted to reach 60.19%-96.74%. Curve fitting results showed that earlier intervention benefits in exponential and linear decrease in prevalence and duration of outbreak respectively. CONCLUSION: Based on past outbreak experience in China, there is a need to implement an internet-based surveillance and monitoring system in order to reinforce health policy, track suspected cases and protect the general public by timely interventions.

PMID: 25467086 [PubMed - as supplied by publisher]
415. Lancet. 2014 Oct 25;384(9953):1499-500. doi: 10.1016/S0140-6736(14)61839-0. Epub 2014 Oct 15.

Ebola control: effect of asymptomatic infection and acquired immunity.

Bellan SE(1), Pulliam JR(2), Dushoff J(3), Meyers LA(4).

Author information: (1)Center for Computational Biology and Bioinformatics, The University of Texas at Austin, Austin, TX 78712, USA. Electronic address: steve.bellan@gmail.com. (2)Department of Biology and Emerging Pathogens Institute, University of Florida, Gainesville, FL, USA; Fogarty International Center, National Institutes of Health, Bethesda, MD, USA. (3)Department of Biology and Institute of Infectious Disease Research, McMaster University, Hamilton, ON, Canada. (4)Department of Integrative Biology, The University of Texas at Austin, Austin, TX 78712, USA; Santa Fe Institute, Santa Fe, NM, USA.
PMID: 25390569 [PubMed - in process]
416. Lancet. 2014 Oct 25;384(9953):1489-90. doi: 10.1016/S0140-6736(14)61906-1. Epub 2014 Oct 22.

US federal health agencies questioned over Ebola response.

Jaffe S.
PMID: 25390564 [PubMed - in process]
417. Vet Rec. 2014 Oct 25;175(16):410. doi: 10.1136/vr.g6353.

Ebola and One Health.

Moore P(1).

Author information: (1)58 Crowtree Lane, Louth, Lincolnshire.
Comment on Vet Rec. 2014 Oct 18;175(15):361.
PMID: 25344047 [PubMed - in process]
418. BMJ. 2014 Oct 24;349:g6466. doi: 10.1136/bmj.g6466.

Vaccine tests to begin in Ebola countries this year.

Gulland A(1).

Author information: (1)London.
PMID: 25344380 [PubMed - in process]
419. BMJ. 2014 Oct 24;349:g6443. doi: 10.1136/bmj.g6443.

What stops healthcare workers volunteering to fight Ebola in west Africa?

Solomon T(1), Turtle L(2), McGill F(2), Matata C(2), Christley R(2).

Author information: (1)Institute of Infection and Global Health, University of Liverpool, Liverpool L69 7BE, UK tsolomon@liv.ac.uk. (2)Institute of Infection and Global Health, University of Liverpool, Liverpool L69 7BE, UK.
PMID: 25344225 [PubMed - in process]
420. BMJ. 2014 Oct 24;349:g6449. doi: 10.1136/bmj.g6449.

NHS staff readied to deal with Ebola cases in hospitals and general practices.

O'Dowd A(1).

Author information: (1)London.
PMID: 25344049 [PubMed - in process]
421. BMJ. 2014 Oct 24;349:g6453. doi: 10.1136/bmj.g6453.

Ebola diagnosed in doctor in New York City.

McCarthy M(1).

Author information: (1)Seattle.

PMID: 25343951 [PubMed - in process]

422. Disaster Med Public Health Prep. 2014 Oct 24:1-6. [Epub ahead of print]

Triage Management, Survival, and the Law in the Age of Ebola.

Burkle FM(1), Burkle CM(2).

Author information: (1)1Harvard Humanitarian Initiative,Harvard University,Cambridge,Massachusetts, andWoodrow Wilson International Center for Scholars,Washington,DC. (2)2Mayo Graduate School of Medicine,Mayo Clinic,Rochester,Minnesota.

Liberia, Sierra Leone, and Guinea lack the public health infrastructure, economic stability, and overall governance to stem the spread of Ebola. Even with robust outside assistance, the epidemiological data have not improved. Vital resource management is haphazard and left to the discretion of individual Ebola treatment units. Only recently has the International Health Regulations (IHR) and World Health Organization (WHO) declared Ebola a Public Health Emergency of International Concern, making this crisis their fifth ongoing level 3 emergency. In particular, the WHO has been severely compromised by post-2003 severe acute respiratory syndrome (SARS) staffing, budget cuts, a weakened IHR treaty, and no unambiguous legal mandate. Population-based triage management under a central authority is indicated to control the transmission and ensure fair and decisive resource allocation across all triage categories. The shared responsibilities critical to global health solutions must be realized and the rightful attention, sustained resources, and properly placed legal authority be assured within the WHO, the IHR, and the vulnerable nations. (Disaster Med Public Health Preparedness. 2014;0:1-6).

PMID: 25343493 [PubMed - as supplied by publisher]

423. Disaster Med Public Health Prep. 2014 Oct 24:1-2. [Epub ahead of print]

Sign Me Up: Rules of the Road for Humanitarian Volunteers During the Ebola Outbreak.

Wildes R(1), Kayden S(2), Goralnick E(3), Niescierenko M(4), Aschkenasy M(5), Kemen KM(6), Vanrooyen M(7), Biddinger P(8), Cranmer H(5).

Author information: (1)1Partners Healthcare Risk and Insurance Services,Boston,Massachusetts. (2)2Division of International Emergency Medicine and Humanitarian Programs,Department of Emergency Medicine,Brigham and Women's Hospital,Boston,Massachusetts. (3)3Brigham and Women's Healthcare,Boston,Massachusetts. (4)4Global Health Program,Boston Children's Hospital,Boston,Massachusetts. (5)5Center for Global Health,Massachusetts General Hospital,Boston,Massachusetts. (6)6Partners HealthCare Emergency Preparedness,Boston,Massachusetts. (7)7Harvard Humanitarian Initiative,Boston,Massachusetts. (8)8Partners Healthcare and Massachusetts General Hospital,Boston,Massachusetts.

The current Ebola outbreak is the worst global public health emergency of our generation, and our global health care community must and will rise to serve those affected. Aid organizations participating in the Ebola response must carefully plan to carry out their responsibility to ensure the health, safety, and security of their responders. At the same time, individual health care workers and their employers must evaluate the ability of an aid organization to protect its workers in the complex environment of this unheralded Ebola outbreak. We present a minimum set of operational standards developed by a consortium of Boston-based hospitals that a professional organization should have in place to ensure the health, safety, and security of its staff in response to the Ebola virus disease outbreak. (Disaster Med Public Health Preparedness. 2014;0:1-2).

PMID: 25343427 [PubMed - as supplied by publisher]

424. MMWR Morb Mortal Wkly Rep. 2014 Oct 24;63(42):959-65.

Control of Ebola virus disease - firestone district, liberia, 2014.

Reaves EJ, Mabande LG, Thoroughman DA, Arwady MA, Montgomery JM.

On March 30, 2014, the Ministry of Health and Social Welfare (MOHSW) of Liberia alerted health officials at Firestone Liberia, Inc. (Firestone) of the first known case of Ebola virus disease (Ebola) inside the Firestone rubber tree plantation of Liberia. The patient, who was the wife of a Firestone employee, had cared for a family member with confirmed Ebola in Lofa County, the epicenter of the Ebola outbreak in Liberia during March-April 2014. To prevent a large outbreak among Firestone's 8,500 employees, their dependents, and the surrounding population, the company responded by 1) establishing an incident management system, 2) instituting procedures for the early recognition and isolation of Ebola patients, 3) enforcing adherence to standard Ebola infection control guidelines, and 4) providing differing levels of management for contacts depending on their exposure, including options for voluntary quarantine in the home or in dedicated facilities. In addition, Firestone created multidisciplinary teams to oversee the outbreak response, address case detection, manage cases in a dedicated unit, and reintegrate convalescent patients into the community. The company also created a robust risk communication, prevention, and social mobilization campaign to boost community awareness of Ebola and how to prevent transmission. During August 1-September 23, a period of intense Ebola transmission in the surrounding areas, 71 cases of Ebola were diagnosed among the approximately 80,000 Liberians for whom Firestone provides health care (cumulative incidence = 0.09%). Fifty-seven (80%) of the cases were laboratory confirmed; 39 (68%) of these cases were fatal. Aspects of Firestone's response appear to have minimized the spread of Ebola in the local population and might be successfully implemented elsewhere to limit the spread of Ebola and prevent transmission to health care workers (HCWs).

PMID: 25340914 [PubMed - indexed for MEDLINE]

425. Philos Ethics Humanit Med. 2014 Oct 24;9(1):15. doi: 10.1186/1747-5341-9-15.

Ebola, epidemics, and ethics - what we have learned.

Donovan GK(1).

Author information: (1)Pellegrino Center for Clinical Bioethics, Georgetown University Medical School, Bldg, D, Rm 236, 4000 Reservoir Road, N.W., Washington, DC 20007-2197, USA. G.Kevin.Donovan@georgetown.edu.

The current Ebola epidemic has presented challenges both medical and ethical. Although we have known epidemics of untreatable diseases in the past, this particular one may be unique in the intensity and rapidity of its spread, as well as ethical challenges that it has created, exacerbated by its geographic location. We will look at the infectious agent and the epidemic it is causing, in order to understand the ethical problems that have arisen.
PMCID: PMC4209768 PMID: 25342227 [PubMed - in process]

426. Science. 2014 Oct 24;346(6208):434. doi: 10.1126/science.346.6208.434-a.

Ebola: social research overlooked.

Guerrier G(1).

Author information: (1)Hôtel-Dieu and Cochin Hospitals, Assistance Publique des Hôpitaux de Paris (AP-HP), Paris Descartes University, 75679, Paris, France. guerriergilles@gmail.com.

Comment on Science. 2014 Sep 12;345(6202):1228-9.

PMID: 25342794 [PubMed - indexed for MEDLINE]

427. Science. 2014 Oct 24;346(6208):433-4. doi: 10.1126/science.346.6208.433-b.

Ebola: public-private partnerships.

Reperant LA(1), van de Burgwal LH(2), Claassen E(3), Osterhaus AD(4).

Author information: (1)Artemis One Health Research Foundation, 3584 CL Utrecht, Netherlands. Department of Viroscience, Erasmus MC, 3000 CA Rotterdam, Netherlands. (2)Athena Institute, Vrije Universiteit Amsterdam, 1081 HV Amsterdam, Netherlands. (3)Artemis One Health Research Foundation, 3584 CL Utrecht, Netherlands. Athena Institute, Vrije Universiteit Amsterdam, 1081 HV Amsterdam, Netherlands. (4)Artemis One Health Research Foundation, 3584 CL Utrecht, Netherlands. Department of Viroscience, Erasmus MC, 3000 CA Rotterdam, Netherlands. a.osterhaus@erasmusmc.nl.

PMID: 25342793 [PubMed - indexed for MEDLINE]

428. Science. 2014 Oct 24;346(6208):433. doi: 10.1126/science.346.6208.433-a.

Ebola: mobility data.

Halloran ME(1), Vespignani A(2), Bharti N(3), Feldstein LR(4), Alexander KA(5), Ferrari M(3), Shaman J(6), Drake JM(7), Porco T(8), Eisenberg JN(9), Del Valle SY(10), Lofgren E(11), Scarpino SV(12), Eisenberg MC(9), Gao D(8), Hyman JM(13), Eubank S(14), Longini IM Jr(15).

Author information: (1)Fred Hutchinson Cancer Research Center, University of Washington, Seattle, WA 98109, USA. Department of Biostatistics, University of Washington, Seattle, WA 98195, USA. betz@u.washington.edu. (2)Department of Physics, Northeastern University, Boston, MA 02115, USA. (3)Department of Biology, Pennsylvania State University, University Park, PA 16802, USA. (4)Fred Hutchinson Cancer Research Center, University of Washington, Seattle, WA 98109, USA. Department of Epidemiology, University of Washington, Seattle, WA 98195, USA. (5)Department of Fish and Wildlife Conservation, Virginia Polytechnic Institute and State University, Blacksburg, VA 24061, USA. (6)Department of Environmental Health Sciences, Mailman School of Public Health, Columbia University, New York, NY 10032, USA. (7)Odum School of Ecology, University of Georgia, Athens, GA 30602, USA. (8)Francis I. Proctor Foundation, University of California, San Francisco, CA 94143, USA. (9)Department of Epidemiology, University of Michigan, Ann Arbor, MI 48109, USA. (10)Los Alamos National Laboratory, Los Alamos, NM 87545, USA. (11)Virginia Bioinformatics Institute, Virginia Polytechnic Institute and State University, Blacksburg, VA 24061, USA. (12)Santa Fe Institute, Santa Fe, NM 87501, USA. (13)Department of Mathematics, Tulane University, New Orleans, LA 70118, USA. (14)Virginia Bioinformatics Institute, Virginia Polytechnic Institute and State University, Blacksburg, VA 24061, USA. Department of Population Health Sciences, Virginia Polytechnic Institute and State University, Blacksburg, VA 24061, USA. (15)Department of Biostatistics, University of Florida, Gainesville, FL 32611, USA.

PMID: 25342792 [PubMed - indexed for MEDLINE]

429. BMJ. 2014 Oct 23;349:g6436. doi: 10.1136/bmj.g6436.

Ebola drug trial is to start next month.

Gulland A(1).

Author information: (1)London.

PMID: 25342503 [PubMed - in process]

430. Cell. 2014 Oct 23;159(3):477-486. doi: 10.1016/j.cell.2014.10.006. Epub 2014 Oct 16

Camouflage and Misdirection: The Full-On Assault of Ebola Virus Disease.

Misasi J(1), Sullivan NJ(2).

Author information: (1)Boston Children's Hospital, Department of Medicine, Division of Infectious Diseases, Boston, MA 02115, USA. (2)Vaccine Research Center, National Institute of Allergy and Infectious Diseases, National Institutes of Health, Bethesda, MD 20892, USA. Electronic address: njsull@mail.nih.gov.

Ebolaviruses cause a severe hemorrhagic fever syndrome that is rapidly fatal to humans and nonhuman primates. Ebola protein interactions with host cellular proteins disrupt type I and type II interferon responses, RNAi antiviral responses, antigen presentation, T-cell-dependent B cell responses, humoral antibodies, and cell-mediated immunity. This multifaceted approach to evasion and suppression of innate and adaptive immune responses in their target hosts leads to the severe immune dysregulation and "cytokine storm" that is characteristic of fatal ebolavirus infection. Here, we highlight some of the processes by which Ebola interacts with its mammalian hosts to evade antiviral defenses.
PMCID: PMC4243531 [Available on 2015/10/23] PMID: 25417101 [PubMed - as supplied by publisher]

431. Euro Surveill. 2014 Oct 23;19(42). pii: 20936.

Assessing the impact of travel restrictions on international spread of the 2014 West African Ebola epidemic.

Poletto C(1), Gomes MF, Pastore y Piontti A, Rossi L, Bioglio L, Chao DL, Longini IM, Halloran ME, Colizza V, Vespignani A.

Author information: (1)INSERM, UMR-S 1136, Institut Pierre Louis d Epidemiologie et de Sante Publique, Paris, France.

The quick spread of an Ebola outbreak in West Africa has led a number of countries and airline companies to issue travel bans to the affected areas. Considering data up to 31 Aug 2014, we assess the impact of the resulting traffic reductions with detailed numerical simulations of the international spread of the epidemic. Traffic reductions are shown to delay by only a few weeks the risk that the outbreak extends to new countries.

PMID: 25358040 [PubMed - in process]

432. N Engl J Med. 2014 Oct 23;371(17):1565-6. doi: 10.1056/NEJMp1411310. Epub 2014 Sep 24.

Doing today's work superbly well--treating Ebola with current tools.

Lamontagne F(1), Clément C, Fletcher T, Jacob ST, Fischer WA 2nd, Fowler RA.

Author information: (1)From the Centre de Recherche Clinique, Centre Hospitalier Universitaire de Sherbrooke, Sherbrooke, QC, Canada (F.L.); Réanimation Médicale, Polyclinique Bordeaux Nord Aquitaine, Bordeaux, France (C.C.); Liverpool School of Tropical Medicine, Liverpool, United Kingdom (T.F.); University of Washington, Seattle (S.T.J.); University of North Carolina at Chapel Hill, Chapel Hill (W.A.F.); and University of Toronto, Toronto (R.A.F.).

PMID: 25251518 [PubMed - indexed for MEDLINE]

433. BMJ. 2014 Oct 22;349:g6417. doi: 10.1136/bmj.g6417.

US revamps domestic Ebola response.

McCarthy M.

PMID: 25338759 [PubMed - indexed for MEDLINE]

434. BMJ. 2014 Oct 22;349:g6418. doi: 10.1136/bmj.g6418.

US issues new guidelines for health workers caring for Ebola patients.

McCarthy M(1).

Author information: (1)Seattle.

PMID: 25338723 [PubMed - indexed for MEDLINE]

435. Disaster Med Public Health Prep. 2014 Oct 22:1-6. [Epub ahead of print]

Hubris: The Recurring Pandemic.

Koch T(1).

Author information: (1)Department of Geography (Medical),University of British Columbia,1984 West Mall,Vancouver,BC,British Columbia,Canada.

The 2014 Ebola outbreak has been seen by many as a "perfect storm" and an unprecedented public health calamity. This article attempts to place this most current of epidemics, one currently struggling for pandemic status, in an historical frame. At least since the 1600s protocols and programs for the containment of epidemic disease have been known, and mapped. And yet it was almost six months after warnings about this epidemic were first sounded that incomplete programs of control and surveillance were instituted. In effect, we have forgotten the basics of what was once common knowledge in public health. Having placed our faith in bacteriology, virology, and pharmacology, we have forgotten the lessons learned, long ago. (Disaster Med Public Health Preparedness. 2014;0:1-6).

PMID: 25335430 [PubMed - as supplied by publisher]

436. Ann Intern Med. 2014 Oct 21. doi: 10.7326/M14-2312. [Epub ahead of print]

The Potential Ebola Virus-Infected Patient in the Ambulatory Care Setting: Preparing for the Worst Without Compromising Care.

Wu HM, Fairley JK, Steinberg J, Kozarsky P.

PMID: 25329137 [PubMed - as supplied by publisher]

437. BMJ. 2014 Oct 21;349:g6390. doi: 10.1136/bmj.g6390.

WHO will review its response to Ebola once outbreak is under control.

Kmietowicz Z(1).

Author information: (1)The BMJ.

PMID: 25336176 [PubMed - indexed for MEDLINE]

438. CMAJ. 2014 Oct 21;186(15):1170. doi: 10.1503/cmaj.114-0074.

Ebola eradication may need wider partnership.

Agoramoorthy G(1), Chakraborty C(1).

Author information: (1)College of Pharmacy and Health Care (Agoramoorthy), Tajen University, Yanpu, Pingtung, Taiwan; Department of Bioinformatics (Chakraborty), Galgotias University, Greater Noida, India.

PMCID: PMC4203610 [Available on 2015/10/21] PMID: 25332426 [PubMed - indexed for MEDLINE]

439. CMAJ. 2014 Oct 21;186(15):1129-30. doi: 10.1503/cmaj.141061. Epub 2014 Aug 19.

Experimental countermeasures against Ebola virus: current progress and an ethical conundrum.

Plummer FA(1), Wong G(2), Kobinger GP(2).

Author information: (1)National Microbiology Laboratory (Plummer, Kobinger), Public Health Agency of Canada; Department of Medical Microbiology (Plummer, Wong, Kobinger), University of Manitoba; Department of Immunology (Kobinger), University of Manitoba, Winnipeg, Man.; Department of Pathology and

Laboratory Medicine (Kobinger), University of Pennsylvania School of Medicine, Philadelphia, Pa. frank.plummer@phac-aspc.gc.ca. (2)National Microbiology Laboratory (Plummer, Kobinger), Public Health Agency of Canada; Department of Medical Microbiology (Plummer, Wong, Kobinger), University of Manitoba; Department of Immunology (Kobinger), University of Manitoba, Winnipeg, Man.; Department of Pathology and Laboratory Medicine (Kobinger), University of Pennsylvania School of Medicine, Philadelphia, Pa.

PMCID: PMC4203593 [Available on 2015/10/21] PMID: 25139506 [PubMed - indexed for MEDLINE]
440. CMAJ. 2014 Oct 21;186(15):E589. doi: 10.1503/cmaj.141010. Epub 2014 Aug 19.

Ebola.

Ibrahim A(1), Lee TC(2).

Author information: (1)Division of Infectious Diseases (Ibrahim, Lee) and Division of General Internal Medicine (Lee), Department of Medicine, McGill University Health Centre; McGill Centre for Quality Improvement (Lee), Montréal, Que. (2)Division of Infectious Diseases (Ibrahim, Lee) and Division of General Internal Medicine (Lee), Department of Medicine, McGill University Health Centre; McGill Centre for Quality Improvement (Lee), Montréal, Que. todd.lee@mcgill.ca.

PMCID: PMC4203626 [Available on 2015/10/21] PMID: 25139505 [PubMed - indexed for MEDLINE]
441. Lancet. 2014 Oct 21. pii: S0140-6736(14)61828-6. doi: 10.1016/S0140-6736(14)61828-6. [Epub ahead of print]

Assessment of the potential for international dissemination of Ebola virus via commercial air travel during the 2014 west African outbreak.

Bogoch II(1), Creatore MI(2), Cetron MS(3), Brownstein JS(4), Pesik N(5), Miniota J(2), Tam T(6), Hu W(2), Nicolucci A(2), Ahmed S(7), Yoon JW(2), Berry I(2), Hay SI(8), Anema A(9), Tatem AJ(10), MacFadden D(11), German M(2), Khan K(12).

Author information: (1)Department of Medicine, Division of Infectious Diseases, University of Toronto, Toronto, ON, Canada; Divisions of Internal Medicine and Infectious Diseases, University Health Network, Toronto, ON, Canada. (2)Centre for Research on Inner City Health, Li Ka Shing Knowledge Institute, St Michael's Hospital, Toronto, ON, Canada. (3)Division of Global Migration and Quarantine, Centers for Disease Control and Prevention, Atlanta, GA, USA. (4)Center for Biomedical Informatics, Harvard Medical School, Boston, MA, USA; Children's Hospital Informatics Program, Boston Children's Hospital Boston, MA, USA. (5)Quarantine and Border Health Services Branch, Division of Global Migration and Quarantine, Centers for Disease Control and Prevention, Atlanta, GA, USA. (6)Health Security Infrastructure Branch, Public Health Agency of Canada, Ottawa, ON, Canada. (7)Schulich School of Medicine & Dentistry, University of Western Ontario, London, ON, Canada. (8)Fogarty International Center, National Institutes of Health, Bethesda, MD, USA; Spatial Ecology and Epidemiology Group, Department of Zoology, University of Oxford, Oxford, UK. (9)Children's Hospital Informatics Program, Boston Children's Hospital Boston, MA, USA; Department of Medicine, Faculty of Medicine, University of British Columbia, Vancouver, BC, Canada. (10)Fogarty International Center, National Institutes of Health, Bethesda, MD, USA; Department of Geography and Environment, University of Southampton, Southampton, UK; Flowminder Foundation, Stockholm, Sweden. (11)Department of Medicine, Division of Infectious Diseases, University of Toronto, Toronto, ON, Canada. (12)Department of Medicine, Division of Infectious Diseases, University of Toronto, Toronto, ON, Canada; Centre for Research on Inner City Health, Li Ka Shing Knowledge Institute, St Michael's Hospital, Toronto, ON, Canada. Electronic address: khank@smh.ca.

BACKGROUND: The WHO declared the 2014 west African Ebola epidemic a public health emergency of international concern in view of its potential for further international spread. Decision makers worldwide are in need of empirical data to inform and implement emergency response measures. Our aim was to assess the potential for Ebola virus to spread across international borders via commercial air travel and assess the relative efficiency of exit versus entry screening of travellers at commercial airports. METHODS: We analysed International Air Transport Association data for worldwide flight schedules between Sept 1, 2014, and Dec 31, 2014, and historic traveller flight itinerary data from 2013 to describe expected global population movements via commercial air travel out of Guinea, Liberia, and Sierra Leone. Coupled with Ebola virus surveillance data, we modelled the expected number of internationally exported Ebola virus infections, the potential effect of air travel restrictions, and the efficiency of airport-based traveller screening at international ports of entry and exit. We deemed individuals initiating travel from any domestic or international airport within these three countries to have possible exposure to Ebola virus. We deemed all other travellers to have no significant risk of exposure to Ebola virus. FINDINGS: Based on epidemic conditions and international flight restrictions to and from Guinea, Liberia, and Sierra Leone as of Sept 1, 2014 (reductions in passenger seats by 51% for Liberia, 66% for Guinea, and 85% for Sierra Leone), our model projects 2·8 travellers infected with Ebola virus departing the above three countries via commercial flights, on average, every month. 91 547 (64%) of all air travellers departing Guinea, Liberia, and Sierra Leone had expected destinations in low-income and lower-middle-income countries. Screening international travellers departing three airports would enable health assessments of all travellers at highest risk of exposure to Ebola virus infection. INTERPRETATION: Decision makers must carefully balance the potential harms from travel restrictions imposed on countries that have Ebola virus activity against any potential reductions in risk from Ebola virus importations. Exit screening of travellers at airports in Guinea, Liberia, and Sierra Leone would be the most efficient frontier at which to assess the health status of travellers at risk of Ebola virus exposure, however, this intervention might require international support to implement effectively. FUNDING: Canadian Institutes of Health Research.

PMID: 25458732 [PubMed - as supplied by publisher]
442. Lancet. 2014 Oct 21. pii: S0140-6736(14)61895-X. doi: 10.1016/S0140-6736(14)61895-X. [Epub ahead of print]

Ebola: worldwide dissemination risk and response priorities.

Cowling BJ(1), Yu H(2).

Author information: (1)School of Public Health, Li Ka Shing Faculty of Medicine, The University of Hong Kong, Hong Kong Special Administrative Region, China. (2)Division of Infectious Disease, Key Laboratory of Surveillance and Early-warning on Infectious Disease, Chinese Center for Disease Control and Prevention, Beijing 102206, China. Electronic address: yuhj@chinacdc.cn.

PMID: 25458730 [PubMed - as supplied by publisher]

443. Nurs Stand. 2014 Oct 21;29(7):9. doi: 10.7748/ns.29.7.9.s6.

British nurses form part of military's latest west African Ebola mission.

Kleebauer A.

Military nurses are part of the British military personnel travelling to west Africa this week to care for healthcare workers with suspected Ebola.

PMID: 25315527 [PubMed - in process]

444. BMJ. 2014 Oct 20;349:g6333. doi: 10.1136/bmj.g6333.

Obama calls for calm as US ramps up domestic Ebola response.

McCarthy M(1).

Author information: (1)Seattle.

PMID: 25330915 [PubMed - indexed for MEDLINE]

445. East Mediterr Health J. 2014 Oct 20;20(10):656-60.

Preventing the introduction of Ebola virus into the Eastern Mediterranean Region: enhanced preparedness is the key.

Malik MR(1), Mahjour J(2), Alwan A(3).

Author information: (1)Regional Adviser, Pandemic and Epidemic Diseases, Department of Communicable Diseases, World Health Organization Regional Office for the Eastern Mediterranean, Cairo Egypt. (2)Director, Department of Communicable Diseases, World Health Organization Regional Office for the Eastern Mediterranean, Cairo Egypt. (3)Regional Director, World Health Organization Regional Office for the Eastern Mediterranean, Cairo Egypt.

PMID: 25356698 [PubMed - in process]

446. Mod Healthc. 2014 Oct 20;44(42):8-9.

CDC and hospitals hit reset on Ebola preparedness.

Kutscher B, Robeznieks A, Rubenfire A.

PMID: 25513690 [PubMed - in process]

447. Lancet. 2014 Oct 18;384(9952):1424. doi: 10.1016/S0140-6736(14)61856-0. Epub 2014 Oct 17.

Ebola crisis: beliefs and behaviours warrant urgent attention.

Bayntun C(1), Houlihan C(2), Edmunds J(2).

Author information: (1)London School of Hygiene & Tropical Medicine, London WC1E 7HT, UK. Electronic address: clairebayntun@doctors.org.uk. (2)London School of Hygiene & Tropical Medicine, London WC1E 7HT, UK.

PMID: 25390320 [PubMed - in process]

448. Lancet. 2014 Oct 18;384(9952):1423-4. doi: 10.1016/S0140-6736(14)61734-7. Epub 2014 Oct 13.

Randomised controlled trials for Ebola: practical and ethical issues.

Adebamowo C(1), Bah-Sow O(2), Binka F(3), Bruzzone R(4), Caplan A(5), Delfraissy JF(6), Heymann D(7), Horby P(8), Kaleebu P(9), Tamfum JJ(10), Olliaro P(11), Piot P(12), Tejan-Cole A(13), Tomori O(14), Toure A(15), Torreele E(16), Whitehead J(17).

Author information: (1)National Health Research Ethics Committee, Abuja, Nigeria. (2)Hôpital National Ignace Deen, Conakry, Guinea. (3)University of Health and Allied Sciences, Ho, Ghana. (4)Hong Kong University-Pasteur Research Pole, School of Public Health, University of Hong Kong, Hong Kong, China. (5)New York University Langone Medical Center, New York, NY, USA. (6)Institut de Microbiologie et Maladies Infectieuses and INSERM, Paris, France. (7)Centre on Global Health Security, Chatham House, London, UK. (8)University of Oxford, Oxford, UK. (9)Medical Research Council, Uganda Virus Research Institute, Entebbe, Uganda. (10)Institut National de Recherche Biomedicale, Kinshasa, DR Congo. (11)WHO, Geneva, Switzerland; University of Oxford, Oxford, UK. Electronic address: piero.olliaro@ndm.ox.ac.uk. (12)London School of Hygiene & Tropical Medicine, London, UK. (13)Open Society Initiative for West Africa, Dakar, Senegal. (14)Nigerian Academy of Science, Lagos, Nigeria. (15)Institut Pasteur Dakar, Dakar, Senegal. (16)Open Society Foundations, New York, NY, USA. (17)Lancaster University, Lancaster, UK.

Comment in Lancet. 2014 Nov 8;384(9955):1667.

PMID: 25390318 [PubMed - in process]

449. Lancet. 2014 Oct 18;384(9952):1409-11.

Controlling Ebola: next steps.

Dhillon RS, Srikrishna D, Sachs J.

PMID: 25308287 [PubMed - in process]

450. Vet Rec. 2014 Oct 18;175(15):361. doi: 10.1136/vr.g6222.

Ebola and dogs: WSAVA calls for testing not automatic euthanasia.

[No authors listed]

Comment in Vet Rec. 2014 Oct 25;175(16):410.

PMID: 25324404 [PubMed - in process]

451. ACS Chem Biol. 2014 Oct 17;9(10):2263-73. doi: 10.1021/cb5006454. Epub 2014 Aug 26

Synthetic antibodies with a human framework that protect mice from lethal Sudan ebolavirus challenge.

Chen G(1), Koellhoffer JF, Zak SE, Frei JC, Liu N, Long H, Ye W, Nagar K, Pan G, Chandran K, Dye JM, Sidhu SS, Lai JR.

Author information: (1)Banting and Best Department of Medical Research, Terrence Donnelly Centre for Cellular and Biomolecular Research, University of Toronto , 160 College Street, Toronto, ON, Canada M5S 3E1.

The ebolaviruses cause severe and rapidly progressing hemorrhagic fever. There are five ebolavirus species; although much is known about Zaire ebolavirus (EBOV) and its neutralization by antibodies, little is known about Sudan ebolavirus (SUDV), which is emerging with increasing frequency. Here we describe monoclonal antibodies containing a human framework that potently inhibit infection by SUDV and protect mice from lethal challenge. The murine antibody 16F6, which binds the SUDV envelope glycoprotein (GP), served as the starting point for design. Sequence and structural alignment revealed similarities between 16F6 and YADS1, a synthetic antibody with a humanized scaffold. A focused phage library was constructed and screened to impart 16F6-like recognition properties onto the YADS1 scaffold. A panel of 17 antibodies were characterized and found to have a range of neutralization potentials against a pseudotype virus infection model. Neutralization correlated with GP binding as determined by ELISA. Two of these clones, E10 and F4, potently inhibited authentic SUDV and conferred protection and memory immunity in mice from lethal SUDV challenge. E10 and F4 were further shown to bind to the same epitope on GP as 16F6 with comparable affinities. These antibodies represent strong immunotherapeutic candidates for treatment of SUDV infection.

PMCID: PMC4201348 PMID: 25140871 [PubMed - in process]

452. BMJ. 2014 Oct 17;349:g6288. doi: 10.1136/bmj.g6288.

Ebola: How well is the UK prepared?

Coombes R(1), Arie S(1).

Author information: (1)The BMJ, London, UK.

PMID: 25354397 [PubMed - in process]

453. BMJ. 2014 Oct 17;349:g6305. doi: 10.1136/bmj.g6305.

Fifteen countries are at risk of Ebola outbreak, says WHO.

Gulland A(1).

Author information: (1)London.

PMID: 25326005 [PubMed - in process]

454. Disaster Med Public Health Prep. 2014 Oct 17:1-5. [Epub ahead of print]

A Primer on Ebola for Clinicians.

Toner E(1), Adalja A(1), Inglesby T(1).

Author information: (1)IUPMC Center for Health Security,Baltimore,Maryland.

The size of the world's largest Ebola outbreak now ongoing in West Africa makes clear that further exportation of Ebola virus disease to other parts of the world will remain a real possibility for the indefinite future. Clinicians outside of West Africa, particularly those who work in emergency medicine, critical care, infectious diseases, and infection control, should be familiar with the fundamentals of Ebola virus disease, including its diagnosis, treatment, and control. In this article we provide basic information on the Ebola virus and its epidemiology and microbiology. We also describe previous outbreaks and draw comparisons to the current outbreak with a focus on the public health measures that have controlled past outbreaks. We review the pathophysiology and clinical features of the disease, highlighting diagnosis, treatment, and hospital infection control issues that are relevant to practicing clinicians. We reference official guidance and point out where important uncertainty or controversy exists. (Disaster Med Public Health Preparedness. 2014;0:1-5).

PMID: 25325294 [PubMed - as supplied by publisher]

455. Disaster Med Public Health Prep. 2014 Oct 17:1-4. [Epub ahead of print]

Ebola Outbreak Response: The Role of Information Resources and the National Library of Medicine.

Love CB(1), Arnesen SJ(1), Phillips SJ(2).

Author information: (1)Disaster Information Management Research Center,Specialized Information Services Division,National Library of Medicine,Bethesda,Maryland. (2)National Library of Medicine,Specialized Information Services,Bethesda,Maryland.

The US National Library of Medicine (NLM) offers Internet-based, no-cost resources useful for responding to the 2014 West Africa Ebola outbreak. Resources for health professionals, planners, responders, and researchers include PubMed, Disaster Lit, the Web page "Ebola Outbreak 2014: Information Resources," and the Virus Variation database of sequences for Ebolavirus. In cooperation with participating publishers, NLM offers free access to full-text articles from over 650 biomedical journals and 4000 online reference books through the Emergency Access Initiative. At the start of a prolonged disaster event or disease outbreak, the documents and information of most immediate use may not be in the peer-reviewed biomedical journal literature. To maintain current awareness may require using any of the following: news outlets; social media; preliminary online data, maps, and situation reports; and documents published by nongovernmental organizations, international associations, and government agencies. Similar to the pattern of interest shown in the news and social media, use of NLM Ebola-related resources is also increasing since the start of the outbreak was first reported in March 2014 (Disaster Med Public Health Preparedness. 2014;0:1-4).

PMID: 25325189 [PubMed - as supplied by publisher]

456. MMWR Morb Mortal Wkly Rep. 2014 Oct 17;63(41):934-6.

Surveillance and preparedness for Ebola virus disease -- New York City, 2014.

Benowitz I, Ackelsberg J, Balter SE, Baumgartner JC, Dentinger C, Fine AD, Harper SA, Jones LE, Laraque F, Lee EH, Merizalde G, Yacisin KA, Varma JK, Layton MC; Centers for Disease Control and Prevention (CDC).

In July 2014, as the Ebola virus disease (Ebola) epidemic expanded in Guinea, Liberia, and Sierra Leone, an air traveler brought Ebola to Nigeria and two American health care workers in West Africa were diagnosed with Ebola and later medically evacuated to a U.S. hospital. New York City (NYC) is a frequent port of entry for travelers from West Africa, a home to communities of West African immigrants who travel back to their home countries, and a home to health care workers who travel to West Africa to treat Ebola patients. Ongoing transmission of Ebolavirus in West Africa could result in an infected person arriving in NYC. The announcement on September 30 of an Ebola case diagnosed in Texas in a person who had recently arrived from an Ebola-affected country further reinforced the need in NYC for local preparedness for Ebola.

PMID: 25321072 [PubMed - indexed for MEDLINE]

457. MMWR Morb Mortal Wkly Rep. 2014 Oct 17;63(41):930-3.

Developing an incident management system to support Ebola response -- Liberia, July-August 2014.

Pillai SK, Nyenswah T, Rouse E, Arwady MA, Forrester JD, Hunter JC, Matanock A, Ayscue P, Monroe B, Schafer IJ, Poblano L, Neatherlin J, Montgomery JM, De Cock KM; Centers for Disease Control and Prevention (CDC).

The ongoing Ebola virus disease (Ebola) outbreak in West Africa is the largest and most sustained Ebola epidemic recorded, with 6,574 cases. Among the five affected countries of West Africa (Liberia, Sierra Leone, Guinea, Nigeria, and Senegal), Liberia has had the highest number cases (3,458). This epidemic has severely strained the public health and health care infrastructure of Liberia, has resulted in restrictions in civil liberties, and has disrupted international travel. As part of the initial response, the Liberian Ministry of Health and Social Welfare (MOHSW) developed a national task force and technical expert committee to oversee the management of the Ebola-related activities. During the third week of July 2014, CDC deployed a team of epidemiologists, data management specialists, emergency management specialists, and health communicators to assist MOHSW in its response to the growing Ebola epidemic. One aspect of CDC's response was to work with MOHSW in instituting incident management system (IMS) principles to enhance the organization of the response. This report describes MOHSW's Ebola response structure as of mid-July, the plans made during the initial assessment of the response structure, the implementation of interventions aimed at improving the system, and plans for further development of the response structure for the Ebola epidemic in Liberia.

PMID: 25321071 [PubMed - indexed for MEDLINE]

458. MMWR Morb Mortal Wkly Rep. 2014 Oct 17;63(41):925-9.

Cluster of Ebola cases among Liberian and U.S. health care workers in an Ebola treatment unit and adjacent hospital -- Liberia, 2014.

Forrester JD, Hunter JC, Pillai SK, Arwady MA, Ayscue P, Matanock A, Monroe B, Schafer IJ, Nyenswah TG, De Cock KM; Centers for Disease Control and Prevention (CDC).

The ongoing Ebola virus disease (Ebola) epidemic in West Africa, like previous Ebola outbreaks, has been characterized by amplification in health care settings and increased risk for health care workers (HCWs), who often do not have access to appropriate personal protective equipment. In many locations, Ebola treatment units (ETUs) have been established to optimize care of patients with Ebola while maintaining infection control procedures to prevent transmission of Ebola virus. These ETUs are considered essential to containment of the epidemic. In July 2014, CDC assisted the Ministry of Health and Social Welfare of Liberia in investigating a cluster of five Ebola cases among HCWs who became ill while working in an ETU, an adjacent general hospital, or both. No common source of exposure or chain of transmission was identified. However, multiple opportunities existed for transmission of Ebola virus to HCWs, including exposure to patients with undetected Ebola in the hospital, inadequate use of personal protective equipment during cleaning and disinfection of environmental surfaces in the hospital, and potential transmission from an ill HCW to another HCW. No evidence was found of a previously unrecognized mode of transmission. Prevention recommendations included reinforcement of existing infection control guidance for both ETUs and general medical care settings, including measures to prevent cross-transmission in co-located facilities.

PMID: 25321070 [PubMed - indexed for MEDLINE]

459. Science. 2014 Oct 17;346(6207):289-90. doi: 10.1126/science.346.6207.289.

Infectious Diseases. Ebola vaccine trials raise ethical issues.

Cohen J, Kupferschmidt K.

PMID: 25324364 [PubMed - indexed for MEDLINE]

460. Viruses. 2014 Oct 17;6(10):3837-54. doi: 10.3390/v6103837.

A loop region in the N-terminal domain of Ebola virus VP40 is important in viral assembly, budding, and egress.

Adu-Gyamfi E(1), Soni SP(2), Jee CS(3), Digman MA(4), Gratton E(5), Stahelin RV(6).

Author information: (1)Department of Chemistry and Biochemistry, the Eck Institute for Global Health, University of Notre Dame, Notre Dame, IN 46556, USA. adugee@gmail.com. (2)Department of Biochemistry and Molecular Biology, Indiana University School of Medicine-South Bend, South Bend, IN 46617, USA. ssoni@iupui.edu. (3)Department of Chemistry and Biochemistry, the Eck Institute for Global Health, University of Notre Dame, Notre Dame, IN 46556, USA. clarasyjee@gmail.com. (4)Department of Biomedical Engineering, University of California, Irvine, CA 92697, USA. mdigman1@gmail.com. (5)Department of Biomedical Engineering, University of California, Irvine, CA 92697, USA. egratton@uci.edu. (6)Department of Chemistry and Biochemistry, the Eck Institute for Global Health, University of Notre Dame, Notre Dame, IN 46556, USA. rstaheli@iu.edu.

Ebola virus (EBOV) causes viral hemorrhagic fever in humans and can have clinical fatality rates of ~60%. The EBOV genome consists of negative sense RNA that encodes seven proteins including viral protein 40 (VP40). VP40 is the major Ebola virus matrix protein and regulates assembly and egress of infectious Ebola virus particles. It is well established that VP40 assembles on the inner leaflet of the plasma membrane of human cells to regulate viral budding where VP40 can produce virus like particles (VLPs) without other Ebola virus proteins present. The mechanistic details, however, of VP40 lipid-interactions and protein-protein interactions that are important for viral release remain to be elucidated. Here, we mutated a loop region in the N-terminal domain of VP40

(Lys127, Thr129, and Asn130) and find that mutations (K127A, T129A, and N130A) in this loop region reduce plasma membrane localization of VP40. Additionally, using total internal reflection fluorescence microscopy and number and brightness analysis we demonstrate these mutations greatly reduce VP40 oligomerization. Lastly, VLP assays demonstrate these mutations significantly reduce VLP release from cells. Taken together, these studies identify an important loop region in VP40 that may be essential to viral egress.

PMCID: PMC4213565 PMID: 25330123 [PubMed - in process]

461. Ann Intern Med. 2014 Oct 16. doi: 10.7326/M14-2289. [Epub ahead of print]

Caring for Patients With Ebola: A Challenge in Any Care Facility.

Kortepeter MG, Smith PW, Hewlett A, Cieslak TJ.

PMID: 25320965 [PubMed - as supplied by publisher]

462. BMJ. 2014 Oct 16;349:g6277. doi: 10.1136/bmj.g6277.

Second US nurse with Ebola had traveled by plane.

McCarthy M(1).

Author information: (1)Seattle.

PMID: 25324208 [PubMed - in process]

463. Immunity. 2014 Oct 16;41(4):515-7. doi: 10.1016/j.immuni.2014.10.001.

New hope in the search for Ebola virus treatments.

Basler CF(1).

Author information: (1)Department of Microbiology, Icahn School of Medicine at Mount Sinai, New York, NY 10029, USA. Electronic address: chris.basler@mssm.edu.

Comment on Nature. 2014 Oct 2;514(7520):47-53.

Because of its lethality, the Ebola virus often appears to be an invincible adversary. In Nature, Qiu et al. (2014) recently described the complete protection of nonhuman primates from deadly Ebola virus disease, even when treatment was begun as late as 5 days after infection.

PMID: 25367568 [PubMed - in process]

464. N Engl J Med. 2014 Oct 16;371(16):1481-95. doi: 10.1056/NEJMoa1411100. Epub 2014 Sep 22.

Ebola virus disease in West Africa--the first 9 months of the epidemic and forward projections.

WHO Ebola Response Team.

Collaborators: Aylward B, Barboza P, Bawo L, Bertherat E, Bilivogui P, Blake I, Brennan R, Briand S, Chakauya JM, Chitala K, Conteh RM, Cori A, Croisier A, Dangou JM, Diallo B, Donnelly CA, Dye C, Eckmanns T, Ferguson NM, Formenty P, Fuhrer C, Fukuda K, Garske T, Gasasira A, Gbanyan S, Graaff P, Heleze E, Jambai A, Jombart T, Kasolo F, Kadiobo AM, Keita S, Kertesz D, Koné M, Lane C, Markoff J, Massaquoi M, Mills H, Mulba JM, Musa E, Myhre J, Nasidi A, Nilles E, Nouvellet P, Nshimirimana D, Nuttall I, Nyenswah T, Olu O, Pendergast S, Perea W, Polonsky J, Riley S, Ronveaux O, Sakoba K, Santhana Gopala Krishnan R, Senga M, Shuaib F, Van Kerkhove MD, Vaz R, Wijekoon Kannangarage N, Yoti Z.

Comment in N Engl J Med. 2014 Oct 16;371(16):1545-6.

BACKGROUND: On March 23, 2014, the World Health Organization (WHO) was notified of an outbreak of Ebola virus disease (EVD) in Guinea. On August 8, the WHO declared the epidemic to be a "public health emergency of international concern." METHODS: By September 14, 2014, a total of 4507 probable and confirmed cases, including 2296 deaths from EVD (Zaire species) had been reported from five countries in West Africa--Guinea, Liberia, Nigeria, Senegal, and Sierra Leone. We analyzed a detailed subset of data on 3343 confirmed and 667 probable Ebola cases collected in Guinea, Liberia, Nigeria, and Sierra Leone as of September 14. RESULTS: The majority of patients are 15 to 44 years of age (49.9% male), and we estimate that the case fatality rate is 70.8% (95% confidence interval [CI], 69 to 73) among persons with known clinical outcome of infection. The course of infection, including signs and symptoms, incubation period (11.4 days), and serial interval (15.3 days), is similar to that reported in previous outbreaks of EVD. On the basis of the initial periods of exponential growth, the estimated basic reproduction numbers (R0) are 1.71 (95% CI, 1.44 to 2.01) for Guinea, 1.83 (95% CI, 1.72 to 1.94) for Liberia, and 2.02 (95% CI, 1.79 to 2.26) for Sierra Leone. The estimated current reproduction numbers (R) are 1.81 (95% CI, 1.60 to 2.03) for Guinea, 1.51 (95% CI, 1.41 to 1.60) for Liberia, and 1.38 (95% CI, 1.27 to 1.51) for Sierra Leone; the corresponding doubling times are 15.7 days (95% CI, 12.9 to 20.3) for Guinea, 23.6 days (95% CI, 20.2 to 28.2) for Liberia, and 30.2 days (95% CI, 23.6 to 42.3) for Sierra Leone. Assuming no change in the control measures for this epidemic, by November 2, 2014, the cumulative reported numbers of confirmed and probable cases are predicted to be 5740 in Guinea, 9890 in Liberia, and 5000 in Sierra Leone, exceeding 20,000 in total. CONCLUSIONS: These data indicate that without drastic improvements in control measures, the numbers of cases of and deaths from EVD are expected to continue increasing from hundreds to thousands per week in the coming months.

PMCID: PMC4235004 [Available on 2015/4/16] PMID: 25244186 [PubMed - indexed for MEDLINE]

465. N Engl J Med. 2014 Oct 16;371(16):1545-6. doi: 10.1056/NEJMe1411471. Epub 2014 Sep 22.

The Ebola emergency--immediate action, ongoing strategy.

Farrar JJ(1), Piot P.

Author information: (1)From the Wellcome Trust (J.J.F.) and the London School of Hygiene and Tropical Medicine (P.P.) - both in London.

Comment on N Engl J Med. 2014 Oct 16;371(16):1481-95.

PMID: 25244185 [PubMed - indexed for MEDLINE]

466. Nature. 2014 Oct 16;514(7522):299-300. doi: 10.1038/514299a.

Ebola: learn from the past.

Heymann DL.

PMID: 25318509 [PubMed - indexed for MEDLINE]

467. Nature. 2014 Oct 16;514(7522):284-5. doi: 10.1038/514284a.

Ebola by the numbers: The size, spread and cost of an outbreak.

Butler D, Morello L.

PMID: 25318501 [PubMed - indexed for MEDLINE]

468. Transfus Apher Sci. 2014 Oct 16;51(2):120-125. doi: 10.1016/j.transci.2014.10.003. [Epub ahead of print]

Ebola virus convalescent blood products: Where we are now and where we may need to go.

Burnouf T(1), Seghatchian J(2).

Author information: (1)Graduate Institute of Biomedical Materials and Tissue Engineering, College of Oral Medicine, Taipei Medical University, Taipei, Taiwan. Electronic address: thburnouf@gmail.com. (2)International Consultancy in Blood Components Quality/Safety Improvements, Audit/Inspection and DDR Strategy, London, UK. Electronic address: jseghatchian@btopenworld.com.

The world is regularly exposed to emerging infections with the potential to burst into a pandemic. One possible way to treat patients, when no other treatment is yet developed, is passive immunization performed by transfusing blood, plasma or plasma immunoglobulin fractions obtained from convalescent donors who have recovered from the disease and have developed protective antibodies. The most recent on-going epidemic is caused by the Ebola virus, a filovirus responsible for Ebola virus disease, a severe, often lethal, hemorrhagic fever. Recently, the use of convalescent blood products was proposed by the WHO as one early option for treating patients with Ebola virus disease. This publication provides an overview of the various convalescent blood products and technological options that could theoretically be considered when there is a need to rely on this therapeutic approach. In countries without access to advanced blood-processing technologies, the choice may initially be restricted to convalescent whole blood or plasma. In technologically advanced countries, additional options for convalescent blood products are available, including virally inactivated plasma and fractionated immunoglobulins. The preparation of minipool immunoglobulins is also a realistic option to consider.

Copyright © 2014 Elsevier Ltd. All rights reserved.

PMID: 25457751 [PubMed - as supplied by publisher]

469. Travel Med Infect Dis. 2014 Oct 16;12(6PA):561-562. doi: 10.1016/j.tmaid.2014.10.008. [Epub ahead of print]

Ebola and travel - Management of imported cases.

Brouqui P(1), Ippolito G(2).

Author information: (1)Southern France Referral Center for EBOLA Care, IHU Méditerranée Infection, Marseille, France; European Network for Highly Infectious Disease (EuroNHID), Italy. (2)National Institute for Infectious Diseases Lazzaro Spallanzani, Rome, Italy; European Network for Highly Infectious Disease (EuroNHID), Italy. Electronic address: giuseppe.ippolito@inmi.it.

PMID: 25459430 [PubMed - as supplied by publisher]

470. BMJ. 2014 Oct 15;349:g6255. doi: 10.1136/bmj.g6255.

WHO hopes Ebola incidence will decline after peaking in December.

Gulland A(1).

Author information: (1)London.

PMID: 25319838 [PubMed - indexed for MEDLINE]

471. BMJ. 2014 Oct 15;349:g6266. doi: 10.1136/bmj.g6266.

US deploys rapid response teams to hospitals with Ebola cases.

McCarthy M(1).

Author information: (1)Seattle.

PMID: 25318993 [PubMed - indexed for MEDLINE]

472. BMJ. 2014 Oct 15;349:g6250. doi: 10.1136/bmj.g6250.

Transferring patients with Ebola from west Africa to "isolation hospitals" in well resourced countries for treatment.

Southall DP(1), MacDonald R(1).

Author information: (1)Maternal and Childhealth Advocacy International (MCAI), Laide IV22 2NL, UK.

PMID: 25318817 [PubMed - indexed for MEDLINE]

473. Ann Intern Med. 2014 Oct 14. doi: 10.7326/M14-2002. [Epub ahead of print]

Drug and Vaccine Access in the Ebola Epidemic: Advising Caution in Compassionate Use.

Hantel A, Olopade CO.

PMID: 25322080 [PubMed - as supplied by publisher]

474. BMJ. 2014 Oct 14;349:g6240. doi: 10.1136/bmj.g6240.

US to "rethink" Ebola infection control after nurse falls ill.

McCarthy M(1).

Author information: (1)Seattle.

PMID: 25316554 [PubMed - indexed for MEDLINE]

475. BMJ. 2014 Oct 14;349:g6202. doi: 10.1136/bmj.g6202.

Airport screening for Ebola.

Mabey D(1), Flasche S(1), Edmunds WJ(1).

Author information: (1)London School of Hygiene and Tropical Medicine, London WC1E 7HT, UK.

Comment in BMJ. 2014;349:g6585. BMJ. 2014;349:g6571.

PMID: 25316030 [PubMed - indexed for MEDLINE]

476. BMJ. 2014 Oct 14;349:g6178. doi: 10.1136/bmj.g6178.

Ebola, Twitter, and misinformation: a dangerous combination?

Oyeyemi SO(1), Gabarron E(2), Wynn R(3).

Author information: (1)Accident and Emergency Department, State Specialist Hospital, Akure, Nigeria femi_oyeyemi@yahoo.com. (2)Norwegian Centre for Integrated Care and Telemedicine, University Hospital of North Norway, Tromsø, Norway. (3)Department of Clinical Medicine, Arctic University of Norway, Tromsø, Norway.

PMID: 25315514 [PubMed - indexed for MEDLINE]

477. BMJ. 2014 Oct 14;349:g6237. doi: 10.1136/bmj.g6237.

Operation Gritrock: first UK army medics fly to Sierra Leone.

Johnston A, Bailey M.

PMID: 25315203 [PubMed - indexed for MEDLINE]

478. Tidsskr Nor Laegeforen. 2014 Oct 14;134(19):1826-7. doi: 10.4045/tidsskr.14.1129. eCollection 2014.

New rules needed to stop the Ebola epidemic.

[Article in English, Norwegian]

Hasle G.

PMID: 25314981 [PubMed - in process]

479. Tidsskr Nor Laegeforen. 2014 Oct 14;134(19):1817. doi: 10.4045/tidsskr.14.1234. eCollection 2014.

Ebola--when will we learn?

[Article in English, Norwegian]

Haug C.

PMID: 25314970 [PubMed - in process]

480. BMJ. 2014 Oct 13;349:g6200. doi: 10.1136/bmj.g6200.

Texas healthcare worker is diagnosed with Ebola.

McCarthy M(1).

Author information: (1)Seattle.

PMID: 25313199 [PubMed - in process]

481. BMJ. 2014 Oct 13;349:g6199. doi: 10.1136/bmj.g6199.

Experts question usefulness of screening travellers to UK for Ebola.

Gulland A(1).

Author information: (1)London.

PMID: 25313188 [PubMed - in process]

482. Nurs Stand. 2014 Oct 13;29(6):33. doi: 10.7748/ns.29.6.33.s44.

Nurses are in the forefront of Ebola virus disease outbreak.

Wiwanitkit V(1).

Author information: (1)Hainan Medical University, China.

PMID: 25294483 [PubMed - in process]

483. Nurs Stand. 2014 Oct 13;29(6):33. doi: 10.7748/ns.29.6.33.s45.

If Ebola were to become airborne, it would be a global catastrophe.

Clark C.

PMID: 25294482 [PubMed - in process]

484. Nurs Stand. 2014 Oct 13;29(6):12. doi: 10.7748/ns.29.6.12.s10.

Ebola nurse calls on world to help.

[No authors listed]

PMID: 25294447 [PubMed - in process]

485. Time. 2014 Oct 13;184(14):38-45.

Racing Ebola. What the world needs to do to stop the deadly virus.

Baker A.

PMID: 25509604 [PubMed - in process]

486. Time. 2014 Oct 13;184(14):34-7.

Now arriving. The deadly Ebola virus lands in America.

Von Drehle D.

PMID: 25509603 [PubMed - in process]

487. Lancet. 2014 Oct 11;384(9951):1323-5. doi: 10.1016/S0140-6736(14)61791-8. Epub 2014 Oct 8.

Ebola: a crisis in global health leadership.

Gostin LO(1), Friedman EA(2).

Author information: (1)O'Neill Institute for National and Global Health Law, Georgetown University Law Center, Washington, DC 20001, USA. Electronic address: gostin@law.georgetown.edu. (2)O'Neill Institute for National and Global Health Law, Georgetown University Law Center, Washington, DC 20001, USA.

PMID: 25306563 [PubMed - in process]

488. Lancet. 2014 Oct 11;384(9951):1321. doi: 10.1016/S0140-6736(14)61697-4. Epub 2014 Oct 8.

Ebola: what lessons for the International Health Regulations?

[No authors listed]

Comment in Lancet. 2014 Dec 6;384(9959):2023.

PMID: 25306562 [PubMed - in process]

489. Lancet. 2014 Oct 11;384(9951):1347-8. doi: 10.1016/S0140-6736(14)61693-7. Epub 2014 Sep 29.

Ebola: a call for blood transfusion strategy in sub-Saharan Africa.

Burnouf T(1), Emmanuel J(2), Mbanya D(3), El-Ekiaby M(4), Murphy W(5), Field S(6), Allain JP(7).

Author information: (1)Graduate Institute of Biomedical Materials and Tissue Engineering Institute, Taipei Medical University, Taipei 11031, Taiwan. Electronic address: thburnouf@gmail.com. (2)National Blood Service, Harare, Zimbabwe. (3)Haematology and Transfusion Service, Centre Hospitalier et Universitaire, Yaounde, Cameroon. (4)Shabrawishi Hospital Blood Bank, Cairo, Egypt. (5)Irish Blood Transfusion Service, Dublin, Ireland. (6)Welsh Blood Service, Pontyclun, Wales, UK. (7)Department of Haematology, University of Cambridge, Cambridge, UK.

PMID: 25277678 [PubMed - in process]

490. Lancet. 2014 Oct 11;384(9951):e49-51. doi: 10.1016/S0140-6736(14)61345-3. Epub 2014 Sep 5.

Ebola: towards an International Health Systems Fund.

Gostin LO(1).

Author information: (1)O'Neill Institute for National and Global Health Law, Georgetown University Law Center, Washington, DC 20001, USA. Electronic address: gostin@law.georgetown.edu.

PMID: 25201591 [PubMed - in process]

491. BMC Med. 2014 Oct 10;12(1):196. [Epub ahead of print]

Transmission dynamics and control of Ebola virus disease (EVD): a review.

Chowell G, Nishiura H.

The complex and unprecedented Ebola epidemic ongoing in West Africa has highlighted the need to review the epidemiological characteristics of Ebola Virus Disease (EVD) as well as our current understanding of the transmission dynamics and the effect of control interventions against Ebola transmission. Here we review key epidemiological data from past Ebola outbreaks and carry out a comparative review of mathematical models of the spread and control of Ebola in the context of past outbreaks and the ongoing epidemic in West Africa. We show that mathematical modeling offers useful insights into the risk of a major epidemic of EVD and the assessment of the impact of basic public health measures on disease spread. We also discuss the critical need to collect detailed epidemiological data in real-time during the course of an ongoing epidemic, carry out further studies to estimate the effectiveness of interventions during past outbreaks and the ongoing epidemic, and develop large-scale modeling studies to study the spread and control of viral hemorrhagic fevers in the context of the highly heterogeneous economic reality of African countries.

PMCID: PMC4207625 PMID: 25300956 [PubMed - as supplied by publisher]

492. BMJ. 2014 Oct 10;349:g6151. doi: 10.1136/bmj.g6151.

Only the military can get the Ebola epidemic under control: MSF head.

Arie S.

PMID: 25304485 [PubMed - in process]

493. Disaster Med Public Health Prep. 2014 Oct 10:1-4. [Epub ahead of print]

Global and Domestic Legal Preparedness and Response: 2014 Ebola Outbreak.

Hodge JG(1).

Author information: (1)Public Health Law and Ethics,Sandra Day O'Connor College of Law,Arizona State University,Tempe,Arizona.

The global rise of Ebola viral diseases in 2014 necessitates legal responses that promote effective public health responses and respect for the health and human rights of populations. Compulsory public health interventions, approval and administration of experimental drugs or vaccines, and allocation of finite resources require difficult choices in law and policy. Crafting legal decisions in real-time emergencies is neither easy nor predictable, but it is essential to controlling epidemics and saving lives.(Disaster Med Public Health Preparedness. 2014;0:1-4).

PMID: 25300952 [PubMed - as supplied by publisher]
494. Int Health. 2014 Oct 10. pii: ihu071. [Epub ahead of print]

Human rabies deaths in Africa: breaking the cycle of indifference.

Dodet B(1), Tejiokem MC(2), Aguemon AR(3), Bourhy H(4).

Author information: (1)AfroREB coordinator, Dodet Bioscience, 6B rue de Verdun, 69300 Caluire et Cuire, France betty.dodet@dodetbioscience.com. (2)Epidemiology and Public Health Service, Centre Pasteur du Cameroun, Yaoundé, Cameroon. (3)Faculté des Sciences de la Santé, 01 BP 188, Cotonou, Bénin. (4)Institut Pasteur, Unité Dynamique des lyssavirus et adaptation à l'hôte, WHO Collaborating Centre for Reference and Research on Rabies, Paris, France.

The current outbreak of Ebola virus disease has mobilized the international community against this deadly disease. However, rabies, another deadly disease, is greatly affecting the African continent, with an estimated 25 000 deaths every year. And yet, the disease can be prevented by a vaccine, if necessary with immunoglobulin, even when administered after exposure to the rabies virus. Rabies victims die because of neglect and ignorance, because they are not aware of these life-saving biologicals, or because they cannot access them or do not have the money to pay for them. Breaking the cycle of indifference of rabies deaths in humans in Africa should be a priority of governments, international organizations and all stakeholders involved.

PMID: 25303941 [PubMed - as supplied by publisher]
495. JAMA Intern Med. 2014 Oct 10. doi: 10.1001/jamainternmed.2014.6235. [Epub ahead of print]

Public Health in the Age of Ebola in West Africa.

Osterholm MT(1), Moore KA(1), Gostin LO(2).

Author information: (1)Center for Infectious Disease Research and Policy, University of Minnesota, Minneapolis. (2)O'Neill Institute for National and Global Health Law, Georgetown Law, Washington, DC.

PMID: 25317856 [PubMed - as supplied by publisher]
496. MMWR Morb Mortal Wkly Rep. 2014 Oct 10;63(40):891-3.

Assessment of ebola virus disease, health care infrastructure, and preparedness - four counties,Southeastern Liberia, august 2014.

Forrester JD, Pillai SK, Beer KD, Neatherlin J, Massaquoi M, Nyenswah TG, Montgomery JM, De Cock K; Centers for Disease Control and Prevention (CDC). Ebola virus disease (Ebola) is a multisystem disease caused by a virus of the genus Ebolavirus. In late March 2014, Ebola cases were described in Liberia, with epicenters in Lofa County and later in Montserrado County. While information about case burden and health care infrastructure was available for the two epicenters, little information was available about remote counties in southeastern Liberia. Over 9 days, August 6-14, 2014, Ebola case burden, health care infrastructure, and emergency preparedness were assessed in collaboration with the Liberian Ministry of Health and Social Welfare in four counties in southeastern Liberia: Grand Gedeh, Grand Kru, River Gee, and Maryland. Data were collected by health care facility visits to three of the four county referral hospitals and by unstructured interviews with county and district health officials, hospital administrators, physicians, nurses, physician assistants, and health educators in all four counties. Local burial practices were discussed with county officials, but no direct observation of burial practices was conducted. Basic information about Ebola surveillance and epidemiology, case investigation, contact tracing, case management, and infection control was provided to local officials.

PMID: 25299605 [PubMed - indexed for MEDLINE]
497. Science. 2014 Oct 10;346(6206):151-2. doi: 10.1126/science.346.6206.151.

Infectious Diseases. Imagining Ebola's next move.

Kupferschmidt K.

PMID: 25301596 [PubMed - indexed for MEDLINE]
498. Artif Cells Nanomed Biotechnol. 2014 Oct 9:1-9. [Epub ahead of print]

A novel nanobiotherapeutic poly-[hemoglobin-superoxide dismutase-catalase-carbonic anhydrase] with no cardiac toxicity for the resuscitation of a rat model with 90 minutes of sustained severe hemorrhagic shock with loss of 2/3 blood volume.

Bian Y(1), Chang TM.

Author information: (1)Artificial Cells and Organs Research Centre, Departments of Physiology, Medicine and Biomedical Engineering, Faculty of Medicine, McGill University , Montreal, QC , Canada.

We crosslink hemoglobin (Hb), superoxide dismutase (SOD), catalase (CAT), and carbonic anhydrase (CA) to form a soluble polyHb-SOD-CAT-CA nanobiotechnological complex. The obtained product is a soluble complex with three enhanced red blood cell (RBC) functions and without blood group antigens. In the present study, 2/3 of blood volume was removed to result in 90-min hemorrhagic shock at mean arterial blood pressure (MAP) of 30 mmHg. This was followed by the reinfusion of different resuscitation fluids, then followed for another 60 min. PolyHb-SOD-CAT-CA maintained the MAP at 87.5 ± 5 mmHg as compared with 3 volumes of lactated Ringer's solution, 43.3 ± 2.8 mmHg; blood, 91.3 ± 3.6 mmHg; polyHb-SOD-CAT, 86.0 ± 4.6 mmHg; poly stroma-free hemolysate (polySFHb), 85.0 ± 2.5 mmHg; and polyHb, 82.6 ± 3.5 mmHg. PolyHb-SOD-CAT-CA was superior to the blood and other fluids based on the following criteria. PolyHb-SOD-CAT-CA reduced tissue pCO_2 from 98 ± 4.5 mmHg to 68.6 ± 3 mmHg. This was significantly ($p < 0.05$) more effective than lactated Ringer's solution (98 ± 4.5 mmHg), polyHb (90.1 ± 4.0 mmHg), polyHb-SOD-CAT (90.9 ± 1.4 mmHg), blood (79.1 ± 4.7 mmHg), and polySFHb (77 ± 5 mmHg). PolyHb-SOD-CAT-CA reduced the elevated ST level to $21.7 \pm 6.7\%$ and is significantly (< 0.05) better than polyHb ($57.7 \pm 8.7\%$), blood ($39.1 \pm 1.5\%$), polySFHb ($38.3\% \pm 2.1\%$), polyHb-SOD-CAT ($27.8 \pm 5.6\%$), and lactated Ringer's solution ($106 \pm 3.1\%$). The plasma cardiac troponin T (cTnT) level of polyHb-SOD-CAT-CA group was significantly (P < 0.05) lower than that of all the other groups. PolyHb-SOD-CAT-CA reduced plasma lactate level from 18 ± 2.3 mM/L to 6.9 ± 0.3 mM/L. It was significantly more effective (P < 0.05) than lactated Ringer's solution (12.4 ± 0.6 mM/L), polyHb (9.6 ± 0.7 mM/L), blood (8.1 ± 0.2 mM/L), polySFHb (8.4 ± 0.1 mM/L), and polyHb-SOD-CAT (7.6 ± 0.3 mM/L). PolyHb-SOD-CAT-CA can be stored for 320 days at room temperature. Lyophilized poly-Hb-SOD-CAT-CA can be heat pasteurized at 68F for 2 h. This can be important if there is a need to inactivate human immunodeficiency virus, Ebola virus, and other infectious organisms.

PMID: 25297052 [PubMed - as supplied by publisher]

499. BMJ. 2014 Oct 9;349:g6145. doi: 10.1136/bmj.g6145.

Liberian man being treated for Ebola in Texas dies.

McCarthy M(1).

Author information: (1)Seattle.

PMID: 25300968 [PubMed - in process]

500. BMJ. 2014 Oct 9;349:g6147. doi: 10.1136/bmj.g6147.

US increases Ebola screening at five airports.

McCarthy M(1).

Author information: (1)Seattle.

PMID: 25300788 [PubMed - in process]

501. Br J Nurs. 2014 Oct 9;23(18):988-91. doi: 10.12968/bjon.2014.23.18.988.

Ebola: where did it come from and where might it go?

Boulton J(1).

Author information: (1)Tutor in Adult Nursing, King's College London, and co-founder and Trustee of UK Friends of the Shepherds' Hospice, Sierra Leone.

Over the last few months, a plethora of headlines have focused on the ebola epidemic sweeping West Africa. On 8 August 2014 this outbreak was defined as a Public Health Event of International Concern by the World Health Organization. Closer to home the focus has been on the possibility of an outbreak in the UK, with calls for specialist nurses to be trained in monitoring travellers at airports. The recent infection of a nurse from Sussex while caring for patients with ebola in Sierra Leone has heightened the interest and need for information on this until now neglected tropical disease. Additionally, an unprecedented collaborative effort to speed up trials on the development of a vaccine has just begun in Oxford. This article discusses the origins of the virus, its symptoms and its modes of transmission. The challenges of managing the virus are discussed, together with current progress on its treatment and prevention, and the implications for nurses in the UK.

PMID: 25302838 [PubMed - in process]

502. Euro Surveill. 2014 Oct 9;19(40):20920.

Transmission dynamics and control of Ebola virus disease outbreak in Nigeria, July to September 2014.

Fasina FO(1), Shittu A, Lazarus D, Tomori O, Simonsen L, Viboud C, Chowell G.

Author information: (1)Department of Production Animal Studies, University of Pretoria, South Africa.

We analyse up-to-date epidemiological data of the Ebola virus disease outbreak in Nigeria as of 1 October 2014 in order to estimate the case fatality rate, the proportion of healthcare workers infected and the transmission tree. We also model the impact of control interventions on the size of the epidemic. Results indicate that Nigeria's quick and forceful implementation of control interventions was determinant in controlling the outbreak rapidly and avoiding a far worse scenario in this country.

PMID: 25323076 [PubMed - in process]

503. Euro Surveill. 2014 Oct 9;19(40):20924.

Describing readmissions to an Ebola case management centre (CMC), Sierra Leone, 2014

Fitzpatrick G(1), Vogt F, Moi Gbabai O, Black B, Santantonio M, Folkesson E, Decroo T, Van Herp M.

Author information: (1)Medecins Sans Frontieres, Dublin, Ireland.

Case management centres (CMCs) are part of the outbreak control plan for Ebola virus disease (EVD). A CMC in Sierra Leone had 33% (138/419) of primary admissions discharged as EVD negative (not a case). Fifteen of these were readmitted within 21 days, nine of which were EVD positive. All readmissions had contact with an Ebola case in the community in the previous 21 days indicating that the infection was likely acquired outside the CMC.

PMID: 25323075 [PubMed - in process]

504. Euro Surveill. 2014 Oct 9;19(40):20925.

Preparedness is crucial for safe care of Ebola patients and to prevent onward transmission in Europe - outbreak control measures are needed at its roots in West Africa.

Sprenger M(1), Coulombier D.

Author information: (1)European Centre for Disease Prevention and Control (ECDC), Stockholm, Sweden.

PMID: 25323074 [PubMed - in process]

505. N Engl J Med. 2014 Oct 9;371(15):1458-9. doi: 10.1056/NEJMe1411378. Epub 2014 Sep 19

Ebola--an ongoing crisis.

Baden LR, Kanapathipillai R, Campion EW, Morrissey S, Rubin EJ, Drazen JM.

PMID: 25237780 [PubMed - indexed for MEDLINE]

506. N Engl J Med. 2014 Oct 9;371(15):1375-8. doi: 10.1056/NEJMp1405314. Epub 2014 May 7

Ebola--a growing threat?

Feldmann H(1).

Author information: (1)From the Laboratory of Virology, Division of Intramural Research, National Institute of Allergy and Infectious Diseases, Rocky Mountain Laboratories, Hamilton, MT.

PMID: 24805988 [PubMed - indexed for MEDLINE]

507. N Engl J Med. 2014 Oct 9;371(15):1418-25. doi: 10.1056/NEJMoa1404505. Epub 2014 Apr 16.

Emergence of Zaire Ebola virus disease in Guinea.

Baize S(1), Pannetier D, Oestereich L, Rieger T, Koivogui L, Magassouba N, Soropogui B, Sow MS, Keïta S, De Clerck H, Tiffany A, Dominguez G, Loua M, Traoré A, Kolié M, Malano ER, Heleze E, Bocquin A, Mély S, Raoul H, Caro V, Cadar D, Gabriel M, Pahlmann M, Tappe D, Schmidt-Chanasit J, Impouma B, Diallo AK, Formenty P, Van Herp M, Günther S.

Author information: (1)The authors' affiliations are listed in the Appendix.

In March 2014, the World Health Organization was notified of an outbreak of a communicable disease characterized by fever, severe diarrhea, vomiting, and a high fatality rate in Guinea. Virologic investigation identified Zaire ebolavirus (EBOV) as the causative agent. Full-length genome sequencing and phylogenetic analysis showed that EBOV from Guinea forms a separate clade in relationship to the known EBOV strains from the Democratic Republic of Congo and Gabon. Epidemiologic investigation linked the laboratory-confirmed cases with the presumed first fatality of the outbreak in December 2013. This study demonstrates the emergence of a new EBOV strain in Guinea.

PMID: 24738640 [PubMed - indexed for MEDLINE]

508. Nature. 2014 Oct 9;514(7521):139. doi: 10.1038/514139a.

Out of Africa.

[No authors listed]

PMID: 25297396 [PubMed - indexed for MEDLINE]

509. BMJ. 2014 Oct 8;349:g6120. doi: 10.1136/bmj.g6120.

Spanish authorities investigate how nurse contracted Ebola.

Gulland A(1).

Author information: (1)London.

PMID: 25297495 [PubMed - in process]

510. Cell Host Microbe. 2014 Oct 8;16(4):419-21. doi: 10.1016/j.chom.2014.09.012.

Portrait of a killer: genome of the 2014 EBOV outbreak strain.

Basler CF(1).

Author information: (1)Icahn School of Medicine at Mount Sinai, Department of Microbiology, Box 1124, 1 Gustave L. Levy Place, New York, NY 10029, USA. Electronic address: chris.basler@mssm.edu.

Comment on Science. 2014 Sep 12;345(6202):1369-72.

A recent study by Gire et al. (2014) identifies differences that make the 2014 West Africa Ebola virus unique and details how the virus spread from Guinea to Sierra Leone. This work highlights the power of new genomic technologies to facilitate rapid public health and scientific responses to the crisis.

Copyright © 2014 Elsevier Inc. All rights reserved.

PMID: 25299323 [PubMed - in process]

511. BMJ. 2014 Oct 7;349:g6094. doi: 10.1136/bmj.g6094.

Obama calls on other nations to step up their efforts to end Ebola outbreak.

McCarthy M(1).

Author information: (1)Seattle.

PMID: 25292171 [PubMed - indexed for MEDLINE]

512. CMAJ. 2014 Oct 7;186(14):E527-8. doi: 10.1503/cmaj.109-4893. Epub 2014 Sep 8.

WHO enters new terrain in Ebola research.

Shuchman M(1).

Author information: (1)Toronto, Ont.

PMCID: PMC4188679 [Available on 2015/10/7] PMID: 25200757 [PubMed - in process]

513. CMAJ. 2014 Oct 7;186(14):E523-4. doi: 10.1503/cmaj.109-4890. Epub 2014 Sep 2.

Ebola epidemic outpacing response: MSF.

Vogel L(1).

Author information: (1)CMAJ.

PMCID: PMC4188676 [Available on 2015/10/7] PMID: 25183725 [PubMed - in process]

514. Disaster Med Public Health Prep. 2014 Oct 7:1. [Epub ahead of print]

The Ebola Epidemic and Translational Public Health.

James JJ.

PMID: 25288342 [PubMed - as supplied by publisher]

515. Disaster Med Public Health Prep. 2014 Oct 7:1-3. [Epub ahead of print]

Operationalizing Public Health Skills to Resource Poor Settings: Is This the Achilles Heel in the Ebola Epidemic Campaign?

Burkle FM(1).

Author information: (1)Harvard Humanitarian Initiative,Harvard University,Cambridge,Massachusetts,and Woodrow Wilson International Center for Scholars,Washington,DC.

Sustainable approaches to crises, especially non-trauma-related public health emergencies, are severely lacking. At present, the Ebola crisis is defining the operational public health skill sets for infectious disease epidemics that are not widely known or appreciated. Indigenous and foreign medical teams will need to adapt to build competency-based curriculum and standards of care for the future that concentrate on public health emergencies. Only by adjusting and adapting specific operational public health skill sets to resource poor environments will it be possible to provide sustainable prevention and preparedness initiatives that work well across cultures and borders.(Diaster Med Public Health Preparedness. 2014;0:1-3).

PMID: 25288216 [PubMed - as supplied by publisher]

516. Nurs Stand. 2014 Oct 7;29(5):35. doi: 10.7748/ns.29.5.35.s46.

Fragile economies in West Africa are being devastated by Ebola.

Lyth N.

Comment on Nurs Stand. 2014 Sep 30;29(4):32-3.

PMID: 25270481 [PubMed - in process]

517. Mod Healthc. 2014 Oct 6;44(40):8.

Dallas error in releasing Ebola patient puts hospitals on alert.

Johnson SR.

PMID: 25509665 [PubMed - in process]

518. Protein Sci. 2014 Oct 6. doi: 10.1002/pro.2578. [Epub ahead of print]

Design and characterization of ebolavirus GP prehairpin intermediate mimics as drug targets.

Clinton TR(1), Weinstock MT, Jacobsen MT, Szabo-Fresnais N, Pandya MJ, Whitby FG, Herbert AS, Prugar LI, McKinnon R, Hill CP, Welch BD, Dye JM, Eckert DM, Kay MS.

Author information: (1)Department of Biochemistry, University of Utah School of Medicine, Salt Lake City, Utah, 84112-5650.

Ebolaviruses are highly lethal filoviruses that cause hemorrhagic fever in humans and nonhuman primates. With no approved treatments or preventatives, the development of an anti-ebolavirus therapy to protect against natural infections and potential weaponization is an urgent global health need. Here, we describe the design, biophysical characterization, and validation of peptide mimics of the ebolavirus N-trimer, a highly conserved region of the GP2 fusion protein, to be used as targets to develop broad-spectrum inhibitors of ebolavirus entry. The N-trimer region of GP2 is 90% identical across all ebolavirus species and forms a critical part of the prehairpin intermediate that is exposed during viral entry. Specifically, we fused designed coiled coils to the N-trimer to present it as a soluble trimeric coiled coil as it appears during membrane fusion. Circular dichroism, sedimentation equilibrium, and X-ray crystallography analyses reveal the helical, trimeric structure of the designed N-trimer mimic targets. Surface plasmon resonance studies validate that the N-trimer mimic binds its native ligand, the C-peptide region of GP2. The longest N-trimer mimic also inhibits virus entry, thereby confirming binding of the C-peptide region during viral entry and the presence of a vulnerable prehairpin intermediate. Using phage display as a model system, we validate the suitability of the N-trimer mimics as drug screening targets. Finally, we describe the foundational work to use the N-trimer mimics as targets in mirror-image phage display, which will be used to identify D-peptide inhibitors of ebolavirus entry.

© 2014 The Protein Society.

PMID: 25287718 [PubMed - as supplied by publisher]

519. Time. 2014 Oct 6;184(13):12.

Liberia struggles in fight against Ebola.

Baker A.

PMID: 25509591 [PubMed - in process]

520. Lancet. 2014 Oct 4;384(9950):1239-40. doi: 10.1016/S0140-6736(14)61694-9.

The Institut Pasteur network: a crucial partner against Ebola.

Ceschia A(1).

Author information: (1)The Lancet, London NW1 7BY, UK.

PMID: 25283561 [PubMed - indexed for MEDLINE]

521. Lancet. 2014 Oct 4;384(9950):e47. doi: 10.1016/S0140-6736(14)61594-4. Epub 2014 Sep 26.

Containment in Sierra Leone: the inability of a state to confront Ebola?

Ozer P(1), Thiry A(2), Fallon C(2), Blocher J(3), de Longueville F(3).

Author information: (1)Department of Environmental Sciences and Management, University of Liege, Arlon, Belgium. Electronic address: pozer@ulg.ac.be. (2)Spiral, University of Liege, Liege, Belgium. (3)Center for Ethnic and Migration Studies, University of Liege, Liege, Belgium.

PMID: 25266710 [PubMed - indexed for MEDLINE]

522. Lancet. 2014 Oct 4;384(9950):1259. doi: 10.1016/S0140-6736(14)61611-1. Epub 2014 Sep 25.

Ebola: an open letter to European governments.

Martin-Moreno JM(1), Ricciardi W(2), Bjegovic-Mikanovic V(3), Maguire P(4), McKee M(5).

Author information: (1)Preventive Medicine and Public Health, University of Valencia, 46010 Valencia, Spain. Electronic address: dr.martinmoreno@gmail.com. (2)European Public Health Association and Catholic University of the Sacred Heart, Rome, Italy. (3)Association of Schools of Public Health in the European Region and University of Belgrade, Institute of Social Medicine, Belgrade, Serbia. (4)European Public Health Alliance, Brussels, Belgium. (5)European Public Health Association and European Centre on Health of Societies in Transition, London School of Hygiene and Tropical Medicine, London, UK.

PMID: 25263575 [PubMed - indexed for MEDLINE]

523. Lancet. 2014 Oct 4;384(9950):1260. doi: 10.1016/S0140-6736(14)61706-2. Epub 2014 Sep 23.

Case fatality rate for Ebola virus disease in west Africa.

Kucharski AJ(1), Edmunds WJ(2).

Author information: (1)Department of Infectious Disease Epidemiology, London School of Hygiene Tropical Medicine, London WC1E 7HT, UK. Electronic address: adam.kucharski@lshtm.ac.uk. (2)Department of Infectious Disease Epidemiology, London School of Hygiene Tropical Medicine, London WC1E 7HT, UK.

PMID: 25260235 [PubMed - indexed for MEDLINE]

524. MMWR Morb Mortal Wkly Rep. 2014 Oct 3;63(39):873-4.

Importation and containment of Ebola virus disease - Senegal, August-September 2014

Mirkovic K, Thwing J, Diack PA; Centers for Disease Control and Prevention (CDC).

Erratum in MMWR Morb Mortal Wkly Rep. 2014 Oct 3;63(39):875.

On August 29, 2014, Senegal confirmed its first case of Ebola virus disease (Ebola) in a Guinean man, aged 21 years, who had traveled from Guinea to Dakar, Senegal, in mid-August to visit family. Senegalese medical and public health personnel were alerted about this patient after public health staff in Guinea contacted his family in Senegal on August 27. The patient had been admitted to a referral hospital in Senegal on August 26. He was promptly isolated, and a blood sample was sent for laboratory confirmation; Ebola was confirmed by reverse transcriptase-polymerase chain reaction at Institut Pasteur Dakar on August 29. The patient's mother and sister had been admitted to an Ebola treatment unit in Guinea on August 26, where they had named the patient as a contact and reported his recent travel to Senegal. Ebola was likely transmitted to the family from the brother of the patient, who had traveled by land from Sierra Leone to Guinea in early August seeking treatment from a traditional healer. The brother died in Guinea on August 10; family members, including the patient, participated in preparing the body for burial.

PMID: 25275333 [PubMed - indexed for MEDLINE]

525. MMWR Morb Mortal Wkly Rep. 2014 Oct 3;63(39):867-72.

Ebola virus disease outbreak - Nigeria, July-September 2014.

Shuaib F, Gunnala R, Musa EO, Mahoney FJ, Oguntimehin O, Nguku PM, Nyanti SB, Knight N, Gwarzo NS, Idigbe O, Nasidi A, Vertefeuille JF; Centers for Disease Control and Prevention (CDC).

On July 20, 2014, an acutely ill traveler from Liberia arrived at the international airport in Lagos, Nigeria, and was confirmed to have Ebola virus disease (Ebola) after being admitted to a private hospital. This index patient potentially exposed 72 persons at the airport and the hospital. The Federal Ministry of Health, with guidance from the Nigeria Centre for Disease Control (NCDC), declared an Ebola emergency. Lagos, (pop. 21 million) is a regional hub for economic, industrial, and travel activities and a setting where communicable diseases can be easily spread and transmission sustained. Therefore, implementing a rapid response using all available public health assets was the highest priority. On July 23, the Federal Ministry of Health, with the Lagos State government and international partners, activated an Ebola Incident Management Center as a precursor to the current Emergency Operations Center (EOC) to rapidly respond to this outbreak. The index patient died on July 25; as of September 24, there were 19 laboratory-confirmed Ebola cases and one probable case in two states, with 894 contacts identified and followed during the response. Eleven patients with laboratory-confirmed Ebola had been discharged, an additional patient was diagnosed at convalescent stage, and eight patients had died (seven with confirmed Ebola; one probable). The isolation wards were empty, and 891 (all but three) contacts had exited follow-up, with the remainder due to exit on October 2. No new cases had occurred since August 31, suggesting that the Ebola outbreak in Nigeria might be contained. The EOC, established quickly and using an Incident Management System (IMS) to coordinate the response and consolidate decision making, is largely credited with helping contain the Nigeria outbreak early. National public health emergency preparedness agencies in the region, including those involved in Ebola responses, should consider including the development of an EOC to improve the ability to rapidly respond to urgent public health threats.

PMID: 25275332 [PubMed - indexed for MEDLINE]

526. MMWR Morb Mortal Wkly Rep. 2014 Oct 3;63(39):865-6.

Ebola virus disease outbreak - West Africa, September 2014.

Incident Management System Ebola Epidemiology Team, CDC; Ministries of Health of Guinea, Sierra Leone, Liberia, Nigeria, and Senegal; Viral Special Pathogens Branch, National Center for Emerging and Zoonotic Infectious Diseases, CDC.

CDC is assisting ministries of health and working with other organizations to control and end the ongoing outbreak of Ebola virus disease (Ebola) in West Africa. The updated data in this report were compiled from ministry of health situation reports and World Health Organization (WHO) sources. Total case counts include all suspected, probable, and confirmed cases as defined by each country. These data reflect reported cases, which make up an unknown proportion of all actual cases. The data also reflect reporting delays that might vary from country to country.

PMID: 25275331 [PubMed - indexed for MEDLINE]

527. Science. 2014 Oct 3;346(6205):17-8. doi: 10.1126/science.346.6205.17. Epub 2014 Oct 2.

Infectious diseases. When Ebola protection fails.

Cohen J.

PMID: 25278588 [PubMed - indexed for MEDLINE]

528. BMJ. 2014 Oct 2;349:g5975. doi: 10.1136/bmj.g5975.

Cuts in aid are linked to Ebola crisis, say MPs.

Gulland A(1).

Author information: (1)London.

PMID: 25277801 [PubMed - indexed for MEDLINE]

529. Nature. 2014 Oct 2;514(7520):15-6. doi: 10.1038/514015a.

Ebola obstructs malaria control.

Check Hayden E.

PMID: 25279895 [PubMed - indexed for MEDLINE]

530. Nature. 2014 Oct 2;514(7520):41-3. doi: 10.1038/nature13746. Epub 2014 Aug 29.

Medical research: Ebola therapy protects severely ill monkeys.

Geisbert TW(1).

Author information: (1)University of Texas Medical Branch at Galveston, Galveston National Laboratory, Galveston, Texas 77550-0610, USA.

Comment on Nature. 2014 Oct 2;514(7520):47-53.

PMID: 25171470 [PubMed - indexed for MEDLINE]

531. Nature. 2014 Oct 2;514(7520):47-53. doi: 10.1038/nature13777. Epub 2014 Aug 29.

Reversion of advanced Ebola virus disease in nonhuman primates with ZMapp.

Qiu X(1), Wong G(2), Audet J(2), Bello A(2), Fernando L(1), Alimonti JB(1), Fausther-Bovendo H(2), Wei H(3), Aviles J(1), Hiatt E(4), Johnson A(4), Morton J(4), Swope K(4), Bohorov O(5), Bohorova N(5), Goodman C(5), Kim D(5), Pauly MH(5), Velasco J(5), Pettitt J(6), Olinger GG(6), Whaley K(5), Xu B(7), Strong JE(8), Zeitlin L(5), Kobinger GP(9).

Author information: (1)National Laboratory for Zoonotic Diseases and Special Pathogens, Public Health Agency of Canada, Winnipeg, Manitoba R3E 3R2, Canada. (2)1] National Laboratory for Zoonotic Diseases and Special Pathogens, Public Health Agency of Canada, Winnipeg, Manitoba R3E 3R2, Canada [2] Department of Medical Microbiology, University of Manitoba, Winnipeg, Manitoba R3E 0J9, Canada. (3)1] National Laboratory for Zoonotic Diseases and Special Pathogens, Public Health Agency of Canada, Winnipeg, Manitoba R3E 3R2, Canada [2] Institute of Infectious Disease, Henan Centre for Disease Control and Prevention, Zhengzhou, 450012 Henan, China. (4)Kentucky BioProcessing, Owensboro, Kentucky 42301, USA. (5)Mapp Biopharmaceutical Inc., San Diego, California 92121, USA. (6)1] United States Army Medical Research Institute of Infectious Diseases (USAMRIID), Frederick, Maryland 21702, USA [2] Integrated Research Facility, National Institute of Allergy and Infectious Diseases, National Institutes of Health, Frederick, Maryland 21702, USA. (7)Institute of Infectious Disease, Henan Centre for Disease Control and Prevention, Zhengzhou, 450012 Henan, China. (8)1] National Laboratory for Zoonotic Diseases and Special Pathogens, Public Health Agency of Canada, Winnipeg, Manitoba R3E 3R2, Canada [2] Department of Medical Microbiology, University of Manitoba, Winnipeg, Manitoba R3E 0J9, Canada [3] Department of Pediatrics and Child Health, University of Manitoba, Winnipeg, Manitoba R3A 1S1, Canada. (9)1] National Laboratory for Zoonotic Diseases and Special Pathogens, Public Health Agency of Canada, Winnipeg, Manitoba R3E 3R2, Canada [2] Department of Medical Microbiology, University of Manitoba, Winnipeg, Manitoba R3E 0J9, Canada [3] Department of Immunology, University of Manitoba, Winnipeg, Manitoba R3E 0T5, Canada [4] Department of Pathology and Laboratory Medicine, University of Pennsylvania School of Medicine, Philadelphia, Pennsylvania 19104, USA.

Comment in Immunity. 2014 Oct 16;41(4):515-7. Nature. 2014 Oct 2;514(7520):41-3.

Without an approved vaccine or treatments, Ebola outbreak management has been limited to palliative care and barrier methods to prevent transmission. These approaches, however, have yet to end the 2014 outbreak of Ebola after its prolonged presence in West Africa. Here we show that a combination of monoclonal antibodies (ZMapp), optimized from two previous antibody cocktails, is able to rescue 100% of rhesus macaques when treatment is initiated up to 5 days post-challenge. High fever, viraemia and abnormalities in blood count and blood chemistry were evident in many animals before ZMapp intervention. Advanced disease, as indicated by elevated liver enzymes, mucosal haemorrhages and generalized petechia could be reversed, leading to full recovery. ELISA and neutralizing antibody assays indicate that ZMapp is cross-reactive with the Guinean variant of Ebola. ZMapp exceeds the efficacy of any other therapeutics described so far, and results warrant further development of this cocktail for clinical use.

PMCID: PMC4214273 [Available on 2015/4/2] PMID: 25171469 [PubMed - indexed for MEDLINE]

532. Acta Obstet Gynecol Scand. 2014 Oct;93(10):957-8. doi: 10.1111/aogs.12493.

Ebola and adverse circumstances.

Geirsson RT.

PMID: 25231284 [PubMed - indexed for MEDLINE]

533. AIDS Rev. 2014 Oct-Dec;16(4):246-7.

RNA Viruses at the Forefront of Human Infections - HIV, Hepatitis C, and Now Ebola.

Soriano V(1), Peña JM(1).

Author information: (1)Infectious Diseases Unit, La Paz Hospital & Autonomous University, Madrid, Spain.

AIDS emerged in 1981, breaking a period of proud medical progresses in controlling infectious diseases with antimicrobials and vaccines. In an unprecedented way, HIV has attracted much attention for three decades, driving the discovery of new extraordinary molecular diagnostic tools and antiviral drugs. As a result, advances in antiretroviral therapy have made it possible to change HIV infection into a chronic illness. However, the prospects for HIV eradication in the short term are not envisioned for the more than 35 million people worldwide estimated to be living with HIV.

PMID: 25373350 [PubMed - in process]

534. Am J Clin Pathol. 2014 Oct;142(4):428-30. doi: 10.1309/AJCPEPQB4G3ECCOP.

When the rubber meets the road: dealing with a returning traveler from West Africa during the Ebola outbreak of 2014.

Guarner J(1).

Author information: (1)From the Department of Pathology and Laboratory Medicine, Emory University School of Medicine, Atlanta, GA.

PMID: 25239405 [PubMed - indexed for MEDLINE]

535. Am J Respir Crit Care Med. 2014 Oct 1;190(7):733-7. doi: 10.1164/rccm.201408-1514CP.

Caring for critically ill patients with ebola virus disease. Perspectives from West Africa.

Fowler RA(1), Fletcher T, Fischer WA 2nd, Lamontagne F, Jacob S, Brett-Major D, Lawler JV, Jacquerioz FA, Houlihan C, O'Dempsey T, Ferri M, Adachi T, Lamah MC, Bah EI, Mayet T, Schieffelin J, McLellan SL, Senga M, Kato Y, Clement C, Mardel S, Vallenas Bejar De Villar RC, Shindo N, Bausch D.

Author information: (1)1 University of Toronto, Toronto, Ontario, Canada.

The largest ever Ebola virus disease outbreak is ravaging West Africa. The constellation of little public health infrastructure, low levels of health literacy, limited acute care and infection prevention and control resources, densely populated areas, and a highly transmissible and lethal viral infection have led to thousands of confirmed, probable, or suspected cases thus far. Ebola virus disease is characterized by a febrile severe illness with profound gastrointestinal manifestations and is complicated by intravascular volume depletion, shock, profound electrolyte abnormalities, and organ dysfunction. Despite no proven Ebola virus-specific medical therapies, the potential effect of supportive care is great for a condition with high baseline mortality and one usually occurring in resource-constrained settings. With more personnel, basic monitoring, and supportive treatment, many of the sickest patients with Ebola virus disease do not need to die. Ebola virus disease represents an illness ready for a paradigm shift in care delivery and outcomes, and the profession of critical care medicine can and should be instrumental in helping this happen.

PMID: 25166884 [PubMed - in process]

536. Aust N Z J Public Health. 2014 Oct;38(5):403-4. doi: 10.1111/1753-6405.12303.

Are we prepared for Ebola and other viral haemorrhagic fevers?

Cheng AC(1), Kelly H.

Author information: (1)Department of Epidemiology and Preventive Medicine, Monash University; Infection Prevention and Healthcare Epidemiology Unit, Alfred Health.

PMID: 25269974 [PubMed - in process]

537. Bioorg Med Chem. 2014 Oct 1;22(19):5315-9. doi: 10.1016/j.bmc.2014.07.051. Epub 2014 Aug 7.

The enantiomers of the 1',6'-isomer of neplanocin A: synthesis and antiviral properties.

Ye W(1), Schneller SW(2).

Author information: (1)Molette Laboratory for Drug Discovery, Department of Chemistry and Biochemistry, Auburn University, Auburn, AL 36849-5312, United States. (2)Molette Laboratory for Drug Discovery, Department of Chemistry and Biochemistry, Auburn University, Auburn, AL 36849-5312, United States. Electronic address: schnest@auburn.edu.

Both enantiomers of 1',6'-isoneplanocin have been prepared from a common substituted cyclopentane epoxide in 7 steps. Both compounds were subjected to DNA and RNA viral assessments with moderate to high activity found for both towards human cytomegalovirus, measles, Ebola, norovirus, and dengue. The D-like congener also showed vaccinia and HBV effectiveness. In many of the other antiviral assays both compounds showed cytotoxicity making, in some cases, an EC50 determination not possible. The S-adenosylhomocysteine hydrolase inhibitory effects showed the D-like target to be equal that of neplanocin itself and better than 3-deazaneplanocin whereas the L-like analogue was 13 to 30 times less inhibitory than 3-deazaneplanocin and neplanocin, respectively.

PMID: 25155914 [PubMed - in process]

538. BMJ. 2014 Oct 1;349:g5980. doi: 10.1136/bmj.g5980.

Ebola is diagnosed in traveler to US.

McCarthy M(1).

Author information: (1)Seattle.

PMID: 25274102 [PubMed - in process]

539. Bull World Health Organ. 2014 Oct 1;92(10):704-5. doi: 10.2471/BLT.14.031014.

Glimmers of hope on the Ebola front.

[No authors listed]

Daniel Bausch has been assisting with patient care during the current Ebola virus disease outbreak in western Africa and - as part of a WHO-led international collaboration - is exploring the possible use of experimental therapies and vaccines. He tells Fiona Fleck why this outbreak is different.

PMCID: PMC4208486 PMID: 25378723 [PubMed - in process]

540. Cardiovasc Diagn Ther. 2014 Oct;4(5):339-40. doi: 10.3978/j.issn.2223-3652.2014.10.02.

Ebola and art.

Schoenhagen P(1), Weiner M(1).

Author information: (1)Cardiovascular Imaging, Cleveland Clinic, Cleveland, Ohio 44195, USA.

PMCID: PMC4221320 PMID: 25414819 [PubMed]

541. Clin Microbiol Infect. 2014 Oct;20(10):O597-9. doi: 10.1111/1469-0691.12781. Epub 2014 Sep 26.

Ebola in West Africa: the outbreak able to change many things.

Leroy EM(1), Labouba I, Maganga GD, Berthet N.

Author information: (1)Centre International de Recherches Médicales, Franceville, Gabon; Institut de Recherche pour le Développement, UMR MIVEGEC 224 'Maladies Infectieuses et Vecteurs: Ecologie, Génétique Evolution et Contrôle, Montpellier, France. eric.leroy@ird.fr.

PMID: 25204860 [PubMed - in process]

542. Drug Discov Ther. 2014 Oct;8(5):229-31.

Drug development for controlling Ebola epidemic - A race against time.

Gao J(1), Yin L.

Author information: (1)Department of Pharmacology, School of Pharmaceutical Sciences, Qingdao University.

The Ebola outbreak in West Africa this year is causing global panic. The high mortality of this disease is largely due to lack of effective preventive vaccines or therapeutic drugs. Realizing the gravity and urgency in controlling the epidemic, governments and drug companies across the world have taken many strong measures to speed up the process of drug development. Several representative candidate drugs that demonstrate potent anti-Ebola activity in preclinical studies have been pushed forward to higher research stages to obtain an earlier official license. It is expected that proven preventive or therapeutic regimens could be established in the near future.

PMID: 25382559 [PubMed - in process]

543. Dtsch Med Wochenschr. 2014 Oct;139(41):2062-3.

[Ebola virus disease: safe management of patients with high risk infections].

[Article in German]

Escher M.

PMID: 25396237 [PubMed - indexed for MEDLINE]

544. ED Manag. 2014 Oct;26(10):109-13.

Public health experts urge U.S. hospitals to be prepared as Ebola outbreak accelerates.

[No authors listed]

With the outbreak of Ebola virus disease (EBD) accelerating in West Africa, public health authorities are urging frontline providers in the United States to be vigilant in questioning patients who present with a suspected infectious disease, and in adhering to infection control practices. Recent travel to West Africa and contact with others who may have been exposed to EVD are key points that need to be covered at triage, say experts. The World Health Organization (WHO) indicates that mortality from the latest outbreak is 55%, although it is as high as 75% in Guinea. Health care workers are particularly vulnerable to EVD, with WHO noting that more than 250 workers in West Africa have contracted EVD and at least 120 have died from the disease. Experts say that one of the greatest times of risk for health care workers is while a patient is at triage because he or she has not yet been placed in isolation precautions. The CDC is recommending that hospitals rigorously apply standard infection control policies at a minimum, and that extra protective equipment may be required when there are body fluids in the patient environment. Hospitals in 27 states have reported dozens of suspected cases of EVD to the CDC, but at press time, none had yet tested positive.

PMID: 25291835 [PubMed - indexed for MEDLINE]

545. Emerg Infect Dis. 2014 Oct;20(10):1683-90. doi: 10.3201/eid2010.140430.

Biomarker correlates of survival in pediatric patients with Ebola virus disease.

McElroy AK, Erickson BR, Flietstra TD, Rollin PE, Nichol ST, Towner JS, Spiropoulou CF.

Outbreaks of Ebola virus disease (EVD) occur sporadically in Africa and are associated with high case-fatality rates. Historically, children have been less affected than adults. The 2000-2001 Sudan virus-associated EVD outbreak in the Gulu district of Uganda resulted in 55 pediatric and 161 adult laboratory-confirmed cases. We used a series of multiplex assays to measure the concentrations of 55 serum analytes in specimens from patients from that outbreak to identify biomarkers specific to pediatric disease. Pediatric patients who survived had higher levels of the chemokine regulated on activation, normal T-cell expressed and secreted marker and lower levels of plasminogen activator inhibitor I, soluble intracellular adhesion molecule, and soluble vascular cell adhesion molecule than did pediatric patients who died. Adult patients had similar levels of these analytes regardless of outcome. Our findings suggest that children with EVD may benefit from different treatment regimens than those for adults.

PMCID: PMC4193175 PMID: 25279581 [PubMed - in process]
546. Epidemiol Mikrobiol Imunol. 2014 Fall;63(3):238-244.

Detection panel for identification of twelve hemorrhagic viruses using real-time RT-PCR.

Fajfr M, Neubauerová V, Pajer P, Kubíčková P, Růžek D.

Background: Viral hemorrhagic fevers are caused by viruses from four viral families and develop diseases with high fatality rates. However, no commercial diagnostic assay for these pathogens is available.Findings: We developed real-time RT-PCR assays for viruses Ebola, Marburg, Lassa, Guanarito, Machupo, Junin, Sabiá, Seoul, Puumala, Hantaan, Crimean-Congo hemorrhagic fever virus and Rift Valley fever virus. The assays were optimized for identical reaction conditions and can be performed using several types of real-time PCR instruments, both capillary and plate, including a portable Ruggedized Advanced Pathogen Identification Device (R.A.P.I.D.) (Idaho Technology, Inc.).Conclusions: In combination with primers and probes from previously published studies, we present a simple system for rapid identification of hemorrhagic filoviruses, arenaviruses and bunyaviruses with sufficient sensitivity for first contact laboratory and diagnosis under field conditions.Keywords: hemorrhagic fever - filovirus - arenavirus - real-time RT-PCR - detection.

PMID: 25412490 [PubMed - as supplied by publisher]
547. Expert Rev Anti Infect Ther. 2014 Oct;12(10):1253-63. doi: 10.1586/14787210.2014.948848. Epub 2014 Aug 28.

Reverse genetics systems as tools for the development of novel therapies against filoviruses.

Hoenen T(1), Feldmann H.

Author information: (1)Division of Intramural Research, Laboratory of Virology, National Institutes of Health, 903 South 4th Street, Hamilton, MT 59840, USA.

Filoviruses cause severe hemorrhagic fevers with case fatality rates of up to 90%, for which no antivirals are currently available. Their categorization as biosafety level 4 agents restricts work with infectious viruses to a few maximum containment laboratories worldwide, which constitutes a significant obstacle for the development of countermeasures. Reverse genetics facilitates the generation of recombinant filoviruses, including reporter-expressing viruses, which have been increasingly used for drug screening and development in recent years. Further, reverse-genetics based lifecycle modeling systems allow modeling of the filovirus lifecycle without the need for a maximum containment laboratory and have recently been optimized for use in high-throughput assays. The availability of these reverse genetics-based tools will significantly improve our ability to find novel antivirals against filoviruses.

PMID: 25169588 [PubMed - in process]
548. Indian J Med Ethics. 2014 Oct-Dec;11(4):200-2.

Ebola virus disease outbreak: incorporating ethical analysis into the health system response.

Saxena A(1).

Author information: (1)Coordinator, Global Health Ethics, KER/HIS, World Health Organization, CH-1211 Geneva 27 Switzerland.

The current outbreak of Ebola in western Africa has been unprecedented for various reasons, mostly because of its magnitude, its expansion across the borders of several countries of the region, and its propagation in capital cities. The outbreak initially involved no more than a few hundred people mainly in the rural parts of Africa, but by mid-September it had affected more than 5800 persons and caused more than 2500 deaths in four countries (mainly in urban locations).

PMID: 25377031 [PubMed - in process]
549. Indian J Med Microbiol. 2014 Oct-Dec;32(4):364-70. doi: 10.4103/0255-0857.142230.

The threat of Ebola: an update.

Mishra B(1).

Author information: (1)Department of Microbiology, All India Institute of Medical Sciences, Bhubaneswar 751 019, Orissa, India.

PMID: 25297018 [PubMed - in process]
550. Indian J Med Microbiol. 2014 Oct-Dec;32(4):363. doi: 10.4103/0255-0857.142229.

Ebola virus re-emergence: is it really knocking at our door?

Dar L(1), Choudhary A.

Author information: (1)Department of Microbiology (LD, AC), All India Institute of Medical Sciences, New Delhi, India.

PMID: 25297017 [PubMed - in process]
551. Int J Infect Dis. 2014 Oct;27:26-31. doi: 10.1016/j.ijid.2014.07.001. Epub 2014 Aug 14.

Mass gathering medicine: 2014 Hajj and Umra preparation as a leading example.

Al-Tawfiq JA(1), Memish ZA(2).

Author information: (1)Johns Hopkins Aramco Healthcare, Dhahran, Saudi Arabia; Indiana University School of Medicine, Indiana, USA. (2)Ministry of Health and Al-Faisal University, PO Box 54146, Riyadh, 11514, Saudi Arabia. Electronic address: zmemish@yahoo.com.

The importation of infectious diseases during a mass gathering may result in outbreaks. Infectious diseases associated with mass gatherings vary depending on the type and location of the mass gathering. The annual Hajj to Makkah in Saudi Arabia is one of the largest annual religious mass gatherings in the world. Preparation for the Hajj encompasses multiple sectors to develop comprehensive plans. These plans include risk assessment, utilizing existing medical infrastructure, developing electronic and paper-based surveillance activity, and the use of information technology. In this review, we describe key features of the preparedness for the 2014 Hajj and Umra, review the recent impact of emerging viruses such as Ebola in West Africa and the Middle East respiratory syndrome coronavirus (MERS-CoV) in affected countries, and highlight the updated requirements and the required vaccines.

PMID: 25128639 [PubMed - in process]

552. J Med Primatol. 2014 Oct;43(5):317-28. doi: 10.1111/jmp.12125. Epub 2014 May 8.

Assessment and improvement of Indian-origin rhesus macaque and Mauritian-origin cynomolgus macaque genome annotations using deep transcriptome sequencing data.

Peng X(1), Pipes L, Xiong H, Green RR, Jones DC, Ruzzo WL, Schroth GP, Mason CE, Palermo RE, Katze MG.

Author information: (1)Department of Microbiology, University of Washington, Seattle, WA, USA; Washington National Primate Research Center, Seattle, WA, USA.

BACKGROUND: The genome annotations of rhesus (Macaca mulatta) and cynomolgus (Macaca fascicularis) macaques, two of the most common non-human primate animal models, are limited. METHODS: We analyzed large-scale macaque RNA-based next-generation sequencing (RNAseq) data to identify un-annotated macaque transcripts. RESULTS: For both macaque species, we uncovered thousands of novel isoforms for annotated genes and thousands of un-annotated intergenic transcripts enriched with non-coding RNAs. We also identified thousands of transcript sequences which are partially or completely 'missing' from current macaque genome assemblies. We showed that many newly identified transcripts were differentially expressed during SIV infection of rhesus macaques or during Ebola virus infection of cynomolgus macaques. CONCLUSIONS: For two important macaque species, we uncovered thousands of novel isoforms and un-annotated intergenic transcripts including coding and non-coding RNAs, polyadenylated and non-polyadenylated transcripts. This resource will greatly improve future macaque studies, as demonstrated by their applications in infectious disease studies.

© 2014 John Wiley & Sons A/S. Published by John Wiley & Sons Ltd.

PMCID: PMC4176519 [Available on 2015/10/1] PMID: 24810475 [PubMed - in process]

553. J Spec Oper Med. 2014 Fall;14(3):93-4.

Ebola hemorrhagic Fever.

Burnett MW.

Ebola hemorrhagic fever is an often-fatal disease caused by a virus of the Filoviridae family, genus Ebolavirus. Initial signs and symptoms of the disease are nonspe-cific, often progressing on to a severe hemorrhagic illness. Special Operations Forces Medical Providers should be aware of this disease, which occurs in sporadic outbreaks throughout Africa. Treatment at the present time is mainly supportive. Special care should be taken to prevent contact with bodily fluids of those infected, which can transmit the virus to caregivers.

2014

PMID: 25344714 [PubMed - in process]

554. JAMA. 2014 Oct 1;312(13):1299-300. doi: 10.1001/jama.2014.12867.

Evaluating novel therapies during the Ebola epidemic.

Joffe S(1).

Author information: (1)Department of Medical Ethics and Health Policy, Perelman School of Medicine, University of Pennsylvania, Philadelphia.

PMID: 25211645 [PubMed - indexed for MEDLINE]

555. JAMA. 2014 Oct 1;312(13):1297-8. doi: 10.1001/jama.2014.12869.

Why should high-income countries help combat Ebola?

Rid A(1), Emanuel EJ(2).

Author information: (1)Department of Social Science, Health & Medicine, King's College London, London, United Kingdom. (2)Department of Medical Ethics and Health Policy, Perelman School of Medicine, University of Pennsylvania, Philadelphia.

PMID: 25210838 [PubMed - indexed for MEDLINE]

556. Lab Med. 2014 Fall;45(4):e146-51. doi: 10.1309/LMTULFM62W3RKMYI.

An integrated approach to laboratory testing for patients with ebola virus disease.

Iwen PC(1), Garrett JL(2), Gibbs SG(3), Lowe JJ(3), Herrera VL(4), Sambol AR(4), Stiles K(4), Wisecarver JL(5), Salerno KJ(2), Pirruccello SJ(5), Hinrichs SH(5).

Author information: (1)Department of Pathology and Microbiology, College of Medicine, Omaha, Nebraska Nebraska Public Health Laboratory, Omaha, Nebraska piwen@unmc.edu. (2)The Nebraska Medical Center, Clinical Laboratory, Omaha, Nebraska (now known as Nebraska Medicine). (3)Department of Environmental, Agricultural, and Occupational Health, College of Public Health, University of Nebraska Medical Center, Omaha, Nebraska. (4)Nebraska Public Health Laboratory, Omaha, Nebraska. (5)Department of Pathology and Microbiology, College of Medicine, Omaha, Nebraska The Nebraska Medical Center, Clinical Laboratory, Omaha, Nebraska (now known as Nebraska Medicine).

PMID: 25348431 [PubMed - in process]

557. Lancet Glob Health. 2014 Oct;2(10):e563-4. doi: 10.1016/S2214-109X(14)70304-3.

Rethinking the development of Ebola treatments.

Gupta R(1).

Author information: (1)Stanford University, Center for Health Policy, Stanford, CA 94305, USA. Electronic address: rguptal@stanford.edu.

Comment on Science. 2014 Aug 15;345(6198):718-9.

PMID: 25304627 [PubMed - in process]

558. Lancet Glob Health. 2014 Oct;2(10):e550. doi: 10.1016/S2214-109X(14)70278-5. Epub 2014 Sep 17.

Ebola: the missing link.

Mullan Z(1).

Author information: (1)Editor, The Lancet Global Health.
PMID: 25304621 [PubMed - in process]
559. Midwifery. 2014 Oct;30(10):1045.

Ebola outbreak and impact on maternity care in Liberia.

[No authors listed]
PMID: 25353047 [PubMed - in process]
560. Nan Fang Yi Ke Da Xue Xue Bao. 2014 Oct;34(10):1519-22.

[Research progress of prevention and treatment of Ebola virus infection].

[Article in Chinese]

Wu W(1), Liu S.

Author information: (1)School of Pharmaceutical Sciences, Southern Medical University, Guangzhou 510515, China.E-mail: wj910103@126.com.

Starting from February 2014, the Ebola virus outbreak had spread across West African countries within a few months and caused great concerns of the World Health Organization. Currently no effective vaccines or drugs have been available for prevention and treatment of Ebola virus infection. This paper gives a brief review of the epidemics and pandemics, the biological characteristics of Ebola virus, the potential antiviral drug targets, and research progress of vaccine and drug development against the virus.

PMID: 25345954 [PubMed - in process]
561. Nat Med. 2014 Oct;20(10):1126-9. doi: 10.1038/nm.3702. Epub 2014 Sep 7.

Chimpanzee adenovirus vaccine generates acute and durable protective immunity against ebolavirus challenge.

Stanley DA(1), Honko AN(2), Asiedu C(3), Trefry JC(4), Lau-Kilby AW(1), Johnson JC(2), Hensley L(2), Ammendola V(5), Abbate A(5), Grazioli F(5), Foulds KE(1), Cheng C(1), Wang L(1), Donaldson MM(1), Colloca S(5), Folgori A(5), Roederer M(1), Nabel GJ(6), Mascola J(1), Nicosia A(7), Cortese R(8), Koup RA(1), Sullivan NJ(1).

Author information: (1)Vaccine Research Center, National Institute of Allergy and Infectious Diseases (NIAID), National Institutes of Health (NIH), Bethesda, Maryland, USA. (2)1 United States Army Medical Research Institute of Infectious Diseases, Fort Detrick, Maryland, USA. [2] Integrated Research Facility, NIAID, NIH, Fort Detrick, Maryland, USA (A.N.H., J.C.J. and L.H.), and Sanofi, Cambridge, Massachusetts, USA (G.J.N.). (3)1 Vaccine Research Center, National Institute of Allergy and Infectious Diseases (NIAID), National Institutes of Health (NIH), Bethesda, Maryland, USA. [2]. (4)United States Army Medical Research Institute of Infectious Diseases, Fort Detrick, Maryland, USA. (5)Okairos, Rome, Italy. (6)1 Vaccine Research Center, National Institute of Allergy and Infectious Diseases (NIAID), National Institutes of Health (NIH), Bethesda, Maryland, USA. [2] Integrated Research Facility, NIAID, NIH, Fort Detrick, Maryland, USA (A.N.H., J.C.J. and L.H.), and Sanofi, Cambridge, Massachusetts, USA (G.J.N.). (7)1 Okairos, Rome, Italy. [2] Centro Ingegneria Genetica (CEINGE), Naples, Italy. [3] Department of Molecular Medicine and Medical Biotechnology, University of Naples Federico II, Naples, Italy. (8)Keires AG, Basel, Switzerland.

Ebolavirus disease causes high mortality, and the current outbreak has spread unabated through West Africa. Human adenovirus type 5 vectors (rAd5) encoding ebolavirus glycoprotein (GP) generate protective immunity against acute lethal Zaire ebolavirus (EBOV) challenge in macaques, but fail to protect animals immune to Ad5, suggesting natural Ad5 exposure may limit vaccine efficacy in humans. Here we show that a chimpanzee-derived replication-defective adenovirus (ChAd) vaccine also rapidly induced uniform protection against acute lethal EBOV challenge in macaques. Because protection waned over several months, we boosted ChAd3 with modified vaccinia Ankara (MVA) and generated, for the first time, durable protection against lethal EBOV challenge.

PMID: 25194571 [PubMed - indexed for MEDLINE]
562. Nat Rev Microbiol. 2014 Oct;12(10):656. doi: 10.1038/nrmicro3355.

Ebola update.

Nunes-Alves C.
PMID: 25226049 [PubMed - indexed for MEDLINE]
563. PLoS Pathog. 2014 Oct 2;10(10):e1004420. doi: 10.1371/journal.ppat.1004420. eCollection 2014.

Characterization of uncultivable bat influenza virus using a replicative synthetic virus.

Zhou B(1), Ma J(2), Liu Q(2), Bawa B(2), Wang W(1), Shabman RS(1), Duff M(2), Lee J(2), Lang Y(2), Cao N(2), Nagy A(2), Lin X(1), Stockwell TB(1), Richt JA(2), Wentworth DE(1), Ma W(2).

Author information: (1)Virology, J. Craig Venter Institute, Rockville, Maryland, United States of America. (2)Department of Diagnostic Medicine/Pathobiology, College of Veterinary Medicine, Kansas State University, Manhattan, Kansas, United States of America.

Bats harbor many viruses, which are periodically transmitted to humans resulting in outbreaks of disease (e.g., Ebola, SARS-CoV). Recently, influenza virus-like sequences were identified in bats; however, the viruses could not be cultured. This discovery aroused great interest in understanding the evolutionary history and pandemic potential of bat-influenza. Using synthetic genomics, we were unable to rescue the wild type bat virus, but could rescue a modified bat-influenza virus that had the HA and NA coding regions replaced with those of A/PR/8/1934 (H1N1). This modified bat-influenza virus replicated efficiently in vitro and in mice, resulting in severe disease. Additional studies using a bat-influenza virus that had the HA and NA of A/swine/Texas/4199-2/1998 (H3N2) showed that the PR8 HA and NA contributed to the pathogenicity in mice. Unlike other influenza viruses, engineering truncations hypothesized to reduce interferon antagonism into the NS1 protein didn't attenuate bat-influenza. In contrast, substitution of a putative virulence mutation from the bat-influenza PB2 significantly attenuated the virus in mice and introduction of a putative virulence mutation increased its pathogenicity. Mini-genome replication studies and virus reassortment experiments demonstrated that bat-influenza has very limited genetic and protein compatibility with Type A or Type B influenza viruses, yet it readily reassorts with another divergent bat-influenza virus, suggesting that the bat-influenza lineage may represent a new Genus/Species within the Orthomyxoviridae family. Collectively, our data indicate that the bat-influenza viruses recently identified are authentic viruses that pose little, if any, pandemic threat to humans; however, they provide new insights into the evolution and basic biology of influenza viruses.

PMCID: PMC4183581 PMID: 25275541 [PubMed - in process]

564. R I Med J (2013). 2014 Oct 1;97(10):63-4.

Professional responsibilities for treatment of patients with Ebola: can a healthcare provider refuse to treat a patient with ebola?

Twardowski L(1), McInnis T(2), Cappuccino CC(3), McDonald J(4), Rhodes J(5).

Author information: (1)President of the Rhode Island State Board of Nursing and Certified School Nurse Teacher (District Coordinator) for the Town of North Kingstown, Rhode Island. (2)Chief Administrative Officer of the Rhode Island Board of Nursing. (3)Chair of the Rhode Island Board of Dentistry. (4)Chief Administrative Officer of the Rhode Island Board of Medical Licensure and Discipline. (5)Chief of Emergency Medical Services, Rhode Island Department of Health.

PMID: 25271667 [PubMed - in process]

565. Sci China Life Sci. 2014 Oct;57(10):973-81. doi: 10.1007/s11427-014-4759-2. Epub 2014 Sep 29.

Identification of Ebola virus microRNAs and their putative pathological function.

Liang H(1), Zhou Z, Zhang S, Zen K, Chen X, Zhang C.

Author information: (1)Jiangsu Engineering Research Center for microRNA Biology and Biotechnology, State Key Laboratory of Pharmaceutical Biotechnology, School of Life Sciences, Nanjing University, Nanjing, 210093, China.

Ebola virus (EBOV), a member of the filovirus family, is an enveloped negative-sense RNA virus that causes lethal infections in humans and primates. Recently, more than 1000 people have been killed by the Ebola virus disease in Africa, yet no specific treatment or diagnostic tests for EBOV are available. In this study, we identified two putative viral microRNA precursors (pre-miRNAs) and three putative mature microRNAs (miRNAs) derived from the EBOV genome. The production of the EBOV miRNAs was further validated in HEK293T cells transfected with a pcDNA6.2-GW/EmGFP-EBOV-pre-miRNA plasmid, indicating that EBOV miRNAs can be produced through the cellular miRNA processing machinery. We also predicted the potential target genes of these EBOV miRNAs and their possible biological functions. Overall, this study reports for the first time that EBOV may produce miRNAs, which could serve as non-invasive biomarkers for the diagnosis and prognosis of EBOV infection and as therapeutic targets for Ebola viral infection treatment.

PMID: 25266153 [PubMed - in process]

566. Sci China Life Sci. 2014 Oct;57(10):982-4. doi: 10.1007/s11427-014-4756-5. Epub 2014 Sep 19.

Potential clinical treatment for Ebola pandemic.

Zhong Y(1), Xu J, Li T, Yu X, Sheng M.

Author information: (1)State Key Laboratory of Medical Molecular Biology, Institute of Basic Medical Sciences, Chinese Academy of Medical Sciences; Department of Biochemistry and Molecular Biology, Peking Union Medical College, Tsinghua University, Beijing, 100005, China.

PMID: 25239448 [PubMed - in process]

567. Sci China Life Sci. 2014 Oct;57(10):985-6. doi: 10.1007/s11427-014-4750-y. Epub 2014 Sep 18.

MicroRNAs: the novel targets for Ebola drugs.

Yan J(1), Gao GF.

Author information: (1)CAS Key Laboratory of Pathogenic Microbiology and Immunology, Institute of Microbiology, Chinese Academy of Sciences, Beijing, 100101, China, yanjh@im.ac.cn.

Comment on Sci China Life Sci. 2014 Oct;57(10):959-72.

PMID: 25234109 [PubMed - in process]

568. Sci China Life Sci. 2014 Oct;57(10):987-8. doi: 10.1007/s11427-014-4746-7. Epub 2014 Sep 13.

Fighting Ebola with ZMapp: spotlight on plant-made antibody.

Zhang Y(1), Li D, Jin X, Huang Z.

Author information: (1)Vaccine Research Center, Institut Pasteur of Shanghai, Chinese Academy of Sciences, Shanghai, 200031, China.

PMID: 25218825 [PubMed - in process]

569. Sci China Life Sci. 2014 Oct;57(10):959-72. doi: 10.1007/s11427-014-4742-y. Epub 2014 Sep 13.

Hsa-miR-1246, hsa-miR-320a and hsa-miR-196b-5p inhibitors can reduce the cytotoxicity of Ebola virus glycoprotein in vitro.

Sheng M(1), Zhong Y, Chen Y, Du J, Ju X, Zhao C, Zhang G, Zhang L, Liu K, Yang N, Xie P, Li D, Zhang MQ, Jiang C.

Author information: (1)State Key Laboratory of Medical Molecular Biology, Institute of Basic Medical Sciences, Chinese Academy of Medical Sciences; Department of Biochemistry and Molecular Biology, Peking Union Medical College, Tsinghua University, Beijing, 100005, China.

Comment in Sci China Life Sci. 2014 Oct;57(10):985-6.

Ebola virus (EBOV) causes a highly lethal hemorrhagic fever syndrome in humans and has been associated with mortality rates of up to 91% in Zaire, the most lethal strain. Though the viral envelope glycoprotein (GP) mediates widespread inflammation and cellular damage, these changes have mainly focused on alterations at the protein level, the role of microRNAs (miRNAs) in the molecular pathogenesis underlying this lethal disease is not fully understood. Here, we report that the mi-RNAs hsa-miR-1246, hsa-miR-320a and hsa-miR-196b-5p were induced in human umbilical vein endothelial cells (HUVECs) following expression of EBOV GP. Among the proteins encoded by predicted targets of these miRNAs, the adhesion-related molecules tissue factor pathway inhibitor

(TFPI), dystroglycan1 (DAG1) and the caspase 8 and FADD-like apoptosis regulator (CFLAR) were significantly downregulated in EBOV GP-expressing HUVECs. Moreover, inhibition of hsa-miR-1246, hsa-miR-320a and hsa-miR-196b-5p, or overexpression of TFPI, DAG1 and CFLAR rescued the cell viability that was induced by EBOV GP. Our results provide a novel molecular basis for EBOV pathogenesis and may contribute to the development of strategies to protect against future EBOV pandemics.

PMID: 25218824 [PubMed - in process]

570. Nurs Stand. 2014 Sep 30;29(4):11. doi: 10.7748/ns.29.4.11.s12.

Former nurse is the first to volunteer for Ebola trial.

[No authors listed]

PMID: 25249086 [PubMed - in process]

571. Vaccine. 2014 Sep 29;32(43):5722-9. doi: 10.1016/j.vaccine.2014.08.028. Epub 2014 Aug 27.

Immunization with vesicular stomatitis virus vaccine expressing the Ebola glycoprotein provides sustained long-term protection in rodents.

Wong G(1), Audet J(1), Fernando L(2), Fausther-Bovendo H(2), Alimonti JB(2), Kobinger GP(3), Qiu X(4).

Author information: (1)Special Pathogens Program, National Microbiology Laboratory, Public Health Agency of Canada, 1015 Arlington Street, Winnipeg, MB, R3E 3R2 Canada; Department of Medical Microbiology, University of Manitoba, Winnipeg, MB, Canada. (2)Special Pathogens Program, National Microbiology Laboratory, Public Health Agency of Canada, 1015 Arlington Street, Winnipeg, MB, R3E 3R2 Canada. (3)Special Pathogens Program, National Microbiology Laboratory, Public Health Agency of Canada, 1015 Arlington Street, Winnipeg, MB, R3E 3R2 Canada; Department of Medical Microbiology, University of Manitoba, Winnipeg, MB, Canada; Department of Immunology, University of Manitoba, Winnipeg, MB, Canada; Department of Pathology and Laboratory Medicine, University of Pennsylvania, School of Medicine, Philadelphia, PA, USA. (4)Special Pathogens Program, National Microbiology Laboratory, Public Health Agency of Canada, 1015 Arlington Street, Winnipeg, MB, R3E 3R2 Canada. Electronic address: xiangguo.qiu@phac-aspc.gc.ca.

Ebola virus (EBOV) infections cause lethal hemorrhagic fever in humans, resulting in up to 90% mortality. EBOV outbreaks are sporadic and unpredictable in nature; therefore, a vaccine that is able to provide durable immunity is needed to protect those who are at risk of exposure to the virus. This study assesses the long-term efficacy of the vesicular stomatitis virus (VSV)-based vaccine (VSVΔG/EBOVGP) in two rodent models of EBOV infection. Mice and guinea pigs were first immunized with $2\times10(4)$ or $2\times10(5)$ plaque forming units (PFU) of VSVΔG/EBOVGP, respectively. Challenge of mice with a lethal dose of mouse-adapted EBOV (MA-EBOV) at 6.5 and 9 months after vaccination provided complete protection, and 80% (12 of 15 survivors) protection at 12 months after vaccination. Challenge of guinea pigs with a lethal dose of guinea pig-adapted EBOV (GA-EBOV) at 7, 12 and 18 months after vaccination resulted in 83% (5 of 6 survivors) at 7 months after vaccination, and 100% survival at 12 and 18 months after vaccination. No weight loss or clinical signs were observed in the surviving animals. Antibody responses were analyzed using sera from individual rodents. Levels of EBOV glycoprotein-specific IgG antibody measured immediately before challenge appeared to correlate with protection. These studies confirm that vaccination with VSVΔG/EBOVGP is able to confer long-term protection against Ebola infection in mice and guinea pigs, and support follow-up studies in non-human primates.

PMID: 25173474 [PubMed - in process]

572. J Vis Exp. 2014 Sep 27;(91):52381. doi: 10.3791/52381.

Modeling the lifecycle of Ebola virus under biosafety level 2 conditions with virus-like particles containing tetracistronic minigenomes.

Hoenen T(1), Watt A(2), Mora A(3), Feldmann H(2).

Author information: (1)Laboratory of Virology, Division of Intramural Research, National Institute of Allergy and Infectious Diseases, National Institutes of Health; thomas.hoenen@nih.gov. (2)Laboratory of Virology, Division of Intramural Research, National Institute of Allergy and Infectious Diseases, National Institutes of Health. (3)Research Technology Branch, Division of Intramural Research, National Institute of Allergy and Infectious Diseases, National Institutes of Health.

Ebola viruses cause severe hemorrhagic fevers in humans and non-human primates, with case fatality rates as high as 90%. There are no approved vaccines or specific treatments for the disease caused by these viruses, and work with infectious Ebola viruses is restricted to biosafety level 4 laboratories, significantly limiting the research on these viruses. Lifecycle modeling systems model the virus lifecycle under biosafety level 2 conditions; however, until recently such systems have been limited to either individual aspects of the virus lifecycle, or a single infectious cycle. Tetracistronic minigenomes, which consist of Ebola virus non-coding regions, a reporter gene, and three Ebola virus genes involved in morphogenesis, budding, and entry (VP40, GP1,2, and VP24), can be used to produce replication and transcription-competent virus-like particles (trVLPs) containing these minigenomes. These trVLPs can continuously infect cells expressing the Ebola virus proteins responsible for genome replication and transcription, allowing us to safely model multiple infectious cycles under biosafety level 2 conditions. Importantly, the viral components of this systems are solely derived from Ebola virus and not from other viruses (as is, for example, the case in systems using pseudotyped viruses), and VP40, GP1,2 and VP24 are not overexpressed in this system, making it ideally suited for studying morphogenesis, budding and entry, although other aspects of the virus lifecycle such as genome replication and transcription can also be modeled with this system. Therefore, the tetracistronic trVLP assay represents the most comprehensive lifecycle modeling system available for Ebola viruses, and has tremendous potential for use in investigating the biology of Ebola viruses in future. Here, we provide detailed information on the use of this system, as well as on expected results.

PMID: 25285674 [PubMed - in process]

573. Lancet. 2014 Sep 27;384(9949):1181. doi: 10.1016/S0140-6736(14)61606-8. Epub 2014 Sep 10.

Ebola: a failure of international collective action.

Philips M(1), Markham A(2).
Author information: (1)Médecins Sans Frontières, Analysis and Advocacy Unit, Brussels 1090, Belgium. Electronic address: mit.philips@brussels.msf.org. (2)Médecins Sans Frontières, Analysis and Advocacy Unit, Brussels 1090, Belgium.
PMID: 25218774 [PubMed - indexed for MEDLINE]

574. Lancet. 2014 Sep 27;384(9949):1181-2. doi: 10.1016/S0140-6736(14)61346-5. Epub 2014 Sep 9.

Ebola control measures and inadequate responses.

Ryschon TW(1).
Author information: (1)Minnechaduza Medical Clinic, Loveland, CO 80538, USA. Electronic address: tim@minnechaduzamedicine.com.

Comment on Lancet. 2014 Sep 6;384(9946):856.

PMID: 25217114 [PubMed - indexed for MEDLINE]

575. BMC Biol. 2014 Sep 26;12(1):80. [Epub ahead of print]

Ebolavirus in West Africa, and the use of experimental therapies or vaccines.

Hoenen T, Feldmann H.

Response to the current ebolavirus outbreak based on traditional control measures has so far been insufficient to prevent the virus from spreading rapidly. This has led to urgent discussions on the use of experimental therapies and vaccines untested in humans and existing in limited quantities, raising political, strategic, technical and ethical questions.

PMCID: PMC4177057 PMID: 25286348 [PubMed - as supplied by publisher]

576. MMWR Surveill Summ. 2014 Sep 26;63 Suppl 3:1-14.

Estimating the future number of cases in the Ebola epidemic--Liberia and Sierra Leone, 2014-2015.

Meltzer MI, Atkins CY, Santibanez S, Knust B, Petersen BW, Ervin ED, Nichol ST, Damon IK, Washington ML; Centers for Disease Control and Prevention (CDC).

The first cases of the current West African epidemic of Ebola virus disease (hereafter referred to as Ebola) were reported on March 22, 2014, with a report of 49 cases in Guinea. By August 31, 2014, a total of 3,685 probable, confirmed, and suspected cases in West Africa had been reported. To aid in planning for additional disease-control efforts, CDC constructed a modeling tool called EbolaResponse to provide estimates of the potential number of future cases. If trends continue without scale-up of effective interventions, by September 30, 2014, Sierra Leone and Liberia will have a total of approximately 8,000 Ebola cases. A potential underreporting correction factor of 2.5 also was calculated. Using this correction factor, the model estimates that approximately 21,000 total cases will have occurred in Liberia and Sierra Leone by September 30, 2014. Reported cases in Liberia are doubling every 15-20 days, and those in Sierra Leone are doubling every 30-40 days. The EbolaResponse modeling tool also was used to estimate how control and prevention interventions can slow and eventually stop the epidemic. In a hypothetical scenario, the epidemic begins to decrease and eventually end if approximately 70% of persons with Ebola are in medical care facilities or Ebola treatment units (ETUs) or, when these settings are at capacity, in a non-ETU setting such that there is a reduced risk for disease transmission (including safe burial when needed). In another hypothetical scenario, every 30-day delay in increasing the percentage of patients in ETUs to 70% was associated with an approximate tripling in the number of daily cases that occur at the peak of the epidemic (however, the epidemic still eventually ends). Officials have developed a plan to rapidly increase ETU capacities and also are developing innovative methods that can be quickly scaled up to isolate patients in non-ETU settings in a way that can help disrupt Ebola transmission in communities. The U.S. government and international organizations recently announced commitments to support these measures. As these measures are rapidly implemented and sustained, the higher projections presented in this report become very unlikely.

PMID: 25254986 [PubMed - indexed for MEDLINE]

577. Science. 2014 Sep 26;345(6204):1549-50. doi: 10.1126/science.345.6204.1549.

Infectious Diseases. Testing new Ebola tests.

Vogel G.

PMID: 25258059 [PubMed - indexed for MEDLINE]

578. N Engl J Med. 2014 Sep 25;371(13):e18. doi: 10.1056/NEJMp1410741.

Ebola virus disease--current knowledge.

Kanapathipillai R.

PMID: 25251632 [PubMed - indexed for MEDLINE]

579. N Engl J Med. 2014 Sep 25;371(13):1185-7. doi: 10.1056/NEJMp1410301. Epub 2014 Sep 3.

A good death---Ebola and sacrifice.

Mugele J(1), Priest C.
Author information: (1)From the Indiana University School of Medicine (J.M., C.P.); and the Indiana University School of Nursing (C.P.) - both in Indianapolis.
PMID: 25184515 [PubMed - indexed for MEDLINE]

580. N Engl J Med. 2014 Sep 25;371(13):1177-80. doi: 10.1056/NEJMp1409903. Epub 2014 Aug 20.

Ebola 2014--new challenges, new global response and responsibility.

Frieden TR(1), Damon I, Bell BP, Kenyon T, Nichol S.
Author information: (1)From the Centers for Disease Control and Prevention, Atlanta.
PMID: 25140858 [PubMed - indexed for MEDLINE]

581. N Engl J Med. 2014 Sep 25;371(13):1183-5. doi: 10.1056/NEJMp1409859. Epub 2014 Aug 20.

Ebola virus disease in West Africa--no early end to the outbreak.

Chan M(1).

Author information: (1)Dr. Chan is the director-general of the World Health Organization, Geneva.

PMID: 25140856 [PubMed - indexed for MEDLINE]

582. N Engl J Med. 2014 Sep 25;371(13):1180-3. doi: 10.1056/NEJMp1409858. Epub 2014 Aug 20.

The international Ebola emergency.

Briand S(1), Bertherat E, Cox P, Formenty P, Kieny MP, Myhre JK, Roth C, Shindo N, Dye C.

Author information: (1)From the World Health Organization, Geneva.

PMID: 25140855 [PubMed - indexed for MEDLINE]

583. Nature. 2014 Sep 25;513(7519):474-7. doi: 10.1038/513474a.

Infectious disease: Ebola's lost ward.

Check Hayden E.

PMID: 25254458 [PubMed - indexed for MEDLINE]

584. Nature. 2014 Sep 25;513(7519):469. doi: 10.1038/513469a.

Global Ebola response kicks into gear at last.

Butler D.

PMID: 25254453 [PubMed - indexed for MEDLINE]

585. Nature. 2014 Sep 25;513(7519):459. doi: 10.1038/513459a.

First response, revisited.

[No authors listed]

PMID: 25254437 [PubMed - indexed for MEDLINE]

586. BMJ. 2014 Sep 24;349:g5866. doi: 10.1136/bmj.g5866.

Liberia and Sierra Leone could see 1.4 million Ebola cases by January.

McCarthy M(1).

Author information: (1)Seattle.

PMID: 25252773 [PubMed - indexed for MEDLINE]

587. Rev Med Suisse. 2014 Sep 24;10(443):1800.

[Ebola: the moral bankruptcy and the irrational].

[Article in French]

Kiefer B.

PMID: 25369709 [PubMed - indexed for MEDLINE]

588. BMJ. 2014 Sep 23;349:g5838. doi: 10.1136/bmj.g5838.

Clinical trials of Ebola treatment to start in Africa.

Gulland A(1).

Author information: (1)London.

PMID: 25248787 [PubMed - indexed for MEDLINE]

589. Nurs Stand. 2014 Sep 23;29(3):8. doi: 10.7748/ns.29.3.8.s4.

Ebola nurse calls on PM for special treatment centres.

[No authors listed]

The British nurse who became the first person in the UK to contract the deadly Ebola virus in Sierra Leone has pledged to return to the country.

PMID: 25227341 [PubMed - in process]

590. Fortune. 2014 Sep 22;170(4):10-2.

How to stop Ebola. The latest epidemic sheds light on a little-known industry that could change the way we treat virus diseases.

Fry E.

PMID: 25509578 [PubMed - in process]

591. Lancet. 2014 Sep 20;384(9948):e45-6.

WHO meeting chooses untried interventions to defeat Ebola.

Maurice J.

PMID: 25247221 [PubMed - indexed for MEDLINE]

592. Elife. 2014 Sep 19;3:e04565. doi: 10.7554/eLife.04565.

Mapping Ebola in wild animals for better disease control.

Funk S(1), Piot P(2).

Author information: (1)Sebastian Funk is in the Centre for the Mathematical Modelling of Infectious Diseases, London School of Hygiene & Tropical Medicine, London, United Kingdom sebastian.funk@lshtm.ac.uk. (2)Peter Piot is in the London School of Hygiene and Tropical Medicine, London, United Kingdom.
Comment on Elife. 2014;3:e04395.

Identifying the regions where wild animal populations could transmit the Ebola virus should help with efforts to prepare at-risk areas for future outbreaks.

PMCID: PMC4166718 PMID: 25238569 [PubMed - in process]

593. Science. 2014 Sep 19;345(6203):1441-2. doi: 10.1126/science.345.6203.1441.

Infectious disease. Ebola vaccine: little and late.

Cohen J.

PMID: 25237082 [PubMed - indexed for MEDLINE]

594. BMJ. 2014 Sep 18;348:g5727. doi: 10.1136/bmj.g5727.

US plans to deploy 3000 army personnel to tackle Ebola in west Africa.

McCarthy M(1).

Author information: (1)Seattle.

PMID: 25234127 [PubMed - indexed for MEDLINE]

595. Euro Surveill. 2014 Sep 18;19(37). pii: 20908.

Feedback from modelling to surveillance of Ebola virus disease.

Nishiura H(1), Chowell G.

Author information: (1)Graduate School of Medicine, The University of Tokyo, Tokyo, Japan.

Comment on Euro Surveill. 2014;19(36). pii: 20894.

PMID: 25259537 [PubMed - in process]

596. Euro Surveill. 2014 Sep 18;19(37). pii: 20907.

Early transmission dynamics of Ebola virus disease (EVD), West Africa, March to August 2014 - Euro surveillance 17 September 2014.

Plachouras D(1), Sudre B, Testa M, Robesyn E, Coulombier D.

Author information: (1)European Centre for Disease Prevention and Control (ECDC), Stockholm, Sweden.

Comment on Euro Surveill. 2014;19(36). pii: 20894.

PMID: 25259536 [PubMed - in process]

597. N Engl J Med. 2014 Sep 18;371(12):1081-3. doi: 10.1056/NEJMp1410179. Epub 2014 Aug 27.

Face to face with Ebola--an emergency care center in Sierra Leone.

Wolz A(1).

Author information: (1)From Médecins sans Frontières, Brussels.

PMID: 25162580 [PubMed - indexed for MEDLINE]

598. N Engl J Med. 2014 Sep 18;371(12):1086-9. doi: 10.1056/NEJMp1409817. Epub 2014 Aug 20.

Studying "secret serums"--toward safe, effective Ebola treatments.

Goodman JL(1).

Author information: (1)From the Department of Medicine, Division of Infectious Diseases, and Center on Medical Product Access, Safety, and Stewardship, Georgetown University; and the Department of Medicine, Division of Infectious Diseases, Veterans Affairs Medical Center - both in Washington, DC.

PMID: 25140857 [PubMed - indexed for MEDLINE]

599. N Engl J Med. 2014 Sep 18;371(12):1084-6. doi: 10.1056/NEJMp1409494. Epub 2014 Aug 13.

Ebola--underscoring the global disparities in health care resources.

Fauci AS(1).

Author information: (1)From the National Institute of Allergy and Infectious Diseases, National Institutes of Health, Bethesda, MD.

PMID: 25119491 [PubMed - indexed for MEDLINE]

600. Nature. 2014 Sep 18;513(7518):315. doi: 10.1038/513315a.

Africa: Ebola virus control needs local buy-in.

Guerrier G(1), D'Ortenzio E(2).

Author information: (1)Hôtel-Dieu and Cochin Hospitals, Paris Descartes University, France. (2)Solthis, France; and Bichat Hospital, Paris, France.

PMID: 25230645 [PubMed - indexed for MEDLINE]

601. JAMA. 2014 Sep 17;312(11):1095-6. doi: 10.1001/jama.2014.11176.

The Ebola epidemic: a global health emergency.

Gostin LO(1), Lucey D(2), Phelan A(1).

Author information: (1)O'Neill Institute for National and Global Health Law, Georgetown University Law Center, Washington, DC. (2)Department of Microbiology and Immunology, Georgetown University Medical Center, Washington, DC.

PMID: 25111044 [PubMed - indexed for MEDLINE]

602. Rev Med Suisse. 2014 Sep 17;10(442):1730-1.

[Ebola: "survivors' blood" gets into the official therapeutic arsenal].

[Article in French]

Nau JY.

PMID: 25322506 [PubMed - in process]

603. Antiviral Res. 2014 Sep 16;111C:143-153. doi: 10.1016/j.antiviral.2014.08.009. [Epub ahead of print]

Meeting report: 27th International conference on antiviral research, in Raleigh, NC, USA.

Vere Hodge RA(1).

Author information: (1)Vere Hodge Antivirals Ltd, Old Denshott, Leigh, Reigate, Surrey, UK.

The 27th International Conference on Antiviral Research (ICAR) was held in Raleigh, North Carolina, USA from May 12 to 16, 2014. This article summarizes the principal invited lectures. John Drach (Elion Award) described the early days of antiviral drugs and their novel modes of action. Piet Herdewijn (Holý Award) used evolutionary pressure to select DNA polymerases that accept nucleoside analogs. Replacing thymine by 5-chlorouracil led to the generation of a new form of Escherichia coli. Adrian Ray (Prusoff Award) demonstrated how prodrugs can markedly improve both the efficacy and safety of potential drugs. The keynote addresses, by David Margolis and Myron Cohen, tackled two emerging areas of HIV research, to find an HIV "cure" and to prevent HIV transmission, respectively. These topics were discussed further in other presentations - a cure seems to be a distant prospect but there are exciting developments for reducing HIV transmission. TDF-containing vaginal rings and GSK-744, as a long-lasting injection, offer great hope. There were three mini-symposia. Although therapy with TDF/FTC gives excellent control of HBV replication, there are only a few patients who achieve a functional cure. Myrcludex, an entry inhibitor, is active against both HBV and HDV. The recent progress with HBV replication in cell cultures has transformed the search for new antiviral compounds. The HBV capsid protein has been recognized as key player in HBV DNA synthesis. Unexpectedly, compounds which enhance capsid formation, markedly reduce HBV DNA synthesis. The development of BCX4430, which is active against Marburg and Ebola viruses, is of great current interest.

Copyright © 2014 The Author. Published by Elsevier B.V. All rights reserved.

PMID: 25218950 [PubMed - as supplied by publisher]

604. CMAJ. 2014 Sep 16;186(13):E477. doi: 10.1503/cmaj.109-4869. Epub 2014 Aug 5.

Canadians leading anti-Ebola research.

Rastogi J(1).

Author information: (1)CMAJ.

PMCID: PMC4162795 [Available on 2015/9/16] PMID: 25096658 [PubMed - indexed for MEDLINE]

605. BMJ. 2014 Sep 15;349:g5597. doi: 10.1136/bmj.g5597.

Ebola in an unprepared Africa.

Tomori O(1).

Author information: (1)Nigerian Academy of Science, University of Lagos Campus, Akoka, Lagos 100213, Nigeria oyewaletomori@yahoo.com.

PMID: 25224647 [PubMed - in process]

606. Med J Aust. 2014 Sep 15;201(6):352-4.

Don't be scared, be angry: the politics and ethics of Ebola.

Hooker LC(1), Mayes C(2), Degeling C(2), Gilbert GL(2), Kerridge IH(2).

Author information: (1)Centre for Values, Ethics and Law in Medicine, University of Sydney, Sydney, NSW, Australia. claire.hooker@sydney.edu.au. (2)Centre for Values, Ethics and Law in Medicine, University of Sydney, Sydney, NSW, Australia.

The current outbreak of Ebola virus disease in West Africa is the worst so far. The unprecedented extent of mortality and morbidity in this outbreak has followed more from imposition of neoliberal economic policies on the countries affected than from the biological virulence of Ebola virus. The lack of vaccines and medications for Ebola virus disease is evidence that markets cannot reliably supply treatments for epidemic diseases. We attribute the current difficulties in containment chiefly to the erosion or non-development of the health and medical infrastructure needed to respond effectively, as a direct result of market-privileging policies imposed in the interests of wealthy nations. These events and responses hold lessons for public health priorities in Australia.

PMID: 25222463 [PubMed - indexed for MEDLINE]

607. Med J Aust. 2014 Sep 15;201(6):320-1.

Vulnerability, hysteria and fear - conquering Ebola virus.

Banerjee A(1), Mor SM(2), Kok J(2), Sorrell TC(2), Hill-Cawthorne GA(2).

Author information: (1)Marie Bashir Institute for Infectious Diseases and Biosecurity, University of Sydney, Sydney, NSW, Australia. grant.hill-cawthorne@sydney.edu.au. (2)Marie Bashir Institute for Infectious Diseases and Biosecurity, University of Sydney, Sydney, NSW, Australia.

PMID: 25222449 [PubMed - indexed for MEDLINE]

608. Med J Aust. 2014 Sep 15;201(6):309.

Doing what's necessary.

Leeder S(1).

Author information: (1)Medical Journal of Australia, Sydney, NSW, Australia. mja@mja.com.au.

PMID: 25222443 [PubMed - indexed for MEDLINE]

609. J Infect Dis. 2014 Sep 14. pii: jiu511. [Epub ahead of print]

Safety and Immunogenicity of DNA Vaccines Encoding Ebolavirus and Marburgvirus Wild-Type Glycoproteins in a Phase I Clinical Trial.

Sarwar UN(1), Costner P(1), Enama ME(1), Berkowitz N(1), Hu Z(2), Hendel CS(1), Sitar S(1), Plummer S(1), Mulangu S(1), Bailer RT(1), Koup RA(1), Mascola JR(1), Nabel GJ(1), Sullivan NJ(1), Graham BS(1), Ledgerwood JE(1); the VRC 206 Study Team.
Author information: (1)Vaccine Research Center. (2)Biostatistics Research Branch, Division of Clinical Research, National Institute of Allergy and Infectious Diseases, National Institutes of Health, Bethesda, Maryland.

BACKGROUND: Ebolavirus and Marburgvirus cause severe hemorrhagic fever with high mortality and are potential bioterrorism agents. There are no available vaccines or therapeutic agents. Previous clinical trials evaluated transmembrane-deleted and point-mutation Ebolavirus glycoproteins (GPs) in candidate vaccines. Constructs evaluated in this trial encode wild-type (WT) GP from Ebolavirus Zaire and Sudan species and the Marburgvirus Angola strain expressed in a DNA vaccine. METHODS: The VRC 206 study evaluated the safety and immunogenicity of these DNA vaccines (4 mg administered intramuscularly by Biojector) at weeks 0, 4, and 8, with a homologous boost at or after week 32. Safety evaluations included solicited reactogenicity and coagulation parameters. Primary immune assessment was done by means of GP-specific enzyme-linked immunosorbent assay. RESULTS: The vaccines were well tolerated, with no serious adverse events; 80% of subjects had positive enzyme-linked immunosorbent assay results (≥30) at week 12. The fourth DNA vaccination boosted the immune responses. CONCLUSIONS: The investigational Ebolavirus and Marburgvirus WT GP DNA vaccines were safe, well tolerated, and immunogenic in this phase I study. These results will further inform filovirus vaccine research toward a goal of inducing protective immunity by using WT GP antigens in candidate vaccine regimens. Clinical Trials Registration.   NCT00605514.

PMID: 25225676 [PubMed - as supplied by publisher]
610. J Infect Dis. 2014 Sep 14. pii: jiu513. [Epub ahead of print]

How the Current West African Ebola Virus Disease Epidemic Is Altering Views on the Need for Vaccines and Is Galvanizing a Global Effort to Field-Test Leading Candidate Vaccines.

Levine MM(1), Tapia M(1), Hill AV(2), Sow SO(3).
Author information: (1)Center for Vaccine Development, University of Maryland School of Medicine, Baltimore. (2)Jenner Institute, Nuffield Department of Medicine, University of Oxford, United Kingdom. (3)Le Centre pour le Développement des Vaccins du Mali, Bamako.

PMID: 25225675 [PubMed - as supplied by publisher]
611. Lancet. 2014 Sep 13;384(9947):930. doi: 10.1016/S0140-6736(14)61613-5.

The silver bullet of resilience.

[No authors listed]

PMID: 25220958 [PubMed - indexed for MEDLINE]
612. Lancet. 2014 Sep 13;384(9947):951. doi: 10.1016/S0140-6736(14)61344-1. Epub 2014 Sep 3.

Taking a religious perspective to contain Ebola.

Bah SM(1), Aljoudi AS(2).
Author information: (1)University of Dammam, Dammam 31441, Saudi Arabia. Electronic address: sbah@ud.edu.sa. (2)University of Dammam, Al Khobar 31952, Saudi Arabia.

PMID: 25194448 [PubMed - indexed for MEDLINE]
613. BMJ. 2014 Sep 12;349:g5647. doi: 10.1136/bmj.g5647.

Cuba pledges 165 health workers to treat Ebola patients in Sierra Leone.

Gulland A(1).
Author information: (1)London.

PMID: 25217171 [PubMed - in process]
614. Elife. 2014 Sep 12;3:e03908. doi: 10.7554/eLife.03908.

Epidemiological dynamics of Ebola outbreaks.

House T(1).
Author information: (1)Warwick Mathematics Institute, University of Warwick, Coventry, United Kingdom.

Ebola is a deadly virus that causes frequent disease outbreaks in the human population. In this study, we analyse its rate of new introductions, case fatality ratio, and potential to spread from person to person. The analysis is performed for all completed outbreaks and for a scenario where these are augmented by a more severe outbreak of several thousand cases. The results show a fast rate of new outbreaks, a high case fatality ratio, and an effective reproductive ratio of just less than 1.

PMID: 25217532 [PubMed - in process]
615. J Infect Dev Ctries. 2014 Sep 12;8(9):1148-59. doi: 10.3855/jidc.4636.

Diagnostic schemes for reducing epidemic size of African viral hemorrhagic fever outbreaks.

Okeke IN(1), Manning RS, Pfeiffer T.
Author information: (1)Haverford College, Haverford, PA, United States. iokeke@haverford.edu.

INTRODUCTION: Viral hemorrhagic fever (VHF) outbreaks, with high mortality rates, have often been amplified in African health institutions due to person-to-person transmission via infected body fluids. By collating and analyzing epidemiological data from documented outbreaks, we observed that diagnostic delay contributes to epidemic size for Ebola and Marburg hemorrhagic fever outbreaks. METHODOLOGY: We used a susceptible-exposed-infectious-removed (SEIR) model and data from the 1995 outbreak in Kikwit, Democratic Republic of Congo, to simulate Ebola hemorrhagic fever epidemics. Our model allows us to describe the dynamics for hospital staff separately from that for the general population, and to implement health worker-specific interventions. RESULTS: The model illustrates that implementing World Health Organization/US Centers for Disease Control and Prevention guidelines of isolating patients who do not respond to antimalarial and antibacterial chemotherapy reduces total outbreak size, from a median of 236, by 90% or more. Routinely employing diagnostic testing in post-mortems of patients that died of refractory fevers reduces the median outbreak size by a further 60%. Even greater reductions in outbreak size were seen when all febrile patients were tested for endemic infections or when febrile health-care workers were tested. The effect of testing strategies was not impaired by the 1-3 day delay that would occur if testing were performed by a reference laboratory. CONCLUSION: In addition to improving the quality of care for common causes of febrile infections, increased and strategic use of laboratory diagnostics for fever could reduce the chance of hospital amplification of VHFs in resource-limited African health systems.
PMID: 25212079 [PubMed - in process]

616. Science. 2014 Sep 12;345(6202):1369-72. doi: 10.1126/science.1259657. Epub 2014 Aug 28.

Genomic surveillance elucidates Ebola virus origin and transmission during the 2014 outbreak.

Gire SK(1), Goba A(2), Andersen KG(3), Sealfon RS(4), Park DJ(5), Kanneh L(6), Jalloh S(6), Momoh M(7), Fullah M(7), Dudas G(8), Wohl S(9), Moses LM(10), Yozwiak NL(1), Winnicki S(1), Matranga CB(5), Malboeuf CM(5), Qu J(5), Gladden AD(5), Schaffner SF(1), Yang X(5), Jiang PP(1), Nekoui M(1), Colubri A(11), Coomber MR(6), Fonnie M(6), Moigboi A(6), Gbakie M(6), Kamara FK(6), Tucker V(6), Konuwa E(6), Saffa S(6), Sellu J(6), Jalloh AA(6), Kovoma A(6), Koninga J(6), Mustapha I(6), Kargbo K(6), Foday M(6), Yillah M(6), Kanneh F(6), Robert W(6), Massally JL(6), Chapman SB(5), Bochicchio J(5), Murphy C(5), Nusbaum C(5), Young S(5), Birren BW(5), Grant DS(6), Scheiffelin JS(10), Lander ES(12), Happi C(13), Gevao SM(14), Gnirke A(5), Rambaut A(15), Garry RF(10), Khan SH(6), Sabeti PC(3).

Author information: (1)Center for Systems Biology, Department of Organismic and Evolutionary Biology, Harvard University, Cambridge, MA 02138, USA. Broad Institute of MIT and Harvard, Cambridge, MA 02142, USA. (2)Kenema Government Hospital, Kenema, Sierra Leone. andersen@broadinstitute.org augstgoba@yahoo.com psabeti@oeb.harvard.edu. (3)Center for Systems Biology, Department of Organismic and Evolutionary Biology, Harvard University, Cambridge, MA 02138, USA. Broad Institute of MIT and Harvard, Cambridge, MA 02142, USA. andersen@broadinstitute.org augstgoba@yahoo.com psabeti@oeb.harvard.edu. (4)Broad Institute of MIT and Harvard, Cambridge, MA 02142, USA. Computer Science and Artificial Intelligence Laboratory, Massachusetts Institute of Technology, Cambridge, MA 02139, USA. (5)Broad Institute of MIT and Harvard, Cambridge, MA 02142, USA. (6)Kenema Government Hospital, Kenema, Sierra Leone. (7)Kenema Government Hospital, Kenema, Sierra Leone. Eastern Polytechnic College, Kenema, Sierra Leone. (8)Institute of Evolutionary Biology, University of Edinburgh, Edinburgh EH9 3JT, UK. (9)Center for Systems Biology, Department of Organismic and Evolutionary Biology, Harvard University, Cambridge, MA 02138, USA. Broad Institute of MIT and Harvard, Cambridge, MA 02142, USA. Systems Biology, Harvard Medical School, Boston, MA 02115, USA. (10)Tulane University Medical Center, New Orleans, LA 70112, USA. (11)Center for Systems Biology, Department of Organismic and Evolutionary Biology, Harvard University, Cambridge, MA 02138, USA. (12)Broad Institute of MIT and Harvard, Cambridge, MA 02142, USA. Systems Biology, Harvard Medical School, Boston, MA 02115, USA. Department of Biology, Massachusetts Institute of Technology, Cambridge, MA 02139, USA. (13)Redeemer's University, Ogun State, Nigeria. (14)University of Sierra Leone, Freetown, Sierra Leone. (15)Institute of Evolutionary Biology, University of Edinburgh, Edinburgh EH9 3JT, UK. Fogarty International Center, National Institutes of Health, Bethesda, MD 20892, USA. Centre for Immunity, Infection and Evolution, University of Edinburgh, Edinburgh EH9 3JT, UK.

Comment in Cell Host Microbe. 2014 Oct 8;16(4):419-21.

In its largest outbreak, Ebola virus disease is spreading through Guinea, Liberia, Sierra Leone, and Nigeria. We sequenced 99 Ebola virus genomes from 78 patients in Sierra Leone to ~2000× coverage. We observed a rapid accumulation of interhost and intrahost genetic variation, allowing us to characterize patterns of viral transmission over the initial weeks of the epidemic. This West African variant likely diverged from central African lineages around 2004, crossed from Guinea to Sierra Leone in May 2014, and has exhibited sustained human-to-human transmission subsequently, with no evidence of additional zoonotic sources. Because many of the mutations alter protein sequences and other biologically meaningful targets, they should be monitored for impact on diagnostics, vaccines, and therapies critical to outbreak response.
PMID: 25214632 [PubMed - indexed for MEDLINE]

617. Science. 2014 Sep 12;345(6202):1229-30. doi: 10.1126/science.345.6202.1229.

Interview. Ebola: 'Wow, that is really tough'.

Aylward B, Roberts L.

PMID: 25214583 [PubMed - indexed for MEDLINE]

618. Science. 2014 Sep 12;345(6202):1228-9. doi: 10.1126/science.345.6202.1228.

Infectious Disease. Ebola vaccines racing forward at record pace.

Cohen J.

Comment in Science. 2014 Oct 24;346(6208):434.

PMID: 25214582 [PubMed - indexed for MEDLINE]

619. Science. 2014 Sep 12;345(6202):1221. doi: 10.1126/science.1260695.

Ebola's perfect storm.

Piot P(1).

Author information: (1)Peter Piot is director and professor of Global Health at the London School of Hygiene & Tropical Medicine, London, UK.

PMID: 25214580 [PubMed - indexed for MEDLINE]

620. Br J Nurs. 2014 Sep 11-24;23(16):886-7. doi: 10.12968/bjon.2014.23.16.886.

Understanding the Ebola threat: the UK government's response.

Glasper A.

PMID: 25203758 [PubMed - indexed for MEDLINE]

621. Br J Nurs. 2014 Sep 11-24;23(16):880. doi: 10.12968/bjon.2014.23.16.880.

Catching the chance to teach infection control.

Jeanes A(1).

Author information: (1)Director of Infection Prevention and Control and Consultant Nurse, University College London Hospitals Foundation Trust, London.

PMID: 25203756 [PubMed - indexed for MEDLINE]

622. Euro Surveill. 2014 Sep 11;19(36). pii: 20894.

Early transmission dynamics of Ebola virus disease (EVD), West Africa, March to August 2014.

Nishiura H(1), Chowell G.

Author information: (1)Graduate School of Medicine, The University of Tokyo, Tokyo, Japan.

Comment in Euro Surveill. 2014;19(37). pii: 20907. Euro Surveill. 2014;19(37). pii: 20908.

PMID: 25232919 [PubMed - in process]

623. Euro Surveill. 2014 Sep 11;19(36). pii: 20899.

Containing Ebola virus infection in West Africa.

Kucharski A(1), Piot P.

Author information: (1)London School of Hygiene & Tropical Medicine, London, United Kingdom.

PMID: 25232918 [PubMed - in process]

624. Nature. 2014 Sep 11;513(7517):145. doi: 10.1038/513145a.

Make diagnostic centres a priority for Ebola crisis.

Kelly JD.

PMID: 25209763 [PubMed - indexed for MEDLINE]

625. Nature. 2014 Sep 11;513(7517):143-4. doi: 10.1038/513143b.

Ebola: time to act.

[No authors listed]

PMID: 25209760 [PubMed - indexed for MEDLINE]

626. JAMA. 2014 Sep 10;312(10):987-9. doi: 10.1001/jama.2014.11170.

Largest-ever outbreak of Ebola virus disease thrusts experimental therapies, vaccines into spotlight.

Hampton T.

PMID: 25162140 [PubMed - indexed for MEDLINE]

627. Rev Med Suisse. 2014 Sep 10;10(441):1684-5.

[Ebola epidemic, mirror of United Nations'powerlessness?].

[Article in French]

Nau JY.

PMID: 25322632 [PubMed - in process]

628. Rev Med Suisse. 2014 Sep 10;10(441):1682-3.

[Ebola: a vaccine on forced accelerated course. Hopes for the ZMapp].

[Article in French]

Nau JY.

PMID: 25322630 [PubMed - in process]

629. BMJ. 2014 Sep 9;349:g5562. doi: 10.1136/bmj.g5562.

Trial of Ebola virus vaccine is due to start next week.

Arie S(1).

Author information: (1)London.

PMID: 25209382 [PubMed - indexed for MEDLINE]

630. BMJ. 2014 Sep 9;349:g5519. doi: 10.1136/bmj.g5519.

NHS contribution to the Ebola epidemic.

Houlihan C(1), Behrens R(2), Moore D(2).
Author information: (1)London School of Hygiene and Tropical Medicine, London, UK catherine.houlihan@lshtm.ac.uk. (2)London School of Hygiene and Tropical Medicine, London, UK.
PMID: 25205392 [PubMed - indexed for MEDLINE]
631. J Med Ethics. 2014 Sep 9. pii: medethics-2014-102434. doi: 10.1136/medethics-2014-102434. [Epub ahead of print]

The Ebola outbreak in Western Africa: ethical obligations for care.

Yakubu A(1), Folayan MO(2), Sani-Gwarzo N(3), Nguku P(4), Peterson K(5), Brown B(6).
Author information: (1)National Health Research Ethics Committee, Federal Ministry of Health, Federal Secretariat, Abuja, Nigeria. (2)Institute of Public Health and Department of Child Dental Health, Obafemi Awolowo University, Ile-Ife, Nigeria. (3)Port Health Services Division, Federal Ministry of Health, Federal Secretariat, Abuja, Nigeria. (4)Nigeria Field Epidemiology & Laboratory Training Program (NFELTP), Haile Selassie St, Asokoro, Abuja, Nigeria. (5)Department of Anthropology, University of California, Irvine, California, USA. (6)Program in Public Health, Department of Population Health & Disease Prevention, University of California, Irvine, California, USA.

The recent wave of the Ebola Virus Disease (EVD) in Western Africa and efforts to control the disease where the health system requires strengthening raises a number of ethical challenges for healthcare workers practicing in these countries. We discuss the implications of weak health systems for controlling EVD and limitations of the ethical obligation to provide care for patients with EVD using Nigeria as a case study. We highlight the right of healthcare workers to protection that should be obligatorily provided by the government. Where the national government cannot meet this obligation, healthcare workers only have a moral and not a professional obligation to provide care to patients with EVD. The national government also has an obligation to adequately compensate healthcare workers that become infected in the course of duty. Institutionalisation of policies that protect healthcare workers are required for effective control of the spread of highly contagious diseases like EVD in a timely manner.

PMID: 25205389 [PubMed - as supplied by publisher]
632. BMJ. 2014 Sep 8;349:g5539. doi: 10.1136/bmj.g5539.

First Ebola treatment is approved by WHO.

Gulland A(1).
Author information: (1)London.
PMID: 25200068 [PubMed - in process]
633. Elife. 2014 Sep 8;3:e04395. doi: 10.7554/eLife.04395.

Mapping the zoonotic niche of Ebola virus disease in Africa.

Pigott DM(1), Golding N(1), Mylne A(1), Huang Z(1), Henry AJ(1), Weiss DJ(1), Brady OJ(1), Kraemer MU(1), Smith DL(1), Moyes CL(1), Bhatt S(1), Gething PW(1), Horby PW(2), Bogoch II(3), Brownstein JS(4), Mekaru SR(5), Tatem AJ(6), Khan K(3), Hay SI(1).
Author information: (1)Spatial Ecology and Epidemiology Group, Department of Zoology, University of Oxford, Oxford, United Kingdom. (2)Epidemic Diseases Research Group, Centre for Tropical Medicine and Global Health, University of Oxford, Oxford, United Kingdom. (3)Department of Medicine, Division of Infectious Diseases, University of Toronto, Toronto, Canada. (4)Department of Pediatrics, Harvard Medical School, Boston, United States. (5)Children's Hospital Informatics Program, Boston Children's Hospital, Boston, United States. (6)Department of Geography and Environment, University of Southampton, Southampton, United Kingdom.
Comment in Elife. 2014;3:e04565.

Ebola virus disease (EVD) is a complex zoonosis that is highly virulent in humans. The largest recorded outbreak of EVD is ongoing in West Africa, outside of its previously reported and predicted niche. We assembled location data on all recorded zoonotic transmission to humans and Ebola virus infection in bats and primates (1976-2014). Using species distribution models, these occurrence data were paired with environmental covariates to predict a zoonotic transmission niche covering 22 countries across Central and West Africa. Vegetation, elevation, temperature, evapotranspiration, and suspected reservoir bat distributions define this relationship. At-risk areas are inhabited by 22 million people; however, the rarity of human outbreaks emphasises the very low probability of transmission to humans. Increasing population sizes and international connectivity by air since the first detection of EVD in 1976 suggest that the dynamics of human-to-human secondary transmission in contemporary outbreaks will be very different to those of the past.
PMCID: PMC4166725 PMID: 25201877 [PubMed - in process]
634. Epidemiol Infect. 2014 Sep 8:1-9. [Epub ahead of print]

Stakeholder prioritization of zoonoses in Japan with analytic hierarchy process method.

Kadohira M(1), Hill G(1), Yoshizaki R(2), Ota S(3), Yoshikawa Y(4).
Author information: (1)Obihiro University of Agriculture and Veterinary Medicine,Obihiro,Japan. (2)Toray Research Center,Tokyo,Japan. (3)Japan Fresh Produce Import and Safety Association,Tokyo,Japan. (4)Chiba Institute of Science,Chiba,Japan.

SUMMARY There exists an urgent need to develop iterative risk assessment strategies of zoonotic diseases. The aim of this study is to develop a method of prioritizing 98 zoonoses derived from animal pathogens in Japan and to involve four major groups of stakeholders: researchers, physicians, public health officials, and citizens. We used a combination of risk profiling and analytic hierarchy process (AHP). Profiling risk was accomplished with semi-quantitative analysis of existing public health data. AHP data collection was performed by administering questionnaires to the four stakeholder groups. Results showed that researchers and public health officials focused on case fatality as the chief important factor, while physicians and citizens placed more weight on diagnosis and prevention, respectively. Most of the six top-ranked diseases were similar among all stakeholders. Transmissible spongiform encephalopathy, severe acute respiratory syndrome, and Ebola fever were ranked first, second, and third, respectively.

PMID: 25195643 [PubMed - as supplied by publisher]

635. Lancet. 2014 Sep 6;384(9946):856. doi: 10.1016/S0140-6736(14)61343-X. Epub 2014 Aug 29.

Is respiratory protection appropriate in the Ebola response?

Martin-Moreno JM(1), Llinás G(2), Hernández JM(3).

Author information: (1)Department of Preventive Medicine and Public Health, University of Valencia, 46010 Valencia, Spain. Electronic address: dr.martinmoreno@gmail.com. (2)Department of Preventive Medicine and Public Health, University of Valencia, 46010 Valencia, Spain. (3)Preventive Medicine and Public Health Service, Hospital La Paz-Carlos III, Madrid, Spain.

Erratum in Lancet. 2014 Sep 6;384(9946):856.

Comment in Lancet. 2014 Sep 27;384(9949):1181-2.

PMID: 25178253 [PubMed - indexed for MEDLINE]

636. BMJ. 2014 Sep 5;349:g5496. doi: 10.1136/bmj.g5496.

World leaders are ignoring worldwide threat of Ebola, says MSF.

Torjesen I(1).

Author information: (1)London.

PMID: 25192726 [PubMed - in process]

637. Science. 2014 Sep 5;345(6201):1108. doi: 10.1126/science.345.6201.1108.

Infectious Disease. Estimating the Ebola epidemic.

Kupferschmidt K.

PMID: 25190771 [PubMed - indexed for MEDLINE]

638. BMJ. 2014 Sep 4;349:g5485. doi: 10.1136/bmj.g5485.

More health staff are needed to contain Ebola outbreak, warns WHO.

Gulland A(1).

Author information: (1)London.

PMID: 25193934 [PubMed - in process]

639. BMJ. 2014 Sep 4;349:g5488. doi: 10.1136/bmj.g5488.

US signs contract with ZMapp maker to accelerate development of the Ebola drug.

McCarthy M(1).

Author information: (1)Seattle.

PMID: 25189475 [PubMed - in process]

640. Euro Surveill. 2014 Sep 4;19(35). pii: 20892.

Association between temperature, humidity and ebolavirus disease outbreaks in Africa, 1976 to 2014.

Ng S(1), Cowling BJ.

Author information: (1)Department of Ecology and Evolutionary Biology, Princeton University, Princeton, New Jersey, United States.

Erratum in Euro Surveill. 2014;19(42):pii/20932. Basta, N E [removed].

Comment in Euro Surveill. 2014;19(41). pii: 20931. Euro Surveill. 2014;19(41). pii: 20930.

Ebolavirus disease (EVD) outbreaks have been occurring sporadically in Central Africa since 1976. In 2014, the first outbreak in West Africa was reported in Guinea. Subsequent outbreaks then appeared in Liberia, Sierra Leone and Nigeria. The study of environmental factors underlying EVD epidemiology may provide useful insights into when and where EVD outbreaks are more likely to occur. In this paper, we aimed to investigate the association between climatic factors and onset of EVD outbreaks in humans. Our results suggest lower temperature and higher absolute humidity are associated with EVD outbreak onset in the previous EVD outbreaks in Africa during 1976 to 2014. Potential mechanisms through which climate may have an influence on ebolavirus infection in the natural host, intermediate hosts and humans are discussed. Current and future surveillance efforts should be supported to further understand ebolavirus transmission events between and within species.

PMID: 25210981 [PubMed - indexed for MEDLINE]

641. Nature. 2014 Sep 4;513(7516):13-4. doi: 10.1038/513013a.

Ebola drug trials set to begin amid crisis.

Butler D.

Erratum in Nature. 2014 Sep 11;513(7517):156.

PMID: 25186878 [PubMed - indexed for MEDLINE]

642. Nurs Times. 2014 Sep 3-9;110(36):3.

Ebola outbreak taking toll on clinicians, warns WHO.

[No authors listed]

PMID: 25318315 [PubMed - indexed for MEDLINE]

643. Rev Med Suisse. 2014 Sep 3;10(440):1634-5.

[Is the World Health Organization guilty of delaying the fight against Ebola?].

[Article in French]

Nau JY.

PMID: 25277008 [PubMed - indexed for MEDLINE]

644. Proc Natl Acad Sci U S A. 2014 Sep 2;111(35):E3699-707. doi: 10.1073/pnas.1404851111. Epub 2014 Aug 18.

TIM-family proteins inhibit HIV-1 release.

Li M(1), Ablan SD(2), Miao C(1), Zheng YM(1), Fuller MS(1), Rennert PD(3), Maury W(4), Johnson MC(1), Freed EO(2), Liu SL(5).

Author information: (1)Department of Molecular Microbiology and Immunology, Bond Life Sciences Center, University of Missouri, Columbia, MO 65211; (2)Virus-Cell Interaction Section, HIV Drug Resistance Program, National Cancer Institute-Frederick, Frederick, MD 21702; (3)Department of Immunotherapy, SugarCone Biotech LLC, Holliston, MA 01746; and. (4)Department of Microbiology, University of Iowa, Iowa City, IA 52245. (5)Department of Molecular Microbiology and Immunology, Bond Life Sciences Center, University of Missouri, Columbia, MO 65211; liushan@missouri.edu.

Accumulating evidence indicates that T-cell immunoglobulin (Ig) and mucin domain (TIM) proteins play critical roles in viral infections. Herein, we report that the TIM-family proteins strongly inhibit HIV-1 release, resulting in diminished viral production and replication. Expression of TIM-1 causes HIV-1 Gag and mature viral particles to accumulate on the plasma membrane. Mutation of the phosphatidylserine (PS) binding sites of TIM-1 abolishes its ability to block HIV-1 release. TIM-1, but to a much lesser extent PS-binding deficient mutants, induces PS flipping onto the cell surface; TIM-1 is also found to be incorporated into HIV-1 virions. Importantly, TIM-1 inhibits HIV-1 replication in CD4-positive Jurkat cells, despite its capability of up-regulating CD4 and promoting HIV-1 entry. In addition to TIM-1, TIM-3 and TIM-4 also block the release of HIV-1, as well as that of murine leukemia virus (MLV) and Ebola virus (EBOV); knockdown of TIM-3 in differentiated monocyte-derived macrophages (MDMs) enhances HIV-1 production. The inhibitory effects of TIM-family proteins on virus release are extended to other PS receptors, such as Axl and RAGE. Overall, our study uncovers a novel ability of TIM-family proteins to block the release of HIV-1 and other viruses by interaction with virion- and cell-associated PS. Our work provides new insights into a virus-cell interaction that is mediated by TIMs and PS receptors.

PMCID: PMC4156686 [Available on 2015/3/2] PMID: 25136083 [PubMed - indexed for MEDLINE]

645. Acta Crystallogr D Biol Crystallogr. 2014 Sep;70(Pt 9):2420-9. doi: 10.1107/S1399004714014710. Epub 2014 Aug 29.

The structure of the C-terminal domain of the Zaire ebolavirus nucleoprotein.

Dziubańska PJ(1), Derewenda U(1), Ellena JF(2), Engel DA(3), Derewenda ZS(1).

Author information: (1)Department of Molecular Physiology and Biological Physics, University of Virginia School of Medicine, Charlottesville, VA 22908-0736, USA. (2)Department of Chemistry, University of Virginia, Charlottesville, VA 22904-4319, USA. (3)Department of Microbiology, Immunology and Cancer Biology, University of Virginia School of Medicine, Charlottesville, VA 22908-0736, USA.

Ebolavirus (EBOV) causes severe hemorrhagic fever with a mortality rate of up to 90%. EBOV is a member of the order Mononegavirales and, like other viruses in this taxonomic group, contains a negative-sense single-stranded (ss) RNA. The EBOV ssRNA encodes seven distinct proteins. One of them, the nucleoprotein (NP), is the most abundant viral protein in the infected cell and within the viral nucleocapsid. Like other EBOV proteins, NP is multifunctional. It is tightly associated with the viral genome and is essential for viral transcription, RNA replication, genome packaging and nucleocapsid assembly prior to membrane encapsulation. NP is unusual among the Mononegavirales in that it contains two distinct regions, or putative domains, the C-terminal of which shows no homology to any known proteins and is purported to be a hub for protein-protein interactions within the nucleocapsid. The atomic structure of NP remains unknown. Here, the boundaries of the N- and C-terminal domains of NP from Zaire EBOV are defined, it is shown that they can be expressed as highly stable recombinant proteins in Escherichia coli, and the atomic structure of the C-terminal domain (residues 641-739) derived from analysis of two distinct crystal forms at 1.98 and 1.75 Å resolution is described. The structure reveals a novel tertiary fold that is distantly reminiscent of the β-grasp architecture.

PMCID: PMC4157450 [Available on 2015/9/1] PMID: 25195755 [PubMed - in process]

646. Acta Med Port. 2014 Sep-Oct;27(5):625-633. Epub 2014 Oct 31.

Ebolavirosis: a 2014 Review for Clinicians.

Nina J(1).

Author information: (1)Serviço de Doenças Infecciosas e Medicina Tropical. Hospital Egas Moniz. Centro Hospitalar Lisboa Ocidental. Lisboa. Portugal. Unidade de Clínica. Instituto de Higiene e Medicina Tropical. Universidade Nova de Lisboa. Lisboa. Portugal.

Ebolavirosis, like Marburgvirosis, are African zoonosis, and for both the primary animal reservoir are bats. It is a typical acute haemorrhagic fever, characterized by a high lethality rate. In an outbreak, the human index case became infected after contact with an infected animal or its blood, in most cases during hunting. Secondary human cases became infected after close contact with another human case, with infected human fluids or with a recent dead corps of a human case. These viruses are easily transmitted by direct contact or by contact with patient body fluids, mainly blood. As such, health professionals working under suboptimal conditions usually constitute a large share of Ebola victims. At the moment, the treatment is only supportive, but several drugs are almost ready to be tried in human trials. There is no vaccine approved, but again there are several very promising in the pipeline.

Publisher: Abstract available from the publisher. PMID: 25409219 [PubMed - as supplied by publisher]

647. Afr Health Sci. 2014 Sep;14(3):i-iii.

Ebola and other issues in the health sector in Africa.

Tumwine JK(1).

Author information: (1)Department of Paediatrics and Child Health, College of Health Sciences, Makerereb University.
PMCID: PMC4209624 PMID: 25352907 [PubMed - in process]
648. Afr Health Sci. 2014 Sep;14(3):495-501. doi: 10.4314/ahs.v14i3.1.

Ebola viral hemorrhagic disease outbreak in West Africa- lessons from Uganda.

Mbonye AK(1), Wamala JF(2), Nanyunja M(3), Opio A(4), Makumbi I(5), Aceng JR(6).

Author information: (1)Associate Professor, School of Public Health- Makerere University &, Commissioner Health Services, Ministry of Health, Box 7272, Kampala, Uganda. (2)Senior Epidemiologist, Epidemiology and Surveillance Division, Ministry of Health, Box 7272, Kampala, Uganda. (3)Disease Prevention and Control Officer, WHO Uganda Country Office, P. O. Box 24578, Kampala. (4)Assistant Commissioner Health Services, Ministry of Health, Box 7272, Kampala, Uganda. (5)Epidemiology and Surveillance Division, Ministry of Health, Box 7272, Kampala, Uganda. (6)Director General of health services, Ministry of Health, Box 7272, Kampala, Uganda.

BACKGROUND: There has been a rapid spread of Ebola Viral Hemorrhagic disease in Guinea, Liberia and Sierra Leone since March 2014. Since this is the first time of a major Ebola outbreak in West Africa; it is possible there is lack of understanding of the epidemic in the communities, lack of experience among the health workers to manage the cases and limited capacities for rapid response. The main objective of this article is to share Uganda's experience in controlling similar Ebola outbreaks and to suggest some lessons that could inform the control of the Ebola outbreak in West Africa. METHODS: The article is based on published papers, reports of previous Ebola outbreaks, response plans and experiences of individuals who have participated in the control of Ebola epidemics in Uganda. Lessons learnt: The success in the control of Ebola epidemics in Uganda has been due to high political support, effective coordination through national and district task forces. In addition there has been active surveillance, strong community mobilization using village health teams and other community resources persons, an efficient laboratory system that has capacity to provide timely results. These have coupled with effective case management and infection control and the involvement of development partners who commit resources with shared responsibility. CONCLUSION: Several factors have contributed to the successful quick containment of Ebola outbreaks in Uganda. West African countries experiencing Ebola outbreaks could draw some lessons from the Uganda experience and adapt them to contain the Ebola epidemic.

PMCID: PMC4209631 PMID: 25352864 [PubMed - in process]
649. Ann Acad Med Singapore. 2014 Sep;43(9):435-6.

Could the devastation from ebola occur in Asia?

Fisher D(1), Salmon S.

Author information: (1)Division of Infectious Diseases, National University Hospital, Singapore.
PMID: 25277081 [PubMed - in process]
650. Antiviral Res. 2014 Sep;109:171-4. doi: 10.1016/j.antiviral.2014.07.004. Epub 2014 Jul 11.

HSPA5 is an essential host factor for Ebola virus infection.

Reid SP(1), Shurtleff AC(1), Costantino JA(1), Tritsch SR(1), Retterer C(1), Spurgers KB(1), Bavari S(2).

Author information: (1)United States Army Medical Research Institute of Infectious Diseases, 1425 Porter Street, Fort Detrick, Frederick, MD 21702-5011, USA. (2)United States Army Medical Research Institute of Infectious Diseases, 1425 Porter Street, Fort Detrick, Frederick, MD 21702-5011, USA. Electronic address: sina.bavari@amedd.army.mil.

Development of novel strategies targeting the highly virulent ebolaviruses is urgently required. A proteomic study identified the ER chaperone HSPA5 as an ebolavirus-associated host protein. Here, we show using the HSPA5 inhibitor (-)- epigallocatechin gallate (EGCG) that the chaperone is essential for virus infection, thereby demonstrating a functional significance for the association. Furthermore, in vitro and in vivo gene targeting impaired viral replication and protected animals in a lethal infection model. These findings demonstrate that HSPA5 is vital for replication and can serve as a viable target for the design of host-based countermeasures.

Published by Elsevier B.V.
PMID: 25017472 [PubMed - in process]
651. Aust Nurs Midwifery J. 2014 Sep;22(3):40.

The challenges faced in infection prevention and control practices.

Roderick A.
PMID: 25286720 [PubMed - indexed for MEDLINE]
652. Br J Hosp Med (Lond). 2014 Sep;75(9):515-22. doi: 10.12968/hmed.2014.75.9.515.

Ebola and other viral haemorrhagic fevers: a local operational approach.

Moore LS(1), Moore M, Sriskandan S.

Author information: (1)NIHR Clinical Research Fellow at the Imperial Biomedical Research Centre, Imperial College London, Hammersmith Campus, London W12 0HS.
PMID: 25216168 [PubMed - indexed for MEDLINE]
653. Bull World Health Organ. 2014 Sep 1;92(9):622. doi: 10.2471/BLT.14.145789.

The 2014 Ebola outbreak: ethical use of unregistered interventions.

Krech R(1), Kieny MP(1).

Author information: (1)World Health Organization, avenue Appia 20, 1211 Geneva 27, Switzerland .

PMCID: PMC4208580 PMID: 25378748 [PubMed - in process]
654. Cent Eur J Public Health. 2014 Sep;22(3):207.

Ebola hemorrhagic fever: case fatality rate 90%?

Allam MF.

PMID: 25507919 [PubMed - in process]
655. Cent Eur J Public Health. 2014 Sep;22(3):207.

Ebola hemorrhagic fever: case fatality rate 90%?

Allam MF.

PMID: 25438402 [PubMed - in process]
656. Emerg Nurse. 2014 Sep;22(5):10-1. doi: 10.7748/en.22.5.10.s10.

Healthcare staff advised to prepare for Ebola cases in UK.

Sprinks J.

EMERGENCY NURSES are accustomed to responding to any kind of presentation, and so should not be alarmed by the latest national guidance on identifying and caring for patients with the Ebola virus.

PMID: 25185907 [PubMed - in process]
657. Germs. 2014 Sep 1;4(3):58. doi: 10.11599/germs.2014.1056. eCollection 2014.

Ebola virus disease - a global threat.

Streinu-Cercel A.

PMCID: PMC4176255 PMID: 25276664 [PubMed]
658. J Korean Med Sci. 2014 Sep;29(9):1185. doi: 10.3346/jkms.2014.29.9.1185.

Preparedness for prevention of Ebola virus disease.

Hwang ES(1).

Author information: (1)Department of Microbiology and Immunology, Seoul National University College of Medicine, and Institute of Endemic Diseases, Seoul National University Medical Research Center, Seoul, Korea.

PMCID: PMC4168168 PMID: 25246733 [PubMed - in process]
659. J Virol. 2014 Sep;88(18):10958-62. doi: 10.1128/JVI.00870-14. Epub 2014 Jul 9.

Spatial localization of the Ebola virus glycoprotein mucin-like domain determined by cryo-electron tomography.

Tran EE(1), Simmons JA(2), Bartesaghi A(1), Shoemaker CJ(2), Nelson E(2), White JM(2), Subramaniam S(3).

Author information: (1)Center for Cancer Research, National Cancer Institute, National Institutes of Health, Bethesda, Maryland, USA. (2)Department of Cell Biology, University of Virginia School of Medicine, Charlottesville, Virginia, USA. (3)Center for Cancer Research, National Cancer Institute, National Institutes of Health, Bethesda, Maryland, USA ss1@nih.gov.

The Ebola virus glycoprotein mucin-like domain (MLD) is implicated in Ebola virus cell entry and immune evasion. Using cryo-electron tomography of Ebola virus-like particles, we determined a three-dimensional structure for the full-length glycoprotein in a near-native state and compared it to that of a glycoprotein lacking the MLD. Our results, which show that the MLD is located at the apex and the sides of each glycoprotein monomer, provide a structural template for analysis of MLD function.

PMCID: PMC4178867 PMID: 25008940 [PubMed - in process]
660. J Virol. 2014 Sep;88(18):10511-24. doi: 10.1128/JVI.01272-14. Epub 2014 Jun 25.

A novel life cycle modeling system for Ebola virus shows a genome length-dependent role of VP24 in virus infectivity.

Watt A(1), Moukambi F(2), Banadyga L(1), Groseth A(3), Callison J(1), Herwig A(2), Ebihara H(1), Feldmann H(4), Hoenen T(5).

Author information: (1)Laboratory of Virology, Division of Intramural Research, National Institute of Allergy and Infectious Diseases, National Institutes of Health, Hamilton, Montana, USA. (2)Institute for Virology, Philipps University Marburg, Marburg, Germany. (3)Laboratory of Virology, Division of Intramural Research, National Institute of Allergy and Infectious Diseases, National Institutes of Health, Hamilton, Montana, USA Institute for Virology, Philipps University Marburg, Marburg, Germany. (4)Laboratory of Virology, Division of Intramural Research, National Institute of Allergy and Infectious Diseases, National Institutes of Health, Hamilton, Montana, USA feldmannh@niaid.nih.gov thomas.hoenen@nih.gov. (5)Laboratory of Virology, Division of Intramural Research, National Institute of Allergy and Infectious Diseases, National Institutes of Health, Hamilton, Montana, USA Institute for Virology, Philipps University Marburg, Marburg, Germany feldmannh@niaid.nih.gov thomas.hoenen@nih.gov.

Work with infectious Ebola viruses is restricted to biosafety level 4 (BSL4) laboratories, presenting a significant barrier for studying these viruses. Life cycle modeling systems, including minigenome systems and transcription- and replication-competent virus-like particle (trVLP) systems, allow modeling of the virus life cycle under BSL2 conditions; however, all current systems model only certain aspects of the virus life cycle, rely on plasmid-based viral protein expression, and have been used to model only single infectious cycles. We have developed a novel life cycle modeling system allowing continuous passaging of infectious trVLPs containing a tetracistronic minigenome that encodes a reporter and the viral proteins VP40, VP24, and GP1,2. This system is ideally suited for studying morphogenesis, budding, and entry, in addition to genome replication and transcription. Importantly, the specific infectivity of trVLPs in this system was ~ 500-fold higher than that in previous systems. Using this system for functional studies of VP24, we showed that, contrary to previous reports, VP24 only very modestly inhibits genome replication and transcription when expressed in a regulated fashion, which we confirmed using infectious Ebola viruses. Interestingly, we also discovered a genome length-dependent effect of VP24 on particle infectivity, which was previously undetected due to the short length of monocistronic minigenomes and which is due at least partially to a previously unknown function of VP24 in RNA packaging. Based on our findings, we propose a model for the function of VP24 that reconciles all currently available data regarding the role of VP24 in nucleocapsid assembly as well as genome replication and transcription.IMPORTANCE: Ebola viruses cause severe hemorrhagic fevers in humans, with no countermeasures currently being available, and must be studied in maximum-containment laboratories. Only a few of these laboratories exist worldwide, limiting our ability to study Ebola viruses and develop countermeasures. Here we report the development of a novel reverse genetics-based system that allows the study of Ebola viruses without maximum-containment laboratories. We used this system to investigate the Ebola virus protein VP24, showing that, contrary to previous reports, it only modestly inhibits virus genome replication and transcription but is important for packaging of genomes into virus particles, which constitutes a previously unknown function of VP24 and a potential antiviral target. We further propose a comprehensive model for the function of VP24 in nucleocapsid assembly. Importantly, on the basis of this approach, it should easily be possible to develop similar experimental systems for other viruses that are currently restricted to maximum-containment laboratories.

PMCID: PMC4178905 [Available on 2015/3/1] PMID: 24965473 [PubMed - in process]
661. J Virol. 2014 Sep 1;88(17):9877-92. doi: 10.1128/JVI.01410-14. Epub 2014 Jun 18.

Ebola virus modulates transforming growth factor β signaling and cellular markers of mesenchyme-like transition in hepatocytes.

Kindrachuk J(1), Wahl-Jensen V(2), Safronetz D(3), Trost B(4), Hoenen T(3), Arsenault R(5), Feldmann F(6), Traynor D(7), Postnikova E(7), Kusalik A(4), Napper S(5), Blaney JE(8), Feldmann H(3), Jahrling PB(9).

Author information: (1)Emerging Viral Pathogens Section, National Institute of Allergy and Infectious Diseases, National Institutes of Health, Bethesda, Maryland, USA Integrated Research Facility, Division of Clinical Research, National Institute of Allergy and Infectious Diseases, National Institutes of Health, Frederick, Maryland, USA kindrachuk.kenneth@nih.gov. (2)Integrated Research Facility, Division of Clinical Research, National Institute of Allergy and Infectious Diseases, National Institutes of Health, Frederick, Maryland, USA National Biodefense Analysis and Countermeasures Center, Frederick, Maryland, USA. (3)Laboratory of Virology, Division of Intramural Research, National Institute of Allergy and Infectious Diseases, National Institutes of Health, Hamilton, Montana, USA. (4)Department of Computer Science, University of Saskatchewan, Saskatoon, Saskatchewan, Canada. (5)Department of Biochemistry, University of Saskatchewan, Saskatoon, Saskatchewan, Canada Vaccine and Infectious Disease Organization, University of Saskatchewan, Saskatoon, Saskatchewan, Canada. (6)Rocky Mountain Veterinary Branch, Division of Intramural Research, National Institute of Allergy and Infectious Diseases, National Institutes of Health, Hamilton, Montana, USA. (7)Integrated Research Facility, Division of Clinical Research, National Institute of Allergy and Infectious Diseases, National Institutes of Health, Frederick, Maryland, USA. (8)Emerging Viral Pathogens Section, National Institute of Allergy and Infectious Diseases, National Institutes of Health, Bethesda, Maryland, USA. (9)Emerging Viral Pathogens Section, National Institute of Allergy and Infectious Diseases, National Institutes of Health, Bethesda, Maryland, USA Integrated Research Facility, Division of Clinical Research, National Institute of Allergy and Infectious Diseases, National Institutes of Health, Frederick, Maryland, USA.

Ebola virus (EBOV) causes a severe hemorrhagic disease in humans and nonhuman primates, with a median case fatality rate of 78.4%. Although EBOV is considered a public health concern, there is a relative paucity of information regarding the modulation of the functional host response during infection. We employed temporal kinome analysis to investigate the relative early, intermediate, and late host kinome responses to EBOV infection in human hepatocytes. Pathway overrepresentation analysis and functional network analysis of kinome data revealed that transforming growth factor (TGF-β)-mediated signaling responses were temporally modulated in response to EBOV infection. Upregulation of TGF-β signaling in the kinome data sets correlated with the upregulation of TGF-β secretion from EBOV-infected cells. Kinase inhibitors targeting TGF-β signaling, or additional cell receptors and downstream signaling pathway intermediates identified from our kinome analysis, also inhibited EBOV replication. Further, the inhibition of select cell signaling intermediates identified from our kinome analysis provided partial protection in a lethal model of EBOV infection. To gain perspective on the cellular consequence of TGF-β signaling modulation during EBOV infection, we assessed cellular markers associated with upregulation of TGF-β signaling. We observed upregulation of matrix metalloproteinase 9, N-cadherin, and fibronectin expression with concomitant reductions in the expression of E-cadherin and claudin-1, responses that are standard characteristics of an epithelium-to-mesenchyme-like transition. Additionally, we identified phosphorylation events downstream of TGF-β that may contribute to this process. From these observations, we propose a model for a broader role of TGF-β-mediated signaling responses in the pathogenesis of Ebola virus disease.IMPORTANCE: Ebola virus (EBOV), formerly Zaire ebolavirus, causes a severe hemorrhagic disease in humans and nonhuman primates and is the most lethal Ebola virus species, with case fatality rates of up to 90%. Although EBOV is considered a worldwide concern, many questions remain regarding EBOV molecular pathogenesis. As it is appreciated that many cellular processes are regulated through kinase-mediated phosphorylation events, we employed temporal kinome analysis to investigate the functional responses of human hepatocytes to EBOV infection. Administration of kinase inhibitors targeting signaling pathway intermediates identified in our kinome analysis inhibited viral replication in vitro and reduced EBOV pathogenesis in vivo. Further analysis of our data also demonstrated that EBOV infection modulated TGF-β-mediated signaling responses and promoted mesenchyme-like phenotypic changes. Taken together, these results demonstrated that EBOV infection specifically modulates TGF-β-mediated signaling responses in epithelial cells and may have broader implications in EBOV pathogenesis.

PMCID: PMC4136307 [Available on 2015/3/1] PMID: 24942569 [PubMed - indexed for MEDLINE]
662. J Zhejiang Univ Sci B. 2014 Sep;15(9):761-5. doi: 10.1631/jzus.B1400222.

Forty years of the war against Ebola.

Zhang L(1), Wang H.

Author information: (1)Tianjin International Joint Academy of Biomedicine, Tianjin 300457, China; Department of Biophysics, Nankai University, Tianjin 300071, China.

Humans have been fighting against the Ebola virus disease (EVD) since its first outbreak in 1976 in southern Sudan and Yambuku in Zaire which lies on the Ebola River. According to the data from the World Health Organization (WHO, 2014b), the first outbreak claimed 431 lives in 1976, and the disease awoke transiently in Sudan three years later and then disappeared for 15 years afterwards. Following that, large outbreaks appeared in 1995 in Zaire with 250 deaths of people, 2001-2002 in Uganda with 224 deaths, 2002-2003 in Congo with 128 deaths, and 2007 in Congo with 187 deaths. In 2014, the most severe and complicated outbreak swept through the West African countries having already taken 1069 lives, with the situation seeming to be out of control. To date, there have been 15 outbreaks in Africa, which have caused 4362 infected cases and claimed 2659 lives. The pandemics of Ebola show obvious independence from any season. Humans are generally susceptible to the Ebola virus without gender or age variation. The natural reservoir of the Ebola virus still remains unclear. During the past 40 years or so, the EVD disappeared after an outbreak in one region and erupted in another region without any warning. The difficulty in understanding the spreading pattern of Ebola was compared to that of the wave-particle duality of light.

PMCID: PMC4162877 PMID: 25183030 [PubMed - in process]

663. Kinderkrankenschwester. 2014 Sep;33(9):336.

[Ebola is not a danger for Europe].

[Article in German]

Schulte-Wissermann H.

PMID: 25291838 [PubMed - indexed for MEDLINE]

664. Lancet Infect Dis. 2014 Sep;14(9):779. doi: 10.1016/S1473-3099(14)70785-6. Epub 2014 Aug 14.

Ebola in West Africa.

The Lancet Infectious Diseases.

PMID: 25131986 [PubMed - indexed for MEDLINE]

665. Med Mal Infect. 2014 Sep;44(9):412-6. doi: 10.1016/j.medmal.2014.08.005. Epub 2014 Sep 2.

Case fatality rates of Ebola virus diseases: a meta-analysis of World Health Organization data.

Lefebvre A(1), Fiet C(1), Belpois-Duchamp C(1), Tiv M(1), Astruc K(1), Aho Glélé LS(2).

Author information: (1)Service d'épidémiologie et d'hygiène hospitalières, hôpital d'enfants, CHU, 14, rue Paul-Gaffarel, BP 77908, 21079 Dijon cedex, France. (2)Service d'épidémiologie et d'hygiène hospitalières, hôpital d'enfants, CHU, 14, rue Paul-Gaffarel, BP 77908, 21079 Dijon cedex, France. Electronic address: Ludwig.aho@chu-dijon.fr.

OBJECTIVE: Our objective was to estimate the case fatality rates of Zaire, Sudan, and Bundibugyo Ebola species, responsible for sometimes-lethal hemorrhagic fevers. METHODS: We performed a meta-analysis of World Health Organization data on outbreaks of infections due to theses species. RESULTS: Twenty outbreaks, including the current one, were studied. The estimated case fatality rate was 65.4% (CI 95% [54.6%; 75.5%]) and varied among the outbreaks. A species effect was identified, with a higher case fatality rate for the Zaire species than for Sudan and Bundibugyo species. The case fatality rate of the Zaire species tended to decrease with time. CONCLUSION: The case fatality rates associated with these 3 species was high. A great variability was observed. It could be explained partly by a species effect and by the decrease of Zaire species case fatality rate, with time.

PMID: 25193630 [PubMed - in process]

666. Med Monatsschr Pharm. 2014 Sep;37(9):324-30; quiz 331-2.

[Marburg and Ebola hemorrhagic fevers--pathogens, epidemiology and therapy].

[Article in German]

Stock I.

Marburg and Ebola hemorrhagic fevers are severe, systemic viral diseases affecting humans and non-human primates. They are characterized by multiple symptoms such as hemorrhages, fever, headache, muscle and abdominal pain, chills, sore throat, nausea, vomiting and diarrhea. Elevated liver-associated enzyme levels and coagulopathy are also associated with these diseases. Marburg and Ebola hemorrhagic fevers are caused by (Lake victoria) Marburg virus and different species of Ebola viruses, respectively. They are enveloped, single-stranded RNA viruses and belong to the family of filoviridae. Case fatality rates of filovirus disease outbreaks are among the highest reported for any human pathogen, ranging from 25 to 90% or more. Outbreaks of Marburg and Ebola hemorrhagic fever occur in certain regions of equatorial Africa at irregular intervals. Since 2000, the number of outbreaks has increased. In 2014, the biggest outbreak of a filovirus-induced hemorrhagic fever that has been documented so far occurred from March to July 2014 in Guinea, Sierra Leone, Liberia and Nigeria. The outbreak was caused by a new variant of Zaire Ebola-Virus, affected more than 2600 people (stated 20 August) and was associated with case-fatality rates of up to 67% (Guinea). Treatment of Marburg and Ebola hemorrhagic fevers is symptomatic and supportive, licensed antiviral agents are currently not available. Recently, BCX4430, a promising synthetic adenosine analogue with high in vitro and in vivo activity against filoviruses and other RNA viruses, has been described. BCX4430 inhibits viral RNA polymerase activity and protects cynomolgus macaques from Marburg virus infection when administered as late as 48 hours after infection. Nucleic acid-based products, recombinant vaccines and antibodies appear to be less suitable for the treatment of Marburg and Ebola hemorrhagic fevers.

PMID: 25282746 [PubMed - indexed for MEDLINE]

667. Med Monatsschr Pharm. 2014 Sep;37(9):313.

[A question of competence].

[Article in German]

Rausch R.

PMID: 25282744 [PubMed - indexed for MEDLINE]

668. Microbiol Immunol. 2014 Sep;58(9):483-91. doi: 10.1111/1348-0421.12181.

Ebola and Marburg virus diseases in Africa: increased risk of outbreaks in previously unaffected areas?

Changula K(1), Kajihara M, Mweene AS, Takada A.

Author information: (1)School of Veterinary Medicine, University of Zambia, Great East Road Campus, Lusaka, Zambia; Southern African Centre for Infectious Disease Surveillance, P.O. Box, 3297, Chuo Kikuu, Morogoro, Tanzania.

Filoviral hemorrhagic fever (FHF) is caused by ebolaviruses and marburgviruses, which both belong to the family Filoviridae. Egyptian fruit bats (Rousettus aegyptiacus) are the most likely natural reservoir for marburgviruses and entry into caves and mines that they stay in has often been associated with outbreaks of MVD. On the other hand, the natural reservoir for ebola viruses remains elusive; however, handling of wild animal carcasses has been associated with some outbreaks of EVD. In the last two decades, there has been an increase in the incidence of FHF outbreaks in Africa, some being caused by a newly found virus and some occurring in previously unaffected areas such as Guinea, Liberia and Sierra Leone, in which the most recent EVD outbreak occurred in 2014. Indeed, the predicted geographic distribution of filoviruses and their potential reservoirs in Africa includes many countries in which FHF has not been reported. To minimize the risk of virus dissemination in previously unaffected areas, there is a need for increased investment in health infrastructure in African countries, policies to facilitate collaboration between health authorities from different countries, implementation of outbreak control measures by relevant multi-disciplinary teams and education of the populations at risk.

PMID: 25040642 [PubMed - in process]

669. Mol Biol Evol. 2014 Sep;31(9):2356-64. doi: 10.1093/molbev/msu185. Epub 2014 Jun 10

Evolutionary origins of human herpes simplex viruses 1 and 2.

Wertheim JO(1), Smith MD(2), Smith DM(3), Scheffler K(4), Kosakovsky Pond SL(5).

Author information: (1)Department of Medicine, University of California, San Diego jwertheim@ucsd.edu. (2)Bioinformatics and Systems Biology Graduate Program, University of California, San Diego. (3)Department of Medicine, University of California, San DiegoVeterans Affairs San Diego Healthcare System, San Diego, CA. (4)Department of Medicine, University of California, San DiegoDepartment of Mathematical Sciences, Stellenbosch University, Stellenbosch, South Africa. (5)Department of Medicine, University of California, San Diego.

Herpesviruses have been infecting and codiverging with their vertebrate hosts for hundreds of millions of years. The primate simplex viruses exemplify this pattern of virus-host codivergence, at a minimum, as far back as the most recent common ancestor of New World monkeys, Old World monkeys, and apes. Humans are the only primate species known to be infected with two distinct herpes simplex viruses: HSV-1 and HSV-2. Human herpes simplex viruses are ubiquitous, with over two-thirds of the human population infected by at least one virus. Here, we investigated whether the additional human simplex virus is the result of ancient viral lineage duplication or cross-species transmission. We found that standard phylogenetic models of nucleotide substitution are inadequate for distinguishing among these competing hypotheses; the extent of synonymous substitutions causes a substantial underestimation of the lengths of some of the branches in the phylogeny, consistent with observations in other viruses (e.g., avian influenza, Ebola, and coronaviruses). To more accurately estimate ancient viral divergence times, we applied a branch-site random effects likelihood model of molecular evolution that allows the strength of natural selection to vary across both the viral phylogeny and the gene alignment. This selection-informed model favored a scenario in which HSV-1 is the result of ancient codivergence and HSV-2 arose from a cross-species transmission event from the ancestor of modern chimpanzees to an extinct Homo precursor of modern humans, around 1.6 Ma. These results provide a new framework for understanding human herpes simplex virus evolution and demonstrate the importance of using selection-informed models of sequence evolution when investigating viral origin hypotheses.

PMCID: PMC4137711 [Available on 2015/9/1] PMID: 24916030 [PubMed - in process]

670. Nat Biotechnol. 2014 Sep;32(9):849-50. doi: 10.1038/nbt0914-849a.

Biotech drugs too little, too late for Ebola outbreak.

Strauss S.

PMID: 25203010 [PubMed - in process]

671. Nat Med. 2014 Sep;20(9):967. doi: 10.1038/nm.3689.

Ebola: a call to action.

[No authors listed]

The size, speed and potential reach of the 2014 Ebola virus outbreak in West Africa presents a wake-up call to the research and pharmaceutical communities - and to federal governments - of the continuing need to invest resources in the study and cure of emerging infectious diseases.

PMID: 25198036 [PubMed - indexed for MEDLINE]

672. Nursing. 2014 Sep;44(9):68-9. doi: 10.1097/01.NURSE.0000453010.02525.ca.

Ebola virus disease: an emerging threat.

Turner C(1).

Author information: (1)Cheryl Turner is an RN at Golisano Children's Hospital in Rochester, N.Y.

PMID: 25140950 [PubMed - in process]

673. Pediatr Ann. 2014 Sep;43(9):332-3. doi: 10.3928/00904481-20140825-01.

What, Ebola here?

Shulman ST.

PMID: 25198438 [PubMed - in process]

674. PLoS Negl Trop Dis. 2014 Sep 18;8(9):e3143. doi: 10.1371/journal.pntd.0003143. eCollection 2014.

A new approach for monitoring ebolavirus in wild great apes.

Reed PE(1), Mulangu S(2), Cameron KN(1), Ondzie AU(1), Joly D(1), Bermejo M(3), Rouquet P(4), Fabozzi G(2), Bailey M(2), Shen Z(2), Keele BF(5), Hahn B(6), Karesh WB(1), Sullivan NJ(2).

Author information: (1)Wildlife Conservation Society, Bronx, New York, New York, United States of America. (2)Vaccine Research Center, National Institute for Allergy and Infectious Disease, National Institutes of Health, Bethesda, Maryland, United States of America. (3)Departamento Biologia Animal (Vertebrados), Facultad de Biologia, Universidad de Barcelona, Barcelona, Spain. (4)ECOFAC, Libreville, Gabon. (5)AIDS and Cancer Virus Program, Frederick National Laboratory, Frederick, Maryland, United States of America. (6)University of Alabama at Birmingham, Birmingham, Alabama, United States of America.

BACKGROUND: Central Africa is a "hotspot" for emerging infectious diseases (EIDs) of global and local importance, and a current outbreak of ebolavirus is affecting multiple countries simultaneously. Ebolavirus is suspected to have caused recent declines in resident great apes. While ebolavirus vaccines have been proposed as an intervention to protect apes, their effectiveness would be improved if we could diagnostically confirm Ebola virus disease (EVD) as the cause of die-offs, establish ebolavirus geographical distribution, identify immunologically naïve populations, and determine whether apes survive virus exposure. METHODOLOGY/PRINCIPAL FINDINGS: Here we report the first successful noninvasive detection of antibodies against Ebola virus (EBOV) from wild ape feces. Using this method, we have been able to identify gorillas with antibodies to EBOV with an overall prevalence rate reaching 10% on average, demonstrating that EBOV exposure or infection is not uniformly lethal in this species. Furthermore, evidence of antibodies was identified in gorillas thought previously to be unexposed to EBOV (protected from exposure by rivers as topological barriers of transmission). CONCLUSIONS/SIGNIFICANCE: Our new approach will contribute to a strategy to protect apes from future EBOV infections by early detection of increased incidence of exposure, by identifying immunologically naïve at-risk populations as potential targets for vaccination, and by providing a means to track vaccine efficacy if such intervention is deemed appropriate. Finally, since human EVD is linked to contact with infected wildlife carcasses, efforts aimed at identifying great ape outbreaks could have a profound impact on public health in local communities, where EBOV causes case-fatality rates of up to 88%.

PMCID: PMC4169258 PMID: 25232832 [PubMed - in process]

675. Public Health. 2014 Sep;128(9):769-70. doi: 10.1016/j.puhe.2014.08.015. Epub 2014 Sep 20.

The rising tide of Ebola.

Sim F(1), Mackie P(2).

Author information: (1)The Royal Society for Public Health, John Snow House, 59 Mansell Street, London E1 8AN, UK. Electronic address: public.health@rsph.org.uk. (2)The Royal Society for Public Health, John Snow House, 59 Mansell Street, London E1 8AN, UK.

PMID: 25246355 [PubMed - indexed for MEDLINE]

676. Rev Prat. 2014 Sep;64(7):905-10.

[Ebola hemorrhagic fever: its extension reflects the African sanitary disaster].

[Article in French]

Bourée P.

Ebola virus, described in 1976 in Zaire, causes severe hemorrhagic fever with a high mortality rate in humans and nonhuman primates. Epidemics occurred since this time to nowadays in Sudan, Gabon, Congo and currently in Guinea, Liberia, Sierra-Leone, Nigeria and Senegal. Specific treatment and vaccine are not available. So, to prevent the virus transmission with live and dead patients, we must use strict individual and collective measures which are not always understood by local populations and make contact tracing; it is the only way to curb the epidemic.

PMID: 25362763 [PubMed - in process]

677. Travel Med Infect Dis. 2014 Sep-Oct;12(5):415-7. doi: 10.1016/j.tmaid.2014.09.003. Epub 2014 Sep 16.

The Hajj in the time of an Ebola outbreak in West Africa.

Memish ZA(1), Al-Tawfiq JA(2).

Author information: (1)Ministry of Health, Riyadh, Kingdom of Saudi Arabia; College of Medicine, Alfaisal University, Riyadh, Kingdom of Saudi Arabia. Electronic address: zmemish@yahoo.com. (2)Johns Hopkins Aramco Healthcare, Dhahran, Kingdom of Saudi Arabia; Indiana University School of Medicine, Indianapolis, IN, USA.

PMID: 25257580 [PubMed - in process]

678. Travel Med Infect Dis. 2014 Sep-Oct;12(5):541-2. doi: 10.1016/j.tmaid.2014.08.002. Epub 2014 Sep 2.

Letters in the time of Ebola.

de Frey A(1).

Author information: (1)iNHEMACO S.A, Geneva, Switzerland. Electronic address: a.defrey@inhemaco.com.
PMID: 25219797 [PubMed - in process]
679. Lancet. 2014 Aug 30;384(9945):740.

Sheik Humarr Khan.

Green A.
PMID: 25184171 [PubMed - indexed for MEDLINE]
680. Virus Res. 2014 Aug 30;189:254-61. doi: 10.1016/j.virusres.2014.06.001. Epub 2014 Jun 12.

A highly immunogenic fragment derived from Zaire Ebola virus glycoprotein elicits effective neutralizing antibody.

Wang Y(1), Liu Z(1), Dai Q(2).

Author information: (1)Beijing Institute of Biotechnology, China. (2)Beijing Institute of Biotechnology, China. Electronic address: qy_dai@yahoo.com.

In order to produce polyvalent vaccines based on single rVSV vector, we investigated the immunogenicity, antibody neutralizing activity, and antigenic determinant domain of Zaire Ebola's fragment MFL (aa 393-556) that contains furin site and internal fusion loop. Both the recombinant protein and the recombinant plasmid of fragment MFL elicited high levels of antibody, similar to those of Zaire Ebola GP (ZGP). The MFL fragment of ZGP also elicited high levels of neutralizing antibody and induced moderate cellular immune response in mice, as revealed by the proliferation and cytokine secretion of splenocytes. Through the analysis of the induction of neutralizing antibody by pVAX1-based recombinant plasmids that expressed truncated fragments of MFL, we found that the domain containing the internal fusion loop and the furin site was the major contributor of fragment MFL's immunogenicity. Furthermore, the rVSV-based bivalent vaccine expressing Sudan Ebola GP (SGP) and MFL fragment elicited efficient cross-immunity against ZGP and SGP with high levels of neutralizing antibody. Our results indicate that fragment MFL is an effective and novel antigen for the production of neutralizing antibody and polyvalent vaccines of Ebola virus.

PMID: 24930448 [PubMed - in process]
681. Science. 2014 Aug 29;345(6200):989-90. doi: 10.1126/science.345.6200.989.

Infectious Disease. Genomes reveal start of Ebola outbreak.

Vogel G.
PMID: 25170128 [PubMed - indexed for MEDLINE]
682. Nature. 2014 Aug 28;512(7515):355-6. doi: 10.1038/512355a.

World struggles to stop Ebola.

Check Hayden E.
PMID: 25164728 [PubMed - indexed for MEDLINE]
683. Nephrol Dial Transplant. 2014 Aug 28. pii: gfu280. [Epub ahead of print]

MicroRNAs in kidney transplantation.

Wilflingseder J(1), Reindl-Schwaighofer R(2), Sunzenauer J(2), Kainz A(1), Heinzel A(3), Mayer B(3), Oberbauer R(1).

Author information: (1)Department of Nephrology and Dialysis, Medical University Vienna, Vienna, Austria Department of Nephrology, KH Elisabethinen, Linz, Austria. (2)Department of Nephrology, KH Elisabethinen, Linz, Austria. (3)emergentec biodevelopment GmbH, Vienna, Austria.

The discovery of novel classes of non-coding RNAs (ncRNAs) has revolutionized medicine. Long thought to be a mere cellular housekeeper, surprising functions have recently been uncovered. MicroRNAs (miRNAs), are a representative of the class of short ncRNAs, play a fundamental role in the control of DNA and protein biosynthesis and activity as well as pathology. Currently, miRNAs are being investigated as diagnostic and prognostic markers and potential therapeutic targets in kidney transplantation for such indolent processes as ischaemia-reperfusion injury, humoral rejection or viral infections. It is realistic to believe that monitoring of renal allograft recipients in the future will include genome-wide miRNA profiling of biological fluids. Based on these individual profiles, an informed decision on therapeutic consequences will be possible. A first success with a specific suppression of miRNAs by antisense oligonucleotides was achieved in experimental studies of reperfusion injury and humoral rejection. Proof of this concept in men comes from studies in such indolent viral infections as Ebola and hepatitis C, where anti-miR therapy led to sustained viral clearance. In this review, we summarize the basis of the recent ncRNA revolution and its implication for kidney transplantation.

PMID: 25170095 [PubMed - as supplied by publisher]
684. BMJ. 2014 Aug 27;349:g5321. doi: 10.1136/bmj.g5321.

Four in 10 US people fear large outbreak of Ebola.

McCarthy M(1).
Author information: (1)Seattle.
PMID: 25163929 [PubMed - in process]
685. Rev Med Suisse. 2014 Aug 27;10(439):1570-1.

[Potential vaccine candidates against Ebola and the first vaccine against chikungunya virus infection].

[Article in French]

Nau JY.

PMID: 25272676 [PubMed - indexed for MEDLINE]

686. Angew Chem Int Ed Engl. 2014 Aug 25;53(35):9222-5. doi: 10.1002/anie.201402698. Epub 2014 Jul 9.

Visual displays that directly interface and provide read-outs of molecular states via molecular graphics processing units.

Poje JE(1), Kastratovic T, Macdonald AR, Guillermo AC, Troetti SE, Jabado OJ, Fanning ML, Stefanovic D, Macdonald J.

Author information: (1)Division of Experimental Therapeutics, Department of Medicine, Columbia University, 630 W 168th St, New York, NY 10032 (USA).

The monitoring of molecular systems usually requires sophisticated technologies to interpret nanoscale events into electronic-decipherable signals. We demonstrate a new method for obtaining read-outs of molecular states that uses graphics processing units made from molecular circuits. Because they are made from molecules, the units are able to directly interact with molecular systems. We developed deoxyribozyme-based graphics processing units able to monitor nucleic acids and output alphanumerical read-outs via a fluorescent display. Using this design we created a molecular 7-segment display, a molecular calculator able to add and multiply small numbers, and a molecular automaton able to diagnose Ebola and Marburg virus sequences. These molecular graphics processing units provide insight for the construction of autonomous biosensing devices, and are essential components for the development of molecular computing platforms devoid of electronics.

© 2014 WILEY-VCH Verlag GmbH & Co. KGaA, Weinheim.

PMID: 25044570 [PubMed - in process]

687. J Infect Dis. 2014 Aug 25. pii: jiu474. [Epub ahead of print]

A Practical Treatment for Patients With Ebola Virus Disease.

Fedson DS(1).

Author information: (1)Sergy Haut, France.

PMID: 25160984 [PubMed - as supplied by publisher]

688. Mod Healthc. 2014 Aug 25;44(34):8.

Do Ebola precautions go far enough?

Johnson SR.

PMID: 25318261 [PubMed - indexed for MEDLINE]

689. Time. 2014 Aug 25;184(7):34-9.

After Ebola. Why the worst outbreak ever is a warning of what could come next.

Walsh B, Sifferlin A.

PMID: 25318249 [PubMed - indexed for MEDLINE]

690. Lancet. 2014 Aug 23;384(9944):649.

Experimental Ebola drugs enter the limelight.

Mullard A.

PMID: 25157386 [PubMed - indexed for MEDLINE]

691. Lancet. 2014 Aug 23;384(9944):637.

Ebola: a failure of international collective action.

[No authors listed]

PMID: 25150744 [PubMed - indexed for MEDLINE]

692. MMW Fortschr Med. 2014 Aug 21;156(14):7.

[Infectiological emergency of worldwide significance. Ebola out of control? (interview by Dr.Robert Bublak)].

[Article in German]

Günther S, Bublak R.

PMID: 25195378 [PubMed - indexed for MEDLINE]

693. Nature. 2014 Aug 21;512(7514):233. doi: 10.1038/512233a.

Scale up the supply of experimental Ebola drugs.

Brady O.

PMID: 25143079 [PubMed - indexed for MEDLINE]

694. JAMA. 2014 Aug 20;312(7):686. doi: 10.1001/jama.2014.10528.

CDC: Ebola risk to US patients is low, but clinicians should be on alert.

Stephenson J.

PMID: 25138319 [PubMed - indexed for MEDLINE]

695. Sci Transl Med. 2014 Aug 20;6(250):250ra116. doi: 10.1126/scitranslmed.3009706.

Marburg virus infection in nonhuman primates: Therapeutic treatment by lipid-encapsulated siRNA.

Thi EP(1), Mire CE(2), Ursic-Bedoya R(1), Geisbert JB(2), Lee AC(1), Agans KN(2), Robbins M(1), Deer DJ(2), Fenton KA(2), MacLachlan I(3), Geisbert TW(4).

Author information: (1)Tekmira Pharmaceuticals, Burnaby, British Columbia V5J 5J8, Canada. (2)Galveston National Laboratory, University of Texas Medical Branch, Galveston, TX 77550, USA. Department of Microbiology and Immunology, University of Texas Medical Branch, Galveston, TX 77550, USA. (3)Tekmira

Pharmaceuticals, Burnaby, British Columbia V5J 5J8, Canada. twgeisbe@utmb.edu lMacLachlan@tekmirapharm.com. (4)Galveston National Laboratory, University of Texas Medical Branch, Galveston, TX 77550, USA. Department of Microbiology and Immunology, University of Texas Medical Branch, Galveston, TX 77550, USA. twgeisbe@utmb.edu lMacLachlan@tekmirapharm.com.

Marburg virus (MARV) and the closely related filovirus Ebola virus cause severe and often fatal hemorrhagic fever (HF) in humans and nonhuman primates with mortality rates up to 90%. There are no vaccines or drugs approved for human use, and no postexposure treatment has completely protected nonhuman primates against MARV-Angola, the strain associated with the highest rate of mortality in naturally occurring human outbreaks. Studies performed with other MARV strains assessed candidate treatments at times shortly after virus exposure, before signs of disease are detectable. We assessed the efficacy of lipid nanoparticle (LNP) delivery of anti-MARV nucleoprotein (NP)-targeting small interfering RNA (siRNA) at several time points after virus exposure, including after the onset of detectable disease in a uniformly lethal nonhuman primate model of MARV-Angola HF. Twenty-one rhesus monkeys were challenged with a lethal dose of MARV-Angola. Sixteen of these animals were treated with LNP containing anti-MARV NP siRNA beginning at 30 to 45 min, 1 day, 2 days, or 3 days after virus challenge. All 16 macaques that received LNP-encapsulated anti-MARV NP siRNA survived infection, whereas the untreated or mock-treated control subjects succumbed to disease between days 7 and 9 after infection. These results represent the successful demonstration of therapeutic anti-MARV-Angola efficacy in nonhuman primates and highlight the substantial impact of an LNP-delivered siRNA therapeutic as a countermeasure against this highly lethal human disease.

PMID: 25143366 [PubMed - in process]

696. Nurs Stand. 2014 Aug 19;28(50):9. doi: 10.7748/ns.28.50.9.s7.

Ebola death toll rises in Africa with at least 14 nurses among the dead.

Duffin C.

At least 14 nurses are among 80 healthcare workers who have died from an outbreak of the Ebola virus spreading across West Africa, declared an international public health emergency last week by the World Health Organization (WHO).

PMID: 25116521 [PubMed - in process]

697. Mod Healthc. 2014 Aug 18;44(33):24.

History and the Ebola outbreak.

Goozner M.

PMID: 25318255 [PubMed - indexed for MEDLINE]

698. BMC Genomics. 2014 Aug 15;15:682. doi: 10.1186/1471-2164-15-682.

Characterisation of novel microRNAs in the Black flying fox (Pteropus alecto) by deep sequencing.

Cowled C(1), Stewart CR, Likic VA, Friedländer MR, Tachedjian M, Jenkins KA, Tizard ML, Cottee P, Marsh GA, Zhou P, Baker ML, Bean AG, Wang LF.

Author information: (1)CSIRO Australian Animal Health Laboratory, 5 Portarlington Rd, Geelong East, Victoria 3220, Australia. chris.cowled@csiro.au.

BACKGROUND: Bats are a major source of new and emerging viral diseases. Despite the fact that bats carry and shed highly pathogenic viruses including Ebola, Nipah and SARS, they rarely display clinical symptoms of infection. Host factors influencing viral replication are poorly understood in bats and are likely to include both pre- and post-transcriptional regulatory mechanisms. MicroRNAs are a major mechanism of post-transcriptional gene regulation, however very little is known about them in bats. RESULTS: This study describes 399 microRNAs identified by deep sequencing of small RNA isolated from tissues of the Black flying fox, Pteropus alecto, a confirmed natural reservoir of the human pathogens Hendra virus and Australian bat lyssavirus. Of the microRNAs identified, more than 100 are unique amongst vertebrates, including a subset containing mutations in critical seed regions. Clusters of rapidly-evolving microRNAs were identified, as well as microRNAs predicted to target genes involved in antiviral immunity, the DNA damage response, apoptosis and autophagy. Closer inspection of the predicted targets for several highly supported novel miRNA candidates suggests putative roles in host-virus interaction. CONCLUSIONS: MicroRNAs are likely to play major roles in regulating virus-host interaction in bats, via dampening of inflammatory responses (limiting the effects of immunopathology), and directly limiting the extent of viral replication, either through restricting the availability of essential factors or by controlling apoptosis. Characterisation of the bat microRNA repertoire is an essential step towards understanding transcriptional regulation during viral infection, and will assist in the identification of mechanisms that enable bats to act as natural virus reservoirs. This in turn will facilitate the development of antiviral strategies for use in humans and other species.

PMCID: PMC4156645 PMID: 25128405 [PubMed - in process]

699. J Biol Chem. 2014 Aug 15;289(33):22723-38. doi: 10.1074/jbc.M114.575050. Epub 2014 Jun 16.

Role of protein phosphatase 1 in dephosphorylation of Ebola virus VP30 protein and its targeting for the inhibition of viral transcription.

Ilinykh PA(1), Tigabu B(1), Ivanov A(2), Ammosova T(3), Obukhov Y(2), Garron T(4), Kumari N(2), Kovalskyy D(5), Platonov MO(5), Naumchik VS(5), Freiberg AN(1), Nekhai S(6), Bukreyev A(7).

Author information: (1)From the Departments of Pathology and Galveston National Laboratory, Galveston, Texas 77555. (2)the Center for Sickle Cell Disease and. (3)the Center for Sickle Cell Disease and Departments of Medicine and. (4)From the Departments of Pathology and Galveston National Laboratory, Galveston, Texas 77555, Microbiology and Immunology, University of Texas Medical Branch at Galveston, Galveston, Texas 77555. (5)Kiev National Taras Shevchenko University, Kiev 01601, Ukraine, and Enamine Ltd., Kiev 01103, Ukraine. (6)Galveston National Laboratory, Galveston, Texas 77555, Departments of Medicine and Microbiology, Howard University, Washington, D. C. 20059, snekhai@howard.edu. (7)From the Departments of Pathology and Galveston National

Laboratory, Galveston, Texas 77555, Microbiology and Immunology, University of Texas Medical Branch at Galveston, Galveston, Texas 77555, alexander.bukreyev@utmb.edu.

The filovirus Ebola (EBOV) causes the most severe hemorrhagic fever known. The EBOV RNA-dependent polymerase complex includes a filovirus-specific VP30, which is critical for the transcriptional but not replication activity of EBOV polymerase; to support transcription, VP30 must be in a dephosphorylated form. Here we show that EBOV VP30 is phosphorylated not only at the N-terminal serine clusters identified previously but also at the threonine residues at positions 143 and 146. We also show that host cell protein phosphatase 1 (PP1) controls VP30 dephosphorylation because expression of a PP1-binding peptide cdNIPP1 increased VP30 phosphorylation. Moreover, targeting PP1 mRNA by shRNA resulted in the overexpression of SIPP1, a cytoplasm-shuttling regulatory subunit of PP1, and increased EBOV transcription, suggesting that cytoplasmic accumulation of PP1 induces EBOV transcription. Furthermore, we developed a small molecule compound, 1E7-03, that targeted a non-catalytic site of PP1 and increased VP30 dephosphorylation. The compound inhibited the transcription but increased replication of the viral genome and completely suppressed replication of EBOV in cultured cells. Finally, mutations of Thr(143) and Thr(146) of VP30 significantly inhibited EBOV transcription and strongly induced VP30 phosphorylation in the N-terminal Ser residues 29-46, suggesting a novel mechanism of regulation of VP30 phosphorylation. Our findings suggest that targeting PP1 with small molecules is a feasible approach to achieve dysregulation of the EBOV polymerase activity. This novel approach may be used for the development of antivirals against EBOV and other filovirus species.
PMCID: PMC4132779 [Available on 2015/8/15] PMID: 24936058 [PubMed - indexed for MEDLINE]

700. J Infect Dis. 2014 Aug 15;210(4):558-66. doi: 10.1093/infdis/jiu088. Epub 2014 Feb 12.

Ebola hemorrhagic Fever: novel biomarker correlates of clinical outcome.

McElroy AK(1), Erickson BR(2), Flietstra TD(2), Rollin PE(2), Nichol ST(2), Towner JS(2), Spiropoulou CF(2).

Author information: (1)Viral Special Pathogens Branch, Centers for Disease Control and Prevention Division of Pediatric Infectious Disease, Emory University School of Medicine, Atlanta, Georgia. (2)Viral Special Pathogens Branch, Centers for Disease Control and Prevention.

BACKGROUND: Ebola hemorrhagic fever (EHF) outbreaks occur sporadically in Africa and result in high rates of death. The 2000-2001 outbreak of Sudan virus-associated EHF in the Gulu district of Uganda led to 425 cases, of which 216 were laboratory confirmed, making it the largest EHF outbreak on record. Serum specimens from this outbreak had been preserved in liquid nitrogen from the time of collection and were available for analysis. METHODS: Available samples were tested using a series of multiplex assays to measure the concentrations of 55 biomarkers. The data were analyzed to identify statistically significant associations between the tested biomarkers and hemorrhagic manifestations, viremia, and/or death. RESULTS: Death, hemorrhage, and viremia were independently associated with elevated levels of several chemokines and cytokines. Death and hemorrhage were associated with elevated thrombomodulin and ferritin levels. Hemorrhage was also associated with elevated levels of soluble intracellular adhesion molecule. Viremia was independently associated with elevated levels of tissue factor and tissue plasminogen activator. Finally, samples from nonfatal cases had higher levels of sCD40L. CONCLUSIONS: These novel associations provide a better understanding of EHF pathophysiology and a starting point for researching new potential targets for therapeutic interventions.
PMCID: PMC4172044 [Available on 2015/8/15] PMID: 24526742 [PubMed - indexed for MEDLINE]

701. Science. 2014 Aug 15;345(6198):718-9. doi: 10.1126/science.345.6198.718.

Infectious diseases. Debate erupts on 'repurposed' drugs for Ebola.

Enserink M.

Comment in Lancet Glob Health. 2014 Oct;2(10):e563-4.
PMID: 25124404 [PubMed - indexed for MEDLINE]

702. BMJ. 2014 Aug 13;349:g5161. doi: 10.1136/bmj.g5161.

WHO gives go ahead for experimental treatments to be used in Ebola outbreak.

Sayburn A(1).

Author information: (1)London.
PMID: 25122051 [PubMed - in process]

703. Cell Host Microbe. 2014 Aug 13;16(2):187-200. doi: 10.1016/j.chom.2014.07.008.

Ebola virus VP24 targets a unique NLS binding site on karyopherin alpha 5 to selectively compete with nuclear import of phosphorylated STAT1.

Xu W(1), Edwards MR(2), Borek DM(3), Feagins AR(2), Mittal A(4), Alinger JB(1), Berry KN(1), Yen B(2), Hamilton J(2), Brett TJ(5), Pappu RV(4), Leung DW(1), Basler CF(2), Amarasinghe GK(6).

Author information: (1)Department of Pathology and Immunology, Washington University School of Medicine, St Louis, MO 63110, USA. (2)Department of Microbiology, Icahn School of Medicine at Mount Sinai, New York, NY 10029, USA. (3)Departments of Biophysics and Biochemistry, University of Texas Southwestern Medical Center at Dallas, Dallas, TX 75390, USA. (4)Department of Biomedical Engineering and Center for Biological Systems Engineering, Washington University, St. Louis, MO 63110, USA. (5)Department of Internal Medicine, Washington University School of Medicine, St. Louis, MO 63110, USA. (6)Department of Pathology and Immunology, Washington University School of Medicine, St Louis, MO 63110, USA. Electronic address: gamarasinghe@path.wustl.edu.

Comment in Cell Host Microbe. 2014 Aug 13;16(2):150-2.

During antiviral defense, interferon (IFN) signaling triggers nuclear transport of tyrosine-phosphorylated STAT1 (PY-STAT1), which occurs via a subset of karyopherin alpha (KPNA) nuclear transporters. Many viruses, including Ebola virus, actively antagonize STAT1 signaling to counteract the antiviral effects of IFN. Ebola virus VP24 protein (eVP24) binds KPNA to inhibit PY-STAT1 nuclear transport and render cells refractory to IFNs. We describe the structure of human KPNA5 C terminus in complex with eVP24. In the complex, eVP24 recognizes a unique nonclassical nuclear localization signal (NLS) binding site on KPNA5 that is necessary for efficient PY-STAT1 nuclear transport. eVP24 binds KPNA5 with very high affinity to effectively compete with and inhibit PY-STAT1 nuclear transport. In contrast, eVP24 binding does not affect the transport of classical NLS cargo. Thus, eVP24 counters cell-intrinsic innate immunity by selectively targeting PY-STAT1 nuclear import while leaving the transport of other cargo that may be required for viral replication unaffected.

PMCID: PMC4188415 [Available on 2015/8/13] PMID: 25121748 [PubMed - in process]

704. Cell Host Microbe. 2014 Aug 13;16(2):150-2. doi: 10.1016/j.chom.2014.07.013.

How a virus blocks a cellular emergency access lane to the nucleus, STAT!

Daugherty MD(1), Malik HS(2).

Author information: (1)Division of Basic Sciences, Fred Hutchinson Cancer Research Center, Seattle, WA 98109, USA; Howard Hughes Medical Institute, Fred Hutchinson Cancer Research Center, Seattle, WA 98109, USA. Electronic address: mdaugher@fhcrc.org. (2)Division of Basic Sciences, Fred Hutchinson Cancer Research Center, Seattle, WA 98109, USA; Howard Hughes Medical Institute, Fred Hutchinson Cancer Research Center, Seattle, WA 98109, USA.

Comment on Cell Host Microbe. 2014 Aug 13;16(2):187-200.

Early in viral infection, the STAT1 transcription factor is rapidly transported into the nucleus using a nonconventional import mechanism to establish an antiviral state. In this issue, Xu et al. (2014) show how the Ebola virus VP24 protein precisely blocks specialized STAT1 import while leaving other cellular import processes intact.

PMID: 25121743 [PubMed - in process]

705. BMJ. 2014 Aug 11;349:g5103. doi: 10.1136/bmj.g5103.

FDA allows second experimental drug to be tested in Ebola patients.

McCarthy M(1).

Author information: (1)Seattle.

PMID: 25113141 [PubMed - in process]

706. BMJ. 2014 Aug 11;349:g5079. doi: 10.1136/bmj.g5079.

Ebola and other viral haemorrhagic fevers.

Fletcher TE(1), Brooks TJ(2), Beeching NJ(3).

Author information: (1)Liverpool School of Tropical Medicine, Liverpool L3 5QA, UK. (2)Rare and Imported Pathogens Laboratory, Public Health England, Porton Down, Salisbury, UK. (3)Liverpool School of Tropical Medicine, Liverpool L3 5QA, UK nicholas.beeching@rlbuht.nhs.uk.

PMID: 25113010 [PubMed - in process]

707. Mod Healthc. 2014 Aug 11;44(32):10.

CDC sends Ebola help to struggling healthcare workers in Africa.

Johnson SR.

PMID: 25318242 [PubMed - indexed for MEDLINE]

708. Lancet. 2014 Aug 9;384(9942):481.

WHO and partners launch Ebola response plan.

Green A.

PMID: 25115001 [PubMed - indexed for MEDLINE]

709. Lancet. 2014 Aug 9;384(9942):470. doi: 10.1016/S0140-6736(14)61319-2.

Ebola: protection of health workers on the front line.

[No authors listed]

PMID: 25110265 [PubMed - indexed for MEDLINE]

710. BMJ. 2014 Aug 8;349:g5089. doi: 10.1136/bmj.g5089.

Ebola outbreak is a public health emergency of international concern, WHO warns.

Hawkes N(1).

Author information: (1)London.

PMID: 25106874 [PubMed - in process]

711. Euro Surveill. 2014 Aug 7;19(31):23.

Information resources and latest news about Ebola virus disease available from ECDC.

Eurosurveillance editorial team.

PMID: 25138973 [PubMed - indexed for MEDLINE]

712. BMJ. 2014 Aug 6;349:g4997. doi: 10.1136/bmj.g4997.

Ebola: an opportunity for a clinical trial?

Arie S.

PMID: 25098954 [PubMed - in process]

713. JAMA. 2014 Aug 6;312(5):476. doi: 10.1001/jama.2014.9757.

Largest-ever Ebola outbreak still simmering in West Africa.

Stephenson J.

PMID: 25096676 [PubMed - indexed for MEDLINE]

714. BMJ. 2014 Aug 4;349:g4987. doi: 10.1136/bmj.g4987.

Courage is treating patients with Ebola.

McCartney M.

PMID: 25092659 [PubMed - in process]

715. Biomed Environ Sci. 2014 Aug;27(8):651-3. doi: 10.3967/bes2014.100.

Ebola virus disease: general characteristics, thoughts, and perspectives.

Cheng Y(1), Li Y(1), Yu HJ(1).

Author information: (1)Division of Infectious Disease, Key Laboratory of Surveillance and Early-warning on Infectious Disease, Chinese Center for Disease Control and Prevention, Beijing 102206, China.

PMID: 25189614 [PubMed - in process]

716. J Antimicrob Chemother. 2014 Aug;69(8):2123-31. doi: 10.1093/jac/dku091. Epub 2014 Apr 7.

The clinically approved drugs amiodarone, dronedarone and verapamil inhibit filovirus cell entry.

Gehring G(1), Rohrmann K(2), Atenchong N(1), Mittler E(3), Becker S(3), Dahlmann F(4), Pöhlmann S(4), Vondran FW(5), David S(6), Manns MP(7), Ciesek S(7), von Hahn T(8).

Author information: (1)Institute for Molecular Biology, Hannover Medical School, Hannover, Germany Department of Gastroenterology, Hepatology and Endocrinology, Hannover Medical School, Hannover, Germany. (2)Institute for Molecular Biology, Hannover Medical School, Hannover, Germany. (3)Institute for Virology, University of Marburg, Marburg, Germany. (4)Infection Biology Unit, German Primate Center, Göttingen, Germany. (5)Department of General, Visceral and Transplant Surgery, Hannover Medical School, Hannover, Germany. (6)Department of Nephrology, Hannover Medical School, Hannover, Germany. (7)Department of Gastroenterology, Hepatology and Endocrinology, Hannover Medical School, Hannover, Germany. (8)Institute for Molecular Biology, Hannover Medical School, Hannover, Germany Department of Gastroenterology, Hepatology and Endocrinology, Hannover Medical School, Hannover, Germany vonhahn.thomas@mh-hannover.de.

OBJECTIVES: Filoviruses such as Ebola virus and Marburg virus cause a severe haemorrhagic fever syndrome in humans for which there is no specific treatment. Since filoviruses use a complex route of cell entry that depends on numerous cellular factors, we hypothesized that there may be drugs already approved for human use for other indications that interfere with signal transduction or other cellular processes required for their entry and hence have anti-filoviral properties. METHODS: We used authentic filoviruses and lentiviral particles pseudotyped with filoviral glycoproteins to identify and characterize such compounds. RESULTS: We discovered that amiodarone, a multi-ion channel inhibitor and adrenoceptor antagonist, is a potent inhibitor of filovirus cell entry at concentrations that are routinely reached in human serum during anti-arrhythmic therapy. A similar effect was observed with the amiodarone-related agent dronedarone and the L-type calcium channel blocker verapamil. Inhibition by amiodarone was concentration dependent and similarly affected pseudoviruses as well as authentic filoviruses. Inhibition of filovirus entry was observed with most but not all cell types tested and was accentuated by the pre-treatment of cells, indicating a host cell-directed mechanism of action. The New World arenavirus Guanarito was also inhibited by amiodarone while the Old World arenavirus Lassa and members of the Rhabdoviridae (vesicular stomatitis virus) and Bunyaviridae (Hantaan) families were largely resistant. CONCLUSIONS: The ion channel blockers amiodarone, dronedarone and verapamil inhibit filoviral cell entry.

© The Author 2014. Published by Oxford University Press on behalf of the British Society for Antimicrobial Chemotherapy. All rights reserved. For Permissions, please e-mail: journals.permissions@oup.com.

PMID: 24710028 [PubMed - in process]

717. J Gen Virol. 2014 Aug;95(Pt 8):1619-24. doi: 10.1099/vir.0.067199-0. Epub 2014 May 2.

The 2014 Ebola virus disease outbreak in West Africa.

Gatherer D(1).

Author information: (1)Division of Biomedical & Life Sciences, Faculty of Health & Medicine, Lancaster University, Lancaster LA1 4YQ, UK d.gatherer@lancaster.ac.uk.

On 23 March 2014, the World Health Organization issued its first communiqué on a new outbreak of Ebola virus disease (EVD), which began in December 2013 in Guinée Forestière (Forested Guinea), the eastern sector of the Republic of Guinea. Located on the Atlantic coast of West Africa, Guinea is the first country in this geographical region in which an outbreak of EVD has occurred, leaving aside the single case reported in Ivory Coast in 1994. Cases have now also been confirmed across Guinea as well as in the neighbouring Republic of Liberia. The appearance of cases in the Guinean capital, Conakry, and the transit of another case through the Liberian capital, Monrovia, presents the first large urban setting for EVD transmission. By 20 April 2014, 242 suspected cases had resulted in a total of 147 deaths in Guinea and Liberia. The causative agent has now been identified as an outlier strain of Zaire Ebola virus. The full geographical extent and

119

degree of severity of the outbreak, its zoonotic origins and its possible spread to other continents are sure to be subjects of intensive discussion over the next months.

© 2014 The Authors.

PMID: 24795448 [PubMed - indexed for MEDLINE]

718. Med Sante Trop. 2014 Aug 1;24(3):229-231.

Ebola virus epidemic in West Africa: facts and prospects.

Rapp C(1).

Author information: (1)Service des maladies infectieuses et tropicales, hôpital d'instruction des armées Bégin, Saint-Mandé, France.

PMID: 25370045 [PubMed - as supplied by publisher]

719. PLoS Negl Trop Dis. 2014 Aug 21;8(8):e3095. doi: 10.1371/journal.pntd.0003095. eCollection 2014.

High content image-based screening of a protease inhibitor library reveals compounds broadly active against Rift Valley fever virus and other highly pathogenic RNA viruses.

Mudhasani R(1), Kota KP(1), Retterer C(1), Tran JP(1), Whitehouse CA(1), Bavari S(1).

Author information: (1)Molecular and Translational Sciences Division, United States Army Medical Research Institute of Infectious Diseases, Frederick, Maryland, United States of America.

High content image-based screening was developed as an approach to test a protease inhibitor small molecule library for antiviral activity against Rift Valley fever virus (RVFV) and to determine their mechanism of action. RVFV is the causative agent of severe disease of humans and animals throughout Africa and the Arabian Peninsula. Of the 849 compounds screened, 34 compounds exhibited ≥ 50% inhibition against RVFV. All of the hit compounds could be classified into 4 distinct groups based on their unique chemical backbone. Some of the compounds also showed broad antiviral activity against several highly pathogenic RNA viruses including Ebola, Marburg, Venezuela equine encephalitis, and Lassa viruses. Four hit compounds (C795-0925, D011-2120, F694-1532 and G202-0362), which were most active against RVFV and showed broad-spectrum antiviral activity, were selected for further evaluation for their cytotoxicity, dose response profile, and mode of action using classical virological methods and high-content imaging analysis. Time-of-addition assays in RVFV infections suggested that D011-2120 and G202-0362 targeted virus egress, while C795-0925 and F694-1532 inhibited virus replication. We showed that D011-2120 exhibited its antiviral effects by blocking microtubule polymerization, thereby disrupting the Golgi complex and inhibiting viral trafficking to the plasma membrane during virus egress. While G202-0362 also affected virus egress, it appears to do so by a different mechanism, namely by blocking virus budding from the trans Golgi. F694-1532 inhibited viral replication, but also appeared to inhibit overall cellular gene expression. However, G202-0362 and C795-0925 did not alter any of the morphological features that we examined and thus may prove to be good candidates for antiviral drug development. Overall this work demonstrates that high-content image analysis can be used to screen chemical libraries for new antivirals and to determine their mechanism of action and any possible deleterious effects on host cellular biology.

PMCID: PMC4140764 PMID: 25144302 [PubMed - in process]

720. Trends Microbiol. 2014 Aug;22(8):456-63. doi: 10.1016/j.tim.2014.04.002. Epub 2014 Apr 30.

Post-exposure therapy of filovirus infections.

Wong G(1), Qiu X(2), Olinger GG(3), Kobinger GP(4).

Author information: (1)Special Pathogens Program, National Microbiology Laboratory, Public Health Agency of Canada, Winnipeg, MB, Canada; Department of Medical Microbiology, University of Manitoba, Winnipeg, MB, Canada. (2)Special Pathogens Program, National Microbiology Laboratory, Public Health Agency of Canada, Winnipeg, MB, Canada. (3)Integrated Research Facility, National Institute of Allergy and Infectious Diseases, National Institutes of Health, Frederick, MD, USA. (4)Special Pathogens Program, National Microbiology Laboratory, Public Health Agency of Canada, Winnipeg, MB, Canada; Department of Medical Microbiology, University of Manitoba, Winnipeg, MB, Canada; Department of Immunology, University of Manitoba, Winnipeg, MB, Canada; Department of Pathology and Laboratory Medicine, University of Pennsylvania School of Medicine, Philadelphia, PA, USA. Electronic address: gary.kobinger@phac-aspc.gc.ca.

Filovirus infections cause fatal hemorrhagic fever characterized by the initial onset of general symptoms before rapid progression to severe disease; the most virulent species can cause death to susceptible hosts within 10 days after the appearance of symptoms. Before the advent of monoclonal antibody (mAb) therapy, infection of nonhuman primates (NHPs) with the most virulent filovirus species was fatal if interventions were not administered within minutes. A novel nucleoside analogue, BCX4430, has since been shown to also demonstrate protective efficacy with a delayed treatment start. This review summarizes and evaluates the potential of current experimental candidates for treating filovirus disease with regard to their feasibility and use in the clinic, and assesses the most promising strategies towards the future development of a pan-filovirus medical countermeasure.

Copyright © 2014 Elsevier Ltd. All rights reserved.

PMID: 24794572 [PubMed - in process]

721. Nature. 2014 Jul 31;511(7511):520. doi: 10.1038/511520a.

Ebola treatments caught in limbo.

Reardon S.

PMID: 25079536 [PubMed - indexed for MEDLINE]

722. Med Clin (Barc). 2014 Jul 30. pii: S0025-7753(14)00457-6. doi: 10.1016/j.medcli.2014.05.031. [Epub ahead of print]

[Chikungunya fever - A new global threat.]

[Article in Spanish]

Montero A(1).

Author information: (1)Miembro de la Carrera del Investigador Científico, Consejo de Investigaciones de la Universidad Nacional de Rosario (CIUNR), Rosario, Santa Fe, Argentina; Centro de Medicina Tropical y Enfermedades Infecciosas Emergentes, Facultad de Ciencias Médicas, Universidad Nacional de Rosario, Rosario, Santa Fe, Argentina. Electronic address: amontero@sede.unr.edu.ar.

The recent onset of epidemics caused by viruses such as Ebola, Marburg, Nipah, Lassa, coronavirus, West-Nile encephalitis, Saint Louis encephalitis, human immunodeficiency virus, dengue, yellow fever and Venezuelan hemorrhagic fever alerts about the risk these agents represent for the global health. Chikungunya virus represents a new threat. Surged from remote African regions, this virus has become endemic in the Indic ocean basin, the Indian subcontinent and the southeast of Asia, causing serious epidemics in Africa, Indic Ocean Islands, Asia and Europe. Due to their epidemiological and biological features and the global presence of their vectors, chikungunya represents a serious menace and could become endemic in the Americas. Although chikungunya infection has a low mortality rate, its high attack ratio may collapse the health system during epidemics affecting a sensitive population. In this paper, we review the clinical and epidemiological features of chikungunya fever as well as the risk of its introduction into the Americas. We remark the importance of the epidemiological control and mosquitoes fighting in order to prevent this disease from being introduced into the Americas.

PMID: 25087211 [PubMed - as supplied by publisher]

723. Soc Sci Med. 2014 Jul 30. pii: S0277-9536(14)00498-5. doi: 10.1016/j.socscimed.2014.07.058. [Epub ahead of print]

Uncovering zoonoses awareness in an emerging disease 'hotspot'

Paige SB(1), Malavé C(2), Mbabazi E(3), Mayer J(4), Goldberg TL(2).

Author information: (1)University of Wisconsin-Madison, USA. Electronic address: spaige1@gmail.com. (2)University of Wisconsin-Madison, USA. (3)Makerere University Biological Field Station, Uganda. (4)University of Washington, USA.

Emerging infectious diseases from animals pose significant and increasing threats to human health; places of risk are simultaneously viewed as conservation and emerging disease 'hotspots'. The One World/One Health paradigm is an 'assemblage' discipline. Extensive research from the natural and social sciences, as well as public health have contributed to designing surveillance and response policy within the One World/One Health framework. However, little research has been undertaken that considers the lives of those who experience risk in hotspots on a daily basis. As a result, policymakers and practitioners are unable to fully comprehend the social and ecological processes that catalyze cross-species pathogen exchange. This study examined local populations' comprehension of zoonotic disease. From October 2008-May 2009 we collected data from people living on the periphery of Kibale National Park, in western Uganda. We administered a survey to 72 individuals and conducted semi-structured, in-depth interviews with 14 individuals. Results from the survey showed respondents had statistically significant awareness that transmission of diseases from animals was possible compared to those who did not think such transmission was possible ($x(2) = 30.68$, df = 1, p

PMID: 25128439 [PubMed - as supplied by publisher]

724. BMJ. 2014 Jul 29;349:g4895. doi: 10.1136/bmj.g4895.

Two doctors die from Ebola and lives of others under threat in West Africa.

Torjesen I(1).

Author information: (1)London.

PMID: 25073968 [PubMed - indexed for MEDLINE]

725. Lancet. 2014 Jul 26;384(9940):303. doi: 10.1016/S0140-6736(14)61119-3. Epub 2014 Jul 4.

Ebola in Sierra Leone: a call for action.

Ansumana R(1), Bonwitt J(1), Stenger DA(2), Jacobsen KH(3).

Author information: (1)Mercy Hospital Research Laboratory, Bo, Sierra Leone. (2)Mercy Hospital Research Laboratory, Bo, Sierra Leone; US Naval Laboratory, Washington, DC, USA. (3)Mercy Hospital Research Laboratory, Bo, Sierra Leone; George Mason University, Global and Community Health, Fairfax, VA 22030, USA. Electronic address: kjacobse@gmu.edu.

PMID: 25002177 [PubMed - indexed for MEDLINE]

726. S Afr Med J. 2014 Jul 25;104(8):555-6. doi: 10.7196/samj.8672.

Ebola virus disease in West Africa - an unprecedented outbreak.

Weyer J(1), Blumberg LH, Paweska JT.

Author information: (1)Centre for Emerging and Zoonotic Diseases, National Institute for Communicable Diseases, National Health Laboratory Service, Sandringham, Johannesburg, South Africa. lucilleb@nicd.ac.za.

Ebola virus disease (EVD) has remained rare since its initial description in 1976. The current outbreak of EVD in West Africa is of particular concern, accounting for more than a third of the cases of EVD ever reported. Indications are that at the time of writing the outbreak is far from over. This is also the first recorded outbreak of EVD in this region of Africa. This editorial comments on the current outbreak, reasons why it has proved challenging to contain, signs, symptoms and transmission of EVD, and implications for South Africa.

PMID: 25213844 [PubMed - in process]

727. Sci Rep. 2014 Jul 25;4:5824. doi: 10.1038/srep05824.

Evaluation of transmission risks associated with in vivo replication of several high containment pathogens in a biosafety level 4 laboratory.

Alimonti J(1), Leung A(1), Jones S(2), Gren J(3), Qiu X(2), Fernando L(2), Balcewich B(4), Wong G(5), Ströher U(1), Grolla A(2), Strong J(6), Kobinger G(7).
Author information: (1)1] Special Pathogens Program, Public Health Agency of Canada, 1015 Arlington St., Winnipeg. Manitoba [2]. (2)Special Pathogens Program, Public Health Agency of Canada, 1015 Arlington St., Winnipeg. Manitoba. (3)Containment Services, Public Health Agency of Canada, 1015 Arlington St., Winnipeg. Manitoba. (4)Bioforensics Assay Development and Diagnostics; Public Health Agency of Canada, 1015 Arlington St., Winnipeg. Manitoba. (5)1] Special Pathogens Program, Public Health Agency of Canada, 1015 Arlington St., Winnipeg. Manitoba [2] Departments of Medical Microbiology, University of Manitoba, Winnipeg, MB, Canada. (6)1] Special Pathogens Program, Public Health Agency of Canada, 1015 Arlington St., Winnipeg. Manitoba [2] Departments of Medical Microbiology, University of Manitoba, Winnipeg, MB, Canada [3] Departments of Pediatrics and Child Health, University of Manitoba, Winnipeg, MB, Canada. (7)1] Special Pathogens Program, Public Health Agency of Canada, 1015 Arlington St., Winnipeg. Manitoba [2] Departments of Medical Microbiology, University of Manitoba, Winnipeg, MB, Canada [3] Departments of Immunology, University of Manitoba, Winnipeg, MB, Canada [4] Department of Pathology and Laboratory Medicine, University of Pennsylvania School of Medicine, Philadelphia, PA, USA.

Containment level 4 (CL4) laboratories studying biosafety level 4 viruses are under strict regulations to conduct nonhuman primate (NHP) studies in compliance of both animal welfare and biosafety requirements. NHPs housed in open-barred cages raise concerns about cross-contamination between animals, and accidental exposure of personnel to infectious materials. To address these concerns, two NHP experiments were performed. One examined the simultaneous infection of 6 groups of NHPs with 6 different viruses (Machupo, Junin, Rift Valley Fever, Crimean-Congo Hemorrhagic Fever, Nipah and Hendra viruses). Washing personnel between handling each NHP group, floor to ceiling biobubble with HEPA filter, and plexiglass between cages were employed for partial primary containment. The second experiment employed no primary containment around open barred cages with Ebola virus infected NHPs 0.3 meters from naïve NHPs. Viral antigen-specific ELISAs, qRT-PCR and TCID50 infectious assays were utilized to determine antibody levels and viral loads. No transmission of virus to neighbouring NHPs was observed suggesting limited containment protocols are sufficient for multi-viral CL4 experiments within one room. The results support the concept that Ebola virus infection is self-contained in NHPs infected intramuscularly, at least in the present experimental conditions, and is not transmitted to naïve NHPs via an airborne route.
PMID: 25059478 [PubMed - in process]

728. Science. 2014 Jul 25;345(6195):364-5. doi: 10.1126/science.345.6195.364.

Infectious diseases. Ebola drugs still stuck in lab.

Enserink M.

PMID: 25061181 [PubMed - indexed for MEDLINE]

729. Clin Infect Dis. 2014 Jul 15;59(2):i.

Ebola virus disease in West Africa-update.

[No authors listed]

PMID: 25105183 [PubMed - in process]

730. Lancet. 2014 Jul 12;384(9938):118.

Ebola emergency meeting establishes new control centre.

Green A.

Erratum in Lancet. 2014 Aug 30;384(9945):746.

PMID: 25025099 [PubMed - indexed for MEDLINE]

731. Nature. 2014 Jul 10;511(7508):126.

Barriers to trust.

[No authors listed]

PMID: 25013881 [PubMed - indexed for MEDLINE]

732. BMJ. 2014 Jul 7;348:g4478. doi: 10.1136/bmj.g4478.

Health ministers in west Africa hold crisis talks on Ebola virus.

Gulland A(1).

Author information: (1)London.

PMID: 25000938 [PubMed - indexed for MEDLINE]

733. J Anim Ecol. 2014 Jul 4. doi: 10.1111/1365-2656.12268. [Epub ahead of print]

How Ebola impacts social dynamics in gorillas: a multistate modelling approach.

Genton C(1), Pierre A, Cristescu R, Lévréro F, Gatti S, Pierre JS, Ménard N, Le Gouar P.
Author information: (1)UMR 6553, ECOBIO: Ecosystems, Biodiversity, Evolution, CNRS/University of Rennes 1, Station Biologique de Paimpont, 35380, Paimpont, France.

Emerging infectious diseases can induce rapid changes in population dynamics and threaten population persistence. In socially structured populations, the transfers of individuals between social units, for example, from breeding groups to non-breeding groups, shape population dynamics. We suggest that diseases may affect these crucial transfers. We aimed to determine how disturbance by an emerging disease affects demographic rates of gorillas, especially transfer rates within populations and immigration rates into populations. We compared social dynamics and key demographic parameters in a gorilla population affected by Ebola using a long-term observation data set including pre-, during and post-outbreak periods. We also studied a population of undetermined epidemiological status in order to assess whether this population was affected by the disease. We developed a multistate model that can handle transition between social units while optimizing the number of states. During the Ebola outbreak, social dynamics displayed increased transfers from a breeding to a non-breeding status for both males and females. Six years after the outbreak, demographic and most of social dynamics parameters had returned to their initial rates, suggesting a certain resilience in the response to disruption. The formation of breeding groups increased just after Ebola, indicating that environmental conditions were still attractive. However, population recovery was likely delayed because compensatory immigration was probably impeded by the potential impact of Ebola in the surrounding areas. The population of undetermined epidemiological status behaved similarly to the other population before Ebola. Our results highlight the need to integrate social dynamics in host-population demographic models to better understand the role of social structure in the sensitivity and the response to disease disturbances.

PMID: 24995485 [PubMed - as supplied by publisher]

734. Ann Glob Health. 2014 July - August;80(4):251-256. doi: 10.1016/j.aogh.2014.09.006. Epub 2014 Nov 25.

Global Occupational Health: Current Challenges and the Need for Urgent Action.

Lucchini RG(1), London L(2).

Author information: (1)Icahn School of Medicine at Mount Sinai, New York, NY and University of Brescia, Brescia, Italy. Electronic address: roberto.lucchini@mssm.edu. (2)Center for Environmental and Occupational Health Research, University of Cape Town, Cape Town, South Africa.

BACKGROUND: Global occupational health and safety (OHS) is strictly linked to the dynamics of economic globalization. As the global market is increasing, the gap between developed and underdeveloped countries, occupational diseases, and injuries affect a vast number of workers worldwide. Global OHS issues also become local in developed countries due to many factors, including untrained migrant workers in the informal sector, construction, and agriculture. OBJECTIVE: To identify the current status and challenges of global occupational health and safety and the needs for preventive action. FINDINGS: Absence of OHS infrastructure amplifies the devastating consequences of infectious outbreaks like the Ebola pandemic and tuberculosis. Interventions in global OHS are urgently needed at various levels: CONCLUSIONS: Following the equation of maximized profits prompted by the inhibition of OHS is an old practice that has proven to cause significant costs to societies in the developed world. It is now an urgent priority to stop this process and promote a harmonized global market where the health of workers is guaranteed in the global perspective.

PMID: 25459325 [PubMed - as supplied by publisher]

735. Antiviral Res. 2014 Jul;107:102-9. doi: 10.1016/j.antiviral.2014.04.014. Epub 2014 May 9.

Pyridinyl imidazole inhibitors of p38 MAP kinase impair viral entry and reduce cytokine induction by Zaire ebolavirus in human dendritic cells.

Johnson JC(1), Martinez O(2), Honko AN(1), Hensley LE(1), Olinger GG(1), Basler CF(3).

Author information: (1)Virology Division, United States Army Medical Research Institute of Infectious Diseases, Ft. Detrick, MD 21702, United States. (2)Dept. of Microbiology, Icahn School of Medicine at Mount Sinai, New York, NY 10029, United States. (3)Dept. of Microbiology, Icahn School of Medicine at Mount Sinai, New York, NY 10029, United States. Electronic address: chris.basler@mssm.edu.

Antigen presenting cells (APCs), including macrophages and dendritic cells, are early and sustained targets of Ebola virus (EBOV) infection in vivo. Because EBOV activates mitogen-activated protein kinase (MAPK) signaling upon infection of APCs, we evaluated the effect of pyridinyl imidazole inhibitors of p38 MAPK on EBOV infection of human APCs and EBOV mediated cytokine production from human DCs. The p38 MAPK inhibitors reduced viral replication in PMA-differentiated macrophage-like human THP-1 cells with an IC50 of 4.73μM (SB202190), 8.26μM (p38kinhIII) and 8.21μM (SB203580) and primary human monocyte-derived dendritic cells (MDDCs) with an IC50 of 2.67μM (SB202190). Furthermore, cytokine production from EBOV-treated MDDCs was inhibited in a dose-dependent manner. A control pyridinyl imidazole compound failed to inhibit either EBOV infection or cytokine induction. Using an established EBOV virus-like particle (VLP) entry assay, we demonstrate that inhibitor pretreatment blocked VLP entry suggesting that the inhibitors blocked infection and replication at least in part by blocking EBOV entry. Taken together, our results indicate that pyridinyl imidazole p38 MAPK inhibitors may serve as leads for the development of therapeutics to treat EBOV infection.

PMCID: PMC4103912 [Available on 2015/7/1] PMID: 24815087 [PubMed - in process]

736. Biosecur Bioterror. 2014 Jul-Aug;12(4):161-2. doi: 10.1089/bsp.2014.1563. Epub 2014 Jul 7.

Ebola in West Africa: a familiar pattern?

Adalja AA(1).

Author information: (1)Amesh A. Adalja, MD, is a Senior Associate, UPMC Center for Health Security , Baltimore, Maryland.

PMID: 24999980 [PubMed - in process]

737. Emerg Infect Dis. 2014 Jul;20(7):1176-82. doi: 10.3201/eid2007.131265.

Undiagnosed acute viral febrile illnesses, Sierra Leone.

Schoepp RJ, Rossi CA, Khan SH, Goba A, Fair JN.

Sierra Leone in West Africa is in a Lassa fever-hyperendemic region that also includes Guinea and Liberia. Each year, suspected Lassa fever cases result in submission of ≈500-700 samples to the Kenema Government Hospital Lassa Diagnostic Laboratory in eastern Sierra Leone. Generally only 30%-40% of samples tested are positive for Lassa virus (LASV) antigen and/or LASV-specific IgM; thus, 60%-70% of these patients have acute diseases of unknown origin. To investigate what other arthropod-borne and hemorrhagic fever viral diseases might cause serious illness in this region and mimic Lassa fever, we tested patient serum samples that were negative for malaria parasites and LASV. Using IgM-capture ELISAs, we evaluated samples for antibodies to arthropod-borne and other hemorrhagic fever viruses. Approximately 25% of LASV-negative patients had IgM to dengue, West Nile, yellow fever, Rift Valley fever, chikungunya, Ebola, and Marburg viruses but not to Crimean-Congo hemorrhagic fever virus.

PMCID: PMC4073864 PMID: 24959946 [PubMed - in process]

738. J Virol. 2014 Jul;88(13):7294-306. doi: 10.1128/JVI.00591-14. Epub 2014 Apr 16.

Small-molecule probes targeting the viral PPxY-host Nedd4 interface block egress of a broad range of RNA viruses.

Han Z(1), Lu J(1), Liu Y(1), Davis B(2), Lee MS(3), Olson MA(4), Ruthel G(1), Freedman BD(1), Schnell MJ(2), Wrobel JE(5), Reitz AB(5), Harty RN(6).

Author information: (1)Department of Pathobiology, School of Veterinary Medicine, University of Pennsylvania, Philadelphia, Pennsylvania, USA. (2)Department of Microbiology and Immunology, Thomas Jefferson University, Philadelphia, Pennsylvania, USA. (3)Integrated Toxicology Division, U.S. Army Medical Research Institute of Infectious Diseases, Fort Detrick, Maryland, USA Simulation Sciences Branch, U.S. Army Research Laboratory, Aberdeen Proving Ground, Maryland, USA. (4)Integrated Toxicology Division, U.S. Army Medical Research Institute of Infectious Diseases, Fort Detrick, Maryland, USA. (5)Fox Chase Chemical Diversity Center, Inc., Doylestown, Pennsylvania, USA. (6)Department of Pathobiology, School of Veterinary Medicine, University of Pennsylvania, Philadelphia, Pennsylvania, USA rharty@vet.upenn.edu.

Budding of filoviruses, arenaviruses, and rhabdoviruses is facilitated by subversion of host proteins, such as Nedd4 E3 ubiquitin ligase, by viral PPxY late (L) budding domains expressed within the matrix proteins of these RNA viruses. As L domains are important for budding and are highly conserved in a wide array of RNA viruses, they represent potential broad-spectrum targets for the development of antiviral drugs. To identify potential competitive blockers, we used the known Nedd4 WW domain-PPxY interaction interface as the basis of an in silico screen. Using PPxY-dependent budding of Marburg (MARV) VP40 virus-like particles (VLPs) as our model system, we identified small-molecule hit 1 that inhibited Nedd4-PPxY interaction and PPxY-dependent budding. This lead candidate was subsequently improved with additional structure-activity relationship (SAR) analog testing which enhanced antibudding activity into the nanomolar range. Current lead compounds 4 and 5 exhibit on-target effects by specifically blocking the MARV VP40 PPxY-host Nedd4 interaction and subsequent PPxY-dependent egress of MARV VP40 VLPs. In addition, lead compounds 4 and 5 exhibited antibudding activity against Ebola and Lassa fever VLPs, as well as vesicular stomatitis and rabies viruses (VSV and RABV, respectively). These data provide target validation and suggest that inhibition of the PPxY-Nedd4 interaction can serve as the basis for the development of a novel class of broad-spectrum, host-oriented antivirals targeting viruses that depend on a functional PPxY L domain for efficient egress.IMPORTANCE: There is an urgent and unmet need for the development of safe and effective therapeutics against biodefense and high-priority pathogens, including filoviruses (Ebola and Marburg) and arenaviruses (e.g., Lassa and Junin) which cause severe hemorrhagic fever syndromes with high mortality rates. We along with others have established that efficient budding of filoviruses, arenaviruses, and other viruses is critically dependent on the subversion of host proteins. As disruption of virus budding would prevent virus dissemination, identification of small-molecule compounds that block these critical viral-host interactions should effectively block disease progression and transmission. Our findings provide validation for targeting these virus-host interactions as we have identified lead inhibitors with broad-spectrum antiviral activity. In addition, such inhibitors might prove useful for newly emerging RNA viruses for which no therapeutics would be available.

PMCID: PMC4054416 [Available on 2015/1/1] PMID: 24741084 [PubMed - in process]

739. Lab Med. 2014 Summer;45(3):e109-11. doi: 10.1309/LMTMW3VVN2OHIFS.

Laboratory test support for ebola patients within a high-containment facility.

Hill CE(1), Burd EM(1), Kraft CS(1), Ryan EL(1), Duncan A(1), Winkler AM(1), Cardella JC(2), Ritchie JC(1), Parslow TG(3).

Author information: (1)Department of Pathology and Laboratory Medicine, Emory University, Atlanta, GA. (2)Department of Pathology and Laboratory Medicine, Emory Medical Laboratories, Atlanta, GA. (3)Department of Pathology and Laboratory Medicine, Emory University, Atlanta, GA tparslo@emory.edu.

PMID: 25184220 [PubMed - in process]

740. PLoS Negl Trop Dis. 2014 Jul 31;8(7):e3061. doi: 10.1371/journal.pntd.0003061. eCollection 2014.

Transcriptional correlates of disease outcome in anticoagulant-treated non-human primates infected with ebolavirus.

Garamszegi S(1), Yen JY(2), Honko AN(3), Geisbert JB(4), Rubins KH(5), Geisbert TW(4), Xia Y(6), Hensley LE(7), Connor JH(8).

Author information: (1)Bioinformatics Program, Boston University, Boston, Massachusetts, University of America. (2)Department of Microbiology, School of Medicine, Boston University, Boston, Massachusetts, University of America; National Emerging Infectious Diseases Laboratories, Boston University, Boston, Massachusetts, University of America. (3)U.S. Army Medical Research Institute of Infectious Diseases, Fort Detrick, Frederick, Maryland, United States of America. (4)Department of Microbiology and Immunology, University of Texas Medical Branch, Galveston, Texas, United States of America. (5)National Aeronautics and Space Administration, Houston, Texas, United States of America. (6)Bioinformatics Program, Boston University, Boston, Massachusetts, University of America; Department of Bioengineering, McGill University, Montreal, Canada. (7)Integrated Research Facility at Fort Detrick, National Institute of Allergy and Infectious Diseases, National Institutes of Health, Fort Detrick, Frederick, Maryland, United States of America. (8)Bioinformatics Program, Boston University, Boston, Massachusetts, University of America; Department of Microbiology, School of Medicine, Boston University, Boston, Massachusetts, University of America; National Emerging Infectious Diseases Laboratories, Boston University, Boston, Massachusetts, University of America.

Ebola virus (EBOV) infection in humans and non-human primates (NHPs) is highly lethal, and there is limited understanding of the mechanisms associated with pathogenesis and survival. Here, we describe a transcriptomic analysis of NHPs that survived lethal EBOV infection, compared to NHPs that did not survive. It has been previously demonstrated that anticoagulant therapeutics increase the survival rate in EBOV-infected NHPs, and that the characteristic transcriptional profile of immune response changes in anticoagulant-treated NHPs. In order to identify transcriptional signatures that correlate with survival following EBOV infection, we compared the mRNA expression profile in peripheral blood mononuclear cells from EBOV-infected NHPs that received anticoagulant treatment, to those that did not receive treatment. We identified a small set of 20 genes that are highly confident predictors and can accurately distinguish between surviving and non-surviving animals. In addition, we identified a larger predictive signature of 238 genes that correlated with disease outcome and treatment; this latter signature was associated with a variety of host responses, such as the inflammatory response, T cell death, and inhibition of viral replication. Notably, among survival-associated genes were subsets of genes that are transcriptionally regulated by (1) CCAAT/enhancer-binding protein alpha, (2) tumor protein 53, and (3) megakaryoblastic leukemia 1 and myocardin-like protein 2. These pathways merit further investigation as potential transcriptional signatures of host immune response to EBOV infection.

PMCID: PMC4117489 PMID: 25079789 [PubMed - in process]

741. PLoS Negl Trop Dis. 2014 Jul 31;8(7):e3056. doi: 10.1371/journal.pntd.0003056. eCollection 2014.

Outbreak of ebola virus disease in Guinea: where ecology meets economy.

Bausch DG(1), Schwarz L(2).

Author information: (1)Tulane School of Public Health and Tropical Medicine, New Orleans, Louisiana, United States of America; United States Naval Medical Research Unit No. 6, Lima, Peru. (2)McGill University, Montreal, Canada.

PMCID: PMC4117598 PMID: 25079231 [PubMed - in process]

742. MMWR Morb Mortal Wkly Rep. 2014 Jun 27;63(25):548-51.

Ebola viral disease outbreak--West Africa, 2014.

Dixon MG, Schafer IJ; Centers for Disease Control and Prevention (CDC).

On March 21, 2014, the Guinea Ministry of Health reported the outbreak of an illness characterized by fever, severe diarrhea, vomiting, and a high case-fatality rate (59%) among 49 persons. Specimens from 15 of 20 persons tested at Institut Pasteur in Lyon, France, were positive for an Ebola virus by polymerase chain reaction. Viral sequencing identified Ebola virus (species Zaïre ebolavirus), one of five viruses in the genus Ebolavirus, as the cause. Cases of Ebola viral disease (EVD) were initially reported in three southeastern districts (Gueckedou, Macenta, and Kissidougou) of Guinea and in the capital city of Conakry. By March 30, cases had been reported in Foya district in neighboring Liberia (1), and in May, the first cases identified in Sierra Leone were reported. As of June 18, the outbreak was the largest EVD outbreak ever documented, with a combined total of 528 cases (including laboratory-confirmed, probable, and suspected cases) and 337 deaths (case-fatality rate = 64%) reported in the three countries. The largest previous outbreak occurred in Uganda during 2000-2001, when 425 cases were reported with 224 deaths (case-fatality rate = 53%). The current outbreak also represents the first outbreak of EVD in West Africa (a single case caused by Taï Forest virus was reported in Côte d'Ivoire in 1994 [3]) and marks the first time that Ebola virus transmission has been reported in a capital city.

PMID: 24964881 [PubMed - indexed for MEDLINE]

743. ACS Nano. 2014 Jun 24;8(6):6047-55. doi: 10.1021/nn501312q. Epub 2014 Jun 4.

Digital sensing and sizing of vesicular stomatitis virus pseudotypes in complex media: a model for ebola and marburg detection.

Daaboul GG(1), Lopez CA, Chinnala J, Goldberg BB, Connor JH, Unlü MS.

Author information: (1)Electrical & Computer Engineering Department, Boston University , Boston, Massachusetts 02215, United States.

Rapid, sensitive, and direct label-free capture and characterization of nanoparticles from complex media such as blood or serum will broadly impact medicine and the life sciences. We demonstrate identification of virus particles in complex samples for replication-competent wild-type vesicular stomatitis virus (VSV), defective VSV, and Ebola- and Marburg-pseudotyped VSV with high sensitivity and specificity. Size discrimination of the imaged nanoparticles (virions) allows differentiation between modified viruses having different genome lengths and facilitates a reduction in the counting of nonspecifically bound particles to achieve a limit-of-detection (LOD) of $5 \times 10(3)$ pfu/mL for the Ebola and Marburg VSV pseudotypes. We demonstrate the simultaneous detection of multiple viruses in a single sample (composed of serum or whole blood) for screening applications and uncompromised detection capabilities in samples contaminated with high levels of bacteria. By employing affinity-based capture, size discrimination, and a "digital" detection scheme to count single virus particles, we show that a robust and sensitive virus/nanoparticle sensing assay can be established for targets in complex samples. The nanoparticle microscopy system is termed the Single Particle Interferometric Reflectance Imaging Sensor (SP-IRIS) and is capable of high-throughput and rapid sizing of large numbers of biological nanoparticles on an antibody microarray for research and diagnostic applications.

PMID: 24840765 [PubMed - in process]

744. Proc Natl Acad Sci U S A. 2014 Jun 17;111(24):8873-6. doi: 10.1073/pnas.1316902111. Epub 2014 May 27.

Vaccinating captive chimpanzees to save wild chimpanzees.

Warfield KL(1), Goetzmann JE(2), Biggins JE(3), Kasda MB(3), Unfer RC(1), Vu H(1), Aman MJ(1), Olinger GG Jr(3), Walsh PD(4).

Author information: (1)Integrated BioTherapeutics, Inc., Gaithersburg, MD 20878; (2)New Iberia Research Center, University of Louisiana at Lafayette, New Iberia, LA 70562-3610; (3)Division of Virology, US Army Medical Research Institute of Infectious Diseases, Fort Detrick, Frederick, MD 21702; and. (4)Department of Archaelogy and Anthropology, University of Cambridge, Cambridge CB2 3QG, United Kingdom pdw36@cam.ac.uk.

Infectious disease has only recently been recognized as a major threat to the survival of Endangered chimpanzees and Critically Endangered gorillas in the wild. One potentially powerful tool, vaccination, has not been deployed in fighting this disease threat, in good part because of fears about vaccine safety. Here we report on what is, to our knowledge, the first trial in which captive chimpanzees were used to test a vaccine intended for use on wild apes rather than humans. We tested a virus-like particle vaccine against Ebola virus, a leading source of death in wild gorillas and chimpanzees. The vaccine was safe and immunogenic. Captive trials of other vaccines and of methods for vaccine delivery hold great potential as weapons in the fight against wild ape extinction.

PMCID: PMC4066532 PMID: 24912183 [PubMed - indexed for MEDLINE]

745. PLoS Curr. 2014 Jun 16;6. pii: ecurrents.outbreaks.c0e035c86d721668a6ad7353f7f6fe86. doi: 10.1371/currents.outbreaks.c0e035c86d721668a6ad7353f7f6fe86.

Clock Rooting Further Demonstrates that Guinea 2014 EBOV is a Member of the Zaïre Lineage.

Calvignac-Spencer S(1), Schulze JM(1), Zickmann F(1), Renard BY(1).

Author information: (1)Robert Koch-Institute, Berlin, Germany.

While initial phylogenetic analyses concluded to Guinea 2014 EBOV falling outside the Zaïre lineage (ZEBOV), a recent re-analysis of the same dataset by Dudas and Rambaut (2014) suggested that Guinea 2014 EBOV actually is ZEBOV. Under the same hypothesis as used by these authors (the molecular clock hypothesis), we reinforce their conclusion by providing a statistical assessment of the location of the root of the Zaïre lineage. Our analysis unambiguously supports Guinea 2014 EBOV as a member of the Zaïre lineage. In addition, we also show that some uncertainty exists so as to the location of the root of the genus Ebolavirus. We release the software we used for these re-analyses. RootAnnotator allows for the easy determination of branch root posterior probability from any posterior sample of clocked trees and is freely available at http://sourceforge.net/projects/rootannotator/.

PMCID: PMC4073806 PMID: 24987574 [PubMed]

746. Lancet. 2014 Jun 7;383(9933):1946. doi: 10.1016/S0140-6736(14)60938-7.

Ebola in west Africa: gaining community trust and confidence.

[No authors listed]

PMID: 24910220 [PubMed - indexed for MEDLINE]

747. Afr J Med Med Sci. 2014 Jun;43(2):87-97.

Outbreaks-of Ebola virus disease in the West African sub-region.

Osungbade KO, Oni AA.

BACKGROUND: Five West African countries, including Nigeria are currently experiencing the largest, most severe, most complex outbreak of Ebola virus disease in history. This paper provided a chronology of outbreaks of Ebola virus disease in the West African sub-region and provided an update on efforts at containing the present outbreak. METHODS: Literature from Pubmed (MEDLINE), AJOL, Google Scholar and Cochrane database were reviewed. RESULTS: Outbreaks of Ebola, virus disease had frequently occurred mainly in Central and East African countries. Occasional outbreaks reported from outside of Africa were due to laboratory contamination and imported monkeys in quarantine facilities. The ongoing outbreak in West Africa is the largest and first in the sub-region; the number of suspected cases and deaths from this single current outbreak is already about three times the total of all cases and deaths from previous known outbreaks in 40 years. Prevention and control efforts are hindered not only by lack of a known vaccine and virus-specific treatment, but also by weak health systems, poor sanitation, poor personal hygiene and cultural beliefs and practices, including myths and misconceptions about Ebola virus disease--all of which are prevalent in affected countries. Constrained by this situation, the World Health Organisation departed from the global standard and recommended the use of not yet proven treatments to treat or prevent the disease in humans on ethical and evidential grounds. CONCLUSION: The large number of people affected by the present outbreak in West Africa and the high case-fatality rate calls for accelerated evaluation and development of the investigational medical interventions for life saving and curbing the epidemic. Meanwhile, existing interventions such as early detection and isolation, contact tracing and monitoring, and adherence to rigorous procedures of infection prevention and control should be intensified.

PMID: 25508762 [PubMed - in process]

748. Afr J Med Med Sci. 2014 Jun;43(2):84.

Outbreak of Ebola virus disease in the West Africa.

Baiyewu O.

PMID: 25508761 [PubMed - in process]

749. Afr J Med Med Sci. 2014 Jun;43(2):87-97.

Outbreaks-of Ebola virus disease in the West African sub-region.

Osungbade KO, Oni AA.

BACKGROUND: Five West African countries, including Nigeria are currently experiencing the largest, most severe, most complex outbreak of Ebola virus disease in history. This paper provided a chronology of outbreaks of Ebola virus disease in the West African sub-region and provided an update on efforts at containing the present outbreak. METHODS: Literature from Pubmed (MEDLINE), AJOL, Google Scholar and Cochrane database were reviewed. RESULTS: Outbreaks of Ebola, virus disease had frequently occurred mainly in Central and East African countries. Occasional outbreaks reported from outside of Africa were due to laboratory contamination and imported monkeys in quarantine facilities. The ongoing outbreak in West Africa is the largest and first in the sub-region; the number of suspected cases and deaths from this single current outbreak is already about three times the total of all cases and deaths from previous known outbreaks in 40 years. Prevention and control efforts are hindered not only by lack of a known vaccine and virus-specific treatment, but also by weak health systems, poor sanitation, poor personal hygiene and cultural beliefs and practices, including myths and misconceptions about Ebola virus disease--all of which are prevalent in affected countries. Constrained by this situation, the World Health Organisation departed from the global standard and recommended the use of not yet proven treatments to treat or prevent the disease in humans on ethical and evidential grounds. CONCLUSION: The large number of people affected by the present outbreak in West Africa and the high case-fatality rate calls for accelerated evaluation and development of the investigational medical interventions for life saving and curbing the epidemic. Meanwhile, existing interventions such as early detection and isolation, contact tracing and monitoring, and adherence to rigorous procedures of infection prevention and control should be intensified.

PMID: 25474983 [PubMed - in process]

750. Afr J Med Med Sci. 2014 Jun;43(2):84.

Outbreak of Ebola virus disease in the West Africa.

Baiyewu O.

PMID: 25474982 [PubMed - in process]

751. Antiviral Res. 2014 Jun;106:86-94. doi: 10.1016/j.antiviral.2014.03.018. Epub 2014 Apr 5.

High-throughput, luciferase-based reverse genetics systems for identifying inhibitors of Marburg and Ebola viruses.

Uebelhoer LS(1), Albariño CG(1), McMullan LK(1), Chakrabarti AK(1), Vincent JP(1), Nichol ST(1), Towner JS(2).

Author information: (1)Centers for Disease Control and Prevention, Atlanta, USA. (2)Centers for Disease Control and Prevention, Atlanta, USA. Electronic address: jit8@cdc.gov.

Marburg virus (MARV) and Ebola virus (EBOV), members of the family Filoviridae, represent a significant challenge to global public health. Currently, no licensed therapies exist to treat filovirus infections, which cause up to 90% mortality in human cases. To facilitate development of antivirals against these viruses, we established two distinct screening platforms based on MARV and EBOV reverse genetics systems that express secreted Gaussia luciferase (gLuc). The first platform is a mini-genome replicon to screen viral replication inhibitors using gLuc quantification in a BSL-2 setting. The second platform is complementary to the first and expresses gLuc as a reporter gene product encoded in recombinant infectious MARV and EBOV, thereby allowing for rapid quantification of viral growth during treatment with antiviral compounds. We characterized these viruses by comparing luciferase activity to virus production, and validated luciferase activity as an authentic real-time measure of viral growth. As proof of concept, we adapt both mini-genome and infectious virus platforms to high-throughput formats, and demonstrate efficacy of several antiviral compounds. We anticipate that both approaches will prove highly useful in the development of anti-filovirus therapies, as well as in basic research on the filovirus life cycle.

Published by Elsevier B.V.

PMID: 24713118 [PubMed - indexed for MEDLINE]

752. Cell Res. 2014 Jun;24(6):647-8. doi: 10.1038/cr.2014.49. Epub 2014 Apr 15.

Possible leap ahead in filovirus therapeutics.

Falzarano D(1), Feldmann H(1).

Author information: (1)Laboratory of Virology, Division of Intramural Research, National Institute of Allergy and Infectious Diseases, National Institutes of Health, Hamilton, MT 59840, USA.

Comment on Nature. 2014 Apr 17;508(7496):402-5.

In a recent study published in Nature, Warren et al. describe the generation of a novel synthetic adenosine analogue, BCX4430, a synthetic drug-like small molecule that provides protection from Ebola and Marburg virus infection in animal models.

PMCID: PMC4042172 [Available on 2015/6/1] PMID: 24732011 [PubMed - in process]

753. Chem Asian J. 2014 Jun;9(6):1436-44. doi: 10.1002/asia.201400133. Epub 2014 Mar 26

Fullerene sugar balls: a new class of biologically active fullerene derivatives.

Nierengarten I(1), Nierengarten JF.

Author information: (1)Laboratoire de Chimie des Matériaux Moléculaires, Université de Strasbourg et CNRS (UMR 7509), Ecole Européenne de Chimie, Polymères et Matériaux, 25 rue Becquerel, 67087 Strasbourg Cedex 2 (France).

Among the large variety of bioactive C60 derivatives, fullerene derivatives substituted with sugar residues, that is, glycofullerenes, are of particular interest. The sugar residues are not only solubilizing groups; their intrinsic biological properties also provide additional appealing features to the conjugates. The most recent advances in the synthesis and the biological applications of glycofullerenes are summarized in the present review article with special emphasis on globular glycofullerenes, that is, fullerene sugar balls, constructed on a hexa-substituted fullerene scaffold. The high local concentration of carbohydrates around the C60 core in fullerene sugar balls is perfectly suited to the binding of lectins through the "glycoside cluster effect", and these compounds are potential anti-adhesive agents against bacterial infection. Moreover, mannosylated fullerene sugar balls have shown antiviral activity in an Ebola pseudotyped infection model. Finally, when substituted with peripheral iminosugars, dramatic multivalent effects have been observed for glycosidase inhibition. These unexpected observations have been rationalized by the interplay of interactions involving the catalytic site of the enzyme and non-glycone binding sites with lectin-like abilities.

© 2014 WILEY-VCH Verlag GmbH & Co. KGaA, Weinheim.

PMID: 24678063 [PubMed - in process]

754. Epidemiol Infect. 2014 Jun;142(6):1138-45. doi: 10.1017/S0950268813002215. Epub 2013 Sep 16.

Evolutionary history of Ebola virus.

Li YH(1), Chen SP(2).

Author information: (1)Center of Hematopoietic Stem Cell Transplantation, Affiliated Hospital of the Academy of Military Medical Sciences, Beijing, PR China. (2)Department of Laboratory Medicine, Affiliated Hospital of the Academy of Military Medical Sciences, Beijing, PR China.

SUMMARY: Since Ebola virus was discovered in 1970s, the virus has persisted in Africa and sporadic fatal outbreaks in humans and non-human primates have been reported. However, the evolutionary history of Ebola virus remains unclear. In this study, 27 Ebola virus strains with complete glycoprotein genes, including five species (Zaire, Sudan, Reston, Tai Forest, Bundibugyo), were analysed. Here, we propose a hypothesis of the evolutionary history of Ebola virus which will be helpful to investigate the molecular evolution of these viruses.

PMID: 24040779 [PubMed - indexed for MEDLINE]
755. Expert Rev Clin Immunol. 2014 Jun;10(6):781-90. doi: 10.1586/1744666X.2014.908705. Epub 2014 Apr 18.

Characterization of host immune responses in Ebola virus infections.

Wong G(1), Kobinger GP, Qiu X.

Author information: (1)Special Pathogens Program, National Microbiology Laboratory, Public Health Agency of Canada, 1015 Arlington Street Winnipeg, MB, R3E 3R2 Canada.

Ebola causes highly lethal hemorrhagic fever in humans with no licensed countermeasures. Its virulence can be attributed to several immunoevasion mechanisms: an early inhibition of innate immunity started by the downregulation of type I interferon, epitope masking and subversion of the adaptive humoural immunity by secreting a truncated form of the viral glycoprotein. Deficiencies in specific and non-specific antiviral responses result in unrestricted viral replication and dissemination in the host, causing death typically within 10 days after the appearance of symptoms. This review summarizes the host immune response to Ebola infection, and highlights the short- and long-term immune responses crucial for protection, which holds implications for the design of future vaccines and therapeutics.

PMID: 24742338 [PubMed - in process]
756. J Interferon Cytokine Res. 2014 Jun;34(6):464-8. doi: 10.1089/jir.2014.0005.

Viral proteins that bind double-stranded RNA: countermeasures against host antiviral responses.

Krug RM(1).

Author information: (1)Molecular Biosciences, Center of Infectious Disease, Institute for Cellular and Molecular Biology, University of Texas at Austin , Austin, Texas.

Several animal viruses encode proteins that bind double-stranded RNA (dsRNA) to counteract host dsRNA-dependent antiviral responses. This article discusses the structure and function of the dsRNA-binding proteins of influenza A virus and Ebola viruses (EBOVs).

PMCID: PMC4046347 [Available on 2015/6/1] PMID: 24905203 [PubMed - in process]
757. J Virol. 2014 Jun;88(12):6636-49. doi: 10.1128/JVI.00396-14. Epub 2014 Apr 2.

Ebolavirus entry requires a compact hydrophobic fist at the tip of the fusion loop.

Gregory SM(1), Larsson P(1), Nelson EA(2), Kasson PM(1), White JM(2), Tamm LK(3).

Author information: (1)Center for Membrane Biology and Department of Molecular Physiology and Biological Physics, University of Virginia, Charlottesville, Virginia, USA. (2)Department of Cell Biology, University of Virginia, Charlottesville, Virginia, USA. (3)Center for Membrane Biology and Department of Molecular Physiology and Biological Physics, University of Virginia, Charlottesville, Virginia, USA lkt2e@virginia.edu.

Ebolavirus is an enveloped virus causing severe hemorrhagic fever. Its surface glycoproteins undergo proteolytic cleavage and rearrangements to permit membrane fusion and cell entry. Here we focus on the glycoprotein's internal fusion loop (FL), critical for low-pH-triggered fusion in the endosome. Alanine mutations at L529 and I544 and particularly the L529 I544 double mutation compromised viral entry and fusion. The nuclear magnetic resonance (NMR) structures of the I544A and L529A I544A mutants in lipid environments showed significant disruption of a three-residue scaffold that is required for the formation of a consolidated fusogenic hydrophobic surface at the tip of the FL. Biophysical experiments and molecular simulation revealed the position of the wild-type (WT) FL in membranes and showed the inability of the inactive double mutant to reach this position. Consolidation of hydrophobic residues at the tip of FLs may be a common requirement for internal FLs of class I, II, and III fusion proteins.IMPORTANCE: Many class I, II, and III viral fusion proteins bear fusion loops for target membrane insertion and fusion. We determined structures of the Ebolavirus fusion loop and found residues critical for forming a consolidated hydrophobic surface, membrane insertion, and viral entry.

PMCID: PMC4054381 PMID: 24696482 [PubMed - indexed for MEDLINE]
758. J Virol. 2014 Jun;88(12):6702-13. doi: 10.1128/JVI.00300-14. Epub 2014 Apr 2.

Characterizing functional domains for TIM-mediated enveloped virus entry.

Moller-Tank S(1), Albritton LM(2), Rennert PD(3), Maury W(4).

Author information: (1)Department of Microbiology, University of Iowa, Iowa City, Iowa, USA. (2)Department of Microbiology, Immunology, and Biochemistry, University of Tennessee Health Science Center, Memphis, Tennessee, USA. (3)SugarCone Biotech LLC, Holliston, Massachusetts, USA. (4)Department of Microbiology, University of Iowa, Iowa City, Iowa, USA wendy-maury@uiowa.edu.

T-cell immunoglobulin and mucin domain I (TIM-1) and other TIM family members were recently identified as phosphatidylserine (PtdSer)-mediated virus entry-enhancing receptors (PVEERs). These proteins enhance entry of Ebola virus (EBOV) and other viruses by binding PtdSer on the viral envelope, concentrating virus on the cell surface, and promoting subsequent internalization. The PtdSer-binding activity of the immunoglobulin-like variable (IgV) domain is essential for both virus binding and internalization by TIM-1. However, TIM-3, whose IgV domain also binds PtdSer, does not effectively enhance virus entry, indicating that other domains of TIM proteins are functionally important. Here, we investigate the domains supporting enhancement of enveloped virus entry, thereby defining the features necessary for a functional PVEER. Using a variety of chimeras and deletion mutants, we found that in addition to a functional PtdSer-binding domain PVEERs require a stalk domain of sufficient length, containing sequences that promote an extended structure. Neither the cytoplasmic nor the transmembrane domain of TIM-1 is essential for enhancing virus entry, provided the protein is still plasma membrane bound. Based on these defined characteristics, we generated a mimic lacking TIM sequences and composed of annexin V, the mucin-like domain of α-dystroglycan, and a glycophosphatidylinositol anchor that functioned as a PVEER to enhance transduction of virions displaying Ebola, Chikungunya, Ross River, or Sindbis virus glycoproteins. This identification of the key features necessary for PtdSer-mediated enhancement of virus entry provides a basis for more effective recognition of unknown PVEERs.IMPORTANCE: T-cell immunoglobulin and mucin domain I (TIM-I) and other TIM family members are recently identified phosphatidylserine (PtdSer)-mediated virus entry-enhancing receptors (PVEERs). These proteins enhance virus entry by binding the phospholipid, PtdSer, present on the viral membrane. While it is known that the PtdSer binding is essential for the PVEER function of TIM-I, TIM-3 shares this binding activity but does not enhance virus entry. No comprehensive studies have been done to characterize the other domains of TIM-I. In this study, using a variety of chimeric proteins and deletion mutants, we define the features necessary for a functional PVEER. With these features in mind, we generated a TIM-I mimic using functionally similar domains from other proteins. This mimic, like TIM-I, effectively enhanced transduction. These studies provide insight into the key features necessary for PVEERs and will allow for more effective identification of unknown PVEERs.

PMCID: PMC4054341 PMID: 24696470 [PubMed - indexed for MEDLINE]

759. Med Anthropol Q. 2014 Jun;28(2):280-303. doi: 10.1111/maq.12092. Epub 2014 Apr 21

Material proximities and hotspots: toward an anthropology of viral hemorrhagic fevers.

Brown H(1), Kelly AH.

Author information: (1)Department of Anthropology, Durham University. hannah.brown@durham.ac.uk.

This article outlines a research program for an anthropology of viral hemorrhagic fevers (collectively known as VHFs). It begins by reviewing the social science literature on Ebola, Marburg, and Lassa fevers and charting areas for future ethnographic attention. We theoretically elaborate the hotspot as a way of integrating analysis of the two routes of VHF infection: from animal reservoirs to humans and between humans. Drawing together recent anthropological investigations of human-animal entanglements with an ethnographic interest in the social production of space, we seek to enrich conceptualizations of viral movement by elaborating the circumstances through which viruses, humans, objects, and animals come into contact. We suggest that attention to the material proximities-between animals, humans, and objects-that constitute the hotspot opens a frontier site for critical and methodological development in medical anthropology and for future collaborations in VHF management and control.

PMID: 24752909 [PubMed - indexed for MEDLINE]

760. Med Sci (Paris). 2014 Jun-Jul;30(6-7):671-3. doi: 10.1051/medsci/20143006018. Epub 2014 Jul 11.

[A first outbreak of Ebola virus in West Africa].

[Article in French]

Reynard O(1), Volchkov V(1), Peyrefitte C(2).

Author information: (1)CIRI-Centre International de Recherche en Infectiologie, Inserm U1111 - CNRS UMR5308, Université Lyon 1, ENS de Lyon, 21, avenue Tony Garnier, 69365 Lyon Cedex 07, France. (2)IRBA-Institut de recherche biomédicale des armées, unité de virologie, ERL, Lyon, France.

PMID: 25014459 [PubMed - indexed for MEDLINE]

761. Nucleic Acid Ther. 2014 Jun;24(3):179-85. doi: 10.1089/nat.2013.0457. Epub 2014 Mar 21.

Induced IL-10 splice altering approach to antiviral drug discovery.

Panchal RG(1), Mourich DV, Bradfute S, Hauck LL, Warfield KL, Iversen PL, Bavari S.

Author information: (1)1 United States Army Medical Research Institute of Infectious Diseases , Fort Detrick, Maryland.

Ebola virus causes an acute hemorrhagic fever lethal in primates and rodents. The contribution of host immune factors to pathogenesis has yet to be determined and may reveal efficacious targets for potential treatment. In this study, we show that the interleukin (IL)-10 signaling pathway modulates Ebola pathogenesis. IL-10(-/-) mice and wild-type mice receiving antisense targeting IL-10 signaling via disrupting expression through aberrant splice altering were resistant to ebola virus infection. IL-10(-/-) mice exhibited reduced viral titers, pathology, and levels of IL-2, IL-6, keratinocyte-derived chemokine (KC), and macrophage inflammatory protein-1 α and increased interferon (IFN)-γ relative to infected wild-type mice. Furthermore, antibody depletion studies in IL-10(-/-) mice suggest a requirement for natural killer cells and IFN-γ for protection. Together, these data demonstrate that resistance to ebola infection is regulated by IL-10 and can be targeted in a prophylactic manner to protect against lethal hemorrhagic virus challenge.

PMID: 24655055 [PubMed - indexed for MEDLINE]

762. Wkly Epidemiol Rec. 2014 May 16;89(20):205-6.

Outbreak news. Ebola virus disease, West Africa.

[Article in English, French]

[No authors listed]

PMID: 24864345 [PubMed - indexed for MEDLINE]

763. J Mol Biol. 2014 May 15;426(10):2045-58. doi: 10.1016/j.jmb.2014.01.010. Epub 2014 Feb 1.

In silico derived small molecules bind the filovirus VP35 protein and inhibit its polymerase cofactor activity.

Brown CS(1), Lee MS(2), Leung DW(3), Wang T(4), Xu W(3), Luthra P(5), Anantpadma M(6), Shabman RS(5), Melito LM(7), MacMillan KS(7), Borek DM(8), Otwinowski Z(8), Ramanan P(9), Stubbs AJ(10), Peterson DS(10), Binning JM(9), Tonelli M(11), Olson MA(12), Davey RA(6), Ready JM(7), Basler CF(5), Amarasinghe GK(13).

Author information: (1)Department of Pathology and Immunology, Washington University School of Medicine, St. Louis, MO 63110, USA; Roy J. Carver Department of Biochemistry, Biophysics and Molecular Biology, Iowa State University, Ames, IA 50011, USA; Biochemistry Undergraduate Program, Iowa State University,

Ames, IA 50011, USA. (2)Simulation Sciences Branch, US Army Research Laboratory, Aberdeen, MD 21005, USA; Department of Cell Biology and Biochemistry, USAMRIID, 1425 Porter St., Fort Detrick, MD 21702, USA. (3)Department of Pathology and Immunology, Washington University School of Medicine, St. Louis, MO 63110, USA. (4)Roy J. Carver Department of Biochemistry, Biophysics and Molecular Biology, Iowa State University, Ames, IA 50011, USA. (5)Department of Microbiology, Icahn School of Medicine at Mount Sinai, New York, NY 10029, USA. (6)Department of Virology and Immunology, Texas Biomedical Research Institute, San Antonio, TX 78227, USA. (7)Department of Biochemistry, UT Southwestern Medical Center at Dallas, Dallas, TX 75390, USA. (8)Department of Biochemistry, UT Southwestern Medical Center at Dallas, Dallas, TX 75390, USA; Department of Biophysics, UT Southwestern Medical Center at Dallas, Dallas, TX 75390, USA; Center for Structural Genomics of Infectious Diseases (CSGID), Chicago, IL, USA. (9)Department of Pathology and Immunology, Washington University School of Medicine, St. Louis, MO 63110, USA; Biochemistry Graduate Program, Iowa State University, Ames, IA 50011, USA. (10)Roy J. Carver Department of Biochemistry, Biophysics and Molecular Biology, Iowa State University, Ames, IA 50011, USA; Biochemistry Undergraduate Program, Iowa State University, Ames, IA 50011, USA. (11)National Magnetic Resonance Facility at Madison, University of Wisconsin, Madison, 433 Babcock Drive, Madison, WI 53706, USA. (12)Department of Cell Biology and Biochemistry, USAMRIID, 1425 Porter St., Fort Detrick, MD 21702, USA. (13)Department of Pathology and Immunology, Washington University School of Medicine, St. Louis, MO 63110, USA. Electronic address: gamarasinghe@path.wustl.edu.

The Ebola virus (EBOV) genome only encodes a single viral polypeptide with enzymatic activity, the viral large (L) RNA-dependent RNA polymerase protein. However, currently, there is limited information about the L protein, which has hampered the development of antivirals. Therefore, antifiloviral therapeutic efforts must include additional targets such as protein-protein interfaces. Viral protein 35 (VP35) is multifunctional and plays important roles in viral pathogenesis, including viral mRNA synthesis and replication of the negative-sense RNA viral genome. Previous studies revealed that mutation of key basic residues within the VP35 interferon inhibitory domain (IID) results in significant EBOV attenuation, both in vitro and in vivo. In the current study, we use an experimental pipeline that includes structure-based in silico screening and biochemical and structural characterization, along with medicinal chemistry, to identify and characterize small molecules that target a binding pocket within VP35. NMR mapping experiments and high-resolution x-ray crystal structures show that select small molecules bind to a region of VP35 IID that is important for replication complex formation through interactions with the viral nucleoprotein (NP). We also tested select compounds for their ability to inhibit VP35 IID-NP interactions in vitro as well as VP35 function in a minigenome assay and EBOV replication. These results confirm the ability of compounds identified in this study to inhibit VP35-NP interactions in vitro and to impair viral replication in cell-based assays. These studies provide an initial framework to guide development of antifiloviral compounds against filoviral VP35 proteins.

PMCID: PMC4163021 [Available on 2015/5/15] PMID: 24495995 [PubMed - indexed for MEDLINE]

764. Vet Pathol. 2014 May 14. pii: 0300985814535612. [Epub ahead of print]

Experimental Aerosolized Guinea Pig-Adapted Zaire Ebolavirus (Variant: Mayinga) Causes Lethal Pneumonia in Guinea Pigs.

Twenhafel NA(1), Shaia CI(2), Bunton TE(2), Shamblin JD(2), Wollen SE(2), Pitt LM(2), Sizemore DR(2), Ogg MM(2), Johnston SC(2).

Author information: (1)US Army Medical Research Institute of Infectious Diseases, Fort Detrick, MD nancy.twenhafel@us.army.mil. (2)US Army Medical Research Institute of Infectious Diseases, Fort Detrick, MD.

Eight guinea pigs were aerosolized with guinea pig-adapted Zaire ebolavirus (variant: Mayinga) and developed lethal interstitial pneumonia that was distinct from lesions described in guinea pigs challenged subcutaneously, nonhuman primates challenged by the aerosol route, and natural infection in humans. Guinea pigs succumbed with significant pathologic changes primarily restricted to the lungs. Intracytoplasmic inclusion bodies were observed in many alveolar macrophages. Perivasculitis was noted within the lungs. These changes are unlike those of documented subcutaneously challenged guinea pigs and aerosolized filoviral infections in nonhuman primates and human cases. Similar to findings in subcutaneously challenged guinea pigs, there were only mild lesions in the liver and spleen. To our knowledge, this is the first report of aerosol challenge of guinea pigs with guinea pig-adapted Zaire ebolavirus (variant: Mayinga). Before choosing this model for use in aerosolized ebolavirus studies, scientists and pathologists should be aware that aerosolized guinea pig-adapted Zaire ebolavirus (variant: Mayinga) causes lethal pneumonia in guinea pigs.

© The Author(s) 2014.

PMID: 24829285 [PubMed - as supplied by publisher]

765. PLoS Curr. 2014 May 2;6. pii: ecurrents.outbreaks.84eefe5ce43ec9dc0bf0670f7b8b417d. doi: 10.1371/currents.outbreaks.84eefe5ce43ec9dc0bf0670f7b8b417d.

Phylogenetic Analysis of Guinea 2014 EBOV Ebolavirus Outbreak.

Dudas G(1), Rambaut A(2).

Author information: (1)Institute of Evolutionary Biology, University of Edinburgh, Edinburgh, UK. (2)University of Edinburgh, Edinburgh, UK.

Members of the genus Ebolavirus have caused outbreaks of haemorrhagic fever in humans in Africa. The most recent outbreak in Guinea, which began in February of 2014, is still ongoing. Recently published analyses of sequences from this outbreak suggest that the outbreak in Guinea is caused by a divergent lineage of Zaire ebolavirus. We report evidence that points to the same Zaire ebolavirus lineage that has previously caused outbreaks in the Democratic Republic of Congo, the Republic of Congo and Gabon as the culprit behind the outbreak in Guinea.

PMCID: PMC4024086 PMID: 24860690 [PubMed]

766. Am J Trop Med Hyg. 2014 May;90(5):790-3. doi: 10.4269/ajtmh.13-0374. Epub 2014 Feb 10.

Emerging filoviral disease in Uganda: proposed explanations and research directions.

Polonsky JA(1), Wamala JF, de Clerck H, Van Herp M, Sprecher A, Porten K, Shoemaker T.

Author information: (1)Epicentre, Paris, France; Ministry of Heath, Kampala, Uganda; Médecins Sans Frontières Operational Centre Brussels, Brussels, Belgium; US Centers for Disease Control and Prevention, Entebbe, Uganda.

Outbreaks of Ebola and Marburg virus diseases have recently increased in frequency in Uganda. This increase is probably caused by a combination of improved surveillance and laboratory capacity, increased contact between humans and the natural reservoir of the viruses, and fluctuations in viral load and prevalence within this reservoir. The roles of these proposed explanations must be investigated in order to guide appropriate responses to the changing epidemiological profile. Other African settings in which multiple filoviral outbreaks have occurred could also benefit from such information.

PMCID: PMC4015565 PMID: 24515940 [PubMed - indexed for MEDLINE]

767. Antiviral Res. 2014 May;105:17-21. doi: 10.1016/j.antiviral.2014.02.014. Epub 2014 Feb 26.

Successful treatment of advanced Ebola virus infection with T-705 (favipiravir) in a small animal model.

Oestereich L(1), Lüdtke A(2), Wurr S(1), Rieger T(1), Muñoz-Fontela C(2), Günther S(3).

Author information: (1)Bernhard-Nocht-Institute for Tropical Medicine, Bernhard-Nocht-Strasse 74, 20359 Hamburg, Germany; German Centre for Infection Research (DZIF), Partner Site Hamburg, Germany. (2)Bernhard-Nocht-Institute for Tropical Medicine, Bernhard-Nocht-Strasse 74, 20359 Hamburg, Germany; Heinrich Pette Institute, Leibniz Institute for Experimental Virology, Martinistrasse 52, 20251 Hamburg, Germany. (3)Bernhard-Nocht-Institute for Tropical Medicine, Bernhard-Nocht-Strasse 74, 20359 Hamburg, Germany; German Centre for Infection Research (DZIF), Partner Site Hamburg, Germany. Electronic address: guenther@bni.uni-hamburg.de.

Outbreaks of Ebola hemorrhagic fever in sub-Saharan Africa are associated with case fatality rates of up to 90%. Currently, neither a vaccine nor an effective antiviral treatment is available for use in humans. Here, we evaluated the efficacy of the pyrazinecarboxamide derivative T-705 (favipiravir) against Zaire Ebola virus (EBOV) in vitro and in vivo. T-705 suppressed replication of Zaire EBOV in cell culture by 4log units with an IC90 of 110μM. Mice lacking the type I interferon receptor (IFNAR(-)(/)(-)) were used as in vivo model for Zaire EBOV-induced disease. Initiation of T-705 administration at day 6 post infection induced rapid virus clearance, reduced biochemical parameters of disease severity, and prevented a lethal outcome in 100% of the animals. The findings suggest that T-705 is a candidate for treatment of Ebola hemorrhagic fever.

PMID: 24583123 [PubMed - indexed for MEDLINE]

768. Arch Virol. 2014 May;159(5):1229-37. doi: 10.1007/s00705-013-1877-2. Epub 2013 Nov 5.

Virus nomenclature below the species level: a standardized nomenclature for filovirus strains and variants rescued from cDNA.

Kuhn JH(1), Bào Y, Bavari S, Becker S, Bradfute S, Brauburger K, Rodney Brister J, Bukreyev AA, Caì Y, Chandran K, Davey RA, Dolnik O, Dye JM, Enterlein S, Gonzalez JP, Formenty P, Freiberg AN, Hensley LE, Hoenen T, Honko AN, Ignatyev GM, Jahrling PB, Johnson KM, Klenk HD, Kobinger G, Lackemeyer MG, Leroy EM, Lever MS, Mühlberger E, Netesov SV, Olinger GG, Palacios G, Patterson JL, Paweska JT, Pitt L, Radoshitzky SR, Ryabchikova EI, Saphire EO, Shestopalov AM, Smither SJ, Sullivan NJ, Swanepoel R, Takada A, Towner JS, van der Groen G, Volchkov VE, Volchkova VA, Wahl-Jensen V, Warren TK, Warfield KL, Weidmann M, Nichol ST.

Author information: (1)Integrated Research Facility at Fort Detrick (IRF-Frederick), Division of Clinical Research (DCR), National Institute of Allergy and Infectious Diseases (NIAID), National Institutes of Health (NIH), B-8200 Research Plaza, Fort Detrick, Frederick, MD, 21702, USA, kuhnjens@mail.nih.gov.

Specific alterations (mutations, deletions, insertions) of virus genomes are crucial for the functional characterization of their regulatory elements and their expression products, as well as a prerequisite for the creation of attenuated viruses that could serve as vaccine candidates. Virus genome tailoring can be performed either by using traditionally cloned genomes as starting materials, followed by site-directed mutagenesis, or by de novo synthesis of modified virus genomes or parts thereof. A systematic nomenclature for such recombinant viruses is necessary to set them apart from wild-type and laboratory-adapted viruses, and to improve communication and collaborations among researchers who may want to use recombinant viruses or create novel viruses based on them. A large group of filovirus experts has recently proposed nomenclatures for natural and laboratory animal-adapted filoviruses that aim to simplify the retrieval of sequence data from electronic databases. Here, this work is extended to include nomenclature for filoviruses obtained in the laboratory via reverse genetics systems. The previously developed template for natural filovirus genetic variant naming, (/)///-, is retained, but we propose to adapt the type of information added to each field for cDNA clone-derived filoviruses. For instance, the full-length designation of an Ebola virus Kikwit variant rescued from a plasmid developed at the US Centers for Disease Control and Prevention could be akin to "Ebola virus H.sapiens-rec/COD/1995/Kikwit-abc1" (with the suffix "rec" identifying the recombinant nature of the virus and "abc1" being a placeholder for any meaningful isolate designator). Such a full-length designation should be used in databases and the methods section of publications. Shortened designations (such as "EBOV H.sap/COD/95/Kik-abc1") and abbreviations (such as "EBOV/Kik-abc1") could be used in the remainder of the text, depending on how critical it is to convey information contained in the full-length name. "EBOV" would suffice if only one EBOV strain/variant/isolate is addressed.

PMCID: PMC4010566 [Available on 2015/5/1] PMID: 24190508 [PubMed - indexed for MEDLINE]

769. Arch Virol. 2014 May;159(5):1129-32. doi: 10.1007/s00705-012-1477-6. Epub 2012 Sep 21.

Reston virus in domestic pigs in China.

Pan Y(1), Zhang W, Cui L, Hua X, Wang M, Zeng Q.

Author information: (1)The College of Veterinary Medicine, Gansu Agricultural University, Lanzhou, People's Republic of China, panyangyang_2007@126.com.

Historically, Reston virus (RESTV) has been found to be associated with outbreaks of disease only in nonhuman primates. Its spread to domestic pigs was reported for the first time in 2008. In this study, we report the discovery, molecular detection, and phylogenetic analysis of Reston virus (RESTV) in domestic pigs in China. A total of 137 spleen specimens from pigs that died after showing typical clinical signs of porcine reproductive and respiratory syndrome (PRRS),

and for which infection with porcine reproductive and respiratory syndrome virus (PRRSV) was confirmed by RT-PCR, were collected from three farms in Shanghai from February to September 2011. Of these samples, 2.92 % (4/137) were found to be positive for RESTV. All of the positive piglets were under the age of 8 weeks and were co-infected with PRRSV. Sequences were found that shared 96.1 %-98.9 % sequence similarity with those of two RESTV variants that had been discovered previously in domestic pigs and cynomolgus macaques from the Philippines. We therefore conclude that RESTV was present in domestic pigs in Shanghai, China.
PMID: 22996641 [PubMed - indexed for MEDLINE]
770. Bing Du Xue Bao. 2014 May;30(3):292-7.

[Characterization of Marburg virus morphology].

[Article in Chinese]

Song JD, Qu JG, Hong T.

Ebola virus (EBOV) and Marburg virus (MARV) belong to the family Filoviridae. Filoviruses cause severe filovirus hemorrhagic fever (FHF) in humans, with high case fatality rates, and represent potential agents for bioterrorism and biological weapons. It is necessary to keep surveillance of filoviruses, even though there is no report of their isolation and patients in China so far. To characterize MARV morphology, the Lake Victoria marburgvirus--Leiden was stained negatively and observed under a transmission electron microscope which is one of important detection methods for filoviruses in emergencies and bioterrorism. MARV showed pleomorphism, with filamentous, rod-shaped, cobra-like, spherical, and branch-shaped particles of uniform diameter but different lengths. Pleomorphism of negatively stained MARV is summarized in this article, so as to provide useful information for possible electron microscopic identification of filoviruses in China.
PMID: 25118385 [PubMed - indexed for MEDLINE]
771. Can J Infect Dis Med Microbiol. 2014 May;25(3):128-9.

Ebola virus disease.

Laupland KB(1), Valiquette L(2).

Author information: (1)Department of Medicine, Royal Inland Hospital, Kamloops, British Columbia; ; Departments of Medicine, Critical Care Medicine, Pathology and Laboratory Medicine and Community Health Sciences, University of Calgary, Calgary, Alberta; (2)Department of Microbiology-Infectious Diseases, Université de Sherbrooke, Sherbrooke, Quebec.
PMCID: PMC4173971 PMID: 25285105 [PubMed]
772. Emerg Infect Dis. 2014 May;20(5):741-5. doi: 10.3201/eid2005.130539.

Bat flight and zoonotic viruses.

O'Shea TJ, Cryan PM, Cunningham AA, Fooks AR, Hayman DT, Luis AD, Peel AJ, Plowright RK, Wood JL.

Bats are sources of high viral diversity and high-profile zoonotic viruses worldwide. Although apparently not pathogenic in their reservoir hosts, some viruses from bats severely affect other mammals, including humans. Examples include severe acute respiratory syndrome coronaviruses, Ebola and Marburg viruses, and Nipah and Hendra viruses. Factors underlying high viral diversity in bats are the subject of speculation. We hypothesize that flight, a factor common to all bats but to no other mammals, provides an intensive selective force for coexistence with viral parasites through a daily cycle that elevates metabolism and body temperature analogous to the febrile response in other mammals. On an evolutionary scale, this host-virus interaction might have resulted in the large diversity of zoonotic viruses in bats, possibly through bat viruses adapting to be more tolerant of the fever response and less virulent to their natural hosts.
PMCID: PMC4012789 PMID: 24750692 [PubMed - indexed for MEDLINE]
773. J Virol. 2014 May;88(9):4736-43. doi: 10.1128/JVI.03757-13. Epub 2014 Feb 12.

A host-oriented inhibitor of Junin Argentine hemorrhagic fever virus egress.

Lu J(1), Han Z, Liu Y, Liu W, Lee MS, Olson MA, Ruthel G, Freedman BD, Harty RN.

Author information: (1)Department of Pathobiology, School of Veterinary Medicine, University of Pennsylvania, Philadelphia, Pennsylvania, USA.
There are currently no U.S. Food and Drug Administration (FDA)-approved vaccines or therapeutics to prevent or treat Argentine hemorrhagic fever (AHF). The causative agent of AHF is Junin virus (JUNV); a New World arenavirus classified as a National Institute of Allergy and Infectious Disease/Centers for Disease Control and Prevention category A priority pathogen. The PTAP late (L) domain motif within JUNV Z protein facilitates virion egress and transmission by recruiting host Tsg101 and other ESCRT complex proteins to promote scission of the virus particle from the plasma membrane. Here, we describe a novel compound (compound 0013) that blocks the JUNV Z-Tsg101 interaction and inhibits budding of virus-like particles (VLPs) driven by ectopic expression of the Z protein and live-attenuated JUNV Candid-1 strain in cell culture. Since inhibition of the PTAP-Tsg101 interaction inhibits JUNV egress, compound 0013 serves as a prototype therapeutic that could reduce virus dissemination and disease progression in infected individuals. Moreover, since PTAP L-domain-mediated Tsg101 recruitment is utilized by other RNA virus pathogens (e.g., Ebola virus and HIV-1), PTAP inhibitors such as compound 0013 have the potential to function as potent broad-spectrum, host-oriented antiviral drugs.IMPORTANCE: There are currently no FDA-approved vaccines or therapeutics to prevent or treat Argentine hemorrhagic fever (AHF). The causative agent of AHF is Junin virus (JUNV); a New World arenavirus classified as an NIAID/CDC category A priority pathogen. Here, we describe a prototype therapeutic that blocks budding of JUNV and has the potential to function as a broad-spectrum antiviral drug.
PMCID: PMC3993831 PMID: 24522922 [PubMed - indexed for MEDLINE]
774. J Virol. 2014 May;88(9):4866-76. doi: 10.1128/JVI.03649-13. Epub 2014 Feb 12.

Middle east respiratory syndrome coronavirus 4a protein is a double-stranded RNA-binding protein that suppresses PACT-induced activation of RIG-I and MDA5 in the innate antiviral response.

Siu KL(1), Yeung ML, Kok KH, Yuen KS, Kew C, Lui PY, Chan CP, Tse H, Woo PC, Yuen KY, Jin DY.
Author information: (1)Department of Biochemistry, University of Hong Kong, Pokfulam, Hong Kong.

Middle East respiratory syndrome coronavirus (MERS-CoV) is an emerging pathogen that causes severe disease in human. MERS-CoV is closely related to bat coronaviruses HKU4 and HKU5. Evasion of the innate antiviral response might contribute significantly to MERS-CoV pathogenesis, but the mechanism is poorly understood. In this study, we characterized MERS-CoV 4a protein as a novel immunosuppressive factor that antagonizes type I interferon production. MERS-CoV 4a protein contains a double-stranded RNA-binding domain capable of interacting with poly(I · C). Expression of MERS-CoV 4a protein suppressed the interferon production induced by poly(I · C) or Sendai virus. RNA binding of MERS-CoV 4a protein was required for IFN antagonism, a property shared by 4a protein of bat coronavirus HKU5 but not by the counterpart in bat coronavirus HKU4. MERS-CoV 4a protein interacted with PACT in an RNA-dependent manner but not with RIG-I or MDA5. It inhibited PACT-induced activation of RIG-I and MDA5 but did not affect the activity of downstream effectors such as RIG-I, MDA5, MAVS, TBK1, and IRF3. Taken together, our findings suggest a new mechanism through which MERS-CoV employs a viral double-stranded RNA-binding protein to circumvent the innate antiviral response by perturbing the function of cellular double-stranded RNA-binding protein PACT. PACT targeting might be a common strategy used by different viruses, including Ebola virus and herpes simplex virus 1, to counteract innate immunity.IMPORTANCE: Middle East respiratory syndrome coronavirus (MERS-CoV) is an emerging and highly lethal human pathogen. Why MERS-CoV causes severe disease in human is unclear, and one possibility is that MERS-CoV is particularly efficient in counteracting host immunity, including the sensing of virus invasion. It will therefore be critical to clarify how MERS-CoV cripples the host proteins that sense viruses and to compare MERS-CoV with its ancestral viruses in bats in the counteraction of virus sensing. This work not only provides a new understanding of the abilities of MERS-CoV and closely related bat viruses to subvert virus sensing but also might prove useful in revealing new strategies for the development of vaccines and antivirals.
PMCID: PMC3993821 PMID: 24522921 [PubMed - indexed for MEDLINE]

775. Lancet Infect Dis. 2014 May;14(5):375.

Ebola haemorrhagic fever in west Africa.

Bagcchi S.

PMID: 24877203 [PubMed - indexed for MEDLINE]

776. Rev Infirm. 2014 May;201:10.

[Ebola vigilance].

[Article in French]

Warnet S.

PMID: 25055582 [PubMed - indexed for MEDLINE]

777. Zh Mikrobiol Epidemiol Immunobiol. 2014 May-Jun;(3):114-24.

[Promising approaches of antiviral therapy of hemorrhagic fevers].

[Article in Russian]

Markin VA.

Acceptable means of therapy and prophylaxis for most of the especially dangerous viral hemorrhagic fevers to present date are lacking. Analysis of the state of this problem shows that creation of a new generation of etiotropic preparations requires selection of additional targets for their effect that may be based on the use of molecular-biological features of pathogenesis of these infections. Literature data analysis has shown that during filovirus infection non-structural and structural proteins of the causative agents serve as pathogens during direct damaging effect of the virus and secondary immune reactions that in general pervert cell and humoral components of immunity converting its destructive effect on cells and tissues of the macro organism. Selection of promising approaches of antiviral therapy is possible based on molecular-biological analysis of interaction of micro- and macro organism with isolation of the most vulnerable for the effect of causative agent aggression factors.
PMID: 25286519 [PubMed - indexed for MEDLINE]

778. Blood. 2014 Apr 24;123(17):2605-13. doi: 10.1182/blood-2013-09-526277. Epub 2014 Mar 14.

Multiple roles of the coagulation protease cascade during virus infection.

Antoniak S(1), Mackman N.

Author information: (1)Thrombosis and Hemostasis Program, Division of Hematology and Oncology, Department of Medicine, University of North Carolina McAllister Heart Institute, University of North Carolina at Chapel Hill, Chapel Hill, NC.

The coagulation cascade is activated during viral infections. This response may be part of the host defense system to limit spread of the pathogen. However, excessive activation of the coagulation cascade can be deleterious. In fact, inhibition of the tissue factor/factor VIIa complex reduced mortality in a monkey model of Ebola hemorrhagic fever. Other studies showed that incorporation of tissue factor into the envelope of herpes simplex virus increases infection of endothelial cells and mice. Furthermore, binding of factor X to adenovirus serotype 5 enhances infection of hepatocytes but also increases the activation of the innate immune response to the virus. Coagulation proteases activate protease-activated receptors (PARs). Interestingly, we and others found that PAR1 and PAR2 modulate the immune response to viral infection. For instance, PAR1 positively regulates TLR3-dependent expression of the antiviral protein interferon β, whereas PAR2 negatively regulates expression during coxsackievirus group B infection. These studies indicate that the coagulation cascade plays multiple roles during viral infections.
PMCID: PMC3999750 [Available on 2015/4/24] PMID: 24632711 [PubMed - indexed for MEDLINE]

779. Nature. 2014 Apr 17;508(7496):402-5. doi: 10.1038/nature13027. Epub 2014 Mar 2.

Protection against filovirus diseases by a novel broad-spectrum nucleoside analogue BCX4430.

Warren TK(1), Wells J(1), Panchal RG(1), Stuthman KS(1), Garza NL(1), Van Tongeren SA(1), Dong L(1), Retterer CJ(1), Eaton BP(1), Pegoraro G(1), Honnold S(1), Bantia S(2), Kotian P(2), Chen X(2), Taubenheim BR(3), Welch LS(1), Minning DM(4), Babu YS(2), Sheridan WP(2), Bavari S(1).

Author information: (1)Division of Molecular and Translational Sciences, Therapeutic Discovery Center, United States Army Medical Research Institute of Infectious Diseases (USAMRIID), Fort Detrick, Maryland 21702, USA. (2)BioCryst Pharmaceuticals Inc., Durham, North Carolina 27703, USA. (3)1] BioCryst Pharmaceuticals Inc., Durham, North Carolina 27703, USA [2] Wilco Consulting, LLC, Durham, North Carolina 27712, USA. (4)MedExpert Consulting, Inc., Indialantic, Florida 32903, USA.

Comment in Cell Res. 2014 Jun;24(6):647-8. Nat Rev Drug Discov. 2014 May;13(5):334.

Filoviruses are emerging pathogens and causative agents of viral haemorrhagic fever. Case fatality rates of filovirus disease outbreaks are among the highest reported for any human pathogen, exceeding 90% (ref. 1). Licensed therapeutic or vaccine products are not available to treat filovirus diseases. Candidate therapeutics previously shown to be efficacious in non-human primate disease models are based on virus-specific designs and have limited broad-spectrum antiviral potential. Here we show that BCX4430, a novel synthetic adenosine analogue, inhibits infection of distinct filoviruses in human cells. Biochemical, reporter-based and primer-extension assays indicate that BCX4430 inhibits viral RNA polymerase function, acting as a non-obligate RNA chain terminator. Post-exposure intramuscular administration of BCX4430 protects against Ebola virus and Marburg virus disease in rodent models. Most importantly, BCX4430 completely protects cynomolgus macaques from Marburg virus infection when administered as late as 48 hours after infection. In addition, BCX4430 exhibits broad-spectrum antiviral activity against numerous viruses, including bunyaviruses, arenaviruses, paramyxoviruses, coronaviruses and flaviviruses. This is the first report, to our knowledge, of non-human primate protection from filovirus disease by a synthetic drug-like small molecule. We provide additional pharmacological characterizations supporting the potential development of BCX4430 as a countermeasure against human filovirus diseases and other viral diseases representing major public health threats.

PMID: 24590073 [PubMed - indexed for MEDLINE]

780. Viruses. 2014 Apr 17;6(4):1759-88. doi: 10.3390/v6041759.

Filoviruses in bats: current knowledge and future directions.

Olival KJ(1), Hayman DT(2).

Author information: (1)EcoHealth Alliance, 460 W. 34th Street, New York, NY 10001, USA. olival@ecohealthalliance.org. (2)Department of Biology, Colorado State University, Fort Collins, CO 80523, USA. davidtshayman@gmail.com.

Filoviruses, including Ebolavirus and Marburgvirus, pose significant threats to public health and species conservation by causing hemorrhagic fever outbreaks with high mortality rates. Since the first outbreak in 1967, their origins, natural history, and ecology remained elusive until recent studies linked them through molecular, serological, and virological studies to bats. We review the ecology, epidemiology, and natural history of these systems, drawing on examples from other bat-borne zoonoses, and highlight key areas for future research. We compare and contrast results from ecological and virological studies of bats and filoviruses with those of other systems. We also highlight how advanced methods, such as more recent serological assays, can be interlinked with flexible statistical methods and experimental studies to inform the field studies necessary to understand filovirus persistence in wildlife populations and cross-species transmission leading to outbreaks. We highlight the need for a more unified, global surveillance strategy for filoviruses in wildlife, and advocate for more integrated, multi-disciplinary approaches to understand dynamics in bat populations to ultimately mitigate or prevent potentially devastating disease outbreaks.

PMCID: PMC4014719 PMID: 24747773 [PubMed - indexed for MEDLINE]

781. Antivir Chem Chemother. 2014 Apr 11;23(5):197-215. doi: 10.3851/IMP2568.

Retinazone inhibits certain blood-borne human viruses including Ebola virus Zaire.

Kesel AJ(1), Huang Z, Murray MG, Prichard MN, Caboni L, Nevin DK, Fayne D, Lloyd DG, Detorio MA, Schinazi RF.

Author information: (1)Chammünsterstr. 47, Munich, Germany. andreas.kesel@gmx.de.

BACKGROUND: Human HBV and HIV integrate their retro-transcribed DNA proviruses into the human host genome. Existing antiretroviral drug regimens fail to directly target these intrachromosomal xenogenomes, leading to persistence of viral genetic information. Retinazone (RTZ) constitutes a novel vitamin A-derived (retinoid) thiosemicarbazone derivative with broad-spectrum antiviral activity versus HIV, HCV, varicella-zoster virus and cytomegalovirus. METHODS: The in vitro inhibitory action of RTZ on HIV-1 strain LAI, human HBV strain ayw, HCV-1b strain ConI, enhanced green fluorescent protein-expressing Ebola virus Zaire 1976 strain Mayinga, wild-type Ebola virus Zaire 1976 strain Mayinga, human herpesvirus 6B and Kaposi's sarcoma-associated herpesvirus replication was investigated. The binding of RTZ to human glucocorticoid receptor was determined. RESULTS: RTZ inhibits blood-borne human HBV multiplication in vitro by covalent inactivation of intragenic and intraexonic viral glucocorticoid response elements, and, in close analogy, RTZ suppresses HIV-1 multiplication in vitro. RTZ disrupts the multiplication of blood-borne human HCV and Ebola Zaire virus at nanomolar concentrations in vitro. RTZ has the capacity to bind to human glucocorticoid receptor, to selectively and covalently bind to intraexonic viral glucocorticoid response elements, and thereby to inactivate human genome-integrated proviral DNA of human HBV and HIV. CONCLUSIONS: RTZ represents the first reported antiviral agent capable of eradicating HIV and HBV proviruses from their human host. Furthermore, RTZ represents a potent and efficacious small-molecule in vitro inhibitor of Ebola virus Zaire 1976 strain Mayinga replication.

PMID: 23636868 [PubMed - in process]

782. Science. 2014 Apr 11;344(6180):140. doi: 10.1126/science.344.6180.140.

Infectious disease. Are bats spreading Ebola across sub-Saharan Africa?

Vogel G.

PMID: 24723589 [PubMed - indexed for MEDLINE]

783. Rev Med Suisse. 2014 Apr 9;10(425):834-5.

[Why does the Ebola virus (which is prevalent in Guinea today) not scare us?].

[Article in French]

Nau JY.

PMID: 24791431 [PubMed - indexed for MEDLINE]

784. Viruses. 2014 Apr 9;6(4):1654-71. doi: 10.3390/v6041654.

Analysis of determinants in filovirus glycoproteins required for tetherin antagonism.

Gnirß K(1), Fiedler M(2), Krämer-Kühl A(3), Bolduan S(4), Mittler E(5), Becker S(6), Schindler M(7), Pöhlmann S(8).

Author information: (1)Infection Biology Unit, German Primate Center, 37077 Göttingen, Germany. KGnirss@dpz.eu. (2)Infection Biology Unit, German Primate Center, 37077 Göttingen, Germany. MFiedler@dpz.eu. (3)Infection Biology Unit, German Primate Center, 37077 Göttingen, Germany. annika.kraemer-kuehl@boehringer-ingelheim.com. (4)Institute of Virology, Helmholtz Center Munich, 85764 Neuherberg, Germany. sebastian.bolduan@helmholtz-muenchen.de. (5)Institute of Virology, Philipps-University-Marburg, 35043 Marburg, Germany. mittlere@staff.uni-marburg.de. (6)Institute of Virology, Philipps-University-Marburg, 35043 Marburg, Germany. becker@staff.uni-marburg.de. (7)Institute of Virology, Helmholtz Center Munich, 85764 Neuherberg, Germany. michael.schindler@helmholtz-muenchen.de. (8)Infection Biology Unit, German Primate Center, 37077 Göttingen, Germany. spoehlmann@dpz.eu.

The host cell protein tetherin can restrict the release of enveloped viruses from infected cells. The HIV-1 protein Vpu counteracts tetherin by removing it from the site of viral budding, the plasma membrane, and this process depends on specific interactions between the transmembrane domains of Vpu and tetherin. In contrast, the glycoproteins (GPs) of two filoviruses, Ebola and Marburg virus, antagonize tetherin without reducing surface expression, and the domains in GP required for tetherin counteraction are unknown. Here, we show that filovirus GPs depend on the presence of their authentic transmembrane domains for virus-cell fusion and tetherin antagonism. However, conserved residues within the transmembrane domain were dispensable for membrane fusion and tetherin counteraction. Moreover, the insertion of the transmembrane domain into a heterologous viral GP, Lassa virus GPC, was not sufficient to confer tetherin antagonism to the recipient. Finally, mutation of conserved residues within the fusion peptide of Ebola virus GP inhibited virus-cell fusion but did not ablate tetherin counteraction, indicating that the fusion peptide and the ability of GP to drive host cell entry are not required for tetherin counteraction. These results suggest that the transmembrane domains of filoviral GPs contribute to tetherin antagonism but are not the sole determinants.

PMCID: PMC4014715 PMID: 24721789 [PubMed - indexed for MEDLINE]

785. BMJ. 2014 Apr 8;348:g2644. doi: 10.1136/bmj.g2644.

Fear spreads as number of Ebola cases in Guinea rises.

Gulland A(1).

Author information: (1)London.

PMID: 24714448 [PubMed - indexed for MEDLINE]

786. Lancet. 2014 Apr 5;383(9924):1196.

West Africa struggles to contain Ebola outbreak.

Green A.

PMID: 24712029 [PubMed - indexed for MEDLINE]

787. J Mol Biol. 2014 Apr 3;426(7):1452-68. doi: 10.1016/j.jmb.2013.12.009. Epub 2013 Dec 12.

Structural characterization of the glycoprotein GP2 core domain from the CAS virus, a novel arenavirus-like species.

Koellhoffer JF(1), Dai Z(1), Malashkevich VN(1), Stenglein MD(2), Liu Y(1), Toro R(1), S Harrison J(3), Chandran K(4), DeRisi JL(5), Almo SC(1), Lai JR(6).

Author information: (1)Department of Biochemistry, Albert Einstein College of Medicine, 1300 Morris Park Avenue, Bronx, NY 10461, USA. (2)Department of Biochemistry and Biophysics, University of California San Francisco, San Francisco, CA 94158-2517, USA. (3)Department of Biochemistry, Albert Einstein College of Medicine, 1300 Morris Park Avenue, Bronx, NY 10461, USA; Department of Biochemistry and Biophysics, University of North Carolina, Chapel Hill, Chapel Hill, NC 27599, USA; Lineberger Comprehensive Cancer Center, University of North Carolina, Chapel Hill, Chapel Hill, NC 27599, USA. (4)Department of Microbiology and Immunology, Albert Einstein College of Medicine, 1300 Morris Park Avenue, Bronx, NY 10461, USA. (5)Department of Biochemistry and Biophysics, University of California San Francisco, San Francisco, CA 94158-2517, USA; Howard Hughes Medical Institute, Chevy Chase, MD 20815-6789, USA. (6)Department of Biochemistry, Albert Einstein College of Medicine, 1300 Morris Park Avenue, Bronx, NY 10461, USA. Electronic address: jon.lai@einstein.yu.edu.

Fusion of the viral and host cell membranes is a necessary first step for infection by enveloped viruses and is mediated by the envelope glycoprotein. The transmembrane subunits from the structurally defined "class I" glycoproteins adopt an α-helical "trimer-of-hairpins" conformation during the fusion pathway. Here, we present our studies on the envelope glycoprotein transmembrane subunit, GP2, of the CAS virus (CASV). CASV was recently identified from annulated tree boas (Corallus annulatus) with inclusion body disease and is implicated in the disease etiology. We have generated and characterized two protein constructs consisting of the predicted CASV GP2 core domain. The crystal structure of the CASV GP2 post-fusion conformation indicates a trimeric α-helical bundle that is highly similar to those of Ebola virus and Marburg virus GP2 despite CASV genome homology to arenaviruses. Denaturation studies demonstrate that the stability of CASV GP2 is pH dependent with higher stability at lower pH; we propose that this behavior is due to a network of interactions among acidic residues that would destabilize the α-helical bundle under conditions where the side chains are deprotonated. The pH-dependent stability of the post-fusion structure has been observed in Ebola virus and Marburg virus GP2, as well as other viruses that enter via the endosome. Infection experiments with CASV and the related Golden Gate virus support a mechanism of entry that requires endosomal acidification. Our results suggest that, despite being primarily arenavirus like, the transmembrane subunit of CASV is extremely similar to the filoviruses.

PMCID: PMC3951589 [Available on 2015/4/3] PMID: 24333483 [PubMed - indexed for MEDLINE]
788. Retrovirology. 2014 Apr 3;11:28. doi: 10.1186/1742-4690-11-28.

Diverse viral glycoproteins as well as CD4 co-package into the same human immunodeficiency virus (HIV-1) particles.

Gregory DA, Olinger GY, Lucas TM, Johnson MC(1).

Author information: (1)Department of Molecular Microbiology and Immunology, University of Missouri, Columbia, MO, USA. marcjohnson@missouri.edu.

BACKGROUND: Retroviruses can acquire not only their own glycoproteins as they bud from the cellular membrane, but also some cellular and foreign viral glycoproteins. Many of these non-native glycoproteins are actively recruited to budding virions, particularly other viral glycoproteins. This observation suggests that there may be a conserved mechanism underlying the recruitment of glycoproteins into viruses. If a conserved mechanism is used, diverse glycoproteins should localize to a single budding retroviral particle. On the other hand, if viral glycoproteins have divergent mechanisms for recruitment, the different glycoproteins could segregate into different particles. RESULTS: To determine if co-packaging occurs among different glycoproteins, we designed an assay that combines virion antibody capture and a determination of infectivity based on a luciferase reporter. Virions were bound to a plate with an antibody against one glycoprotein, and then the infectivity was measured with cells that allow entry only with a second glycoprotein. We tested pairings of glycoproteins from HIV, murine leukemia virus (MLV), Rous sarcoma virus (RSV), vesicular stomatitis virus (VSV), and Ebola virus. The results showed that glycoproteins that were actively recruited into virions were co-packaged efficiently with each other. We also tested cellular proteins and found CD4 also had a similar correlation between active recruitment and efficient co-packaging, but other cellular proteins did not. CONCLUSION: Glycoproteins that are actively incorporated into HIV-1 virions are efficiently co-packaged into the same virus particles, suggesting that the same general mechanism for recruitment may act in many viruses.

PMCID: PMC3985584 PMID: 24708808 [PubMed - indexed for MEDLINE]
789. Acta Crystallogr F Struct Biol Commun. 2014 Apr;70(Pt 4):457-60. doi: 10.1107/S2053230X14003811. Epub 2014 Mar 25.

Structure of the Reston ebolavirus VP30 C-terminal domain.

Clifton MC(1), Kirchdoerfer RN(2), Atkins K(1), Abendroth J(1), Raymond A(1), Grice R(1), Barnes S(1), Moen S(1), Lorimer D(1), Edwards TE(1), Myler PJ(1), Saphire EO(2).

Author information: (1)Seattle Structural Genomics Center for Infectious Disease (SSGCID), 307 Westlake Avenue North, Suite 500, Seattle, WA 98109, USA. (2)Department of Immunology and Microbial Science, The Scripps Research Institute, 10550 North Torrey Pines Road, IMM-21, La Jolla, CA 92037, USA.

The ebolaviruses can cause severe hemorrhagic fever. Essential to the ebolavirus life cycle is the protein VP30, which serves as a transcriptional cofactor. Here, the crystal structure of the C-terminal, NP-binding domain of VP30 from Reston ebolavirus is presented. Reston VP30 and Ebola VP30 both form homodimers, but the dimeric interfaces are rotated relative to each other, suggesting subtle inherent differences or flexibility in the dimeric interface.

PMCID: PMC3976061 PMID: 24699737 [PubMed - indexed for MEDLINE]
790. Antiviral Res. 2014 Apr;104:153-5. doi: 10.1016/j.antiviral.2014.01.012. Epub 2014 Jan 24.

Post-exposure efficacy of oral T-705 (Favipiravir) against inhalational Ebola virus infection in a mouse model.

Smither SJ(1), Eastaugh LS(2), Steward JA(2), Nelson M(2), Lenk RP(3), Lever MS(2).

Author information: (1)Biomedical Sciences Department, Defence Science and Technology Laboratory (Dstl), Porton Down, Salisbury, Wiltshire SP4 0JQ, UK. Electronic address: sjsmither@dstl.gov.uk. (2)Biomedical Sciences Department, Defence Science and Technology Laboratory (Dstl), Porton Down, Salisbury, Wiltshire SP4 0JQ, UK. (3)MediVector, Inc., Two International Place, 22nd Floor, Boston, MA 02110, United States.

Filoviruses cause disease with high case fatality rates and are considered biological threat agents. Licensed post-exposure therapies that can be administered by the oral route are desired for safe and rapid distribution and uptake in the event of exposure or outbreaks. Favipiravir or T-705 has broad antiviral activity and has already undergone phase II and is undergoing phase III clinical trials for influenza. Here we report the first use of T-705 against Ebola virus. T-705 gave 100% protection against aerosol Ebola virus E718 infection; protection was shown in immune-deficient mice after 14 days of twice-daily dosing. T-705 was also shown to inhibit Ebola virus infection in cell culture. T-705 is likely to be licensed for use against influenza in the near future and could also be used with a new indication for filovirus infection.

PMID: 24462697 [PubMed - indexed for MEDLINE]
791. Assay Drug Dev Technol. 2014 Apr;12(3):155-61. doi: 10.1089/adt.2013.567.

A BSL-4 high-throughput screen identifies sulfonamide inhibitors of Nipah virus.

Tigabu B(1), Rasmussen L, White EL, Tower N, Saeed M, Bukreyev A, Rockx B, LeDuc JW, Noah JW.

Author information: (1)I Department of Microbiology & Immunology, Galveston National Laboratory, The University of Texas Medical Branch , Galveston, Texas.

Nipah virus is a biosafety level 4 (BSL-4) pathogen that causes severe respiratory illness and encephalitis in humans. To identify novel small molecules that target Nipah virus replication as potential therapeutics, Southern Research Institute and Galveston National Laboratory jointly developed an automated high-throughput screening platform that is capable of testing 10,000 compounds per day within BSL-4 biocontainment. Using this platform, we screened a 10,080-compound library using a cell-based, high-throughput screen for compounds that inhibited the virus-induced cytopathic effect. From this pilot effort, 23 compounds were identified with EC50 values ranging from 3.9 to 20.0 μM and selectivities >10. Three sulfonamide compounds with EC50 values

PMCID: PMC3994909 [Available on 2015/4/1] PMID: 24735442 [PubMed - indexed for MEDLINE]

792. Expert Rev Vaccines. 2014 Apr;13(4):521-31. doi: 10.1586/14760584.2014.885841. Epub 2014 Feb 27.

Ebola virus vaccines: an overview of current approaches.

Marzi A(1), Feldmann H.

Author information: (1)Laboratory of Virology, Division of Intramural Research, National Institute of Allergy and Infectious Diseases, National Institutes of Health, Rocky Mountain Laboratories, Hamilton, Montana 59840, MT, USA.

Ebola hemorrhagic fever is one of the most fatal viral diseases worldwide affecting humans and nonhuman primates. Although infections only occur frequently in Central Africa, the virus has the potential to spread globally and is classified as a category A pathogen that could be misused as a bioterrorism agent. As of today there is no vaccine or treatment licensed to counteract Ebola virus infections. DNA, subunit and several viral vector approaches, replicating and non-replicating, have been tested as potential vaccine platforms and their protective efficacy has been evaluated in nonhuman primate models for Ebola virus infections, which closely resemble disease progression in humans. Though these vaccine platforms seem to confer protection through different mechanisms, several of them are efficacious against lethal disease in nonhuman primates attesting that vaccination against Ebola virus infections is feasible.

PMID: 24575870 [PubMed - indexed for MEDLINE]

793. Hum Vaccin Immunother. 2014 Apr;10(4):964-7. Epub 2014 Feb 6.

Antibody therapy for Ebola: is the tide turning around?

Qiu X(1), Kobinger GP(2).

Author information: (1)National Microbiology Laboratory; Public Health Agency of Canada; Winnipeg, MB Canada. (2)National Microbiology Laboratory; Public Health Agency of Canada; Winnipeg, MB Canada; Department of Medical Microbiology; University of Manitoba; Winnipeg, MB Canada; Department of Immunology; University of Manitoba; Winnipeg, MB Canada; Department of Pathology and Laboratory Medicine; University of Pennsylvania School of Medicine; Philadelphia, PA USA.

Ebola viruses can cause severe hemorrhagic fever in humans and nonhuman primates with fatality rates up to 90%, and are identified as biosafety level 4 pathogens and CDC Category A Agents of Bioterrorism. To date, there are no approved therapies and vaccines available to treat these infections. Antibody therapy was estimated to be an effective and powerful treatment strategy against infectious pathogens in the late 19th, early 20th centuries but has fallen short to meet expectations to widely combat infectious diseases. Passive immunization for Ebola virus was successful in 2012, after over 15 years of failed attempts leading to skepticism that the approach would ever be of potential benefit. Currently, monoclonal antibody (mAbs)-based therapies are the most efficient at reversing the progression of a lethal Ebola virus infection in nonhuman primates, which recapitulate the human disease with the highest similarity. Novel combinations of mAbs can even fully cure lethally infected animals after clinical symptoms and circulating virus have been detected, days into the infection. These new developments have reopened the door for using antibody-based therapies for filovirus infections. Furthermore, they are reigniting hope that these strategies will contribute to better control the spread of other infectious agents and provide new tools against infectious diseases.

PMID: 24503566 [PubMed - in process]

794. J Virol. 2014 Apr;88(8):4353-65. doi: 10.1128/JVI.03050-13. Epub 2014 Feb 5.

Identification of a broad-spectrum antiviral small molecule against severe acute respiratory syndrome coronavirus and Ebola, Hendra, and Nipah viruses by using a novel high-throughput screening assay.

Elshabrawy HA(1), Fan J, Haddad CS, Ratia K, Broder CC, Caffrey M, Prabhakar BS.

Author information: (1)Department of Microbiology and Immunology, College of Medicine, University of Illinois at Chicago, Chicago, Illinois, USA.

Severe acute respiratory syndrome coronavirus (SARS-CoV) and Ebola, Hendra, and Nipah viruses are members of different viral families and are known causative agents of fatal viral diseases. These viruses depend on cathepsin L for entry into their target cells. The viral glycoproteins need to be primed by protease cleavage, rendering them active for fusion with the host cell membrane. In this study, we developed a novel high-throughput screening assay based on peptides, derived from the glycoproteins of the aforementioned viruses, which contain the cathepsin L cleavage site. We screened a library of 5,000 small molecules and discovered a small molecule that can inhibit the cathepsin L cleavage of all viral peptides with minimal inhibition of cleavage of a host protein-derived peptide (pro-neuropeptide Y). The small molecule inhibited the entry of all pseudotyped viruses in vitro and the cleavage of SARS-CoV spike glycoprotein in an in vitro cleavage assay. In addition, the Hendra and Nipah virus fusion glycoproteins were not cleaved in the presence of the small molecule in a cell-based cleavage assay. Furthermore, we demonstrate that the small molecule is a mixed inhibitor of cathepsin L. Our broad-spectrum antiviral small molecule appears to be an ideal candidate for future optimization and development into a potent antiviral against SARS-CoV and Ebola, Hendra, and Nipah viruses.IMPORTANCE: We developed a novel high-throughput screening assay to identify small molecules that can prevent cathepsin L cleavage of viral glycoproteins derived from SARS-CoV and Ebola, Hendra, and Nipah viruses that are required for their entry into the host cell. We identified a novel broad-spectrum small molecule that could block cathepsin L-mediated cleavage and thus inhibit the entry of pseudotypes bearing the glycoprotein derived from SARS-CoV or Ebola, Hendra, or Nipah virus. The small molecule can be further optimized and developed into a potent broad-spectrum antiviral drug.

PMCID: PMC3993759 PMID: 24501399 [PubMed - indexed for MEDLINE]

795. J Virol. 2014 Apr;88(8):4275-90. doi: 10.1128/JVI.03287-13. Epub 2014 Jan 29.

Role of phosphatidylserine receptors in enveloped virus infection.

Morizono K(1), Chen IS.

Author information: (1)Division of Hematology and Oncology, Department of Medicine, David Geffen School of Medicine, University of California, Los Angeles, California, USA.

We recently demonstrated that a soluble protein, Gas6, can facilitate viral entry by bridging viral envelope phosphatidylserine to Axl, a receptor tyrosine kinase expressed on target cells. The interaction between phosphatidylserine, Gas6, and Axl was originally shown to be a molecular mechanism through which phagocytes recognize phosphatidylserine exposed on dead cells. Since our initial report, several groups have confirmed that Axl/Gas6, as well as other phosphatidylserine receptors, facilitate entry of dengue, West Nile, and Ebola viruses. Virus binding by viral envelope phosphatidylserine is now a viral entry mechanism generalized to many families of viruses. In addition to Axl/Gas6, various molecules are known to recognize phosphatidylserine; however, the effects of these molecules on virus binding and entry have not been comprehensively evaluated and compared. In this study, we examined most of the known human phosphatidylserine-recognizing molecules, including MFG-E8, TIM-1, -3, and -4, CD300a, BAI1, and stabilin-1 and -2, for their abilities to facilitate virus binding and infection. Using pseudotyped lentiviral vectors, we found that a soluble phosphatidylserine-binding protein, MFG-E8, enhances transduction. Cell surface receptors TIM-1 and -4 also enhance virus binding/transduction. The extent of enhancement by these molecules varies, depending on the type of pseudotyping envelope proteins. Mutated MFG-E8, which binds viral envelope phosphatidylserine without bridging virus to cells, but, surprisingly, not annexin V, which has been used to block phagocytosis of dead cells by concealing phosphatidylserine, efficiently blocks these phosphatidylserine-dependent viral entry mechanisms. These results provide insight into understanding the role of viral envelope phosphatidylserine in viral infection.IMPORTANCE: Envelope phosphatidylserine has previously been shown to be important for replication of various envelope viruses, but details of this mechanism(s) were unclear. We were the first to report that a bifunctional serum protein, Gas6, bridges envelope phosphatidylserine to a cell surface receptor, Axl. Recent studies demonstrated that many envelope viruses, including vaccinia, dengue, West Nile, and Ebola viruses, utilize Axl/Gas6 to facilitate their entry, suggesting that the phosphatidylserine-mediated viral entry mechanism can be shared by various enveloped viruses. In addition to Axl/Gas6, various molecules are known to recognize phosphatidylserine; however, the effects of these molecules on virus binding and entry have not been comprehensively evaluated and compared. In this study, we examined most human phosphatidylserine-recognizing molecules for their abilities to facilitate viral infection. The results provide insights into the role(s) of envelope phosphatidylserine in viral infection, which can be applicable to the development of novel antiviral reagents that block phosphatidylserine-mediated viral entry.

PMCID: PMC3993771 PMID: 24478428 [PubMed - indexed for MEDLINE]

796. Sci Am. 2014 Apr;310(4):52-9.

The RNA revolution.

Gorman C, Maron DF.

PMID: 24712124 [PubMed - indexed for MEDLINE]

797. BMJ. 2014 Mar 31;348:g2473. doi: 10.1136/bmj.g2473.

Ebola outbreak claims more than 60 lives.

Gulland A(1).

Author information: (1)London.

PMID: 24687456 [PubMed - indexed for MEDLINE]

798. Cell Rep. 2014 Mar 27;6(6):1017-25. doi: 10.1016/j.celrep.2014.01.043. Epub 2014 Mar 13.

The Marburg virus VP24 protein interacts with Keap1 to activate the cytoprotective antioxidant response pathway.

Edwards MR(1), Johnson B(2), Mire CE(3), Xu W(2), Shabman RS(1), Speller LN(2), Leung DW(2), Geisbert TW(3), Amarasinghe GK(2), Basler CF(4).

Author information: (1)Department Microbiology, Icahn School of Medicine, Mount Sinai, New York, NY 10029, USA. (2)Department of Pathology and Immunology, Washington University School of Medicine, St. Louis, MO 63110, USA. (3)Galveston National Laboratory, Department of Microbiology and Immunology, University of Texas Medical Branch, Galveston, TX 77555, USA. (4)Department Microbiology, Icahn School of Medicine, Mount Sinai, New York, NY 10029, USA. Electronic address: chris.basler@mssm.edu.

Comment in Nat Rev Microbiol. 2014 May;12(5):311.

Kelch-like ECH-associated protein 1 (Keap1) is a ubiquitin E3 ligase specificity factor that targets transcription factor nuclear factor (erythroid-derived 2)-like 2 (Nrf2) for ubiquitination and degradation. Disrupting Keap1-Nrf2 interaction stabilizes Nrf2, resulting in Nrf2 nuclear accumulation, binding to antioxidant response elements (AREs), and transcription of cytoprotective genes. Marburg virus (MARV) is a zoonotic pathogen that likely uses bats as reservoir hosts. We demonstrate that MARV protein VP24 (mVP24) binds the Kelch domain of either human or bat Keap1. This binding is of high affinity and 1:1 stoichiometry and activates Nrf2. Modeling based on the Zaire ebolavirus (EBOV) VP24 (eVP24) structure identified in mVP24 an acidic loop (K-loop) critical for Keap1 interaction. Transfer of the K-loop to eVP24, which otherwise does not bind Keap1, confers Keap1 binding and Nrf2 activation, and infection by MARV, but not EBOV, activates ARE gene expression. Therefore, MARV targets Keap1 to activate Nrf2-induced cytoprotective responses during infection.

PMCID: PMC3985291 [Available on 2015/3/27] PMID: 24630991 [PubMed - in process]

799. Lancet. 2014 Mar 22;383(9922):1098. doi: 10.1016/S0140-6736(14)60262-2.

Kikuchi-Fujimoto disease.

Dalton J(1), Shaw R(2), Democratis J(3).

Author information: (1)Royal Berkshire Hospital, Reading, UK. Electronic address: j.dalton@doctors.org.uk. (2)John Radcliffe Hospital, Oxford, UK. (3)Wexham Park Hospital, Slough, UK.

PMID: 24656202 [PubMed - indexed for MEDLINE]

800. Infect Genet Evol. 2014 Mar;22:250-6. doi: 10.1016/j.meegid.2013.06.022. Epub 2013 Jul 2.

Trypanosome species in neo-tropical bats: biological, evolutionary and epidemiological implications.

Ramírez JD(1), Tapia-Calle G(1), Muñoz-Cruz G(2), Poveda C(1), Rendón LM(1), Hincapié E(2), Guhl F(3).

Author information: (1)Centro de Investigaciones en Microbiología y Parasitología Tropical, CIMPAT, Universidad de los Andes, Bogotá, Colombia. (2)Grupo de Investigaciones entomológicas de la Orinoquía Colombiana, GIENOC, Unitropico, Yopal, Colombia. (3)Centro de Investigaciones en Microbiología y Parasitología Tropical, CIMPAT, Universidad de los Andes, Bogotá, Colombia. Electronic address: fguhl@uniandes.edu.co.

Bats (Chiroptera) are the only mammals naturally able to fly. Due to this characteristic they play a relevant ecological role in the niches they inhabit. These mammals spread infectious diseases from enzootic to domestic foci. Rabbies, SARS, fungi, ebola and trypanosomes are the most common pathogens these animals may host. We conducted intensive sampling of bats from the phyllostomidae, vespertilionidae and emballonuridae families in six localities from Casanare department in eastern Colombia. Blood-EDTA samples were obtained and subsequently submitted to analyses of mitochondrial and nuclear genetic markers in order to conduct barcoding analyses to discriminate trypanosome species. The findings according to the congruence of the three molecular markers suggest the occurrence of Trypanosoma cruzi cruzi (51%), T. c. marinkellei (9%), T. dionisii (13%), T. rangeli (21%), T. evansi (4%) and T. theileri (2%) among 107 positive bat specimens. Regarding the T. cruzi DTUs, we observed the presence of TcI (60%), TcII (15%), TcIII (7%), TcIV (7%) and TcBAT (11%) being the first evidence to our concern of the foreseen genotype TcBAT in Colombia. These results allowed us to propose reliable hypotheses regarding the ecology and biology of the bats circulating in the area including the enigmatic question whether TcBAT should be considered a novel DTU. The epidemiological and evolutionary implications of these findings are herein discussed.

PMID: 23831017 [PubMed - indexed for MEDLINE]

801. J Virol. 2014 Mar;88(6):3255-72. doi: 10.1128/JVI.03814-13. Epub 2014 Jan 3.

Feline immunodeficiency virus envelope glycoproteins antagonize tetherin through a distinctive mechanism that requires virion incorporation.

Morrison JH(1), Guevara RB, Marcano AC, Saenz DT, Fadel HJ, Rogstad DK, Poeschla EM.

Author information: (1)Department of Molecular Medicine, Mayo Clinic College of Medicine, Rochester, Minnesota, USA.

BST2/tetherin inhibits the release of enveloped viruses from cells. Primate lentiviruses have evolved specific antagonists (Vpu, Nef, and Env). Here we characterized tetherin proteins of species representing both branches of the order Carnivora. Comparison of tiger and cat (Feliformia) to dog and ferret (Caniformia) genes demonstrated that the tiger and cat share a start codon mutation that truncated most of the tetherin cytoplasmic tail early in the Feliformia lineage (19 of 27 amino acids, including the dual tyrosine motif). Alpha interferon (IFN-α) induced tetherin and blocked feline immunodeficiency virus (FIV) replication in lymphoid and nonlymphoid feline cells. Budding of bald FIV and HIV particles was blocked by carnivore tetherins. However, infectious FIV particles were resistant, and spreading FIV replication was uninhibited. Antagonism mapped to the envelope glycoprotein (Env), which rescued FIV from carnivore tetherin restriction when expressed in trans but, in contrast to known antagonists, did not rescue noncognate particles. Also unlike the primate lentiviral antagonists, but similar to the Ebola virus glycoprotein, FIV Env did not reduce intracellular or cell surface tetherin levels. Furthermore, FIV-enveloped FIV particles actually required tetherin for optimal release from cells. The results show that FIV Envs mediate a distinctive tetherin evasion. Well adapted to a phylogenetically ancient tetherin tail truncation in the Felidae, it requires functional virion incorporation of Env, and it shields the budding particle without downregulating plasma membrane tetherin. Moreover, FIV has evolved dependence on this protein: particles containing FIV Env need tetherin for optimal release from the cell, while Env(-) particles do not.IMPORTANCE: HIV-1 antagonizes the restriction factor tetherin with the accessory protein Vpu, while HIV-2 and the filovirus Ebola use their envelope (Env) glycoproteins for this purpose. It turns out that the FIV tetherin antagonist is also its Env protein, but the mechanism is distinctive. Unlike other tetherin antagonists, FIV Env cannot act in trans to rescue vpu-deficient HIV-1. It must be incorporated specifically into FIV virions to be active. Also unlike other retroviral antagonists, but similar to Ebola virus Env, it does not act by downregulating or degrading tetherin. FIV Env might exclude tetherin locally or direct assembly to tetherin-negative membrane domains. Other distinctive features are apparent, including evidence that this virus evolved an equilibrium in which tetherin is both restriction factor and cofactor, as FIV requires tetherin for optimal particle release.

PMCID: PMC3957917 PMID: 24390322 [PubMed - indexed for MEDLINE]

802. Virology. 2014 Mar;452-453:324-33. doi: 10.1016/j.virol.2013.03.028. Epub 2014 Jan 24.

Vaccination with recombinant adenoviruses expressing Ebola virus glycoprotein elicits protection in the interferon alpha/beta receptor knock-out mouse.

O'Brien LM(1), Stokes MG(2), Lonsdale SG(2), Maslowski DR(2), Smither SJ(2), Lever MS(2), Laws TR(2), Perkins SD(2).

Author information: (1)Biomedical Sciences Department, Defence Science and Technology Laboratory (Dstl), Porton Down, Salisbury, Wiltshire SP4 0JQ, United Kingdom. Electronic address: lmobrien@dstl.gov.uk. (2)Biomedical Sciences Department, Defence Science and Technology Laboratory (Dstl), Porton Down, Salisbury, Wiltshire SP4 0JQ, United Kingdom.

The resistance of adult immunocompetent mice to infection with ebolaviruses has led to the development of alternative small animal models that utilise immunodeficient mice, for example the interferon α/β receptor knock-out mouse (IFNR(-/-)). IFNR(-/-) mice have been shown to be susceptible to infection with ebolaviruses by multiple routes but it is not known if this murine model is suitable for testing therapeutics that rely on the generation of an immune response for efficacy. We have tested recombinant adenovirus vectors for their ability to protect IFNR(-/-) mice from challenge with Ebola virus and have analysed the humoral response generated after immunisation. The recombinant vaccines elicited good levels of protection in the knock-out mouse and the antibody response in IFNR(-/-) mice was similar to that observed in vaccinated wild-type mice. These results indicate that the IFNR(-/-) mouse is a relevant small animal model for studying ebolavirus-specific therapeutics.

PMID: 24461913 [PubMed - indexed for MEDLINE]
803. Viruses. 2014 Feb 19;6(2):927-37. doi: 10.3390/v6020927.

Clinical documentation and data transfer from Ebola and Marburg virus disease wards in outbreak settings: health care workers' experiences and preferences.

Bühler S(1), Roddy P(2), Nolte E(3), Borchert M(4).

Author information: (1)London School of Hygiene and Tropical Medicine, Keppel Street, London WC1E 7HT, UK. silja.buehler@ifspm.uzh.ch. (2)Médecins Sans Frontières - Spain, Nou de la Rambla, 26, Barcelona 08001, Spain. paul.roddy@barcelona.msf.org. (3)London School of Hygiene and Tropical Medicine, Keppel Street, London WC1E 7HT, UK. enolte@rand.org. (4)London School of Hygiene and Tropical Medicine, Keppel Street, London WC1E 7HT, UK. Matthias.Borchert@charite.de.

Understanding human filovirus hemorrhagic fever (FHF) clinical manifestations and evaluating treatment strategies require the collection of clinical data in outbreak settings, where clinical documentation has been limited. Currently, no consensus among filovirus outbreak-response organisations guides best practice for clinical documentation and data transfer. Semi-structured interviews were conducted with health care workers (HCWs) involved in FHF outbreaks in sub-Saharan Africa, and with HCWs experienced in documenting and transferring data from high-risk areas (isolation wards or biosafety level 4 laboratories). Methods for data documentation and transfer were identified, described in detail and categorised by requirement for electricity and ranked by interviewee preference. Some methods involve removing paperwork and other objects from the filovirus disease ward without disinfection. We believe that if done properly, these methods are reasonably safe for certain settings. However, alternative methods avoiding the removal of objects, or involving the removal of paperwork or objects after non-damaging disinfection, are available. These methods are not only safer, they are also perceived as safer and likely more acceptable to health workers and members of the community. The use of standardised clinical forms is overdue. Experiments with by sunlight disinfection should continue, and non-damaging disinfection of impregnated paper, suitable tablet computers and underwater cameras should be evaluated under field conditions.

PMCID: PMC3939489 PMID: 24556792 [PubMed - indexed for MEDLINE]
804. Acta Crystallogr F Struct Biol Commun. 2014 Feb;70(Pt 2):248-51. doi: 10.1107/S2053230X14000430. Epub 2014 Jan 22.

Expression, purification, crystallization and preliminary X-ray analysis of full-length human RIG-I.

Kwok J(1), Hui KP(2), Lescar J(3), Kotaka M(1).

Author information: (1)Department of Physiology, Li Ka Shing Faculty of Medicine, University of Hong Kong, Hong Kong. (2)Department of Microbiology, Li Ka Shing Faculty of Medicine, University of Hong Kong, Hong Kong. (3)Division of Structural Biology and Biochemistry, School of Biological Sciences, Nanyang Technological University, Singapore 138673, Singapore.

The human innate immune system can detect invasion by microbial pathogens through pattern-recognition receptors that recognize structurally conserved pathogen-associated molecular patterns. Retinoic acid-inducible gene I (RIG-I)-like helicases (RLHs) are one of the two major families of pattern-recognition receptors that can detect viral RNA. RIG-I, belonging to the RLH family, is capable of recognizing intracellular viral RNA from RNA viruses, including influenza virus and Ebola virus. Here, full-length human RIG-I (hRIG-I) was cloned in Escherichia coli and expressed in a recombinant form with a His-SUMO tag. The protein was purified and crystallized at 291 K using the hanging-drop vapour-diffusion method. X-ray diffraction data were collected to 2.85 Å resolution; the crystal belonged to space group F23, with unit-cell parameters a = b = c = 216.43 Å, $\alpha = \beta = \gamma = 90^\circ$.

PMID: 24637767 [PubMed - indexed for MEDLINE]
805. Expert Opin Ther Targets. 2014 Feb;18(2):115-20. doi: 10.1517/14728222.2014.863877. Epub 2013 Nov 28.

Could the Ebola virus matrix protein VP40 be a drug target?

Stahelin RV(1).

Author information: (1)Indiana University School of Medicine-South Bend, Department of Biochemistry and Molecular Biology , South Bend, IN 46617 , USA.

Filoviruses are filamentous lipid-enveloped viruses and include Ebola (EBOV) and Marburg, which are morphologically identical but antigenically distinct. These viruses can be very deadly with outbreaks of EBOV having clinical fatality as high as 90%. In 2012 there were two separate Ebola outbreaks in the Democratic Republic of Congo and Uganda that resulted in 25 and 4 fatalities, respectively. The lack of preventive vaccines and FDA-approved therapeutics has struck fear that the EBOV could become a pandemic threat. The Ebola genome encodes only seven genes, which mediate the entry, replication, and egress of the virus from the host cell. The EBOV matrix protein is VP40, which is found localized under the lipid envelope of the virus where it bridges the viral lipid envelope and nucleocapsid. VP40 is effectively a peripheral protein that mediates the plasma membrane binding and budding of the virus prior to egress. A number of studies have demonstrated specific deletions or mutations of VP40 to abrogate viral egress but to date pharmacological inhibition of VP40 has not been demonstrated. This editorial highlights VP40, which is the most abundantly expressed protein of the virus and discusses VP40 as a potential therapeutic target.

PMID: 24283270 [PubMed - indexed for MEDLINE]
806. J Interferon Cytokine Res. 2014 Feb;34(2):79-89. doi: 10.1089/jir.2013.0035. Epub 2013 Oct 8.

Ebola virus-like particles stimulate type I interferons and proinflammatory cytokine expression through the toll-like receptor and interferon signaling pathways.

Ayithan N(1), Bradfute SB, Anthony SM, Stuthman KS, Dye JM, Bavari S, Bray M, Ozato K.

Author information: (1)1 Program in Genomics of Differentiation, National Institute of Child Health and Human Development , National Institutes of Health, Bethesda, Maryland.

Ebola viruses (EBOV) can cause severe hemorrhagic disease with high case fatality rates. Currently, no vaccines or therapeutics are approved for use in humans. Ebola virus-like particles (eVLP) comprising of virus protein (VP40), glycoprotein, and nucleoprotein protect rodents and nonhuman primates from lethal EBOV infection, representing as a candidate vaccine for EBOV infection. Previous reports have shown that eVLP stimulate the expression of proinflammatory cytokines in dendritic cells (DCs) and macrophages (MΦs) in vitro. However, the molecular mechanisms and signaling pathways through which eVLP induce innate immune responses remain obscure. In this study, we show that eVLP stimulate not only the expression of proinflammatory cytokines but also the expression of type I interferons (IFNs) and IFN-stimulated genes (ISGs) in murine bone marrow-derived DCs (BMDCs) and MΦs. Our data indicate that eVLP trigger host responses through toll-like receptor (TLR) pathway utilizing 2 distinct adaptors, MyD88 and TRIF. More interestingly, eVLP activated the IFN signaling pathway by inducing a set of potent antiviral ISGs. Last, eVLP and synthetic adjuvants, Poly I:C and CpG DNA, cooperatively increased the expression of cytokines and ISGs. Further supporting this synergy, eVLP when administered together with Poly I:C conferred mice enhanced protection against EBOV infection. These results indicate that eVLP stimulate early innate immune responses through TLR and type I IFN signaling pathways to protect the host from EBOV infection.

PMCID: PMC3924795 [Available on 2015/2/1] PMID: 24102579 [PubMed - indexed for MEDLINE]
807. MBio. 2014 Jan 28;5(1):e00862-13. doi: 10.1128/mBio.00862-13.

Comprehensive functional analysis of N-linked glycans on Ebola virus GP1.

Lennemann NJ, Rhein BA, Ndungo E, Chandran K, Qiu X, Maury W.

Ebola virus (EBOV) entry requires the virion surface-associated glycoprotein (GP) that is composed of a trimer of heterodimers (GP1/GP2). The GP1 subunit contains two heavily glycosylated domains, the glycan cap and the mucin-like domain (MLD). The glycan cap contains only N-linked glycans, whereas the MLD contains both N- and O-linked glycans. Site-directed mutagenesis was performed on EBOV GP1 to systematically disrupt N-linked glycan sites to gain an understanding of their role in GP structure and function. All 15 N-glycosylation sites of EBOV GP1 could be removed without compromising the expression of GP. The loss of these 15 glycosylation sites significantly enhanced pseudovirion transduction in Vero cells, which correlated with an increase in protease sensitivity. Interestingly, exposing the receptor-binding domain (RBD) by removing the glycan shield did not allow interaction with the endosomal receptor, NPC1, indicating that the glycan cap/MLD domains mask RBD residues required for binding. The effects of the loss of GP1 N-linked glycans on Ca(2+)-dependent (C-type) lectin (CLEC)-dependent transduction were complex, and the effect was unique for each of the CLECs tested. Surprisingly, EBOV entry into murine peritoneal macrophages was independent of GP1 N-glycans, suggesting that CLEC-GP1 N-glycan interactions are not required for entry into this important primary cell. Finally, the removal of all GP1 N-glycans outside the MLD enhanced antiserum and antibody sensitivity. In total, our results provide evidence that the conserved N-linked glycans on the EBOV GP1 core protect GP from antibody neutralization despite the negative impact the glycans have on viral entry efficiency.IMPORTANCE: Filovirus outbreaks occur sporadically throughout central Africa, causing high fatality rates among the general public and health care workers. These unpredictable hemorrhagic fever outbreaks are caused by multiple species of Ebola viruses, as well as Marburg virus. While filovirus vaccines and therapeutics are being developed, there are no licensed products. The sole viral envelope glycoprotein, which is a principal immunogenic target, contains a heavy shield of glycans surrounding the conserved receptor-binding domain. We find that disruption of this shield through targeted mutagenesis leads to an increase in cell entry, protease sensitivity, and antiserum/antibody sensitivity but is not sufficient to allow virion binding to the intracellular receptor NPC1. Therefore, our studies provide evidence that filoviruses maintain glycoprotein glycosylation to protect against proteases and antibody neutralization at the expense of efficient entry. Our results unveil interesting insights into the unique entry process of filoviruses and potential immune evasion tactics of the virus.

PMCID: PMC3950510 PMID: 24473128 [PubMed - indexed for MEDLINE]
808. Ann Ist Super Sanita. 2014;50(4):307-8.DOI: 10.4415/ANN_14_04_01.

Ebola: when a nightmare becomes reality. Editorial.

Rezza G(1).

Author information: (1)Dipartimento di Malattie Infettive, Parassitarie ed Immunomediate, Istituto Superiore di Sanità, Rome, Italy.

PMID: 25522067 [PubMed - in process]
809. Antimicrob Agents Chemother. 2014;58(1):120-7. doi: 10.1128/AAC.01407-13. Epub 2013 Oct 21.

Activity of and effect of subcutaneous treatment with the broad-spectrum antiviral lectin griffithsin in two laboratory rodent models.

Barton C(1), Kouokam JC, Lasnik AB, Foreman O, Cambon A, Brock G, Montefiori DC, Vojdani F, McCormick AA, O'Keefe BR, Palmer KE.

Author information: (1)Department of Pharmacology and Toxicology and James Graham Brown Cancer Center, University of Louisville School of Medicine, Louisville, Kentucky, USA.

Griffithsin (GRFT) is a red-alga-derived lectin that binds the terminal mannose residues of N-linked glycans found on the surface of human immunodeficiency virus type 1 (HIV-1), HIV-2, and other enveloped viruses, including hepatitis C virus (HCV), severe acute respiratory syndrome coronavirus (SARS-CoV), and Ebola virus. GRFT displays no human T-cell mitogenic activity and does not induce production of proinflammatory cytokines in treated human cell lines. However, despite the growing evidence showing the broad-spectrum nanomolar or better antiviral activity of GRFT, no study has reported a comprehensive assessment of GRFT safety as a potential systemic antiviral treatment. The results presented in this work show that minimal toxicity was induced by a range of single and repeated daily subcutaneous doses of GRFT in two rodent species, although we noted treatment-associated increases in spleen and liver mass suggestive of an antidrug immune response. The drug is systemically distributed, accumulating to high levels in the serum and plasma after subcutaneous delivery. Further, we showed that serum from GRFT-treated animals retained antiviral activity against HIV-1-enveloped pseudoviruses in a cell-based neutralization assay. Overall, our data presented here show that GRFT accumulates to relevant therapeutic concentrations which are tolerated with minimal toxicity. These studies support further development of GRFT as a systemic antiviral therapeutic agent against enveloped viruses, although deimmunizing the molecule may be necessary if it is to be used in long-term treatment of chronic viral infections.

PMCID: PMC3910741 PMID: 24145548 [PubMed - indexed for MEDLINE]

810. Biochim Biophys Acta. 2014 Jan;1838(1 Pt B):117-26. doi: 10.1016/j.bbamem.2013.09.003. Epub 2013 Sep 18.

Structure and orientation study of Ebola fusion peptide inserted in lipid membrane models.

Agopian A(1), Castano S.

Author information: (1)CBMN-UMR 5248 CNRS, Université de Bordeaux, IPB, Allée Geoffroy Saint Hilaire, 33600 Pessac, France.

The fusion peptide of Ebola virus comprises a highly hydrophobic sequence located downstream from the N-terminus of the glycoprotein GP2 responsible for virus-host membrane fusion. The internal fusion peptide of GP2 inserts into membranes of infected cell to mediate the viral and the host cell membrane fusion. Since the sequence length of Ebola fusion peptide is still not clear, we study in the present work the behavior of two fusion peptides of different lengths which were named EBO17 and EBO24 referring to their amino acid length. The secondary structure and orientation of both peptides in lipid model systems made of DMPC:DMPG:cholesterol:DMPE (6:2:5:3) were investigated using PMIRRAS and polarized ATR spectroscopy coupled with Brewster angle microscopy. The infrared results showed a structural flexibility of both fusion peptides which are able to transit reversibly from an α-helix to antiparallel β-sheets. Ellipsometry results corroborate together with isotherm measurements that EBO peptides interacting with lipid monolayer highly affected the lipid organization. When interacting with a single lipid bilayer, at low peptide content, EBO peptides insert as mostly α-helices mainly perpendicular into the lipid membrane thus tend to organize the lipid acyl chains. Inserted in multilamellar vesicles at higher peptide content, EBO peptides are mostly in β-sheet structures and induce a disorganization of the lipid chain order. In this paper, we show that the secondary structure of the Ebola fusion peptide is reversibly flexible between α-helical and β-sheet conformations, this feature being dependent on its concentration in lipids, eventually inducing membrane fusion. © 2013.

PMID: 24055820 [PubMed - indexed for MEDLINE]

811. Biomark Med. 2014;8(9):1053-6. doi: 10.2217/bmm.14.75.

Biomarkers for understanding Ebola virus disease.

McElroy AK(1), Spiropoulou CF.

Author information: (1)Viral Special Pathogens Branch, US Centers for Disease Control & Prevention, Atlanta, GA 30333, USA.

PMID: 25402574 [PubMed - in process]

812. BMC Bioinformatics. 2014;15 Suppl 4:S1. doi: 10.1186/1471-2105-15-S4-S1. Epub 2014 Mar 19.

Integrated assessment of predicted MHC binding and cross-conservation with self reveals patterns of viral camouflage.

He L, De Groot AS, Gutierrez AH, Martin WD, Moise L, Bailey-Kellogg C.

BACKGROUND: Immune recognition of foreign proteins by T cells hinges on the formation of a ternary complex sandwiching a constituent peptide of the protein between a major histocompatibility complex (MHC) molecule and a T cell receptor (TCR). Viruses have evolved means of "camouflaging" themselves, avoiding immune recognition by reducing the MHC and/or TCR binding of their constituent peptides. Computer-driven T cell epitope mapping tools have been used to evaluate the degree to which particular viruses have used this means of avoiding immune response, but most such analyses focus on MHC-facing 'agretopes'. Here we set out a new means of evaluating the TCR faces of viral peptides in addition to their agretopes, integrating evaluations of both sides of the ternary complex in a single analysis. METHODS: This paper develops what we call the Janus Immunogenicity Score (JIS), bringing together a well-established method for predicting MHC binding, with a novel assessment of the potential for TCR binding based on similarity with self. Intuitively, both good MHC binding and poor self-similarity are required for high immunogenicity (i.e., a robust T effector response). RESULTS: Focusing on the class II antigen-processing pathway, we show that the JIS of T effector epitopes and null or regulatory epitopes deposited in a large database of epitopes (Immune Epitope Database) are significantly different. We then show that different types of viruses display significantly different patterns of scores over their constituent peptides, with viruses causing chronic infection (Epstein-Barr and cytomegalovirus) strongly shifted to lower scores relative to those causing acute infection (Ebola and Marburg). Similarly we find distinct patterns among influenza proteins in H1N1 (a strain against which human populations rapidly developed immunity) and H5N1 and H7N9 (highly pathogenic avian flu strains, with significantly greater case mortality rates). CONCLUSION: The Janus Immunogenicity Score, which integrates MHC binding and TCR cross-reactivity, provides a new tool for studying immunogenicity of pathogens and may improve the selection and optimization of antigenic elements for vaccine design.

PMCID: PMC4094998 PMID: 25104221 [PubMed - indexed for MEDLINE]

813. Clin Ophthalmol. 2014 Nov 21;8:2355-7. doi: 10.2147/OPTH.S73583. eCollection 2014

What we know about ocular manifestations of Ebola.

Moshirfar M(1), Fenzl CR(2), Li Z(3).

Author information: (1)Department of Ophthalmology, Francis I Proctor Foundation, University of California San Francisco, San Francisco, CA, USA. (2)John A Moran Eye Center, University of Utah, Salt Lake City, UT, USA. (3)University of Nevada School of Medicine, Reno, NV, USA.

Ebola hemorrhagic fever is a deadly disease caused by several species of ebolavirus. The current outbreak of 2014 is unique in that it has affected a greater number of people than ever before. It also has an unusual geographic distribution. Nonspecific findings such as fever and generalized weakness have traditionally been very common early in the acute phase. Ophthalmic manifestations have also been reported in significant numbers. Conjunctival injection has been identified in both the acute and late phases. Subconjunctival hemorrhage and excessive lacrimation have also been reported. Various forms of uveitis have been associated with the convalescent phase of the disease. When identified in conjunction with other signs such as fever, acute findings such as

conjunctivitis may contribute to the diagnosis of Ebola hemorrhagic fever. Ideally, serologic testing should be performed prior to isolation and treatment of these individuals. Considering the prevalence of the current outbreak and the threat of transcontinental spread, ophthalmic health professionals need to be aware of the ocular manifestations of Ebola hemorrhagic fever as well as the associated signs and symptoms in order to prevent further spread.
PMCID: PMC4247133 PMID: 25473261 [PubMed]

814. Curr Top Microbiol Immunol. 2014;375:107-26. doi: 10.1007/82_2012_240.

Emerging antibody-based products.

Whaley KJ(1), Morton J, Hume S, Hiatt E, Bratcher B, Klimyuk V, Hiatt A, Pauly M, Zeitlin L.

Author information: (1)Mapp Biopharmaceutical Inc, 6160 Lusk Blvd, Suite C105, San Diego, CA, 92121, USA, Kevin.whaley@mappbio.com.

Antibody-based products are not widely available to address many global health challenges due to high costs, limited manufacturing capacity, and long manufacturing lead times. There are now tremendous opportunities to address these industrialization challenges as a result of revolutionary advances in plant virus-based transient expression. This review focuses on some antibody-based products that are in preclinical and clinical development, and have scaled up manufacturing and purification (mg of purified mAb/kg of biomass). Plant virus-based antibody products provide lower upfront cost, shorter time to clinical and market supply, and lower cost of goods (COGs). Further, some plant virus-based mAbs may provide improvements in pharmacokinetics, safety and efficacy.

PMID: 22772797 [PubMed - indexed for MEDLINE]

815. Epidemiol Health. 2014 Aug 28;36:e2014015. doi: 10.4178/epih/e2014015. eCollection 2014.

Ebola, fear and preparedness.

Wiwanitkit V(1).

Author information: (1)Wiwanitkit House, Bangkhae, Bangkok, Thailand.
PMCID: PMC4162143 PMID: 25220146 [PubMed]

816. Epidemiol Health. 2014 Aug 18;36:e2014014. doi: 10.4178/epih/e2014014. eCollection 2014.

What do we really fear? The epidemiological characteristics of Ebola and our preparedness.

Ki M(1).

Author information: (1)Department of Cancer Control and Policy, Graduated School of Cancer Science and Policy, National Cancer Center, Goyang, Korea.
Ebola virus disease (hereafter Ebola) has a high fatality rate; currently lacks a treatment or vaccine with proven safety and efficacy, and thus many people fear this infection. As of August 13, 2014, 2,127 patients across four West African countries have been infected with the Ebola virus over the past nine months. Among these patients, approximately 1 in 2 has subsequently died from the disease. In response, the World Health Organization has declared the Ebola outbreak in West Africa to be a Public Health Emergency of International Concern. However, Ebola is only transmitted by patients who already present symptoms of the disease, and infection only occurs upon direct contact with the blood or body fluids of an Ebola patient. Consequently, transmission of the outbreak can be contained through careful monitoring for fever among persons who have visited, or come into contact with persons from, the site of the outbreak. Thus, patients suspected of presenting symptoms characteristic of Ebola should be quarantined. To date, South Korea is not equipped with the special containment clinical units and biosafety level 4 facilities required to contain the outbreak of a fatal virus disease, such as Ebola. Therefore, it is necessary for South Korea to make strategies to the outbreak by using present facilities as quickly as possible. It is also imperative that the government establish suitable communication with its citizens to prevent the spread of uninformed fear and anxiety regarding the Ebola outbreak.
PMCID: PMC4153011 PMID: 25132130 [PubMed]

817. Front Immunol. 2014 Oct 27;5:562. doi: 10.3389/fimmu.2014.00562. eCollection 2014

A dead-end host: is there a way out? A position piece on the ebola virus outbreak by the international union of immunology societies.

Gray CM(1), Addo M(2), Schmidt RE(3); Clinical Immunology Committee of the IUIS.

Author information: (1)Division of Immunology, Institute of Infectious Diseases and Molecular Medicine, National Health Laboratory Services, University of Cape Town , Cape Town , South Africa. (2)Division of Emerging Infections/Tropical Medicine, Department of Medicine, University Medical Center Hamburg-Eppendorf , Hamburg , Germany. (3)Division of Immunology and Rheumatology, University of Hannover , Hannover , Germany.
PMCID: PMC4213834 PMID: 25400640 [PubMed]

818. Front Microbiol. 2014 Jun 18;5:300. doi: 10.3389/fmicb.2014.00300. eCollection 2014

Membrane binding and bending in Ebola VP40 assembly and egress.

Stahelin RV(1).

Author information: (1)Department of Biochemistry and Molecular Biology, Indiana University School of Medicine-South Bend South Bend, IN, USA ; Department of Chemistry and Biochemistry, Eck Institute for Global Health, University of Notre Dame Notre Dame, IN, USA.
Lipid-enveloped viruses contain a lipid bilayer coat that protects their genome and helps to facilitate entry into the host cell. Filoviruses are lipid-enveloped viruses that have up to 90% clinical fatality and include Marbug (MARV) and Ebola (EBOV). These pleomorphic filamentous viruses enter the host cell through their membrane-embedded glycoprotein and then replicate using just seven genes encoded in their negative-sense RNA genome. EBOV budding occurs from the inner leaflet of the plasma membrane (PM) and is driven by the matrix protein VP40, which is the most abundantly expressed protein of the virus. VP40 expressed in mammalian cells alone can trigger budding of filamentous virus-like particles (VLPs) that are nearly indistinguishable from authentic EBOV. VP40, such as matrix proteins from other viruses, has been shown to bind anionic lipid membranes. However, how VP40 selectively interacts with the inner leaflet of

the PM and assembles into a filamentous lipid enveloped particle is mostly unknown. This article describes what is known regarding VP40 membrane interactions and what answers will fill the gaps.

PMCID: PMC4061899 PMID: 24995005 [PubMed]

819. Front Public Health. 2014 Dec 1;2:263. doi: 10.3389/fpubh.2014.00263. eCollection 2014

Ebola viral disease outbreak-2014: implications and pitfalls.

Acharya M(1).

Author information: (1)Independent Researcher , Kathmandu , Nepal.

PMCID: PMC4249494 PMID: 25520949 [PubMed]

820. Front Public Health. 2014 Nov 3;2:218. doi: 10.3389/fpubh.2014.00218. eCollection 2014

The importance of veterinary policy in preventing the emergence and re-emergence of zoonotic disease: examining the case of human african trypanosomiasis in Uganda.

Okello AL(1), Welburn SC(1).

Author information: (1)Division of Pathway Medicine, Centre for Infectious Diseases, School of Biomedical Sciences, College of Medicine and Veterinary Medicine, The University of Edinburgh , Edinburgh , UK.

Rapid changes in human behavior, resource utilization, and other extrinsic environmental factors continue to threaten the current distribution of several endemic and historically neglected zoonoses in many developing regions worldwide. There are numerous examples of zoonotic diseases which have circulated within relatively localized geographical areas for some time, before emerging into new regions as a result of changing human, environmental, or behavioral dynamics. While the world's focus is currently on the Ebola virus gaining momentum in western Africa, another pertinent example of this phenomenon is zoonotic human African trypanosomiasis (HAT), endemic to south and eastern Africa, and spread via infected cattle. In recent years, the ongoing northwards spread of this disease in the country has posed a serious public health threat to the human population of Uganda, increasing the pressure on both individual families and government services to control the disease. Moreover, the emergence of HAT into new areas of Uganda in recent years exemplifies the important role of veterinary policy in mitigating the severe human health and economic impacts of zoonotic disease. The systemic challenges surrounding the development and enforcement of veterinary policy described here are similar across sub-Saharan Africa, highlighting the necessity to consider and support zoonotic disease control in broader human and animal health systems strengthening and associated development programs on the continent.

PMCID: PMC4217318 PMID: 25405148 [PubMed]

821. Glob Health Action. 2014 Nov 17;7:26356. doi: 10.3402/gha.v7.26356. eCollection 2014

Black market blood transfusions for Ebola: potential for increases in other infections.

Folayan MO(1), Brown B(2), Yakubu A(3).

Author information: (1)Obafemi Awolowo University, Ile-Ife, Nigeria; Department of Child Dental Health, Obafemi Awolowo University, Ile-Ife, Nigeria. (2)Department of Population Health & Disease Prevention, University of California, Irvine, CA, USA; brandon.brown@uci.edu. (3)Department of Health Planning and Research, Federal Ministry of Health, Abuja, Nigeria.

PMCID: PMC4236640 PMID: 25406794 [PubMed - in process]

822. Glob Health Action. 2014 Nov 7;7:26058. doi: 10.3402/gha.v7.26058. eCollection 2014

Addressing Ebola-related stigma: lessons learned from HIV/AIDS.

Davtyan M(1), Brown B(2), Folayan MO(3).

Author information: (1)Department of Population Health & Disease Prevention, University of California, Irvine, CA, USA. (2)Department of Population Health & Disease Prevention, University of California, Irvine, CA, USA; brandon.brown@uci.edu. (3)Department of Child Dental Health, Institute of Public Health, Obafemi Awolowo University, Ile-Ife, Nigeria.

BACKGROUND: HIV/AIDS and Ebola Virus Disease (EVD) are contemporary epidemics associated with significant social stigma in which communities affected suffer from social rejection, violence, and diminished quality of life. OBJECTIVE: To compare and contrast stigma related to HIV/AIDS and EVD, and strategically think how lessons learned from HIV stigma can be applied to the current EVD epidemic. METHODS: To identify relevant articles about HIV/AIDS and EVD-related stigma, we conducted an extensive literature review using multiple search engines. PubMed was used to search for relevant peer-reviewed journal articles and Google for online sources. We also consulted the websites of the World Health Organization (WHO), Centers for Disease Control and Prevention (CDC), and the National Institutes of Health to retrieve up-to-date information about EVD and HIV/AIDS. RESULTS: Many stigmatizing attitudes and behaviors directed towards those with EVD are strikingly similar to those with HIV/AIDS but there are significant differences worthy of discussion. Both diseases are life-threatening and there is no medical cure. Additionally misinformation about affected groups and modes of transmission runs rampant. Unlike in persons with EVD, historically criminalized and marginalized populations carry a disproportionately higher risk for HIV infection. Moreover, mortality due to EVD occurs within a shorter time span as compared to HIV/AIDS. CONCLUSIONS: Stigma disrupts quality of life, whether it is associated with HIV infection or EVD. When addressing EVD, we must think beyond the immediate clinical therapeutic response, to possible HIV implications of serum treatment. There are emerging social concerns of stigma associated with EVD infection and double stigma associated with EVD and HIV infection. Drawing upon lessons learned from HIV, we must work to empower and mobilize prominent members of the community, those who recovered from the disease, and organizations working at the grassroots level to disseminate clear and accurate information about EVD transmission and prevention while promoting stigma reduction in the process. In the long run, education, prevention, and a therapeutic vaccine will be the optimal solutions for reducing the stigma associated with both EVD and HIV.

PMCID: PMC4225220 PMID: 25382685 [PubMed - in process]

823. Glob Health Action. 2014 Oct 10;7:25287. doi: 10.3402/gha.v7.25287. eCollection 2014
The interconnected and cross-border nature of risks posed by infectious diseases.

Suk JE(1), Van Cangh T(2), Beauté J(2), Bartels C(2), Tsolova S(2), Pharris A(2), Ciotti M(2), Semenza JC(2).

Author information: (1)European Centre for Disease Prevention and Control, Stockholm, Sweden; Global Public Health Unit, School of Social and Political Science, University of Edinburgh, Edinburgh, UK; jonathan.suk@ecdc.europa.eu. (2)European Centre for Disease Prevention and Control, Stockholm, Sweden.

Infectious diseases can constitute public health emergencies of international concern when a pathogen arises, acquires new characteristics, or is deliberately released, leading to the potential for loss of human lives as well as societal disruption. A wide range of risk drivers are now known to lead to and/or exacerbate the emergence and spread of infectious disease, including global trade and travel, the overuse of antibiotics, intensive agriculture, climate change, high population densities, and inadequate infrastructures, such as water treatment facilities. Where multiple risk drivers interact, the potential impact of a disease outbreak is amplified. The varying temporal and geographic frequency with which infectious disease events occur adds yet another layer of complexity to the issue. Mitigating the emergence and spread of infectious disease necessitates mapping and prioritising the interdependencies between public health and other sectors. Conversely, during an international public health emergency, significant disruption occurs not only to healthcare systems but also to a potentially wide range of sectors, including trade, tourism, energy, civil protection, transport, agriculture, and so on. At the same time, dealing with a disease outbreak may require a range of critical sectors for support. There is a need to move beyond narrow models of risk to better account for the interdependencies between health and other sectors so as to be able to better mitigate and respond to the risks posed by emerging infectious disease.

PMCID: PMC4195207 PMID: 25308818 [PubMed - in process]

824. Infect Dis Poverty. 2014 Aug 5;3:29. doi: 10.1186/2049-9957-3-29. eCollection 2014.
Need of surveillance response systems to combat Ebola outbreaks and other emerging infectious diseases in African countries.

Tambo E(1), Ugwu EC(2), Ngogang JY(3).

Author information: (1)Sydney Brenner Institute for Molecular Bioscience, Wits 21st Century Institute, Faculty of Health Sciences, University of the Witwatersrand, Johannesburg, South Africa ; Center for Sustainable Malaria Control, Department of Biochemistry, Faculty of Natural and Agricultural Sciences, University of Pretoria, Pretoria, South Africa ; National Institute of Parasitic Diseases, Chinese Center for Disease Control and Prevention, and the WHO Collaborating Centre on Malaria, Schisostomiasis and Filariasis, Shanghai 200025, PR China. (2)Faculty of Basic Medical Sciences, Department of Human Biochemistry, Nnamdi Azikiwe University Awka, Nnewi Campus, Nigeria ; National Institute of Parasitic Diseases, Chinese Center for Disease Control and Prevention, and the WHO Collaborating Centre on Malaria, Schisostomiasis and Filariasis, Shanghai 200025, PR China. (3)Faculté des Sciences Biomédicales, Département de Biochimie, Université de Yaoundé, Yaoundé, République du Cameroun.

There is growing concern in Sub-Saharan Africa about the spread of the Ebola virus disease (EVD), formerly known as Ebola haemorrhagic fever, and the public health burden that it ensues. Since 1976, there have been 885,343 suspected and laboratory confirmed cases of EVD and the disease has claimed 2,512 cases and 932 fatality in West Africa. There are certain requirements that must be met when responding to EVD outbreaks and this process could incur certain challenges. For the purposes of this paper, five have been identified: (i) the deficiency in the development and implementation of surveillance response systems against Ebola and others infectious disease outbreaks in Africa; (ii) the lack of education and knowledge resulting in an EVD outbreak triggering panic, anxiety, psychosocial trauma, isolation and dignity impounding, stigmatisation, community ostracism and resistance to associated socio-ecological and public health consequences; (iii) limited financial resources, human technical capacity and weak community and national health system operational plans for prevention and control responses, practices and management; (iv) inadequate leadership and coordination; and (v) the lack of development of new strategies, tools and approaches, such as improved diagnostics and novel therapies including vaccines which can assist in preventing, controlling and containing Ebola outbreaks as well as the spread of the disease. Hence, there is an urgent need to develop and implement an active early warning alert and surveillance response system for outbreak response and control of emerging infectious diseases. Understanding the unending risks of transmission dynamics and resurgence is essential in implementing rapid effective response interventions tailored to specific local settings and contexts.THEREFORE, THE FOLLOWING ACTIONS ARE RECOMMENDED: (i) national and regional inter-sectorial and trans-disciplinary surveillance response systems that include early warnings, as well as critical human resources development, must be quickly adopted by allied ministries and organisations in African countries in epidemic and pandemic responses; (ii) harnessing all stakeholders commitment and advocacy in sustained funding, collaboration, communication and networking including community participation to enhance a coordinated responses, as well as tracking and prompt case management to combat challenges; (iii) more research and development in new drug discovery and vaccines; and (iv) understanding the involvement of global health to promote the establishment of public health surveillance response systems with functions of early warning, as well as monitoring and evaluation in upholding research-action programmes and innovative interventions.

PMCID: PMC4130433 PMID: 25120913 [PubMed]

825. Inquiry. 2014 Jan 1;51. pii: 0046958014564055. doi: 10.1177/0046958014564055. Print 2014.
Ebola crisis in the United States: a glimpse of its larger shadow.

Patwardhan AR(1).

Author information: (1)George Mason University, Fairfax, VA, USA apatward@gmu.edu.

This article is about readiness of the U.S. health care system to deal with crises. Using the Ebola crisis as a reference, first it examines the response to the current challenge. However, that is the smaller objective of the article. Lately, we are also being challenged to deal with other kinds of epidemics like obesity, mental health diseases, and violence. These crises are not dramatic like the Ebola crisis. However, these are no less insidious than Ebola. If we are not ready for them, then these crises have the potential to undermine the long-term health and prosperity of our society. In this context, and therefore mainly, this article is about two major long-standing systemic problems in the U.S. health care system that the unfolding of the Ebola crisis has bared. One is about how the inherent problem in the design of American federalist system regarding state autonomy on health matters is creating a dysfunctional health care system. The other is about the inertia of the research industry in the health care system in clinging to an archaic outdated inefficient mind-set and methodology that fails to generate the right information required for an appropriate decision making in matters of health care delivery, including crises. These problems are not small, nor their solutions easy. However, no matter how uncomfortable and tedious, facing them is necessary and inevitable. The discussions and arguments in this article are to outline their nature broadly and to make a call to further a dialogue.

© The Author(s) 2014.

PMID: 25512226 [PubMed - in process]

826. J Immunol Res. 2014;2014:237043. doi: 10.1155/2014/237043. Epub 2014 Sep 16.

The impact of "omic" and imaging technologies on assessing the host immune response to biodefence agents.

Tree JA(1), Flick-Smith H(2), Elmore MJ(1), Rowland CA(2).

Author information: (1)Biodefence and PreClinical Evaluation Group, Public Health England (PHE), Porton Down, Salisbury, Wiltshire, SP5 3NU, UK. (2)Biomedical Sciences Department, Defence Science and Technology Laboratory (Dstl), Porton Down, Salisbury, Wiltshire, SP4 0JQ, UK.

Understanding the interactions between host and pathogen is important for the development and assessment of medical countermeasures to infectious agents, including potential biodefence pathogens such as Bacillus anthracis, Ebola virus, and Francisella tularensis. This review focuses on technological advances which allow this interaction to be studied in much greater detail. Namely, the use of omic technologies (next generation sequencing, DNA, and protein microarrays) for dissecting the underlying host response to infection at the molecular level; optical imaging techniques (flow cytometry and fluorescence microscopy) for assessing cellular responses to infection; and biophotonic imaging for visualising the infectious disease process. All of these technologies hold great promise for important breakthroughs in the rational development of vaccines and therapeutics for biodefence agents.

PMCID: PMC4182007 PMID: 25333059 [PubMed - in process]

827. J Int AIDS Soc. 2014 Dec 1;17:19896. doi: 10.7448/IAS.17.1.19896. eCollection 2014

HIV and Ebola: similarities and differences.

Wainberg MA(1), Kippax S(2), Bras M(3), Sow PS(4).

Author information: (1)McGill University AIDS Centre, Jewish General Hospital, Montreal, Quebec, Canada; Journal of the International AIDS Society, Geneva, Switzerland; (2)Journal of the International AIDS Society, Geneva, Switzerland;; Social Policy Research Centre, University of New South Wales, Sydney, Australia. (3)Journal of the International AIDS Society, Geneva, Switzerland; (4)Journal of the International AIDS Society, Geneva, Switzerland;; Department of Infectious Diseases, University of Dakar, Dakar, Senegal.

PMCID: PMC4252165 PMID: 25466882 [PubMed - in process]

828. J Spec Oper Med. 2014 Winter;14(4):113-21.

Bites, stings, and rigors: clinical considerations in african operations.

Lynch JH, Verlo AR, Givens ML, Munoz CE.

The natural health threats in Africa pose daunting clinical challenges for any provider, as evidenced by the current Ebola epidemic in West Africa, but the threat is multiplied for the Special Operations provider on the continent who faces these challenges with limited resources and the tyranny of distance. The majority of operationally significant health risks can be mitigated by strict adherence to a comprehensive force health protection plan. The simplest, yet most effective, technique for preventing mosquito-borne diseases is the prevention of mosquito bites with repellent, bed nets, and appropriate clothing in addition to chemoprophylaxis. Some of the more likely or lethal infectious diseases encountered on the continent include malaria, Chikungunya, dengue, human immunodeficiency virus, and Ebola. Venomous snakes pose a particular challenge since the treatment can be as deadly as the injury. Providers supporting African operations should educate themselves on the clinical characteristics of possible envenomations in their area while promoting snake avoidance as the primary mitigation measure. To succeed in Africa, the Special Operations provider must consider how to meet these challenges in an environment where there may not be reliable evacuation, hospitalization, or logistics channels.

2014

PMID: 25399379 [PubMed - in process]

829. J Venom Anim Toxins Incl Trop Dis. 2014 Oct 3;20(1):44. doi: 10.1186/1678-9199-20-44. eCollection 2014.

Outbreaks of Ebola virus disease in Africa: the beginnings of a tragic saga.

Chippaux JP(1).

Author information: (1)UMR 216, Mother and Child Facing Tropical Diseases, Institut de Recherche pour le Développement (IRD), Cotonou, Bénin ; Sorbonne Paris Cité, Faculté de Pharmacie, Université Paris Descartes, Paris, France.

The tremendous outbreak of Ebola virus disease occurring in West Africa since the end of 2013 surprises by its remoteness from previous epidemics and dramatic extent. This review aims to describe the 27 manifestations of Ebola virus that arose after its discovery in 1976. It provides an update on research on the ecology of Ebola viruses, modes of contamination and human transmission of the disease that are mainly linked to close contact with an infected animal or a patient suffering from the disease. The recommendations to contain the epidemic and challenges to achieve it are reminded.

PMCID: PMC4197285 PMID: 25320574 [PubMed]

830. J Virol. 2014 Jan;88(1):99-109. doi: 10.1128/JVI.02265-13. Epub 2013 Oct 16.

Characterization of the envelope glycoprotein of a novel filovirus, lloviu virus.

Maruyama J(1), Miyamoto H, Kajihara M, Ogawa H, Maeda K, Sakoda Y, Yoshida R, Takada A.

Author information: (1)Division of Global Epidemiology, Research Center for Zoonosis Control, Hokkaido University, Sapporo, Japan.

Lloviu virus (LLOV), a novel filovirus detected in bats, is phylogenetically distinct from viruses in the genera Ebolavirus and Marburgvirus in the family Filoviridae. While filoviruses are known to cause severe hemorrhagic fever in humans and/or nonhuman primates, LLOV is biologically uncharacterized, since infectious LLOV has never been isolated. To examine the properties of LLOV, we characterized its envelope glycoprotein (GP), which likely plays a key role in viral tropism and pathogenicity. We first found that LLOV GP principally has the same primary structure as the other filovirus GPs. Similar to the other filoviruses, virus-like particles (VLPs) produced by transient expression of LLOV GP, matrix protein, and nucleoprotein in 293T cells had densely arrayed GP spikes on a filamentous particle. Mouse antiserum to LLOV VLP was barely cross-reactive to viruses of the other genera, indicating that LLOV is serologically distinct from the other known filoviruses. For functional study of LLOV GP, we utilized a vesicular stomatitis virus (VSV) pseudotype system and found that LLOV GP requires low endosomal pH and cathepsin L, and that human C-type lectins act as attachment factors for LLOV entry into cells. Interestingly, LLOV GP-pseudotyped VSV infected particular bat cell lines more efficiently than viruses bearing other filovirus GPs. These results suggest that LLOV GP mediates cellular entry in a manner similar to that of the other filoviruses while showing preferential tropism for some bat cells.

PMCID: PMC3911722 PMID: 24131711 [PubMed - indexed for MEDLINE]

831. Krankenpfl Soins Infirm. 2014;107(10):59.

[Diabolical affair].

[Article in French]

Taillens F.

PMID: 25345206 [PubMed - indexed for MEDLINE]

832. Laeknabladid. 2014 Oktober;100(10):503.

[Ebola and us[Editorial].]

[Article in Icelandic]

Gudmundsson S.

PMID: 25310037 [PubMed - as supplied by publisher]

833. Ned Tijdschr Geneeskd. 2014;158(0):A8575.

[Is the caregiver fit to help Ebola patient?].

[Article in Dutch]

Jungbauer FH(1), Wulp PB.

Author information: (1)UMCG, afd. Arbeid en Gezondheid, Groningen.

Ebola is an exceptionally risky infection and safety measures are therefore unprecedentedly strict. However, despite stringent measures infection of health care providers by the Ebola virus cannot be excluded. Strict barrier care is physically and mentally demanding for the care provider. Before undertaking care for Ebola patients, 'fit for the job'screening is necessary. We should only expose our care givers if we know that they are physically and mentally up to the task.

PMID: 25492738 [PubMed - in process]

834. Ned Tijdschr Geneeskd. 2014;158:A8448.

[Ebola and the hypocrisy of the Western world].

[Article in Dutch]

van den Brink R(1).

Author information: (1)NOS Nieuws, Hilversum.

The response to the Ebola outbreak in West Africa of the governments of Guinea, Sierra Leone and Liberia, local WHO representatives, international organisations with WHO at the helm, and the international community has been much too slow. The help that is now at last being given has come much too late, and, with a few notable exceptions, it is far too little. The European Union, including the Netherlands, is distinguishing itself by its absence. It does not appear to have got through to Europe that, even if it is only in its own interest, it must offer far more help to Guinea, Sierra Leone and Liberia - and quickly.

PMID: 25351388 [PubMed - in process]

835. Ned Tijdschr Geneeskd. 2014;158:A8402.

[The embarrassing lessons of Ebola: scientific knowledge comes too late].

[Article in Dutch]

Murk JL(1), Bonten M.

Author information: (1)Universitair Medisch Centrum Utrecht, afd. Medische Microbiologie en Julius Centrum voor Gezondheidswetenschappen en Huisartsgeneeskunde, Utrecht.

The current Ebola epidemic in Western Africa painfully illustrates both the devastating power of a deadly virus once introduced into a severely compromised health care system, and the unpreparedness of Western countries to respond appropriately. After at least 3857 casualties there has still been hardly any scientific evaluation of therapeutic or preventive treatments. The first uncontrolled observations of a new cocktail of monoclonal antibodies look promising, but given the size of the epidemic, only large-scale vaccination might be sufficient for effective control.

PMID: 25351387 [PubMed - in process]

836. PeerJ. 2014 Sep 2;2:e556. doi: 10.7717/peerj.556. eCollection 2014.

Evidence that ebolaviruses and cuevaviruses have been diverging from marburgviruses since the Miocene.

Taylor DJ(1), Ballinger MJ(1), Zhan JJ(1), Hanzly LE(1), Bruenn JA(1).
Author information: (1)Department of Biological Sciences, The State University of New York at Buffalo , Buffalo, NY , USA.

An understanding of the timescale of evolution is critical for comparative virology but remains elusive for many RNA viruses. Age estimates based on mutation rates can severely underestimate divergences for ancient viral genes that are evolving under strong purifying selection. Paleoviral dating, however, can provide minimum age estimates for ancient divergence, but few orthologous paleoviruses are known within clades of extant viruses. For example, ebolaviruses and marburgviruses are well-studied mammalian pathogens, but their comparative biology is difficult to interpret because the existing estimates of divergence are controversial. Here we provide evidence that paleoviral elements of two genes (ebolavirus-like VP35 and NP) in cricetid rodent genomes originated after the divergence of ebolaviruses and cuevaviruses from marburgviruses. We provide evidence of orthology by identifying common paleoviral insertion sites among the rodent genomes. Our findings indicate that ebolaviruses and cuevaviruses have been diverging from marburgviruses since the early Miocene.
PMCID: PMC4157239 PMID: 25237605 [PubMed]

837. PLoS One. 2014 Nov 14;9(11):e112617. doi: 10.1371/journal.pone.0112617. eCollection 2014.

Sequencing, Annotation and Analysis of the Syrian Hamster (Mesocricetus auratus) Transcriptome.

Tchitchek N(1), Safronetz D(2), Rasmussen AL(1), Martens C(3), Virtaneva K(3), Porcella SF(3), Feldmann H(2), Ebihara H(2), Katze MG(4).
Author information: (1)Department of Microbiology, University of Washington, Seattle, Washington, United States of America. (2)Laboratory of Virology, Division of Intramural Research, National Institute of Allergy and Infectious Diseases, National Institutes of Health, Rocky Mountain Laboratories, Hamilton, Montana, United States of America. (3)Genomics Unit, Research Technologies Section, National Institute of Allergy and Infectious Diseases, National Institutes of Health, Rocky Mountain Laboratories, Hamilton, Montana, United States of America. (4)Department of Microbiology, University of Washington, Seattle, Washington, United States of America; Washington National Primate Research Center, University of Washington, Seattle, Washington, United States of America.

BACKGROUND: The Syrian hamster (golden hamster, Mesocricetus auratus) is gaining importance as a new experimental animal model for multiple pathogens, including emerging zoonotic diseases such as Ebola. Nevertheless there are currently no publicly available transcriptome reference sequences or genome for this species. RESULTS: A cDNA library derived from mRNA and snRNA isolated and pooled from the brains, lungs, spleens, kidneys, livers, and hearts of three adult female Syrian hamsters was sequenced. Sequence reads were assembled into 62,482 contigs and 111,796 reads remained unassembled (singletons). This combined contig/singleton dataset, designated as the Syrian hamster transcriptome, represents a total of 60,117,204 nucleotides. Our Mesocricetus auratus Syrian hamster transcriptome mapped to 11,648 mouse transcripts representing 9,562 distinct genes, and mapped to a similar number of transcripts and genes in the rat. We identified 214 quasi-complete transcripts based on mouse annotations. Canonical pathways involved in a broad spectrum of fundamental biological processes were significantly represented in the library. The Syrian hamster transcriptome was aligned to the current release of the Chinese hamster ovary (CHO) cell transcriptome and genome to improve the genomic annotation of this species. Finally, our Syrian hamster transcriptome was aligned against 14 other rodents, primate and laurasiatheria species to gain insights about the genetic relatedness and placement of this species. CONCLUSIONS: This Syrian hamster transcriptome dataset significantly improves our knowledge of the Syrian hamster's transcriptome, especially towards its future use in infectious disease research. Moreover, this library is an important resource for the wider scientific community to help improve genome annotation of the Syrian hamster and other closely related species. Furthermore, these data provide the basis for development of expression microarrays that can be used in functional genomics studies.
PMCID: PMC4232415 PMID: 25398096 [PubMed - in process]

838. PLoS One. 2014 Sep 26;9(9):e108770. doi: 10.1371/journal.pone.0108770. eCollection 2014.

RIG-I self-oligomerization is either dispensable or very transient for signal transduction.

Louber J(1), Kowalinski E(2), Bloyet LM(1), Brunel J(1), Cusack S(2), Gerlier D(1).
Author information: (1)Centre International de Recherche en Infectiologie, INSERM, U1111, CNRS, UMR5308, Université Lyon I, ENS Lyon, Lyon, France. (2)European Molecular Biology Laboratory, Grenoble Outstation, Grenoble Cedex 9, France; Unit of Virus Host-Cell Interactions, UJF-EMBL-CNRS, UMI 3265, Grenoble Cedex 9, France.

Effective host defence against viruses depends on the rapid triggering of innate immunity through the induction of a type I interferon (IFN) response. To this end, microbe-associated molecular patterns are detected by dedicated receptors. Among them, the RIG-I-like receptors RIG-I and MDA5 activate IFN gene expression upon sensing viral RNA in the cytoplasm. While MDA5 forms long filaments in vitro upon activation, RIG-I is believed to oligomerize after RNA binding in order to transduce a signal. Here, we show that in vitro binding of synthetic RNA mimicking that of Mononegavirales (Ebola, rabies and measles viruses) leader sequences to purified RIG-I does not induce RIG-I oligomerization. Furthermore, in cells devoid of endogenous functional RIG-I-like receptors, after activation of exogenous Flag-RIG-I by a 62-mer-5'ppp-dsRNA or by polyinosinic:polycytidylic acid, a dsRNA analogue, or by measles virus infection, anti-Flag immunoprecipitation and specific elution with Flag peptide indicated a monomeric form of RIG-I. Accordingly, when using the Gaussia Luciferase-Based Protein Complementation Assay (PCA), a more sensitive in cellula assay, no RIG-I oligomerization could be detected upon RNA stimulation. Altogether our data indicate that the need for self-oligomerization of RIG-I for signal transduction is either dispensable or very transient.
PMCID: PMC4178188 PMID: 25259935 [PubMed - in process]

839. PLoS One. 2014 Sep 10;9(9):e107007. doi: 10.1371/journal.pone.0107007. eCollection 2014.

Development and evaluation of a panel of filovirus sequence capture probes for pathogen detection by next-generation sequencing.

Koehler JW(1), Hall AT(1), Rolfe PA(2), Honko AN(3), Palacios GF(4), Fair JN(5), Muyembe JJ(6), Mulembekani P(7), Schoepp RJ(1), Adesokan A(2), Minogue TD(1).
Author information: (1)Diagnostic Systems Division, United States Army Medical Research Institute of Infectious Diseases, Fort Detrick, Maryland, United States of America. (2)Pathogenica, Inc., Boston, Massachusetts, United States of America. (3)Virology Division, United States Army Medical Research Institute of

Infectious Diseases, Fort Detrick, Maryland, United States of America. (4)Center for Genomic Sciences, United States Army Medical Research Institute of Infectious Diseases, Fort Detrick, Maryland, United States of America. (5)Metabiota, San Francisco, California, United States of America. (6)Institut National de Recherche Biomédicale, Kinshasa, Democratic Republic of the Congo. (7)Kinshasa School of Public Health, Kinshasa, Democratic Republic of the Congo.

A detailed understanding of the circulating pathogens in a particular geographic location aids in effectively utilizing targeted, rapid diagnostic assays, thus allowing for appropriate therapeutic and containment procedures. This is especially important in regions prevalent for highly pathogenic viruses co-circulating with other endemic pathogens such as the malaria parasite. The importance of biosurveillance is highlighted by the ongoing Ebola virus disease outbreak in West Africa. For example, a more comprehensive assessment of the regional pathogens could have identified the risk of a filovirus disease outbreak earlier and led to an improved diagnostic and response capacity in the region. In this context, being able to rapidly screen a single sample for multiple pathogens in a single tube reaction could improve both diagnostics as well as pathogen surveillance. Here, probes were designed to capture identifying filovirus sequence for the ebolaviruses Sudan, Ebola, Reston, Taï Forest, and Bundibugyo and the Marburg virus variants Musoke, Ci67, and Angola. These probes were combined into a single probe panel, and the captured filovirus sequence was successfully identified using the MiSeq next-generation sequencing platform. This panel was then used to identify the specific filovirus from nonhuman primates experimentally infected with Ebola virus as well as Bundibugyo virus in human sera samples from the Democratic Republic of the Congo, thus demonstrating the utility for pathogen detection using clinical samples. While not as sensitive and rapid as real-time PCR, this panel, along with incorporating additional sequence capture probe panels, could be used for broad pathogen screening and biosurveillance.
PMCID: PMC4160210 PMID: 25207553 [PubMed - in process]

840. PLoS One. 2014 Jul 9;9(7):e100333. doi: 10.1371/journal.pone.0100333. eCollection 2014

Ebola outbreak response; experience and development of screening tools for viral haemorrhagic fever (VHF) in a HIV center of excellence near to VHF epicentres.

Parkes-Ratanshi R(1), Elbireer A(2), Mbambu B(1), Mayanja F(1), Coutinho A(1), Merry C(3).

Author information: (1)Infectious Diseases Institute, Makerere College of Health Sciences, Kampala, Uganda. (2)Infectious Diseases Institute, Makerere College of Health Sciences, Kampala, Uganda; Johns Hopkins University, School of Medicine, Baltimore, Maryland, United States of America. (3)Infectious Diseases Institute, Makerere College of Health Sciences, Kampala, Uganda; Trinity College Dublin, Dublin, Ireland; Northwestern University, Chicago, Illinois, United States of America.

INTRODUCTION: There have been 3 outbreaks of viral hemorrhagic fever (VHF) in Uganda in the last 2 years. VHF often starts with non-specific symptoms prior to the onset of haemorrhagic signs. HIV clinics in VHF outbreak countries such as Uganda see large numbers of patients with HIV 1/2 infection presenting with non-specific symptoms every day. Whilst there are good screening tools for general health care facilities expecting VHF suspects, we were unable to find tools for use in HIV or other non-acute clinics. METHODS: We designed tools to help with communication to staff, infection control and screening of HIV patients with non-specific symptoms in a large HIV clinic during the outbreaks in Uganda. We describe our experiences in using these tools in 2 Ebola Virus Disease outbreaks in Uganda. RESULTS: During the Ebola Virus Disease (EVD) outbreaks, enhanced infection control and communication procedures were implemented within 24 hours of the WHO/Ministry of Health announcement of the outbreaks. During course of these outbreaks the clinic saw 12,544 patients with HIV 1/2 infection, of whom 3,713 attended without an appointment, suggesting new symptoms. Of these 4 were considered at risk of EVD and seen with full infection procedures; 3 were sent home after further investigation. One patient was referred to the National Referral Hospital VHF unit, but discharged on the same day. One additional VHF suspect was identified outside of a VHF outbreak; he was transferred to the National Referral Hospital and placed in isolation within 2 hours of arriving at the HIV clinic. DISCUSSION: Use of simple screening tools can be helpful in managing large numbers of symptomatic patients attending for routine and non-routine medical care (including HIV care) within a country experiencing a VHF outbreak, and can raise medical staff awareness of VHF outside of the epidemics.
PMCID: PMC4090118 PMID: 25007269 [PubMed - in process]

841. PLoS One. 2014 Jun 10;9(6):e96360. doi: 10.1371/journal.pone.0096360. eCollection 2014

Identification of continuous human B-cell epitopes in the VP35, VP40, nucleoprotein and glycoprotein of Ebola virus.

Becquart P(1), Mahlaköiv T(2), Nkoghe D(2), Leroy EM(1).

Author information: (1)UMR 264 MIVEGEC, Institut de Recherche pour le Développement (IRD). Montpellier, France; Centre International de Recherches Médicales de Franceville, Franceville, Gabon. (2)Centre International de Recherches Médicales de Franceville, Franceville, Gabon.

Ebola virus (EBOV) is a highly virulent human pathogen. Recovery of infected patients is associated with efficient EBOV-specific immunoglobulin G (IgG) responses, whereas fatal outcome is associated with defective humoral immunity. As B-cell epitopes on EBOV are poorly defined, we sought to identify specific epitopes in four EBOV proteins (Glycoprotein (GP), Nucleoprotein (NP), and matrix Viral Protein (VP)40 and VP35). For the first time, we tested EBOV IgG+ sera from asymptomatic individuals and symptomatic Gabonese survivors, collected during the early humoral response (seven days after the end of symptoms) and the late memory phase (7-12 years post-infection). We also tested sera from EBOV-seropositive patients who had never had clinical signs of hemorrhagic fever or who lived in non-epidemic areas (asymptomatic subjects). We found that serum from asymptomatic individuals was more strongly reactive to VP40 peptides than to GP, NP or VP35. Interestingly, anti-EBOV IgG from asymptomatic patients targeted three immunodominant regions of VP40 reported to play a crucial role in virus assembly and budding. In contrast, serum from most survivors of the three outbreaks, collected a few days after the end of symptoms, reacted mainly with GP peptides. However, in asymptomatic subjects the longest immunodominant domains were identified in GP, and analysis of the GP crystal structure revealed that these domains covered a larger surface area of the chalice bowl formed by three GP1 subunits. The B-cell epitopes we identified in the EBOV VP35, VP40, NP and GP proteins may represent important tools for understanding the humoral response to this virus and for developing new antibody-based therapeutics or detection methods.

PMCID: PMC4051576 PMID: 24914933 [PubMed - in process]
842. PLoS One. 2014 Apr 23;9(4):e94355. doi: 10.1371/journal.pone.0094355. eCollection 2014

Durability of a vesicular stomatitis virus-based marburg virus vaccine in nonhuman primates.

Mire CE(1), Geisbert JB(1), Agans KN(1), Satterfield BA(1), Versteeg KM(1), Fritz EA(1), Feldmann H(2), Hensley LE(3), Geisbert TW(1).

Author information: (1)Galveston National Laboratory, University of Texas Medical Branch, Galveston, Texas, United States of America; Department of Microbiology and Immunology, University of Texas Medical Branch, Galveston, Texas, United States of America. (2)Laboratory of Virology, Division of Intramural Research, National Institute of Allergy and Infectious Diseases, National Institutes of Health, Hamilton, Montana, United States of America. (3)Integrated Research Facility at Fort Detrick, Division of Clinical Research, National Institute of Allergy and Infectious Diseases, National Institutes of Health, Frederick, Maryland, United States of America.

The filoviruses, Marburg virus (MARV) and Ebola virus, causes severe hemorrhagic fever with high mortality in humans and nonhuman primates. A promising filovirus vaccine under development is based on a recombinant vesicular stomatitis virus (rVSV) that expresses individual filovirus glycoproteins (GPs) in place of the VSV glycoprotein (G). These vaccines have shown 100% efficacy against filovirus infection in nonhuman primates when challenge occurs 28-35 days after a single injection immunization. Here, we examined the ability of a rVSV MARV-GP vaccine to provide protection when challenge occurs more than a year after vaccination. Cynomolgus macaques were immunized with rVSV-MARV-GP and challenged with MARV approximately 14 months after vaccination. Immunization resulted in the vaccine cohort of six animals having anti-MARV GP IgG throughout the pre-challenge period. Following MARV challenge none of the vaccinated animals showed any signs of clinical disease or viremia and all were completely protected from MARV infection. Two unvaccinated control animals exhibited signs consistent with MARV infection and both succumbed. Importantly, these data are the first to show 100% protective efficacy against any high dose filovirus challenge beyond 8 weeks after final vaccination. These findings demonstrate the durability of VSV-based filovirus vaccines.

PMCID: PMC3997383 PMID: 24759889 [PubMed - in process]
843. PLoS One. 2014 Feb 24;9(2):e89735. doi: 10.1371/journal.pone.0089735. eCollection 2014

Toll-like receptor agonist augments virus-like particle-mediated protection from Ebola virus with transient immune activation.

Martins KA(1), Steffens JT(1), van Tongeren SA(1), Wells JB(1), Bergeron AA(1), Dickson SP(2), Dye JM(3), Salazar AM(4), Bavari S(1).

Author information: (1)Molecular and Translational Sciences, United States Army Medical Research Institute of Infectious Diseases, Fort Detrick, Maryland, United States of America. (2)Office of Regulated Studies, United States Army Medical Research Institute of Infectious Diseases, Fort Detrick, Maryland, United States of America. (3)Virology Division, United States Army Medical Research Institute of Infectious Diseases, Fort Detrick, Maryland, United States of America. (4)Oncovir Inc., Washington, DC, United States of America.

Identifying safe and effective adjuvants is critical for the advanced development of protein-based vaccines. Pattern recognition receptor (PRR) agonists are increasingly being explored as potential adjuvants, but there is concern that the efficacy of these molecules may be dependent on potentially dangerous levels of non-specific immune activation. The filovirus virus-like particle (VLP) vaccine protects mice, guinea pigs, and nonhuman primates from viral challenge. In this study, we explored the impact of a stabilized dsRNA mimic, polyICLC, on VLP vaccination of C57BL/6 mice and Hartley guinea pigs. We show that at dose levels as low as 100 ng, the adjuvant increased the efficacy of the vaccine in mice. Antigen-specific, polyfunctional CD4 and CD8 T cell responses and antibody responses increased significantly upon inclusion of adjuvant. To determine whether the efficacy of polyICLC correlated with systemic immune activation, we examined serum cytokine levels and cellular activation in the draining lymph node. PolyICLC administration was associated with increases in TNFα, IL6, MCP1, MIP1α, KC, and MIP1β levels in the periphery and with the activation of dendritic cells (DCs), NK cells, and B cells. However, this activation resolved within 24 to 72 hours at efficacious adjuvant dose levels. These studies are the first to examine the polyICLC-induced enhancement of antigen-specific immune responses in the context of non-specific immune activation, and they provide a framework from which to consider adjuvant dose levels.

PMCID: PMC3933660 PMID: 24586996 [PubMed - in process]
844. Rev Environ Health. 2014;29(3):221-31. doi: 10.1515/reveh-2014-0054.

Environmental airborne contact dermatoses.

Lachapelle JM.

This chapter is complementary to Chapter 4 published in the same series. Airborne contact dermatitis (ABCD) is considered a prototype in the field of environmental dermatology. It is often underestimated in most textbooks of general dermatology, despite its frequent occurrence in daily life. ABCD may be irritant, allergic, phototoxic, or photoallergic. Airborne contact urticaria is another example. A particular clinical aspect is the "head and neck dermatitis", which occurs in atopic adult patients. Occupational ABCD represents a most difficult issue in terms of diagnostic procedures. It is obvious that non-occupational ABCD cases involve similar problems, usually easier to solve, and our comments refer to both conditions. Two examples of potentially airborne skin infections (e.g., anthrax and Ebola virus hemorrhagic fever) are also described because they are closely related to the same problematics. A new example of airborne irritant contact dermatitis, not reported so far, is linked with the use of continuous airway pressure in the treatment of obstructive sleep apnea.

PMID: 25252746 [PubMed - in process]
845. Z Evid Fortbild Qual Gesundhwes. 2014;108(10):604-5. doi: 10.1016/j.zefq.2014.10.026. Epub 2014 Nov 7.

Ebola - contradictions between knowledge and communication.

Antes G(1).

Author information: (1)Director of German Cochrane Centre, Universitätsklinikum Freiburg, Freiburg, Germany. Electronic address: antes@cochrane.de.

PMID: 25499115 [PubMed - in process]
846. J Mol Biol. 2013 Dec 13;425(24):4937-55. doi: 10.1016/j.jmb.2013.09.024. Epub 2013 Sep 25.

IFITMs restrict the replication of multiple pathogenic viruses.

Perreira JM(1), Chin CR, Feeley EM, Brass AL.

Author information: (1)Microbiology and Physiological Systems (MaPS) Department, University of Massachusetts Medical School, Albert Sherman Center 8 1001, 368 Plantation Street, Worcester, MA 01655, USA.

The interferon-inducible transmembrane protein (IFITM) family inhibits a growing number of pathogenic viruses, among them influenza A virus, dengue virus, hepatitis C virus, and Ebola virus. This review covers recent developments in our understanding of the IFITM's molecular determinants, potential mechanisms of action, and impact on pathogenesis.

© 2013.
PMCID: PMC4121887 PMID: 24076421 [PubMed - indexed for MEDLINE]

847. Antiviral Res. 2013 Dec;100(3):615-35. doi: 10.1016/j.antiviral.2013.10.002. Epub 2013 Oct 12.

Strategies of highly pathogenic RNA viruses to block dsRNA detection by RIG-I-like receptors: hide, mask, hit.

Zinzula L(1), Tramontano E.

Author information: (1)Department of Life and Environmental Sciences, University of Cagliari, Cittadella di Monserrato, SS554, 09042 Monserrato (Cagliari), Italy. Electronic address: lucazinzula@unica.it.

Double-stranded RNA (dsRNA) is synthesized during the course of infection by RNA viruses as a byproduct of replication and transcription and acts as a potent trigger of the host innate antiviral response. In the cytoplasm of the infected cell, recognition of the presence of viral dsRNA as a signature of "non-self" nucleic acid is carried out by RIG-I-like receptors (RLRs), a set of dedicated helicases whose activation leads to the production of type I interferon α/β (IFN-α/β). To overcome the innate antiviral response, RNA viruses encode suppressors of IFN-α/β induction, which block RLRs recognition of dsRNA by means of different mechanisms that can be categorized into: (i) dsRNA binding and/or shielding ("hide"), (ii) dsRNA termini processing ("mask") and (iii) direct interaction with components of the RLRs pathway ("hit"). In light of recent functional, biochemical and structural findings, we review the inhibition mechanisms of RLRs recognition of dsRNA displayed by a number of highly pathogenic RNA viruses with different disease phenotypes such as haemorrhagic fever (Ebola, Marburg, Lassa fever, Lujo, Machupo, Junin, Guanarito, Crimean-Congo, Rift Valley fever, dengue), severe respiratory disease (influenza, SARS, Hendra, Hantaan, Sin Nombre, Andes) and encephalitis (Nipah, West Nile).

Copyright © 2013 Elsevier B.V. All rights reserved.
PMID: 24129118 [PubMed - indexed for MEDLINE]

848. BioDrugs. 2013 Dec;27(6):565-83. doi: 10.1007/s40259-013-0046-1.

Emerging targets and novel approaches to Ebola virus prophylaxis and treatment.

Choi JH(1), Croyle MA.

Author information: (1)Division of Pharmaceutics, The University of Texas at Austin, College of Pharmacy, PHR 4.214D, 2409 W. University Ave., 1 University Station #A1920, Austin, TX, 78712-1074, USA.

Ebola is a highly virulent pathogen causing severe hemorrhagic fever with a high case fatality rate in humans and non-human primates (NHPs). Although safe and effective vaccines or other medicinal agents to block Ebola infection are currently unavailable, a significant effort has been put forth to identify several promising candidates for the treatment and prevention of Ebola hemorrhagic fever. Among these, recombinant adenovirus-based vectors have been identified as potent vaccine candidates, with some affording both pre- and post-exposure protection from the virus. Recently, Investigational New Drug (IND) applications have been approved by the US Food and Drug Administration (FDA) and phase I clinical trials have been initiated for two small-molecule therapeutics: anti-sense phosphorodiamidate morpholino oligomers (PMOs: AVI-6002, AVI-6003) and lipid nanoparticle/small interfering RNA (LNP/siRNA: TKM-Ebola). These potential alternatives to vector-based vaccines require multiple doses to achieve therapeutic efficacy, which is not ideal with regard to patient compliance and outbreak scenarios. These concerns have fueled a quest for even better vaccination and treatment strategies. Here, we summarize recent advances in vaccines or post-exposure therapeutics for prevention of Ebola hemorrhagic fever. The utility of novel pharmaceutical approaches to refine and overcome barriers associated with the most promising therapeutic platforms are also discussed.

PMCID: PMC3833964 PMID: 23813435 [PubMed - indexed for MEDLINE]

849. J Virol. 2013 Dec;87(24):13795-802. doi: 10.1128/JVI.02422-13. Epub 2013 Oct 9.

The cytoprotective enzyme heme oxygenase-1 suppresses Ebola virus replication.

Hill-Batorski L(1), Halfmann P, Neumann G, Kawaoka Y.

Author information: (1)Department of Pathobiological Sciences, School of Veterinary Medicine, Influenza Research Institute, University of Wisconsin-Madison, Madison, Wisconsin, USA.

Ebola virus (EBOV) is the causative agent of a severe hemorrhagic fever in humans with reported case fatality rates as high as 90%. There are currently no licensed vaccines or antiviral therapeutics to combat EBOV infections. Heme oxygenase-1 (HO-1), an enzyme that catalyzes the rate-limiting step in heme degradation, has antioxidative properties and protects cells from various stresses. Activated HO-1 was recently shown to have antiviral activity, potently inhibiting the replication of viruses such as hepatitis C virus and human immunodeficiency virus. However, the effect of HO-1 activation on EBOV replication remains unknown. To determine whether the upregulation of HO-1 attenuates EBOV replication, we treated cells with cobalt protoporphyrin (CoPP), a selective HO-1 inducer, and assessed its effects on EBOV replication. We found that CoPP treatment, pre- and postinfection, significantly suppressed EBOV replication in a manner dependent upon HO-1 upregulation and activity. In addition, stable overexpression of HO-1 significantly attenuated EBOV growth. Although the exact mechanism behind the antiviral properties of HO-1 remains to be elucidated, our data show that HO-1 upregulation does not attenuate EBOV entry or budding but specifically targets EBOV transcription/replication. Therefore, modulation of the cellular enzyme HO-1 may represent a novel therapeutic strategy against EBOV infection.

PMCID: PMC3838215 PMID: 24109237 [PubMed - indexed for MEDLINE]

850. J Virol. 2013 Dec;87(24):13141-9. doi: 10.1128/JVI.02564-13. Epub 2013 Sep 25.

Suppression of PACT-induced type I interferon production by herpes simplex virus 1 Us11 protein.

Kew C(1), Lui PY, Chan CP, Liu X, Au SW, Mohr I, Jin DY, Kok KH.

Author information: (1)Department of Biochemistry, Li Ka Shing Faculty of Medicine, The University of Hong Kong, Pokfulam, Hong Kong.

Herpes simplex virus 1 (HSV-1) Us11 protein is a double-stranded RNA-binding protein that suppresses type I interferon production through the inhibition of the cytoplasmic RNA sensor RIG-I. Whether additional cellular mediators are involved in this suppression remains to be determined. In this study, we report on the requirement of cellular double-stranded RNA-binding protein PACT for Us11-mediated perturbation of type I interferon production. Us11 associates with PACT tightly to prevent it from binding with and activating RIG-I. The Us11-deficient HSV-1 was indistinguishable from the Us11-proficient virus in the suppression of interferon production when PACT was compromised. More importantly, HSV-1-induced activation of interferon production was abrogated in PACT knockout murine embryonic fibroblasts. Our findings suggest a new mechanism for viral evasion of innate immunity through which a viral double-stranded RNA-binding protein interacts with PACT to circumvent type I interferon production. This mechanism might also be used by other PACT-binding viral interferon-antagonizing proteins such as Ebola virus VP35 and influenza A virus NS1.

PMCID: PMC3838286 PMID: 24067967 [PubMed - indexed for MEDLINE]

851. Biochem Biophys Res Commun. 2013 Nov 29;441(4):994-8. doi: 10.1016/j.bbrc.2013.11.018. Epub 2013 Nov 12.

Suppression of Fas-mediated apoptosis via steric shielding by filovirus glycoproteins.

Noyori O(1), Nakayama E, Maruyama J, Yoshida R, Takada A.

Author information: (1)Division of Global Epidemiology, Hokkaido University Research Center for Zoonosis Control, Sapporo 001-0020, Japan.

Apoptotic death of virus-infected cells is generally thought to be a defense mechanism to limit the spread of infectious virions by eliminating virus-producing cells in host animals. On the other hand, several viruses have been shown to have anti-apoptotic mechanisms to facilitate efficient viral replication and transmission. In this study, we found that the filovirus glycoprotein (GP) expressed on cell surfaces formed a steric shield over the Fas molecule and that GP-expressing cells showed resistance to cell death induced by a Fas agonistic antibody. These results suggest that filovirus GP-mediated steric shielding may interfere with the Fas-induced apoptotic signal transduction in infected cells and serve as an immune evasion mechanism for filoviruses.

Copyright © 2013 Elsevier Inc. All rights reserved.

PMID: 24239546 [PubMed - indexed for MEDLINE]

852. Sci Rep. 2013 Nov 28;3:3365. doi: 10.1038/srep03365.

Sustained protection against Ebola virus infection following treatment of infected nonhuman primates with ZMAb.

Qiu X(1), Audet J, Wong G, Fernando L, Bello A, Pillet S, Alimonti JB, Kobinger GP.

Author information: (1)National Microbiology Laboratory, Public Health Agency of Canada, Winnipeg, Manitoba R3E 3R2, Canada.

Ebola virus (EBOV) is one of the most lethal filoviruses, with mortality rates of up to 90% in humans. Previously, we demonstrated 100% and 50% survival of EBOV-infected cynomolgus macaques with a combination of 3 EBOV-GP-specific monoclonal antibodies (ZMAb) administered at 24 or 48 hours post-exposure, respectively. The survivors demonstrated EBOV-GP-specific humoral and cell-mediated immune responses. In order to evaluate whether the immune response induced in NHPs during the ZMAb treatment and EBOV challenge is sufficient to protect survivors against a subsequent exposure, animals that survived the initial challenge were rechallenged at 10 or 13 weeks after the initial challenge. The animals rechallenged at 10 weeks all survived whereas 4 of 6 animals survived a rechallenge at 13 weeks. The data indicate that a robust immune response was generated during the successful treatment of EBOV-infected NHPs with EBOV, which resulted in sustained protection against a second lethal exposure.

PMCID: PMC3842534 PMID: 24284388 [PubMed - in process]

853. Biochemistry. 2013 Nov 26;52(47):8406-19. doi: 10.1021/bi400704d. Epub 2013 Nov 14

Development of RNA aptamers targeting Ebola virus VP35.

Binning JM(1), Wang T, Luthra P, Shabman RS, Borek DM, Liu G, Xu W, Leung DW, Basler CF, Amarasinghe GK.

Author information: (1)Department of Pathology and Immunology, Washington University School of Medicine , St. Louis, Missouri 63110, United States.

Viral protein 35 (VP35), encoded by filoviruses, is a multifunctional dsRNA binding protein that plays important roles in viral replication, innate immune evasion, and pathogenesis. The multifunctional nature of these proteins also presents opportunities to develop countermeasures that target distinct functional regions. However, functional validation and the establishment of therapeutic approaches toward such multifunctional proteins, particularly for nonenzymatic targets, are often challenging. Our previous work on filoviral VP35 proteins defined conserved basic residues located within its C-terminal dsRNA binding interferon (IFN) inhibitory domain (IID) as important for VP35 mediated IFN antagonism and viral polymerase cofactor functions. In the current study, we used a combination of structural and functional data to determine regions of Ebola virus (EBOV) VP35 (eVP35) to target for aptamer selection using SELEX. Select aptamers, representing, two distinct classes, were further characterized based on their interaction properties to eVP35 IID. These results revealed that these aptamers bind to distinct regions of eVP35 IID with high affinity (10-50 nM) and specificity. These aptamers can compete with dsRNA for binding to eVP35 and disrupt the eVP35-nucleoprotein (NP) interaction. Consistent with the ability to antagonize the eVP35-NP interaction, select aptamers can inhibit the function of the EBOV polymerase complex reconstituted by the expression of select viral proteins. Taken together, our results support the identification of two aptamers that bind filoviral VP35 proteins with high affinity and specificity and have the capacity to potentially function as filoviral VP35 protein inhibitors.

PMCID: PMC3909728 PMID: 24067086 [PubMed - indexed for MEDLINE]
854. J Am Chem Soc. 2013 Nov 13;135(45):16785-8. doi: 10.1021/ja4085397. Epub 2013 Oct 29

A multistage volumetric bar chart chip for visualized quantification of DNA.

Song Y(1), Wang Y, Qin L.

Author information: (1)Department of Nanomedicine, Houston Methodist Research Institute , Houston, Texas 77030, United States.

Nucleic acid detection is critical in disease diagnosis as well as in the environmental assays of harmful bacteria or viruses and forensic applications. Current methods for visualized quantification of DNA require costly and sophisticated instruments. Here, we report a multistage propelled volumetric bar chart chip (MV-Chip) for multiplexing and quantitative detection of DNA. Because of its "rocket-like" propelling reaction, the predeposited platinum films could perform cascade amplification and detect as low as 20 pM DNA targets after three stages of platinum-catalyzed propulsion. The resulting ink bar charts can be directly read out by the naked eye, and the signal shows little interference from serum. Single-nucleotide polymorphism and multiplex DNA detection were carried out to demonstrate this powerful application.

PMCID: PMC3875332 PMID: 24160770 [PubMed - indexed for MEDLINE]
855. Virol J. 2013 Nov 9;10:331. doi: 10.1186/1743-422X-10-331.

Recombinant lentogenic Newcastle disease virus expressing Ebola virus GP infects cells independently of exogenous trypsin and uses macropinocytosis as the major pathway for cell entry.

Wen Z, Zhao B, Song K, Hu X, Chen W, Kong D, Ge J, Bu Z(1).

Author information: (1)State Key Laboratory of Veterinary Biotechnology, Harbin Veterinary Research Institute, Chinese Academy of Agricultural Sciences, 427 Maduan Street, Harbin 150001, People's Republic of China. zgbu@yahoo.com.

BACKGROUND: Using reverse genetics, we generated a recombinant low-pathogenic LaSota strain Newcastle disease virus (NDV) expressing the glycoprotein (GP) of Ebola virus (EBOV), designated rLa-EBOVGP, and evaluated its biological characteristic in vivo and in vitro. RESULTS: The introduction and expression of the EBOV GP gene did not increase the virulence of the NDV vector in poultry or mice. EBOV GP was incorporated into the particle of the vector virus and the recombinant virus rLa-EBOVGP infected cells and spread within them independently of exogenous trypsin. rLa-EBOVGP is more resistant to NDV antiserum than the vector NDV and is moderately sensitive to EBOV GP antiserum. More importantly, infection with rLa-EBOVGP was markedly inhibited by IPA3, indicating that rLa-EBOVGP uses macropinocytosis as the major internalization pathway for cell entry. CONCLUSIONS: The results demonstrate that EBOV GP in recombinant NDV particles functions independently to mediate the viral infection of the host cells and alters the cell-entry pathway.

PMCID: PMC3826533 PMID: 24209904 [PubMed - indexed for MEDLINE]
856. Immunotherapy. 2013 Nov;5(11):1221-33. doi: 10.2217/imt.13.124.

An update on the use of antibodies against the filoviruses.

Saphire EO(1).

Author information: (1)Department of Immunology & Microbial Science & The Skaggs Institute of Chemical Biology, The Scripps Research Institute, La Jolla, CA 92037, USA. erica@scripps.edu.

Multiple recent, independent studies have confirmed that passively administered antibodies can provide effective postexposure therapy in nonhuman primates after exposure to an otherwise lethal dose of Ebola virus or Marburg virus. In this article, we review composition and performance of the antibody cocktails tested thus far, what is known about antibody epitopes on the viral glycoprotein target and ongoing research questions in further development of such cocktails for pre-exposure or emergency postexposure use.

PMID: 24188676 [PubMed - indexed for MEDLINE]
857. Trends Microbiol. 2013 Nov;21(11):583-93. doi: 10.1016/j.tim.2013.08.001. Epub 2013 Sep 4.

How do filovirus filaments bend without breaking?

Booth TF(1), Rabb MJ, Beniac DR.

Author information: (1)National Microbiology Laboratory, Winnipeg, Canada; Department of Medical Microbiology, University of Manitoba, Winnipeg, Canada. Electronic address: tim_booth@phac-aspc.gc.ca.

Viruses of the Mononegavirales have helical nucleocapsids containing a single-stranded negative-sense RNA genome complexed with the nucleoprotein and several other virus-encoded proteins. This RNA-protein complex acts as the template for replication and transcription during infection. Recent structural data has advanced our understanding of how these functions are achieved in filoviruses, which include dangerous pathogens such as Ebola virus. Polyploid filoviruses package multiple genome copies within strikingly long filamentous viral envelopes, which must be flexible to avoid breakage of the 19kb non-segmented genomic RNA. We review how the structure of filoviruses and paramyxoviruses permits this morphological flexibility in comparison to rhabdoviruses that have short, bullet-shaped virions with relatively rigid envelopes.

PMID: 24011860 [PubMed - indexed for MEDLINE]
858. Virology. 2013 Nov;446(1-2):152-61. doi: 10.1016/j.virol.2013.07.029. Epub 2013 Aug 28.

Differential potential for envelope glycoprotein-mediated steric shielding of host cell surface proteins among filoviruses.

Noyori O(1), Matsuno K, Kajihara M, Nakayama E, Igarashi M, Kuroda M, Isoda N, Yoshida R, Takada A.

Author information: (1)Division of Global Epidemiology, Hokkaido University Research Center for Zoonosis Control, Kita-20, Nishi-10, Kita-ku, Sapporo 001-0020, Japan.

The viral envelope glycoprotein (GP) is thought to play important roles in the pathogenesis of filovirus infection. It is known that GP expressed on the cell surface forms a steric shield over host proteins such as major histocompatibility complex class I and integrin β1, which may result in the disorder of cell-to-cell contacts and/or inhibition of the immune response. However, it is not clarified whether this phenomenon contributes to the pathogenicity of filoviruses. In this study, we found that the steric shielding efficiency differed among filovirus strains and was correlated with the difference in their relative pathogenicities. While the highly glycosylated mucin-like region of GP was indispensable, the differential shielding efficiency did not necessarily depend on the primary structure of the mucin-like region, suggesting the importance of the overall properties (e.g., flexibility and stability) of the GP molecule for efficient shielding of host proteins.

PMID: 24074577 [PubMed - indexed for MEDLINE]

859. Sci Transl Med. 2013 Oct 16;5(207):207ra143. doi: 10.1126/scitranslmed.3006605.

mAbs and Ad-vectored IFN-α therapy rescue Ebola-infected nonhuman primates when administered after the detection of viremia and symptoms.

Qiu X(1), Wong G, Fernando L, Audet J, Bello A, Strong J, Alimonti JB, Kobinger GP.

Author information: (1)Special Pathogens Program, National Microbiology Laboratory, Public Health Agency of Canada, Winnipeg, Manitoba R3E 3R2, Canada.

ZMAb is a promising treatment against Ebola virus (EBOV) disease that has been shown to protect 50% (two of four) of nonhuman primates (NHPs) when administered 2 days post-infection (dpi). To extend the treatment window and improve protection, we combined ZMAb with adenovirus-vectored interferon-α (Ad-IFN) and evaluated efficacy in EBOV-infected NHPs. Seventy-five percent (three of four) and 100% (four of four) of cynomolgus and rhesus macaques survived, respectively, when treatment was initiated after detection of viremia at 3 dpi. Fifty percent (two of four) of the cynomolgus macaques survived when Ad-IFN was given at 1 dpi, followed by ZMAb starting at 4 dpi, after positive diagnosis. The treatment was able to suppress viremia reaching ~10(5) TCID50 (median tissue culture infectious dose) per milliliter, leading to survival and robust specific immune responses. This study describes conditions capable of saving 100% of EBOV-infected NHPs when initiated after the presence of detectable viremia along with symptoms.

PMID: 24132638 [PubMed - indexed for MEDLINE]

860. JAMA. 2013 Oct 2;310(13):1327-8. doi: 10.1001/jama.2013.278188.

Malaria vaccine, Ebola therapy promising in early studies.

Kuehn BM.

PMID: 24084902 [PubMed - indexed for MEDLINE]

861. Biochemistry. 2013 Oct 1;52(39):6779-89. doi: 10.1021/bi401029q. Epub 2013 Sep 19

Fine modulation of the respiratory syncytial virus M2-1 protein quaternary structure by reversible zinc removal from its Cys(3)-His(1) motif.

Esperante SA(1), Noval MG, Altieri TA, de Oliveira GA, Silva JL, de Prat-Gay G.

Author information: (1)Protein Structure-Function and Engineering Laboratory, Fundación Instituto Leloir and IIBA-Conicet , Patricias Argentinas 435, (1405) Buenos Aires, Argentina.

Human respiratory syncytial virus (hRSV) is a worldwide distributed pathogen that causes respiratory disease mostly in infants and the elderly. The M2-1 protein of hRSV functions as a transcription antiterminator and partakes in virus particle budding. It is present only in Pneumovirinae, namely, Pneumovirus (RSV) and Metapneumovirus, making it an interesting target for specific antivirals. hRSV M2-1 is a tight tetramer bearing a Cys3-His1 zinc-binding motif, present in Ebola VP30 protein and some eukaryotic proteins, whose integrity was shown to be essential for protein function but without a biochemical mechanistic basis. We showed that removal of the zinc atom causes dissociation to a monomeric apo-M2-1 species. Surprisingly, the secondary structure and stability of the apo-monomer is indistinguishable from that of the M2-1 tetramer. Dissociation reported by a highly sensitive tryptophan residue is much increased at pH 5.0 compared to pH 7.0, suggesting a histidine protonation cooperating in zinc removal. The monomeric apo form binds RNA at least as well as the tetramer, and this interaction is outcompeted by the phosphoprotein P, the RNA polymerase cofactor. The role of zinc goes beyond stabilization of local structure, finely tuning dissociation to a fully folded and binding competent monomer. Removal of zinc is equivalent to the disruption of the motif by mutation, only that the former is potentially reversible in the cellular context. Thus, this process could be triggered by a natural chelator such as glutathione or thioneins, where reversibility strongly suggests a modulatory role in the participation of M2-1 in the assembly of the polymerase complex or in virion budding.

PMID: 23984912 [PubMed - indexed for MEDLINE]

862. Bioorg Med Chem Lett. 2013 Oct 1;23(19):5356-60. doi: 10.1016/j.bmcl.2013.07.056. Epub 2013 Aug 2.

C-peptide inhibitors of Ebola virus glycoprotein-mediated cell entry: effects of conjugation to cholesterol and side chain-side chain crosslinking.

Higgins CD(1), Koellhoffer JF, Chandran K, Lai JR.

Author information: (1)Department of Biochemistry, Albert Einstein College of Medicine, Bronx, NY 10461, USA.

We previously described potent inhibition of Ebola virus entry by a 'C-peptide' based on the GP2 C-heptad repeat region (CHR) targeted to endosomes ('Tat-Ebo'). Here, we report the synthesis and evaluation of C-peptides conjugated to cholesterol, and Tat-Ebo analogs containing covalent side chain-side chain crosslinks to promote α-helical conformation. We found that the cholesterol-conjugated C-peptides were potent inhibitors of Ebola virus glycoprotein (GP)-mediated cell entry (~10(3)-fold reduction in infection at 40 μM). However, this mechanism of inhibition is somewhat non-specific because the cholesterol-conjugated peptides also inhibited cell entry mediated by vesicular stomatitis virus glycoprotein G. One side chain-side chain crosslinked peptide had moderately higher activity than the parent compound Tat-Ebo. Circular dichroism revealed that the cholesterol-conjugated peptides unexpectedly formed a strong α-helical conformation that was independent of concentration. Side chain-side chain crosslinking enhanced α-helical stability of the Tat-Ebo variants, but only at neutral pH. These result provide insight into mechanisms of C-peptide inhibiton of Ebola virus GP-mediated cell entry.

PMCID: PMC3822755 PMID: 23962564 [PubMed - indexed for MEDLINE]

863. Biotechnol J. 2013 Oct;8(10):1193-202. doi: 10.1002/biot.201300162. Epub 2013 Jul 15

Plant-derived pharmaceuticals for the developing world.

Hefferon K(1).

Author information: (1)Cell and Systems Biology, University of Toronto, Toronto, Ontario, Canada; Cornell University, Ithaca, NY, USA. kathleen.hefferon@utoronto.ca.

Plant-produced vaccines and therapeutic agents offer enormous potential for providing relief to developing countries by reducing the incidence of infant mortality caused by infectious diseases. Vaccines derived from plants have been demonstrated to effectively elicit an immune response. Biopharmaceuticals produced in plants are inexpensive to produce, require fewer expensive purification steps, and can be stored at ambient temperatures for prolonged periods of time. As a result, plant-produced biopharmaceuticals have the potential to be more accessible to the rural poor. This review describes current progress with respect to plant-produced biopharmaceuticals, with a particular emphasis on those that target developing countries. Specific emphasis is given to recent research on the production of plant-produced vaccines toward human immunodeficiency virus, malaria, tuberculosis, hepatitis B virus, Ebola virus, human papillomavirus, rabies virus and common diarrheal diseases. Production platforms used to express vaccines in plants, including nuclear and chloroplast transformation, and the use of viral expression vectors, are described in this review. The review concludes by outlining the next steps for plant-produced vaccines to achieve their goal of providing safe, efficacious and inexpensive vaccines to the developing world.

PMID: 23857915 [PubMed - indexed for MEDLINE]

864. Front Microbiol. 2013 Sep 5;4:267. doi: 10.3389/fmicb.2013.00267.

Animal models for Ebola and Marburg virus infections.

Nakayama E(1), Saijo M.

Author information: (1)Department of Virology 1, National Institute of Infectious Diseases Tokyo, Japan.

Ebola and Marburg hemorrhagic fevers (EHF and MHF) are caused by the Filoviridae family, Ebolavirus and Marburgvirus (ebolavirus and marburgvirus), respectively. These severe diseases have high mortality rates in humans. Although EHF and MHF are endemic to sub-Saharan Africa. A novel filovirus, Lloviu virus, which is genetically distinct from ebolavirus and marburgvirus, was recently discovered in Spain where filoviral hemorrhagic fever had never been reported. The virulence of this virus has not been determined. Ebolavirus and marburgvirus are classified as biosafety level-4 (BSL-4) pathogens and Category A agents, for which the US government requires preparedness in case of bioterrorism. Therefore, preventive measures against these viral hemorrhagic fevers should be prepared, not only in disease-endemic regions, but also in disease-free countries. Diagnostics, vaccines, and therapeutics need to be developed, and therefore the establishment of animal models for EHF and MHF is invaluable. Several animal models have been developed for EHF and MHF using non-human primates (NHPs) and rodents, which are crucial to understand pathophysiology and to develop diagnostics, vaccines, and therapeutics. Rhesus and cynomolgus macaques are representative models of filovirus infection as they exhibit remarkably similar symptoms to those observed in humans. However, the NHP models have practical and ethical problems that limit their experimental use. Furthermore, there are no inbred and genetically manipulated strains of NHP. Rodent models such as mouse, guinea pig, and hamster, have also been developed. However, these rodent models require adaptation of the virus to produce lethal disease and do not mirror all symptoms of human filovirus infection. This review article provides an outline of the clinical features of EHF and MHF in animals, including humans, and discusses how the animal models have been developed to study pathophysiology, vaccines, and therapeutics.

PMCID: PMC3763195 PMID: 24046765 [PubMed]

865. Mol Pharm. 2013 Sep 3;10(9):3342-55. doi: 10.1021/mp4001316. Epub 2013 Aug 19.

Modeling pre-existing immunity to adenovirus in rodents: immunological requirements for successful development of a recombinant adenovirus serotype 5-based ebola vaccine.

Choi JH(1), Schafer SC, Zhang L, Juelich T, Freiberg AN, Croyle MA.

Author information: (1)Division of Pharmaceutics, College of Pharmacy, The University of Texas at Austin , Austin, Texas 78712, United States.

Pre-existing immunity (PEI) to human adenovirus serotype 5 (Ad5) worldwide is the primary limitation to routine clinical use of Ad5-based vectors in immunization platforms. Using systemic and mucosal PEI induction models in rodents (mice and guinea pigs), we assessed the influence of PEI on the type of adaptive immune response elicited by an Ad5-based vaccine for Ebola with respect to immunization route. Splenocytes isolated from vaccinated animals revealed that immunization by the same route in which PEI was induced significantly compromised Ebola Zaire glycoprotein (ZGP)-specific IFN-γ+ CD8+ T cells and ZGP-specific multifunctional CD8+ T cell populations. ZGP-specific IgG1 antibody levels were also significantly reduced and a sharp increase in serum anti-Ad5 neutralizing antibody (NAB) titers were noted following immunization. These immune parameters correlated with poor survival after lethal challenge with rodent-adapted Ebola Zaire virus (ZEBOV). Although the number of IFN-γ+ CD8+ T cells was reduced in animals given the vaccine by a different route from that used for PEI induction, the multifunctional CD8+ T cell response was not compromised. Survival rates in these groups were higher than when PEI was induced by the same route as immunization. These results suggest that antigen-specific multifunctional CD8(+) T cell and Th2 type antibody responses compromised by PEI to Ad5 are required for protection from Ebola. They also illustrate that methods for induction of PEI used in preclinical studies must be carefully evaluated for successful development of novel Ad5-based vaccines.

PMCID: PMC3948217 PMID: 23915419 [PubMed - indexed for MEDLINE]

866. Antimicrob Agents Chemother. 2013 Sep;57(9):4114-27. doi: 10.1128/AAC.02594-12. Epub 2013 Jun 17.

Myxomavirus-derived serpin prolongs survival and reduces inflammation and hemorrhage in an unrelated lethal mouse viral infection.

Chen H(1), Zheng D, Abbott J, Liu L, Bartee MY, Long M, Davids J, Williams J, Feldmann H, Strong J, Grau KR, Tibbetts S, Macaulay C, McFadden G, Thoburn R, Lomas DA, Spinale FG, Virgin HW, Lucas A.

Author information: (1)Divisions of Cardiology and Rheumatology, Department of Medicine, University of Florida, Gainesville, Florida, USA.

Lethal viral infections produce widespread inflammation with vascular leak, clotting, and bleeding (disseminated intravascular coagulation [DIC]), organ failure, and high mortality. Serine proteases in clot-forming (thrombotic) and clot-dissolving (thrombolytic) cascades are activated by an inflammatory cytokine storm and also can induce systemic inflammation with loss of normal serine protease inhibitor (serpin) regulation. Myxomavirus secretes a potent anti-inflammatory serpin, Serp-1, that inhibits clotting factor X (fX) and thrombolytic tissue- and urokinase-type plasminogen activators (tPA and uPA) with anti-inflammatory activity in multiple animal models. Purified serpin significantly improved survival in a murine gammaherpesvirus 68 (MHV68) infection in gamma interferon receptor (IFN-γR) knockout mice, a model for lethal inflammatory vasculitis. Treatment of MHV68-infected mice with neuroserpin, a mammalian serpin that inhibits only tPA and uPA, was ineffective. Serp-1 reduced virus load, lung hemorrhage, and aortic, lung, and colon inflammation in MHV68-infected mice and also reduced virus load. Neuroserpin suppressed a wide range of immune spleen cell responses after MHV68 infection, while Serp-1 selectively increased CD11c(+) splenocytes (macrophage and dendritic cells) and reduced CD11b(+) tissue macrophages. Serp-1 altered gene expression for coagulation and inflammatory responses, whereas neuroserpin did not. Serp-1 treatment was assessed in a second viral infection, mouse-adapted Zaire ebolavirus in wild-type BALB/c mice, with improved survival and reduced tissue necrosis. In summary, treatment with this unique myxomavirus-derived serpin suppresses systemic serine protease and innate immune responses caused by unrelated lethal viral infections (both RNA and DNA viruses), providing a potential new therapeutic approach for treatment of lethal viral sepsis.

PMCID: PMC3754305 PMID: 23774438 [PubMed - indexed for MEDLINE]

867. Antiviral Res. 2013 Sep;99(3):207-13. doi: 10.1016/j.antiviral.2013.05.017. Epub 2013 Jun 7.

A novel Ebola virus expressing luciferase allows for rapid and quantitative testing of antivirals.

Hoenen T(1), Groseth A, Callison J, Takada A, Feldmann H.

Author information: (1)Laboratory of Virology, Division of Intramural Research, National Institute of Allergy and Infectious Diseases, National Institutes of Health, Hamilton, MT, USA. Electronic address: thomas.hoenen@nih.gov.

Ebola virus (EBOV) causes a severe hemorrhagic fever with case fatality rates of up to 90%, for which no antiviral therapies are available. Antiviral screening is hampered by the fact that development of cytopathic effect, the easiest means to detect infection with wild-type EBOV, is relatively slow. To overcome this problem we generated a recombinant EBOV carrying a luciferase reporter. Using this virus we show that EBOV entry is rapid, with viral protein expression detectable within 2 h after infection. Further, luminescence-based assays were developed to allow highly sensitive titer determination within 48 h. As a proof-of-concept for its utility in antiviral screening we used this virus to assess neutralizing antibodies and siRNAs, with significantly faster screening times than currently available wild-type or recombinant viruses. The availability of this recombinant virus will allow for more rapid and quantitative evaluation of antivirals against EBOV, as well as the study of details of the EBOV life cycle.

Published by Elsevier B.V.

PMCID: PMC3787978 PMID: 23751367 [PubMed - indexed for MEDLINE]

868. J Virol. 2013 Sep;87(18):10385-8. doi: 10.1128/JVI.01452-13. Epub 2013 Jul 3.

Ebolavirus VP35 coats the backbone of double-stranded RNA for interferon antagonism.

Bale S(1), Julien JP, Bornholdt ZA, Krois AS, Wilson IA, Saphire EO.

Author information: (1)Department of Immunology and Microbial Science, The Scripps Research Institute, La Jolla, California, USA.

Recognition of viral double-stranded RNA (dsRNA) activates interferon production and immune signaling in host cells. Crystal structures of ebolavirus VP35 show that it caps dsRNA ends to prevent sensing by pattern recognition receptors such as RIG-I. In contrast, structures of marburgvirus VP35 show that it primarily coats the dsRNA backbone. Here, we demonstrate that ebolavirus VP35 also coats the dsRNA backbone in solution, although binding to the dsRNA ends probably constitutes the initial binding event.

PMCID: PMC3753998 PMID: 23824825 [PubMed - indexed for MEDLINE]

869. Mol Biol (Mosk). 2013 Sep-Oct;47(5):707-16.

[Mechanisms of retroviral immunosuppressive domain-induced immune modulation].

[Article in Russian]

[No authors listed]

Immunosuppressive domains (ISD) of viral envelope glycoproteins provide highly pathogenic phenotypes of various retroviruses. ISD interaction with immune cells leads to an inhibition of a response. In the 1980s it was shown that the fragment of ISD comprising of 17 amino acids (named CKS-17) is carrying out such immune modulation. However the underlying mechanisms were not known. The years of thorough research allowed to identify the regulation of Ras-Raf-MEK-MAPK and PI3K-AKT-mTOR cellular pathways as a result of ISD interaction with immune cells. By the way, this leads to decrease of secretion of stimulatory cytokines (e.g., IL-12) and increase of inhibitory, anti-inflammatory ones (e.g., IL-10). One of the receptor tyrosine kinases inducing signal in these pathways acts as the primary target of ISD while other key regulators--cAMP and diacylglycerol (DAG), act as secondary messengers of signal transduction. Immunosuppressive-like domains can be found not only in retroviruses; the presence of ISD within Ebola viral envelope glycoproteins caused extremely hard clinical course of virus-induced hemorrhagic fever. A number of retroviral-origin fragments encoding ISD can be found in the human genome. These regions are expressed in the placenta within genes of syncytins providing a tolerance of mother's immune system to an embryo. The present review is devoted to molecular aspects of retroviral ISD-induced modulation of host immune system.

PMID: 25509343 [PubMed - in process]

870. Virus Res. 2013 Sep;176(1-2):83-90. doi: 10.1016/j.virusres.2013.05.004. Epub 2013 May 20.

Mapping of conserved and species-specific antibody epitopes on the Ebola virus nucleoprotein.

Changula K(1), Yoshida R, Noyori O, Marzi A, Miyamoto H, Ishijima M, Yokoyama A, Kajihara M, Feldmann H, Mweene AS, Takada A.

Author information: (1)School of Veterinary Medicine, The University of Zambia, Great East Road Campus, Lusaka, Zambia.

Filoviruses (viruses in the genus Ebolavirus and Marburgvirus in the family Filoviridae) cause severe haemorrhagic fever in humans and nonhuman primates. Rapid, highly sensitive, and reliable filovirus-specific assays are required for diagnostics and outbreak control. Characterisation of antigenic sites in viral proteins can aid in the development of viral antigen detection assays such immunochromatography-based rapid diagnosis. We generated a panel of mouse monoclonal antibodies (mAbs) to the nucleoprotein (NP) of Ebola virus belonging to the species Zaire ebolavirus. The mAbs were divided into seven groups based on the profiles of their specificity and cross-reactivity to other species in the Ebolavirus genus. Using synthetic peptides corresponding to the Ebola virus NP sequence, the mAb binding sites were mapped to seven antigenic regions in the C-terminal half of the NP, including two highly conserved regions among all five Ebolavirus species currently known. Furthermore, we successfully produced species-specific rabbit antisera to synthetic peptides predicted to represent unique filovirus B-cell epitopes. Our data provide useful information for the development of Ebola virus antigen detection assays.

Copyright © 2013 Elsevier B.V. All rights reserved.

PMCID: PMC3787873 PMID: 23702199 [PubMed - indexed for MEDLINE]

871. Proc Natl Acad Sci U S A. 2013 Aug 27;110(35):14402-7. doi: 10.1073/pnas.1307681110. Epub 2013 Aug 12.

Live-cell imaging of Marburg virus-infected cells uncovers actin-dependent transport of nucleocapsids over long distances.

Schudt G(1), Kolesnikova L, Dolnik O, Sodeik B, Becker S.

Author information: (1)Institut für Virologie, Philipps-Universität Marburg, D-35043 Marburg, Germany.

Transport of large viral nucleocapsids from replication centers to assembly sites requires contributions from the host cytoskeleton via cellular adaptor and motor proteins. For the Marburg and Ebola viruses, related viruses that cause severe hemorrhagic fevers, the mechanism of nucleocapsid transport remains poorly understood. Here we developed and used live-cell imaging of fluorescently labeled viral and host proteins to characterize the dynamics and molecular requirements of nucleocapsid transport in Marburg virus-infected cells under biosafety level 4 conditions. The study showed a complex actin-based transport of nucleocapsids over long distances from the viral replication centers to the budding sites. Only after the nucleocapsids had associated with the matrix viral protein VP40 at the plasma membrane were they recruited into filopodia and cotransported with host motor myosin 10 toward the budding sites at the tip or side of the long cellular protrusions. Three different transport modes and velocities were identified: (i) Along actin filaments in the cytosol, nucleocapsids were transported at ~200 nm/s; (ii) nucleocapsids migrated from one actin filament to another at ~400 nm/s; and (iii) VP40-associated nucleocapsids moved inside filopodia at 100 nm/s. Unique insights into the spatiotemporal dynamics of nucleocapsids and their interaction with the cytoskeleton and motor proteins can lead to novel classes of antivirals that interfere with the trafficking and subsequent release of the Marburg virus from infected cells.

PMCID: PMC3761630 PMID: 23940347 [PubMed - indexed for MEDLINE]

872. Sci Transl Med. 2013 Aug 21;5(199):199ra113. doi: 10.1126/scitranslmed.3006608.

Therapeutic intervention of Ebola virus infection in rhesus macaques with the MB-003 monoclonal antibody cocktail.

Pettitt J(1), Zeitlin L, Kim do H, Working C, Johnson JC, Bohorov O, Bratcher B, Hiatt E, Hume SD, Johnson AK, Morton J, Pauly MH, Whaley KJ, Ingram MF, Zovanyi A, Heinrich M, Piper A, Zelko J, Olinger GG.

Author information: (1)Division of Virology, U.S. Army Medical Research Institute of Infectious Diseases, 1425 Porter Street, Frederick, MD 21702, USA.

Ebola virus (EBOV) remains one of the most lethal transmissible infections and is responsible for high fatality rates and substantial morbidity during sporadic outbreaks. With increasing human incursions into endemic regions and the reported possibility of airborne transmission, EBOV is a high-priority public health threat for which no preventive or therapeutic options are currently available. Recent studies have demonstrated that cocktails of monoclonal antibodies are effective at preventing morbidity and mortality in nonhuman primates (NHPs) when administered as a post-exposure prophylactic within 1 or 2 days of challenge. To test whether one of these cocktails (MB-003) demonstrates efficacy as a therapeutic (after the onset of symptoms), we challenged NHPs with EBOV and initiated treatment upon confirmation of infection according to a diagnostic protocol for U.S. Food and Drug Administration Emergency Use Authorization and observation of a documented fever. Of the treated animals, 43% survived challenge, whereas both the controls and all historical controls with the same challenge stock succumbed to infection. These results represent successful therapy of EBOV infection in NHPs.

PMID: 23966302 [PubMed - indexed for MEDLINE]

873. Cell. 2013 Aug 15;154(4):763-74. doi: 10.1016/j.cell.2013.07.015.

Structural rearrangement of ebola virus VP40 begets multiple functions in the virus life cycle.

Bornholdt ZA(1), Noda T, Abelson DM, Halfmann P, Wood MR, Kawaoka Y, Saphire EO.

Author information: (1)Department of Immunology and Microbial Science, The Scripps Research Institute, La Jolla, CA 92037, USA.

Proteins, particularly viral proteins, can be multifunctional, but the mechanisms behind multifunctionality are not fully understood. Here, we illustrate through multiple crystal structures, biochemistry, and cellular microscopy that VP40 rearranges into different structures, each with a distinct function required for the ebolavirus life cycle. A butterfly-shaped VP40 dimer traffics to the cellular membrane. Once there, electrostatic interactions trigger rearrangement of the polypeptide into a linear hexamer. These hexamers construct a multilayered, filamentous matrix structure that is critical for budding and resembles

157

tomograms of authentic virions. A third structure of VP40, formed by a different rearrangement, is not involved in virus assembly but instead uniquely binds RNA to regulate viral transcription inside infected cells. These results provide a functional model for ebolavirus matrix assembly and the other roles of VP40 in the virus life cycle and demonstrate how a single wild-type, unmodified polypeptide can assemble into different structures for different functions.

PMCID: PMC4138722 PMID: 23953110 [PubMed - indexed for MEDLINE]

874. J Cell Sci. 2013 Aug 1;126(Pt 15):3462-74. doi: 10.1242/jcs.129270. Epub 2013 May 31

Late endosomal transport and tethering are coupled processes controlled by RILP and the cholesterol sensor ORP1L.

van der Kant R(1), Fish A, Janssen L, Janssen H, Krom S, Ho N, Brummelkamp T, Carette J, Rocha N, Neefjes J.

Author information: (1)Division of Cell Biology II, The Netherlands Cancer Institute, Plesmanlaan 121, 1066CX Amsterdam, The Netherlands.

Late endosomes and lysosomes are dynamic organelles that constantly move and fuse to acquire cargo from early endosomes, phagosomes and autophagosome. Defects in lysosomal dynamics cause severe neurodegenerative and developmental diseases, such as Niemann-Pick type C disease and ARC syndrome, yet little is known about the regulation of late endosomal fusion in a mammalian system. Mammalian endosomes destined for fusion need to be transported over very long distances before they tether to initiate contact. Here, we describe that lysosomal tethering and transport are combined processes co-regulated by one multi-protein complex: RAB7-RILP-ORP1L. We show that RILP directly and concomitantly binds the tethering HOPS complex and the p150(Glued) subunit of the dynein motor. ORP1L then functions as a cholesterol-sensing switch controlling RILP-HOPS-p150(Glued) interactions. We show that RILP and ORP1L control Ebola virus infection, a process dependent on late endosomal fusion. By combining recruitment and regulation of both the dynein motor and HOPS complex into a single multiprotein complex, the RAB7-RILP-ORP1L complex efficiently couples and regulates the timing of microtubule minus-end transport and fusion, two major events in endosomal biology.

PMID: 23729732 [PubMed - indexed for MEDLINE]

875. J Virol. 2013 Aug;87(15):8327-41. doi: 10.1128/JVI.01025-13. Epub 2013 May 22.

Role of the phosphatidylserine receptor TIM-1 in enveloped-virus entry.

Moller-Tank S(1), Kondratowicz AS, Davey RA, Rennert PD, Maury W.

Author information: (1)Department of Microbiology, University of Iowa, Iowa City, Iowa, USA.

The cell surface receptor T cell immunoglobulin mucin domain 1 (TIM-1) dramatically enhances filovirus infection of epithelial cells. Here, we showed that key phosphatidylserine (PtdSer) binding residues of the TIM-1 IgV domain are critical for Ebola virus (EBOV) entry through direct interaction with PtdSer on the viral envelope. PtdSer liposomes but not phosphatidylcholine liposomes competed with TIM-1 for EBOV pseudovirion binding and transduction. Further, annexin V (AnxV) substituted for the TIM-1 IgV domain, supporting a PtdSer-dependent mechanism. Our findings suggest that TIM-1-dependent uptake of EBOV occurs by apoptotic mimicry. Additionally, TIM-1 enhanced infection of a wide range of enveloped viruses, including alphaviruses and a baculovirus. As further evidence of the critical role of enveloped-virion-associated PtdSer in TIM-1-mediated uptake, TIM-1 enhanced internalization of pseudovirions and virus-like proteins (VLPs) lacking a glycoprotein, providing evidence that TIM-1 and PtdSer-binding receptors can mediate virus uptake independent of a glycoprotein. These results provide evidence for a broad role of TIM-1 as a PtdSer-binding receptor that mediates enveloped-virus uptake. Utilization of PtdSer-binding receptors may explain the wide tropism of many of these viruses and provide new avenues for controlling their virulence.

PMCID: PMC3719829 PMID: 23698310 [PubMed - indexed for MEDLINE]

876. J Virol. 2013 Aug;87(16):8862-9. doi: 10.1128/JVI.03544-12. Epub 2013 May 8.

DNA topoisomerase I facilitates the transcription and replication of the Ebola virus genome.

Takahashi K(1), Halfmann P, Oyama M, Kozuka-Hata H, Noda T, Kawaoka Y.

Author information: (1)Division of Virology, Department of Microbiology and Immunology, Institute of Medical Science, University of Tokyo, Tokyo, Japan.

Ebola virus (EBOV) protein L (EBOL) acts as a viral RNA-dependent RNA polymerase. To better understand the mechanisms underlying the transcription and replication of the EBOV genome, we sought to identify cellular factors involved in these processes via their coimmunoprecipitation with EBOL and by mass spectrometry. Of 65 candidate proteins identified, we focused on DNA topoisomerase I (TOP1), which localizes to the nucleus and unwinds helical DNA. We found that in the presence of EBOL, TOP1 colocalizes and interacts with EBOL in the cytoplasm, where transcription and replication of the EBOV genome occur. Knockdown of TOP1 markedly reduced virus replication and viral polymerase activity. We also found that the phosphodiester bridge-cleaving and recombination activities of TOP1 are required for the polymerase activity of EBOL. These results demonstrate that TOP1 is an important cellular factor for the transcription and replication of the EBOV genome and, as such, plays a key role in the EBOV life cycle.

PMCID: PMC3754039 PMID: 23658456 [PubMed - indexed for MEDLINE]

877. N Engl J Med. 2013 Aug 1;369(5):492-3. doi: 10.1056/NEJMc1300266.

Persistent immune responses after Ebola virus infection.

Sobarzo A, Ochayon DE, Lutwama JJ, Balinandi S, Guttman O, Marks RS, Kuehne AI, Dye JM, Yavelsky V, Lewis EC, Lobel L.

PMID: 23902512 [PubMed - indexed for MEDLINE]

878. S Afr Med J. 2013 Aug;103(8):500.

Ebola outbreak in Uganda: what we can and can not see from query trends.

Carrillo-Larco RM.

PMID: 24046848 [PubMed - indexed for MEDLINE]

879. Cell Host Microbe. 2013 Jul 17;14(1):74-84. doi: 10.1016/j.chom.2013.06.010.

Mutual antagonism between the Ebola virus VP35 protein and the RIG-I activator PACT determines infection outcome.

Luthra P(1), Ramanan P, Mire CE, Weisend C, Tsuda Y, Yen B, Liu G, Leung DW, Geisbert TW, Ebihara H, Amarasinghe GK, Basler CF.

Author information: (1)Department of Microbiology, Icahn School of Medicine at Mount Sinai School, New York, NY 10029, USA.

Comment in Cell Host Microbe. 2013 Jul 17;14(1):5-6.

The cytoplasmic pattern recognition receptor RIG-I is activated by viral RNA and induces type I IFN responses to control viral replication. The cellular dsRNA binding protein PACT can also activate RIG-I. To counteract innate antiviral responses, some viruses, including Ebola virus (EBOV), encode proteins that antagonize RIG-I signaling. Here, we show that EBOV VP35 inhibits PACT-induced RIG-I ATPase activity in a dose-dependent manner. The interaction of PACT with RIG-I is disrupted by wild-type VP35, but not by VP35 mutants that are unable to bind PACT. In addition, PACT-VP35 interaction impairs the association between VP35 and the viral polymerase, thereby diminishing viral RNA synthesis and modulating EBOV replication. PACT-deficient cells are defective in IFN induction and are insensitive to VP35 function. These data support a model in which the VP35-PACT interaction is mutually antagonistic and plays a fundamental role in determining the outcome of EBOV infection.

PMCID: PMC3875338 PMID: 23870315 [PubMed - indexed for MEDLINE]

880. Cell Host Microbe. 2013 Jul 17;14(1):5-6. doi: 10.1016/j.chom.2013.07.004.

Balance of power in host-virus arms races.

Kok KH(1), Jin DY.

Author information: (1)Department of Biochemistry and State Key Laboratory for Liver Research, The University of Hong Kong, 21 Sassoon Road, Pokfulam, Hong Kong.

Comment on Cell Host Microbe. 2013 Jul 17;14(1):74-84.

The sensing of viral RNA by the host innate immune system is mediated by RIG-I and its partner PACT. In this issue of Cell Host & Microbe, Luthra et al. (2013) show that the Ebola virus VP35 protein counteracts the action of PACT at the cost of compromising its own function in viral replication.

PMID: 23870307 [PubMed - indexed for MEDLINE]

881. J Infect Dis. 2013 Jul 15;208(2):299-309. doi: 10.1093/infdis/jit162. Epub 2013 Apr 12.

Profile and persistence of the virus-specific neutralizing humoral immune response in human survivors of Sudan ebolavirus (Gulu).

Sobarzo A(1), Groseth A, Dolnik O, Becker S, Lutwama JJ, Perelman E, Yavelsky V, Muhammad M, Kuehne AI, Marks RS, Dye JM, Lobel L.

Author information: (1)Department of Virology, Ben-Gurion University of the Negev, Beer-Sheva, Israel.

To better understand humoral immunity following ebolavirus infection, a serological study of the humoral immune response against the individual viral proteins of Sudan ebolavirus (Gulu) in human survivors was performed. An enzyme-linked immunosorbent assay specific for full-length recombinant viral proteins NP, VP30, VP40, and GPI-649 (GP lacking the transmembrane domain) of Sudan ebolavirus (Gulu) was used as well as a plaque reduction neutralization test. Serum samples from human survivors, which were collected up to 10 years following recovery, were screened and analyzed. Results demonstrate that samples obtained 10 years following infection contain virus-specific antibodies that can neutralize virus. Neutralization correlates well with immunoreactivity against the viral proteins NP, VP30, and GPI-649. Sera from individuals who died or those with no documented infection but immunoreactive to ebolavirus did not neutralize. This work provides insight into the duration, profile of immunoreactivity, and neutralization capacity of the humoral immune response in ebolavirus survivors.

PMID: 23585686 [PubMed - indexed for MEDLINE]

882. J Infect Dis. 2013 Jul 15;208(2):310-8. doi: 10.1093/infdis/jis921. Epub 2012 Dec 18

Interferon-β therapy prolongs survival in rhesus macaque models of Ebola and Marburg hemorrhagic fever.

Smith LM(1), Hensley LE, Geisbert TW, Johnson J, Stossel A, Honko A, Yen JY, Geisbert J, Paragas J, Fritz E, Olinger G, Young HA, Rubins KH, Karp CL.

Author information: (1)Whitehead Institute for Biomedical Research, Cambridge, Massachusetts, USA.

There is a clear need for novel, effective therapeutic approaches to hemorrhagic fever due to filoviruses. Ebola virus hemorrhagic fever is associated with robust interferon (IFN)-α production, with plasma concentrations of IFN-α that greatly (60- to 100-fold) exceed those seen in other viral infections, but little IFN-β production. While all of the type I IFNs signal through the same receptor complex, both quantitative and qualitative differences in biological activity are observed after stimulation of the receptor complex with different type I IFNs. Taken together, this suggested potential for IFN-β therapy in filovirus infection. Here we show that early postexposure treatment with IFN-β significantly increased survival time of rhesus macaques infected with a lethal dose of Ebola virus, although it failed to alter mortality. Early treatment with IFN-β also significantly increased survival time after Marburg virus infection. IFN-β may have promise as an adjunctive postexposure therapy in filovirus infection.

PMCID: PMC3685222 PMID: 23255566 [PubMed - indexed for MEDLINE]

883. Virology. 2013 Jul 5;441(2):135-45. doi: 10.1016/j.virol.2013.03.013. Epub 2013 Apr 11.

The L-VP35 and L-L interaction domains reside in the amino terminus of the Ebola virus L protein and are potential targets for antivirals.

Trunschke M(1), Conrad D, Enterlein S, Olejnik J, Brauburger K, Mühlberger E.

Author information: (1)Department of Virology, Philipps University of Marburg, Hans-Meerwein-Strβe 2, 35043 Marburg, Germany.

The Ebola virus (EBOV) RNA-dependent RNA polymerase (RdRp) complex consists of the catalytic subunit of the polymerase, L, and its cofactor VP35. Using immunofluorescence analysis and coimmunoprecipitation assays, we mapped the VP35 binding site on L. A core binding domain spanning amino acids 280-370 of L was sufficient to mediate weak interaction with VP35, while the entire N-terminus up to amino acid 380 was required for strong VP35-L binding. Interestingly, the VP35 binding site overlaps with an N-terminal L homo-oligomerization domain in a non-competitive manner. N-terminal L deletion mutants containing the VP35 binding site were able to efficiently block EBOV replication and transcription in a minigenome system suggesting the VP35 binding site on L as a potential target for the development of antivirals.

PMCID: PMC3773471 PMID: 23582637 [PubMed - indexed for MEDLINE]
884. J Virol. 2013 Jul;87(13):7777-80. doi: 10.1128/JVI.00470-13. Epub 2013 May 1.

Host IQGAP1 and Ebola virus VP40 interactions facilitate virus-like particle egress.

Lu J(1), Qu Y, Liu Y, Jambusaria R, Han Z, Ruthel G, Freedman BD, Harty RN.

Author information: (1)Department of Pathobiology, School of Veterinary Medicine, University of Pennsylvania, Philadelphia, Pennsylvania, USA.

We have identified host IQGAP1 as an interacting partner for Ebola virus (EBOV) VP40, and its expression is required for EBOV VP40 virus-like particle (VLP) budding. IQGAP1 is involved in actin cytoskeletal remodeling during cell migration and formation of filopodia. The physical interaction and the functional requirement for IQGAP1 in EBOV VP40 VLP egress link virus budding to the cytoskeletal remodeling machinery. Consequently, this interaction represents a novel target for development of therapeutics to block budding and transmission of filoviruses.

PMCID: PMC3700276 PMID: 23637409 [PubMed - indexed for MEDLINE]
885. J Virol. 2013 Jul;87(13):7471-85. doi: 10.1128/JVI.03316-12. Epub 2013 Apr 24.

The lack of maturation of Ebola virus-infected dendritic cells results from the cooperative effect of at least two viral domains.

Lubaki NM(1), Ilinykh P, Pietzsch C, Tigabu B, Freiberg AN, Koup RA, Bukreyev A.

Author information: (1)Department of Pathology, University of Texas Medical Branch, Galveston, Texas, USA.

Erratum in J Virol. 2013 Nov;87(22):12506.

Ebola virus (EBOV) infections are characterized by deficient T lymphocyte responses, T lymphocyte apoptosis, and lymphopenia in the absence of direct infection of T lymphocytes. In contrast, dendritic cells (DC) are infected but fail to mature appropriately, thereby impairing the T cell response. We investigated the contributions of EBOV proteins in modulating DC maturation by generating recombinant viruses expressing enhanced green fluorescent protein and carrying mutations affecting several potentially immunomodulating domains. They included envelope glycoprotein (GP) domains, as well as innate response antagonist domains (IRADs) previously identified in the VP24 and VP35 proteins. GP expressed by an unrelated vector, but not the wild-type EBOV, was found to strongly induce DC maturation, and infections with recombinant EBOV carrying mutations disabling GP functional domains did not restore DC maturation. In contrast, each of the viruses carrying mutations disabling any IRAD in VP35 induced a dramatic upregulation of DC maturation markers. This was dependent on infection, but not interaction with GP. Disabling of IRADs also resulted in up to a several hundredfold increase in secretion of cytokines and chemokines. Furthermore, these mutations induced formation of homotypic DC clusters, which represent close correlates of their maturation and presumably facilitate transfer of antigen from migratory DC to lymph node DC. Thus, an individual IRAD is insufficient to suppress DC maturation; rather, the suppression of DC maturation and the "immune paralysis" observed during EBOV infections results from a cooperative effect of two or more individual IRADs.

PMCID: PMC3700277 PMID: 23616668 [PubMed - indexed for MEDLINE]
886. J Virol. 2013 Jul;87(13):7754-7. doi: 10.1128/JVI.00173-13. Epub 2013 Apr 24.

Monoclonal antibodies combined with adenovirus-vectored interferon significantly extend the treatment window in Ebola virus-infected guinea pigs.

Qiu X(1), Wong G, Fernando L, Ennis J, Turner JD, Alimonti JB, Yao X, Kobinger GP.

Author information: (1)Special Pathogens Program, National Microbiology Laboratory, Public Health Agency of Canada, Winnipeg, Manitoba, Canada. xiangguo_qiu@phac-aspc.ga.ca

Monoclonal antibodies (MAbs) are currently a promising treatment strategy against Ebola virus infection. This study combined MAbs with an adenovirus-vectored interferon (DEF201) to evaluate the efficacy in guinea pigs and extend the treatment window obtained with MAbs alone. Initiating the combination therapy at 3 days postinfection (d.p.i.) provided 100% survival, a significant improvement over survival with either treatment alone. The administration of DEF201 within 2 d.p.i. permits later MAb use, with protective efficacy observed up to 8 d.p.i.

PMCID: PMC3700280 PMID: 23616649 [PubMed - indexed for MEDLINE]
887. Mol Ther. 2013 Jul;21(7):1432-44. doi: 10.1038/mt.2013.61. Epub 2013 May 14.

Induction of broad cytotoxic T cells by protective DNA vaccination against Marburg and Ebola.

Shedlock DJ(1), Aviles J, Talbott KT, Wong G, Wu SJ, Villarreal DO, Myles DJ, Croyle MA, Yan J, Kobinger GP, Weiner DB.

Author information: (1)Department of Pathology & Laboratory Medicine, Perelman School of Medicine, University of Pennsylvania, Philadelphia, Pennsylvania, USA.

Marburg and Ebola hemorrhagic fevers have been described as the most virulent viral diseases known to man due to associative lethality rates of up to 90%. Death can occur within days to weeks of exposure and there is currently no licensed vaccine or therapeutic. Recent evidence suggests an important role for antiviral T cells in conferring protection, but little detailed analysis of this response as driven by a protective vaccine has been reported. We developed a synthetic polyvalent-filovirus DNA vaccine against Marburg marburgvirus (MARV), Zaire ebolavirus (ZEBOV), and Sudan ebolavirus (SUDV). Preclinical efficacy studies were performed in guinea pigs and mice using rodent-adapted viruses, whereas murine T-cell responses were extensively analyzed using a novel modified assay described herein. Vaccination was highly potent, elicited robust neutralizing antibodies, and completely protected against MARV and ZEBOV challenge. Comprehensive T-cell analysis revealed cytotoxic T lymphocytes (CTLs) of great magnitude, epitopic breadth, and Th1-type marker expression. This

model provides an important preclinical tool for studying protective immune correlates that could be applied to existing platforms. Data herein support further evaluation of this enhanced gene-based approach in nonhuman primate studies for in depth analyses of T-cell epitopes in understanding protective efficacy.
PMCID: PMC3705942 PMID: 23670573 [PubMed - indexed for MEDLINE]

888. Soc Sci Med. 2013 Jul;88:10-7. doi: 10.1016/j.socscimed.2013.03.017. Epub 2013 Mar 26.

The social and political lives of zoonotic disease models: narratives, science and policy.

Leach M(1), Scoones I.

Author information: (1)STEPS Centre, Institute of Development Studies, University of Sussex, Falmer, Brighton BN1 9RE, UK. m.leach@ids.ac.uk

Zoonotic diseases currently pose both major health threats and complex scientific and policy challenges, to which modelling is increasingly called to respond. In this article we argue that the challenges are best met by combining multiple models and modelling approaches that elucidate the various epidemiological, ecological and social processes at work. These models should not be understood as neutral science informing policy in a linear manner, but as having social and political lives: social, cultural and political norms and values that shape their development and which they carry and project. We develop and illustrate this argument in relation to the cases of H5N1 avian influenza and Ebola, exploring for each the range of modelling approaches deployed and the ways they have been co-constructed with a particular politics of policy. Addressing the complex, uncertain dynamics of zoonotic disease requires such social and political lives to be made explicit in approaches that aim at triangulation rather than integration, and plural and conditional rather than singular forms of policy advice.
PMID: 23702205 [PubMed - indexed for MEDLINE]

889. PLoS One. 2013 Jun 27;8(6):e67584. Print 2013.

Duration of Maternal Antibodies against Canine Distemper Virus and Hendra Virus in Pteropid Bats.

Epstein JH(1), Baker ML, Zambrana-Torrelio C, Middleton D, Barr JA, Dubovi E, Boyd V, Pope B, Todd S, Crameri G, Walsh A, Pelican K, Fielder MD, Davies AJ, Wang LF, Daszak P.

Author information: (1)EcoHealth Alliance, New York, New York, United States of America ; Faculty of Science, Engineering and Computing, Kingston University, Kingston-Upon-Thames, United Kingdom.

Old World frugivorous bats have been identified as natural hosts for emerging zoonotic viruses of significant public health concern, including henipaviruses (Nipah and Hendra virus), Ebola virus, and Marburg virus. Epidemiological studies of these viruses in bats often utilize serology to describe viral dynamics, with particular attention paid to juveniles, whose birth increases the overall susceptibility of the population to a viral outbreak once maternal immunity wanes. However, little is understood about bat immunology, including the duration of maternal antibodies in neonates. Understanding duration of maternally derived immunity is critical for characterizing viral dynamics in bat populations, which may help assess the risk of spillover to humans. We conducted two separate studies of pregnant Pteropus bat species and their offspring to measure the half-life and duration of antibodies to 1) canine distemper virus antigen in vaccinated captive Pteropus hypomelanus; and 2) Hendra virus in wild-caught, naturally infected Pteropus alecto. Both of these pteropid bat species are known reservoirs for henipaviruses. We found that in both species, antibodies were transferred from dam to pup. In P. hypomelanus pups, titers against CDV waned over a mean period of 228.6 days (95% CI: 185.4-271.8) and had a mean terminal phase half-life of 96.0 days (CI 95%: 30.7-299.7). In P. alecto pups, antibodies waned over 255.13 days (95% CI: 221.0-289.3) and had a mean terminal phase half-life of 52.24 days (CI 95%: 33.76-80.83). Each species showed a duration of transferred maternal immunity of between 7.5 and 8.5 months, which was longer than has been previously estimated. These data will allow for more accurate interpretation of age-related Henipavirus serological data collected from wild pteropid bats.
PMCID: PMC3695084 PMID: 23826322 [PubMed - as supplied by publisher]

890. Sci Transl Med. 2013 Jun 19;5(190):190ra79. doi: 10.1126/scitranslmed.3005471.

FDA-approved selective estrogen receptor modulators inhibit Ebola virus infection.

Johansen LM(1), Brannan JM, Delos SE, Shoemaker CJ, Stossel A, Lear C, Hoffstrom BG, Dewald LE, Schornberg KL, Scully C, Lehár J, Hensley LE, White JM, Olinger GG.

Author information: (1)Zalicus Inc., 245 First Street, Cambridge, MA 02142, USA. ljohansen@zalicus.com

Ebola viruses remain a substantial threat to both civilian and military populations as bioweapons, during sporadic outbreaks, and from the possibility of accidental importation from endemic regions by infected individuals. Currently, no approved therapeutics exist to treat or prevent infection by Ebola viruses. Therefore, we performed an in vitro screen of Food and Drug Administration (FDA)- and ex-US-approved drugs and selected molecular probes to identify drugs with antiviral activity against the type species Zaire ebolavirus (EBOV). From this screen, we identified a set of selective estrogen receptor modulators (SERMs), including clomiphene and toremifene, which act as potent inhibitors of EBOV infection. Anti-EBOV activity was confirmed for both of these SERMs in an in vivo mouse infection model. This anti-EBOV activity occurred even in the absence of detectable estrogen receptor expression, and both SERMs inhibited virus entry after internalization, suggesting that clomiphene and toremifene are not working through classical pathways associated with the estrogen receptor. Instead, the response appeared to be an off-target effect where the compounds interfere with a step late in viral entry and likely affect the triggering of fusion. These data support the screening of readily available approved drugs to identify therapeutics for the Ebola viruses and other infectious diseases. The SERM compounds described in this report are an immediately actionable class of approved drugs that can be repurposed for treatment of filovirus infections.
PMCID: PMC3955358 PMID: 23785035 [PubMed - indexed for MEDLINE]

891. Antiviral Res. 2013 Jun;98(3):432-40. doi: 10.1016/j.antiviral.2013.03.023. Epub 2013 Apr 8.

Small molecule inhibitors of ER α-glucosidases are active against multiple hemorrhagic fever viruses.

Chang J(1), Warren TK, Zhao X, Gill T, Guo F, Wang L, Comunale MA, Du Y, Alonzi DS, Yu W, Ye H, Liu F, Guo JT, Mehta A, Cuconati A, Butters TD, Bavari S, Xu X, Block TM.

Author information: (1)Drexel Institute for Biotechnology and Virology Research, Department of Microbiology and Immunology, Drexel University College of Medicine, Doylestown, PA 18902, United States. jinhong.chang@drexelmed.edu

Host cellular endoplasmic reticulum α-glucosidases I and II are essential for the maturation of viral glycosylated envelope proteins that use the calnexin mediated folding pathway. Inhibition of these glycan processing enzymes leads to the misfolding and degradation of these viral glycoproteins and subsequent reduction in virion secretion. We previously reported that, CM-10-18, an imino sugar α-glucosidase inhibitor, efficiently protected the lethality of dengue virus infection of mice. In the current study, through an extensive structure-activity relationship study, we have identified three CM-10-18 derivatives that demonstrated superior in vitro antiviral activity against representative viruses from four viral families causing hemorrhagic fever. Moreover, the three novel imino sugars significantly reduced the mortality of two of the most pathogenic hemorrhagic fever viruses, Marburg virus and Ebola virus, in mice. Our study thus proves the concept that imino sugars are promising drug candidates for the management of viral hemorrhagic fever caused by variety of viruses.

PMCID: PMC3663898 PMID: 23578725 [PubMed - indexed for MEDLINE]
892. Biochem J. 2013 Jun 1;452(2):359-65. doi: 10.1042/BJ20121873.

Ebola virus VP35 induces high-level production of recombinant TPL-2-ABIN-2-NF-κB1 p105 complex in co-transfected HEK-293 cells.

Gantke T(1), Boussouf S, Janzen J, Morrice NA, Howell S, Mühlberger E, Ley SC.

Author information: (1)Division of Immune Cell Biology, MRC National Institute for Medical Research, Mill Hill, London NW7 1AA, UK.

Activation of PKR (double-stranded-RNA-dependent protein kinase) by DNA plasmids decreases translation, and limits the amount of recombinant protein produced by transiently transfected HEK (human embryonic kidney)-293 cells. Co-expression with Ebola virus VP35 (virus protein 35), which blocked plasmid activation of PKR, substantially increased production of recombinant TPL-2 (tumour progression locus 2)-ABIN-2 [A20-binding inhibitor of NF-κB (nuclear factor κB) 2]-NF-κB1 p105 complex. VP35 also increased expression of other co-transfected proteins, suggesting that VP35 could be employed generally to boost recombinant protein production by HEK-293 cells.

PMCID: PMC3727213 PMID: 23557442 [PubMed - indexed for MEDLINE]
893. East Afr J Public Health. 2013 Jun;10(2):397-402.

A descriptive overview of the burden, distribution and characteristics of epidemics in Uganda.

Mayega RW, Musenero M, Nabukenya I, Kiguli J, Bazeyo W.

BACKGROUND: Although Uganda is a high burden country for epidemics of infectious diseases, the pattern of epidemics has not yet been adequately documented. The purpose of this study was to describe the distribution, magnitude and characteristics of recent epidemics in Uganda, as a basis for informing policy on priorities for targeted prevention of epidemics. METHODS: Qualitative and quantitative data was collected from the Epidemiological Surveillance Division of the Ministry of Health and the African Field Epidemiology Network through key informant interviews and a documents review. RESULTS: Acute outbreaks that have occurred since 2002 are: Cholera, Meningitis, Malaria, Viral Hemorrhagic Fevers (Ebola, Marburg), arboviruses (yellow-fever), Anthrax, Hepatitis E, Measles, Polio, Influenza A viruses, dysentery and other diarrheal diseases. Chronic outbreaks include: Propagated epidemics of cholera, head nodding disease, Hepatitis B, Hepatitis E, HIV and Typhoid Fever. Thirty-one districts had a high incidence of cholera. Most of the epidemic prone diseases are preventable through appropriate behavior change and sanitation measures. However, current focus is mainly on prevention, low focus on prevention. Community involvement in resilience and early detection is inadequate. CONCLUSION: Uganda has a high burden of preventable epidemic prone diseases. There is need to invest in surveillance, early detection and sustainable prevention through appropriate technology and behavior change involving individuals, families, communities and policy makers.

PMID: 25130019 [PubMed - indexed for MEDLINE]
894. Biochemistry. 2013 May 21;52(20):3393-404. doi: 10.1021/bi400040v. Epub 2013 May 7

Conformational properties of peptides corresponding to the ebolavirus GP2 membrane-proximal external region in the presence of micelle-forming surfactants and lipids.

Regula LK(1), Harris R, Wang F, Higgins CD, Koellhoffer JF, Zhao Y, Chandran K, Gao J, Girvin ME, Lai JR.

Author information: (1)Department of Biochemistry and ‡Department of Microbiology and Immunology, Albert Einstein College of Medicine , 1300 Morris Park Avenue, Bronx, New York 10461, United States.

Ebola virus and Sudan virus are members of the family Filoviridae of nonsegmented negative-strand RNA viruses ("filoviruses") that cause severe hemorrhagic fever with fatality rates as high as 90%. Infection by filoviruses requires membrane fusion between the host and the virus; this process is facilitated by the two subunits of the envelope glycoprotein, GP1 (the surface subunit) and GP2 (the transmembrane subunit). The membrane-proximal external region (MPER) is a Trp-rich segment that immediately precedes the transmembrane domain of GP2. In the analogous glycoprotein for HIV-1 (gp41), the MPER is critical for membrane fusion and is the target of several neutralizing antibodies. However, the role of the MPER in filovirus GP2 and its importance in membrane fusion have not been established. Here, we characterize the conformational properties of peptides representing the GP MPER segments of Ebola virus and Sudan virus in the presence of micelle-forming surfactants and lipids, at pH 7 and 4.6. Circular dichroism spectroscopy and tryptophan fluorescence indicate that the GP2 MPER peptides bind to micelles of sodium dodecyl sulfate and dodecylphosphocholine (DPC). Nuclear magnetic resonance spectroscopy of the Sudan virus MPER peptide revealed that residues 644-651 interact directly with DPC, and that this interaction enhances the helical conformation of the peptide. The Sudan virus MPER peptide was found to moderately inhibit cell entry by a GP-pseudotyped vesicular stomatitis virus but did not induce leakage of a fluorescent

162

molecule from a large unilammellar vesicle comprised of 1-palmitoyl-2-oleoylphosphatidylcholine or cause hemolysis. Taken together, this analysis suggests the filovirus GP2 MPER binds and inserts shallowly into lipid membranes.

PMCID: PMC3772975 PMID: 23650881 [PubMed - indexed for MEDLINE]

895. Biophys J. 2013 May 7;104(9):1940-9. doi: 10.1016/j.bpj.2013.03.021.

The Ebola virus matrix protein deeply penetrates the plasma membrane: an important step in viral egress.

Soni SP(1), Adu-Gyamfi E, Yong SS, Jee CS, Stahelin RV.

Author information: (1)Department of Biochemistry and Molecular Biology, Indiana University School of Medicine-South Bend, South Bend, Indiana, USA.

Ebola virus, from the Filoviridae family has a high fatality rate in humans and nonhuman primates and to date, to the best of our knowledge, has no FDA approved vaccines or therapeutics. Viral protein 40 (VP40) is the major Ebola virus matrix protein that regulates assembly and egress of infectious Ebola virus particles. It is well established that VP40 assembles on the inner leaflet of the plasma membrane; however, the mechanistic details of VP40 membrane binding that are important for viral release remain to be elucidated. In this study, we used fluorescence quenching of a tryptophan on the membrane-binding interface with brominated lipids along with mutagenesis of VP40 to understand the depth of membrane penetration into lipid bilayers. Experimental results indicate that VP40 penetrates 8.1 Å into the hydrocarbon core of the plasma membrane bilayer. VP40 also induces substantial changes to membrane curvature as it tubulates liposomes and induces vesiculation into giant unilamellar vesicles, effects that are abrogated by hydrophobic mutations. This is a critical step in viral egress as cellular assays demonstrate that hydrophobic residues that penetrate deeply into the plasma membrane are essential for plasma membrane localization and virus-like particle formation and release from cells.

PMCID: PMC3647161 PMID: 23663837 [PubMed - indexed for MEDLINE]

896. Expert Rev Anti Infect Ther. 2013 May;11(5):475-8. doi: 10.1586/eri.13.30.

A novel mechanism of immune evasion mediated by Ebola virus soluble glycoprotein.

Basler CF(1).

Author information: (1)Department of Microbiology, Icahn School of Medicine at Mount Sinai, New York, NY 10029, USA. chris.basler@mssm.edu

Comment on PLoS Pathog. 2012;8(12):e1003065.

Ebola viruses encode two glycoproteins (GPs): a membrane-associated GP that is present in the viral membrane and mediates viral attachment and entry into host cells; and a secreted, nonstructural glycoprotein (sGP) that is identical to GP over approximately 90% of its length. A recent study by Mohan and colleagues attributes a novel immune evasion mechanism dubbed 'antigenic subversion' to sGP. Using DNA immunization in mice, the authors demonstrate that sGP elicits antibodies that crossreact with GP, but these antibodies are non-neutralizing. Coimmunization with sGP plus GP or sequential immunizations with GP and sGP direct the host antibody response toward non-neutralizing epitopes. Therefore, the production of sGP may prevent effective neutralization of the virus during Ebola virus infection, and may reduce the effectiveness of vaccines that rely upon neutralizing antibody responses.

PMID: 23627853 [PubMed]

897. Immunotherapy. 2013 May;5(5):441-3. doi: 10.2217/imt.13.29.

Do therapeutic antibodies hold the key to an effective treatment for Ebola hemorrhagic fever?

Takada A.

PMID: 23638738 [PubMed - indexed for MEDLINE]

898. J Gen Virol. 2013 May;94(Pt 5):1028-38. doi: 10.1099/vir.0.049759-0. Epub 2013 Jan 30.

Coronaviruses in bats from Mexico.

Anthony SJ(1), Ojeda-Flores R, Rico-Chávez O, Navarrete-Macias I, Zambrana-Torrelio CM, Rostal MK, Epstein JH, Tipps T, Liang E, Sanchez-Leon M, Sotomayor-Bonilla J, Aguirre AA, Ávila-Flores R, Medellín RA, Goldstein T, Suzán G, Daszak P, Lipkin WI.

Author information: (1)Center for Infection and Immunity, Mailman School of Public Health, Columbia University, 722 West 168th Street, NY, USA. sja2127@columbia.edu

Bats are reservoirs for a wide range of human pathogens including Nipah, Hendra, rabies, Ebola, Marburg and severe acute respiratory syndrome coronavirus (CoV). The recent implication of a novel beta (β)-CoV as the cause of fatal respiratory disease in the Middle East emphasizes the importance of surveillance for CoVs that have potential to move from bats into the human population. In a screen of 606 bats from 42 different species in Campeche, Chiapas and Mexico City we identified 13 distinct CoVs. Nine were alpha (α)-CoVs; four were β-CoVs. Twelve were novel. Analyses of these viruses in the context of their hosts and ecological habitat indicated that host species is a strong selective driver in CoV evolution, even in allopatric populations separated by significant geographical distance; and that a single species/genus of bat can contain multiple CoVs. A β-CoV with 96.5% amino acid identity to the β-CoV associated with human disease in the Middle East was found in a Nyctinomops laticaudatus bat, suggesting that efforts to identify the viral reservoir should include surveillance of the bat families Molossidae/Vespertilionidae, or the closely related Nycteridae/Emballonuridae. While it is important to investigate unknown viral diversity in bats, it is also important to remember that the majority of viruses they carry will not pose any clinical risk, and bats should not be stigmatized ubiquitously as significant threats to public health.

PMCID: PMC3709589 PMID: 23364191 [PubMed - indexed for MEDLINE]

899. J Virol. 2013 May;87(10):5384-96. doi: 10.1128/JVI.01461-12. Epub 2013 Mar 6.

Ebola virus does not block apoptotic signaling pathways.

Olejnik J(1), Alonso J, Schmidt KM, Yan Z, Wang W, Marzi A, Ebihara H, Yang J, Patterson JL, Ryabchikova E, Mühlberger E.

163

Author information: (1)Department of Microbiology, Boston University School of Medicine, Boston, Massachusetts, USA.

Since viruses rely on functional cellular machinery for efficient propagation, apoptosis is an important mechanism to fight viral infections. In this study, we sought to determine the mechanism of cell death caused by Ebola virus (EBOV) infection by assaying for multiple stages of apoptosis and hallmarks of necrosis. Our data indicate that EBOV does not induce apoptosis in infected cells but rather leads to a nonapoptotic form of cell death. Ultrastructural analysis confirmed necrotic cell death of EBOV-infected cells. To investigate if EBOV blocks the induction of apoptosis, infected cells were treated with different apoptosis-inducing agents. Surprisingly, EBOV-infected cells remained sensitive to apoptosis induced by external stimuli. Neither receptor- nor mitochondrion-mediated apoptosis signaling was inhibited in EBOV infection. Although double-stranded RNA (dsRNA)-induced activation of protein kinase R (PKR) was blocked in EBOV-infected cells, induction of apoptosis mediated by dsRNA was not suppressed. When EBOV-infected cells were treated with dsRNA-dependent caspase recruiter (dsCARE), an antiviral protein that selectively induces apoptosis in cells containing dsRNA, virus titers were strongly reduced. These data show that the inability of EBOV to block apoptotic pathways may open up new strategies toward the development of antiviral therapeutics.

PMCID: PMC3648168 PMID: 23468487 [PubMed - indexed for MEDLINE]
900. J Virol. 2013 May;87(9):4952-64. doi: 10.1128/JVI.03361-12. Epub 2013 Feb 13.

Venezuelan equine encephalitis virus replicon particle vaccine protects nonhuman primates from intramuscular and aerosol challenge with ebolavirus.

Herbert AS(1), Kuehne AI, Barth JF, Ortiz RA, Nichols DK, Zak SE, Stonier SW, Muhammad MA, Bakken RR, Prugar LI, Olinger GG, Groebner JL, Lee JS, Pratt WD, Custer M, Kamrud KI, Smith JF, Hart MK, Dye JM.
Author information: (1)U.S. Army Medical Research Institute of Infectious Diseases, Fort Detrick, Frederick, Maryland, USA.

There are no vaccines or therapeutics currently approved for the prevention or treatment of ebolavirus infection. Previously, a replicon vaccine based on Venezuelan equine encephalitis virus (VEEV) demonstrated protective efficacy against Marburg virus in nonhuman primates. Here, we report the protective efficacy of Sudan virus (SUDV)- and Ebola virus (EBOV)-specific VEEV replicon particle (VRP) vaccines in nonhuman primates. VRP vaccines were developed to express the glycoprotein (GP) of either SUDV or EBOV. A single intramuscular vaccination of cynomolgus macaques with VRP expressing SUDV GP provided complete protection against intramuscular challenge with SUDV. Vaccination against SUDV and subsequent survival of SUDV challenge did not fully protect cynomolgus macaques against intramuscular EBOV back-challenge. However, a single simultaneous intramuscular vaccination with VRP expressing SUDV GP combined with VRP expressing EBOV GP did provide complete protection against intramuscular challenge with either SUDV or EBOV in cynomolgus macaques. Finally, intramuscular vaccination with VRP expressing SUDV GP completely protected cynomolgus macaques when challenged with aerosolized SUDV, although complete protection against aerosol challenge required two vaccinations with this vaccine.

PMCID: PMC3624300 PMID: 23408633 [PubMed - indexed for MEDLINE]
901. Vet Pathol. 2013 May;50(3):514-29. doi: 10.1177/0300985812469636. Epub 2012 Dec 23

Pathology of experimental aerosol Zaire ebolavirus infection in rhesus macaques.

Twenhafel NA(1), Mattix ME, Johnson JC, Robinson CG, Pratt WD, Cashman KA, Wahl-Jensen V, Terry C, Olinger GG, Hensley LE, Honko AN.
Author information: (1)Pathology Division, US Army Medical Research Institute of Infectious Diseases, 1425 Porter St, Fort Detrick, MD 21702-5011, USA.
nancy.twenhafel@us.army.mil

There is limited knowledge of the pathogenesis of human ebolavirus infections and no reported human cases acquired by the aerosol route. There is a threat of ebolavirus as an aerosolized biological weapon, and this study evaluated the pathogenesis of aerosol infection in 18 rhesus macaques. Important and unique findings include early infection of the respiratory lymphoid tissues, early fibrin deposition in the splenic white pulp, and perivasculitis and vasculitis in superficial dermal blood vessels of haired skin with rash. Initial infection occurred in the respiratory lymphoid tissues, fibroblastic reticular cells, dendritic cells, alveolar macrophages, and blood monocytes. Virus spread to regional lymph nodes, where significant viral replication occurred. Virus secondarily infected many additional blood monocytes and spread from the respiratory tissues to multiple organs, including the liver and spleen. Viremia, increased temperature, lymphocytopenia, neutrophilia, thrombocytopenia, and increased alanine aminotransferase, aspartate aminotransferase, γ-glutamyl transpeptidase, total bilirubin, serum urea nitrogen, creatinine, and hypoalbuminemia were measurable mid to late infection. Infection progressed rapidly with whole-body destruction of lymphoid tissues, hepatic necrosis, vasculitis, hemorrhage, and extravascular fibrin accumulation. Hypothermia and thrombocytopenia were noted in late stages with the development of disseminated intravascular coagulation and shock. This study provides unprecedented insight into pathogenesis of human aerosol Zaire ebolavirus infection and suggests development of a medical countermeasure to aerosol infection will be a great challenge due to massive early infection of respiratory lymphoid tissues. Rhesus macaques may be used as a model of aerosol infection that will allow the development of lifesaving medical countermeasures under the Food and Drug Administration's animal rule.

PMID: 23262834 [PubMed - indexed for MEDLINE]
902. PLoS One. 2013 Apr 23;8(4):e61904. doi: 10.1371/journal.pone.0061904. Print 2013.

Immunopathogenesis of severe acute respiratory disease in Zaire ebolavirus-infected pigs.

Nfon CK(1), Leung A, Smith G, Embury-Hyatt C, Kobinger G, Weingartl HM.
Author information: (1)National Center for Foreign Animal Disease, Canadian Food Inspection Agency, Winnipeg, Manitoba, Canada.
Charles.nfon@inspection.gc.ca

Ebola viruses (EBOV) are filamentous single-stranded RNA viruses of the family Filoviridae. Zaire ebolavirus (ZEBOV) causes severe haemorrhagic fever in humans, great apes and non-human primates (NHPs) with high fatality rates. In contrast, Reston ebolavirus (REBOV), the only species found outside Africa, is lethal to some NHPs but has never been linked to clinical disease in humans despite documented exposure. REBOV was isolated from pigs in the Philippines and subsequent experiments confirmed the susceptibility of pigs to both REBOV and ZEBOV with predilection for the lungs. However, only ZEBOV caused severe lung pathology in 5-6 weeks old pigs leading to respiratory distress. To further elucidate the mechanisms for lung pathology, microarray analysis of changes in gene expression was performed on lung tissue from ZEBOV-infected pigs. Furthermore, systemic effects were monitored by looking at changes in peripheral blood leukocyte subsets and systemic cytokine responses. Following oro-nasal challenge, ZEBOV replicated mainly in the respiratory tract, causing severe inflammation of the lungs and consequently rapid and difficult breathing. Neutrophils and macrophages infiltrated the lungs but only the latter were positive for ZEBOV antigen. Genes for proinflammatory cytokines, chemokines and acute phase proteins, known to attract immune cells to sites of infection, were upregulated in the lungs, causing the heavy influx of cells into this site. Systemic effects included a decline in the proportion of monocyte/dendritic and B cells and a mild proinflammatory cytokine response. Serum IgM was detected on day 5 and 6 post infection. In conclusion, a dysregulation/over-activation of the pulmonary proinflammatory response may play a crucial role in the pathogenesis of ZEBOV infection in 5-6 weeks old pigs by attracting inflammatory cells to the lungs.

PMCID: PMC3633953 PMID: 23626748 [PubMed - indexed for MEDLINE]

903. J Biol Chem. 2013 Apr 19;288(16):11165-74. doi: 10.1074/jbc.M113.461285. Epub 2013 Mar 14.

Phosphorylation of Ebola virus VP30 influences the composition of the viral nucleocapsid complex: impact on viral transcription and replication.

Biedenkopf N(1), Hartlieb B, Hoenen T, Becker S.

Author information: (1)Institut für Virologie, Philipps-Universität Marburg, Hans-Meerwein-Str. 2, 35043 Marburg, Germany.

Ebola virus is a non-segmented negative-sense RNA virus causing severe hemorrhagic fever with high fatality rates in humans and nonhuman primates. For transcription of the viral genome four viral proteins are essential: the nucleoprotein NP, the polymerase L, the polymerase cofactor VP35, and VP30. VP30 represents an essential Ebola virus-specific transcription factor whose activity is regulated via its phosphorylation state. In contrast to viral transcription, VP30 is not required for viral replication. Using a minigenome assay, we show that phosphorylation of VP30 inhibits viral transcription while viral replication is increased. Concurrently, phosphorylation of VP30 reciprocally regulates a newly described interaction of VP30 with VP35, and strengthens the interaction with NP. Our results indicate a critical role of VP30 phosphorylation for viral transcription and replication, suggesting a mechanism by which VP30 phosphorylation modulates the composition of the viral polymerase complex presumably forming a transcriptase in the presence of non-phosphorylated VP30 or a replicase in the presence of phosphorylated VP30.

PMCID: PMC3630872 PMID: 23493393 [PubMed - indexed for MEDLINE]

904. J Clin Microbiol. 2013 Apr;51(4):1110-7. doi: 10.1128/JCM.02704-12. Epub 2013 Jan 23

Development of a panel of recombinase polymerase amplification assays for detection of biothreat agents.

Euler M(1), Wang Y, Heidenreich D, Patel P, Strohmeier O, Hakenberg S, Niedrig M, Hufert FT, Weidmann M.

Author information: (1)University Medical Center, Department of Virology, Göttingen, Germany.

Syndromic panels for infectious disease have been suggested to be of value in point-of-care diagnostics for developing countries and for biodefense. To test the performance of isothermal recombinase polymerase amplification (RPA) assays, we developed a panel of 10 RPAs for biothreat agents. The panel included RPAs for Francisella tularensis, Yersinia pestis, Bacillus anthracis, variola virus, and reverse transcriptase RPA (RT-RPA) assays for Rift Valley fever virus, Ebola virus, Sudan virus, and Marburg virus. Their analytical sensitivities ranged from 16 to 21 molecules detected (probit analysis) for the majority of RPA and RT-RPA assays. A magnetic bead-based total nucleic acid extraction method was combined with the RPAs and tested using inactivated whole organisms spiked into plasma. The RPA showed comparable sensitivities to real-time RCR assays in these extracts. The run times of the assays at 42°C ranged from 6 to 10 min, and they showed no cross-detection of any of the target genomes of the panel nor of the human genome. The RPAs therefore seem suitable for the implementation of syndromic panels onto microfluidic platforms.

PMCID: PMC3666764 PMID: 23345286 [PubMed - indexed for MEDLINE]

905. J Gen Virol. 2013 Apr;94(Pt 4):876-83. doi: 10.1099/vir.0.049114-0. Epub 2013 Jan 3

Novel mutations in Marburg virus glycoprotein associated with viral evasion from antibody mediated immune pressure.

Kajihara M(1), Nakayama E, Marzi A, Igarashi M, Feldmann H, Takada A.

Author information: (1)Division of Global Epidemiology, Hokkaido University Research Center for Zoonosis Control, Sapporo 001-0020, Japan.

Marburg virus (MARV) and Ebola virus, members of the family Filoviridae, cause lethal haemorrhagic fever in humans and non-human primates. Although the outbreaks are concentrated mainly in Central Africa, these viruses are potential agents of imported infectious diseases and bioterrorism in non-African countries. Recent studies demonstrated that non-human primates passively immunized with virus-specific antibodies were successfully protected against fatal filovirus infection, highlighting the important role of antibodies in protective immunity for this disease. However, the mechanisms underlying potential evasion from antibody mediated immune pressure are not well understood. To analyse possible mutations involved in immune evasion in the MARV envelope glycoprotein (GP) which is the major target of protective antibodies, we selected escape mutants of recombinant vesicular stomatitis virus (rVSV) expressing MARV GP (rVSVΔG/MARVGP) by using two GP-specific mAbs, AGP127-8 and MGP72-17, which have been previously shown to inhibit MARV budding. Interestingly, several rVSVΔG/MARVGP variants escaping from the mAb pressure-acquired amino acid substitutions in the furin-cleavage site rather than in the mAb-specific epitopes, suggesting that these epitopes are recessed, not exposed on the uncleaved GP molecule, and therefore inaccessible to the mAbs. More surprisingly, some variants escaping mAb MGP72-17 lacked a large proportion of the mucin-like region of GP, indicating that these mutants efficiently escaped the selective pressure by deleting the mucin-like region including the mAb-specific epitope. Our data demonstrate that MARV GP possesses the potential to evade antibody mediated immune pressure due to extraordinary structural flexibility and variability.

PMCID: PMC3709686 PMID: 23288419 [PubMed - indexed for MEDLINE]

906. J Immunol. 2013 Apr 1;190(7):3399-409. doi: 10.4049/jimmunol.1203173. Epub 2013 Mar 4.

The context of gene expression defines the immunodominance hierarchy of cytomegalovirus antigens.

Dekhtiarenko I(1), Jarvis MA, Ruzsics Z, Čičin-Šain L.

Author information: (1)Department of Vaccinology, Helmholtz Center for Infection Research, Braunschweig 38124, Germany.

Natural immunity to CMV dominates the CD4 and CD8 memory compartments of the CMV-seropositive host. This property has been recently exploited for experimental CMV-based vaccine vector strategies, and it has shown promise in animal models of AIDS and Ebola disease. Although it is generally agreed that CMV-based vaccine vectors may induce highly protective and persistent memory T cells, the influence of the gene expression context on Ag-specific T cell memory responses and immune protection induced by CMV vectors is not known. Using murine CMV (MCMV) recombinants expressing a single CD8 T cell epitope from HSV-1 fused to different MCMV genes, we show that magnitude and kinetics of T cell responses induced by CMV are dependent on the gene expression of CMV Ags. Interestingly, the kinetics of the immune response to the HSV-1 epitope was paralleled by a reciprocal depression of immune responses to endogenous MCMV Ags. Infection with a recombinant MCMV inducing a vigorous initial immune response to the recombinant peptide resulted in a depressed early response to endogenous MCMV Ag. Another recombinant virus, which induced a slowly developing "inflationary" T cell response to the HSV-1 peptide, induced weaker long-term responses to endogenous CMV Ags. Importantly, both mutants were able to protect mice from a challenge with HSV-1, mediating strong sterilizing immunity. Our data suggest that the context of gene expression markedly influences the T cell immunodominance hierarchy of CMV Ags, but the immune protection against HSV-1 does not require inflationary CD8 responses against the recombinant CMV-expressed epitope.

PMID: 23460738 [PubMed - indexed for MEDLINE]

907. J Virol. 2013 Apr;87(7):3801-14. doi: 10.1128/JVI.02695-12. Epub 2013 Jan 23.

Ebola virus exploits a monocyte differentiation program to promote its entry.

Martinez O(1), Johnson JC, Honko A, Yen B, Shabman RS, Hensley LE, Olinger GG, Basler CF.

Author information: (1)Icahn School of Medicine at Mount Sinai, New York, New York, USA.

Antigen-presenting cells (APCs) are critical targets of Ebola virus (EBOV) infection in vivo. However, the susceptibility of monocytes to infection is controversial. Studies indicate productive monocyte infection, and yet monocytes are also reported to be resistant to EBOV GP-mediated entry. In contrast, monocyte-derived macrophages and dendritic cells are permissive for both EBOV entry and replication. Here, freshly isolated monocytes are demonstrated to indeed be refractory to ERNV entry. However, EBOV binds monocytes, and delayed entry occurs during monocyte differentiation. Cultured monocytes spontaneously downregulate the expression of viral entry restriction factors such as interferon-inducible transmembrane proteins, while upregulating the expression of critical EBOV entry factors cathepsin B and NPC1. Moreover, these processes are accelerated by EBOV infection. Finally, ectopic expression of NPC1 is sufficient to rescue entry into an undifferentiated, normally nonpermissive monocytic cell line. These results define the molecular basis for infection of APCs and suggest means to limit APC infection.

PMCID: PMC3624207 PMID: 23345511 [PubMed - indexed for MEDLINE]

908. J Virol. 2013 Apr;87(7):3668-77. doi: 10.1128/JVI.02864-12. Epub 2013 Jan 9.

Airway delivery of an adenovirus-based Ebola virus vaccine bypasses existing immunity to homologous adenovirus in nonhuman primates.

Richardson JS(1), Pillet S, Bello AJ, Kobinger GP.

Author information: (1)Special Pathogens Department, National Microbiology Laboratory, Public Health Agency of Canada, Winnipeg, Manitoba, Canada.

Anti-adenovirus serotype 5 antibodies are capable of neutralizing adenovirus serotype 5-based vaccines. In mice and guinea pigs, intranasal delivery of adenovirus serotype 5-based vaccine bypasses induced adenovirus serotype 5 preexisting immunity, resulting in protection against species-adapted Ebola virus challenge. In this study, nonhuman primates were vaccinated with adenovirus serotype 5-based vaccine either intramuscularly or via the airway route (intranasally/intratracheally) in the presence or absence of adenovirus serotype 5 preexisting immunity. Immune responses were evaluated to determine the effect of both the vaccine delivery route and preexisting immunity before and after a lethal Ebola virus (Zaïre strain Kikwit 95) challenge. Intramuscular vaccination fully protected nonhuman primates in the absence of preexisting immunity, whereas the presence of preexisting immunity abrogated vaccine efficacy and resulted in complete mortality. In contrast, the presence of preexisting immunity to adenovirus serotype 5 did not alter the survival rate of nonhuman primates receiving the adenovirus serotype 5-based Ebola virus vaccine in the airway. This study shows that airway vaccination with adenovirus serotype 5-based Ebola virus vaccine can efficiently bypass preexisting immunity to adenovirus serotype 5 and induce protective immune responses, albeit at lower efficacy than that using an intramuscular vaccine delivery route.

PMCID: PMC3624216 PMID: 23302894 [PubMed - indexed for MEDLINE]

909. Traffic. 2013 Apr;14(4):458-69. doi: 10.1111/tra.12046. Epub 2013 Feb 20.

The cytosolic adaptor AP-1A is essential for the trafficking and function of Niemann-Pick type C proteins.

Poirier S(1), Mayer G, Murphy SR, Garver WS, Chang TY, Schu P, Seidah NG.

Author information: (1)Laboratory of Biochemical Neuroendocrinology, Clinical Research Institute of Montreal, Montréal, QC, Canada.

Niemann-Pick type C (NPC) disease is a fatal neurodegenerative disorder characterized by over-accumulation of low-density lipoprotein-derived cholesterol and glycosphingolipids in late endosomes/lysosomes (LE/L) throughout the body. Human mutations in either NPC1 or NPC2 genes have been directly associated with impaired cholesterol efflux from LE/L. Independent from its role in cholesterol homeostasis and its NPC2 partner, NPC1 was unexpectedly identified as a critical player controlling intracellular entry of filoviruses such as Ebola. In this study, a yeast three-hybrid system revealed that the NPC1 cytoplasmic tail directly interacts with the clathrin adaptor protein AP-1 via its acidic/di-leucine motif. Consequently, a nonfunctional AP-1A cytosolic complex resulted in a typical NPC-like phenotype mainly due to a direct impairment of NPC1 trafficking to LE/L and a partial secretion of NPC2. Furthermore, the mislocalization of

NPCl was not due to cholesterol accumulation in LE/L, as it was not rescued upon treatment with Mβ-cyclodextrin, which almost completely eliminated intracellular free cholesterol. Our cumulative data demonstrate that the cytosolic clathrin adaptor AP-IA is essential for the lysosomal targeting and function of NPCl and NPC2.

PMCID: PMC3607445 PMID: 23350547 [PubMed - indexed for MEDLINE]
910. Virol Sin. 2013 Apr;28(2):71-80. doi: 10.1007/s12250-013-3313-x. Epub 2013 Apr 11

Human monoclonal antibodies as candidate therapeutics against emerging viruses and HIV-1.

Zhu Z(1), Prabakaran P, Chen W, Broder CC, Gong R, Dimitrov DS.

Author information: (1)Protein Interactions Group, National Cancer Institute, National Institutes of Health, Frederick, MD 21702, USA.

More than 40 monoclonal antibodies (mAbs) have been approved for a number of disease indications with only one of these (Synagis) - for a viral disease, and not for therapy but for prevention. However, in the last decade novel potent mAbs have been discovered and characterized with potential as therapeutics against viruses of major importance for public health and biosecurity including Hendra virus (HeV), Nipah virus (NiV), severe acute respiratory syndrome coronavirus (SARS-CoV), Ebola virus (EBOV), West Nile virus (WNV), influenza virus (IFV) and human immunodeficiency virus type I (HIV-1). Here, we review such mAbs with an emphasis on antibodies of human origin, and highlight recent results as well as technologies and mechanisms related to their potential as therapeutics.

PMID: 23575729 [PubMed - indexed for MEDLINE]
911. Chem Biol. 2013 Mar 21;20(3):424-33. doi: 10.1016/j.chembiol.2013.02.011.

Identification of a broad-spectrum inhibitor of viral RNA synthesis: validation of a prototype virus-based approach.

Filone CM(1), Hodges EN, Honeyman B, Bushkin GG, Boyd K, Platt A, Ni F, Strom K, Hensley L, Snyder JK, Connor JH.

Author information: (1)Department of Microbiology, School of Medicine, Boston University, Boston, MA 02118, USA.

There are no approved therapeutics for the most deadly nonsegmented negative-strand (NNS) RNA viruses, including Ebola (EBOV). To identify chemical scaffolds for the development of broad-spectrum antivirals, we undertook a prototype-based lead identification screen. Using the prototype NNS virus, vesicular stomatitis virus (VSV), multiple inhibitory compounds were identified. Three compounds were investigated for broad-spectrum activity and inhibited EBOV infection. The most potent, CMLDBU3402, was selected for further study. CMLDBU3402 did not show significant activity against segmented negative-strand RNA viruses, suggesting proscribed broad-spectrum activity. Mechanistic analysis indicated that CMLDBU3402 blocked VSV viral RNA synthesis and inhibited EBOV RNA transcription, demonstrating a consistent mechanism of action against genetically distinct viruses. The identification of this chemical backbone as a broad-spectrum inhibitor of viral RNA synthesis offers significant potential for the development of new therapies for highly pathogenic viruses.

PMCID: PMC3712830 PMID: 23521799 [PubMed - indexed for MEDLINE]
912. Med Res Rev. 2013 Mar 11. doi: 10.1002/med.21281. [Epub ahead of print]

A Cutting-Edge View on the Current State of Antiviral Drug Development.

De Clercq E(1).

Author information: (1)Rega Institute for Medical Research, KU Leuven, B-3000, Leuven, Belgium.

Prominent in the current stage of antiviral drug development are: (i) for human immunodeficiency virus (HIV), the use of fixed-dose combinations (FDCs), the most recent example being Stribild(TM) ; (ii) for hepatitis C virus (HCV), the pleiade of direct-acting antivirals (DAAs) that should be formulated in the most appropriate combinations so as to obtain a cure of the infection; (iii)-(v) new strategies (i.e., AIC316, AIC246, and FV-100) for the treatment of herpesvirus infections: herpes simplex virus (HSV), cytomegalovirus (CMV), and varicella-zoster virus (VZV), respectively; (vi) the role of a new tenofovir prodrug, tenofovir alafenamide (TAF) (GS-7340) for the treatment of HIV infections; (vii) the potential use of poxvirus inhibitors (CMX001 and ST-246); (viii) the usefulness of new influenza virus inhibitors (peramivir and laninamivir octanoate); (ix) the position of the hepatitis B virus (HBV) inhibitors [lamivudine, adefovir dipivoxil, entecavir, telbivudine, and tenofovir disoproxil fumarate (TDF)]; and (x) the potential of new compounds such as FGI-103, FGI-104, FGI-106, dUY11, and LJ-001 for the treatment of filoviruses (i.e., Ebola). Whereas for HIV and HCV therapy is aimed at multiple-drug combinations, for all other viruses, HSV, CMV, VZV, pox, influenza, HBV, and filoviruses, current strategies are based on the use of single compounds.

PMID: 23495004 [PubMed - as supplied by publisher]
913. Bing Du Xue Bao. 2013 Mar;29(2):233-7.

[Research progress on ebola virus glycoprotein].

[Article in Chinese]

Ding GY(1), Wang ZY, Gao L, Jiang BF.

Author information: (1)School of Public Health, Taishan Medical College, Taian 271016, China. dgy153@126.com

Ebola virus (EBOV) causes outbreaks of a highly lethal hemorrhagic fever in humans and there are no effective therapeutic or prophylactic treatments available. The glycoprotein (GP) of EBOV is a transmembrane envelope protein known to play multiple functions including virus attachment and entry, cell rounding and cytotoxicity, down-regulation of host surface proteins, and enhancement of virus assembly and budding. GP is the primary target of protective immunity and the key target for developing neutralizing antibodies. In this paper, the research progress on genetic structure, pathogenesis and immunogenicity of EBOV GP in the last 5 years is reviewed.

PMID: 23757858 [PubMed - indexed for MEDLINE]
914. J Hosp Infect. 2013 Mar;83(3):185-92. doi: 10.1016/j.jhin.2012.10.013. Epub 2013 Jan 16.

Viral haemorrhagic fevers in healthcare settings.

Ftika L(1), Maltezou HC.

Author information: (1)Department for Interventions in Healthcare Facilities, Hellenic Centre for Disease Control and Prevention, Athens, Greece.

Viral haemorrhagic fevers (VHFs) typically manifest as rapidly progressing acute febrile syndromes with profound haemorrhagic manifestations and very high fatality rates. VHFs that have the potential for human-to-human transmission and onset of large nosocomial outbreaks include Crimean-Congo haemorrhagic fever, Ebola haemorrhagic fever, Marburg haemorrhagic fever and Lassa fever. Nosocomial outbreaks of VHFs are increasingly reported nowadays, which likely reflects the dynamics of emergence of VHFs. Such outbreaks are associated with an enormous impact in terms of human lives and costs for the management of cases, contact tracing and containment. Surveillance, diagnostic capacity, infection control and the overall preparedness level for management of a hospital-based VHF event are very limited in most endemic countries. Diagnostic capacities for VHFs should increase in the field and become affordable. Availability of appropriate protective equipment and education of healthcare workers about safe clinical practices and infection control is the mainstay for the prevention of nosocomial spread of VHFs.

PMID: 23333147 [PubMed - indexed for MEDLINE]
915. J Virol. 2013 Mar;87(6):3324-34. doi: 10.1128/JVI.01598-12. Epub 2013 Jan 9.

A mutation in the Ebola virus envelope glycoprotein restricts viral entry in a host species- and cell-type-specific manner.

Martinez O(1), Ndungo E, Tantral L, Miller EH, Leung LW, Chandran K, Basler CF.

Author information: (1)Icahn School of Medicine at Mount Sinai, New York, NY, USA.

Zaire Ebola virus (EBOV) is a zoonotic pathogen that causes severe hemorrhagic fever in humans. A single viral glycoprotein (GP) mediates viral attachment and entry. Here, virus-like particle (VLP)-based entry assays demonstrate that a GP mutant, GP-F88A, which is defective for entry into a variety of human cell types, including antigen-presenting cells (APCs), such as macrophages and dendritic cells, can mediate viral entry into mouse CD11b(+) APCs. Like that of wild-type GP (GP-wt), GP-F88A-mediated entry occurs via a macropinocytosis-related pathway and requires endosomal cysteine proteases and an intact fusion peptide. Several additional hydrophobic residues lie in close proximity to GP-F88, including L111, I113, L122, and F225. GP mutants in which these residues are mutated to alanine displayed preferential and often impaired entry into several cell types, although not in a species-specific manner. Niemann-Pick C1 (NPC1) protein is an essential filovirus receptor that binds directly to GP. Overexpression of NPC1 was recently demonstrated to rescue GP-F88A-mediated entry. A quantitative enzyme-linked immunosorbent assay (ELISA) demonstrated that while the F88A mutation impairs GP binding to human NPC1 by 10-fold, it has little impact on GP binding to mouse NPC1. Interestingly, not all mouse macrophage cell lines permit GP-F88A entry. The IC-21 cell line was permissive, whereas RAW 264.7 cells were not. Quantitative reverse transcription (RT)-PCR assays demonstrate higher NPC1 levels in GP-F88A permissive IC-21 cells and mouse peritoneal macrophages than in RAW 264.7 cells. Cumulatively, these studies suggest an important role for NPC1 in the differential entry of GP-F88A into mouse versus human APCs.

PMCID: PMC3592116 PMID: 23302883 [PubMed - indexed for MEDLINE]
916. J Virol. 2013 Mar;87(5):2735-43. doi: 10.1128/JVI.03015-12. Epub 2012 Dec 19.

ZAP inhibits murine gammaherpesvirus 68 ORF64 expression and is antagonized by RTA.

Xuan Y(1), Gong D, Qi J, Han C, Deng H, Gao G.

Author information: (1)CAS Key Laboratory of Infection and Immunity, Institute of Biophysics, Chinese Academy of Sciences, Chaoyang District, Beijing, China.

Zinc finger antiviral protein (ZAP) is an interferon-inducible host antiviral factor that specifically inhibits the replication of certain viruses, including HIV-1 and Ebola virus. ZAP functions as a dimer formed through intermolecular interactions of its N-terminal tails. ZAP binds directly to specific viral mRNAs and inhibits their expression by repressing translation and/or promoting degradation of the target mRNA. ZAP is not a universal antiviral factor, since some viruses grow normally in ZAP-expressing cells. It is not fully understood what determines whether a virus is susceptible to ZAP. We explored the interaction between ZAP and murine gammaherpesvirus 68 (MHV-68), whose life cycle has latent and lytic phases. We previously reported that ZAP inhibits the expression of M2, which is expressed mainly in the latent phase, and regulates MHV-68 latency in cultured cells. Here, we report that ZAP inhibits the expression of ORF64, a tegument protein that is expressed in the lytic phase and is essential for lytic replication. MHV-68 infection induced ZAP expression. However, ZAP did not inhibit lytic replication of MHV-68. We provide evidence showing that the antiviral activity of ZAP is antagonized by MHV-68 RTA, a critical viral transactivator expressed in the lytic phase. We further show that RTA inhibits the antiviral activity of ZAP by disrupting the N-terminal intermolecular interaction of ZAP. Our results provide an example of how a virus can escape ZAP-mediated immunity.

PMCID: PMC3571413 PMID: 23255809 [PubMed - indexed for MEDLINE]
917. J Virol. 2013 Mar;87(5):2608-16. doi: 10.1128/JVI.03118-12. Epub 2012 Dec 19.

Molecular evolution of viruses of the family Filoviridae based on 97 whole-genome sequences.

Carroll SA(1), Towner JS, Sealy TK, McMullan LK, Khristova ML, Burt FJ, Swanepoel R, Rollin PE, Nichol ST.

Author information: (1)Viral Special Pathogens Branch, Centers for Disease Control and Prevention, Atlanta, Georgia, USA.

Viruses in the Ebolavirus and Marburgvirus genera (family Filoviridae) have been associated with large outbreaks of hemorrhagic fever in human and nonhuman primates. The first documented cases occurred in primates over 45 years ago, but the amount of virus genetic diversity detected within bat populations, which have recently been identified as potential reservoir hosts, suggests that the filoviruses are much older. Here, detailed Bayesian coalescent phylogenetic analyses are performed on 97 whole-genome sequences, 55 of which are newly reported, to comprehensively examine molecular evolutionary rates and estimate dates of common ancestry for viruses within the family Filoviridae. Molecular evolutionary rates for viruses belonging to different species range from $0.46 \times 10(-4)$ nucleotide substitutions/site/year for Sudan ebolavirus to $8.21 \times 10(-4)$ nucleotide substitutions/site/year for Reston ebolavirus. Most recent common ancestry can be traced back only within the last 50 years for Reston ebolavirus and Zaire ebolavirus species and suggests that viruses within these species may have undergone recent genetic bottlenecks. Viruses within Marburg marburgvirus and Sudan ebolavirus species can be traced back further and share most recent common ancestors approximately 700 and 850 years before the present, respectively. Examination of the whole family suggests that members of the Filoviridae, including the recently described Lloviu virus, shared a most recent common ancestor approximately 10,000 years ago. These data will be valuable for understanding the evolution of filoviruses in the context of natural history as new reservoir hosts are identified and, further, for determining mechanisms of emergence, pathogenicity, and the ongoing threat to public health.

PMCID: PMC3571414 PMID: 23255795 [PubMed - indexed for MEDLINE]

918. Mol Biol Evol. 2013 Mar;30(3):669-88. doi: 10.1093/molbev/mss258. Epub 2012 Dec 11.

Bayesian selection of nucleotide substitution models and their site assignments.

Wu CH(1), Suchard MA, Drummond AJ.

Author information: (1)Department of Computer Science, University of Auckland, Auckland, New Zealand.

Probabilistic inference of a phylogenetic tree from molecular sequence data is predicated on a substitution model describing the relative rates of change between character states along the tree for each site in the multiple sequence alignment. Commonly, one assumes that the substitution model is homogeneous across sites within large partitions of the alignment, assigns these partitions a priori, and then fixes their underlying substitution model to the best-fitting model from a hierarchy of named models. Here, we introduce an automatic model selection and model averaging approach within a Bayesian framework that simultaneously estimates the number of partitions, the assignment of sites to partitions, the substitution model for each partition, and the uncertainty in these selections. This new approach is implemented as an add-on to the BEAST 2 software platform. We find that this approach dramatically improves the fit of the nucleotide substitution model compared with existing approaches, and we show, using a number of example data sets, that as many as nine partitions are required to explain the heterogeneity in nucleotide substitution process across sites in a single gene analysis. In some instances, this improved modeling of the substitution process can have a measurable effect on downstream inference, including the estimated phylogeny, relative divergence times, and effective population size histories.

PMCID: PMC3563969 PMID: 23233462 [PubMed - indexed for MEDLINE]

919. PLoS Pathog. 2013 Mar;9(3):e1003232. doi: 10.1371/journal.ppat.1003232. Epub 2013 Mar 28.

TIM-family proteins promote infection of multiple enveloped viruses through virion-associated phosphatidylserine.

Jemielity S(1), Wang JJ, Chan YK, Ahmed AA, Li W, Monahan S, Bu X, Farzan M, Freeman GJ, Umetsu DT, Dekruyff RH, Choe H.

Author information: (1)Division of Respiratory Diseases Children's Hospital Boston, Harvard Medical School, Boston, Massachusetts, United States of America.

Human T-cell Immunoglobulin and Mucin-domain containing proteins (TIM1, 3, and 4) specifically bind phosphatidylserine (PS). TIM1 has been proposed to serve as a cellular receptor for hepatitis A virus and Ebola virus and as an entry factor for dengue virus. Here we show that TIM1 promotes infection of retroviruses and virus-like particles (VLPs) pseudotyped with a range of viral entry proteins, in particular those from the filovirus, flavivirus, New World arenavirus and alphavirus families. TIM1 also robustly enhanced the infection of replication-competent viruses from the same families, including dengue, Tacaribe, Sindbis and Ross River viruses. All interactions between TIM1 and pseudoviruses or VLPs were PS-mediated, as demonstrated with liposome blocking and TIM1 mutagenesis experiments. In addition, other PS-binding proteins, such as Axl and TIM4, promoted infection similarly to TIM1. Finally, the blocking of PS receptors on macrophages inhibited the entry of Ebola VLPs, suggesting that PS receptors can contribute to infection in physiologically relevant cells. Notably, infection mediated by the entry proteins of Lassa fever virus, influenza A virus and SARS coronavirus was largely unaffected by TIM1 expression. Taken together our data show that TIM1 and related PS-binding proteins promote infection of diverse families of enveloped viruses, and may therefore be useful targets for broad-spectrum antiviral therapies.

PMCID: PMC3610696 PMID: 23555248 [PubMed - indexed for MEDLINE]

920. J Biol Chem. 2013 Feb 22;288(8):5779-89. doi: 10.1074/jbc.M112.443960. Epub 2013 Jan 6.

The Ebola virus matrix protein penetrates into the plasma membrane: a key step in viral protein 40 (VP40) oligomerization and viral egress.

Adu-Gyamfi E(1), Soni SP, Xue Y, Digman MA, Gratton E, Stahelin RV.

Author information: (1)Department of Chemistry and Biochemistry, the Eck Institute for Global Health, and the Center for Rare and Neglected Diseases, University of Notre Dame, South Bend, Indiana 46556, USA.

Ebola, a fatal virus in humans and non-human primates, has no Food and Drug Administration-approved vaccines or therapeutics. The virus from the Filoviridae family causes hemorrhagic fever, which rapidly progresses and in some cases has a fatality rate near 90%. The Ebola genome encodes seven genes, the most abundantly expressed of which is viral protein 40 (VP40), the major Ebola matrix protein that regulates assembly and egress of the virus. It is well established that VP40 assembles on the inner leaflet of the plasma membrane; however, the mechanistic details of plasma membrane association by VP40 are not well understood. In this study, we used an array of biophysical experiments and cellular assays along with mutagenesis of VP40 to investigate the role of membrane penetration in VP40 assembly and egress. Here we demonstrate that VP40 is able to penetrate specifically into the plasma membrane through an interface enriched in hydrophobic residues in its C-terminal domain. Mutagenesis of this hydrophobic region consisting of Leu(213), Ile(293), Leu(295), and Val(298) demonstrated that membrane penetration is critical to plasma membrane localization, VP40 oligomerization, and viral particle egress. Taken together, VP40 membrane penetration is an important step in the plasma membrane localization of the matrix protein where oligomerization and budding are defective in the absence of key hydrophobic interactions with the membrane.

PMCID: PMC3581432 PMID: 23297401 [PubMed - indexed for MEDLINE]

921. ACS Med Chem Lett. 2013 Feb 14;4(2):239-243. Epub 2012 Dec 19.

Inhibition of Ebola Virus Infection: Identification of Niemann-Pick C1 as the Target by Optimization of a Chemical Probe.

Lee K(1), Ren T, Côté M, Gholamreza B, Misasi J, Bruchez A, Cunningham J.

Author information: (1)New England Regional Center of Excellence for Biodefense and Emerging Infectious Diseases, Harvard Medical School, Boston, Massachusetts 02115, USA.

A high throughput screen identified adamantane dipeptide 1 as an inhibitor of Ebola virus (EboV) infection. Hit-to-lead optimization to determine the structure-activity relationship (SAR) identified the more potent EboV inhibitor 2 and a photoaffinity labeling agent 3. These anti-viral compounds were employed to identify the target as Niemann-Pick C1 (NPC1), a host protein that binds the EboV glycoprotein and is essential for infection. These studies establish NPC1 as a promising target for anti-viral therapy.

PMCID: PMC3601783 PMID: 23526644 [PubMed]

922. Biomacromolecules. 2013 Feb 11;14(2):431-7. doi: 10.1021/bm3016658. Epub 2013 Jan 10

Glycofullerenes inhibit viral infection.

Luczkowiak J(1), Muñoz A, Sánchez-Navarro M, Ribeiro-Viana R, Ginieis A, Illescas BM, Martín N, Delgado R, Rojo J.

Author information: (1)Glycosystems Laboratory, Instituto de Investigaciones Químicas (IIQ), CSIC-Universidad de Sevilla, Av. Américo Vespucio 49, Seville, Spain.

Water-soluble glycofullerenes based on a hexakis-adduct of [60]fullerene with an octahedral addition pattern are very attractive compounds providing a spherical presentation of carbohydrates. These tools have been recently described and they have been used to interact with lectins in a multivalent manner. Here, we present the use of these glycofullerenes, including new members with 36 mannoses, as compounds able to inhibit a DC-SIGN-dependent cell infection by pseudotyped viral particles. The results obtained in these experiments demonstrate for the first time that these glycoconjugates are adequate to inhibit efficiently an infection process, and therefore, they can be considered as very promising and interesting tools to interfere in biological events where lectins such as DC-SIGN are involved.

PMID: 23281578 [PubMed - indexed for MEDLINE]

923. Antiviral Res. 2013 Feb;97(2):108-11. doi: 10.1016/j.antiviral.2012.11.003. Epub 2012 Nov 16.

Catheterized guinea pigs infected with Ebola Zaire virus allows safer sequential sampling to determine the pharmacokinetic profile of a phosphatidylserine-targeting monoclonal antibody.

Dowall S(1), Taylor I, Yeates P, Smith L, Rule A, Easterbrook L, Bruce C, Cook N, Corbin-Lickfett K, Empig C, Schlunegger K, Graham V, Dennis M, Hewson R.

Author information: (1)Health Protection Agency, Porton Down, Salisbury, Wiltshire, UK. stuart.dowall@hpa.org.uk

Sequential sampling from animals challenged with highly pathogenic organisms, such as haemorrhagic fever viruses, is required for many pharmaceutical studies. Using the guinea pig model of Ebola virus infection, a catheterized system was used which had the benefits of allowing repeated sampling of the same cohort of animals, and also a reduction in the use of sharps at high biological containment. Levels of a PS-targeting antibody (Bavituximab) were measured in Ebola-infected animals and uninfected controls. Data showed that the pharmacokinetics were similar in both groups, therefore Ebola virus infection did not have an observable effect on the half-life of the antibody.

PMID: 23165089 [PubMed - indexed for MEDLINE]

924. Curr Opin Virol. 2013 Feb;3(1):84-91. doi: 10.1016/j.coviro.2012.11.006. Epub 2012 Dec 21.

Bats and their virome: an important source of emerging viruses capable of infecting humans.

Smith I(1), Wang LF.

Author information: (1)CSIRO Australian Animal Health Laboratory, Geelong, Victoria 3220, Australia.

Bats are being increasingly recognized as an important reservoir of zoonotic viruses of different families, including SARS coronavirus, Nipah virus, Hendra virus and Ebola virus. Several recent studies hypothesized that bats, an ancient group of flying mammals, are the major reservoir of several important RNA virus families from which other mammalian viruses of livestock and humans were derived. Although this hypothesis needs further investigation, the premise that bats carry a large number of viruses is commonly accepted. The question of whether bats have unique biological features making them ideal reservoir hosts has been the subject of several recent reviews. In this review, we will focus on the public health implications of bat derived zoonotic viral disease outbreaks, examine the drivers and risk factors of past disease outbreaks and outline research directions for better control of future disease events.

PMID: 23265969 [PubMed - indexed for MEDLINE]

925. Emerg Infect Dis. 2013 Feb;19(2):270-3. doi: 10.3201/eid1902.120524.

Ebola virus antibodies in fruit bats, bangladesh.

Olival KJ(1), Islam A, Yu M, Anthony SJ, Epstein JH, Khan SA, Khan SU, Crameri G, Wang LF, Lipkin WI, Luby SP, Daszak P.

Author information: (1)EcoHealth Alliance, New York, New York 10001, USA. olival@ecohealthalliance.org

To determine geographic range for Ebola virus, we tested 276 bats in Bangladesh. Five (3.5%) bats were positive for antibodies against Ebola Zaire and Reston viruses; no virus was detected by PCR. These bats might be a reservoir for Ebola or Ebola-like viruses, and extend the range of filoviruses to mainland Asia.
PMCID: PMC3559038 PMID: 23343532 [PubMed - indexed for MEDLINE]

926. Proc Natl Acad Sci U S A. 2013 Jan 29;110(5):1893-8. doi: 10.1073/pnas.1209591110. Epub 2013 Jan 14.

Antibodies are necessary for rVSV/ZEBOV-GP-mediated protection against lethal Ebola virus challenge in nonhuman primates.

Marzi A(1), Engelmann F, Feldmann F, Haberthur K, Shupert WL, Brining D, Scott DP, Geisbert TW, Kawaoka Y, Katze MG, Feldmann H, Messaoudi I.

Author information: (1)Laboratory of Virology, Rocky Mountain Laboratories, Division of Intramural Research, National Institute of Allergy and Infectious Diseases, National Institutes of Health, Hamilton, MT 59840, USA.

Ebola viruses cause hemorrhagic disease in humans and nonhuman primates with high fatality rates. These viruses pose a significant health concern worldwide due to the lack of approved therapeutics and vaccines as well as their potential misuse as bioterrorism agents. Although not licensed for human use, recombinant vesicular stomatitis virus (rVSV) expressing the filovirus glycoprotein (GP) has been shown to protect macaques from Ebola virus and Marburg virus infections, both prophylactically and postexposure in a homologous challenge setting. However, the immune mechanisms of protection conferred by this vaccine platform remain poorly understood. In this study, we set out to investigate the role of humoral versus cellular immunity in rVSV vaccine-mediated protection against lethal Zaire ebolavirus (ZEBOV) challenge. Groups of cynomolgus macaques were depleted of CD4+ T, CD8+ T, or CD20+ B cells before and during vaccination with rVSV/ZEBOV-GP. Unfortunately, CD20-depleted animals generated a robust IgG response. Therefore, an additional group of vaccinated animals were depleted of CD4+ T cells during challenge. All animals were subsequently challenged with a lethal dose of ZEBOV. Animals depleted of CD8+ T cells survived, suggesting a minimal role for CD8+ T cells in vaccine-mediated protection. Depletion of CD4+ T cells during vaccination caused a complete loss of glycoprotein-specific antibodies and abrogated vaccine protection. In contrast, depletion of CD4+ T cells during challenge resulted in survival of the animals, indicating a minimal role for CD4+ T-cell immunity in rVSV-mediated protection. Our results suggest that antibodies play a critical role in rVSV-mediated protection against ZEBOV.

PMCID: PMC3562844 PMID: 23319647 [PubMed - indexed for MEDLINE]

927. Science. 2013 Jan 25;339(6118):456-60. doi: 10.1126/science.1230835. Epub 2012 Dec 20.

Comparative analysis of bat genomes provides insight into the evolution of flight and immunity.

Zhang G(1), Cowled C, Shi Z, Huang Z, Bishop-Lilly KA, Fang X, Wynne JW, Xiong Z, Baker ML, Zhao W, Tachedjian M, Zhu Y, Zhou P, Jiang X, Ng J, Yang L, Wu L, Xiao J, Feng Y, Chen Y, Sun X, Zhang Y, Marsh GA, Crameri G, Broder CC, Frey KG, Wang LF, Wang J.

Author information: (1)BGI-Shenzhen, Shenzhen, 518083, China. zhanggj@genomics.org.cn

Bats are the only mammals capable of sustained flight and are notorious reservoir hosts for some of the world's most highly pathogenic viruses, including Nipah, Hendra, Ebola, and severe acute respiratory syndrome (SARS). To identify genetic changes associated with the development of bat-specific traits, we performed whole-genome sequencing and comparative analyses of two distantly related species, fruit bat Pteropus alecto and insectivorous bat Myotis davidii. We discovered an unexpected concentration of positively selected genes in the DNA damage checkpoint and nuclear factor κB pathways that may be related to the origin of flight, as well as expansion and contraction of important gene families. Comparison of bat genomes with other mammalian species has provided new insights into bat biology and evolution.

PMID: 23258410 [PubMed - indexed for MEDLINE]

928. Annu Rev Pathol. 2013 Jan 24;8:411-40. doi: 10.1146/annurev-pathol-020712-164041. Epub 2012 Nov 1.

Pathogenesis of the viral hemorrhagic fevers.

Paessler S(1), Walker DH.

Author information: (1)Department of Pathology, University of Texas Medical Branch at Galveston, Galveston, TX 77555, USA. slpaessl@utmb.edu

Four families of enveloped RNA viruses, filoviruses, flaviviruses, arenaviruses, and bunyaviruses, cause hemorrhagic fevers. These viruses are maintained in specific natural cycles involving nonhuman primates, bats, rodents, domestic ruminants, humans, mosquitoes, and ticks. Vascular instability varies from mild to fatal shock, and hemorrhage ranges from none to life threatening. The pathogenic mechanisms are extremely diverse and include deficiency of hepatic synthesis of coagulation factors owing to hepatocellular necrosis, cytokine storm, increased permeability by vascular endothelial growth factor, complement activation, and disseminated intravascular coagulation in one or more hemorrhagic fevers. The severity of disease caused by these agents varies tremendously; there are extremely high fatality rates in Ebola and Marburg hemorrhagic fevers, and asymptomatic infection predominates in yellow fever and dengue viral infections. Although ineffective immunity and high viral loads are characteristic of several viral hemorrhagic fevers, severe plasma leakage occurs at the time of viral clearance and defervescence in dengue hemorrhagic fever.

PMID: 23121052 [PubMed - indexed for MEDLINE]

929. J Infect Dis. 2013 Jan 15;207(2):306-18. doi: 10.1093/infdis/jis626. Epub 2012 Oct 8.

A Syrian golden hamster model recapitulating ebola hemorrhagic fever.

Ebihara H(1), Zivcec M, Gardner D, Falzarano D, LaCasse R, Rosenke R, Long D, Haddock E, Fischer E, Kawaoka Y, Feldmann H.

Author information: (1)Laboratory of Virology, Division of Intramural Research, National Institute of Allergy and Infectious Diseases (NIAID), National Institutes of Health (NID), Rocky Mountain Laboratories (RML), Hamilton, Montana 59840, USA. ebiharah@niaid.nih.gov

Ebola hemorrhagic fever (EHF) is a severe viral infection for which no effective treatment or vaccine is currently available. While the nonhuman primate (NHP) model is used for final evaluation of experimental vaccines and therapeutic efficacy, rodent models have been widely used in ebolavirus research because of their convenience. However, the validity of rodent models has been questioned given their low predictive value for efficacy testing of vaccines and therapeutics, a result of the inconsistent manifestation of coagulopathy seen in EHF. Here, we describe a lethal Syrian hamster model of EHF using mouse-adapted Ebola virus. Infected hamsters displayed most clinical hallmarks of EHF, including severe coagulopathy and uncontrolled host immune responses. Thus, the hamster seems to be superior to the existing rodent models, offering a better tool for understanding the critical processes in pathogenesis and providing a new model for evaluating prophylactic and postexposure interventions prior to testing in NHPs.

PMCID: PMC3532827 PMID: 23045629 [PubMed - indexed for MEDLINE]

930. Bing Du Xue Bao. 2013 Jan;29(1):71-5.

[Research progress of the molecule mechanisms of Ebola virus infection of cells].

[Article in Chinese]

Shi M(1), Shen YQ.

Author information: (1)Medical School of Southeast University, Nanjing 210009, China. shimingseu@hotmail.com

Ebola virus can cause severe Ebola hemorrhagic fever. The mortality rate is 90 percent. Up till now, there is no effective vaccine or treatment of Ebola virus infection. Relaed researches on Ebola virus have become a hot topic in virology. The understanding of molecular mechanisms of Ebola virus infection of cells are important for the development of vaccine and anti-virus drugs. Therefore, this review summarized the recent research progress on the mechanisms of Ebola virus infection.

PMID: 23547383 [PubMed - indexed for MEDLINE]

931. Bioinformation. 2013;9(6):286-92. doi: 10.6026/97320630009286. Epub 2013 Mar 19.

High-throughput virtual screening and docking studies of matrix protein vp40 of ebola virus.

Tamilvanan T(1), Hopper W.

Author information: (1)Department of Bioinformatics, School of Bioengineering, Faculty of Engineering & Technology, SRM University, Kattankulathur, 603203, Tamil Nadu, India.

Ebolavirus, a member of the Filoviridae family of negative-sense RNA viruses, causes severe haemorrhagic fever leading up to 90% lethality. Ebolavirus matrix protein VP40 is involved in the virus assembly and budding process. The RNA binding pocket of VP40 is considered as the drug target site for structure based drug design. High Throughput Virtual Screening and molecular docking studies were employed to find the suitable inhibitors against VP40. Ten compounds showing good glide score and glide energy as well as interaction with specific amino acid residues were short listed as drug leads. These small molecule inhibitors could be potent inhibitors for VP40 matrix protein by blocking virus assembly and budding process.

PMCID: PMC3607187 PMID: 23559747 [PubMed]

932. Biomed Res Int. 2013;2013:467078. doi: 10.1155/2013/467078. Epub 2013 Jul 24.

A universal model for predicting dynamics of the epidemics caused by special pathogens.

Bachinsky AG(1), Nizolenko LP.

Author information: (1)State Research Center of Virology and Biotechnology Vector, Russian Federation, Koltsovo, Novosibirsk 630559, Russia.

A universal model intended primarily for predicting dynamics of the mass epidemics (outbreaks) caused by special pathogens is being developed at the State Research Center of Virology and Biotechnology Vector. The model includes the range of major countermeasures: preventive and emergency mass vaccination, vaccination of risk groups as well as search for and isolation/observation of infected cases, contacts, and suspects, and quarantine. The intensity of interventions depends on the availability of the relevant resources. The effect of resource limitations on the development of a putative epidemic of Ebola hemorrhagic fever is demonstrated. The modeling results allow for estimation of the material and human resources necessary for eradication of an epidemic.

PMCID: PMC3741903 PMID: 23998125 [PubMed - indexed for MEDLINE]

933. Curr Top Microbiol Immunol. 2013;365:337-53. doi: 10.1007/82_2012_304.

Men, primates, and germs: an ongoing affair.

Gonzalez JP(1), Prugnolle F, Leroy E.

Author information: (1)International Center for Medical Research of Franceville, Franceville, Gabon, jean-paul.gonzalez@ird.fr.

Humans and nonhuman primates are phylogenetically (i.e., genetically) related and share pathogens that can jump from one species to another. The specific strategies of three groups of pathogens for crossing the species barrier among primates will be discussed. In Africa, gorillas and chimpanzees have succumbed for years to simultaneous epizootics (i.e.. "multi-emergence") of Ebola virus in places where they are in contact with Chiropters, which could be animal reservoirs of these viruses. Human epidemics often follow these major outbreaks. Simian immunodeficiency viruses (SIVs) have an ancient history of coevolution and many interspecific exchanges with their natural hosts. Chimpanzee and gorilla SIVs have crossed the species barrier at different times and places, leading to the emergence of HIV-1 and HIV-2. Other retroviruses, such as the Simian T-Lymphotropic Viruses and Foamiviruses, have also a unique ancient or recent history of crossing the species barrier. The identification of gorilla Plasmodium parasites that are genetically close to P. falciparum suggests that gorillas were the source of the deadly human P. falciparum. Nonhuman plasmodium species that can infect humans represent an underestimated risk.

PMID: 23239237 [PubMed - indexed for MEDLINE]

934. Dev Biol (Basel). 2013;135:211-8. doi: 10.1159/000178495. Epub 2013 May 14.

Review of Ebola virus infections in domestic animals.

Weingartl HM(1), Nfon C, Kobinger G.

Author information: (1)National Centre for Foreign Animal Disease (NCFAD), Canadian Food Inspection Agency (CFIA), Canadian Science Centre for Human and Animal Health, Winnipeg, Canada.

Ebola viruses (EBOV; genus Ebolavirus, family Filoviridae) cause often fatal, hemorrhagic fever in several species of simian primates including human. While fruit bats are considered a natural reservoir, the involvement of other species in the EBOV transmission cycle is unclear, especially for domesticated animals. Dogs and pigs are so far the only domestic animals identified as species that can be infected with EBOV. In 2009 Reston-EBOV was the first EBOV reported to infect swine with indicated transmission to humans; and a survey in Gabon found over 30% seroprevalence for EBOV in dogs during the Ebola outbreak in 2001-2002. While infections in dogs appear to be asymptomatic, pigs experimentally infected with EBOV can develop clinical disease, depending on the virus species and possibly the age of the infected animals. In the experimental settings, pigs can transmit Zaire-Ebola virus to naive pigs and macaques; however, their role during Ebola outbreaks in Africa needs to be clarified. Attempts at virus and antibody detection require as a prerequisite validation of viral RNA and antibody detection methods especially for pigs, as well as the development of a sampling strategy. Significant issues about disease development remain to be resolved for EBOV. Evaluation of current human vaccine candidates or development of veterinary vaccines de novo for EBOV might need to be considered, especially if pigs or dogs are implicated in the transmission of an African species of EBOV to humans.

PMID: 23689899 [PubMed - indexed for MEDLINE]

935. Dev Biol (Basel). 2013;135:201-9. doi: 10.1159/000190049. Epub 2013 May 14.

Ebola: facing a new transboundary animal disease?

Feldmann F(1), Feldmann H.

Author information: (1)Office of Operations Management, Division of Intramural Research, National Institute of Allergy and Infectious Diseases, National Institutes of Health, Rocky Mountain Laboratories, Hamilton, Montana, USA.

Ebola viruses are zoonotic pathogens with the potential of causing severe viral hemorrhagic fever in humans and nonhuman primates. Bats have been identified as a reservoir for Ebola viruses but it remains unclear if transmission to an end host involves intermediate hosts. Recently, one of the Ebola species has been found in Philippine pigs raising concerns regarding animal health and food safety. Diagnostics have so far focused on human application, but enhanced pig surveillance and diagnostics, particularly in Asia, for Ebola virus infections seem to be needed to establish reasonable guidelines for public and animal health and food safety. Livestock vaccination against Ebola seems currently not justified but proper preparedness may include experimental vaccine approaches.

PMID: 23689898 [PubMed - indexed for MEDLINE]

936. Infect Dis (Auckl). 2013 Feb 28;6:1-5. doi: 10.4137/IDRT.S11205. eCollection 2013

Ethical dilemmas in protecting individual rights versus public protection in the case of infectious diseases.

Phua KL(1).

Author information: (1)Monash University, Sunway Campus, Selangor, Malaysia.

Infectious diseases-including emerging and re-emerging diseases such as Ebola and tuberculosis-continue to be important causes of morbidity and mortality in the globalizing, contemporary world. This article discusses the ethical issues associated with protecting the rights of individuals versus the protection of the health of populations in the case of infectious diseases. The discussion uses the traditional medical ethics approach together with the public health approach presented by Faden and Shebaya.3 Infectious diseases such as Ebola hemorrhagic fever, Nipah virus and HIV/AIDS (together with tuberculosis) will be used to illustrate particular points in the discussion.

PMCID: PMC3988619 PMID: 24847171 [PubMed]

937. J Pharm Biomed Anal. 2013 Jan;72:231-9. doi: 10.1016/j.jpba.2012.08.025. Epub 2012 Aug 27.

Correlation between structure, retention, property, and activity of biologically relevant 1,7-bis(aminoalkyl)diazachrysene derivatives.

Šegan S(1), Trifković J, Verbić T, Opsenica D, Zlatović M, Burnett J, Šolaja B, Milojković-Opsenica D.

Author information: (1)Institute of Chemistry, Technology and Metallurgy, University of Belgrade, Njegoševa 12, 11000 Belgrade, Serbia.

The physicochemical properties, retention parameters (R(M)(0)), partition coefficients (logP(OW)), and pK(a) values for a series of thirteen 1,7-bis(aminoalkyl) diazachrysene (1,7-DAAC) derivatives were determined in order to reveal the characteristics responsible for their biological behavior. The investigated compounds inhibit three unrelated pathogens (the Botulinum neurotoxin serotype A light chain (BoNT/A LC), Plasmodium falciparum malaria, and Ebola filovirus) via three different mechanisms of action. To determine the most influential factors governing the retention and activities of the investigated diazachrysenes, R(M)(0), logP(OW), and biological activity values were correlated with 2D and 3D molecular descriptors, using a partial least squares regression. The resulting quantitative structure-retention (property) relationships indicate the importance of descriptors related to the hydrophobicity of the molecules (e.g., predicted partition coefficients and hydrophobic surface area). Quantitative structure-activity relationship models for describing biological activity against the BoNT/A LC and malarial strains also include overall compound polarity, electron density distribution, and proton donor/acceptor potential. Furthermore, models for Ebola filovirus inhibition are presented qualitatively to provide insights into parameters that may contribute to the compounds' antiviral activities. Overall, the models form the basis for selecting structural features that significantly affect the compound's absorption, distribution, metabolism, excretion, and toxicity profiles.

Copyright © 2012 Elsevier B.V. All rights reserved.

PMID: 22985530 [PubMed - indexed for MEDLINE]

938. J Virol. 2013 Jan;87(2):746-55. doi: 10.1128/JVI.01634-12. Epub 2012 Oct 31.

AMP-activated protein kinase is required for the macropinocytic internalization of ebolavirus.

Kondratowicz AS(1), Hunt CL, Davey RA, Cherry S, Maury WJ.

Author information: (1)Department of Microbiology, University of Iowa, Iowa City, IA, USA.

Identification of host factors that are needed for Zaire Ebolavirus (EBOV) entry provides insights into the mechanism(s) of filovirus uptake, and these factors may serve as potential antiviral targets. In order to identify novel host genes and pathways involved in EBOV entry, gene array findings in the National Cancer Institute's NCI-60 panel of human tumor cell lines were correlated with permissivity for EBOV glycoprotein (GP)-mediated entry. We found that the gene encoding the $\gamma 2$ subunit of AMP-activated protein kinase (AMPK) strongly correlated with EBOV transduction in the tumor panel. The AMPK inhibitor compound C inhibited infectious EBOV replication in Vero cells and diminished EBOV GP-dependent, but not Lassa fever virus GPC-dependent, entry into a variety of cell lines in a dose-dependent manner. Compound C also prevented EBOV GP-mediated infection of primary human macrophages, a major target of filoviral replication in vivo. Consistent with a role for AMPK in filovirus entry, time-of-addition studies demonstrated that compound C abrogated infection when it was added at early time points but became progressively less effective when added later. Compound C prevented EBOV pseudovirion internalization at 37°C as cell-bound particles remained susceptible to trypsin digestion in the presence of the inhibitor but not in its absence. Mouse embryonic fibroblasts lacking the AMPKα1 and AMPKα2 catalytic subunits were significantly less permissive to EBOV GP-mediated infection than their wild-type counterparts, likely due to decreased macropinocytic uptake. In total, these findings implicate AMPK in macropinocytic events needed for EBOV GP-dependent entry and identify a novel cellular target for new filoviral antivirals.

PMCID: PMC3554099 PMID: 23115293 [PubMed - indexed for MEDLINE]

939. J Virol Methods. 2013 Jan;187(1):159-65. doi: 10.1016/j.jviromet.2012.10.003. Epub 2012 Oct 13.

Multiple phosphorylable sites in the Zaire Ebolavirus nucleoprotein evidenced by high resolution tandem mass spectrometry.

Peyrol J(1), Thizon C, Gaillard JC, Marchetti C, Armengaud J, Rollin-Genetet F.

Author information: (1)Commissariat à l'Energie Atomique, iBEB/SBTN/LDCAE, Bagnols-sur-Cèze, France.

The 739-amino-acid nucleoprotein (NP) of Zaire Ebolavirus (ZEBOV) plays a key role in Ebola virion formation and replication. A stable HEK-293 cell line capable of producing an N-ter 6His-tagged recombinant form of NP - ZEBOV was created. Production of this protein was triggered in batch culture using microcarriers. Because NP Ebola phosphorylation has been shown to occur but localization of the modified residues remained to be established, the phosphorylation status of recombinant NP - ZEBOV was investigated through extensive characterization by high-resolution tandem mass spectrometry. The NP - ZEBOV sequence may well be covered by the use of multiple proteases. NP was found to be phosphorylated in two different amino acid stretches: [561-594] and [636-653]. Furthermore, residues Thr(563), Ser(581), Ser(587) and Ser(647) were accurately identified as phosphorylated sites. These data highlight how high resolution tandem mass spectrometry is a method of choice for characterizing post-translational modifications of viral proteins. Because these four phosphorylable sites are conserved among Ebolavirus and Marburgvirus NPs, their modification may play a modulatory role in viral RNA synthesis.

Copyright © 2012 Elsevier B.V. All rights reserved.

PMID: 23068963 [PubMed - indexed for MEDLINE]

940. Mol Phylogenet Evol. 2013 Jan;66(1):126-37. doi: 10.1016/j.ympev.2012.09.028. Epub 2012 Oct 10.

Molecular systematics and phylogeography of the tribe Myonycterini (Mammalia, Pteropodidae) inferred from mitochondrial and nuclear markers.

Nesi N(1), Kadjo B, Pourrut X, Leroy E, Pongombo Shongo C, Cruaud C, Hassanin A.

Author information: (1)Unité Origine, Structure et Evolution de la Biodiversité, Département Systématique et Evolution, Muséum National d'Histoire Naturelle, CP 51, 55 rue Buffon, 75005 Paris Cedex 05, France.

The tribe Myonycterini comprises five fruit bat species of the family Pteropodidae, which are endemic to tropical Africa. Previous studies have produced conflicting results about their interspecific relationships. Here, we performed a comparative phylogeographic analysis based on 148 complete cytochrome b gene sequences from the three species distributed in West Africa and Central Africa (Myonycteris torquata, Lissonycteris angolensis and Megaloglossus woermanni). In addition, we investigated phylogenetic relationships within the tribe Myonycterini, using a matrix including 29 terminal taxa and 7235 nucleotide characters, corresponding to an alignment of two mitochondrial genes and seven nuclear introns. Our phylogenetic analyses confirmed that the genus Megaloglossus belongs to the tribe Myonycterini. Further, the genus Rousettus is paraphyletic, with R. lanosus, sometimes placed in the genus Stenonycteris, being the sister-group of the tribes Myonycterini and Epomophorini. Our phylogeographic results showed that populations of Myonycteris torquata and Megaloglossus woermanni from the Upper Guinea Forest are highly divergent from those of the Congo Basin Forest. Based on our molecular data, we recommended several taxonomic changes. First, Stenonycteris should be recognized as a separate genus from Rousettus and composed of S. lanosus. This genus should be elevated to a new tribe, Stenonycterini, within the subfamily Epomophorinae. This result shows that the evolution of lingual echolocation was more complicated than previously accepted. Second, the genus Lissonycteris is synonymised with Myonycteris. Third, the populations from West Africa formerly included in Myonycteris torquata and Megaloglossus woermanni are now placed in two distinct species, respectively, Myonycteris leptodon and Megaloglossus azagnyi sp. nov. Our molecular dating estimates show that the three phases of taxonomic diversification detected within the tribe Myonycterini can be related to three distinct decreases in tree cover vegetation, at 6.5-6, 2.7-2.5, and 1.8-1.6Ma. Our results suggest that the high nucleotide distance between Ebolavirus Côte d'Ivoire and Ebolavirus Zaire can be correlated with the Plio/Pleistocene divergence between their putative reservoir host species, i.e., Myonycteris leptodon and Myonycteris torquata, respectively.

Copyright © 2012 Elsevier Inc. All rights reserved.

PMID: 23063885 [PubMed - indexed for MEDLINE]

941. PLoS Negl Trop Dis. 2013 Dec 19;7(12):e2600. doi: 10.1371/journal.pntd.0002600. eCollection 2013.

Vesicular stomatitis virus-based vaccines protect nonhuman primates against Bundibugyo ebolavirus.

Mire CE(1), Geisbert JB(1), Marzi A(2), Agans KN(1), Feldmann H(2), Geisbert TW(1).

Author information: (1)Galveston National Laboratory, University of Texas Medical Branch, Galveston, Texas, United States of America ; Department of Microbiology and Immunology, University of Texas Medical Branch, Galveston, Texas, United States of America. (2)Laboratory of Virology, Division of Intramural Research, National Institute of Allergy and Infectious Diseases, National Institutes of Health, Hamilton, Montana, United States of America.

Ebola virus (EBOV) causes severe and often fatal hemorrhagic fever in humans and nonhuman primates (NHPs). Currently, there are no licensed vaccines or therapeutics for human use. Recombinant vesicular stomatitis virus (rVSV)-based vaccine vectors, which encode an EBOV glycoprotein in place of the VSV glycoprotein, have shown 100% efficacy against homologous Sudan ebolavirus (SEBOV) or Zaire ebolavirus (ZEBOV) challenge in NHPs. In addition, a single injection of a blend of three rVSV vectors completely protected NHPs against challenge with SEBOV, ZEBOV, the former Côte d'Ivoire ebolavirus, and Marburg virus. However, recent studies suggest that complete protection against the newly discovered Bundibugyo ebolavirus (BEBOV) using several different heterologous filovirus vaccines is more difficult and presents a new challenge. As BEBOV caused nearly 50% mortality in a recent outbreak any filovirus vaccine advanced for human use must be able to protect against this new species. Here, we evaluated several different strategies against BEBOV using rVSV-based vaccines. Groups of cynomolgus macaques were vaccinated with a single injection of a homologous BEBOV vaccine, a single injection of a blended heterologous vaccine (SEBOV/ZEBOV), or a prime-boost using heterologous SEBOV and ZEBOV vectors. Animals were challenged with BEBOV 29-36 days after initial vaccination. Macaques vaccinated with the homologous BEBOV vaccine or the prime-boost showed no overt signs of illness and survived challenge. In contrast, animals vaccinated with the heterologous blended vaccine and unvaccinated control animals developed severe clinical symptoms consistent with BEBOV infection with 2 of 3 animals in each group succumbing. These data show that complete protection against BEBOV will likely require incorporation of BEBOV glycoprotein into the vaccine or employment of a prime-boost regimen. Fortunately, our results demonstrate that heterologous rVSV-based filovirus vaccine vectors employed in the prime-boost approach can provide protection against BEBOV using an abbreviated regimen, which may have utility in outbreak settings.

PMCID: PMC3868506 PMID: 24367715 [PubMed - indexed for MEDLINE]

942. PLoS Negl Trop Dis. 2013 Sep 19;7(9):e2435. doi: 10.1371/journal.pntd.0002435. eCollection 2013.

Hospital-based surveillance for viral hemorrhagic fevers and hepatitides in Ghana.

Bonney JH(1), Osei-Kwasi M, Adiku TK, Barnor JS, Amesiya R, Kubio C, Ahadzie L, Olschläger S, Lelke M, Becker-Ziaja B, Pahlmann M, Günther S.

Author information: (1)Virology Department, Noguchi Memorial Institute of Medical Research, University of Ghana, Legon, Ghana ; Department of Virology, Bernhard-Nocht-Institute for Tropical Medicine, Hamburg, Germany.

BACKGROUND: Viral hemorrhagic fevers (VHF) are acute diseases associated with bleeding, organ failure, and shock. VHF may hardly be distinguished clinically from other diseases in the African hospital, including viral hepatitis. This study was conducted to determine if VHF and viral hepatitis contribute to hospital morbidity in the Central and Northern parts of Ghana. METHODOLOGY/PRINCIPAL FINDINGS: From 2009 to 2011, blood samples of 258 patients with VHF symptoms were collected at 18 hospitals in Ashanti, Brong-Ahafo, Northern, Upper West, and Upper East regions. Patients were tested by PCR for Lassa, Rift Valley, Crimean-Congo, Ebola/Marburg, and yellow fever viruses; hepatitis A (HAV), B (HBV), C (HCV), and E (HEV) viruses; and by ELISA for serological hepatitis markers. None of the patients tested positive for VHF. However, 21 (8.1%) showed anti-HBc IgM plus HBV DNA and/or HBsAg; 37 (14%) showed HBsAg and HBV DNA without anti-HBc IgM; 26 (10%) showed anti-HAV IgM and/or HAV RNA; and 20 (7.8%) were HCV RNA-positive. None was positive for HEV RNA or anti-HEV IgM plus IgG. Viral genotypes were determined as HAV-IB, HBV-A and E, and HCV-1, 2, and 4. CONCLUSIONS/SIGNIFICANCE: VHFs do not cause significant hospital morbidity in the study area. However, the incidence of acute hepatitis A and B, and hepatitis B and C with active virus replication is high. These infections may mimic VHF and need to be considered if VHF is suspected. The data may help decision makers to allocate resources and focus surveillance systems on the diseases of relevance in Ghana.

PMCID: PMC3777898 PMID: 24069490 [PubMed - indexed for MEDLINE]

943. PLoS Negl Trop Dis. 2013 Sep 12;7(9):e2430. doi: 10.1371/journal.pntd.0002430. eCollection 2013.

A fusion-inhibiting peptide against Rift Valley fever virus inhibits multiple, diverse viruses.

Koehler JW(1), Smith JM, Ripoll DR, Spik KW, Taylor SL, Badger CV, Grant RJ, Ogg MM, Wallqvist A, Guttieri MC, Garry RF, Schmaljohn CS.

Author information: (1)United States Army Medical Research Institute of Infectious Diseases, Virology Division, Fort Detrick, Maryland, United States of America.

For enveloped viruses, fusion of the viral envelope with a cellular membrane is critical for a productive infection to occur. This fusion process is mediated by at least three classes of fusion proteins (Class I, II, and III) based on the protein sequence and structure. For Rift Valley fever virus (RVFV), the glycoprotein Gc (Class II fusion protein) mediates this fusion event following entry into the endocytic pathway, allowing the viral genome access to the cell cytoplasm. Here, we show that peptides analogous to the RVFV Gc stem region inhibited RVFV infectivity in cell culture by inhibiting the fusion process. Further, we show that infectivity can be inhibited for diverse, unrelated RNA viruses that have Class I (Ebola virus), Class II (Andes virus), or Class III (vesicular stomatitis virus) fusion proteins using this single peptide. Our findings are consistent with an inhibition mechanism similar to that proposed for stem peptide fusion inhibitors of dengue virus in which the RVFV inhibitory peptide first binds to both the virion and cell membranes, allowing it to traffic with the virus into the endocytic pathway. Upon acidification and rearrangement of Gc, the peptide is then able to specifically bind to Gc and prevent fusion of the viral and endocytic membranes, thus inhibiting viral infection. These results could provide novel insights into conserved features among the three classes of viral fusion proteins and offer direction for the future development of broadly active fusion inhibitors.

PMCID: PMC3772029 PMID: 24069485 [PubMed - indexed for MEDLINE]

944. PLoS One. 2013;8(4):e61232. doi: 10.1371/journal.pone.0061232. Epub 2013 Apr 5.

Ebolavirus nucleoprotein C-termini potently attract single domain antibodies enabling monoclonal affinity reagent sandwich assay (MARSA) formulation.

Sherwood LJ(1), Hayhurst A.
Author information: (1)Department of Virology and Immunology, Texas Biomedical Research Institute, San Antonio, Texas, USA.

BACKGROUND: Antigen detection assays can play an important part in environmental surveillance and diagnostics for emerging threats. We are interested in accelerating assay formulation; targeting the agents themselves to bypass requirements for a priori genome information or surrogates. Previously, using in vitro affinity reagent selection on Marburg virus we rapidly established monoclonal affinity reagent sandwich assay (MARSA) where one recombinant antibody clone was both captor and tracer for polyvalent nucleoprotein (NP). Hypothesizing that the closely related Ebolavirus genus may share the same Achilles' heel, we redirected the scheme to see whether similar assays could be delivered and began to explore their mechanism. METHODS AND FINDINGS: In parallel we selected panels of llama single domain antibodies (sdAb) from a semi-synthetic library against Zaire, Sudan, Ivory Coast, and Reston Ebola viruses. Each could perform as both captor and tracer in the same antigen sandwich capture assay thereby forming MARSAs. All sdAb were specific for NP and those tested required the C-terminal domain for recognition. Several clones were cross-reactive, indicating epitope conservation across the Ebolavirus genus. Analysis of two immune shark sdAb revealed they also targeted the C-terminal domain, and could be similarly employed, yet were less sensitive than a comparable llama sdAb despite stemming from immune selections. CONCLUSIONS: The C-terminal domain of Ebolavirus NP is a strong attractant for antibodies and enables sensitive sandwich immunoassays to be rapidly generated using a single antibody clone. The polyvalent nature of nucleocapsid borne NP and display of the C-terminal region likely serves as a bountiful affinity sink during selections, and a highly avid target for subsequent immunoassay capture. Combined with the high degree of amino acid conservation through 37 years and across wide geographies, this domain makes an ideal handle for monoclonal affinity reagent driven antigen sandwich assays for the Ebolavirus genus.
PMCID: PMC3618483 PMID: 23577211 [PubMed - indexed for MEDLINE]
945. PLoS One. 2013;8(4):e60579. doi: 10.1371/journal.pone.0060579. Epub 2013 Apr 5.

A systematic screen of FDA-approved drugs for inhibitors of biological threat agents.

Madrid PB(1), Chopra S, Manger ID, Gilfillan L, Keepers TR, Shurtleff AC, Green CE, Iyer LV, Dilks HH, Davey RA, Kolokoltsov AA, Carrion R Jr, Patterson JL, Bavari S, Panchal RG, Warren TK, Wells JB, Moos WH, Burke RL, Tanga MJ.
Author information: (1)Center for Infectious Disease and Biodefense Research, SRI International, Menlo Park, California, USA. peter.madrid@sri.com

BACKGROUND: The rapid development of effective medical countermeasures against potential biological threat agents is vital. Repurposing existing drugs that may have unanticipated activities as potential countermeasures is one way to meet this important goal, since currently approved drugs already have well-established safety and pharmacokinetic profiles in patients, as well as manufacturing and distribution networks. Therefore, approved drugs could rapidly be made available for a new indication in an emergency. METHODOLOGY/PRINCIPAL FINDINGS: A large systematic effort to determine whether existing drugs can be used against high containment bacterial and viral pathogens is described. We assembled and screened 1012 FDA-approved drugs for off-label broad-spectrum efficacy against Bacillus anthracis; Francisella tularensis; Coxiella burnetii; and Ebola, Marburg, and Lassa fever viruses using in vitro cell culture assays. We found a variety of hits against two or more of these biological threat pathogens, which were validated in secondary assays. As expected, antibiotic compounds were highly active against bacterial agents, but we did not identify any non-antibiotic compounds with broad-spectrum antibacterial activity. Lomefloxacin and erythromycin were found to be the most potent compounds in vivo protecting mice against Bacillus anthracis challenge. While multiple virus-specific inhibitors were identified, the most noteworthy antiviral compound identified was chloroquine, which disrupted entry and replication of two or more viruses in vitro and protected mice against Ebola virus challenge in vivo. CONCLUSIONS/SIGNIFICANCE: The feasibility of repurposing existing drugs to face novel threats is demonstrated and this represents the first effort to apply this approach to high containment bacteria and viruses.
PMCID: PMC3618516 PMID: 23577127 [PubMed - indexed for MEDLINE]
946. PLoS One. 2013;8(4):e60838. doi: 10.1371/journal.pone.0060838. Epub 2013 Apr 2.

Lectin-dependent enhancement of Ebola virus infection via soluble and transmembrane C-type lectin receptors.

Brudner M(1), Karpel M, Lear C, Chen L, Yantosca LM, Scully C, Sarraju A, Sokolovska A, Zariffard MR, Eisen DP, Mungall BA, Kotton DN, Omari A, Huang IC, Farzan M, Takahashi K, Stuart L, Stahl GL, Ezekowitz AB, Spear GT, Olinger GG, Schmidt EV, Michelow IC.
Author information: (1)Programs of Developmental Immunology, Department of Pediatrics, Massachusetts General Hospital, Boston, Massachusetts, United States of America.

Mannose-binding lectin (MBL) is a key soluble effector of the innate immune system that recognizes pathogen-specific surface glycans. Surprisingly, low-producing MBL genetic variants that may predispose children and immunocompromised individuals to infectious diseases are more common than would be expected in human populations. Since certain immune defense molecules, such as immunoglobulins, can be exploited by invasive pathogens, we hypothesized that MBL might also enhance infections in some circumstances. Consequently, the low and intermediate MBL levels commonly found in human populations might be the result of balancing selection. Using model infection systems with pseudotyped and authentic glycosylated viruses, we demonstrated that MBL indeed enhances infection of Ebola, Hendra, Nipah and West Nile viruses in low complement conditions. Mechanistic studies with Ebola virus (EBOV) glycoprotein pseudotyped lentiviruses confirmed that MBL binds to N-linked glycan epitopes on viral surfaces in a specific manner via the MBL carbohydrate recognition domain, which is necessary for enhanced infection. MBL mediates lipid-raft-dependent macropinocytosis of EBOV via a pathway that appears to require less actin or early endosomal processing compared with the filovirus canonical endocytic pathway. Using a validated RNA interference screen, we identified C1QBP (gC1qR) as a candidate surface receptor that mediates MBL-dependent enhancement of EBOV infection. We also identified dectin-2 (CLEC6A) as a potentially novel candidate attachment factor for EBOV. Our findings support the concept of an innate immune haplotype that represents critical interactions between MBL and complement component C4 genes and that may modify susceptibility or resistance to certain glycosylated pathogens. Therefore, higher levels of native or exogenous MBL could be deleterious in the setting of relative hypocomplementemia which can occur genetically or because of immunodepletion during active infections. Our findings confirm our hypothesis that the pressure of infectious diseases may have contributed in part to evolutionary selection of MBL mutant haplotypes.

PMCID: PMC3614905 PMID: 23573288 [PubMed - indexed for MEDLINE]

947. PLoS One. 2013;8(3):e60289. doi: 10.1371/journal.pone.0060289. Epub 2013 Mar 20.

Expression of concern: Serological evidence of Ebola virus infection in Indonesian orangutans.

PLOS ONE Editors.

Comment on PLoS One. 2012;7(7):e40740.

PMCID: PMC3603915 PMID: 23527312 [PubMed - indexed for MEDLINE]

948. PLoS One. 2013;8(2):e56265. doi: 10.1371/journal.pone.0056265. Epub 2013 Feb 18.

Multiple cationic amphiphiles induce a Niemann-Pick C phenotype and inhibit Ebola virus entry and infection.

Shoemaker CJ(1), Schornberg KL, Delos SE, Scully C, Pajouhesh H, Olinger GG, Johansen LM, White JM.

Author information: (1)Departmentof Cell Biology, University of Virginia, Charlottesville, Virginia, United States of America.

Erratum in PLoS One. 2013;8(10). doi:10.1371/annotation/76780c06-ac81-48a3-8cce-509da6858fe5.

Ebola virus (EBOV) is an enveloped RNA virus that causes hemorrhagic fever in humans and non-human primates. Infection requires internalization from the cell surface and trafficking to a late endocytic compartment, where viral fusion occurs, providing a conduit for the viral genome to enter the cytoplasm and initiate replication. In a concurrent study, we identified clomiphene as a potent inhibitor of EBOV entry. Here, we screened eleven inhibitors that target the same biosynthetic pathway as clomiphene. From this screen we identified six compounds, including U18666A, that block EBOV infection (IC(50) 1.6 to 8.0 µM) at a late stage of entry. Intriguingly, all six are cationic amphiphiles that share additional chemical features. U18666A induces phenotypes, including cholesterol accumulation in endosomes, associated with defects in Niemann-Pick C1 protein (NPC1), a late endosomal and lysosomal protein required for EBOV entry. We tested and found that all six EBOV entry inhibitors from our screen induced cholesterol accumulation. We further showed that higher concentrations of cationic amphiphiles are required to inhibit EBOV entry into cells that overexpress NPC1 than parental cells, supporting the contention that they inhibit EBOV entry in an NPC1-dependent manner. A previously reported inhibitor, compound 3.47, inhibits EBOV entry by blocking binding of the EBOV glycoprotein to NPC1. None of the cationic amphiphiles tested had this effect. Hence, multiple cationic amphiphiles (including several FDA approved agents) inhibit EBOV entry in an NPC1-dependent fashion, but by a mechanism distinct from that of compound 3.47. Our findings suggest that there are minimally two ways of perturbing NPC1-dependent pathways that can block EBOV entry, increasing the attractiveness of NPC1 as an anti-filoviral therapeutic target.

PMCID: PMC3575416 PMID: 23441171 [PubMed - indexed for MEDLINE]

949. PLoS Pathog. 2013;9(10):e1003677. doi: 10.1371/journal.ppat.1003677. Epub 2013 Oct 17.

Ebola virus RNA editing depends on the primary editing site sequence and an upstream secondary structure.

Mehedi M(1), Hoenen T, Robertson S, Ricklefs S, Dolan MA, Taylor T, Falzarano D, Ebihara H, Porcella SF, Feldmann H.

Author information: (1)Department of Medical Microbiology, University of Manitoba, Winnipeg, Manitoba, Canada ; Laboratory of Virology, Rocky Mountain Laboratories, Division of Intramural Research, National Institute of Allergy and Infectious Diseases, National Institutes of Health, Hamilton, Montana, United States of America.

Ebolavirus (EBOV), the causative agent of a severe hemorrhagic fever and a biosafety level 4 pathogen, increases its genome coding capacity by producing multiple transcripts encoding for structural and nonstructural glycoproteins from a single gene. This is achieved through RNA editing, during which non-template adenosine residues are incorporated into the EBOV mRNAs at an editing site encoding for 7 adenosine residues. However, the mechanism of EBOV RNA editing is currently not understood. In this study, we report for the first time that minigenomes containing the glycoprotein gene editing site can undergo RNA editing, thereby eliminating the requirement for a biosafety level 4 laboratory to study EBOV RNA editing. Using a newly developed dual-reporter minigenome, we have characterized the mechanism of EBOV RNA editing, and have identified cis-acting sequences that are required for editing, located between 9 nt upstream and 9 nt downstream of the editing site. Moreover, we show that a secondary structure in the upstream cis-acting sequence plays an important role in RNA editing. EBOV RNA editing is glycoprotein gene-specific, as a stretch encoding for 7 adenosine residues located in the viral polymerase gene did not serve as an editing site, most likely due to an absence of the necessary cis-acting sequences. Finally, the EBOV protein VP30 was identified as a trans-acting factor for RNA editing, constituting a novel function for this protein. Overall, our results provide novel insights into the RNA editing mechanism of EBOV, further understanding of which might result in novel intervention strategies against this viral pathogen.

PMCID: PMC3798607 PMID: 24146620 [PubMed - indexed for MEDLINE]

950. PLoS Pathog. 2013;9(5):e1003389. doi: 10.1371/journal.ppat.1003389. Epub 2013 May 30

Antibody quality and protection from lethal Ebola virus challenge in nonhuman primates immunized with rabies virus based bivalent vaccine.

Blaney JE(1), Marzi A, Willet M, Papaneri AB, Wirblich C, Feldmann F, Holbrook M, Jahrling P, Feldmann H, Schnell MJ.

Author information: (1)Emerging Viral Pathogens Section, National Institute of Allergy and Infectious Diseases, National Institutes of Health, Bethesda, MD, USA.

We have previously described the generation of a novel Ebola virus (EBOV) vaccine platform based on (a) replication-competent rabies virus (RABV), (b) replication-deficient RABV, or (c) chemically inactivated RABV expressing EBOV glycoprotein (GP). Mouse studies demonstrated safety, immunogenicity, and protective efficacy of these live or inactivated RABV/EBOV vaccines. Here, we evaluated these vaccines in nonhuman primates. Our results indicate that all three vaccines do induce potent immune responses against both RABV and EBOV, while the protection of immunized animals against EBOV was largely dependent on the quality of humoral immune response against EBOV GP. We also determined if the induced antibodies against EBOV GP differ in their target, affinity, or the isotype. Our results show that IgG1-biased humoral responses as well as high levels of GP-specific antibodies were beneficial for the control of

EBOV infection after immunization. These results further support the concept that a successful EBOV vaccine needs to induce strong antibodies against EBOV. We also showed that a dual vaccine against RABV and filoviruses is achievable; therefore addressing concerns for the marketability of this urgently needed vaccine.

PMCID: PMC3667758 PMID: 23737747 [PubMed - indexed for MEDLINE]

951. PLoS Pathog. 2013;9(5):e1003258. doi: 10.1371/journal.ppat.1003258. Epub 2013 May 16

The secret life of viral entry glycoproteins: moonlighting in immune evasion.

Cook JD(1), Lee JE.

Author information: (1)Department of Laboratory Medicine and Pathobiology, Faculty of Medicine, University of Toronto, Toronto, Ontario, Canada.

PMCID: PMC3656028 PMID: 23696729 [PubMed - indexed for MEDLINE]

952. PLoS Pathog. 2013 Jan;9(1):e1003147. doi: 10.1371/journal.ppat.1003147. Epub 2013 Jan 31.

An upstream open reading frame modulates ebola virus polymerase translation and virus replication.

Shabman RS(1), Hoenen T, Groseth A, Jabado O, Binning JM, Amarasinghe GK, Feldmann H, Basler CF.

Author information: (1)Department of Microbiology, Mount Sinai School of Medicine, New York, New York, United States of America.

Ebolaviruses, highly lethal zoonotic pathogens, possess longer genomes than most other non-segmented negative-strand RNA viruses due in part to long 5' and 3' untranslated regions (UTRs) present in the seven viral transcriptional units. To date, specific functions have not been assigned to these UTRs. With reporter assays, we demonstrated that the Zaire ebolavirus (EBOV) 5'-UTRs lack internal ribosomal entry site function. However, the 5'-UTRs do differentially regulate cap-dependent translation when placed upstream of a GFP reporter gene. Most dramatically, the 5'-UTR derived from the viral polymerase (L) mRNA strongly suppressed translation of GFP compared to a β-actin 5'-UTR. The L 5'-UTR is one of four viral genes to possess upstream AUGs (uAUGs), and ablation of each uAUG enhanced translation of the primary ORF (pORF), most dramatically in the case of the L 5'-UTR. The L uAUG was sufficient to initiate translation, is surrounded by a "weak" Kozak sequence and suppressed pORF translation in a position-dependent manner. Under conditions where eIF2α was phosphorylated, the presence of the uORF maintained translation of the L pORF, indicating that the uORF modulates L translation in response to cellular stress. To directly address the role of the L uAUG in virus replication, a recombinant EBOV was generated in which the L uAUG was mutated to UCG. Strikingly, mutating two nucleotides outside of previously-defined protein coding and cis-acting regulatory sequences attenuated virus growth to titers 10-100-fold lower than a wild-type virus in Vero and A549 cells. The mutant virus also exhibited decreased viral RNA synthesis as early as 6 hours post-infection and enhanced sensitivity to the stress inducer thapsigargin. Cumulatively, these data identify novel mechanisms by which EBOV regulates its polymerase expression, demonstrate their relevance to virus replication and identify a potential therapeutic target.

PMCID: PMC3561295 PMID: 23382680 [PubMed - indexed for MEDLINE]

953. Sci Rep. 2013;3:1206. doi: 10.1038/srep01206. Epub 2013 Feb 4.

The spatio-temporal distribution dynamics of Ebola virus proteins and RNA in infected cells.

Nanbo A(1), Watanabe S, Halfmann P, Kawaoka Y.

Author information: (1)Influenza Research Institute, Department of Pathobiological Sciences, University of Wisconsin-Madison, Madison, WI 53711, USA. nanboa@pharm.hokudai.ac.jp

Here, we used a biologically contained Ebola virus system to characterize the spatio-temporal distribution of Ebola virus proteins and RNA during virus replication. We found that viral nucleoprotein (NP), the polymerase cofactor VP35, the major matrix protein VP40, the transcription activator VP30, and the minor matrix protein VP24 were distributed in cytoplasmic inclusions. These inclusions enlarged near the nucleus, became smaller pieces, and subsequently localized near the plasma membrane. GP was distributed in the cytoplasm and transported to the plasma membrane independent of the other viral proteins. We also found that viral RNA synthesis occurred within the inclusions. Newly synthesized negative-sense RNA was distributed inside the inclusions, whereas positive-sense RNA was distributed both inside and outside. These findings provide useful insights into Ebola virus replication.

PMCID: PMC3563031 PMID: 23383374 [PubMed - indexed for MEDLINE]

954. Viruses. 2012 Dec 14;4(12):3754-84. doi: 10.3390/v4123754.

Use of the Syrian hamster as a new model of ebola virus disease and other viral hemorrhagic fevers.

Wahl-Jensen V(1), Bollinger L, Safronetz D, de Kok-Mercado F, Scott DP, Ebihara H.

Author information: (1)Integrated Research Facility at Fort Detrick, National Institute of Allergy and Infectious Diseases (NIAID), National Institutes of Health (NIH), National Interagency Biodefense Campus, B-8200 Research Plaza, Fort Detrick, Frederick, Maryland 21702, USA. victoria.jensen@nih.gov

Historically, mice and guinea pigs have been the rodent models of choice for therapeutic and prophylactic countermeasure testing against Ebola virus disease (EVD). Recently, hamsters have emerged as a novel animal model for the in vivo study of EVD. In this review, we discuss the history of the hamster as a research laboratory animal, as well as current benefits and challenges of this model. Availability of immunological reagents is addressed. Salient features of EVD in hamsters, including relevant pathology and coagulation parameters, are compared directly with the mouse, guinea pig and nonhuman primate models.

PMCID: PMC3528289 PMID: 23242370 [PubMed - indexed for MEDLINE]

955. Proc Natl Acad Sci U S A. 2012 Dec 11;109(50):20661-6. doi: 10.1073/pnas.1213559109. Epub 2012 Nov 26.

Structural basis for Marburg virus VP35-mediated immune evasion mechanisms.

Ramanan P(1), Edwards MR, Shabman RS, Leung DW, Endlich-Frazier AC, Borek DM, Otwinowski Z, Liu G, Huh J, Basler CF, Amarasinghe GK.

Author information: (1)Department of Pathology and Immunology, Washington University School of Medicine, St. Louis, MO 63110, USA.

Filoviruses, marburgvirus (MARV) and ebolavirus (EBOV), are causative agents of highly lethal hemorrhagic fever in humans. MARV and EBOV share a common genome organization but show important differences in replication complex formation, cell entry, host tropism, transcriptional regulation, and immune evasion. Multifunctional filoviral viral protein (VP) 35 proteins inhibit innate immune responses. Recent studies suggest double-stranded (ds)RNA sequestration is a potential mechanism that allows EBOV VP35 to antagonize retinoic-acid inducible gene-I (RIG-I) like receptors (RLRs) that are activated by viral pathogen-associated molecular patterns (PAMPs), such as double-strandedness and dsRNA blunt ends. Here, we show that MARV VP35 can inhibit IFN production at multiple steps in the signaling pathways downstream of RLRs. The crystal structure of MARV VP35 IID in complex with 18-bp dsRNA reveals that despite the similar protein fold as EBOV VP35 IID, MARV VP35 IID interacts with the dsRNA backbone and not with blunt ends. Functional studies show that MARV VP35 can inhibit dsRNA-dependent RLR activation and interferon (IFN) regulatory factor 3 (IRF3) phosphorylation by IFN kinases TRAF family member-associated NFkb activator (TANK) binding kinase-I (TBK-I) and IFN kB kinase e (IKKe) in cell-based studies. We also show that MARV VP35 can only inhibit RIG-I and melanoma differentiation associated gene 5 (MDA5) activation by double strandedness of RNA PAMPs (coating backbone) but is unable to inhibit activation of RLRs by dsRNA blunt ends (end capping). In contrast, EBOV VP35 can inhibit activation by both PAMPs. Insights on differential PAMP recognition and inhibition of IFN induction by a similar filoviral VP35 fold, as shown here, reveal the structural and functional plasticity of a highly conserved virulence factor.
PMCID: PMC3528546 PMID: 23185024 [PubMed - indexed for MEDLINE]

956. Wkly Epidemiol Rec. 2012 Dec 7;87(49/50):493.

Outbreak news. Ebola haemorrhagic fever, Uganda – update.

[Article in English, French]

[No authors listed]

PMID: 23311004 [PubMed - indexed for MEDLINE]

957. Viruses. 2012 Dec 6;4(12):3511-30. doi: 10.3390/v4123511.

Standardization of the filovirus plaque assay for use in preclinical studies.

Shurtleff AC(1), Biggins JE, Keeney AE, Zumbrun EE, Bloomfield HA, Kuehne A, Audet JL, Alfson KJ, Griffiths A, Olinger GG, Bavari S; Filovirus Animal Nonclinical Group (FANG) Assay Working Group.

Collaborators: Garges S, Kolhekar A, Bruce C, Smither S, Kurnat R.

Author information: (1)Integrated Toxicology Division, United States Army Medical Research Institute of Infectious Diseases, 1425 Porter Street, Frederick, MD 21702, USA. amy.c.shurtleff.ctr@us.army.mil

The filovirus plaque assay serves as the assay of choice to measure infectious virus in a cell culture, blood, or homogenized tissue sample. It has been in use for more than 30 years and is the generally accepted assay used to titrate virus in samples from animals treated with a potential antiviral therapeutic or vaccine. As these animal studies are required for the development of vaccines and therapeutics under the FDA Animal Rule, it is essential to have a standardized assay to compare their efficacies against the various filoviruses. Here, we present an evaluation of the conditions under which the filovirus plaque assay performs best for the Ebola virus Kikwit variant and the Angola variant of Marburg virus. The indicator cell type and source, inoculum volumes, length of incubation and general features of filovirus biology as visualized in the assay are addressed in terms of the impact on the sample viral titer calculations. These optimization studies have resulted in a plaque assay protocol which can be used for preclinical studies, and as a standardized protocol for use across institutions, to aid in data comparison. This protocol will be validated for use in GLP studies supporting advanced development of filovirus therapeutics and vaccines.
PMCID: PMC3528277 PMID: 23223188 [PubMed - indexed for MEDLINE]

958. Virology. 2012 Dec 5;434(1):18-26. doi: 10.1016/j.virol.2012.07.020. Epub 2012 Aug 11.

A replication-deficient rabies virus vaccine expressing Ebola virus glycoprotein is highly attenuated for neurovirulence.

Papaneri AB(1), Wirblich C, Cann JA, Cooper K, Jahrling PB, Schnell MJ, Blaney JE.

Author information: (1)Emerging Viral Pathogens Section, National Institute of Allergy and Infectious Diseases, National Institutes of Health, Fort Detrick, MD 21702, USA.

We are developing inactivated and live-attenuated rabies virus (RABV) vaccines expressing Ebola virus (EBOV) glycoprotein for use in humans and endangered wildlife, respectively. Here, we further characterize the pathogenesis of the live-attenuated RABV/EBOV vaccine candidates in mice in an effort to define their growth properties and potential for safety. RABV vaccines expressing GP (RV-GP) or a replication-deficient derivative with a deletion of the RABV G gene (RVΔG-GP) are both avirulent after intracerebral inoculation of adult mice. Furthermore, RVΔG-GP is completely avirulent upon intracerebral inoculation of suckling mice unlike parental RABV vaccine or RV-GP. Analysis of RVΔG-GP in the brain by quantitative PCR, determination of virus titer, and immunohistochemistry indicated greatly restricted virus replication. In summary, our findings indicate that RV-GP retains the attenuation phenotype of the live-attenuated RABV vaccine, and RVΔG-GP would appear to be an even safer alternative for use in wildlife or consideration for human use.
Published by Elsevier Inc.

PMCID: PMC3484205 PMID: 22889613 [PubMed - indexed for MEDLINE]

959. Viruses. 2012 Dec 3;4(12):3468-93. doi: 10.3390/v4123468.

Development of a murine model for aerosolized ebolavirus infection using a panel of recombinant inbred mice.

Zumbrun EE(1), Abdeltawab NF, Bloomfield HA, Chance TB, Nichols DK, Harrison PE, Kotb M, Nalca A.

Author information: (1)Center for Aerobiological Sciences, U.S. Army Medical Research Institute of Infectious Diseases (USAMRIID), 1425 Porter Street, Fort Detrick, Maryland 21702, USA. Elizabeth.Zumbrun@us.army.mil

Countering aerosolized filovirus infection is a major priority of biodefense research. Aerosol models of filovirus infection have been developed in knock-out mice, guinea pigs and non-human primates; however, filovirus infection of immunocompetent mice by the aerosol route has not been reported. A murine model of aerosolized filovirus infection in mice should be useful for screening vaccine candidates and therapies. In this study, various strains of wild-type and immunocompromised mice were exposed to aerosolized wild-type (WT) or mouse-adapted (MA) Ebola virus (EBOV). Upon exposure to aerosolized WT-EBOV, BALB/c, C57BL/6 (B6), and DBA/2 (D2) mice were unaffected, but 100% of severe combined immunodeficiency (SCID) and 90% of signal transducers and activators of transcription (Stat1) knock-out (KO) mice became moribund between 7–9 days post-exposure (dpe). Exposure to MA-EBOV caused 15% body weight loss in BALB/c, but all mice recovered. In contrast, 10–30% lethality was observed in B6 and D2 mice exposed to aerosolized MA-EBOV, and 100% of SCID, Stat1 KO, interferon (IFN)-γ KO and Perforin KO mice became moribund between 7–14 dpe. In order to identify wild-type, inbred, mouse strains in which exposure to aerosolized MA-EBOV is uniformly lethal, 60 BXD (C57BL/6 crossed with DBA/2) recombinant inbred (RI) and advanced RI (ARI) mouse strains were exposed to aerosolized MA-EBOV, and monitored for disease severity. A complete spectrum of disease severity was observed. All BXD strains lost weight but many recovered. However, infection was uniformly lethal within 7 to 12 days post-exposure in five BXD strains. Aerosol exposure of these five BXD strains to 10-fold less MA-EBOV resulted in lethality ranging from 0% in two strains to 90–100% lethality in two strains. Analysis of post-mortem tissue from BXD strains that became moribund and were euthanized at the lower dose of MA-EBOV, showed liver damage in all mice as well as lung lesions in two of the three strains. The two BXD strains that exhibited 90–100% mortality, even at a low dose of airborne MA-EBOV will be useful mouse models for testing vaccines and therapies. Additionally, since disease susceptibility is affected by complex genetic traits, a systems genetics approach was used to identify preliminary gene loci modulating disease severity among the panel BXD strains. Preliminary quantitative trait loci (QTLs) were identified that are likely to harbor genes involved in modulating differential susceptibility to Ebola infection.

PMCID: PMC3528275 PMID: 23207275 [PubMed - indexed for MEDLINE]

960. Afr Health Sci. 2012 Dec;12(4):579-83.

Repeated outbreaks of viral hemorrhagic fevers in Uganda.

Mbonye A(1), Wamala J, Winyi-Kaboyo, Tugumizemo V, Aceng J, Makumbi I.

Author information: (1)Ministry of Health Head Quarters, P.O Box 7272 Kampala, Uganda. vpadmn@infocom.co.ug

BACKGROUND: Since the year 2000, Uganda has experienced repeated outbreaks of viral hemorrhagic fevers (VHF). Ebola VHF outbreak occurred in the districts of Gulu in 2000, Bundibugyo, 2007, Luwero, 2011, Kibaale in July 2012, Luwero in November 2012. Marburg VHF was earlier reported in Ibanda in 2007. More recently in 2012, two outbreaks of Marburg VHF have occurred in Ibanda and Kabale districts. OBJECTIVE: To present the epidemiological picture of the Marburg VHF recently reported in Ibanda and Kabale districts and propose research questions to generate evidence to mitigate future epidemics. METHODS: A case definition for a VHF was developed. A frequency distribution of symptoms of confirmed and probable cases was done. Descriptive analyses of reported cases using simple percentages, percent distributions and computation of means was performed. RESULTS: The Marburg epidemic was reported in early September and by November 2012, a cumulative of 14 cases (9 confirmed and 5 probable) including 7 deaths had been registered, giving a case fatality rate (CFR) of 50%. A total of 202 contacts had been listed; out of which 193 had completed the 21-day follow-up period. The index case was a 33-year old male, a teacher at Nyakatukura Secondary School in Ibanda district. He travelled to Ibanda from Kabale, his home district on 31st August 2012, reportedly healthy. He fell sick on 3rd September 2012 with complaints of fever, headache, loss of appetite and general body weakness. Overall, the dominant symptoms for all cases were fever, vomiting, loss of appetite, headache, abdominal pain, fatigue, diarrhea, and the least in occurrence was bleeding which accounted for 35.5% of all the cases. CONCLUSION: The source of infection for all the five Ebola Hemorrhagic fever outbreaks in Uganda and the recent Marburg VHF outbreak in Ibanda and Kabale is not known. Currently there is suspicion that there could be an animal reservoir of the Ebola and Marburg viruses from where occasional spillage into the human population occurs resulting in disease outbreaks. This and other hypotheses require further investigation.

PMCID: PMC3598306 PMID: 23516123 [PubMed - indexed for MEDLINE]

961. J Virol. 2012 Dec;86(24):13467-74. doi: 10.1128/JVI.01896-12. Epub 2012 Oct 3.

Inhibition of Marburg virus budding by nonneutralizing antibodies to the envelope glycoprotein.

Kajihara M(1), Marzi A, Nakayama E, Noda T, Kuroda M, Manzoor R, Matsuno K, Feldmann H, Yoshida R, Kawaoka Y, Takada A.

Author information: (1)Division of Global Epidemiology, Hokkaido University Research Center for Zoonosis Control, Sapporo, Japan.

The envelope glycoprotein (GP) of Marburg virus (MARV) and Ebola virus (EBOV) is responsible for virus entry into host cells and is known as the only target of neutralizing antibodies. While knowledge about EBOV-neutralizing antibodies and the mechanism for the neutralization of infectivity is being accumulated gradually, little is known about antibodies that can efficiently regulate MARV infectivity. Here we show that MARV GP-specific monoclonal antibodies AGP127-8 (IgG1) and MGP72-17 (IgM), which do not inhibit the GP-mediated entry of MARV into host cells, drastically reduced the budding and release of progeny viruses from infected cells. These antibodies similarly inhibited the formation of virus-like particles (VLPs) consisting of GP, the viral matrix protein, and nucleoprotein, whereas the Fab fragment of AGP127-8 showed no inhibitory effect. Morphological analyses revealed that filamentous VLPs were bunched on the surface of VLP-producing cells cultured in the presence of the antibodies. These results demonstrate a novel mechanism of the antibody-mediated inhibition of MARV budding, in which antibodies arrest unformed virus particles on the cell surface. Our data lead to the idea that such antibodies, like classical neutralizing antibodies, contribute to protective immunity against MARV and that the classical neutralizing activity is not the only indicator of a protective antibody that may be available for prophylactic and therapeutic use.

PMCID: PMC3503067 PMID: 23035224 [PubMed - indexed for MEDLINE]

962. Klin Mikrobiol Infekc Lek. 2012 Dec;18(6):180-3.

[Highly contagious diseases with human-to-human transmission].

[Article in Czech]

Rybka A(1), Szanyi J, Kapla J, Plíšek S.
Author information: (1)Department of Infectious Diseases, Charles University, Czech Republic. ales.rybka@fnhk.cz

Highly contagious diseases are caused by various biological agents that pose a risk to individuals and may have a potential for public health impact. They result in high mortality and morbidity rates, might cause public panic and therefore require special measures. The pathogens that can be easily disseminated or transmitted from person to person are the riskiest for clinicians (Ebola virus, Marburg virus, Lassa virus, Crimean-Congo hemorrhagic fever virus, Variola major, SARS virus and Yersinia pestis). Human-to-human transmission has not been confirmed for the other biological agents and therefore they pose a very low risk for population.

PMID: 23386507 [PubMed - indexed for MEDLINE]
963. Chembiochem. 2012 Nov 26;13(17):2549-57. doi: 10.1002/cbic.201200493. Epub 2012 Oct 30.

Two synthetic antibodies that recognize and neutralize distinct proteolytic forms of the ebola virus envelope glycoprotein.

Koellhoffer JF(1), Chen G, Sandesara RG, Bale S, Saphire EO, Chandran K, Sidhu SS, Lai JR.
Author information: (1)Department of Biochemistry, Albert Einstein College of Medicine, 1300 Morris Park Avenue, Bronx, NY 10461, USA.

Ebola virus (EBOV) is a highly pathogenic member of the Filoviridae family of viruses that causes severe hemorrhagic fever. Infection proceeds through fusion of the host cell and viral membranes, a process that is mediated by the viral envelope glycoprotein (GP). Following endosomal uptake, a key step in viral entry is the proteolytic cleavage of GP by host endosomal cysteine proteases. Cleavage exposes a binding site for the host cell receptor Niemann-Pick C1 (NPC1) and may induce conformational changes in GP leading to membrane fusion. However, the precise details of the structural changes in GP associated with proteolysis and the role of these changes in viral entry have not been established. Here, we have employed synthetic antibody technology to identify antibodies targeting EBOV GP prior to and following proteolysis (i.e. in the "uncleaved" [GP(UNCL)] and cleaved [GP(CL)] forms). We identified antibodies with distinct recognition profiles: Fab(CL) bound preferentially to GP(CL) (EC(50)=1.7 nM), whereas Fab(UNCL) bound specifically to GP(UNCL) (EC(50)=75 nM). Neutralization assays with GP-containing pseudotyped viruses indicated that these antibodies inhibited GP(CL)- or GP(UNCL)-mediated viral entry with specificity matching their recognition profiles (IC(50): 87 nM for IgG(CL); 1 μM for Fab(UNCL)). Competition ELISAs indicate that Fab(CL) binds an epitope distinct from that of KZ52, a well-characterized EBOV GP antibody, and from that of the luminal domain of NPC1. The binding epitope of Fab(UNCL) was also distinct from that of KZ52, suggesting that Fab(UNCL) binds a novel neutralization epitope on GP(UNCL). Furthermore, the neutralizing ability of Fab(CL) suggests that there are targets on GP(CL) available for neutralization. This work showcases the applicability of synthetic antibody technology to the study of viral membrane fusion, and provides new tools for dissecting intermediates of EBOV entry.

PMCID: PMC3684266 PMID: 23111988 [PubMed - indexed for MEDLINE]
964. BMC Public Health. 2012 Nov 21;12:1014. doi: 10.1186/1471-2458-12-1014.

Guidance for contact tracing of cases of Lassa fever, Ebola or Marburg haemorrhagic fever on an airplane: results of a European expert consultation.

Gilsdorf A(1), Morgan D, Leitmeyer K.
Author information: (1)Department for Infectious Disease Epidemiology, Robert Koch Institute, Berlin, Germany. GilsdorfA@rki.de

BACKGROUND: Travel from countries where viral haemorrhagic fevers (VHF) are endemic has increased significantly over the past decades. In several reported VHF events on airplanes, passenger trace back was initiated but the scale of the trace back differed considerably. The absence of guidance documents to help the decision on necessity and scale of the trace back contributed to this variation.This article outlines the recommendations of an expert panel on Lassa fever, Ebola and Marburg haemorrhagic fever to the wider scientific community in order to advise the relevant stakeholders in the decision and scale of a possible passenger trace back. METHOD: The evidence was collected through review of published literature and through the views of an expert panel. The guidance was agreed by consensus. RESULTS: Only a few events of VHF cases during air travel are reported in literature, with no documented infection in followed up contacts, so that no evidence of transmission of VHF during air travel exists to date. Based on this and the expert opinion, it was recommended that passenger trace back was undertaken only if: the index case had symptoms during the flight; the flight was within 21 days after detection of the event; and for Lassa fever if exposure of body fluid has been reported. The trace back should only be done after confirmation of the index case. Passengers and crew with direct contact, seat neighbours (+/- 1 seat), crew and cleaning personal of the section of the index case should be included in the trace back. CONCLUSION: No evidence has been found for the transmission of VHF in airplanes. This information should be taken into account, when a trace back decision has to be taken, because such a measure produces an enormous work load. The procedure suggested by the expert group can guide decisions made in future events, where a patient with suspected VHF infection travelled on a plane. However, the actual decision on start and scale of a trace back always lies in the hands of the responsible people taking all relevant information into account.

PMCID: PMC3533809 PMID: 23170851 [PubMed - indexed for MEDLINE]
965. Infect Dis (Auckl). 2012 Nov 19;5:59-64.

In Vivo Replication and Pathogenesis of Vesicular Stomatitis Virus Recombinant M40 Containing Ebola Virus L-Domain Sequences.

Irie T(1), Carnero E, García-Sastre A, Harty RN.
Author information: (1)Department of Virology, Institute of Biomedical and Health Sciences, Hiroshima University, Hiroshima, Japan.

The M40 VSV recombinant was engineered to contain overlapping PTAP and PPxY L-domain motifs and flanking residues from the VP40 protein of Ebola virus. Replication of M40 in cell culture is virtually indistinguishable from that of control viruses. However, the presence of the Ebola PTAP motif in the M40

recombinant enabled this virus to interact with and recruit host Tsg101, which was packaged into M40 virions. In this brief report, we compared replication and the pathogenic profiles of M40 and the parental virus M51R in mice to determine whether the presence of the Ebola L-domains and flanking residues altered in vivo characteristics of the virus. Overall, the in vivo characteristics of M40 were similar to those of the parental M51R virus, indicating that the Ebola sequences did not alter pathogenesis of VSV in this small animal model of infection.
PMCID: PMC3686127 PMID: 23794798 [PubMed]
966. Lancet. 2012 Nov 17;380(9855):1726.

Uganda battles Marburg fever outbreak.
Green A.
PMID: 23166919 [PubMed - indexed for MEDLINE]
967. Science. 2012 Nov 9;338(6108):750-2. doi: 10.1126/science.1225893.

Epidemiology. Emerging disease or diagnosis?
Gire SK(1), Stremlau M, Andersen KG, Schaffner SF, Bjornson Z, Rubins K, Hensley L, McCormick JB, Lander ES, Garry RF, Happi C, Sabeti PC.
Author information: (1)Center for Systems Biology, Department of Organismic and Evolutionary Biology, Harvard University, Cambridge, MA, USA. sgire@oeb.harvard.edu
PMID: 23139320 [PubMed - indexed for MEDLINE]
968. Biophys J. 2012 Nov 7;103(9):L41-3. doi: 10.1016/j.bpj.2012.09.026.

Single-particle tracking demonstrates that actin coordinates the movement of the Ebola virus matrix protein.
Adu-Gyamfi E(1), Digman MA, Gratton E, Stahelin RV.
Author information: (1)Department of Chemistry & Biochemistry and the Eck Institute for Global Health, University of Notre Dame, Notre Dame, Indiana, USA.
The Ebola virus causes severe hemorrhagic fever and has a mortality rate that can be as high as 90%, yet no vaccines or approved therapeutics, to our knowledge, are available. To replicate and egress the infected host cell the Ebola virus uses VP40, its major matrix protein to assemble at the inner leaflet of the plasma membrane. The assembly and budding of VP40 from the plasma membrane of host cells seem still poorly understood. We investigated the assembly and egress of VP40 at the plasma membrane of human cells using single-particle tracking. Our results demonstrate that actin coordinates the movement and assembly of VP40, a critical step in viral egress. These findings underscore the ability of single-molecule techniques to investigate the interplay of VP40 and host proteins in viral replication.
PMCID: PMC3491695 PMID: 23199932 [PubMed - indexed for MEDLINE]
969. Viruses. 2012 Nov 6;4(11):2806-30. doi: 10.3390/v4112806.

Discovery and early development of AVI-7537 and AVI-7288 for the treatment of Ebola virus and Marburg virus infections.
Iversen PL(1), Warren TK, Wells JB, Garza NL, Mourich DV, Welch LS, Panchal RG, Bavari S.
Author information: (1)Sarepta Therapeutics, Bothell, Washington 98021, USA. piversen@sareptatherapeutics.com
There are no currently approved treatments for filovirus infections. In this study we report the discovery process which led to the development of antisense Phosphorodiamidate Morpholino Oligomers (PMOs) AVI-6002 (composed of AVI-7357 and AVI-7539) and AVI-6003 (composed of AVI-7287 and AVI-7288) targeting Ebola virus and Marburg virus respectively. The discovery process involved identification of optimal transcript binding sites for PMO based RNA-therapeutics followed by screening for effective viral gene target in mouse and guinea pig models utilizing adapted viral isolates. An evolution of chemical modifications were tested, beginning with simple Phosphorodiamidate Morpholino Oligomers (PMO) transitioning to cell penetrating peptide conjugated PMOs (PPMO) and ending with PMOplus containing a limited number of positively charged linkages in the PMO structure. The initial lead compounds were combinations of two agents targeting separate genes. In the final analysis, a single agent for treatment of each virus was selected, AVI-7537 targeting the VP24 gene of Ebola virus and AVI-7288 targeting NP of Marburg virus, and are now progressing into late stage clinical development as the optimal therapeutic candidates.
PMCID: PMC3509674 PMID: 23202506 [PubMed - indexed for MEDLINE]
970. Wkly Epidemiol Rec. 2012 Nov 2;87(44):421.

Outbreak news. Ebola, Democratic Republic of the Congo.
[Article in English, French]
[No authors listed]
PMID: 23139950 [PubMed - indexed for MEDLINE]
971. Clin Vaccine Immunol. 2012 Nov;19(11):1844-52. doi: 10.1128/CVI.00363-12. Epub 2012 Sep 19.

Profiling the native specific human humoral immune response to Sudan Ebola virus strain Gulu by chemiluminescence enzyme-linked immunosorbent assay.
Sobarzo A(1), Perelman E, Groseth A, Dolnik O, Becker S, Lutwama JJ, Dye JM, Yavelsky V, Lobel L, Marks RS.
Author information: (1)Department of Virology & Developmental Genetics, Ben-Gurion University of the Negev, Beer-Sheva, Israel.
Ebolavirus, a member of the family Filoviridae, causes high lethality in humans and nonhuman primates. Research focused on protection and therapy for Ebola virus infection has investigated the potential role of antibodies. Recent evidence suggests that antibodies can be effective in protection from lethal challenge with Ebola virus in nonhuman primates. However, despite these encouraging results, studies have not yet determined the optimal antibodies and composition of an antibody cocktail, if required, which might serve as a highly effective and efficient prophylactic. To better understand optimal antibodies and their targets,

which might be important for protection from Ebola virus infection, we sought to determine the profile of viral protein-specific antibodies generated during a natural cycle of infection in humans. To this end, we characterized the profile of antibodies against individual viral proteins of Sudan Ebola virus (Gulu) in human survivors and nonsurvivors of the outbreak in Gulu, Uganda, in 2000-2001. We developed a unique chemiluminescence enzyme-linked immunosorbent assay (ELISA) for this purpose based on the full-length recombinant viral proteins NP, VP30, and VP40 and two recombinant forms of the viral glycoprotein (GP(1-294) and GP(1-649)) of Sudan Ebola virus (Gulu). Screening results revealed that the greatest immunoreactivity was directed to the viral proteins NP and GP(1-649), followed by VP40. Comparison of positive immunoreactivity between the viral proteins NP, GP(1-649), and VP40 demonstrated a high correlation of immunoreactivity between these viral proteins, which is also linked with survival. Overall, our studies of the profile of immunorecognition of antibodies against four viral proteins of Sudan Ebola virus in human survivors may facilitate development of effective monoclonal antibody cocktails in the future.

PMCID: PMC3491549 PMID: 22993411 [PubMed - indexed for MEDLINE]

972. Hum Vaccin Immunother. 2012 Nov 1;8(11):1703-6. doi: 10.4161/hv.21873. Epub 2012 Aug 24.

A multiagent filovirus DNA vaccine delivered by intramuscular electroporation completely protects mice from ebola and Marburg virus challenge.

Grant-Klein RJ(1), Van Deusen NM, Badger CV, Hannaman D, Dupuy LC, Schmaljohn CS.

Author information: (1)U.S. Army Medical Research Institute of Infectious Diseases, Fort Detrick, MD, USA. Rebecca.J.Klein@us.army.mil

We evaluated the immunogenicity and protective efficacy of DNA vaccines expressing the codon-optimized envelope glycoprotein genes of Zaire ebolavirus, Sudan ebolavirus, and Marburg marburgvirus (Musoke and Ravn). Intramuscular or intradermal delivery of the vaccines in BALB/c mice was performed using the TriGrid™ electroporation device. Mice that received DNA vaccines against the individual viruses developed robust glycoprotein-specific antibody titers as determined by ELISA and survived lethal viral challenge with no display of clinical signs of infection. Survival curve analysis revealed there was a statistically significant increase in survival compared to the control groups for both the Ebola and Ravn virus challenges. These data suggest that further analysis of the immune responses generated in the mice and additional protection studies in nonhuman primates are warranted.

PMCID: PMC3601145 PMID: 22922764 [PubMed - indexed for MEDLINE]

973. J Virol. 2012 Nov;86(21):11779-88. doi: 10.1128/JVI.01525-12. Epub 2012 Aug 22.

Inclusion bodies are a site of ebolavirus replication.

Hoenen T(1), Shabman RS, Groseth A, Herwig A, Weber M, Schudt G, Dolnik O, Basler CF, Becker S, Feldmann H.

Author information: (1)Laboratory for Virology, Division of Intramural Research, National Institute of Allergy and Infectious Diseases, National Institutes of Health, Rocky Mountain Laboratories, Hamilton, Montana, USA.

Inclusion bodies are a characteristic feature of ebolavirus infections in cells. They contain large numbers of preformed nucleocapsids, but their biological significance has been debated, and they have been suggested to be aggregates of viral proteins without any further biological function. However, recent data for other viruses that produce similar structures have suggested that inclusion bodies might be involved in genome replication and transcription. In order to study filovirus inclusion bodies, we fused mCherry to the ebolavirus polymerase L, which is found in inclusion bodies. The resulting L-mCherry fusion protein was functional in minigenome assays and incorporated into virus-like particles. Importantly, L-mCherry fluorescence in transfected cells was readily detectable and distributed in a punctate pattern characteristic for inclusion bodies. A recombinant ebolavirus encoding L-mCherry instead of L was rescued and showed virtually identical growth kinetics and endpoint titers to those for wild-type virus. Using this virus, we showed that the onset of inclusion body formation corresponds to the onset of viral genome replication, but that viral transcription occurs prior to inclusion body formation. Live-cell imaging further showed that inclusion bodies are highly dynamic structures and that they can undergo dramatic reorganization during cell division. Finally, by labeling nascent RNAs using click technology we showed that inclusion bodies are indeed the site of viral RNA synthesis. Based on these data we conclude that, rather than being inert aggregates of nucleocapsids, ebolavirus inclusion bodies are in fact complex and dynamic structures and an important site at which viral RNA replication takes place.

PMCID: PMC3486333 PMID: 22915810 [PubMed - indexed for MEDLINE]

974. Sheng Wu Gong Cheng Xue Bao. 2012 Nov;28(11):1317-27.

Generation and epitope mapping of a monoclonal antibody against nucleoprotein of Ebola virus.

Wang X(1), Liu Y, Wang H, Shi Z, Zhao F, Wei J, Shao D, Ma Z.

Author information: (1)Forestry and Biotechnology School, Zhejiang Agriculture and Forestry University, Lin'an 311300, Zhejiang, China. xiaoduwang@163.com

Ebola virus (EBOV) causes highly lethal hemorrhagic fever in humans and nonhuman primates and has a significant impact on public health. The nucleoprotein (NP) of EBOV (EBOV-NP) plays a central role in virus replication and has been used as a target molecule for disease diagnosis. In this study, we generated a monoclonal antibody (MAb) against EBOV-NP and mapped the epitope motif required for recognition by the MAb. The MAb generated via immunization of mice with prokaryotically expressed recombinant NP of the Zaire Ebola virus (ZEBOV-NP) was specific to ZEBOV-NP and able to recognize ZEBOV-NP expressed in prokaryotic and eukaryotic cells. The MAb cross-reacted with the NP of the Reston Ebola virus (REBOV), the Cote-d'Ivoire Ebola virus (CIEBOV) and the Bundibugyo Ebola virus (BEBOV) but not with the NP of the Sudan Ebola virus (SEBOV) or the Marburg virus (MARV). The minimal epitope sequence required for recognition by the MAb was the motif PPLESD, which is located between amino acid residues 583 and 588 at the C-terminus of ZEBOV-NP and well conserved among all 16 strains of ZEBOV, CIEBOV and BEBOV deposited in GenBank. The epitope motif is conserved in four out of five strains of REBOV.

PMID: 23457784 [PubMed - indexed for MEDLINE]

975. Vopr Virusol. 2012 Nov-Dec;57(6):5-8.

[Immunosuppression at pregnancy and flu].

[Article in Russian]

Kiselev OI.

The hypothesis of the development of immunosuppression at the pregnancy is put forward in this review. This hypothesis is explaining the complicated character of the pandemic H1N1pdm09 infection among pregnant women. Physiological immunosuppression at pregnancy is based on suppression of various T-lymphocyte subpopulations using a unique mechanism: dimerization blockade of TcR receptors by special domains known as immunosuppressive sequences. These protein sequences were recognized in placentary Syntcytins and in proteins of pathogenic viruses, including Ebola virus and retroviruses. Among H5N1 and H1N1pdm09 influenza virus homologs of immunosuppressive domains are revealed and identified as the pathogenicity factors. Synthetic peptides, homologs of these domains, suppress an antigen-induced T-lymphocyte proliferation by inhibiting of TcR and NKG2D receptor activation. Integration of immunosuppressive domains into T-lymphocyte membrane leads to electrostatic pair formation and dimerization through interaction with transmembrane domains of TcR and NKG2D receptors.

PMID: 23477246 [PubMed - indexed for MEDLINE]

976. Zh Mikrobiol Epidemiol Immunobiol. 2012 Nov-Dec;(6):103-6.

[Evaluation of safety of prophylactic use of immunoglobulins against viral hemorrhagic fevers from horse blood sera].

[Article in Russian]

Khmelev AL, Borisevich IV, Chernikova NK, Makhlaĭ AA, Mikhaĭlov VV, Iakovlev AK, Podkuĭko VN, Krasnianskiĭ VP, Borisevich SV, Bondarev VP.

AIM: Evaluate safety of prophylaxis of viral hemorrhagic fevers by specific heterologous immunoglobulins. MATERIALS AND METHODS: Clinical-laboratory examination of 24 individuals after intramuscular administration of heterologous Ebola immunoglobulin was carried out. Anaphylactogenicity of the immunoglobulins was studied by WD 42-28-8-89 in guinea pigs compared with commercial preparations. RESULTS: Immediate type reactions were not observed. In individuals with normal anamnesis the number of local reactions was 31%, general in the form of lung serum disease - 13%. In individuals with unfavorable anamnesis against the background of desensitization therapy there were almost no reactions; without it local reactions were present in 50%, mild severity serum lung disease - in 17%, medium - in 33%. Immunoglobulins against especially dangerous viral agents by anaphylactogenic properties did not differ from commercial heterologous preparations. CONCLUSION: Application of specific immunoglobulins from horse blood sera (the main means of protection from dangerous and especially dangerous exotic viral infections) with compliance by desensitization principles is relatively safe. Safe level of sensitization properties is characterized by anaphylaxis index up to 3.7 for guinea pigs.

PMID: 23297643 [PubMed - indexed for MEDLINE]

977. Sci Transl Med. 2012 Oct 31;4(158):158ra146. doi: 10.1126/scitranslmed.3004582.

Immune parameters correlate with protection against ebola virus infection in rodents and nonhuman primates.

Wong G(1), Richardson JS, Pillet S, Patel A, Qiu X, Alimonti J, Hogan J, Zhang Y, Takada A, Feldmann H, Kobinger GP.

Author information: (1)Special Pathogens Program, National Microbiology Laboratory, Public Health Agency of Canada, Winnipeg, Manitoba R3E 3R2, Canada.

Ebola virus causes severe hemorrhagic fever in susceptible hosts. Currently, no licensed vaccines or treatments are available; however, several experimental vaccines have been successful in protecting rodents and nonhuman primates (NHPs) from the lethal Zaire ebolavirus (ZEBOV) infection. The objective of this study was to evaluate immune responses correlating with survival in these animals after lethal challenge with ZEBOV. Knockout mice with impaired ability to generate normal T and/or B cell responses were vaccinated and challenged with ZEBOV. Vaccine-induced protection in mice was mainly mediated by B cells and CD4(+) T cells. Vaccinated, outbred guinea pigs and NHPs demonstrated the highest correlation between survival and levels of total immunoglobulin G (IgG) specific to the ZEBOV glycoprotein (ZGP). These results highlight the relevance of total ZGP-specific IgG levels as a meaningful correlate of protection against ZEBOV exposure.

PMCID: PMC3789651 PMID: 23115355 [PubMed - indexed for MEDLINE]

978. Proc Natl Acad Sci U S A. 2012 Oct 30;109(44):18030-5. doi: 10.1073/pnas.1213709109. Epub 2012 Oct 15.

Delayed treatment of Ebola virus infection with plant-derived monoclonal antibodies provides protection in rhesus macaques.

Olinger GG Jr(1), Pettitt J, Kim D, Working C, Bohorov O, Bratcher B, Hiatt E, Hume SD, Johnson AK, Morton J, Pauly M, Whaley KJ, Lear CM, Biggins JE, Scully C, Hensley L, Zeitlin L.

Author information: (1)Division of Virology, United States Army Medical Research Institute of Infectious Diseases, Frederick, MD 21702, USA. olinger@us.army.mil

Filovirus infections can cause a severe and often fatal disease in humans and nonhuman primates, including great apes. Here, three anti-Ebola virus mouse/human chimeric mAbs (c13C6, h-13F6, and c6D8) were produced in Chinese hamster ovary and in whole plant (Nicotiana benthamiana) cells. In pilot experiments testing a mixture of the three mAbs (MB-003), we found that MB-003 produced in both manufacturing systems protected rhesus macaques from lethal challenge when administered 1 h postinfection. In a pivotal follow-up experiment, we found significant protection (P < 0.05) when MB-003 treatment began 24 or 48 h postinfection (four of six survived vs. zero of two controls). In all experiments, surviving animals that received MB-003 experienced little to no viremia and had few, if any, of the clinical symptoms observed in the controls. The results represent successful postexposure in vivo efficacy by a mAb mixture and suggest that this immunoprotectant should be further pursued as a postexposure and potential therapeutic for Ebola virus exposure.

PMCID: PMC3497800 PMID: 23071322 [PubMed - indexed for MEDLINE]

979. Viruses. 2012 Oct 25;4(11):2471-84. doi: 10.3390/v4112471.

Niemann-Pick C1 (NPC1)/NPC1-like1 chimeras define sequences critical for NPC1's function as a flovirus entry receptor.

Krishnan A(1), Miller EH, Herbert AS, Ng M, Ndungo E, Whelan SP, Dye JM, Chandran K.

Author information: (1)Department of Microbiology and Immunology, Albert Einstein College of Medicine, 1300 Morris Park Ave, Bronx, NY 10461, USA. anuja@immindia.org

We recently demonstrated that Niemann-Pick C1 (NPC1), a ubiquitous 13-pass cellular membrane protein involved in lysosomal cholesterol transport, is a critical entry receptor for filoviruses. Here we show that Niemann-Pick C1-like1 (NPC1L1), an NPC1 paralog and hepatitis C virus entry factor, lacks filovirus receptor activity. We exploited the structural similarity between NPC1 and NPC1L1 to construct and analyze a panel of chimeras in which NPC1L1 sequences were replaced with cognate sequences from NPC1. Only one chimera, NPC1L1 containing the second luminal domain (C) of NPC1 in place of its own, bound to the viral glycoprotein, GP. This engineered protein mediated authentic filovirus infection nearly as well as wild-type NPC1, and more efficiently than did a minimal NPC1 domain C-based receptor recently described by us. A reciprocal chimera, NPC1 containing NPC1L1's domain C, was completely inactive. Remarkably, an intra-domain NPC1L1-NPC1 chimera bearing only a ~130-amino acid N-terminal region of NPC1 domain C could confer substantial viral receptor activity on NPC1L1. Taken together, these findings account for the failure of NPC1L1 to serve as a filovirus receptor, highlight the central role of the luminal domain C of NPC1 in filovirus entry, and reveal the direct involvement of N-terminal domain C sequences in NPC1's function as a filovirus receptor.

PMCID: PMC3509659 PMID: 23202491 [PubMed - indexed for MEDLINE]

980. Viruses. 2012 Oct 23;4(10):2400-16. doi: 10.3390/v4102400.

The Baboon (Papio spp.) as a model of human Ebola virus infection.

Perry DL(1), Bollinger L, White GL.

Author information: (1)Integrated Research Facility, Division of Clinical Research, NIAID, NIH, Frederick, MD, USA. perrydl@niaid.nih.gov

Baboons are susceptible to natural Ebola virus (EBOV) infection and share 96% genetic homology with humans. Despite these characteristics, baboons have rarely been utilized as experimental models of human EBOV infection to evaluate the efficacy of prophylactics and therapeutics in the United States. This review will summarize what is known about the pathogenesis of EBOV infection in baboons compared to EBOV infection in humans and other Old World nonhuman primates. In addition, we will discuss how closely the baboon model recapitulates human EBOV infection. We will also review some of the housing requirements and behavioral attributes of baboons compared to other Old World nonhuman primates. Due to the lack of data available on the pathogenesis of Marburg virus (MARV) infection in baboons, discussion of the pathogenesis of MARV infection in baboons will be limited.

PMCID: PMC3497058 PMID: 23202470 [PubMed - indexed for MEDLINE]

981. Philos Trans R Soc Lond B Biol Sci. 2012 Oct 19;367(1604):2881-92. doi: 10.1098/rstb.2012.0228.

A framework for the study of zoonotic disease emergence and its drivers: spillover of bat pathogens as a case study.

Wood JL(1), Leach M, Waldman L, Macgregor H, Fooks AR, Jones KE, Restif O, Dechmann D, Hayman DT, Baker KS, Peel AJ, Kamins AO, Fahr J, Ntiamoa-Baidu Y, Suu-Ire R, Breiman RF, Epstein JH, Field HE, Cunningham AA.

Author information: (1)Disease Dynamics Unit, University of Cambridge, Madingley Road, Cambridge CB3 0ES, UK. jlnw2@cam.ac.uk

Many serious emerging zoonotic infections have recently arisen from bats, including Ebola, Marburg, SARS-coronavirus, Hendra, Nipah, and a number of rabies and rabies-related viruses, consistent with the overall observation that wildlife are an important source of emerging zoonoses for the human population. Mechanisms underlying the recognized association between ecosystem health and human health remain poorly understood and responding appropriately to the ecological, social and economic conditions that facilitate disease emergence and transmission represents a substantial societal challenge. In the context of disease emergence from wildlife, wildlife and habitat should be conserved, which in turn will preserve vital ecosystem structure and function, which has broader implications for human wellbeing and environmental sustainability, while simultaneously minimizing the spillover of pathogens from wild animals into human beings. In this review, we propose a novel framework for the holistic and interdisciplinary investigation of zoonotic disease emergence and its drivers, using the spillover of bat pathogens as a case study. This study has been developed to gain a detailed interdisciplinary understanding, and it combines cutting-edge perspectives from both natural and social sciences, linked to policy impacts on public health, land use and conservation.

PMCID: PMC3427567 PMID: 22966143 [PubMed - indexed for MEDLINE]

982. Viruses. 2012 Oct 15;4(10):2115-36. doi: 10.3390/v4102115.

A characterization of aerosolized Sudan virus infection in African green monkeys, cynomolgus macaques, and rhesus macaques.

Zumbrun EE(1), Bloomfield HA, Dye JM, Hunter TC, Dabisch PA, Garza NL, Bramel NR, Baker RJ, Williams RD, Nichols DK, Nalca A.

Author information: (1)Center for Aerobiological Sciences, US Army Medical Research Institute of Infectious Diseases, Fort Detrick, Maryland 21702, USA.

Filoviruses are members of the genera Ebolavirus, Marburgvirus, and "Cuevavirus". Because they cause human disease with high lethality and could potentially be used as a bioweapon, these viruses are classified as CDC Category A Bioterrorism Agents. Filoviruses are relatively stable in aerosols, retain virulence after lyophilization, and can be present on contaminated surfaces for extended periods of time. This study explores the characteristics of aerosolized Sudan virus (SUDV) Boniface in non-human primates (NHP) belonging to three different species. Groups of cynomolgus macaques (cyno), rhesus macaques (rhesus), and African green monkeys (AGM) were challenged with target doses of 50 or 500 plaque-forming units (pfu) of aerosolized SUDV. Exposure to either viral dose resulted in increased body temperatures in all three NHP species beginning on days 4-5 post-exposure. Other clinical findings for all three NHP species included leukocytosis, thrombocytopenia, anorexia, dehydration, and lymphadenopathy. Disease in all of the NHPs was severe beginning on day 6 post-exposure, and all animals except one surviving rhesus macaque were euthanized by day 14. Serum alanine transaminase (ALT) and aspartate transaminase (AST) concentrations were elevated during the course of disease in all three species; however, AGMs had significantly higher ALT and AST concentrations than cynos and rhesus. While all three species had detectable viral load by days 3-4 post exposure, Rhesus had lower average peak viral load than cynos or AGMs. Overall, the results indicate that the disease course after exposure to aerosolized SUDV is similar for all three species of NHP.

PMCID: PMC3497044 PMID: 23202456 [PubMed - indexed for MEDLINE]

983. Virol J. 2012 Oct 13;9:236. doi: 10.1186/1743-422X-9-236.

Serological evidence of ebolavirus infection in bats, China.

Yuan J(1), Zhang Y, Li J, Zhang Y, Wang LF, Shi Z.
Author information: (1)State Key Laboratory of Virology, Wuhan Institute of Virology-Chinese Academy of Sciences, Wuhan, Hubei 430071, P R China.

BACKGROUND: The genus Ebolavirus of the family Filoviridae currently consists of five species. All species, with the exception of Reston ebolavirus, have been found in Africa and caused severe human diseases. Bats have been implicated as reservoirs for ebolavirus. Reston ebolavirus, discovered in the Philippines, is the only ebolavirus species identified in Asia to date. Whether this virus is prevalent in China is unknown. FINDINGS: In this study, we developed an enzyme linked immunosorbent assay (ELISA) for ebolavirus using the recombinant nucleocapsid protein and performed sero-surveillance for the virus among Chinese bat populations. Our results revealed the presence of antibodies to ebolavirus in 32 of 843 bat sera samples and 10 of 16 were further confirmed by western blot analysis. CONCLUSION: To our knowledge, this is the first report of any filovirus infection in China.

PMCID: PMC3492202 PMID: 23062147 [PubMed - indexed for MEDLINE]

984. BMC Vet Res. 2012 Oct 11;8:189. doi: 10.1186/1746-6148-8-189.

Analysis of the humoral immune responses among cynomolgus macaque naturally infected with Reston virus during the 1996 outbreak in the Philippines.

Taniguchi S(1), Sayama Y, Nagata N, Ikegami T, Miranda ME, Watanabe S, Iizuka I, Fukushi S, Mizutani T, Ishii Y, Saijo M, Akashi H, Yoshikawa Y, Kyuwa S, Morikawa S.
Author information: (1)Special Pathogens Laboratory, Department of Virology 1, National Institute of Infectious Diseases, 4-7-1 Gakuen, Musashimurayama, Tokyo, 208-0011, Japan.

BACKGROUND: Ebolaviruses induce lethal viral hemorrhagic fevers (VHFs) in humans and non-human primates, with the exceptions of Reston virus (RESTV), which is not pathogenic for humans. In human VHF cases, extensive analyses of the humoral immune responses in survivors and non-survivors have shown that the IgG responses to nucleoprotein (NP) and other viral proteins are associated with asymptomatic and survival outcomes, and that the neutralizing antibody responses targeting ebolaviruses glycoprotein (GP1,2) are the major indicator of protective immunity. On the other hand, the immune responses in non-human primates, especially naturally infected ones, have not yet been elucidated in detail, and the significance of the antibody responses against NP and GP1,2 in RESTV-infected cynomolgus macaques is still unclear. In this study, we analyzed the humoral immune responses of cynomolgus macaque by using serum specimens obtained from the RESTV epizootic in 1996 in the Philippines to expand our knowledge on the immune responses in naturally RESTV-infected non-human primates. RESULTS: The antibody responses were analyzed using IgG-ELISA, an indirect immunofluorescent antibody assay (IFA), and a pseudotyped VSV-based neutralizing (NT) assay. Antigen-capture (Ag)-ELISA was also performed to detect viral antigens in the serum specimens. We found that the anti-GP1,2 responses, but not the anti-NP responses, closely were correlated with the neutralization responses, as well as the clearance of viremia in the sera of the RESTV-infected cynomolgus macaques. Additionally, by analyzing the cytokine/chemokine concentrations of these serum specimens, we found high concentrations of proinflammatory cytokines/chemokines, such as IFNγ, IL8, IL-12, and MIP1α, in the convalescent phase sera. CONCLUSIONS: These results imply that both the antibody response to GP1,2 and the proinflammatory innate responses play significant roles in the recovery from RESTV infection in cynomolgus macaques.

PMCID: PMC3528628 PMID: 23057674 [PubMed - indexed for MEDLINE]

985. Euro Surveill. 2012 Oct 11;17(41):20295.

The Hajj: updated health hazards and current recommendations for 2012.

Al-Tawfiq JA(1), Memish ZA.
Author information: (1)Saudi Aramco Medical Services Organization, Dhahran, Kingdom of Saudi Arabia.

This year the Hajj will take place during 24-29 October. Recent outbreaks of Ebola haemorrhagic fever in Uganda and the Democratic Republic of the Congo, cholera in Sierra Leone, and infections associated with a novel coronavirus in Saudi Arabia and Qatar required review of the health recommendations of the 2012 Hajj. Current guidelines foresee mandatory vaccination with quadrivalent meningococcal vaccine for all pilgrims, and yellow fever and poliomyelitis vaccine for pilgrims from high-risk countries. Influenza vaccine is strongly recommended.

PMID: 23078811 [PubMed - indexed for MEDLINE]

986. Virology. 2012 Oct 10;432(1):20-8. doi: 10.1016/j.virol.2012.05.018. Epub 2012 Jun 21.

Chinese hamster ovary cell lines selected for resistance to ebolavirus glycoprotein mediated infection are defective for NPC1 expression.

Haines KM(1), Vande Burgt NH, Francica JR, Kaletsky RL, Bates P.
Author information: (1)Department of Microbiology, Perelman School of Medicine, University of Pennsylvania, Philadelphia, PA 19104-6076, USA.

Ebolavirus causes severe hemorrhagic fever in humans and non-human primates. Entry of ebolavirus is mediated by the viral glycoprotein, GP; however, the required host factors have not been fully elucidated. A screen utilizing a recombinant Vesicular Stomatitis Virus (VSV) encoding Zaire ebolavirus GP identified four Chinese Hamster Ovary (CHO) cell lines resistant to GP-mediated viral entry. Susceptibility to vectors carrying SARS coronavirus S or VSV-G glycoproteins suggests that endocytic and processing pathways utilized by other viruses are intact in these cells. A cathepsin-activated form of the ebolaviral glycoprotein did not overcome the entry restriction, nor did expression of several host factors previously described as important for ebolavirus entry. Conversely, expression of the recently described ebolavirus host entry factor Niemann-Pick Type C1 (NPC1) restored infection. Resistant cells encode distinct mutations in the NPC1 gene, resulting in loss of protein expression. These studies reinforce the importance of NPC1 for ebolavirus entry.

PMCID: PMC3402687 PMID: 22726751 [PubMed - indexed for MEDLINE]

987. Biochemistry. 2012 Oct 2;51(39):7665-75. doi: 10.1021/bi300976m. Epub 2012 Sep 19

Crystal structure of the Marburg virus GP2 core domain in its postfusion conformation.

Koellhoffer JF(1), Malashkevich VN, Harrison JS, Toro R, Bhosle RC, Chandran K, Almo SC, Lai JR.

Author information: (1)Department of Biochemistry, Albert Einstein College of Medicine, Bronx, New York 10461, United States.

Marburg virus (MARV) and Ebola virus (EBOV) are members of the family Filoviridae ("filoviruses") and cause severe hemorrhagic fever with human case fatality rates of up to 90%. Filovirus infection requires fusion of the host cell and virus membranes, a process that is mediated by the envelope glycoprotein (GP). GP contains two subunits, the surface subunit (GP1), which is responsible for cell attachment, and the transmembrane subunit (GP2), which catalyzes membrane fusion. The GP2 ectodomain contains two heptad repeat regions, N-terminal and C-terminal (NHR and CHR, respectively), that adopt a six-helix bundle during the fusion process. The refolding of this six-helix bundle provides the thermodynamic driving force to overcome barriers associated with membrane fusion. Here we report the crystal structure of the MARV GP2 core domain in its postfusion (six-helix bundle) conformation at 1.9 Å resolution. The MARV GP2 core domain backbone conformation is virtually identical to that of EBOV GP2 (reported previously), and consists of a central NHR core trimeric coiled coil packed against peripheral CHR α-helices and an intervening loop and helix-turn-helix segments. We previously reported that the stability of the MARV GP2 postfusion structure is highly pH-dependent, with increasing stability at lower pH [Harrison, J. S., Koellhoffer, J. K., Chandran, K., and Lai, J. R. (2012) Biochemistry51, 2515-2525]. We hypothesized that this pH-dependent stability provides a mechanism for conformational control such that the postfusion six-helix bundle is promoted in the environments of appropriately mature endosomes. In this report, a structural rationale for this pH-dependent stability is described and involves a high-density array of core and surface acidic side chains at the midsection of the structure, termed the "anion stripe". In addition, many surface-exposed salt bridges likely contribute to the stabilization of the postfusion structure at low pH. These results provide structural insights into the mechanism of MARV GP2-mediated membrane fusion.

PMCID: PMC3464016 PMID: 22935026 [PubMed - indexed for MEDLINE]

988. Expert Opin Drug Discov. 2012 Oct;7(10):935-54. Epub 2012 Aug 8.

Therapeutics for filovirus infection: traditional approaches and progress towards in silico drug design.

Shurtleff AC(1), Nguyen TL, Kingery DA, Bavari S.

Author information: (1)U.S. Army Medical Research Institute of Infectious Diseases, Integrated Toxicology Division, Fort Detrick, 1425 Porter Street, Frederick, MD 21702, USA. amy.c.shurtleff.ctr@us.army.mil

INTRODUCTION: Ebolaviruses and marburgviruses cause severe and often lethal human hemorrhagic fevers. As no FDA-approved therapeutics are available for these infections, efforts to discover new therapeutics are important, especially because these pathogens are considered biothreats and emerging infectious diseases. All methods for discovering new therapeutics should be considered, including compound library screening in vitro against virus and in silico structure-based drug design, where possible, if sufficient biochemical and structural information is available. AREAS COVERED: This review covers the structure and function of filovirus proteins, as they have been reported to date, as well as some of the current antiviral screening approaches. The authors discuss key studies mapping small-molecule modulators that were found through library and in silico screens to potential sites on viral proteins or host proteins involved in virus trafficking and pathogenesis. A description of ebolavirus and marburgvirus diseases and available animal models is also presented. EXPERT OPINION: To discover novel therapeutics with potent efficacy using sophisticated computational methods, more high-resolution crystal structures of filovirus proteins and more details about the protein functions and host interaction will be required. Current compound screening efforts are finding active antiviral compounds, but an emphasis on discovery research to investigate protein structures and functions enabling in silico drug design would provide another avenue for finding antiviral molecules. Additionally, targeting of protein-protein interactions may be a future avenue for drug discovery since disrupting catalytic sites may not be possible for all proteins.

PMID: 22873527 [PubMed - indexed for MEDLINE]

989. Expert Rev Anti Infect Ther. 2012 Oct;10(10):1129-38. doi: 10.1586/eri.12.104.

Development of novel entry inhibitors targeting emerging viruses.

Zhou Y(1), Simmons G.

Author information: (1)Blood Systems Research Institute and Department of Laboratory Medicine, University of California, San Francisco, 270 Masonic Avenue, San Francisco, CA 94118, USA.

Emerging viral diseases pose a unique risk to public health, and thus there is a need to develop therapies. A current focus of funding agencies, and hence research, is the development of broad-spectrum antivirals, and in particular, those targeting common cellular pathways. The scope of this article is to review screening strategies and recent advances in this area, with a particular emphasis on antivirals targeting the step of viral entry for emerging lipid-enveloped viruses such as Ebola virus and SARS-coronavirus.

PMCID: PMC3587779 PMID: 23199399 [PubMed - indexed for MEDLINE]

990. J Wildl Dis. 2012 Oct;48(4):888-98. doi: 10.7589/2011-11-341.

Maximizing nonhuman primate fecal sampling in the Republic of Congo.

Olson SH(1), Cameron K, Reed P, Ondzie A, Joly D.

Author information: (1)Wildlife Conservation Society, 900 Fifth Street, Building 373, Nanaimo, BC V9R 5S5, Canada.

Techniques for detection of pathogens in wildlife feces allow disease surveillance of species that are difficult to locate and capture (e.g., great apes). However, optimal strategies for detection of feces in logistically challenging environments, such as the forests of Central Africa, have not been developed. We modeled fecal gorilla sampling in the Republic of Congo with computer simulations to explore the performance of different fecal sampling designs in large tropical landscapes. We simulated directed reconnaissance walk (recce) and line-transect distance-sampling survey designs and combinations thereof to maximize the number of fecal samples collected, while also estimating relative ape density on a virtual landscape. We analyzed the performance of different sampling designs across different densities and distributions of ape populations, assessing each for accuracy as well as cost and time efficiencies. Past ape density surveys and fecal deposition rates were used to parameterize the simulated fecal sampling designs. Our results showed that a mixed sampling design that combines traditional transect and a directed reconnaissance sampling design maximized the number of fecal samples collected and estimates of species density. Targeted sampling produced strongly biased estimates of population abundance but maximized efficiency. This research will help design the fecal sampling component of a larger study relating great ape density to Ebola fecal antibody prevalence.

PMID: 23060490 [PubMed - indexed for MEDLINE]

991. Virol Sin. 2012 Oct;27(5):273-7. doi: 10.1007/s12250-012-3252-y. Epub 2012 Sep 21

Rapid detection of filoviruses by real-time TaqMan polymerase chain reaction assays.

Huang Y(1), Wei H, Wang Y, Shi Z, Raoul H, Yuan Z.

Author information: (1)State Key Laboratory of Virology, Wuhan Institute of Virology, Chinese Academy of Sciences, Wuhan 430071, China.

Ebola virus (EBOV) and Marburg virus (MARV) are causative agents of severe hemorrhagic fever with high mortality rates in humans and non-human primates and there is currently no licensed vaccine or therapeutics. To date, there is no specific laboratory diagnostic test in China, while there is a national need to provide differential diagnosis during outbreaks and for instituting acceptable quarantine procedures. In this study, the TaqMan RT-PCR assays targeting the nucleoprotein genes of the Zaire Ebolavirus (ZEBOV) and MARV were developed and their sensitivities and specificities were investigated. Our results indicated that the assays were able to make reliable diagnosis over a wide range of virus copies from $10(3)$ to $10(9)$, corresponding to the threshold of a standard RNA transcript. The results showed that there were about $10(10)$ RNA copies per milliliter of virus culture supernatant, equivalent to 10,000 RNA molecules per infectious virion, suggesting the presence of many non-infectious particles. These data indicated that the TaqMan RT-PCR assays developed in this study will be suitable for future surveillance and specific diagnosis of ZEBOV and MARV in China.

PMID: 23001480 [PubMed - indexed for MEDLINE]

992. Viruses. 2012 Sep 25;4(10):1865-77. doi: 10.3390/v4101865.

High content image based analysis identifies cell cycle inhibitors as regulators of Ebola virus infection.

Kota KP(1), Benko JG, Mudhasani R, Retterer C, Tran JP, Bavari S, Panchal RG.

Author information: (1)PerkinElmer, 940 Waltham, MA 02451, USA. krishna.kota@amedd.army.mil

Viruses modulate a number of host biological responses including the cell cycle to favor their replication. In this study, we developed a high-content imaging (HCI) assay to measure DNA content and identify different phases of the cell cycle. We then investigated the potential effects of cell cycle arrest on Ebola virus (EBOV) infection. Cells arrested in G1 phase by serum starvation or G1/S phase using aphidicolin or G2/M phase using nocodazole showed much reduced EBOV infection compared to the untreated control. Release of cells from serum starvation or aphidicolin block resulted in a time-dependent increase in the percentage of EBOV infected cells. The effect of EBOV infection on cell cycle progression was found to be cell-type dependent. Infection of asynchronous MCF-10A cells with EBOV resulted in a reduced number of cells in G2/M phase with concomitant increase of cells in G1 phase. However, these effects were not observed in HeLa or A549 cells. Together, our studies suggest that EBOV requires actively proliferating cells for efficient replication. Furthermore, multiplexing of HCI based assays to detect viral infection, cell cycle status and other phenotypic changes in a single cell population will provide useful information during screening campaigns using siRNA and small molecule therapeutics.

PMCID: PMC3497033 PMID: 23202445 [PubMed - indexed for MEDLINE]

993. Vaccine. 2012 Sep 21;30(43):6136-41. doi: 10.1016/j.vaccine.2012.07.073. Epub 2012 Aug 8.

Further characterization of the immune response in mice to inactivated and live rabies vaccines expressing Ebola virus glycoprotein.

Papaneri AB(1), Wirblich C, Cooper K, Jahrling PB, Schnell MJ, Blaney JE.

Author information: (1)Emerging Viral Pathogens Section, National Institute of Allergy and Infectious Diseases, National Institutes of Health, Fort Detrick, MD 21702, USA.

We have previously developed (a) replication-competent, (b) replication-deficient, and (c) chemically inactivated rabies virus (RABV) vaccines expressing Ebola virus (EBOV) glycoprotein (GP) that induce humoral immunity against each virus and confer protection from both lethal RABV and mouse-adapted EBOV challenge in mice. Here, we expand our investigation of the immunogenic properties of these bivalent vaccines in mice. Both live and killed vaccines induced primary EBOV GP-specific T-cells and a robust recall response as measured by interferon-γ ELISPOT assay. In addition to cellular immunity, an effective filovirus vaccine will likely require a multivalent humoral immune response against multiple virus species. As a proof-of-principle experiment, we demonstrated that inactivated RV-GP could be formulated with another inactivated RABV vaccine expressing the nontoxic fragment of botulinum neurotoxin A heavy chain (HC50) without a reduction in immunity to each component. Finally, we demonstrated that humoral immunity to GP could be induced by immunization of mice with inactivated RV-GP in the presence of pre-existing immunity to RABV. The ability of these novel vaccines to induce strong humoral and cellular immunity indicates that they should be further evaluated in additional animal models of infection.

Published by Elsevier Ltd.

PMCID: PMC3434297 PMID: 22884661 [PubMed - indexed for MEDLINE]

994. Wkly Epidemiol Rec. 2012 Sep 21;87(38):357.

Outbreak news. Ebola, Democratic Republic of Congo – update.

[Article in English, French]

[No authors listed]

PMID: 23061101 [PubMed - indexed for MEDLINE]

995. Wkly Epidemiol Rec. 2012 Sep 7;87(36):339.

Outbreak news. Ebola haemorrhagic fever, Uganda.

[Article in English, French]

[No authors listed]

PMID: 22977950 [PubMed - indexed for MEDLINE]

996. Wkly Epidemiol Rec. 2012 Sep 7;87(36):338-9.

Outbreak news. Ebola haemorrhagic fever, Democratic Republic of the Congo.

[Article in English, French]

[No authors listed]

PMID: 22977949 [PubMed - indexed for MEDLINE]

997. Am J Trop Med Hyg. 2012 Sep;87(3):576-8. doi: 10.4269/ajtmh.2012.11-0416. Epub 2012 Jul 16.

Detection of Nipah virus RNA in fruit bat (Pteropus giganteus) from India.

Yadav PD(1), Raut CG, Shete AM, Mishra AC, Towner JS, Nichol ST, Mourya DT.

Author information: (1)Microbial Containment Complex, National Institute of Virology, Pune, India.

The study deals with the survey of different bat populations (Pteropus giganteus, Cynopterus sphinx, and Megaderma lyra) in India for highly pathogenic Nipah virus (NiV), Reston Ebola virus, and Marburg virus. Bats (n = 140) from two states in India (Maharashtra and West Bengal) were tested for IgG (serum samples) against these viruses and for virus RNAs. Only NiV RNA was detected in a liver homogenate of P. giganteus captured in Myanaguri, West Bengal. Partial sequence analysis of nucleocapsid, glycoprotein, fusion, and phosphoprotein genes showed similarity with the NiV sequences from earlier outbreaks in India. A serum sample of this bat was also positive by enzyme-linked immunosorbent assay for NiV-specific IgG. This is the first report on confirmation of Nipah viral RNA in Pteropus bat from India and suggests the possible role of this species in transmission of NiV in India.

PMCID: PMC3435367 PMID: 22802440 [PubMed - indexed for MEDLINE]

998. Bing Du Xue Bao. 2012 Sep;28(5):567-71.

[Development of SYBR Green I real-time RT-PCR for the detection of Ebola virus].

[Article in Chinese]

Liu Y(1), Shi ZX, Ma YK, Wang HT, Wang ZY, Shao DH, Wei JC, Wang SH, Li BB, Wang SM, Liu XH, Ma ZY.

Author information: (1)Department of Veterinary Public Health, Shanghai Veterinary Research Institute, Chinese Academy of Agricultural Sciences, Shanghai 200241, China.

In order to establish a rapid and accurate method for the detection of Ebola virus (EBOV), the primers used in SYBR Green I real-time RT-PCR were designed based on the EBOV NP gene sequences published in GenBank. The SYBR Green I real-time RT-PCR was established and optimized for the detection of EBOV. The EBOV RNA that was transcribed in vitro was used as a template. The sensitivity of this method was found to reach $1.0 \times 10(2)$ copies/microL and the detection range was $10(2) - 10(10)$. No cross reaction with RNA samples from Marburg virus, Dengue virus, Xinjiang hemorrhagic fever virus, Japanese encephalitis virus, Influenza virus (H1N1 and H3N2) and Porcine reproductive and respiratory syndrome virus E genomic RNA was found. The method would be useful for the detection and monitoring of EBOV in China.

PMID: 23233935 [PubMed - indexed for MEDLINE]

999. Emerg Infect Dis. 2012 Sep;18(9):1480-3. doi: 10.3201/eid1809.111536.

Reemerging Sudan Ebola virus disease in Uganda, 2011.

Shoemaker T(1), MacNeil A, Balinandi S, Campbell S, Wamala JF, McMullan LK, Downing R, Lutwama J, Mbidde E, Ströher U, Rollin PE, Nichol ST.

Author information: (1)US Centers for Disease Control and Prevention, Entebbe, Uganda.

Two large outbreaks of Ebola hemorrhagic fever occurred in Uganda in 2000 and 2007. In May 2011, we identified a single case of Sudan Ebola virus disease in Luwero District. The establishment of a permanent in-country laboratory and cooperation between international public health entities facilitated rapid outbreak response and control activities.

PMCID: PMC3437705 PMID: 22931687 [PubMed - indexed for MEDLINE]

1000. Int J Dermatol. 2012 Sep;51(9):1037-43. doi: 10.1111/j.1365-4632.2011.05379.x.

Cutaneous manifestations of filovirus infections.

Nkoghe D(1), Leroy EM, Toung-Mve M, Gonzalez JP.

Author information: (1)Centre International de Recherches Médicales de Franceville (CIRMF), Franceville, Gabon Ministry of Health, Libreville, Gabon. dnkoghe@hotmail.com

Ebolavirus and Marburgvirus, two filoviruses belonging to the Filoviridae family, are among the most virulent pathogens for humans and non-human primates, causing outbreaks of fulminant hemorrhagic fever (HF) in Central African countries with case fatality rates of up to 90%. Fruit bats are the likely reservoir, and human infection occurs through contact with bats or infected large-animal carcasses or by person-to-person contact (through body fluids, medical care, and burial practices). Schematically, clinical manifestations occur in three successive phases and include general, gastrointestinal, and mucocutaneous disorders. Death usually results from hemorrhagic complications. Cutaneous manifestations rarely make a major contribution to disease severity but can assist with the diagnosis. Rash, the main cutaneous disorder, is nonspecific and cannot guide the differential diagnosis. Immunohistochemical examination of skin biopsy or necropsy specimens can confirm the diagnosis.

© 2012 The International Society of Dermatology.

PMID: 22909355 [PubMed - indexed for MEDLINE]

1001. Nat Med. 2012 Sep;18(9):1312. doi: 10.1038/nm0912-1312b.

Stop-work order creates uncertainty for Ebola drug research.

Raven K.

PMID: 22961145 [PubMed - indexed for MEDLINE]

1002. Natl Med J India. 2012 Sep-Oct;25(5):317.

Twin Ebola outbreaks in Africa: Uganda and Democratic Republic of Congo affected.

Bhaumik S.

PMID: 23448651 [PubMed - indexed for MEDLINE]

1003. PLoS Pathog. 2012 Sep;8(9):e1002916. doi: 10.1371/journal.ppat.1002916. Epub 2012 Sep 13.

Marburg virus VP35 can both fully coat the backbone and cap the ends of dsRNA for interferon antagonism.

Bale S(1), Julien JP, Bornholdt ZA, Kimberlin CR, Halfmann P, Zandonatti MA, Kunert J, Kroon GJ, Kawaoka Y, MacRae IJ, Wilson IA, Saphire EO.

Author information: (1)Department of Immunology and Microbial Science, The Scripps Research Institute, La Jolla, California, USA.

Filoviruses, including Marburg virus (MARV) and Ebola virus (EBOV), cause fatal hemorrhagic fever in humans and non-human primates. All filoviruses encode a unique multi-functional protein termed VP35. The C-terminal double-stranded (ds)RNA-binding domain (RBD) of VP35 has been implicated in interferon antagonism and immune evasion. Crystal structures of the VP35 RBD from two ebolaviruses have previously demonstrated that the viral protein caps the ends of dsRNA. However, it is not yet understood how the expanses of dsRNA backbone, between the ends, are masked from immune surveillance during filovirus infection. Here, we report the crystal structure of MARV VP35 RBD bound to dsRNA. In the crystal structure, molecules of dsRNA stack end-to-end to form a pseudo-continuous oligonucleotide. This oligonucleotide is continuously and completely coated along its sugar-phosphate backbone by the MARV VP35 RBD. Analysis of dsRNA binding by dot-blot and isothermal titration calorimetry reveals that multiple copies of MARV VP35 RBD can indeed bind the dsRNA sugar-phosphate backbone in a cooperative manner in solution. Further, MARV VP35 RBD can also cap the ends of the dsRNA in solution, although this arrangement was not captured in crystals. Together, these studies suggest that MARV VP35 can both coat the backbone and cap the ends, and that for MARV, coating of the dsRNA backbone may be an essential mechanism by which dsRNA is masked from backbone-sensing immune surveillance molecules.

PMCID: PMC3441732 PMID: 23028316 [PubMed - indexed for MEDLINE]

1004. Viruses. 2012 Sep;4(9):1668-86. doi: 10.3390/v4091668. Epub 2012 Sep 21.

Clinical management of filovirus-infected patients.

Clark DV(1), Jahrling PB, Lawler JV.

Author information: (1)NIH/NIAID Integrated Research Facility, Fort Detrick, MD, USA. Danielle.clark.ctr@med.navy.mil

Filovirus infection presents many unique challenges to patient management. Currently no approved treatments are available, and the recommendations for supportive care are not evidence based. The austere clinical settings in which patients often present and the sporadic and at times explosive nature of filovirus outbreaks have effectively limited the information available to evaluate potential management strategies. This review will summarize the management approaches used in filovirus outbreaks and provide recommendations for collecting the information necessary for evaluating and potentially improving patient outcomes in the future.

PMCID: PMC3499825 PMID: 23170178 [PubMed - indexed for MEDLINE]

1005. Viruses. 2012 Sep;4(9):1619-50. doi: 10.3390/v4091619. Epub 2012 Sep 21.

Potential vaccines and post-exposure treatments for filovirus infections.

Friedrich BM(1), Trefry JC, Biggins JE, Hensley LE, Honko AN, Smith DR, Olinger GG.

Author information: (1)United States Army Medical Research Institute of Infectious Diseases, Division of Virology, Frederick, MD 21702, USA. brian.m.friedrich.ctr@us.army.mil

Viruses of the family Filoviridae represent significant health risks as emerging infectious diseases as well as potentially engineered biothreats. While many research efforts have been published offering possibilities toward the mitigation of filoviral infection, there remain no sanctioned therapeutic or vaccine strategies. Current progress in the development of filovirus therapeutics and vaccines is outlined herein with respect to their current level of testing, evaluation, and proximity toward human implementation, specifically with regard to human clinical trials, nonhuman primate studies, small animal studies, and in vitro development. Contemporary methods of supportive care and previous treatment approaches for human patients are also discussed.

PMCID: PMC3499823 PMID: 23170176 [PubMed - indexed for MEDLINE]

1006. Viruses. 2012 Sep;4(9):1592-604. doi: 10.3390/v4091592. Epub 2012 Sep 13.

Filovirus research in Gabon and equatorial Africa: the experience of a research center in the heart of Africa.

Leroy E(1), Gonzalez JP.

Author information: (1)Centre International de Recherches Médicales de Franceville (Franceville International Center for Medical Research), CIRMF, Libreville BP 2105, Gabon. eric.leroy@ird.fr

Health research programs targeting the population of Gabon and Equatorial Africa at the International Center for Medical Research in Franceville (CIRMF), Gabon, have evolved during the years since its inception in 1979 in accordance with emerging diseases. Since the reemergence of Ebola virus in Central Africa, the CIRMF "Emerging Viral Disease Unit" developed diagnostic tools and epidemiologic strategies and transfers of such technology to support the response of the National Public Health System and the World Health Organization to epidemics of Ebola virus disease. The Unit carries out a unique investigation program on the natural history of the filoviruses, emergence of epidemics, and Ebola virus pathogenesis. In addition, academic training is provided at all levels to regional and international students covering emerging conditions (host factors, molecular biology, genetics) that favor the spread of viral diseases.

PMCID: PMC3499821 PMID: 23170174 [PubMed - indexed for MEDLINE]

1007. Viruses. 2012 Sep;4(9):1477-508. doi: 10.3390/v4091477. Epub 2012 Sep 7.

Mouse models for filovirus infections.

Bradfute SB(1), Warfield KL, Bray M.

Author information: (1)Molecular Genetics and Microbiology, University of New Mexico, Albuquerque, NM 87131, USA. sbradfute@salud.unm.edu

The filoviruses marburg- and ebolaviruses can cause severe hemorrhagic fever (HF) in humans and nonhuman primates. Because many cases have occurred in geographical areas lacking a medical research infrastructure, most studies of the pathogenesis of filoviral HF, and all efforts to develop drugs and vaccines, have been carried out in biocontainment laboratories in non-endemic countries, using nonhuman primates (NHPs), guinea pigs and mice as animal models. NHPs appear to closely mirror filoviral HF in humans (based on limited clinical data), but only small numbers may be used in carefully regulated experiments; much research is therefore done in rodents. Because of their availability in large numbers and the existence of a wealth of reagents for biochemical and immunological testing, mice have become the preferred small animal model for filovirus research. Since the first experiments following the initial 1967 marburgvirus outbreak, wild-type or mouse-adapted viruses have been tested in immunocompetent or immunodeficient mice. In this paper, we review how these types of studies have been used to investigate the pathogenesis of filoviral disease, identify immune responses to infection and evaluate antiviral drugs and vaccines. We also discuss the strengths and weaknesses of murine models for filovirus research, and identify important questions for further study.

PMCID: PMC3499815 PMID: 23170168 [PubMed - indexed for MEDLINE]

1008. Viruses. 2012 Sep;4(9):1425-37. doi: 10.3390/v4091425. Epub 2012 Aug 31.

Genetics-based classification of filoviruses calls for expanded sampling of genomic sequences.

Lauber C(1), Gorbalenya AE.

Author information: (1)Molecular Virology Laboratory, Department of Medical Microbiology, Leiden University Medical Center, 2333 ZA Leiden, The Netherlands. c.lauber@lumc.nl

We have recently developed a computational approach for hierarchical, genome-based classification of viruses of a family (DEmARC). In DEmARC, virus clusters are delimited objectively by devising a universal family-wide threshold on intra-cluster genetic divergence of viruses that is specific for each level of the classification. Here, we apply DEmARC to a set of 56 filoviruses with complete genome sequences and compare the resulting classification to the ICTV taxonomy of the family Filoviridae. We find in total six candidate taxon levels two of which correspond to the species and genus ranks of the family. At these two levels, the six filovirus species and two genera officially recognized by ICTV, as well as a seventh tentative species for Lloviu virus and prototyping a third genus, are reproduced. DEmARC lends the highest possible support for these two as well as the four other levels, implying that the actual number of valid taxon levels remains uncertain and the choice of levels for filovirus species and genera is arbitrary. Based on our experience with other virus families, we conclude that the current sampling of filovirus genomic sequences needs to be considerably expanded in order to resolve these uncertainties in the framework of genetics-based classification.

PMCID: PMC3499813 PMID: 23170166 [PubMed - indexed for MEDLINE]

1009. Zoonoses Public Health. 2012 Sep;59 Suppl 2:151-7. doi: 10.1111/j.1863-2378.2012.01477.x.

Flexibility of mobile laboratory unit in support of patient management during the 2007 Ebola-Zaire outbreak in the Democratic Republic of Congo.

Grolla A(1), Jones S, Kobinger G, Sprecher A, Girard G, Yao M, Roth C, Artsob H, Feldmann H, Strong JE.

Author information: (1)Special Pathogens, National Microbiology Laboratory, Public Health Agency of Canada, Winnipeg, Canada

The mobile laboratory provides a safe, rapid and flexible platform to provide effective diagnosis of Ebola virus as well as additional differential diagnostic agents in remote settings of equatorial Africa. During the 2007 Democratic Republic of Congo outbreak of Ebola-Zaire, the mobile laboratory was set up in two different locations by two separate teams within a day of equipment arriving in each location. The first location was in Mweka where our laboratory took over the diagnostic laboratory space of the local hospital, whereas the second location, approximately 50 km south near Kampungu at the epicentre of the outbreak, required local labour to fabricate a tent structure as a suitable pre-existing structure was not available. In both settings, the laboratory was able to quickly set up, providing accurate and efficient molecular diagnostics (within 3 h of receiving samples) for 67 individuals, including four cases of Ebola, seven cases of Shigella and 13 cases of malaria. This rapid turn-around time provides an important role in the support of patient management and epidemiological surveillance.

© 2012 Blackwell Verlag GmbH.

PMID: 22958259 [PubMed - indexed for MEDLINE]

1010. Zoonoses Public Health. 2012 Sep;59 Suppl 2:116-31. doi: 10.1111/j.1863-2378.2012.01454.x.

How Ebola virus counters the interferon system.

Kühl A(1), Pöhlmann S.

Author information: (1)Institute of Virology, Hannover Medical School, Hannover, Germany. kuehl.annika@mh-hannover.de

Zoonotic transmission of Ebola virus (EBOV) to humans causes a severe haemorrhagic fever in afflicted individuals with high case-fatality rates. Neither vaccines nor therapeutics are at present available to combat EBOV infection, making the virus a potential threat to public health. To devise antiviral strategies, it is important to understand which components of the immune system could be effective against EBOV infection. The interferon (IFN) system constitutes a key innate defence against viral infections and prevents development of lethal disease in mice infected with EBOV strains not adapted to this host. Recent research revealed that expression of the host cell IFN-inducible transmembrane proteins 1-3 (IFITM1-3) and tetherin is induced by IFN and restricts EBOV infection, at least in cell culture model systems. IFITMs, tetherin and other effector molecules of the IFN system could thus pose a potent barrier against EBOV spread in humans. However, EBOV interferes with signalling events required for human cells to express these proteins. Here, we will review the strategies employed by EBOV to fight the IFN system, and we will discuss how IFITM proteins and tetherin inhibit EBOV infection.
© 2012 Blackwell Verlag GmbH.
PMID: 22958256 [PubMed - indexed for MEDLINE]
1011. Nature. 2012 Aug 16;488(7411):265-6. doi: 10.1038/488265a.
Ebola outbreak tests local surveillance.
Callaway E.
PMID: 22895312 [PubMed - indexed for MEDLINE]
1012. Virulence. 2012 Aug 15;3(5):440-5. doi: 10.4161/viru.21302. Epub 2012 Aug 15.
The ebolavirus VP24 interferon antagonist: know your enemy.
Zhang AP(1), Abelson DM, Bornholdt ZA, Liu T, Woods VL Jr, Saphire EO.
Author information: (1)Department of Immunology and Microbial Science, The Scripps Research Institute, La Jolla, CA, USA.
Suppression during the early phases of the immune system often correlates directly with a fatal outcome for the host. The ebolaviruses, some of the most lethal viruses known, appear to cripple initial stages of the host defense network via multiple distinct paths. Two of the eight viral proteins are critical for immunosuppression. One of these proteins is VP35, which binds double-stranded RNA and antagonizes several antiviral signaling pathways. The other protein is VP24, which binds transporter molecules to prevent STAT1 translocation. A more recent discovery is that VP24 also binds STAT1 directly, suggesting that VP24 may operate in at least two separate branches of the interferon pathway. New crystal structures of VP24 derived from pathogenic and nonpathogenic ebolaviruses reveal its novel, pyramidal fold, upon which can be mapped sites required for virulence and for STAT1 binding. These structures of VP24, and new information about its direct binding to STAT1, provide avenues by which we may explore its many roles in the viral life cycle, and reasons for differences in pathogenesis among the ebolaviruses.
PMCID: PMC3485981 PMID: 23076242 [PubMed - indexed for MEDLINE]
1013. BMJ. 2012 Aug 1;345:e5210. doi: 10.1136/bmj.e5210.
Uganda gears up to contain Ebola epidemic as fears of spread cause panic.
Wasswa H.
PMID: 22859784 [PubMed - indexed for MEDLINE]
1014. Ecol Evol. 2012 Aug;2(8):1826-33. doi: 10.1002/ece3.297. Epub 2012 Jul 1.
Phylogenetic assessment of filoviruses: how many lineages of Marburg virus?
Peterson AT(1), Holder MT.
Author information: (1)Department of Ecology and Evolutionary Biology, The University of Kansas Lawrence, Kansas, 66045.
Filoviruses have to date been considered as consisting of one diverse genus (Ebola viruses) and one undifferentiated genus (Marburg virus). We reconsider this idea by means of detailed phylogenetic analyses of sequence data available for the Filoviridae: using coalescent simulations, we ascertain that two Marburg isolates (termed the "RAVN" strain) represent a quite-distinct lineage that should be considered in studies of biogeography and host associations, and may merit recognition at the level of species. In contrast, filovirus isolates recently obtained from bat tissues are not distinct from previously known strains, and should be considered as drawn from the same population. Implications for understanding the transmission geography and host associations of these viruses are discussed.
PMCID: PMC3433987 PMID: 22957185 [PubMed]
1015. Eur J Pharm Biopharm. 2012 Aug;81(3):486-97. doi: 10.1016/j.ejpb.2012.03.021. Epub 2012 Apr 6.
Novel thermal-sensitive hydrogel enhances both humoral and cell-mediated immune responses by intranasal vaccine delivery.
Wu Y(1), Wu S, Hou L, Wei W, Zhou M, Su Z, Wu J, Chen W, Ma G.
Author information: (1)National Key Laboratory of Biochemical Engineering, Institute of Process Engineering, Chinese Academy of Sciences, Beijing, PR China.
A novel thermal sensitive hydrogel was formulated with N-[(2-hydroxy-3-trimethylammonium) propyl] chitosan chloride (HTCC) and α, β-glycerophosphate (α, β-GP). A serial of hydrogels containing different amount of GP and HTCC with diverse quarternize degree (QD, 41%, 59%, 79.5%, and 99%) were prepared and characterized by rheological method. The hydrogel was subsequently evaluated for intranasal vaccine delivery with adenovirus based Zaire Ebola virus glycoprotein antigen (Ad-GPZ). Results showed that moderate quarternized HTCC (60% and 79.5%) hydrogel/antigen formulations induced highest IgG, IgG1, and IgG2a antibody titers in serum, as well as mucosal IgA responses in lung wash, which may attributed to the prolonged antigen residence time due to the thermal-sensitivity of this hydrogel. Furthermore, CD8(+) splenocytes for IFN-γ positive cell assay and the release profile of Th1/Th2 type cytokines (IFN-γ, IL-2, IL-10, and IL-4) showed that hydrogel/Ad-GPZ generated an overwhelmingly enhanced Th1 biased cellular immune response. In addition, this hydrogel

displayed low toxicity to nasal tissue and epithelial cells even by frequently intranasal dosing of hydrogel. All these results strongly supported this hydrogel as a safe and effective delivery system for nasal immunization.

PMID: 22507968 [PubMed - indexed for MEDLINE]

1016. Med Mal Infect. 2012 Aug;42(8):335-43. doi: 10.1016/j.medmal.2012.05.011. Epub 2012 Jul 4.

Microparticles and infectious diseases.

Delabranche X(1), Berger A, Boisramé-Helms J, Meziani F.

Author information: (1)Service de réanimation médicale, nouvel hôpital civil, hôpitaux universitaires de Strasbourg, 1, place de l'Hôpital, 67091 Strasbourg cedex, France.

Membrane shedding with microvesicle (MV) release after membrane budding due to cell stimulation is a highly conserved intercellular interplay. MV can be released by micro-organisms or by host cells in the course of infectious diseases. Host MVs are divided according to cell compartment origin in microparticles (MPs) from plasma membrane and exosomes from intracellular membranes. MPs are cell fragments resulting from plasma membrane reorganization characterized by phosphatidylserine (PhtdSer) content and parental cell antigens on membrane. The role of MPs in physiology and pathophysiology is not yet well elucidated; they are a pool of bioactive molecules able to transmit a pro-inflammatory message to neighboring or target cells. The first acknowledged function of MP was the dissemination of a procoagulant potential via PhtdSer and it is now obvious than MPs bear tissue factor (TF). Such MPs have been implicated in the coagulation disorders observed during sepsis and septic shock. MPs have been implicated in the regulation of vascular tone and cardiac dysfunction in experimental sepsis. Beside a non-specific role, pathogens such as Neisseria meningitidis and Ebola Virus can specifically activate blood coagulation after TF-bearing MPs release in the bloodstream with disseminated intravascular coagulopathy and Purpura fulminans. The role of MPs in host-pathogen interactions is also fundamental in Chagas disease, where MPs could allow immune evasion by inhibiting C3 convertase. During cerebral malaria, MPs play a complex role facilitating the activation of brain endothelium that contributes to amplify vascular obstruction by parasitized erythrocytes. Phagocytosis of HIV induced MPs expressing PhtdSer by monocytes/macrophages results in cellular infection and non-inflammatory response via up-regulation of TGF-β.

PMID: 22766273 [PubMed - indexed for MEDLINE]

1017. Virology. 2012 Aug 1;429(2):155-62. doi: 10.1016/j.virol.2012.04.008. Epub 2012 May 8.

A facile quantitative assay for viral particle genesis reveals cooperativity in virion assembly and saturation of an antiviral protein.

Yadav SS(1), Wilson SJ, Bieniasz PD.

Author information: (1)Howard Hughes Medical Institute, Laboratory of Retrovirology, Aaron Diamond AIDS Research Center, The Rockefeller University, 455 First Avenue, New York, NY 10016, USA.

Conventional assays of viral particle assembly and release are time consuming and laborious. We have developed an enzymatic virus-like particle (VLP) genesis assay that rapid and quantitative and is also versatile and applicable to diverse viruses including HIV-1 and Ebola virus. Using this assay, which has a dynamic range of several orders of magnitude, we show that the efficiency of VLP assembly and release, i.e., the fraction of the expressed protein that is assembled into extracellular particles, is dependent on the absolute level of expression of either HIV-1 Gag or Ebola virus VP40. We also demonstrate that the activity of the antiviral factor tetherin is dependent on the level of HIV-1 Gag expression and the numbers of VLPs generated, and appears to become saturated as these parameters are increased.

PMCID: PMC3419437 PMID: 22575053 [PubMed - indexed for MEDLINE]

1018. Viruses. 2012 Aug;4(8):1279-88. Epub 2012 Aug 15.

A limited structural modification results in a significantly more efficacious diazachrysene-based filovirus inhibitor.

Selakovic Z(1), Opsenica D, Eaton B, Retterer C, Bavari S, Burnett JC, Solaja BA, Panchal RG.

Author information: (1)University of Belgrade, Studentski trg 16, P.O. Box 51, Belgrade 11158, Serbia. zivota.selakovic@gmail.com

Ebola (EBOV) and Marburg (MARV) filoviruses are highly infectious pathogens causing deadly hemorrhagic fever in humans and non-human primates. Promising vaccine candidates providing immunity against filoviruses have been reported. However, the sporadic nature and swift progression of filovirus disease underlines the need for the development of small molecule therapeutics providing immediate antiviral effects. Herein we describe a brief structural exploration of two previously reported diazachrysene (DAAC)-based EBOV inhibitors. Specifically, three analogs were prepared to examine how slight substituent modifications would affect inhibitory efficacy and inhibitor-mediated toxicity during not only EBOV, but also MARV cellular infection. Of the three analogs, one was highly efficacious, providing IC(50) values of 0.696 µM ± 0.13 µM and 2.76 µM ± 0.21 µM against EBOV and MARV infection, respectively, with little or no associated cellular toxicity. Overall, the structure-activity and structure-toxicity results from this study provide a framework for the future development of DAAC-based filovirus inhibitors that will be both active and non-toxic in vivo.

PMCID: PMC3446762 PMID: 23012625 [PubMed - indexed for MEDLINE]

1019. Zhonghua Shi Yan He Lin Chuang Bing Du Xue Za Zhi. 2012 Aug;26(4):313-5.

[Multiplex real-time PCR method for rapid detection of Marburg virus and Ebola virus].

[Article in Chinese]

Yang Y(1), Bai L, Hu KX, Yang ZH, Hu JP, Wang J.

Author information: (1)Chinese Academy of Inspection and Quarantine, Beijing 100123, China.+

OBJECTIVE: Marburg virus and Ebola virus are acute infections with high case fatality rates. A rapid, sensitive detection method was established to detect Marburg virus and Ebola virus by multiplex real-time fluorescence quantitative PCR. METHODS: Designing primers and Taqman probes from highly conserved sequences of Marburg virus and Ebola virus through whole genome sequences alignment, Taqman probes labeled by FAM and Texas Red, the sensitivity of the multiplex real-time quantitative PCR assay was optimized by evaluating the different concentrations of primers and Probes. RESULTS: We have developed a real-time PCR method with the sensitivity of 30.5 copies/microl for Marburg virus positive plasmid and 28.6 copies/microl for Ebola virus positive plasmids, Japanese encephalitis virus, Yellow fever virus, Dengue virus were using to examine the specificity. CONCLUSIONS: The Multiplex real-time PCR assays provide a sensitive, reliable and efficient method to detect Marburg virus and Ebola virus simultaneously.
PMID: 23189855 [PubMed - indexed for MEDLINE]

1020. J Vis Exp. 2012 Jul 31;(65). pii: 4041. doi: 10.3791/4041.

A convenient and general expression platform for the production of secreted proteins from human cells.

Aydin H(1), Azimi FC, Cook JD, Lee JE.

Author information: (1)Department of Laboratory Medicine and Pathobiology, University of Toronto.

Recombinant protein expression in bacteria, typically E. coli, has been the most successful strategy for milligram quantity expression of proteins. However, prokaryotic hosts are often not as appropriate for expression of human, viral or eukaryotic proteins due to toxicity of the foreign macromolecule, differences in the protein folding machinery, or due to the lack of particular co- or post-translational modifications in bacteria. Expression systems based on yeast (P. pastoris or S. cerevisiae) (1,2), baculovirus-infected insect (S. frugiperda or T. ni) cells (3), and cell-free in vitro translation systems (2,4) have been successfully used to produce mammalian proteins. Intuitively, the best match is to use a mammalian host to ensure the production of recombinant proteins that contain the proper post-translational modifications. A number of mammalian cell lines (Human Embryonic Kidney (HEK) 293, CV-1 cells in Origin carrying the SV40 larget T-antigen (COS), Chinese Hamster Ovary (CHO), and others) have been successfully utilized to overexpress milligram quantities of a number of human proteins (5-9). However, the advantages of using mammalian cells are often countered by higher costs, requirement of specialized laboratory equipment, lower protein yields, and lengthy times to develop stable expression cell lines. Increasing yield and producing proteins faster, while keeping costs low, are major factors for many academic and commercial laboratories. Here, we describe a time- and cost-efficient, two-part procedure for the expression of secreted human proteins from adherent HEK 293T cells. This system is capable of producing microgram to milligram quantities of functional protein for structural, biophysical and biochemical studies. The first part, multiple constructs of the gene of interest are produced in parallel and transiently transfected into adherent HEK 293T cells in small scale. The detection and analysis of recombinant protein secreted into the cell culture medium is performed by western blot analysis using commercially available antibodies directed against a vector-encoded protein purification tag. Subsequently, suitable constructs for large-scale protein production are transiently transfected using polyethyleneimine (PEI) in 10-layer cell factories. Proteins secreted into litre-volumes of conditioned medium are concentrated into manageable amounts using tangential flow filtration, followed by purification by anti-HA affinity chromatography. The utility of this platform is proven by its ability to express milligram quantities of cytokines, cytokine receptors, cell surface receptors, intrinsic restriction factors, and viral glycoproteins. This method was also successfully used in the structural determination of the trimeric ebolavirus glycoprotein (5,10). In conclusion, this platform offers ease of use, speed and scalability while maximizing protein quality and functionality. Moreover, no additional equipment, other than a standard humidified CO_2 incubator, is required. This procedure may be rapidly expanded to systems of greater complexity, such as co-expression of protein complexes, antigens and antibodies, production of virus-like particles for vaccines, or production of adenoviruses or lentiviruses for transduction of difficult cell lines.

PMCID: PMC3476395 PMID: 22872008 [PubMed - indexed for MEDLINE]

1021. Chem Commun (Camb). 2012 Jul 28;48(59):7416-8. doi: 10.1039/c2cc33249c. Epub 2012 Jun 20.

A universal platform for amplified multiplexed DNA detection based on exonuclease III-coded magnetic microparticle probes.

Luo M(1), Xiang X, Xiang D, Yang S, Ji X, He Z.

Author information: (1)Key Laboratory of Analytical Chemistry for Biology and Medicine (Ministry of Education), College of Chemistry and Molecular Sciences, Wuhan University, Wuhan 430072, PR China.

An amplified multiplexed DNA detection biosensor has been developed, which combines the unique cleavage function of exonuclease III (Exo III) with the separating ability of magnetic microparticles (MMPs). By using different fluorophores, the multiplexed detection of DNA is demonstrated.

PMID: 22714662 [PubMed - indexed for MEDLINE]

1022. Emerg Infect Dis. 2012 Jul;18(7):1207-9. doi: 10.3201/eid1807.111654.

Ebola virus antibodies in fruit bats, Ghana, West Africa.

Hayman DT, Yu M, Crameri G, Wang LF, Suu-Ire R, Wood JL, Cunningham AA.

PMCID: PMC3376795 PMID: 22710257 [PubMed - indexed for MEDLINE]

1023. Expert Opin Biol Ther. 2012 Jul;12(7):859-72. doi: 10.1517/14712598.2012.685152. Epub 2012 May 5.

Current ebola vaccines.

Hoenen T(1), Groseth A, Feldmann H.

Author information: (1)National Institute of Allergy and Infectious Diseases, National Institutes of Health, Division of Intramural Research, Rocky Mountain Laboratories, Disease Modelling and Transmission Unit - Laboratory of Virology , 2A120A, 903 S 4th St, Hamilton, MT, USA. thomas.hoenen@nih.gov

INTRODUCTION: Ebolaviruses cause severe viral hemorrhagic fever in humans and non-human primates (NHPs), with case fatality rates of up to 90%. Currently, neither a specific treatment nor a vaccine licensed for use in humans is available. However, a number of vaccine candidates have been developed in the last decade that are highly protective in NHPs, the gold standard animal model for ebola hemorrhagic fever. AREAS COVERED: This review analyzes a number of scenarios for the use of ebolavirus vaccines, discusses the requirements for ebolavirus vaccines in these scenarios and describes current ebolavirus vaccines. Among these vaccines are recombinant adenoviruses, recombinant vesicular stomatitis viruses (VSVs), recombinant human parainfluenza viruses and virus-like particles. Interestingly, one of these vaccine platforms, based on recombinant VSVs, has also demonstrated post-exposure protection in NHPs. EXPERT OPINION: The most pressing remaining challenge is now to move these vaccine candidates forward into human trials and toward licensure. In order to achieve this, it will be necessary to establish the mechanisms and correlates of protection for these vaccines, and to continue to demonstrate their safety, particularly in potentially immunocompromised populations. However, already now there is sufficient evidence that, from a scientific perspective, a vaccine protective against ebolaviruses is possible.

PMCID: PMC3422127 PMID: 22559078 [PubMed - indexed for MEDLINE]
1024. J Infect. 2012 Jul;65(1):1-16. doi: 10.1016/j.jinf.2012.03.019. Epub 2012 Apr 4.

Encephalitis due to emerging viruses: CNS innate immunity and potential therapeutic targets.

Denizot M(1), Neal JW, Gasque P.

Author information: (1)GRI, Immunopathology and Infectious Disease Research Grouping (IRG, GRI), University of La Reunion, Reunion.

The emerging viruses represent a group of pathogens that are intimately connected to a diverse range of animal vectors. The recent escalation of air travel climate change and urbanization has meant humans will have increased risk of contacting these pathogens resulting in serious CNS infections. Many RNA viruses enter the CNS by evading the BBB due to axonal transport from the periphery. The systemic adaptive and CNS innate immune systems express pattern recognition receptors PRR (TLRs, RiG-I and MDA-5) that detect viral nucleic acids and initiate host antiviral response. However, several emerging viruses (West Nile Fever, Influenza A, Enterovirus 71 Ebola) are recognized and internalized by host cell receptors (TLR, MMR, DC-SIGN, CD162 and Scavenger receptor B) and escape immuno surveillance by the host systemic and innate immune systems. Many RNA viruses express viral proteins WNF (E protein), Influenza A (NS1), EV71 (protein 3C), Rabies (Glycoprotein), Ebola proteins (VP24 and VP 35) that inhibit the host cell anti-virus Interferon type I response promoting virus replication and encephalitis. The therapeutic use of RNA interference methodologies to silence gene expression of viral peptides and treat emerging virus infection of the CNS is discussed.

PMID: 22484271 [PubMed - indexed for MEDLINE]
1025. J Virol. 2012 Jul;86(14):7473-83. doi: 10.1128/JVI.00136-12. Epub 2012 May 9.

Ebolavirus requires acid sphingomyelinase activity and plasma membrane sphingomyelin for infection.

Miller ME(1), Adhikary S, Kolokoltsov AA, Davey RA.

Author information: (1)Department of Microbiology and Immunology, University of Texas Medical Branch, Galveston, TX, USA.

Acid sphingomyelinase (ASMase) converts the lipid sphingomyelin (SM) to phosphocholine and ceramide and has optimum activity at acidic pH. Normally, ASMase is located in lysosomes and endosomes, but membrane damage or the interaction with some bacterial and viral pathogens can trigger its recruitment to the plasma membrane. Rhinovirus and measles viruses each require ASMase activity during early stages of infection. Both sphingomyelin and ceramide are important components of lipid rafts and are potent signaling molecules. Each plays roles in mediating macropinocytosis, which has been shown to be important for ebolavirus (EBOV) infection. Here, we investigated the role of ASMase and its substrate, SM, in EBOV infection. The work was performed at biosafety level 4 with wild-type virus with specificity and mechanistic analysis performed using virus pseudotypes and virus-like particles. We found that virus particles strongly associate with the SM-rich regions of the cell membrane and depletion of SM reduces EBOV infection. ASM-specific drugs and multiple small interfering RNAs strongly inhibit the infection by EBOV and EBOV glycoprotein pseudotyped viruses but not by the pseudotypes bearing the glycoprotein of vesicular stomatitis virus. Interestingly, the binding of virus-like particles to cells is strongly associated with surface-localized ASMase as well as SM-enriched sites. Our work suggests that ASMase activity and SM presence are necessary for efficient infection of cells by EBOV. The inhibition of this pathway may provide new avenues for drug treatment.

PMCID: PMC3416309 PMID: 22573858 [PubMed - indexed for MEDLINE]
1026. Jpn J Infect Dis. 2012 Jul;65(4):279-88.

On case-fatality rate: review and hypothesis.

Yoshikura H(1).

Author information: (1)National Institute of Infectious Diseases, Tokyo, Japan. yoshikura-hiroshi@mhlw.go.jp

The relationship between log cumulative number of patients (X) and that of deaths (Y) in an epidemic follows the equation $\log Y = k \log X - k \log N(0)$, where k is a constant determining the slope and N(0) is the value of X when Y = 1. Diseases with k = 1 are Ebola hemorrhagic fever, avian influenza H5N1, cholera, and hand, foot, and mouth disease; those with k > 1 are the influenza H1N1 2009 pandemic in countries other than Mexico and the SARS epidemic in some countries; and those with k < 1 include the influenza H1N1 2009 pandemic in Mexico. Epidemics with k > 1 can be simulated by postulating two subpopulations (normal population [NP] and vulnerable population [VP]), where the epidemic proceeds at higher speed and at higher mortality in VP than in NP. Epidemics with k < 1 can be simulated by postulating coexisting high virulence virus (HVV) and low virulence virus (LVV), with the former being propagated at slower speed and with a higher mortality rate than the latter. An epidemic with k > 1 was simulated using parameters that are fractions of subpopulations NP or VP from the total population (f) and NP- or VP-specific patient multiplication (M) and mortality (D) rates. An epidemic with k < 1 was simulated using parameters that are fractions of HVV- or LVV-infected human populations (f), and HVV- or LVV-specific M and D.

PMID: 22814148 [PubMed - indexed for MEDLINE]
1027. J Biol Chem. 2012 Jun 29;287(27):22882-8. doi: 10.1074/jbc.M111.306373. Epub 2012 Apr 18.

195

Glycogen synthase kinase 3β (GSK3β) modulates antiviral activity of zinc-finger antiviral protein (ZAP).

Sun L(1), Lv F, Guo X, Gao G.

Author information: (1)Key Laboratory of Infection and Immunity, Institute of Biophysics, Chinese Academy of Sciences, Beijing 100101, China.

Zinc-finger antiviral protein (ZAP) is a host factor that specifically inhibits the replication of certain viruses, including HIV-1, Ebola virus, and Sindbis virus. ZAP binds directly to specific viral mRNAs and recruits cellular mRNA degradation machinery to degrade the target RNA. ZAP has also been suggested to repress translation of the target mRNA. In this study, we report that ZAP is phosphorylated by glycogen synthase kinase 3β (GSK3β). GSK3β sequentially phosphorylated Ser-270, Ser-266, Ser-262, and Ser-257 of rat ZAP. Inhibition of GSK3β by inhibitor SB216763 or down-regulation of GSK3β by RNAi reduced the antiviral activity of ZAP. These results indicate that phosphorylation of ZAP by GSK3β modulates ZAP activity.

PMCID: PMC3391094 PMID: 22514281 [PubMed - indexed for MEDLINE]

1028. BMC Genomics. 2012 Jun 20;13:261. doi: 10.1186/1471-2164-13-261.

The immune gene repertoire of an important viral reservoir, the Australian black flying fox.

Papenfuss AT(1), Baker ML, Feng ZP, Tachedjian M, Crameri G, Cowled C, Ng J, Janardhana V, Field HE, Wang LF.

Author information: (1)The Walter and Eliza Hall Institute of Medical Research, Parkville, Melbourne, VIC 3052, Australia.

BACKGROUND: Bats are the natural reservoir host for a range of emerging and re-emerging viruses, including SARS-like coronaviruses, Ebola viruses, henipaviruses and Rabies viruses. However, the mechanisms responsible for the control of viral replication in bats are not understood and there is little information available on any aspect of antiviral immunity in bats. Massively parallel sequencing of the bat transcriptome provides the opportunity for rapid gene discovery. Although the genomes of one megabat and one microbat have now been sequenced to low coverage, no transcriptomic datasets have been reported from any bat species. In this study, we describe the immune transcriptome of the Australian flying fox, Pteropus alecto, providing an important resource for identification of genes involved in a range of activities including antiviral immunity. RESULTS: Towards understanding the adaptations that have allowed bats to coexist with viruses, we have de novo assembled transcriptome sequence from immune tissues and stimulated cells from P. alecto. We identified about 18,600 genes involved in a broad range of activities with the most highly expressed genes involved in cell growth and maintenance, enzyme activity, cellular components and metabolism and energy pathways. 3.5% of the bat transcribed genes corresponded to immune genes and a total of about 500 immune genes were identified, providing an overview of both innate and adaptive immunity. A small proportion of transcripts found no match with annotated sequences in any of the public databases and may represent bat-specific transcripts. CONCLUSIONS: This study represents the first reported bat transcriptome dataset and provides a survey of expressed bat genes that complement existing bat genomic data. In addition, these data provide insight into genes relevant to the antiviral responses of bats, and form a basis for examining the roles of these molecules in immune response to viral infection.

PMCID: PMC3436859 PMID: 22716473 [PubMed - indexed for MEDLINE]

1029. Onderstepoort J Vet Res. 2012 Jun 20;79(2):451. doi: 10.4102/ojvr.v79i2.451.

Ebola virus outbreaks in Africa: past and present.

Muyembe-Tamfum JJ(1), Mulangu S, Masumu J, Kayembe JM, Kemp A, Paweska JT.

Author information: (1)Institut national de Recherche Biomédicale, Kinshasa 1. justin.masumu@sacids.org.

Ebola haemorrhagic fever (EHF) is a zoonosis affecting both human and non-human primates (NHP). Outbreaks in Africa occur mainly in the Congo and Nile basins. The first outbreaks of EHF occurred nearly simultaneously in 1976 in the Democratic Republic of the Congo (DRC, former Zaire) and Sudan with very high case fatality rates of 88% and 53%, respectively. The two outbreaks were caused by two distinct species of Ebola virus named Zaire ebolavirus (ZEBOV) and Sudan ebolavirus (SEBOV). The source of transmission remains unknown. After a long period of silence (1980-1993), EHF outbreaks in Africa caused by the two species erupted with increased frequency and new species were discovered, namely Côte d'Ivoire ebolavirus (CIEBOV) in 1994 in the Ivory Coast and Bundibugyo ebolavirus (BEBOV) in 2007 in Uganda. The re-emergence of EHF outbreaks in Gabon and Republic of the Congo were concomitant with an increase in mortality amongst gorillas and chimpanzees infected with ZEBOV. The human outbreaks were related to multiple, unrelated index cases who had contact with dead gorillas or chimpanzees. However, in areas where NHP were rare or absent, as in Kikwit (DRC) in 1995, Mweka (DRC) in 2007, Gulu (Uganda) in 2000 and Yambio (Sudan) in 2004, the hunting and eating of fruit bats may have resulted in the primary transmission of Ebola virus to humans. Human-to-human transmission is associated with direct contact with body fluids or tissues from an infected subject or contaminated objects. Despite several, often heroic field studies, the epidemiology and ecology of Ebola virus, including identification of its natural reservoir hosts, remains a formidable challenge for public health and scientific communities.

PMID: 23327370 [PubMed - in process]

1030. BMC Vet Res. 2012 Jun 18;8;82. doi: 10.1186/1746-6148-8-82.

A seroepidemiologic study of Reston ebolavirus in swine in the Philippines.

Sayama Y(1), Demetria C, Saito M, Azul RR, Taniguchi S, Fukushi S, Yoshikawa T, Iizuka I, Mizutani T, Kurane I, Malbas FF Jr, Lupisan S, Catbagan DP, Animas SB, Morales RG, Lopez EL, Dazo KR, Cruz MS, Olveda R, Saijo M, Oshitani H, Morikawa S.

Author information: (1)Department of Virology 1, National Institute of Infectious Diseases, 4-7-1 Gakuen, Musashimurayama, Tokyo, 208-0011, Japan.

BACKGROUND: Ebola viruses cause viral hemorrhagic fever in humans and non-human primates and are endemic in Africa. Reston ebolavirus (REBOV) has caused several epizootics in cynomolgus monkeys (Macaca fascicularis) but is not associated with any human disease. In late 2008, REBOV infections were identified in swine for the first time in the Philippines. METHODS: A total of 215 swine sera collected at two REBOV-affected farms in 2008, in Pangasinan and Bulacan, were tested for the presence of REBOV-specific antibodies using multiple serodiagnosis systems. A total of 98 swine sera collected in a non-epizootic region, Tarlac, were also tested to clarify the prevalence of REBOV infection in the general swine population in the Philippines. RESULTS: Some 70 % of swine sera at the affected farms were positive for REBOV antibodies in the multiple serodiagnosis systems. On the other hand, none of the swine sera collected in Tarlac showed positive reactions in any of the diagnosis systems. CONCLUSIONS: The high prevalence of REBOV infection in swine in the affected farms in 2008 suggests that swine is susceptible for REBOV infection. The multiple serological assays used in the study are thought to be useful for future surveillance of REOBV infection in swine in the Philippines.

PMCID: PMC3433389 PMID: 22709971 [PubMed - indexed for MEDLINE]

1031. Global Health. 2012 Jun 13;8:15. doi: 10.1186/1744-8603-8-15.

A time of fear: local, national, and international responses to a large Ebola outbreak in Uganda.

Kinsman J(1).

Author information: (1)Umeå Centre for Global Health Research, Epidemiology and Global Health Unit, Department of Public Health and Clinical Medicine, Umeå University, 901 85, Umeå, Sweden. john.kinsman@epiph.umu.se

BACKGROUND: This paper documents and analyses some of the responses to the largest Ebola outbreak on record, which took place in Uganda between September 2000 and February 2001. Four hundred and twenty five people developed clinical symptoms in three geographically distinct parts of the country (Gulu, Masindi, and Mbarara), of whom 224 (53%) died. Given the focus of previous social scientific Ebola research on experiences in communities that have been directly affected, this article expands the lens to include responses to the outbreak in local, national, and international contexts over the course of the outbreak. METHODS: Responses to the outbreak were gauged through the articles, editorials, cartoons, and letters that were published in the country's two main English language daily national newspapers: the New Vision and the Monitor (now the Daily Monitor). All the relevant pieces from these two sources over the course of the epidemic were cut out, entered onto a computer, and the originals filed. The three a priori codes, based on the local, national, and international levels, were expanded into six, to include issues that emerged inductively during analysis. The data within each code were subsequently worked into coherent, chronological narratives. RESULTS: A total of 639 cuttings were included in the analysis. Strong and varied responses to the outbreak were identified from across the globe. These included, among others: confusion, anger, and serious stigma in affected communities; medical staff working themselves to exhaustion, with some quitting their posts; patients fleeing from hospitals; calls on spiritual forces for protection against infection; a well-coordinated national control strategy; and the imposition of some international travel restrictions. Responses varied both quantitatively and qualitatively according to the level (i.e. local, national, or international) at which they were manifested. CONCLUSIONS: The Ugandan experience of 2000/2001 demonstrates that responses to an Ebola outbreak can be very dramatic, but perhaps disproportionate to the actual danger presented. An important objective for any future outbreak control strategy must be to prevent excessive fear, which, it is expected, would reduce stigma and other negative outcomes. To this end, the value of openness in the provision of public information, and critically, of being seen to be open, cannot be overstated.

PMCID: PMC3477054 PMID: 22695277 [PubMed - indexed for MEDLINE]

1032. Sci Transl Med. 2012 Jun 13;4(138):138ra81. doi: 10.1126/scitranslmed.3003876.

Successful treatment of ebola virus-infected cynomolgus macaques with monoclonal antibodies.

Qiu X(1), Audet J, Wong G, Pillet S, Bello A, Cabral T, Strong JE, Plummer F, Corbett CR, Alimonti JB, Kobinger GP.

Author information: (1)National Microbiology Laboratory, Public Health Agency of Canada, Winnipeg, Manitoba R3E 3R2, Canada.

Ebola virus (EBOV) is considered one of the most aggressive infectious agents and is capable of causing death in humans and nonhuman primates (NHPs) within days of exposure. Recent strategies have succeeded in preventing acquisition of infection in NHPs after treatment; however, these strategies are only successful when administered before or minutes after infection. The present work shows that a combination of three neutralizing monoclonal antibodies (mAbs) directed against the Ebola envelope glycoprotein (GP) resulted in complete survival (four of four cynomolgus macaques) with no apparent side effects when three doses were administered 3 days apart beginning at 24 hours after a lethal challenge with EBOV. The same treatment initiated 48 hours after lethal challenge with EBOV resulted in two of four cynomolgus macaques fully recovering. The survivors demonstrated an EBOV-GP-specific humoral and cell-mediated immune response. These data highlight the important role of antibodies to control EBOV replication in vivo, and support the use of mAbs against a severe filovirus infection.

PMID: 22700957 [PubMed - indexed for MEDLINE]

1033. Virol J. 2012 Jun 13;9:111. doi: 10.1186/1743-422X-9-111.

Prediction and identification of mouse cytotoxic T lymphocyte epitopes in Ebola virus glycoproteins.

Wu S(1), Yu T, Song X, Yi S, Hou L, Chen W.

Author information: (1)State Key Laboratory of Pathogens and Biosecurity, Beijing Institute of Microbiology and Epidemiology, No.20 Dongdajie Street, Fengtai district, Beijing 100071, People's Republic of China.

BACKGROUND: Ebola viruses (EBOVs) cause severe hemorrhagic fever with a high mortality rate. At present, there are no licensed vaccines or efficient therapies to combat EBOV infection. Previous studies have shown that both humoral and cellular immune responses are crucial for controlling Ebola infection. CD8+ T cells play an important role in mediating vaccine-induced protective immunity. The objective of this study was to identify H-2d-specific T cell epitopes in EBOV glycoproteins (GPs). RESULTS: Computer-assisted algorithms were used to predict H-2d-specific T cell epitopes in two species of EBOV (Sudan and Zaire) GP. The predicted peptides were synthesized and identified in BALB/c mice immunized with replication-deficient adenovirus vectors expressing the EBOV GP. Enzyme-linked immunospot assays and intracellular cytokine staining showed that the peptides RPHTPQFLF (Sudan EBOV), GPCAGDFAF and LYDRLASTV (Zaire EBOV) could stimulate splenocytes in immunized mice to produce large amounts of interferon-gamma. CONCLUSION: Three peptides within the GPs of two EBOV strains were identified as T cell epitopes. The identification of these epitopes should facilitate the evaluation of vaccines based on the Ebola virus glycoprotein in a BALB/c mouse model.

PMCID: PMC3411508 PMID: 22695180 [PubMed - indexed for MEDLINE]
1034. Biophys J. 2012 Jun 6;102(11):2517-25. doi: 10.1016/j.bpj.2012.04.022. Epub 2012 Jun 5.

Investigation of Ebola VP40 assembly and oligomerization in live cells using number and brightness analysis.

Adu-Gyamfi E(1), Digman MA, Gratton E, Stahelin RV.

Author information: (1)Department of Chemistry and Biochemistry and the Eck Institute for Global Health, University of Notre Dame, Notre Dame, Indiana, USA.

Ebola virus assembles and buds from the inner leaflet of the plasma membrane of mammalian cells, which is primarily attributed to its major matrix protein VP40. Oligomerization of VP40 has been shown to be essential to the life cycle of the virus including formation of virions from infected cells. To date, VP40 oligomerization has mainly been assessed by chemical cross-linking following cell fractionation studies with VP40 transfected cells. This has made it difficult to discern the spatial and temporal dynamics of VP40 oligomerization. To gain a better understanding of the VP40 assembly and oligomerization process in live cells, we have employed real-time imaging of enhanced green fluorescent protein tagged VP40. Here, we use both confocal and total internal reflection microscopy coupled with number and brightness analysis to show that VP40 oligomers are localized on the plasma membrane and are highly enriched at sites of membrane protrusion, consistent with sites of viral budding. These filamentous plasma membrane protrusion sites harbor VP40 hexamers, octamers, and higher order oligomers. Consistent with previous reports, abrogation of VP40 oligomerization through mutagenesis greatly diminished VP40 egress and also abolished membrane protrusion sites enriched with VP40. In sum, real-time single-molecule imaging of fluorescently labeled Ebola VP40 is able to resolve the spatial and temporal dynamics of VP40 oligomerization.

PMCID: PMC3368128 PMID: 22713567 [PubMed - indexed for MEDLINE]
1035. Curr Opin Virol. 2012 Jun;2(3):324-9. doi: 10.1016/j.coviro.2012.04.003. Epub 2012 May 4.

Ebolavirus vaccines for humans and apes.

Fausther-Bovendo H(1), Mulangu S, Sullivan NJ.

Author information: (1)VRC/NIAID/NIH, 40 Convent Drive, Bethesda, MD 20892, USA.

Because of high case fatality proportions, person-to-person transmission, and potential use in bioterrorism, the development of a vaccine against ebolavirus remains a top priority. Although no licensed vaccine or treatment against ebolavirus is currently available, progress in preclinical testing of countermeasures has been made. Here, we will review ebolavirus vaccine candidates and considerations for their use in humans and wild apes.

PMCID: PMC3397659 PMID: 22560007 [PubMed - indexed for MEDLINE]
1036. PLoS Negl Trop Dis. 2012 Jun;6(6):e1546. doi: 10.1371/journal.pntd.0001546. Epub 2012 Jun 26.

Ebola and Marburg hemorrhagic fevers: neglected tropical diseases?

MacNeil A(1), Rollin PE.

Author information: (1)Viral Special Pathogens Branch, the Centers for Disease Control and Prevention, Atlanta, GA, USA. aho3@cdc.gov

Ebola hemorrhagic fever (EHF) and Marburg hemorrhagic fever (MHF) are rare viral diseases, endemic to central Africa. The overall burden of EHF and MHF is small in comparison to the more common protozoan, helminth, and bacterial diseases typically referred to as neglected tropical diseases (NTDs). However, EHF and MHF outbreaks typically occur in resource-limited settings, and many aspects of these outbreaks are a direct consequence of impoverished conditions. We will discuss aspects of EHF and MHF disease, in comparison to the "classic" NTDs, and examine potential ways forward in the prevention and control of EHF and MHF in sub-Saharan Africa, as well as examine the potential for application of novel vaccines or antiviral drugs for prevention or control of EHF and MHF among populations at highest risk for disease.

PMCID: PMC3385614 PMID: 22761967 [PubMed - indexed for MEDLINE]
1037. J Virol. 2012 May;86(10):5467-80. doi: 10.1128/JVI.06280-11. Epub 2012 Mar 7.

Anti-tetherin activities of HIV-1 Vpu and Ebola virus glycoprotein do not involve removal of tetherin from lipid rafts.

Lopez LA(1), Yang SJ, Exline CM, Rengarajan S, Haworth KG, Cannon PM.

Author information: (1)Department of Molecular Microbiology and Immunology, Keck School of Medicine of the University of Southern California, Los Angeles, California, USA.

BST-2/tetherin is an interferon-inducible host restriction factor that blocks the release of newly formed enveloped viruses. It is enriched in lipid raft membrane microdomains, which are also the sites of assembly of several enveloped viruses. Viral anti-tetherin factors, such as the HIV-1 Vpu protein, typically act by removing tetherin from the cell surface. In contrast, the Ebola virus glycoprotein (GP) is unusual in that it blocks tetherin restriction without apparently altering its cell surface localization. We explored the possibility that GP acts to exclude tetherin from the specific sites of virus assembly without overtly removing it from the cell surface and that lipid raft exclusion is the mechanism involved. However, we found that neither GP nor Vpu had any effect on tetherin's distribution within lipid raft domains. Furthermore, GP did not prevent the colocalization of tetherin and budding viral particles. Contrary to previous reports, we also found no evidence that GP is itself a raft protein. Together, our data indicate that the exclusion of tetherin from lipid rafts is not the mechanism used by either HIV-1 Vpu or Ebola virus GP to counteract tetherin restriction.

PMCID: PMC3347301 PMID: 22398279 [PubMed - indexed for MEDLINE]
1038. EMBO J. 2012 Apr 18;31(8):1947-60. doi: 10.1038/emboj.2012.53. Epub 2012 Mar 6.

Ebola virus entry requires the host-programmed recognition of an intracellular receptor.

Miller EH(1), Obernosterer G, Raaben M, Herbert AS, Deffieu MS, Krishnan A, Ndungo E, Sandesara RG, Carette JE, Kuehne AI, Ruthel G, Pfeffer SR, Dye JM, Whelan SP, Brummelkamp TR, Chandran K.
Author information: (1)Department of Microbiology and Immunology, Albert Einstein College of Medicine, Bronx, NY, USA.
Ebola and Marburg filoviruses cause deadly outbreaks of haemorrhagic fever. Despite considerable efforts, no essential cellular receptors for filovirus entry have been identified. We showed previously that Niemann-Pick C1 (NPC1), a lysosomal cholesterol transporter, is required for filovirus entry. Here, we demonstrate that NPC1 is a critical filovirus receptor. Human NPC1 fulfills a cardinal property of viral receptors: it confers susceptibility to filovirus infection when expressed in non-permissive reptilian cells. The second luminal domain of NPC1 binds directly and specifically to the viral glycoprotein, GP, and a synthetic single-pass membrane protein containing this domain has viral receptor activity. Purified NPC1 binds only to a cleaved form of GP that is generated within cells during entry, and only viruses containing cleaved GP can utilize a receptor retargeted to the cell surface. Our findings support a model in which GP cleavage by endosomal cysteine proteases unmasks the binding site for NPC1, and GP-NPC1 engagement within lysosomes promotes a late step in entry proximal to viral escape into the host cytoplasm. NPC1 is the first known viral receptor that recognizes its ligand within an intracellular compartment and not at the plasma membrane.
PMCID: PMC3343336 PMID: 22395071 [PubMed - indexed for MEDLINE]
1039. Nat Rev Microbiol. 2012 Apr 11;10(5):317-22. doi: 10.1038/nrmicro2764.

A new player in the puzzle of filovirus entry.

White JM(1), Schornberg KL.
Author information: (1)Department of Cell Biology, University of Virginia, 1340 Jefferson Park Avenue, Charlottesville, Virginia 22908-20732, USA. jw7g@virginia.edu
Viruses of the genera Ebolavirus and Marburgvirus are filoviruses that cause haemorrhagic fever in primates, with extremely high fatality rates. Studies have focused on elucidating how these viruses enter host cells, with the aim of developing therapeutics. The ebolavirus glycoprotein has been found to play key parts in all steps of entry. Furthermore, recent studies have identified Niemann-Pick C1 (NPC1), a protein that resides deep in the endocytic pathway, as an important host factor in this process.
PMCID: PMC3540776 PMID: 22491356 [PubMed - indexed for MEDLINE]
1040. Antiviral Res. 2012 Apr;94(1):80-8. doi: 10.1016/j.antiviral.2012.02.004. Epub 2012 Feb 14.

Advanced morpholino oligomers: a novel approach to antiviral therapy.

Warren TK(1), Shurtleff AC, Bavari S.
Author information: (1)United States Army Medical Research Institute of Infectious Diseases, Fort Detrick, MD 21769, USA.
Phosphorodiamidate morpholino oligomers (PMOs) are synthetic antisense oligonucleotide analogs that are designed to interfere with translational processes by forming base-pair duplexes with specific RNA sequences. Positively charged PMOs (PMOplus™) are effective for the postexposure protection of two fulminant viral diseases, Ebola and Marburg hemorrhagic fever in nonhuman primates, and this class of antisense agent may also have possibilities for treatment of other viral diseases. PMOs are highly stable, are effective by a variety of routes of administration, can be readily formulated in common isotonic delivery vehicles, and can be rapidly designed and synthesized. These are properties which may make PMOs good candidates for use during responses to emerging or reemerging viruses that may be insensitive to available therapies or for use during outbreaks, especially in regions that lack a modern medical infrastructure. While the efficacy of sequence-specific therapies can be limited by target-site sequence variations that occur between variants or by the emergence of resistant mutants during infections, various PMO design strategies can minimize these impacts. These strategies include the use of promiscuous bases such as inosine to compensate for predicted base-pair mismatches, the use of sequences that target conserved sites between viral strains, and the use of sequences that target host products that viruses utilize for infection.
PMID: 22353544 [PubMed - indexed for MEDLINE]
1041. Curr Opin Virol. 2012 Apr;2(2):151-6. doi: 10.1016/j.coviro.2012.01.003. Epub 2012 Jan 28.

Hiding the evidence: two strategies for innate immune evasion by hemorrhagic fever viruses.

Hastie KM(1), Bale S, Kimberlin CR, Saphire EO.
Author information: (1)Dept. of Immunology and Microbial Science, The Scripps Research Institute, La Jolla, CA 92037, USA.
The innate immune system is one of the first lines of defense against invading pathogens. Pathogens have, in turn, evolved different strategies to counteract these responses. Recent studies have illuminated how the hemorrhagic fever viruses Ebola and Lassa fever prevent host sensing of double-stranded RNA (dsRNA), a key hallmark of viral infection. The ebolavirus protein VP35 adopts a unique bimodal configuration to mask key cellular recognition sites on dsRNA. Conversely, the Lassa fever virus nucleoprotein actually digests the dsRNA signature. Collectively, these structural and functional studies shed new light on the mechanisms of pathogenesis of these viruses and provide new targets for therapeutic intervention.
PMCID: PMC3758253 PMID: 22482712 [PubMed - indexed for MEDLINE]
1042. Viruses. 2012 Apr;4(4):447-70. doi: 10.3390/v4040447. Epub 2012 Apr 5.

Structural basis for differential neutralization of ebolaviruses.

Bale S(1), Dias JM, Fusco ML, Hashiguchi T, Wong AC, Liu T, Keuhne AI, Li S, Woods VL Jr, Chandran K, Dye JM, Saphire EO.
Author information: (1)Dept. of Immunology and Microbial Science, The Scripps Research Institute, La Jolla, CA 92037, USA.

There are five antigenically distinct ebolaviruses that cause hemorrhagic fever in humans or non-human primates (Ebola virus, Sudan virus, Reston virus, Taï Forest virus, and Bundibugyo virus). The small handful of antibodies known to neutralize the ebolaviruses bind to the surface glycoprotein termed $GP_{1,2}$. Curiously, some antibodies against them are known to neutralize in vitro but not protect in vivo, whereas other antibodies are known to protect animal models in vivo, but not neutralize in vitro. A detailed understanding of what constitutes a neutralizing and/or protective antibody response is critical for development of novel therapeutic strategies. Here, we show that paradoxically, a lower affinity antibody with restricted access to its epitope confers better neutralization than a higher affinity antibody against a similar epitope, suggesting that either subtle differences in epitope, or different characteristics of the $GP_{1,2}$ molecules themselves, confer differential neutralization susceptibility. Here, we also report the crystal structure of trimeric, prefusion $GP_{1,2}$ from the original 1976 Boniface variant of Sudan virus complexed with 16F6, the first antibody known to neutralize Sudan virus, and compare the structure to that of Sudan virus, variant Gulu. We discuss new structural details of the GP_1-GP_2 clamp, thermal motion of various regions in $GP_{1,2}$ across the two viruses visualized, details of differential interaction of the crystallized neutralizing antibodies, and their relevance for virus neutralization.
PMCID: PMC3347318 PMID: 22590681 [PubMed - indexed for MEDLINE]

1043. Biochemistry. 2012 Mar 27;51(12):2515-25. doi: 10.1021/bi3000353. Epub 2012 Mar 12

Marburg virus glycoprotein GP2: pH-dependent stability of the ectodomain α-helical bundle.

Harrison JS(1), Koellhoffer JF, Chandran K, Lai JR.

Author information: (1)Department of Biochemistry, Albert Einstein College of Medicine, Bronx, New York 10461, United States.

Marburg virus (MARV) and Ebola virus (EBOV) constitute the family Filoviridae of enveloped viruses (filoviruses) that cause severe hemorrhagic fever. Infection by MARV requires fusion between the host cell and viral membranes, a process that is mediated by the two subunits of the envelope glycoprotein, GP1 (surface subunit) and GP2 (transmembrane subunit). Upon viral attachment and uptake, it is believed that the MARV viral fusion machinery is triggered by host factors and environmental conditions found in the endosome. Next, conformational rearrangements in the GP2 ectodomain result in the formation of a highly stable six-helix bundle; this refolding event provides the energetic driving force for membrane fusion. Both GP1 and GP2 from EBOV have been extensively studied, but there is little information available for the MARV glycoproteins. Here we have expressed two variants of the MARV GP2 ectodomain in Escherichia coli and analyzed their biophysical properties. Circular dichroism indicates that the MARV GP2 ectodomain adopts an α-helical conformation, and one variant sediments as a trimer by equilibrium analytical ultracentrifugation. Denaturation studies indicate the α-helical structure is highly stable at pH 5.3 (unfolding energy, ΔG(unf,H(2)0), of 33.4 ± 2.5 kcal/mol and melting temperature, T(m), of 75.3 ± 2.1 °C for one variant). Furthermore, we found the α-helical stability to be strongly dependent on pH, with higher stability under lower-pH conditions (T(m) values ranging from ~92 °C at pH 4.0 to ~38 °C at pH 8.0). Mutational analysis suggests two glutamic acid residues (E579 and E580) are partially responsible for this pH-dependent behavior. On the basis of these results, we hypothesize that the pH-dependent folding stability of the MARV GP2 ectodomain provides a mechanism for controlling conformational preferences such that the six-helix bundle "postfusion" state is preferred under conditions of appropriately matured endosomes.
PMCID: PMC3314129 PMID: 22369502 [PubMed - indexed for MEDLINE]

1044. Proc Natl Acad Sci U S A. 2012 Mar 27;109(13):5034-9. doi: 10.1073/pnas.1200409109. Epub 2012 Mar 12.

Postexposure antibody prophylaxis protects nonhuman primates from filovirus disease.

Dye JM(1), Herbert AS, Kuehne AI, Barth JF, Muhammad MA, Zak SE, Ortiz RA, Prugar LI, Pratt WD.

Author information: (1)Division of Virology, US Army Medical Research Institute for Infectious Diseases, Frederick, MD 21702, USA. john.m.dye1@us.army.mil

Antibody therapies to prevent or limit filovirus infections have received modest interest in recent years, in part because of early negative experimental evidence. We have overcome the limitations of this approach, leveraging the use of antibody from nonhuman primates (NHPs) that survived challenge to filoviruses under controlled conditions. By using concentrated, polyclonal IgG antibody from these survivors, we treated filovirus-infected NHPs with multiple doses administered over the clinical phase of disease. In the first study, Marburg virus (MARV)-infected NHPs were treated 15 to 30 min postexposure with virus-specific IgG, with additional treatments on days 4 and 8 postexposure. The postexposure IgG treatment was completely protective, with no signs of disease or detectable viremia. MARV-specific IgM antibody responses were generated, and all macaques survived rechallenge with MARV, suggesting that they generated an immune response to virus replication. In the next set of studies, NHPs were infected with MARV or Ebola virus (EBOV), and treatments were delayed 48 h, with additional treatments on days 4 and 8 postexposure. The delayed treatments protected both MARV- and EBOV-challenged NHPs. In both studies, two of the three IgG-treated NHPs had no clinical signs of illness, with the third NHP developing mild and delayed signs of disease followed by full recovery. These studies clearly demonstrate that postexposure antibody treatments can protect NHPs and open avenues for filovirus therapies for human use using established Food and Drug Administration-approved polyclonal or monoclonal antibody technologies.
PMCID: PMC3323977 PMID: 22411795 [PubMed - indexed for MEDLINE]

1045. Proc Natl Acad Sci U S A. 2012 Mar 13;109(11):4275-80. doi: 10.1073/pnas.1120453109. Epub 2012 Feb 27.

Structural dissection of Ebola virus and its assembly determinants using cryo-electron tomography.

Bharat TA(1), Noda T, Riches JD, Kraehling V, Kolesnikova L, Becker S, Kawaoka Y, Briggs JA.

Author information: (1)Structural and Computational Biology Unit, European Molecular Biology Laboratory, 69117 Heidelberg, Germany.

Ebola virus is a highly pathogenic filovirus causing severe hemorrhagic fever with high mortality rates. It assembles heterogenous, filamentous, enveloped virus particles containing a negative-sense, single-stranded RNA genome packaged within a helical nucleocapsid (NC). We have used cryo-electron microscopy and tomography to visualize Ebola virus particles, as well as Ebola virus-like particles, in three dimensions in a near-native state. The NC within the virion forms a left-handed helix with an inner nucleoprotein layer decorated with protruding arms composed of VP24 and VP35. A comparison with the closely related Marburg virus shows that the N-terminal region of nucleoprotein defines the inner diameter of the Ebola virus NC, whereas the RNA genome defines its length.

Binding of the nucleoprotein to RNA can assemble a loosely coiled NC-like structure; the loose coil can be condensed by binding of the viral matrix protein VP40 to the C terminus of the nucleoprotein, and rigidified by binding of VP24 and VP35 to alternate copies of the nucleoprotein. Four proteins (NP, VP24, VP35, and VP40) are necessary and sufficient to mediate assembly of an NC with structure, symmetry, variability, and flexibility indistinguishable from that in Ebola virus particles released from infected cells. Together these data provide a structural and architectural description of Ebola virus and define the roles of viral proteins in its structure and assembly.

PMCID: PMC3306676 PMID: 22371572 [PubMed - indexed for MEDLINE]

1046. Antiviral Res. 2012 Mar;93(3):416-28. doi: 10.1016/j.antiviral.2012.01.011. Epub 2012 Feb 8.

The role of antigen-presenting cells in filoviral hemorrhagic fever: gaps in current knowledge.

Martinez O(1), Leung LW, Basler CF.

Author information: (1)Department of Microbiology, Mount Sinai School of Medicine, New York, NY 10029, USA.

The filoviruses, Ebola virus (EBOV) and Marburg virus (MARV), are highly lethal zoonotic agents of concern as emerging pathogens and potential bioweapons. Antigen-presenting cells (APCs), particularly macrophages and dendritic cells, are targets of filovirus infection in vivo. Infection of these cell types has been proposed to contribute to the inflammation, activation of coagulation cascades and ineffective immune responses characteristic of filovirus hemorrhagic fever. However, many aspects of filovirus-APC interactions remain to be clarified. Among the unanswered questions: What determines the ability of filoviruses to replicate in different APC subsets? What are the cellular signaling pathways that sense infection and lead to production of copious quantities of cytokines, chemokines and tissue factor? What are the mechanisms by which innate antiviral responses are disabled by these viruses, and how may these mechanisms contribute to inadequate adaptive immunity? A better understanding of these issues will clarify the pathogenesis of filoviral hemorrhagic fever and provide new avenues for development of therapeutics.

PMCID: PMC3299938 PMID: 22333482 [PubMed - indexed for MEDLINE]

1047. Antiviral Res. 2012 Mar;93(3):354-63. doi: 10.1016/j.antiviral.2012.01.005. Epub 2012 Jan 25.

dsRNA binding characterization of full length recombinant wild type and mutants Zaire ebolavirus VP35.

Zinzula L(1), Esposito F, Pala D, Tramontano E.

Author information: (1)Department of Life and Environmental Sciences, University of Cagliari, Cittadella di Monserrato SS554, 09042 Monserrato, Cagliari, Italy.

The Ebola viruses (EBOVs) VP35 protein is a multifunctional major virulence factor involved in EBOVs replication and evasion of the host immune system. EBOV VP35 is an essential component of the viral RNA polymerase, it is a key participant of the nucleocapsid assembly and it inhibits the innate immune response by antagonizing RIG-I like receptors through its dsRNA binding function and, hence, by suppressing the host type I interferon (IFN) production. Insights into the VP35 dsRNA recognition have been recently revealed by structural and functional analysis performed on its C-terminus protein. We report the biochemical characterization of the Zaire ebolavirus (ZEBOV) full-length recombinant VP35 (rVP35)-dsRNA binding function. We established a novel in vitro magnetic dsRNA binding pull down assay, determined the rVP35 optimal dsRNA binding parameters, measured the rVP35 equilibrium dissociation constant for heterologous in vitro transcribed dsRNA of different length and short synthetic dsRNA of 8bp, and validated the assay for compound screening by assessing the inhibitory ability of auryntricarboxylic acid (IC(50) value of 50µg/mL). Furthermore, we compared the dsRNA binding properties of full length wt rVP35 with those of R305A, K309A and R312A rVP35 mutants, which were previously reported to be defective in dsRNA binding-mediated IFN inhibition, showing that the latter have measurably increased K(d) values for dsRNA binding and modified migration patterns in mobility shift assays with respect to wt rVP35. Overall, these results provide the first characterization of the full-length wt and mutants VP35-dsRNA binding functions.

PMID: 22289166 [PubMed - indexed for MEDLINE]

1048. J Virol. 2012 Mar;86(6):3284-92. doi: 10.1128/JVI.06346-11. Epub 2012 Jan 11.

Filoviruses require endosomal cysteine proteases for entry but exhibit distinct protease preferences.

Misasi J(1), Chandran K, Yang JY, Considine B, Filone CM, Côté M, Sullivan N, Fabozzi G, Hensley L, Cunningham J.

Author information: (1)Division of Hematology, Department of Medicine, Brigham & Women's Hospital, Boston, Massachusetts, USA.

Filoviruses are enveloped viruses that cause sporadic outbreaks of severe hemorrhagic fever [CDC, MMWR Morb. Mortal. Wkly. Rep. 50:73-77, 2001; Colebunders and Borchert, J. Infect. 40:16-20, 2000; Colebunders et al., J. Infect. Dis. 196(Suppl. 2):S148-S153, 2007; Geisbert and Jahrling, Nat. Med. 10:S110-S121, 2004]. Previous studies revealed that endosomal cysteine proteases are host factors for ebolavirus Zaire (Chandran et al., Science 308:1643-1645, 2005; Schornberg et al., J. Virol. 80:4174-4178, 2006). In this report, we show that infection mediated by glycoproteins from other phylogenetically diverse filoviruses are also dependent on these proteases and provide additional evidence indicating that they cleave GP1 and expose the binding domain for the critical host factor Niemann-Pick C1. Using selective inhibitors and knockout-derived cell lines, we show that the ebolaviruses Zaire and Cote d'Ivoire are strongly dependent on cathepsin B, while the ebolaviruses Sudan and Reston and Marburg virus are not. Taking advantage of previous studies of cathepsin B inhibitor-resistant viruses (Wong et al., J. Virol. 84:163-175, 2010), we found that virus-specific differences in the requirement for cathepsin B are correlated with sequence polymorphisms at residues 47 in GP1 and 584 in GP2. We applied these findings to the analysis of additional ebolavirus isolates and correctly predicted that the newly identified ebolavirus species Bundibugyo, containing D47 and I584, is cathepsin B dependent and that ebolavirus Zaire-1995, the single known isolate of ebolavirus Zaire that lacks D47, is not. We also obtained evidence for virus-specific differences in the role of cathepsin L, including cooperation with cathepsin B. These studies strongly suggest that the use of endosomal cysteine proteases as host factors for entry is a general property of members of the family Filoviridae.

PMCID: PMC3302294 PMID: 22238307 [PubMed - indexed for MEDLINE]
1049. J Virol. 2012 Mar;86(6):3038-49. doi: 10.1128/JVI.05741-11. Epub 2012 Jan 11.

Characterization of the RNA silencing suppression activity of the Ebola virus VP35 protein in plants and mammalian cells.

Zhu Y(1), Cherukuri NC, Jackel JN, Wu Z, Crary M, Buckley KJ, Bisaro DM, Parris DS.

Author information: (1)Department of Molecular Virology, Immunology and Medical Genetics, The Ohio State University, Columbus, Ohio, USA.

Ebola virus (EBOV) causes a lethal hemorrhagic fever for which there is no approved effective treatment or prevention strategy. EBOV VP35 is a virulence factor that blocks innate antiviral host responses, including the induction of and response to alpha/beta interferon. VP35 is also an RNA silencing suppressor (RSS). By inhibiting microRNA-directed silencing, mammalian virus RSSs have the capacity to alter the cellular environment to benefit replication. A reporter gene containing specific microRNA target sequences was used to demonstrate that prior expression of wild-type VP35 was able to block establishment of microRNA silencing in mammalian cells. In addition, wild-type VP35 C-terminal domain (CTD) protein fusions were shown to bind small interfering RNA (siRNA). Analysis of mutant proteins demonstrated that reporter activity in RSS assays did not correlate with their ability to antagonize double-stranded RNA (dsRNA)-activated protein kinase R (PKR) or bind siRNA. The results suggest that enhanced reporter activity in the presence of VP35 is a composite of nonspecific translational enhancement and silencing suppression. Moreover, most of the specific RSS activity in mammalian cells is RNA binding independent, consistent with VP35's proposed role in sequestering one or more silencing complex proteins. To examine RSS activity in a system without interferon, VP35 was tested in well-characterized plant silencing suppression assays. VP35 was shown to possess potent plant RSS activity, and the activities of mutant proteins correlated strongly, but not exclusively, with RNA binding ability. The results suggest the importance of VP35-protein interactions in blocking silencing in a system (mammalian) that cannot amplify dsRNA.

PMCID: PMC3302343 PMID: 22238300 [PubMed - indexed for MEDLINE]
1050. J Virol. 2012 Mar;86(5):2809-16. doi: 10.1128/JVI.05549-11. Epub 2011 Dec 14.

Structure of an antibody in complex with its mucin domain linear epitope that is protective against Ebola virus.

Olal D(1), Kuehne AI, Bale S, Halfmann P, Hashiguchi T, Fusco ML, Lee JE, King LB, Kawaoka Y, Dye JM Jr, Saphire EO.

Author information: (1)Department of Immunology and Microbial Science, The Scripps Research Institute, La Jolla, California, USA.

Antibody 14G7 is protective against lethal Ebola virus challenge and recognizes a distinct linear epitope in the prominent mucin-like domain of the Ebola virus glycoprotein GP. The structure of 14G7 in complex with its linear peptide epitope has now been determined to 2.8 Å. The structure shows that this GP sequence forms a tandem β-hairpin structure that binds deeply into a cleft in the antibody-combining site. A key threonine at the apex of one turn is critical for antibody interaction and is conserved among all Ebola viruses. This work provides further insight into the mechanism of protection by antibodies that target the protruding, highly accessible mucin-like domain of Ebola virus and the structural framework for understanding and characterizing candidate immunotherapeutics.

PMCID: PMC3302272 PMID: 22171276 [PubMed - indexed for MEDLINE]
1051. Virology. 2012 Mar 1;424(1):3-10. doi: 10.1016/j.virol.2011.11.031. Epub 2012 Jan 4

Cathepsins B and L activate Ebola but not Marburg virus glycoproteins for efficient entry into cell lines and macrophages independent of TMPRSS2 expression.

Gnirss K(1), Kühl A, Karsten C, Glowacka I, Bertram S, Kaup F, Hofmann H, Pöhlmann S.

Author information: (1)Institute of Virology, Hannover Medical School, Hannover, Germany.

Ebola (EBOV) and Marburg virus (MARV) cause severe hemorrhagic fever. The host cell proteases cathepsin B and L activate the Zaire ebolavirus glycoprotein (GP) for cellular entry and constitute potential targets for antiviral intervention. However, it is unclear if different EBOV species and MARV equally depend on cathepsin B/L activity for infection of cell lines and macrophages, important viral target cells. Here, we show that cathepsin B/L inhibitors markedly reduce 293T cell infection driven by the GPs of all EBOV species, independent of the type II transmembrane serine protease TMPRSS2, which cleaved but failed to activate EBOV-GPs. Similarly, a cathepsin B/L inhibitor blocked macrophage infection mediated by different EBOV-GPs. In contrast, MARV-GP-driven entry exhibited little dependence on cathepsin B/L activity. Still, MARV-GP-mediated entry was efficiently blocked by leupeptin. These results suggest that cathepsins B/L promote entry of EBOV while MARV might employ so far unidentified proteases for GP activation.

PMID: 22222211 [PubMed - indexed for MEDLINE]
1052. Vopr Virusol. 2012 Mar-Apr;57(2):14-9.

[Development of methodology for predictably significant evaluation of the protective efficacy of antiviral agents].

[Article in Russian]

Markin VA.

The paper provides a theoretical analysis for determining whether the antiviral nonspecific drugs being tested are promising to solve biosafety problems in the treatment of exotic viral infections. The essence of the proposed concept of evaluation of protective effectiveness is to analyze the effect of a test drug on the pathogenesis of experimental infection from the fact that it is effective in adequately eliminating the animal-simulated leading syndrome of human disease. The given approaches to using adequacy criteria to select the species of animals meeting the goals of tests in terms of pathogenetic and pharmacological parameters determine a new methodology for evaluating the efficacy of protective agents. Basic requirements for a testing procedure are presented. The prognostic value of evaluation of the protective efficacy of antiviral agents for man will depend on the approximation of the pathogenetic features and external manifestation of disease in the selected animal species to human Infection. The paper also covers the comparative characteristics of the course of Ebola fever and Venezuelan equine encephalomyelitis in man and some species of monkey.

PMID: 22834141 [PubMed - indexed for MEDLINE]

1053. Sci Transl Med. 2012 Feb 29;4(123):123ra24. doi: 10.1126/scitranslmed.3003500.

Productive replication of Ebola virus is regulated by the c-Abl1 tyrosine kinase.

García M(1), Cooper A, Shi W, Bornmann W, Carrion R, Kalman D, Nabel GJ.

Author information: (1)Vaccine Research Center, National Institute of Allergy and Infectious Diseases, National Institutes of Health, Bethesda, MD 20892, USA. Ebola virus causes a fulminant infection in humans resulting in diffuse bleeding, vascular instability, hypotensive shock, and often death. Because of its high mortality and ease of transmission from human to human, Ebola virus remains a biological threat for which effective preventive and therapeutic interventions are needed. An understanding of the mechanisms of Ebola virus pathogenesis is critical for developing antiviral therapeutics. Here, we report that productive replication of Ebola virus is modulated by the c-Abl1 tyrosine kinase. Release of Ebola virus-like particles (VLPs) in a cell culture cotransfection system was inhibited by c-Abl1-specific small interfering RNA (siRNA) or by Abl-specific kinase inhibitors and required tyrosine phosphorylation of the Ebola matrix protein VP40. Expression of c-Abl1 stimulated an increase in phosphorylation of tyrosine 13 (Y(13)) of VP40, and mutation of Y(13) to alanine decreased the release of Ebola VLPs. Productive replication of the highly pathogenic Ebola virus Zaire strain was inhibited by c-Abl1-specific siRNAs or by the Abl-family inhibitor nilotinib by up to four orders of magnitude. These data indicate that c-Abl1 regulates budding or release of filoviruses through a mechanism involving phosphorylation of VP40. This step of the virus life cycle therefore may represent a target for antiviral therapy.

PMID: 22378924 [PubMed - indexed for MEDLINE]

1054. Virology. 2012 Feb 20;423(2):119-24. doi: 10.1016/j.virol.2011.11.027. Epub 2011 Dec 23.

Serology and cytokine profiles in patients infected with the newly discovered Bundibugyo ebolavirus.

Gupta M(1), MacNeil A, Reed ZD, Rollin PE, Spiropoulou CF.

Author information: (1)Viral Special Pathogens Branch, NCEZID, DHCPP, Centers for Disease Control and Prevention, Atlanta, GA 30033, USA. mgupta@cdc.gov
A new species of Ebolavirus, Bundibugyo ebolavirus, was discovered in an outbreak in western Uganda in November 2007. To study the correlation between fatal infection and immune response in Bundibugyo ebolavirus infection, viral antigen, antibodies, and 17 soluble factors important for innate immunity were examined in 44 patient samples. Using Luminex assays, we found that fatal infection was associated with high levels of viral antigen, low levels of pro-inflammatory cytokines, such as IL-1α, IL-1β, IL-6, TNF-α, and high levels of immunosuppressor cytokines like IL-10. Also, acute infected patients died in spite of generating high levels of antibodies against the virus. Thus, our results imply that disease severity in these patients is not due to the multi-organ failure and septic shock caused by a flood of inflammatory cytokines, as seen in infections with other Ebolavirus species.

Published by Elsevier Inc.

PMID: 22197674 [PubMed - indexed for MEDLINE]

1055. Expert Rev Vaccines. 2012 Feb;11(2):163-6. doi: 10.1586/erv.11.179.

A strategy to simultaneously eradicate the natural reservoirs of rabies and Ebola virus.

Wong G(1), Kobinger G.

Author information: (1)Special Pathogens Program, National Microbiology Laboratory, Public Health Agency of Canada, 1015 Arlington Street, Winnipeg, MB, R3E 3R2, Canada.

Comment on J Virol. 2011 Oct;85(20):10605-16.

The efficacy of a recombinant live-attenuated or chemically inactivated bivalent vaccine against rabies virus (RABV) and Ebola virus (EBOV) infection was evaluated in a lethal mouse model of infection. The vaccines were derived from the live-attenuated Street Alabama Dufferin B19 RABV platform already approved for veterinary use, where intramuscular, intranasal and intraperitoneal administration of the recombinant vaccines were avirulent in adult mice. Significant levels of serum RABV- and EBOV-specific antibodies were observed postvaccination, with levels that correlated with protection in vaccinated mice post-RABV or -EBOV challenge. These results justify further studies in guinea pigs and nonhuman primates, and highlight a promising strategy to eradicate the natural reservoirs of RABV and EBOV.

PMID: 22309665 [PubMed]

1056. Gene Ther. 2012 Feb;19(2):201-9. doi: 10.1038/gt.2011.83. Epub 2011 Jun 9.

Jaagsiekte sheep retrovirus pseudotyped lentiviral vector-mediated gene transfer to fetal ovine lung.

Davey MG(1), Zoltick PW, Todorow CA, Limberis MP, Ruchelli ED, Hedrick HL, Flake AW.

Author information: (1)The Children's Center for Fetal Research, The Children's Hospital of Philadelphia, Philadelphia, PA 19104, USA. daveym@email.chop.edu
Viral vector-mediated gene transfer to the postnatal respiratory epithelium has, in general, been of low efficiency due to physical and immunological barriers, non-apical location of cellular receptors critical for viral uptake and limited transduction of resident stem/progenitor cells. These obstacles may be overcome using a prenatal strategy. In this study, HIV-1-based lentiviral vectors (LVs) pseudotyped with the envelope glycoproteins of Jaagsiekte sheep retrovirus (JSRV-LV), baculovirus GP64 (GP64-LV), Ebola Zaire-LV or vesicular stomatitis virus (VSVg-LV) and the adeno-associated virus-2/6.2 (AAV2/6.2) were compared for in utero transfer of a green fluorescent protein (GFP) reporter gene to ovine lung epithelium between days 65 and 78 of gestation. GFP expression was examined on day 85 or 136 of gestation (term is ~145 days). The percentage of the respiratory epithelial cells expressing GFP in fetal sheep that received the JSRV-LV (3.18 × 10(8)-6.85 × 10(9) viral particles per fetus) was 24.6±0.9% at 3 weeks postinjection (day 85) and 29.9±4.8% at 10 weeks postinjection (day 136). Expression was limited to the surface epithelium lining fetal airways

PMID: 21654824 [PubMed - indexed for MEDLINE]

1057. Hepatology. 2012 Feb;55(2):354-63. doi: 10.1002/hep.24686. Epub 2011 Dec 16.

CD59 incorporation protects hepatitis C virus against complement-mediated destruction.

Amet T(1), Ghabril M, Chalasani N, Byrd D, Hu N, Grantham A, Liu Z, Qin X, He JJ, Yu Q.

Author information: (1)Department of Microbiology and Immunology, Indiana University School of Medicine, Indianapolis, IN 46202, USA.

Several enveloped viruses including human immunodeficiency virus type 1 (HIV-1), cytomegalovirus (CMV), herpes simplex virus 1 (HSV-1), Ebola virus, vaccinia virus, and influenza virus have been found to incorporate host regulators of complement activation (RCA) into their viral envelopes and, as a result, escape antibody-dependent complement-mediated lysis (ADCML). Hepatitis C virus (HCV) is an enveloped virus of the family Flaviviridae and incorporates more than 10 host lipoproteins. Patients chronically infected with HCV develop high-titer and crossreactive neutralizing antibodies (nAbs), yet fail to clear the virus, raising the possibility that HCV may also use the similar strategy of RCA incorporation to escape ADCML. The current study was therefore undertaken to determine whether HCV virions incorporate biologically functional CD59, a key member of RCA. Our experiments provided several lines of evidence demonstrating that CD59 was associated with the external membrane of HCV particles derived from either Huh7.5.1 cells or plasma samples from HCV-infected patients. First, HCV particles were captured by CD59-specific Abs. Second, CD59 was detected in purified HCV particles by immunoblot analysis and in the cell-free supernatant from HCV-infected Huh7.5.1 cells, but not from uninfected or adenovirus serotype 5 (Ad5) (a nonenveloped cytolytic virus)-infected Huh7.5.1 cells by enzyme-linked immunosorbent assay. Last, abrogation of CD59 function with its blockers increased the sensitivity of HCV virions to ADCML, resulting in a significant reduction of HCV infectivity. Additionally, direct addition of CD59 blockers into plasma samples from HCV-infected patients increased autologous virolysis.CONCLUSION: Our study, for the first time, demonstrates that CD59 is incorporated into both cell line-derived and plasma primary HCV virions at levels that protect against ADCML. This is also the first report to show that direct addition of RCA blockers into plasma from HCV-infected patients renders endogenous plasma virions sensitive to ADCML.

Copyright © 2011 American Association for the Study of Liver Diseases.

PMCID: PMC3417136 PMID: 21932413 [PubMed - indexed for MEDLINE]

1058. PLoS Pathog. 2012 Feb;8(2):e1002550. doi: 10.1371/journal.ppat.1002550. Epub 2012 Feb 23.

The ebola virus interferon antagonist VP24 directly binds STAT1 and has a novel, pyramidal fold.

Zhang AP(1), Bornholdt ZA, Liu T, Abelson DM, Lee DE, Li S, Woods VL Jr, Saphire EO.

Author information: (1)Department of Immunology and Microbial Science, The Scripps Research Institute, La Jolla, California, USA.

Erratum in PLoS Pathog. 2013 Dec;9(12). doi:10.1371/annotation/360ddc68-0313-4eae-af24-043cc040c52d.

Ebolaviruses cause hemorrhagic fever with up to 90% lethality and in fatal cases, are characterized by early suppression of the host innate immune system. One of the proteins likely responsible for this effect is VP24. VP24 is known to antagonize interferon signaling by binding host karyopherin α proteins, thereby preventing them from transporting the tyrosine-phosphorylated transcription factor STAT1 to the nucleus. Here, we report that VP24 binds STAT1 directly, suggesting that VP24 can suppress at least two distinct branches of the interferon pathway. Here, we also report the first crystal structures of VP24, derived from different species of ebolavirus that are pathogenic (Sudan) and nonpathogenic to humans (Reston). These structures reveal that VP24 has a novel, pyramidal fold. A site on a particular face of the pyramid exhibits reduced solvent exchange when in complex with STAT1. This site is above two highly conserved pockets in VP24 that contain key residues previously implicated in virulence. These crystal structures and accompanying biochemical analysis map differences between pathogenic and nonpathogenic viruses, offer templates for drug design, and provide the three-dimensional framework necessary for biological dissection of the many functions of VP24 in the virus life cycle.

PMCID: PMC3285596 PMID: 22383882 [PubMed - indexed for MEDLINE]

1059. Viruses. 2012 Feb;4(2):258-75. doi: 10.3390/v4020258. Epub 2012 Feb 7.

Filovirus entry: a novelty in the viral fusion world.

Hunt CL(1), Lennemann NJ, Maury W.

Author information: (1)Department of Microbiology, University of Iowa, Iowa City, IA 52242, USA. catherine-l-miller@uiowa.edu

Ebolavirus (EBOV) and Marburgvirus (MARV) that compose the filovirus family of negative strand RNA viruses infect a broad range of mammalian cells. Recent studies indicate that cellular entry of this family of viruses requires a series of cellular protein interactions and molecular mechanisms, some of which are unique to filoviruses and others are commonly used by all viral glycoproteins. Details of this entry pathway are highlighted here. Virus entry into cells is initiated by the interaction of the viral glycoprotein(1) subunit (GP(1)) with both adherence factors and one or more receptors on the surface of host cells. On epithelial cells, we recently demonstrated that TIM-1 serves as a receptor for this family of viruses, but the cell surface receptors in other cell types remain unidentified. Upon receptor binding, the virus is internalized into endosomes primarily via macropinocytosis, but perhaps by other mechanisms as well. Within the acidified endosome, the heavily glycosylated GP(1) is cleaved to a smaller form by the low pH-dependent cellular proteases Cathepsin L and B, exposing residues in the receptor binding site (RBS). Details of the molecular events following cathepsin-dependent trimming of GP(1) are currently incomplete; however, the processed GP(1) specifically interacts with endosomal/lysosomal membranes that contain the Niemann Pick C1 (NPC1) protein and expression of NPC1 is required for productive infection, suggesting that GP/NPC1 interactions may be an important late step in the entry process. Additional events such as further GP(1) processing and/or reducing events may also be required to generate a fusion-ready form of the glycoprotein. Once this has been achieved, sequences in the filovirus GP(2) subunit mediate viral/cellular membrane fusion via mechanisms similar to those previously described for other enveloped viruses. This multi-step entry pathway highlights the complex and highly orchestrated path of internalization and fusion that appears unique for filoviruses.

PMCID: PMC3315215 PMID: 22470835 [PubMed - indexed for MEDLINE]

1060. Virol J. 2012 Jan 25;9:32. doi: 10.1186/1743-422X-9-32.

Induction of ebolavirus cross-species immunity using retrovirus-like particles bearing the Ebola virus glycoprotein lacking the mucin-like domain.

Ou W(1), Delisle J, Jacques J, Shih J, Price G, Kuhn JH, Wang V, Verthelyi D, Kaplan G, Wilson CA.

Author information: (1)Division of Cellular and Gene Therapies, Center for Biologics Evaluation and Research, Bldg, 29B, Room 5NN22, 8800 Rockville Pike, Bethesda, MD 20892, USA.

BACKGROUND: The genus Ebolavirus includes five distinct viruses. Four of these viruses cause hemorrhagic fever in humans. Currently there are no licensed vaccines for any of them; however, several vaccines are under development. Ebola virus envelope glycoprotein (GP1,2) is highly immunogenic, but antibodies frequently arise against its least conserved mucin-like domain (MLD). We hypothesized that immunization with MLD-deleted GP1,2 (GPΔMLD) would induce cross-species immunity by making more conserved regions accessible to the immune system. METHODS: To test this hypothesis, mice were immunized with retrovirus-like particles (retroVLPs) bearing Ebola virus GPΔMLD, DNA plasmids (plasmo-retroVLP) that can produce such retroVLPs in vivo, or plasmo-retroVLP followed by retroVLPs. RESULTS: Cross-species neutralizing antibody and GP1,2-specific cellular immune responses were successfully induced. CONCLUSION: Our findings suggest that GPΔMLD presented through retroVLPs may provide a strategy for development of a vaccine against multiple ebolaviruses. Similar vaccination strategies may be adopted for other viruses whose envelope proteins contain highly variable regions that may mask more conserved domains from the immune system.

PMCID: PMC3284443 PMID: 22273269 [PubMed - indexed for MEDLINE]

1061. Virology. 2012 Jan 5;422(1):1-5. doi: 10.1016/j.virol.2011.08.024. Epub 2011 Oct 2

Using next generation sequencing to identify yellow fever virus in Uganda.

McMullan LK(1), Frace M, Sammons SA, Shoemaker T, Balinandi S, Wamala JF, Lutwama JJ, Downing RG, Stroeher U, MacNeil A, Nichol ST.

Author information: (1)Virus Special Pathogens Branch, Centers for Disease Control and Prevention, Atlanta, GA 30329, USA.

In October and November 2010, hospitals in northern Uganda reported patients with suspected hemorrhagic fevers. Initial tests for Ebola viruses, Marburg virus, Rift Valley fever virus, and Crimean Congo hemorrhagic fever virus were negative. Unbiased PCR amplification of total RNA extracted directly from patient sera and next generation sequencing resulted in detection of yellow fever virus and generation of 98% of the virus genome sequence. This finding demonstrated the utility of next generation sequencing and a metagenomic approach to identify an etiological agent and direct the response to a disease outbreak.

Copyright © 2011. Published by Elsevier Inc.

PMID: 21962764 [PubMed - indexed for MEDLINE]

1062. Antiviral Res. 2012 Jan;93(1):23-9. doi: 10.1016/j.antiviral.2011.10.011. Epub 2011 Oct 18.

Identification of an antioxidant small-molecule with broad-spectrum antiviral activity.

Panchal RG(1), Reid SP, Tran JP, Bergeron AA, Wells J, Kota KP, Aman J, Bavari S.

Author information: (1)United States Army Medical Research Institute of Infectious Diseases, 1425 Porter Street, Fort Detrick, Frederick, MD 21702-5011, USA.

The highly lethal filoviruses, Ebola and Marburg cause severe hemorrhagic fever in humans and non-human primates. To date there are no licensed vaccines or therapeutics to counter these infections. Identifying novel pathways and host targets that play an essential role during infection will provide potential targets to develop therapeutics. Small molecule chemical screening for Ebola virus inhibitors resulted in identification of a compound NSC 62914. The compound was found to exhibit anti-filovirus activity in cell-based assays and in vivo protected mice following challenge with Ebola or Marburg viruses. Additionally, the compound was found to inhibit Rift Valley fever virus, Lassa virus and Venezuelan equine encephalitis virus in cell-based assays. Investigation of the mechanism of action of the compound revealed that it had antioxidant properties. Specifically, compound NSC 62914 was found to act as a scavenger of reactive oxygen species, and to up-regulate oxidative stress-induced genes. However, four known antioxidant compounds failed to inhibit filovirus infection, thus suggesting that the mechanistic basis of the antiviral function of the antioxidant NSC 62914 may involve modulation of multiple signaling pathways/targets.

Published by Elsevier B.V.

PMID: 22027648 [PubMed - indexed for MEDLINE]

1063. Arch Virol. 2012 Jan;157(1):121-7. doi: 10.1007/s00705-011-1115-8. Epub 2011 Sep 25

Inhibition of Lassa virus and Ebola virus infection in host cells treated with the kinase inhibitors genistein and tyrphostin.

Kolokoltsov AA(1), Adhikary S, Garver J, Johnson L, Davey RA, Vela EM.

Author information: (1)Department of Microbiology and Immunology, The University of Texas Medical Branch, Galveston, TX 77555, USA.

Arenaviruses and filoviruses are capable of causing hemorrhagic fever syndrome in humans. Limited therapeutic and/or prophylactic options are available for humans suffering from viral hemorrhagic fever. In this report, we demonstrate that pre-treatment of host cells with the kinase inhibitors genistein and tyrphostin AG1478 leads to inhibition of infection or transduction in cells infected with Ebola virus, Marburg virus, and Lassa virus. In all, the results demonstrate that a kinase inhibitor cocktail consisting of genistein and tyrphostin AG1478 is a broad-spectrum antiviral that may be used as a therapeutic or prophylactic against arenavirus and filovirus hemorrhagic fever.

PMID: 21947546 [PubMed - indexed for MEDLINE]

1064. Curr Med Chem. 2012;19(7):992-1007.

DC-SIGN antagonists, a potential new class of anti-infectives.

Anderluh M(1), Jug G, Svajger U, Obermajer N.

Author information: (1)Department of Medicinal Chemistry, University of Ljubljana, Ljubljana, Slovenia. marko.anderluh@ffa.uni-lj.si

DC-SIGN (Dendritic Cell-Specific Intercellular adhesion molecule-3-Grabbing Non-integrin) is a type II C-type lectin that functions as an adhesion molecule located on dendritic cells (DCs). It enables some of the functions of DCs, including migration, pathogen recognition, internalisation and processing, and their binding to T cells. HIV-I has been reported to enter DCs by being bound to DC-SIGN, escaping the normal lytic pathway in DCs' endosomes and avoiding the immune system defence system. A very similar mechanism of survival has been observed for some other pathogens. This makes DC-SIGN a receptor of interest in the design of distinctive anti-infectives that would inhibit DC-SIGN-pathogen interaction by blocking the very first step in pathogen infection. In this review we outline the development of DC-SIGN antagonists, focusing mainly on a glycomimetic approach. Based on the fact that DCSIGN binds mannose- and fucose-based oligo- and polysaccharides, their structural mimics have been designed and proved to inhibit pathogen-DC-SIGN interaction. Furthermore, recent in vitro studies have demonstrated that DC-SIGN antagonists block effectively the transmission of pathogens like HIV-I and Ebola to CD4+ T cells. Although DC-SIGN has not been validated in vivo as a druggable target yet, we await future DC-SIGN antagonists as a new and highly promising group of novel anti-infectives.

PMID: 22257062 [PubMed - indexed for MEDLINE]

1065. Ecol Evol. 2012 Jan;3(1):80-8. doi: 10.1002/ece3.422. Epub 2012 Dec 6.

Genetic diversity of North American captive-born gorillas (Gorilla gorilla gorilla).

Simons ND(1), Wagner RS, Lorenz JG.

Author information: (1)Primate Behavior Program, Central Washington University Ellensburg, Washington.

Western lowland gorillas (Gorilla gorilla gorilla) are designated as critically endangered and wild populations are dramatically declining as a result of habitat destruction, fragmentation, diseases (e.g., Ebola) and the illegal bushmeat trade. As wild populations continue to decline, the genetic management of the North American captive western lowland gorilla population will be an important component of the long-term conservation of the species. We genotyped 26 individuals from the North American captive gorilla collection at 11 autosomal microsatellite loci in order to compare levels of genetic diversity to wild populations, investigate genetic signatures of a population bottleneck and identify the genetic structure of the captive-born population. Captive gorillas had significantly higher levels of allelic diversity ($t(7) = 4.49$, $P = 0.002$) and heterozygosity ($t(7) = 4.15$, $P = 0.004$) than comparative wild populations, yet the population has lost significant allelic diversity while in captivity when compared to founders ($t(7) = 2.44$, $P = 0.04$). Analyses suggested no genetic evidence for a population bottleneck of the captive population. Genetic structure results supported the management of North American captive gorillas as a single population. Our results highlight the utility of genetic management approaches for endangered nonhuman primate species.

PMCID: PMC3568845 PMID: 23403930 [PubMed]

1066. Emerg Health Threats J. 2012;5. doi: 10.3402/ehtj.v5i0.9134. Epub 2012 Apr 30.

Dead or alive: animal sampling during Ebola hemorrhagic fever outbreaks in humans.

Olson SH(1), Reed P, Cameron KN, Ssebide BJ, Johnson CK, Morse SS, Karesh WB, Mazet JA, Joly DO.

Author information: (1)Wildlife Health Program, Wildlife Conservation Society, Nanaimo, BC, Canada.

There are currently no widely accepted animal surveillance guidelines for human Ebola hemorrhagic fever (EHF) outbreak investigations to identify potential sources of Ebolavirus (EBOV) spillover into humans and other animals. Animal field surveillance during and following an outbreak has several purposes, from helping identify the specific animal source of a human case to guiding control activities by describing the spatial and temporal distribution of wild circulating EBOV, informing public health efforts, and contributing to broader EHF research questions. Since 1976, researchers have sampled over 10,000 individual vertebrates from areas associated with human EHF outbreaks and tested for EBOV or antibodies. Using field surveillance data associated with EHF outbreaks, this review provides guidance on animal sampling for resource-limited outbreak situations, target species, and in some cases which diagnostics should be prioritized to rapidly assess the presence of EBOV in animal reservoirs. In brief, EBOV detection was 32.7% (18/55) for carcasses (animals found dead) and 0.2% (13/5309) for live captured animals. Our review indicates that for the purposes of identifying potential sources of transmission from animals to humans and isolating suspected virus in an animal in outbreak situations, (1) surveillance of free-ranging non-human primate mortality and morbidity should be a priority, (2) any wildlife morbidity or mortality events should be investigated and may hold the most promise for locating virus or viral genome sequences, (3) surveillance of some bat species is worthwhile to isolate and detect evidence of exposure, and (4) morbidity, mortality, and serology studies of domestic animals should prioritize dogs and pigs and include testing for virus and previous exposure.

PMCID: PMC3342678 PMID: 22558004 [PubMed]

1067. Front Microbiol. 2012 Apr 2;3:111. doi: 10.3389/fmicb.2012.00111. eCollection 2012

Ebolavirus Replication and Tetherin/BST-2.

Yasuda J(1).

Author information: (1)Department of Emerging Infectious Diseases, Institute of Tropical Medicine, Nagasaki University Nagasaki, Japan.

Ebolavirus (EBOV) is an enveloped, non-segmented, negative-stranded RNA virus, which consists of five species: Zaire ebolavirus, Sudan ebolavirus, Tai Forest ebolavirus, Bundibugyo ebolavirus, and Reston ebolavirus. EBOV causes a lethal hemorrhagic fever in both humans and non-human primates. The EBOV RNA genome encodes seven viral proteins: NP, VP35, VP40, GP, VP30, VP24, and L. VP40 is a matrix protein and is essential for virus assembly and release from host cells. Expression of VP40 in mammalian cells is sufficient to generate extracellular virus-like particles, which resemble authentic virions. Tetherin/BST-2, which was identified as an effective cellular factor that prevents human immunodeficiency virus-I release in the absence of viral accessory protein Vpu, has been reported to inhibit ZEBOV VP40-induced VLP release. Tetherin/BST-2 appears to inhibit virus release by physically tethering viral particles to the cell surface via its N-terminal transmembrane domain and C-terminal glycosylphosphatidylinositol anchor. Replication of ZEBOV is not inhibited by tetherin/BST-2 expression, although tetherin/BST-2 was expected to inhibit EBOV release as well as VLP release. Recently, it was reported that viral glycoprotein of EBOV, GP, antagonizes the antiviral effect of tetherin/BST-2. However, the mechanism by which GP antagonizes the antiviral activity of tetherin/BST-2 and whether GP of the other EBOV species function as antagonists of tetherin/BST-2 remain unclear.

PMCID: PMC3316994 PMID: 22485110 [PubMed]

1068. Front Microbiol. 2012 Feb 6;3:34. doi: 10.3389/fmicb.2012.00034. eCollection 2012

Filovirus tropism: cellular molecules for viral entry.

Takada A(1).

Author information: (1)Division of Global Epidemiology, Research Center for Zoonosis Control, Hokkaido University Sapporo, Japan.

In human and non-human primates, filoviruses (Ebola and Marburg viruses) cause severe hemorrhagic fever. Recently, other animals such as pigs and some species of fruit bats have also been shown to be susceptible to these viruses. While having a preference for some cell types such as hepatocytes, endothelial cells, dendritic cells, monocytes, and macrophages, filoviruses are known to be pantropic in infection of primates. The envelope glycoprotein (GP) is responsible for both receptor binding and fusion of the virus envelope with the host cell membrane. It has been demonstrated that filovirus GP interacts with multiple molecules for entry into host cells, whereas none of the cellular molecules so far identified as a receptor/co-receptor fully explains filovirus tissue tropism and host range. Available data suggest that the mucin-like region (MLR) on GP plays an important role in attachment to the preferred target cells, whose infection is likely involved in filovirus pathogenesis, whereas the MLR is not essential for the fundamental function of the GP in viral entry into cells in vitro. Further studies elucidating the mechanisms of cellular entry of filoviruses may shed light on the development of strategies for prophylaxis and treatment of Ebola and Marburg hemorrhagic fevers.

PMCID: PMC3277274 PMID: 22363323 [PubMed]

1069. Future Microbiol. 2012 Jan;7(1):1-4. doi: 10.2217/fmb.11.110.

Ebolavirus: a brief review of novel therapeutic targets.

Kondratowicz AS, Maury WJ.

PMID: 22191439 [PubMed - indexed for MEDLINE]

1070. Intervirology. 2012;55(6):488-90. doi: 10.1159/000337026. Epub 2012 May 3.

Isolation of a novel adenovirus from Rousettus leschenaultii bats from India.

Raut CG(1), Yadav PD, Towner JS, Amman BR, Erickson BR, Cannon DL, Sivaram A, Basu A, Nichol ST, Mishra AC, Mourya DT.

Author information: (1)Microbial Containment Complex, National Institute of Virology, Pune, India.

Surveillance work was initiated to study the presence of highly infectious diseases like Ebola-Reston, Marburg, Nipah and other possible viruses that are known to be found in the bat species and responsible for causing diseases in humans. A novel adenovirus was isolated from a common species of fruit bat (Rousettus leschenaultii) captured in Maharashtra State, India. Partial sequence analysis of the DNA polymerase gene shows this isolate to be a newly recognized member of the genus Mastadenovirus (family Adenoviridae), approximately 20% divergent at the nucleotide level from Japanese BatAdV, its closest known relative.

Copyright © 2012 S. Karger AG, Basel.

PMID: 22572722 [PubMed - indexed for MEDLINE]

1071. J Glob Infect Dis. 2012 Jan;4(1):69-74. doi: 10.4103/0974-777X.93765.

Infection control during filoviral hemorrhagic Fever outbreaks.

Raabea VN(1), Borcherta M.

Author information: (1)Departments of Internal Medicine and Pediatrics, University of California San Diego, 200 West Arbor Drive, San Diego, CA, USA.

Breaking the human-to-human transmission cycle remains the cornerstone of infection control during filoviral (Ebola and Marburg) hemorrhagic fever outbreaks. This requires effective identification and isolation of cases, timely contact tracing and monitoring, proper usage of barrier personal protection gear by health workers, and safely conducted burials. Solely implementing these measures is insufficient for infection control; control efforts must be culturally sensitive and conducted in a transparent manner to promote the necessary trust between the community and infection control team in order to succeed. This article provides a review of the literature on infection control during filoviral hemorrhagic fever outbreaks focusing on outbreaks in a developing setting and lessons learned from previous outbreaks. The primary search database used to review the literature was PUBMED, the National Library of Medicine website.

PMCID: PMC3326963 PMID: 22529631 [PubMed]

1072. J Med Microbiol. 2012 Jan;61(Pt 1):8-15. doi: 10.1099/jmm.0.036210-0. Epub 2011 Aug 18.

Lethality and pathogenesis of airborne infection with filoviruses in A129 α/β -/- interferon receptor-deficient mice.

Lever MS(1), Piercy TJ, Steward JA, Eastaugh L, Smither SJ, Taylor C, Salguero FJ, Phillpotts RJ.

Author information: (1)Defence Science and Technology Laboratories (Dstl), Porton Down, Salisbury, Wiltshire, UK. mslever@dstl.gov.uk

Normal immunocompetent mice are not susceptible to non-adapted filoviruses. There are therefore two strategies available to establish a murine model of filovirus infection: adaptation of the virus to the host or the use of genetically modified mice that are susceptible to the virus. A number of knockout (KO) strains of mice with defects in either their adaptive or innate immunity are susceptible to non-adapted filoviruses. In this study, A129 α/β -/- interferon receptor-deficient KO mice, strain A129 IFN-α/β -/-, were used to determine the lethality of a range of filoviruses, including Lake Victoria marburgvirus (MARV), Zaire ebolavirus (ZEBOV), Sudan ebolavirus (SEBOV), Reston ebolavirus (REBOV) and Côte d'Ivoire ebolavirus (CIEBOV), administered by using intraperitoneal (IP) or aerosol routes of infection. One hundred percent mortality was observed in all groups of KO mice that were administered with a range of challenge doses of MARV and ZEBOV by either IP or aerosol routes. Mean time to death for both routes was dose-dependent and ranged from 5.4 to 7.4 days in the IP injection challenge, and from 10.2 to 13 days in the aerosol challenge. The lethal dose (50 % tissue culture infective dose, TCID(50)) of ZEBOV for KO mice was

PMID: 21852521 [PubMed - indexed for MEDLINE]

1073. J Virol. 2012 Jan;86(1):364-72. doi: 10.1128/JVI.05708-11. Epub 2011 Oct 26.

Cathepsin cleavage potentiates the Ebola virus glycoprotein to undergo a subsequent fusion-relevant conformational change.

Brecher M(1), Schornberg KL, Delos SE, Fusco ML, Saphire EO, White JM.

Author information: (1)Department of Microbiology, University of Virginia, Charlottesville, Virginia, USA.

Cellular entry of Ebola virus (EBOV), a deadly hemorrhagic fever virus, is mediated by the viral glycoprotein (GP). The receptor-binding subunit of GP must be cleaved (by endosomal cathepsins) in order for entry and infection to proceed. Cleavage appears to proceed through 50-kDa and 20-kDa intermediates, ultimately generating a key 19-kDa core. How 19-kDa GP is subsequently triggered to bind membranes and induce fusion remains a mystery. Here we show that 50-kDa GP cannot be triggered to bind to liposomes in response to elevated temperature but that 20-kDa and 19-kDa GP can. Importantly, 19-kDa GP can be triggered at temperatures ~10°C lower than 20-kDa GP, suggesting that it is the most fusion ready form. Triggering by heat (or urea) occurs only at pH 5, not pH 7.5, and involves the fusion loop, as a fusion loop mutant is defective in liposome binding. We further show that mild reduction (preferentially at low pH) triggers 19-kDa GP to bind to liposomes, with the wild-type protein being triggered to a greater extent than the fusion loop mutant. Moreover, mild reduction inactivates pseudovirion infection, suggesting that reduction can also trigger 19-kDa GP on virus particles. Our results support the hypothesis that priming of EBOV GP, specifically to the 19-kDa core, potentiates GP to undergo subsequent fusion-relevant conformational changes. Our findings also indicate that low pH and an additional endosomal factor (possibly reduction or possibly a process mimicked by reduction) act as fusion triggers.

PMCID: PMC3255896 PMID: 22031933 [PubMed - indexed for MEDLINE]

1074. Med Hist. 2012 Jan;56(1):72-93. doi: 10.1017/S0025727300000284.

Showers, sweating and suing: Legionnaires' disease and 'new' infections in Britain, 1977-90.

Macfarlane JT(1), Worboys M.

Author information: (1)Professor of Respiratory Medicine, University of Nottingham, and Visiting Professor, Centre for the History of Science, Technology and Medicine and Wellcome Unit for the History of Medicine, Faculty of Life Sciences, University of Manchester, c/o Watergate Barn, Loweswater, Cumbria CA13 0RU, UK. jtmacfarlane@gmail.com

Legionnaires' disease is now routinely discussed as an 'emerging infectious disease' (EID) and is said to be one of the earliest such diseases to be recognised. It first appeared in 1976 and its cause was identified in 1977, the same year that Ebola fever, Hantaan virus and Campylobacter jejuni arrived. The designation of Legionnaires' disease as an EID was retrospective; it was not and could not be otherwise as the category only gained currency in the early 1990s. In this article we reflect on the changing medical understanding and social profile of Legionnaires' disease in the decade or so from its recognition to the creation of EIDs, especially its ambivalent position between public health and clinical medicine. However, we question any simple opposition, between public health experts who approached Legionnaires' disease as a new and worrying environmental threat that could be prevented, and clinicians who saw it as another cause of pneumonia that could be managed by improved diagnosis and treatment. We argue that in the British context of public spending cuts and the reform of public health, the category of 'new' diseases, in which Legionnaires' disease was central, was mobilised ahead of the EID lobby of the early 1990s, by interested groups in medicine to defend infectious diseases services.

PMCID: PMC3314898 PMID: 23752984 [PubMed - indexed for MEDLINE]

1075. Methods Mol Biol. 2012;824:271-303. doi: 10.1007/978-1-61779-433-9_14.

Plasmid DNA production for therapeutic applications.

Lara AR(1), Ramírez OT, Wunderlich M.

Author information: (1)Departamento de Procesos y Tecnología, Universidad Autónoma Metropolitana-Cuajimalpa, Mexico City, Mexico. alara@correo.cua.uam.mx

Erratum in Methods Mol Biol. 2012;824:E1. Wunderlich, Martin [added].

Plasmid DNA (pDNA) is the base for promising DNA vaccines and gene therapies against many infectious, acquired, and genetic diseases, including HIV-AIDS, Ebola, Malaria, and different types of cancer, enteric pathogens, and influenza. Compared to conventional vaccines, DNA vaccines have many advantages such as high stability, not being infectious, focusing the immune response to only those antigens desired for immunization and long-term persistence of the vaccine protection. Especially in developing countries, where conventional effective vaccines are often unavailable or too expensive, there is a need for both new and improved vaccines. Therefore the demand of pDNA is expected to rise significantly in the near future. Since the injection of pDNA usually only leads to a weak immune response, several milligrams of DNA vaccine are necessary for immunization protection. Hence, there is a special interest to raise the product yield in order to reduce manufacturing costs. In this chapter, the different stages of plasmid DNA production are reviewed, from the vector design to downstream operation options. In particular, recent advances on cell engineering for improving plasmid DNA production are discussed.

PMID: 22160904 [PubMed - indexed for MEDLINE]

1076. Mol Cell Proteomics. 2012 Jan;11(1):M111.008730. doi: 10.1074/mcp.M111.008730. Epub 2011 Oct 10.

Tumor biomarker glycoproteins in the seminal plasma of healthy human males are endogenous ligands for DC-SIGN.

Clark GF(1), Grassi P, Pang PC, Panico M, Lafrenz D, Drobnis EZ, Baldwin MR, Morris HR, Haslam SM, Schedin-Weiss S, Sun W, Dell A.

Author information: (1)Division of Reproductive and Perinatal Research, Department of Obstetrics, Gynecology and Women's Health, University of Missouri, Columbia, Missouri 65211, USA. clarkgf@health.missouri.edu

DC-SIGN is an immune C-type lectin that is expressed on both immature and mature dendritic cells associated with peripheral and lymphoid tissues in humans. It is a pattern recognition receptor that binds to several pathogens including HIV-1, Ebola virus, Mycobacterium tuberculosis, Candida albicans, Helicobacter pylori, and Schistosoma mansoni. Evidence is now mounting that DC-SIGN also recognizes endogenous glycoproteins, and that such interactions play a major role in maintaining immune homeostasis in humans and mice. Autoantigens (neoantigens) are produced for the first time in the human testes and other organs of the male urogenital tract under androgenic stimulus during puberty. Such antigens trigger autoimmune orchitis if the immune response is not tightly regulated within this system. Endogenous ligands for DC-SIGN could play a role in modulating such responses. Human seminal plasma glycoproteins express a high level of terminal Lewis(x) and Lewis(y) carbohydrate antigens. These epitopes react specifically with the lectin domains of DC-SIGN. However, because the expression of these sequences is necessary but not sufficient for interaction with DC-SIGN, this study was undertaken to determine if any seminal plasma glycoproteins are also endogenous ligands for DC-SIGN. Glycoproteins bearing terminal Lewis(x) and Lewis(y) sequences were initially isolated by lectin affinity chromatography. Protein sequencing established that three tumor biomarker glycoproteins (clusterin, galectin-3 binding glycoprotein, prostatic acid phosphatase) and protein C inhibitor were purified by using this affinity method. The binding of DC-SIGN to these seminal plasma glycoproteins was demonstrated in both Western blot and immunoprecipitation studies. These findings have confirmed that human seminal plasma contains endogenous glycoprotein ligands for DC-SIGN that could play a role in maintaining immune homeostasis both in the male urogenital tract and the vagina after coitus.
PMCID: PMC3270097 PMID: 21986992 [PubMed - indexed for MEDLINE]

1077. Mol Pharm. 2012 Jan 1;9(1):156-67. doi: 10.1021/mp200392g. Epub 2011 Dec 15.

A single sublingual dose of an adenovirus-based vaccine protects against lethal Ebola challenge in mice and guinea pigs.

Choi JH(1), Schafer SC, Zhang L, Kobinger GP, Juelich T, Freiberg AN, Croyle MA.

Author information: (1)Division of Pharmaceutics, College of Pharmacy, The University of Texas at Austin, Austin, Texas 78712, United States.

Sublingual (SL) delivery, a noninvasive immunization method that bypasses the intestinal tract for direct entry into the circulation, was evaluated with an adenovirus (Ad5)-based vaccine for Ebola. Mice and guinea pigs were immunized via the intramuscular (IM), nasal (IN), oral (PO) and SL routes. SL immunization elicited strong transgene expression in and attracted CD11c(+) antigen presenting cells to the mucosa. A SL dose of 1×10^8 infectious particles induced Ebola Zaire glycoprotein (ZGP)-specific IFN-γ^+ T cells in spleen, bronchoalveolar lavage, mesenteric lymph nodes and submandibular lymph nodes (SMLN) of naive mice in a manner similar to the same dose given IN. Ex vivo CFSE and in vivo cytotoxic T lymphocyte (CTL) assays confirmed that SL immunization elicits a notable population of effector memory CD8+ T cells and strong CTL responses in spleen and SMLN. SL immunization induced significant ZGP-specific Th1 and Th2 type responses unaffected by pre-existing immunity (PEI) that protected mice and guinea pigs from lethal challenge. SL delivery protected more mice with PEI to Ad5 than IM injection. SL immunization also reduced systemic anti-Ad5 T and B cell responses in naive mice and those with PEI, suggesting that secondary immunizations could be highly effective for both populations.
PMCID: PMC3358355 PMID: 22149096 [PubMed - indexed for MEDLINE]

1078. Nat Commun. 2012;3:1303. doi: 10.1038/ncomms2302.

Virus-like glycodendrinanoparticles displaying quasi-equivalent nested polyvalency upon glycoprotein platforms potently block viral infection.

Ribeiro-Viana R(1), Sánchez-Navarro M, Luczkowiak J, Koeppe JR, Delgado R, Rojo J, Davis BG.

Author information: (1)Department of Chemistry, University of Oxford, Chemistry Research Laboratory, 12 Mansfield Road, Oxford OX1 3TA, UK.

Erratum in Nat Commun. 2013;4:1459.

Ligand polyvalency is a powerful modulator of protein-receptor interactions. Host-pathogen infection interactions are often mediated by glycan ligand-protein interactions, yet its interrogation with very high copy number ligands has been limited to heterogenous systems. Here we report that through the use of nested layers of multivalency we are able to assemble the most highly valent glycodendrimeric constructs yet seen (bearing up to 1,620 glycans). These constructs are pure and well-defined single entities that at diameters of up to 32 nm are capable of mimicking pathogens both in size and in their highly glycosylated surfaces. Through this mimicry these glyco-dendri-protein-nano-particles are capable of blocking (at picomolar concentrations) a model of the infection of T-lymphocytes and human dendritic cells by Ebola virus. The high associated polyvalency effects ($\beta>10(6)$, $\beta/N \sim 10(2)-10(3)$) displayed on an unprecedented surface area by precise clusters suggest a general strategy for modulation of such interactions.
PMCID: PMC3535419 PMID: 23250433 [PubMed - indexed for MEDLINE]

1079. Plant Biotechnol J. 2012 Jan;10(1):95-104. doi: 10.1111/j.1467-7652.2011.00649.x. Epub 2011 Aug 26.

Robust production of virus-like particles and monoclonal antibodies with geminiviral replicon vectors in lettuce.

Lai H(1), He J, Engle M, Diamond MS, Chen Q.

Author information: (1)The Biodesign Institute and College of Technology and Innovation, Arizona State University, Tempe, AZ, USA.

Pharmaceutical protein production in plants has been greatly promoted by the development of viral-based vectors and transient expression systems. Tobacco and related Nicotiana species are currently the most common host plants for the generation of plant-made pharmaceutical proteins (PMPs). Downstream processing of target PMPs from these plants, however, is hindered by potential technical and regulatory difficulties owing to the presence of high levels of phenolics and toxic alkaloids. Here, we explored the use of lettuce, which grows quickly yet produces low levels of secondary metabolites and viral vector-based transient expression systems to develop a robust PMP production platform. Our results showed that a geminiviral replicon system based on the bean yellow dwarf virus permits high-level expression in lettuce of virus-like particles (VLP) derived from the Norwalk virus capsid protein and therapeutic monoclonal antibodies (mAbs) against Ebola and West Nile viruses. These vaccine and therapeutic candidates can be readily purified from lettuce leaves with scalable processing methods while fully retaining functional activity. Furthermore, this study also demonstrated the feasibility of using commercially produced lettuce for high-level PMP production. This allows our production system to have access to unlimited quantities of inexpensive plant material for large-scale production. These results establish a new production platform for biological pharmaceutical agents that are effective, safe, low cost, and amenable to large-scale manufacturing.

PMCID: PMC3232331 PMID: 21883868 [PubMed - indexed for MEDLINE]
1080. PLoS Negl Trop Dis. 2012;6(12):e1923. doi: 10.1371/journal.pntd.0001923. Epub 2012 Dec 6.

Cathepsin B & L are not required for ebola virus replication.

Marzi A(1), Reinheckel T, Feldmann H.
Author information: (1)Laboratory of Virology, Division of Intramural Research, National Institute of Allergy and Infectious Diseases, National Institutes of Health, Hamilton, Montana, United States of America.

Ebola virus (EBOV), family Filoviridae, emerged in 1976 on the African continent. Since then it caused several outbreaks of viral hemorrhagic fever in humans with case fatality rates up to 90% and remains a serious Public Health concern and biothreat pathogen. The most pathogenic and best-studied species is Zaire ebolavirus (ZEBOV). EBOV encodes one viral surface glycoprotein (GP), which is essential for replication, a determinant of pathogenicity and an important immunogen. GP mediates viral entry through interaction with cellular surface molecules, which results in the uptake of virus particles via macropinocytosis. Later in this pathway endosomal acidification activates the cysteine proteases Cathepsin B and L (CatB, CatL), which have been shown to cleave ZEBOV-GP leading to subsequent exposure of the putative receptor-binding and fusion domain and productive infection. We studied the effect of CatB and CatL on in vitro and in vivo replication of EBOV. Similar to previous findings, our results show an effect of CatB, but not CatL, on ZEBOV entry into cultured cells. Interestingly, cell entry by other EBOV species (Bundibugyo, Côte d'Ivoire, Reston and Sudan ebolavirus) was independent of CatB or CatL as was EBOV replication in general. To investigate whether CatB and CatL have a role in vivo during infection, we utilized the mouse model for ZEBOV. Wild-type (control), catB(-/-) and catL(-/-) mice were equally susceptible to lethal challenge with mouse-adapted ZEBOV with no difference in virus replication and time to death. In conclusion, our results show that CatB and CatL activity is not required for EBOV replication. Furthermore, EBOV glycoprotein cleavage seems to be mediated by an array of proteases making targeted therapeutic approaches difficult.

PMCID: PMC3516577 PMID: 23236527 [PubMed - indexed for MEDLINE]
1081. PLoS Negl Trop Dis. 2012;6(3):e1575. doi: 10.1371/journal.pntd.0001575. Epub 2012 Mar 20.

Ebola GP-specific monoclonal antibodies protect mice and guinea pigs from lethal Ebola virus infection.

Qiu X(1), Fernando L, Melito PL, Audet J, Feldmann H, Kobinger G, Alimonti JB, Jones SM.
Author information: (1)Special Pathogens Program, National Microbiology Laboratory, Public Health Agency of Canada, Winnipeg, Manitoba, Canada.
xiangguo.qiu@phac-aspc.gc.ca

Ebola virus (EBOV) causes acute hemorrhagic fever in humans and non-human primates with mortality rates up to 90%. So far there are no effective treatments available. This study evaluates the protective efficacy of 8 monoclonal antibodies (MAbs) against Ebola glycoprotein in mice and guinea pigs. Immunocompetent mice or guinea pigs were given MAbs i.p. in various doses individually or as pools of 3-4 MAbs to test their protection against a lethal challenge with mouse- or guinea pig-adapted EBOV. Each of the 8 MAbs (100 μg) protected mice from a lethal EBOV challenge when administered 1 day before or after challenge. Seven MAbs were effective 2 days post-infection (dpi), with 1 MAb demonstrating partial protection 3 dpi. In the guinea pigs each MAb showed partial protection at 1 dpi, however the mean time to death was significantly prolonged compared to the control group. Moreover, treatment with pools of 3-4 MAbs completely protected the majority of animals, while administration at 2-3 dpi achieved 50-100% protection. This data suggests that the MAbs generated are capable of protecting both animal species against lethal Ebola virus challenge. These results indicate that MAbs particularly when used as an oligoclonal set are a potential therapeutic for post-exposure treatment of EBOV infection.

PMCID: PMC3308939 PMID: 22448295 [PubMed - indexed for MEDLINE]
1082. PLoS Negl Trop Dis. 2012;6(3):e1567. doi: 10.1371/journal.pntd.0001567. Epub 2012 Mar 20.

Recombinant vesicular stomatitis virus vaccine vectors expressing filovirus glycoproteins lack neurovirulence in nonhuman primates.

Mire CE(1), Miller AD, Carville A, Westmoreland SV, Geisbert JB, Mansfield KG, Feldmann H, Hensley LE, Geisbert TW.
Author information: (1)Galveston National Laboratory, University of Texas Medical Branch, Galveston, Texas, USA.

The filoviruses, Marburg virus and Ebola virus, cause severe hemorrhagic fever with high mortality in humans and nonhuman primates. Among the most promising filovirus vaccines under development is a system based on recombinant vesicular stomatitis virus (rVSV) that expresses an individual filovirus glycoprotein (GP) in place of the VSV glycoprotein (G). The main concern with all replication-competent vaccines, including the rVSV filovirus GP vectors, is their safety. To address this concern, we performed a neurovirulence study using 21 cynomolgus macaques where the vaccines were administered intrathalamically. Seven animals received a rVSV vector expressing the Zaire ebolavirus (ZEBOV) GP; seven animals received a rVSV vector expressing the Lake Victoria marburgvirus (MARV) GP; three animals received rVSV-wild type (wt) vector, and four animals received vehicle control. Two of three animals given rVSV-wt showed severe neurological symptoms whereas animals receiving vehicle control, rVSV-ZEBOV-GP, or rVSV-MARV-GP did not develop these symptoms. Histological analysis revealed major lesions in neural tissues of all three rVSV-wt animals; however, no significant lesions were observed in any animals from the filovirus vaccine or vehicle control groups. These data strongly suggest that rVSV filovirus GP vaccine vectors lack the neurovirulence properties associated with the rVSV-wt parent vector and support their further development as a vaccine platform for human use.

PMCID: PMC3308941 PMID: 22448291 [PubMed - indexed for MEDLINE]
1083. PLoS One. 2012;7(12):e52986. doi: 10.1371/journal.pone.0052986. Epub 2012 Dec 28.

Clinical manifestations and case management of Ebola haemorrhagic fever caused by a newly identified virus strain, Bundibugyo, Uganda, 2007-2008.

Roddy P(1), Howard N, Van Kerkhove MD, Lutwama J, Wamala J, Yoti Z, Colebunders R, Palma PP, Sterk E, Jeffs B, Van Herp M, Borchert M.

Author information: (1)Medical Departments of Médecins Sans Frontières, Barcelona, Spain. roddypd@gmail.com

A confirmed Ebola haemorrhagic fever (EHF) outbreak in Bundibugyo, Uganda, November 2007-February 2008, was caused by a putative new species (Bundibugyo ebolavirus). It included 93 putative cases, 56 laboratory-confirmed cases, and 37 deaths (CFR=25%). Study objectives are to describe clinical manifestations and case management for 26 hospitalised laboratory-confirmed EHF patients. Clinical findings are congruous with previously reported EHF infections. The most frequently experienced symptoms were non-bloody diarrhoea (81%), severe headache (81%), and asthenia (77%). Seven patients reported or were observed with haemorrhagic symptoms, six of whom died. Ebola care remains difficult due to the resource-poor setting of outbreaks and the infection-control procedures required. However, quality data collection is essential to evaluate case definitions and therapeutic interventions, and needs improvement in future epidemics. Organizations usually involved in EHF case management have a particular responsibility in this respect.

PMCID: PMC3532309 PMID: 23285243 [PubMed - indexed for MEDLINE]

1084. PLoS One. 2012;7(12):e51112. doi: 10.1371/journal.pone.0051112. Epub 2012 Dec 12.

Effects of epidemic diseases on the distribution of bonobos.

Inogwabini BI(1), Leader-Williams N.

Author information: (1)Durrell Institute for Conservation and Ecology, University of Kent, Canterbury, United Kingdom. bi4@kentforlife.net

This study examined how outbreaks and the occurrence of Anthrax, Ebola, Monkeypox and Trypanosomiasis may differentially affect the distribution of bonobos (Pan paniscus). Using a combination of mapping, Jaccard overlapping coefficients and binary regressions, the study determined how each disease correlated with the extent of occurrence of, and the areas occupied by, bonobos. Anthrax has only been reported to occur outside the range of bonobos and so was not considered further. Ebola, Monkeypox and Trypanosomiasis were each reported within the area of occupancy of bonobos. Their respective overlap coefficients were: $J = 0.10$; $Q(\alpha = 0.05) = 2.00$ (odds ratios = 0.0001, 95% CI = 0.0057; Z =-19.41, significant) for Ebola; $J = 1.00$; $Q(\alpha = 0.05) = 24.0$ (odds ratios = 1.504, 95% CI = 0.5066-2.6122) for Monkeypox; and, $J = 0.33$; $Q(\alpha = 0.05) = 11.5$ (Z = 1.14, significant) for Trypanosomiasis. There were significant relationships for the presence and absence of Monkeypox and Trypanosomiasis and the known extent of occurrence of bonobos, based on the equations $y = 0.2368Ln(x)+0.8006$ $(R(2) = 0.9772)$ and $y = -0.2942Ln(x)+0.7155$ $(R(2) = 0.698)$, respectively. The positive relationship suggested that bonobos tolerated the presence of Monkeypox. In contrast, the significant negative coefficient suggested that bonobos were absent in areas where Trypanosomiasis is endemic. Our results suggest that large rivers may have prevented Ebola from spreading into the range of bonobos. Meanwhile, Trypanosomiasis has been recorded among humans within the area of occurrence of bonobos, and appears the most important disease in shaping the area of occupancy of bonobos within their overall extent of occupancy.

PMCID: PMC3521019 PMID: 23251431 [PubMed - indexed for MEDLINE]

1085. PLoS One. 2012;7(12):e44115. doi: 10.1371/journal.pone.0044115. Epub 2012 Dec 6.

Ad35 and ad26 vaccine vectors induce potent and cross-reactive antibody and T-cell responses to multiple filovirus species.

Zahn R(1), Gillisen G, Roos A, Koning M, van der Helm E, Spek D, Weijtens M, Grazia Pau M, Radošević K, Weverling GJ, Custers J, Vellinga J, Schuitemaker H, Goudsmit J, Rodríguez A.

Author information: (1)Crucell Holland BV, Leiden, The Netherlands.

Filoviruses cause sporadic but highly lethal outbreaks of hemorrhagic fever in Africa in the human population. Currently, no drug or vaccine is available for treatment or prevention. A previous study with a vaccine candidate based on the low seroprevalent adenoviruses 26 and 35 (Ad26 and Ad35) was shown to provide protection against homologous Ebola Zaire challenge in non human primates (NHP) if applied in a prime-boost regimen. Here we have aimed to expand this principle to construct and evaluate Ad26 and Ad35 vectors for development of a vaccine to provide universal filovirus protection against all highly lethal strains that have caused major outbreaks in the past. We have therefore performed a phylogenetic analysis of filovirus glycoproteins to select the glycoproteins from two Ebola species (Ebola Zaire and Ebola Sudan/Gulu,), two Marburg strains (Marburg Angola and Marburg Ravn) and added the more distant non-lethal Ebola Ivory Coast species for broadest coverage. Ad26 and Ad35 vectors expressing these five filovirus glycoproteins were evaluated to induce a potent cellular and humoral immune response in mice. All adenoviral vectors induced a humoral immune response after single vaccination in a dose dependent manner that was cross-reactive within the Ebola and Marburg lineages. In addition, both strain-specific as well as cross-reactive T cell responses could be detected. A heterologous Ad26-Ad35 prime-boost regime enhanced mainly the humoral and to a lower extend the cellular immune response against the transgene. Combination of the five selected filovirus glycoproteins in one multivalent vaccine potentially elicits protective immunity in man against all major filovirus strains that have caused lethal outbreaks in the last 20 years.

PMCID: PMC3516506 PMID: 23236343 [PubMed - indexed for MEDLINE]

1086. PLoS One. 2012;7(11):e50316. doi: 10.1371/journal.pone.0050316. Epub 2012 Nov 28.

Ebola virus genome plasticity as a marker of its passaging history: a comparison of in vitro passaging to non-human primate infection.

Kugelman JR(1), Lee MS, Rossi CA, McCarthy SE, Radoshitzky SR, Dye JM, Hensley LE, Honko A, Kuhn JH, Jahrling PB, Warren TK, Whitehouse CA, Bavari S, Palacios G.

Author information: (1)Genomics Division, United States Army Medical Research Institute of Infectious Diseases (USAMRIID), Fort Detrick, Maryland, United States of America.

To identify polymorphic sites that could be used as biomarkers of Ebola virus passage history, we repeatedly amplified Ebola virus (Kikwit variant) in vitro and in vivo and performed deep sequencing analysis of the complete genomes of the viral subpopulations. We then determined the sites undergoing selection during passage in Vero E6 cells. Four locations within the Ebola virus Kikwit genome were identified that together segregate cell culture-passaged virus and virus obtained from infected non-human primates. Three of the identified sites are located within the glycoprotein gene (GP) sequence: the poly-U (RNA editing) site at position 6925, as well as positions 6677, and 6179. One site was found in the VP24 gene at position 10833. In all cases, in vitro and in vivo, both populations (majority and minority variants) were maintained in the viral swarm, with rapid selections occurring after a few passages or infections. This analysis approach will be useful to differentiate whether filovirus stocks with unknown history have been passaged in cell culture and may support filovirus stock standardization for medical countermeasure development.

PMCID: PMC3509072 PMID: 23209706 [PubMed - indexed for MEDLINE]

1087. PLoS One. 2012;7(10):e44769. doi: 10.1371/journal.pone.0044769. Epub 2012 Oct 3.

Designing and testing broadly-protective filoviral vaccines optimized for cytotoxic T-lymphocyte epitope coverage.

Fenimore PW(1), Muhammad MA, Fischer WM, Foley BT, Bakken RR, Thurmond JR, Yusim K, Yoon H, Parker M, Hart MK, Dye JM, Korber B, Kuiken C.

Author information: (1)Theoretical Biology and Biophysics Group, Los Alamos National Laboratory, Los Alamos, New Mexico, United States of America. paulf@lanl.gov

We report the rational design and in vivo testing of mosaic proteins for a polyvalent pan-filoviral vaccine using a computational strategy designed for the Human Immunodeficiency Virus type 1 (HIV-1) but also appropriate for Hepatitis C virus (HCV) and potentially other diverse viruses. Mosaics are sets of artificial recombinant proteins that are based on natural proteins. The recombinants are computationally selected using a genetic algorithm to optimize the coverage of potential cytotoxic T lymphocyte (CTL) epitopes. Because evolutionary history differs markedly between HIV-1 and filoviruses, we devised an adapted computational technique that is effective for sparsely sampled taxa; our first significant result is that the mosaic technique is effective in creating high-quality mosaic filovirus proteins. The resulting coverage of potential epitopes across filovirus species is superior to coverage by any natural variants, including current vaccine strains with demonstrated cross-reactivity. The mosaic cocktails are also robust: mosaics substantially outperformed natural strains when computationally tested against poorly sampled species and more variable genes. Furthermore, in a computational comparison of cross-reactive potential a design constructed prior to the Bundibugyo outbreak performed nearly as well against all species as an updated design that included Bundibugyo. These points suggest that the mosaic designs would be more resilient than natural-variant vaccines against future Ebola outbreaks dominated by novel viral variants. We demonstrate in vivo immunogenicity and protection against a heterologous challenge in a mouse model. This design work delineates the likely requirements and limitations on broadly-protective filoviral CTL vaccines.

PMCID: PMC3463593 PMID: 23056184 [PubMed - indexed for MEDLINE]

1088. PLoS One. 2012;7(7):e40740. doi: 10.1371/journal.pone.0040740. Epub 2012 Jul 18.

Serological evidence of Ebola virus infection in Indonesian orangutans.

Nidom CA(1), Nakayama E, Nidom RV, Alamudi MY, Daulay S, Dharmayanti IN, Dachlan YP, Amin M, Igarashi M, Miyamoto H, Yoshida R, Takada A.

Author information: (1)Avian Influenza-zoonosis Research Center, Airlangga University, Surabaya, Indonesia. nidomca@unair.ac.id

Comment in PLoS One. 2013;8(3):e60289.

Ebola virus (EBOV) and Marburg virus (MARV) belong to the family Filoviridae and cause severe hemorrhagic fever in humans and nonhuman primates. Despite the discovery of EBOV (Reston virus) in nonhuman primates and domestic pigs in the Philippines and the serological evidence for its infection of humans and fruit bats, information on the reservoirs and potential amplifying hosts for filoviruses in Asia is lacking. In this study, serum samples collected from 353 healthy Bornean orangutans (Pongo pygmaeus) in Kalimantan Island, Indonesia, during the period from December 2005 to December 2006 were screened for filovirus-specific IgG antibodies using a highly sensitive enzyme-linked immunosorbent assay (ELISA) with recombinant viral surface glycoprotein (GP) antigens derived from multiple species of filoviruses (5 EBOV and 1 MARV species). Here we show that 18.4% (65/353) and 1.7% (6/353) of the samples were seropositive for EBOV and MARV, respectively, with little cross-reactivity among EBOV and MARV antigens. In these positive samples, IgG antibodies to viral internal proteins were also detected by immunoblotting. Interestingly, while the specificity for Reston virus, which has been recognized as an Asian filovirus, was the highest in only 1.4% (5/353) of the serum samples, the majority of EBOV-positive sera showed specificity to Zaire, Sudan, Cote d'Ivoire, or Bundibugyo viruses, all of which have been found so far only in Africa. These results suggest the existence of multiple species of filoviruses or unknown filovirus-related viruses in Indonesia, some of which are serologically similar to African EBOVs, and transmission of the viruses from yet unidentified reservoir hosts into the orangutan populations. Our findings point to the need for risk assessment and continued surveillance of filovirus infection of human and nonhuman primates, as well as wild and domestic animals, in Asia.

PMCID: PMC3399888 PMID: 22815803 [PubMed - indexed for MEDLINE]

1089. PLoS One. 2012;7(7):e39978. doi: 10.1371/journal.pone.0039978. Epub 2012 Jul 5.

Assembly of Ebola virus matrix protein VP40 is regulated by latch-like properties of N and C terminal tails.

Silva LP(1), Vanzile M, Bavari S, Aman JM, Schriemer DC.

Author information: (1)Department of Biochemistry and Molecular Biology, University of Calgary, Calgary, Alberta, Canada.

The matrix protein VP40 coordinates numerous functions in the viral life cycle of the Ebola virus. These range from the regulation of viral transcription to morphogenesis, packaging and budding of mature virions. Similar to the matrix proteins of other nonsegmented, negative-strand RNA viruses, VP40 proceeds through intermediate states of assembly (e.g. octamers) but it remains unclear how these intermediates are coordinated with the various stages of the life cycle. In this study, we investigate the molecular basis of synchronization as governed by VP40. Hydrogen/deuterium exchange mass spectrometry was used to follow induced structural and conformational changes in VP40. Together with computational modeling, we demonstrate that both extreme N and C terminal tail regions stabilize the monomeric state through a direct association. The tails appear to function as a latch, released upon a specific molecular trigger such as RNA ligation. We propose that triggered release of the tails permits the coordination of late-stage events in the viral life cycle, at the inner membrane of the host cell. Specifically, N-tail release exposes the L-domain motifs PTAP/PPEY to the transport and budding complexes, whereas triggered C-tail release could improve association with the site of budding.

PMCID: PMC3390324 PMID: 22792204 [PubMed - indexed for MEDLINE]

1090. PLoS One. 2012;7(5):e37106. doi: 10.1371/journal.pone.0037106. Epub 2012 May 23.

Recovery potential of a western lowland gorilla population following a major Ebola outbreak: results from a ten year study.

Genton C(1), Cristescu R, Gatti S, Levréro F, Bigot E, Caillaud D, Pierre JS, Ménard N.

Author information: (1)UMR 6553, ECOBIO: Ecosystems, Biodiversity, Evolution, CNRS/University of Rennes 1, Biological Station of Paimpont, Paimpont, France. celine.genton@yahoo.fr

Investigating the recovery capacity of wildlife populations following demographic crashes is of great interest to ecologists and conservationists. Opportunities to study these aspects are rare due to the difficulty of monitoring populations both before and after a demographic crash. Ebola outbreaks in central Africa have killed up to 95% of the individuals in affected western lowland gorilla (Gorilla gorilla gorilla) populations. Assessing whether and how fast affected populations recover is essential for the conservation of this critically endangered taxon. The gorilla population visiting Lokoué forest clearing, Odzala-Kokoua National Park, Republic of the Congo, has been monitored before, two years after and six years after Ebola affected it in 2004. This allowed us to describe Ebola's short-term and long-term impacts on the structure of the population. The size of the population, which included around 380 gorillas before the Ebola outbreak, dropped to less than 40 individuals after the outbreak. It then remained stable for six years after the outbreak. However, the demographic structure of this small population has significantly changed. Although several solitary males have disappeared, the immigration of adult females, the formation of new breeding groups, and several birth events suggest that the population is showing potential to recover. During the outbreak, surviving adult and subadult females joined old solitary silverbacks. Those females were subsequently observed joining young silverbacks, forming new breeding groups where they later gave birth. Interestingly, some females were observed joining silverbacks that were unlikely to have sired their infant, but no infanticide was observed. The consequences of the Ebola outbreak on the population structure were different two years and six years after the outbreak. Therefore, our results could be used as demographic indicators to detect and date outbreaks that have happened in other, non-monitored gorilla populations.

PMCID: PMC3359368 PMID: 22649511 [PubMed - indexed for MEDLINE]

1091. PLoS One. 2012;7(4):e36192. doi: 10.1371/journal.pone.0036192. Epub 2012 Apr 27.

Protective efficacy of neutralizing monoclonal antibodies in a nonhuman primate model of Ebola hemorrhagic fever.

Marzi A(1), Yoshida R, Miyamoto H, Ishijima M, Suzuki Y, Higuchi M, Matsuyama Y, Igarashi M, Nakayama E, Kuroda M, Saijo M, Feldmann F, Brining D, Feldmann H, Takada A.

Author information: (1)Laboratory of Virology, Rocky Mountain Laboratories, Division of Intramural Research, National Institute of Allergy and Infectious Diseases, National Institutes of Health, Hamilton, Montana, USA.

Ebola virus (EBOV) is the causative agent of severe hemorrhagic fever in primates, with human case fatality rates up to 90%. Today, there is neither a licensed vaccine nor a treatment available for Ebola hemorrhagic fever (EHF). Single monoclonal antibodies (MAbs) specific for Zaire ebolavirus (ZEBOV) have been successfully used in passive immunization experiments in rodent models, but have failed to protect nonhuman primates from lethal disease. In this study, we used two clones of human-mouse chimeric MAbs (ch133 and ch226) with strong neutralizing activity against ZEBOV and evaluated their protective potential in a rhesus macaque model of EHF. Reduced viral loads and partial protection were observed in animals given MAbs ch133 and ch226 combined intravenously at 24 hours before and 24 and 72 hours after challenge. MAbs circulated in the blood of a surviving animal until virus-induced IgG responses were detected. In contrast, serum MAb concentrations decreased to undetectable levels at terminal stages of disease in animals that succumbed to infection, indicating substantial consumption of these antibodies due to virus replication. Accordingly, the rapid decrease of serum MAbs was clearly associated with increased viremia in non-survivors. Our results indicate that EBOV neutralizing antibodies, particularly in combination with other therapeutic strategies, might be beneficial in reducing viral loads and prolonging disease progression during EHF.

PMCID: PMC3338609 PMID: 22558378 [PubMed - indexed for MEDLINE]

1092. PLoS One. 2012;7(1):e29608. doi: 10.1371/journal.pone.0029608. Epub 2012 Jan 11.

The organisation of Ebola virus reveals a capacity for extensive, modular polyploidy.

Beniac DR(1), Melito PL, Devarennes SL, Hiebert SL, Rabb MJ, Lamboo LL, Jones SM, Booth TF.

Author information: (1)Viral Diseases Division, National Microbiology Laboratory, Public Health Agency of Canada, Winnipeg, Manitoba, Canada.

BACKGROUND: Filoviruses, including Ebola virus, are unusual in being filamentous animal viruses. Structural data on the arrangement, stoichiometry and organisation of the component molecules of filoviruses has until now been lacking, partially due to the need to work under level 4 biological containment. The present study provides unique insights into the structure of this deadly pathogen. METHODOLOGY AND PRINCIPAL FINDINGS: We have investigated the structure of Ebola virus using a combination of cryo-electron microscopy, cryo-electron tomography, sub-tomogram averaging, and single particle image processing. Here we report the three-dimensional structure and architecture of Ebola virus and establish that multiple copies of the RNA genome can be packaged to produce polyploid virus particles, through an extreme degree of length polymorphism. We show that the helical Ebola virus inner nucleocapsid containing RNA and nucleoprotein is stabilized by an outer layer of VP24-VP35 bridges. Elucidation of the structure of the membrane-associated glycoprotein in its native state indicates that the putative receptor-binding site is occluded within the molecule, while a major neutralizing epitope is exposed on its surface proximal to the viral envelope. The matrix protein VP40 forms a regular lattice within the envelope, although its contacts with the nucleocapsid are irregular. CONCLUSIONS: The results of this study demonstrate a modular organization in Ebola virus that accommodates a well-ordered, symmetrical nucleocapsid within a flexible, tubular membrane envelope.

PMCID: PMC3256159 PMID: 22247782 [PubMed - indexed for MEDLINE]

1093. PLoS Pathog. 2012;8(12):e1003065. doi: 10.1371/journal.ppat.1003065. Epub 2012 Dec 13.

Antigenic subversion: a novel mechanism of host immune evasion by Ebola virus.

Mohan GS(1), Li W, Ye L, Compans RW, Yang C.

Author information: (1)Department of Microbiology and Immunology, Emory University, Atlanta, Georgia, United States of America.

Comment in Expert Rev Anti Infect Ther. 2013 May;11(5):475-8.

In addition to its surface glycoprotein (GP(1,2)), Ebola virus (EBOV) directs the production of large quantities of a truncated glycoprotein isoform (sGP) that is secreted into the extracellular space. The generation of secreted antigens has been studied in several viruses and suggested as a mechanism of host immune evasion through absorption of antibodies and interference with antibody-mediated clearance. However such a role has not been conclusively determined for the Ebola virus sGP. In this study, we immunized mice with DNA constructs expressing GP(1,2) and/or sGP, and demonstrate that sGP can efficiently compete for anti-GP(12) antibodies, but only from mice that have been immunized by sGP. We term this phenomenon "antigenic subversion", and propose a model whereby sGP redirects the host antibody response to focus on epitopes which it shares with membrane-bound GP(1,2), thereby allowing it to absorb anti-GP(1,2) antibodies. Unexpectedly, we found that sGP can also subvert a previously immunized host's anti-GP(1,2) response resulting in strong cross-reactivity with sGP. This finding is particularly relevant to EBOV vaccinology since it underscores the importance of eliciting robust immunity that is sufficient to rapidly clear an infection before antigenic subversion can occur. Antigenic subversion represents a novel virus escape strategy that likely helps EBOV evade host immunity, and may represent an important obstacle to EBOV vaccine design.

PMCID: PMC3521666 PMID: 23271969 [PubMed - indexed for MEDLINE]

1094. PLoS Pathog. 2012;8(8):e1002847. doi: 10.1371/journal.ppat.1002847. Epub 2012 Aug 2

The Ebola virus glycoprotein contributes to but is not sufficient for virulence in vivo.

Groseth A(1), Marzi A, Hoenen T, Herwig A, Gardner D, Becker S, Ebihara H, Feldmann H.

Author information: (1)Laboratory of Virology, Division of Intramural Research, National Institute of Allergy and Infectious Diseases, National Institutes of Health, Hamilton, Montana, USA.

Among the Ebola viruses most species cause severe hemorrhagic fever in humans; however, Reston ebolavirus (REBOV) has not been associated with human disease despite numerous documented infections. While the molecular basis for this difference remains unclear, in vitro evidence has suggested a role for the glycoprotein (GP) as a major filovirus pathogenicity factor, but direct evidence for such a role in the context of virus infection has been notably lacking. In order to assess the role of GP in EBOV virulence, we have developed a novel reverse genetics system for REBOV, which we report here. Together with a previously published full-length clone for Zaire ebolavirus (ZEBOV), this provides a unique possibility to directly investigate the role of an entire filovirus protein in pathogenesis. To this end we have generated recombinant ZEBOV (rZEBOV) and REBOV (rREBOV), as well as chimeric viruses in which the glycoproteins from these two virus species have been exchanged (rZEBOV-RGP and rREBOV-ZGP). All of these viruses could be rescued and the chimeras replicated with kinetics similar to their parent virus in tissue culture, indicating that the exchange of GP in these chimeric viruses is well tolerated. However, in a mouse model of infection rZEBOV-RGP demonstrated markedly decreased lethality and prolonged time to death when compared to rZEBOV, confirming that GP does indeed contribute to the full expression of virulence by ZEBOV. In contrast, rREBOV-ZGP did not show any signs of virulence, and was in fact slightly attenuated compared to rREBOV, demonstrating that GP alone is not sufficient to confer a lethal phenotype or exacerbate disease in this model. Thus, while these findings provide direct evidence that GP contributes to filovirus virulence in vivo, they also clearly indicate that other factors are needed for the acquisition of full virulence.

PMCID: PMC3410889 PMID: 22876185 [PubMed - indexed for MEDLINE]

1095. PLoS Pathog. 2012;8(5):e1002734. doi: 10.1371/journal.ppat.1002734. Epub 2012 May 31

Structure and functional analysis of the RNA- and viral phosphoprotein-binding domain of respiratory syncytial virus M2-1 protein.

Blondot ML(1), Dubosclard V, Fix J, Lassoued S, Aumont-Nicaise M, Bontems F, Eléouët JF, Sizun C.

Author information: (1)Unité de Virologie et Immunologie Moléculaires (UR892), INRA, Jouy-en-Josas, France.

Respiratory syncytial virus (RSV) protein M2-1 functions as an essential transcriptional cofactor of the viral RNA-dependent RNA polymerase (RdRp) complex by increasing polymerase processivity. M2-1 is a modular RNA binding protein that also interacts with the viral phosphoprotein P, another component of the RdRp complex. These binding properties are related to the core region of M2-1 encompassing residues S58 to K177. Here we report the NMR structure of the RSV M2-1(58-177) core domain, which is structurally homologous to the C-terminal domain of Ebola virus VP30, a transcription co-factor sharing functional similarity with M2-1. The partial overlap of RNA and P interaction surfaces on M2-1(58-177), as determined by NMR, rationalizes the previously observed competitive behavior of RNA versus P. Using site-directed mutagenesis, we identified eight residues located on these surfaces that are critical for an efficient transcription activity of the RdRp complex. Single mutations of these residues disrupted specifically either P or RNA binding to M2-1 in vitro. M2-1 recruitment to cytoplasmic inclusion bodies, which are regarded as sites of viral RNA synthesis, was impaired by mutations affecting only binding to P, but not to RNA, suggesting that M2-1 is associated to the holonucleocapsid by interacting with P. These results reveal that RNA and P binding to M2-1 can be uncoupled and that both are critical for the transcriptional antitermination function of M2-1.

PMCID: PMC3364950 PMID: 22675274 [PubMed - indexed for MEDLINE]

1096. Sci Rep. 2012;2:811. doi: 10.1038/srep00811. Epub 2012 Nov 15.

Transmission of Ebola virus from pigs to non-human primates.

Weingartl HM(1), Embury-Hyatt C, Nfon C, Leung A, Smith G, Kobinger G.

Author information: (1)National Centre for Foreign Animal Disease, Canadian Food Inspection Agency, 1015 Arlington St. Winnipeg, Manitoba, R3E 3M4, Canada. hana.weingartl@inspection.gc.ca

Ebola viruses (EBOV) cause often fatal hemorrhagic fever in several species of simian primates including human. While fruit bats are considered natural reservoir, involvement of other species in EBOV transmission is unclear. In 2009, Reston-EBOV was the first EBOV detected in swine with indicated transmission to humans. In-contact transmission of Zaire-EBOV (ZEBOV) between pigs was demonstrated experimentally. Here we show ZEBOV transmission from pigs to cynomolgus macaques without direct contact. Interestingly, transmission between macaques in similar housing conditions was never observed. Piglets inoculated oro-nasally with ZEBOV were transferred to the room housing macaques in an open inaccessible cage system. All macaques became infected. Infectious virus was detected in oro-nasal swabs of piglets, and in blood, swabs, and tissues of macaques. This is the first report of experimental interspecies virus transmission, with the macaques also used as a human surrogate. Our finding may influence prevention and control measures during EBOV outbreaks.

PMCID: PMC3498927 PMID: 23155478 [PubMed - indexed for MEDLINE]

1097. Sci Rep. 2012;2:807. doi: 10.1038/srep00807. Epub 2012 Nov 12.

Hapten mediated display and pairing of recombinant antibodies accelerates assay assembly for biothreat countermeasures.

Sherwood LJ(1), Hayhurst A.

Author information: (1)Department of Virology and Immunology, Texas Biomedical Research Institute, San Antonio, Texas, USA.

A bottle-neck in recombinant antibody sandwich immunoassay development is pairing, demanding protein purification and modification to distinguish captor from tracer. We developed a simple pairing scheme using microliter amounts of E. coli osmotic shockates bearing site-specific biotinylated antibodies and demonstrated proof of principle with a single domain antibody (sdAb) that is both captor and tracer for polyvalent Marburgvirus nucleoprotein. The system could also host pairs of different sdAb specific for the 7 botulinum neurotoxin (BoNT) serotypes, enabling recognition of the cognate serotype. Inducible supE co-expression enabled sdAb populations to be propagated as either phage for more panning from repertoires or expressed as soluble sdAb for screening within a single host strain. When combined with streptavidin-g3p fusions, a novel transdisplay system was formulated to retrofit a semi-synthetic sdAb library which was mined for an anti-Ebolavirus sdAb which was immediately immunoassay ready, thereby speeding up the recombinant antibody discovery and utilization processes.

PMCID: PMC3495282 PMID: 23150778 [PubMed - indexed for MEDLINE]

1098. Uirusu. 2012;62(2):197-208.

[Filoviruses].

[Article in Japanese]

Takada A(1).

Author information: (1)Hokkaido University Research Center for Zoonosis Control.

Filoviruses (Ebola and Marburg viruses) cause severe hemorrhagic fever in humans and nonhuman primates. No effective prophylaxis or treatment for filovirus diseases is yet commercially available. Recent studies have advanced our knowledge of filovirus protein functions and interaction between viral and host factors in the replication cycle. Current findings on the ecology of filoviruses (i.e., natural infection of nonprimate animals and discovery of a new member of filoviruses in Europe) have also provided new insights into the epidemiology of Ebola and Marburg hemorrhagic fever. This article reviews the fundamental aspects of filovirus biology and the latest topics on filovirus research.

PMID: 24153230 [PubMed - indexed for MEDLINE]

1099. BMC Infect Dis. 2011 Dec 28;11:357. doi: 10.1186/1471-2334-11-357.

Ebola haemorrhagic fever outbreak in Masindi District, Uganda: outbreak description and lessons learned.

Borchert M(1), Mutyaba I, Van Kerkhove MD, Lutwama J, Luwaga H, Bisoborwa G, Turyagaruka J, Pirard P, Ndayimirije N, Roddy P, Van Der Stuyft P.

Author information: (1)Unit of Epidemiology and Disease Control, Institute of Tropical Medicine, Antwerp, Belgium. matthias.borchert@charite.de

BACKGROUND: Ebola haemorrhagic fever (EHF) is infamous for its high case-fatality proportion (CFP) and the ease with which it spreads among contacts of the diseased. We describe the course of the EHF outbreak in Masindi, Uganda, in the year 2000, and report on response activities. METHODS: We analysed surveillance records, hospital statistics, and our own observations during response activities. We used Fisher's exact tests for differences in proportions, t-tests for differences in means, and logistic regression for multivariable analysis. RESULTS: The response to the outbreak consisted of surveillance, case management, logistics and public mobilisation. Twenty-six EHF cases (24 laboratory confirmed, two probable) occurred between October 21st and December 22nd, 2000. CFP was 69% (18/26). Nosocomial transmission to the index case occurred in Lacor hospital in Gulu, outside the Ebola ward. After returning home to Masindi district the index case became the origin of a transmission chain within her own extended family (18 further cases), from index family members to health care workers (HCWs, 6 cases), and from HCWs to their household contacts (1 case). Five out of six occupational cases of EHF in HCWs occurred after the introduction of barrier nursing, probably due to breaches of barrier nursing principles. CFP was initially very high (76%) but decreased (20%) due to better case management after reinforcing the response team. The mobilisation of the community for the response efforts was challenging at the beginning, when fear, panic and mistrust had to be countered by the response team. CONCLUSIONS: Large scale transmission in the community beyond the index family was prevented by early case identification and isolation as well as quarantine imposed by the community. The high number of occupational EHF after implementing barrier nursing points at the need to strengthen training and supervision of local HCWs. The difference in CFP before and after reinforcing the response team together with observations on the ward suggest a critical role for intensive supportive treatment. Collecting high quality clinical data is a priority for future outbreaks in order to identify the best possible FHF treatment regime under field conditions.

PMCID: PMC3276451 PMID: 22204600 [PubMed - indexed for MEDLINE]

1100. Proc Natl Acad Sci U S A. 2011 Dec 20;108(51):20690-4. doi: 10.1073/pnas.1108360108. Epub 2011 Dec 5.

Enhanced potency of a fucose-free monoclonal antibody being developed as an Ebola virus immunoprotectant.

Zeitlin L(1), Pettitt J, Scully C, Bohorova N, Kim D, Pauly M, Hiatt A, Ngo L, Steinkellner H, Whaley KJ, Olinger GG.

Author information: (1)Mapp Biopharmaceutical, San Diego, CA 92121, USA. larry.zeitlin@mappbio.com

No countermeasures currently exist for the prevention or treatment of the severe sequelae of Filovirus (such as Ebola virus; EBOV) infection. To overcome this limitation in our biodefense preparedness, we have designed monoclonal antibodies (mAbs) which could be used in humans as immunoprotectants for EBOV, starting with a murine mAb (13F6) that recognizes the heavily glycosylated mucin-like domain of the virion-attached glycoprotein (GP). Point mutations were introduced into the variable region of the murine mAb to remove predicted human T-cell epitopes, and the variable regions joined to human constant regions to generate a mAb (h-13F6) appropriate for development for human use. We have evaluated the efficacy of three variants of h-13F6 carrying different glycosylation patterns in a lethal mouse EBOV challenge model. The pattern of glycosylation of the various mAbs was found to correlate to level of protection, with aglycosylated h-13F6 providing the least potent efficacy (ED(50) = 33 µg). A version with typical heterogenous mammalian glycoforms (ED(50) = 11 µg) had similar potency to the original murine mAb. However, h-13F6 carrying complex N-glycosylation lacking core fucose exhibited superior potency (ED(50) = 3 µg). Binding studies using Fcγ receptors revealed enhanced binding of nonfucosylated h-13F6 to mouse and human FcγRIII. Together the results indicate the presence of Fc N-glycans enhances the protective efficacy of h-13F6, and that mAbs manufactured with uniform glycosylation and a higher potency glycoform offer promise as biodefense therapeutics.

PMCID: PMC3251097 PMID: 22143789 [PubMed - indexed for MEDLINE]

1101. Proc Natl Acad Sci U S A. 2011 Dec 20;108(51):20695-700. doi: 10.1073/pnas.1117715108. Epub 2011 Dec 5.

A nonreplicating subunit vaccine protects mice against lethal Ebola virus challenge.

Phoolcharoen W(1), Dye JM, Kilbourne J, Piensook K, Pratt WD, Arntzen CJ, Chen Q, Mason HS, Herbst-Kralovetz MM.

Author information: (1)Center of Infectious Disease and Vaccinology, Biodesign Institute, Arizona State University, Tempe, AZ 85287, USA.

Ebola hemorrhagic fever is an acute and often deadly disease caused by Ebola virus (EBOV). The possible intentional use of this virus against human populations has led to design of vaccines that could be incorporated into a national stockpile for biological threat reduction. We have evaluated the immunogenicity and efficacy of an EBOV vaccine candidate in which the viral surface glycoprotein is biomanufactured as a fusion to a monoclonal antibody that recognizes an epitope in glycoprotein, resulting in the production of Ebola immune complexes (EICs). Although antigen-antibody immune complexes are known to be efficiently processed and presented to immune effector cells, we found that codelivery of the EIC with Toll-like receptor agonists elicited a more robust antibody response in mice than did EIC alone. Among the compounds tested, polyinosinic:polycytidylic acid (PIC, a Toll-like receptor 3 agonist) was highly effective as an adjuvant agent. After vaccinating mice with EIC plus PIC, 80% of the animals were protected against a lethal challenge with live EBOV (30,000 LD(50) of mouse adapted virus). Surviving animals showed a mixed Th1/Th2 response to the antigen, suggesting this may be important for protection. Survival after vaccination with EIC plus PIC was statistically equivalent to that achieved with an alternative viral vector vaccine candidate reported in the literature. Because nonreplicating subunit vaccines offer the possibility of formulation for cost-effective, long-term storage in biothreat reduction repositories, EIC is an attractive option for public health defense measures.

PMCID: PMC3251076 PMID: 22143779 [PubMed - indexed for MEDLINE]

1102. Virology. 2011 Dec 20;421(2):129-40. doi: 10.1016/j.virol.2011.09.016. Epub 2011 Oct 19.

Simian hemorrhagic fever virus infection of rhesus macaques as a model of viral hemorrhagic fever: clinical characterization and risk factors for severe disease.

Johnson RF(1), Dodd LE, Yellayi S, Gu W, Cann JA, Jett C, Bernbaum JG, Ragland DR, St Claire M, Byrum R, Paragas J, Blaney JE, Jahrling PB.

Author information: (1)Emerging Viral Pathogens Section, National Institute of Allergy and Infectious Diseases, National Institutes of Health, Bethesda, MD 20892, USA. johnsonreed@mail.nih.gov

Simian Hemorrhagic Fever Virus (SHFV) has caused sporadic outbreaks of hemorrhagic fevers in macaques at primate research facilities. SHFV is a BSL-2 pathogen that has not been linked to human disease; as such, investigation of SHFV pathogenesis in non-human primates (NHPs) could serve as a model for hemorrhagic fever viruses such as Ebola, Marburg, and Lassa viruses. Here we describe the pathogenesis of SHFV in rhesus macaques inoculated with doses ranging from 50 PFU to 500,000 PFU. Disease severity was independent of dose with an overall mortality rate of 64% with signs of hemorrhagic fever and multiple organ system involvement. Analyses comparing survivors and non-survivors were performed to identify factors associated with survival revealing differences in the kinetics of viremia, immunosuppression, and regulation of hemostasis. Notable similarities between the pathogenesis of SHFV in NHPs and hemorrhagic fever viruses in humans suggest that SHFV may serve as a suitable model of BSL-4 pathogens.

Published by Elsevier Inc.

PMCID: PMC3210905 PMID: 22014505 [PubMed - indexed for MEDLINE]

1103. Am J Epidemiol. 2011 Dec 1;174(11 Suppl):S97-112. doi: 10.1093/aje/kwr312.

Fifty-five years of international epidemic-assistance investigations conducted by CDC's disease detectives.

Rolle IV(1), Pearson ML, Nsubuga P.

Author information: (1)Division of Public Health Systems and Workforce Development, Center for Global Health, CDC, 1600 Clifton Road NE, Mailstop E-93, Atlanta, GA 30333, USA. irolle@cdc.gov

For more than 60 years, the Centers for Disease Control and Prevention (CDC) has used its scientific expertise to help people throughout the world live healthier, safer, longer lives through science-based health action. In 1951, CDC officially established the Epidemic Intelligence Service to help build public health capacity. During 1950-2005, CDC's Epidemic Intelligence Service officers conducted 462 international epidemiologic field investigations in 131 foreign countries and 7 territories. Investigations have included responding to emerging infectious and noninfectious disease outbreaks, assisting in disaster response, and evaluating core components of public health programs worldwide. Approximately 81% of investigations were responses to infectious disease outbreaks, but the proportion of investigations related to chronic and other noninfectious conditions increased 7-fold (6%-45%). These investigations have contributed to detecting and characterizing new pathogens (e.g., severe acute respiratory syndrome-associated coronavirus) and conditions, provided insights regarding factors that cause or contribute to disease acquisition (e.g., Ebola hemorrhagic fever), led to development of new diagnostics and surveillance technologies, and provided information upon which global health policies and regulations can be based. CDC's disease detectives will undoubtedly continue to play a critical role in global health and in responding to emerging global disease threats.

PMID: 22135398 [PubMed - indexed for MEDLINE]

1104. Biol Trace Elem Res. 2011 Dec;143(3):1325-36. doi: 10.1007/s12011-011-8977-1. Epub 2011 Feb 12.

Review: micronutrient selenium deficiency influences evolution of some viral infectious diseases.

Harthill M(1).

Author information: (1)Geochemistry and Health International, Inc., Frederick, MD 21705-3523, USA. mharthill@gmail.com

Recently emerged viral infectious diseases (VIDs) include HIV/AIDS, influenzas H5N1 and 2009 H1N1, SARS, and Ebola hemorrhagic fevers. Earlier research determined metabolic oxidative stress in hosts deficient in antioxidant selenium (Se) (

PMID: 21318622 [PubMed - indexed for MEDLINE]

1105. Biosecur Bioterror. 2011 Dec;9(4):361-71. doi: 10.1089/bsp.2011.0051. Epub 2011 Nov 9.

Evaluation of perceived threat differences posed by filovirus variants.

Kuhn JH(1), Dodd LE, Wahl-Jensen V, Radoshitzky SR, Bavari S, Jahrling PB.

Author information: (1)National Institutes of Health, National Institute of Allergy and Infectious Diseases, Division of Clinical Research, Integrated Research Facility at Fort Detrick, Frederick, Maryland, USA.

In the United States, filoviruses (ebolaviruses and marburgviruses) are listed as National Institute of Allergy and Infectious Diseases (NIAID) Category A Priority Pathogens, Select Agents, and Centers for Disease Control and Prevention (CDC) Category A Bioterrorism Agents. In recent months, U.S. biodefense professionals and policy experts have initiated discussions on how to optimize filovirus research in regard to medical countermeasure (ie, diagnostics, antiviral, and vaccine) development. Standardized procedures and reagents could accelerate the independent verification of research results across government agencies and establish baselines for the development of animal models acceptable to regulatory entities, such as the Food and Drug Administration (FDA), while being fiscally responsible. At the root of standardization lies the question of which filovirus strains, variants, or isolates ought to be the prototypes for product development, evaluation, and validation. Here we discuss a rationale for their selection. We conclude that, based on currently available data, filovirus biodefense research ought to focus on the classical taxonomic filovirus prototypes: Marburg virus Musoke in the case of marburgviruses and Ebola virus Mayinga in the case of Zaire ebolaviruses. Arguments have been made in various committees in favor of other variants, such as Marburg virus Angola, Ci67 or Popp, or Ebola virus Kikwit, but these rationales seem to be largely based on anecdotal or unpublished and unverified data, or they may reflect a lack of awareness of important facts about the variants' isolation history and genomic properties.

PMCID: PMC3233913 PMID: 22070137 [PubMed - indexed for MEDLINE]

1106. Curr Opin Virol. 2011 Dec;1(6):649-57. doi: 10.1016/j.coviro.2011.10.013. Epub 2011 Nov 9.

Mass extinctions, biodiversity and mitochondrial function: are bats 'special' as reservoirs for emerging viruses?

Wang LF(1), Walker PJ, Poon LL.

Author information: (1)CSIRO Livestock Industries, Australian Animal Health Laboratory, Geelong, Victoria 3216, Australia. linfa.wang@csiro.au

For the past 10-15 years, bats have attracted growing attention as reservoirs of emerging zoonotic viruses. This has been due to a combination of factors including the emergence of highly virulent zoonotic pathogens, such as Hendra, Nipah, SARS and Ebola viruses, and the high rate of detection of a large number of previously unknown viral sequences in bat specimens. As bats have ancient evolutionary origins and are the only flying mammals, it has been hypothesized that some of their unique biological features may have made them especially suitable hosts for different viruses. So the question 'Are bats different, special or exceptional?' has become a focal point in the field of virology, bat biology and virus-host co-evolution. In this brief review, we examine the topic in a relatively unconventional way, that is, our discussion will be based on both scientific discoveries and theoretical predictions. This approach was chosen partially because the data in this field are so limited that it is impossible to conduct a useful review based on published results only and also because we believe it is important to provoke original, speculative or even controversial ideas or theories in this important field of research.

PMID: 22440923 [PubMed - indexed for MEDLINE]

1107. J Gen Virol. 2011 Dec;92(Pt 12):2900-5. doi: 10.1099/vir.0.036863-0. Epub 2011 Sep 7.

Genus-specific recruitment of filovirus ribonucleoprotein complexes into budding particles.

Spiegelberg L(1), Wahl-Jensen V, Kolesnikova L, Feldmann H, Becker S, Hoenen T.

Author information: (1)Department of Virology, Philipps University Marburg, Hans-Meerwein-Str. 2, 35043 Marburg, Germany.

The filoviral matrix protein VP40 orchestrates virus morphogenesis and budding. To do this it interacts with both the glycoprotein (GP1,2) and the ribonucleoprotein (RNP) complex components; however, these interactions are still not well understood. Here we show that for efficient VP40-driven formation of transcription and replication-competent virus-like particles (trVLPs), which contain both an RNP complex and GP1,2, the RNP components and VP40, but not GP1,2 and VP40, must be from the same genus. trVLP preparations contained both spherical and filamentous particles, but only the latter were able to infect target cells and to lead to genome replication and transcription. Interestingly, the genus specificity of the VP40-RNP interactions was specific to the formation of filamentous trVLPs, but not to spherical particles. These results not only further our understanding of VP40 interactions, but also suggest that special care is required when using trVLP or VLP systems to model virus morphogenesis.
PMCID: PMC3352568 PMID: 21900424 [PubMed - indexed for MEDLINE]
1108. J Pharm Sci. 2011 Dec;100(12):5156-73. doi: 10.1002/jps.22724. Epub 2011 Aug 19.

Biophysical characterization and conformational stability of Ebola and Marburg virus-like particles.

Hu L(1), Trefethen JM, Zeng Y, Yee L, Ohtake S, Lechuga-Ballesteros D, Warfield KL, Aman MJ, Shulenin S, Unfer R, Enterlein SG, Truong-Le V, Volkin DB, Joshi SB, Middaugh CR.

Author information: (1)Department of Pharmaceutical Chemistry, University of Kansas, Lawrence, Kansas 66047, USA.

The filoviruses, Ebola virus and Marburg virus, cause severe hemorrhagic fever with up to 90% human mortality. Virus-like particles of EBOV (eVLPs) and MARV (mVLPs) are attractive vaccine candidates. For the development of stable vaccines, the conformational stability of these two enveloped VLPs produced in insect cells was characterized by various spectroscopic techniques over a wide pH and temperature range. Temperature-induced aggregation of the VLPs at various pH values was monitored by light scattering. Temperature/pH empirical phase diagrams (EPDs) of the two VLPs were constructed to summarize the large volume of data generated. The EPDs show that both VLPs lose their conformational integrity above about 50°C-60°C, depending on solution pH. The VLPs were maximally thermal stable in solution at pH 7-8, with a significant reduction in stability at pH 5 and 6. They were much less stable in solution at pH 3-4 due to increased susceptibility of the VLPs to aggregation. The characterization data and conformational stability profiles from these studies provide a basis for selection of optimized solution conditions for further vaccine formulation and long-term stability studies of eVLPs and mVLPs.

PMID: 21858822 [PubMed - indexed for MEDLINE]
1109. Mol Biol Evol. 2011 Dec;28(12):3355-65. doi: 10.1093/molbev/msr170. Epub 2011 Jun 24

Purifying selection can obscure the ancient age of viral lineages.

Wertheim JO(1), Kosakovsky Pond SL.

Author information: (1)Department of Pathology, University of California, San Diego, CA, USA. jwertheim@ucsd.edu

Statistical methods for molecular dating of viral origins have been used extensively to infer the time of most common recent ancestor for many rapidly evolving pathogens. However, there are a number of cases, in which epidemiological, historical, or genomic evidence suggests much older viral origins than those obtained via molecular dating. We demonstrate how pervasive purifying selection can mask the ancient origins of recently sampled pathogens, in part due to the inability of nucleotide-based substitution models to properly account for complex patterns of spatial and temporal variability in selective pressures. We use codon-based substitution models to infer the length of branches in viral phylogenies; these models produce estimates that are often considerably longer than those obtained with traditional nucleotide-based substitution models. Correcting the apparent underestimation of branch lengths suggests substantially older origins for measles, Ebola, and avian influenza viruses. This work helps to reconcile some of the inconsistencies between molecular dating and other types of evidence concerning the age of viral lineages.
PMCID: PMC3247791 PMID: 21705379 [PubMed - indexed for MEDLINE]
1110. Virus Res. 2011 Dec;162(1-2):100-9. doi: 10.1016/j.virusres.2011.09.012. Epub 2011 Sep 16.

An unconventional pathway of mRNA cap formation by vesiculoviruses.

Ogino T(1), Banerjee AK.

Author information: (1)Department of Molecular Genetics, Section of Virology, Lerner Research Institute, Cleveland Clinic, Cleveland, OH 44195, USA. oginot@ccf.org

mRNAs of vesicular stomatitis virus (VSV), a prototype of nonsegmented negative strand (NNS) RNA viruses (e.g., rabies, measles, mumps, Ebola, and Borna disease viruses), possess the 5'-terminal cap structure identical to that of eukaryotic mRNAs, but the mechanism of mRNA cap formation is distinctly different from the latter. The elucidation of the unconventional capping of VSV mRNA remained elusive for three decades since the discovery of the cap structure in some viral and eukaryotic mRNAs in 1975. Only recently our biochemical studies revealed an unexpected strategy employed by vesiculoviruses (VSV and Chandipura virus, an emerging arbovirus) to generate the cap structure. This article summarizes the historical and current research that led to the discovery of the novel vesiculoviral mRNA capping reaction.

PMCID: PMC3221763 PMID: 21945214 [PubMed - indexed for MEDLINE]
1111. Virus Res. 2011 Dec;162(1-2):148-61. doi: 10.1016/j.virusres.2011.09.005. Epub 2011 Sep 10.

Progress in recombinant DNA-derived vaccines for Lassa virus and filoviruses.

Grant-Klein RJ(1), Altamura LA, Schmaljohn CS.

Author information: (1)U.S. Army Medical Research Institute of Infectious Diseases, Fort Detrick, MD 21702, USA.

Developing vaccines for highly pathogenic viruses such as those causing Lassa, Ebola, and Marburg hemorrhagic fevers is a daunting task due to both scientific and logistical constraints. Scientific hurdles to overcome include poorly defined relationships between pathogenicity and protective immune responses, genetic diversity of viruses, and safety in a target population that includes a large number of individuals with compromised immune systems. Logistical obstacles include the requirement for biosafety level-4 containment to study the authentic viruses, the poor public health infrastructure of the endemic disease areas, and the cost of developing these vaccines for use in non-lucrative markets. Recombinant DNA-based vaccine approaches offer promise of overcoming some of these issues. In this review, we consider the status of various recombinant DNA candidate vaccines against Lassa virus and filoviruses which have been tested in animals.

Published by Elsevier B.V.

PMID: 21925552 [PubMed - indexed for MEDLINE]
1112. Virology. 2011 Nov 25;420(2):117-24. doi: 10.1016/j.virol.2011.08.022. Epub 2011 Sep 28.

A small nonhuman primate model for filovirus-induced disease.

Carrion R Jr(1), Ro Y, Hoosien K, Ticer A, Brasky K, de la Garza M, Mansfield K, Patterson JL.

Author information: (1)Department of Virology and Immunology, Texas Biomedical Research Institute, 7620 NW Loop 410, San Antonio, TX 78227, USA. carrion@TxBiomed.org

Ebolavirus and Marburgvirus are members of the filovirus family and induce a fatal hemorrhagic disease in humans and nonhuman primates with 90% case fatality. To develop a small nonhuman primate model for filovirus disease, common marmosets (Callithrix jacchus) were intramuscularly inoculated with wild type Marburgvirus Musoke or Ebolavirus Zaire. The infection resulted in a systemic fatal disease with clinical and morphological features closely resembling human infection. Animals experienced weight loss, fever, high virus titers in tissue, thrombocytopenia, neutrophilia, high liver transaminases and phosphatases and disseminated intravascular coagulation. Evidence of a severe disseminated viral infection characterized principally by multifocal to coalescing hepatic necrosis was seen in EBOV animals. MARV-infected animals displayed only moderate fibrin deposition in the spleen. Lymphoid necrosis and lymphocytic depletion observed in spleen. These findings provide support for the use of the common marmoset as a small nonhuman primate model for filovirus induced hemorrhagic fever.

Copyright © 2011 Elsevier Inc. All rights reserved.

PMCID: PMC3195836 PMID: 21959017 [PubMed - indexed for MEDLINE]
1113. Nat Struct Mol Biol. 2011 Nov 20;18(12):1424-7. doi: 10.1038/nsmb.2150.

A shared structural solution for neutralizing ebolaviruses.

Dias JM(1), Kuehne AI, Abelson DM, Bale S, Wong AC, Halfmann P, Muhammad MA, Fusco ML, Zak SE, Kang E, Kawaoka Y, Chandran K, Dye JM, Saphire EO.

Author information: (1)Department of Immunology and Microbial Science, The Scripps Research Institute, La Jolla, California, USA.

Sudan virus (genus Ebolavirus) is lethal, yet no monoclonal antibody is known to neutralize it. We here describe antibody 16F6 that neutralizes Sudan virus and present its structure bound to the trimeric viral glycoprotein. Unexpectedly, the 16F6 epitope overlaps that of KZ52, the only other antibody against the GP(1,2) core to be visualized to date. Furthermore, both antibodies against this crucial epitope bridging GP1-GP2 neutralize at a post-internalization step--probably fusion.

PMCID: PMC3230659 PMID: 22101933 [PubMed - indexed for MEDLINE]
1114. BMC Evol Biol. 2011 Nov 17;11:336. doi: 10.1186/1471-2148-11-336.

Evolutionary maintenance of filovirus-like genes in bat genomes.

Taylor DJ(1), Dittmar K, Ballinger MJ, Bruenn JA.

Author information: (1)Department of Biological Sciences, The State University of New York at Buffalo, Buffalo, NY 14260, USA. djtaylor@buffalo.edu

BACKGROUND: Little is known of the biological significance and evolutionary maintenance of integrated non-retroviral RNA virus genes in eukaryotic host genomes. Here, we isolated novel filovirus-like genes from bat genomes and tested for evolutionary maintenance. We also estimated the age of filovirus VP35-like gene integrations and tested the phylogenetic hypotheses that there is a eutherian mammal clade and a marsupial/ebolavirus/Marburgvirus dichotomy for filoviruses. RESULTS: We detected homologous copies of VP35-like and NP-like gene integrations in both Old World and New World species of Myotis (bats). We also detected previously unknown VP35-like genes in rodents that are positionally homologous. Comprehensive phylogenetic estimates for filovirus NP-like and VP35-like loci support two main clades with a marsupial and a rodent grouping within the ebolavirus/Lloviu virus/Marburgvirus clade. The concordance of VP35-like, NP-like and mitochondrial gene trees with the expected species tree supports the notion that the copies we examined are orthologs that predate the global spread and radiation of the genus Myotis. Parametric simulations were consistent with selective maintenance for the open reading frame (ORF) of VP35-like genes in Myotis. The ORF of the filovirus-like VP35 gene has been maintained in bat genomes for an estimated 13. 4 MY. ORFs were disrupted for the NP-like genes in Myotis. Likelihood ratio tests revealed that a model that accommodates positive selection is a significantly better fit to the data than a model that does not allow for positive selection for VP35-like sequences. Moreover, site-by-site analysis of selection using two methods indicated at least 25 sites in the VP35-like alignment are under positive selection in Myotis. CONCLUSIONS: Our results indicate that filovirus-like elements have significance beyond genomic imprints of prior infection. That is, there appears to be, or have been, functionally maintained copies of such genes in mammals. "Living fossils" of filoviruses appear to be selectively maintained in a diverse mammalian genus (Myotis).

PMCID: PMC3229293 PMID: 22093762 [PubMed - indexed for MEDLINE]
1115. Clin Immunol. 2011 Nov;141(2):218-27. doi: 10.1016/j.clim.2011.08.008. Epub 2011 Aug 31.

Characterization of Zaire ebolavirus glycoprotein-specific monoclonal antibodies.

Qiu X(1), Alimonti JB, Melito PL, Fernando L, Ströher U, Jones SM.
Author information: (1)Special Pathogens Program, National Microbiology Laboratory, Public Health Agency of Canada, Winnipeg, Manitoba, Canada. xiangguo.qiu@phac-aspc.gc.ca

Zaire ebolavirus (ZEBOV) can be transmitted by human-to-human contact and causes acute haemorrhagic fever with case fatality rates up to 90%. There are no effective therapeutic or prophylactic treatments available. The sole transmembrane glycoprotein (GP) is the key target for developing neutralizing antibodies. In this study, recombinant VSVΔG/ZEBOVGP was used to generate monoclonal antibodies (MAbs) against the ZEBOV GP. A total of 8 MAbs were produced using traditional hybridoma cell fusion technology, and then characterized by ELISA using ZEBOV VLPs, Western blotting, an immunofluorescence assay, and immunoprecipitation. All 8 MAbs worked in IFA and IP, suggesting that they are all conformational MAbs, however six of them recognized linearized epitopes by WB. ELISA results demonstrated that one MAb bound to a secreted GP (sGP 1-295aa); three bind to a part of the mucin domain (333-458aa); three MAbs recognized epitopes on the C-terminal domain of GP1 (296-501aa); and one bound to full length GP (VLPs/GP1,2 ΔTm). Using a mouse model these MAbs were evaluated for their therapeutic capacity during a lethal infection. All 8 MAb improved survival rates by 33%-100% against a high dose lethal challenge with mouse-adapted ZEBOV. This work has important implications for further development of vaccines and immunotherapies for ZEBOV infection.

PMID: 21925951 [PubMed - indexed for MEDLINE]
1116. J Infect Dis. 2011 Nov;204 Suppl 3:S840-9. doi: 10.1093/infdis/jir306.

Comparative analysis of Ebola virus glycoprotein interactions with human and bat cells.

Kühl A(1), Hoffmann M, Müller MA, Munster VJ, Gnirss K, Kiene M, Tsegaye TS, Behrens G, Herrler G, Feldmann H, Drosten C, Pöhlmann S.
Author information: (1)Institute of Virology, Hannover Medical School, Germany.

Infection with Ebola virus (EBOV) causes hemorrhagic fever in humans with high case-fatality rates. The EBOV-glycoprotein (EBOV-GP) facilitates viral entry and promotes viral release from human cells. African fruit bats are believed not to develop disease upon EBOV infection and have been proposed as a natural reservoir of EBOV. We compared EBOV-GP interactions with human cells and cells from African fruit bats. We found that susceptibility to EBOV-GP-dependent infection was not limited to bat cells from potential reservoir species, and we observed that GP displayed similar biological properties in human and bat cells. The only exception was GP localization, which was to a greater extent intracellular in bat cells as compared to human cells. Collectively, our results suggest that GP interactions with fruit bat and human cells are similar and do not limit EBOV tropism for certain bat species.

PMCID: PMC3189982 PMID: 21987760 [PubMed - indexed for MEDLINE]
1117. J Infect Dis. 2011 Nov;204 Suppl 3:S991-9. doi: 10.1093/infdis/jir336.

Host response dynamics following lethal infection of rhesus macaques with Zaire ebolavirus.

Ebihara H(1), Rockx B, Marzi A, Feldmann F, Haddock E, Brining D, LaCasse RA, Gardner D, Feldmann H.
Author information: (1)Laboratory of Virology, Rocky Mountain Veterinary Branch, Division of Intramural Research, National Institute of Allergy and Infectious Diseases, National Institutes of Health, Rocky Mountain Laboratories, Hamilton, Montana 59840, USA. ebiharah@niaid.nih.gov

To gain further insight into the interdependent pathogenic processes in Ebola hemorrhagic fever (EHF), we have examined the dynamics of host responses in individual rhesus macaques infected with Zaire ebolavirus over the entire disease course. Examination of coagulation parameters revealed that decreased coagulation inhibitor activity triggered severe coagulopathy as indicated by prolonged coagulation times and decreased fibrinogen levels. This has been proposed as one of the significant mechanisms underlying disseminated intravascular coagulation in EHF patients. Furthermore, monitoring of expression levels for cytokines/chemokines suggested a mixed anti-inflammatory response syndrome (MARS), which indicates that a catastrophic uncontrolled immunological status contributes to the development of fatal hemorrhagic fever. These results highlight the pathological analogies between EHF and severe sepsis and not only contribute to our understanding of the pathogenic process, but will also help to establish novel postexposure treatment modalities.

PMCID: PMC3189992 PMID: 21987781 [PubMed - indexed for MEDLINE]
1118. J Infect Dis. 2011 Nov;204 Suppl 3:S986-90. doi: 10.1093/infdis/jir335.

Filovirus infection of STAT-1 knockout mice.

Raymond J(1), Bradfute S, Bray M.
Author information: (1)Department of Veterinary Pathology, Armed Forces Institutes of Pathology, Washington, District of Columbia, USA.

We evaluated the susceptibility to Ebola and Marburg virus infection of mice that cannot respond to interferon (IFN)-α/β and IFN-γ because of deletion of the STAT-1 gene. A mouse-adapted Zaire ebolavirus (ZEBOV) caused rapidly lethal disease; wild-type ZEBOV and Sudan Ebolavirus and 4 different Marburg virus strains produced severe, but more slowly progressive illness; and Reston Ebolavirus caused mild disease that was late in onset. The virulence of each agent was mirrored by the pace and severity of pathologic changes in the liver and lymphoid tissues. A virus-like particle vaccine elicited strong antibody responses but did not protect against mouse-adapted ZEBOV challenge.

PMID: 21987780 [PubMed - indexed for MEDLINE]
1119. J Infect Dis. 2011 Nov;204 Suppl 3:S978-85. doi: 10.1093/infdis/jir334.

Antibody-dependent enhancement of Marburg virus infection.

Nakayama E(1), Tomabechi D, Matsuno K, Kishida N, Yoshida R, Feldmann H, Takada A.
Author information: (1)Department of Global Epidemiology, Hokkaido University Research Center for Zoonosis Control, Sapporo, Japan.

BACKGROUND: Marburg virus (MARV) and Ebola virus (EBOV) cause severe hemorrhagic fever in primates. Earlier studies demonstrated that antibodies to particular epitopes on the glycoprotein (GP) of EBOV enhanced virus infectivity in vitro. METHODS: To investigate this antibody-dependent enhancement (ADE) in MARV infection, we produced mouse antisera and monoclonal antibodies (mAbs) to the GPs of MARV strains Angola and Musoke. RESULTS: The infectivity of vesicular stomatitis virus pseudotyped with Angola GP in K562 cells was significantly enhanced in the presence of Angola GP antisera, whereas only minimal ADE activity was seen with Musoke GP antisera. This difference correlated with the percentage of hybridoma clones producing infectivity-enhancing mAbs. Using mAbs to MARV GP, we identified 3 distinct ADE epitopes in the mucinlike region on Angola GP. Interestingly, some of these antibodies bound to both Angola and Musoke GPs but showed significantly higher ADE activity for strain Angola. ADE activity depended on epitopes in the mucinlike region and glycine at amino acid position 547, present in the Angola but absent in the Musoke GP. CONCLUSIONS: These results suggest a possible link between ADE and MARV pathogenicity and provide new insights into the mechanisms underlying ADE entry of filoviruses.
PMCID: PMC3189991 PMID: 21987779 [PubMed - indexed for MEDLINE]

1120. J Infect Dis. 2011 Nov;204 Suppl 3:S973-7. doi: 10.1093/infdis/jir331.

Ebola virus failure to stimulate plasmacytoid dendritic cell interferon responses correlates with impaired cellular entry.

Leung LW(1), Martinez O, Reynard O, Volchkov VE, Basler CF.

Author information: (1)Department of Microbiology, Mount Sinai School of Medicine, One Gustave L. Levy Place, New York, New York 10029, USA.

We examined the ability of the Ebola virus to elicit an antiviral response from plasmacytoid dendritic cells (pDCs). Exposure of pDCs to Ebola virus did not result in significantly higher levels of interferon-α production than the levels in mock-infected cells. After inoculation with Ebola virus under the same conditions, conventional dendritic cells expressed viral proteins whereas pDCs did not, suggesting that the latter cells were not infected. Assessment of the entry of Ebola virus-like particles into pDCs revealed that pDCs are highly impaired for viral entry in comparison with conventional dendritic cells. These observations identify a novel means by which Ebola virus can avoid triggering an antiviral response.

PMCID: PMC3189990 PMID: 21987778 [PubMed - indexed for MEDLINE]

1121. J Infect Dis. 2011 Nov;204 Suppl 3:S968-72. doi: 10.1093/infdis/jir330.

Assessment of rodents as animal models for Reston ebolavirus.

de Wit E(1), Munster VJ, Metwally SA, Feldmann H.

Author information: (1)Laboratory of Virology, Division of Intramural Research, National Institute of Allergy and Infectious Diseases, National Institutes of Health, Hamilton, Montana, USA.

The emergence of Reston ebolavirus (REBOV) in domestic swine in the Philippines has caused a renewed interest in REBOV pathogenicity. Here, the use of different rodent species as animal disease models for REBOV was investigated. BALB/c and STAT1(-)(/-) mice, Hartley guinea pigs, and Syrian hamsters were inoculated intraperitoneally with REBOV strain Pennsylvania or Reston08-A. Although virus replication occurred in guinea pigs, hamsters, and STAT1(-/-) mice, progression to disease was only observed in STAT1(-)(/-) mice. Moreover, REBOV Pennsylvania was more pathogenic than REBOV Reston08-A in this model. Thus, STAT1(-)(/-) mice may be used for research of REBOV pathogenicity and intervention strategies.

PMCID: PMC3189989 PMID: 21987777 [PubMed - indexed for MEDLINE]

1122. J Infect Dis. 2011 Nov;204 Suppl 3:S957-67. doi: 10.1093/infdis/jir326.

Ebola virus enters host cells by macropinocytosis and clathrin-mediated endocytosis.

Aleksandrowicz P(1), Marzi A, Biedenkopf N, Beimforde N, Becker S, Hoenen T, Feldmann H, Schnittler HJ.

Author information: (1)Institute of Anatomy and Vascular Biology, Westfälische Wilhelms University Muenster, Vesaliusweg, Germany.

Virus entry into host cells is the first step of infection and a crucial determinant of pathogenicity. Here we show that Ebola virus-like particles (EBOV-VLPs) composed of the glycoprotein GP(1,2) and the matrix protein VP40 use macropinocytosis and clathrin-mediated endocytosis to enter cells. EBOV-VLPs applied to host cells induced actin-driven ruffling and enhanced FITC-dextran uptake, which indicated macropinocytosis as the main entry mechanism. This was further supported by inhibition of entry through inhibitors of actin polymerization (latrunculin A), Na(+)/H(+)-exchanger (EIPA), and PI3-kinase (wortmannin). A fraction of EBOV-VLPs, however, colocalized with clathrin heavy chain (CHC), and VLP uptake was reduced by CHC small interfering RNA transfection and expression of the dominant negative dynamin II-K44A mutant. In contrast, we found no evidence that EBOV-VLPs enter cells via caveolae. This work identifies macropinocytosis as the major, and clathrin-dependent endocytosis as an alternative, entry route for EBOV particles. Therefore, EBOV seems to utilize different entry pathways depending on both cell type and virus particle size.

PMCID: PMC3189988 PMID: 21987776 [PubMed - indexed for MEDLINE]

1123. J Infect Dis. 2011 Nov;204 Suppl 3:S953-6. doi: 10.1093/infdis/jir325.

The Ebolavirus VP24 protein blocks phosphorylation of p38 mitogen-activated protein kinase.

Halfmann P(1), Neumann G, Kawaoka Y.

Author information: (1)Department of Pathobiological Sciences, School of Veterinary Medicine, Influenza Research Institute, University of Wisconsin-Madison, WI, USA.

Type I interferon (IFN) signaling is mediated through several signaling pathways, including the Janus kinase and signal transducer and activator (JAK-STAT) and p38 mitogen-activated protein (MAP) kinase pathways. The VP24 protein of Ebolavirus is an IFN antagonist, blocking type I IFN signaling through the JAK-STAT pathway. Here, we show that, in 293 cells, VP24 also interferes with the p38 MAP kinase pathway by blocking IFN-β-stimulated phosphorylation of p38-α. Similar inhibition was not observed in HeLa cells, suggesting cell type-specific differences in signal transduction.

PMCID: PMC3189987 PMID: 21987775 [PubMed - indexed for MEDLINE]

1124. J Infect Dis. 2011 Nov;204 Suppl 3:S947-52. doi: 10.1093/infdis/jir322.

The Ebola virus soluble glycoprotein (sGP) does not affect lymphocyte apoptosis and adhesion to activated endothelium.

Wolf K(1), Beimforde N, Falzarano D, Feldmann H, Schnittler HJ.

Author information: (1)Institut für Physiologie, Technische-Universität Dresden, Dresden, Germany.

Ebola virus infection is associated with the release of a soluble glycoprotein (sGP) from infected cells. The sGP has been proposed to modulate Ebola virus pathogenesis in primates but little is known about the role of this protein during infection and disease manifestation. So far sGP has been shown to revert the effect of tumor necrosis factor α (TNF-α) on endothelial permeability, indicating that the function of sGP might be antiinflammatory. Since bystander apoptosis of lymphocytes has been demonstrated in Ebola virus infections, we aimed to investigate the ability of sGP to modulate lymphocyte apoptosis and adhesion of lymphocytes to activated endothelium. Recombinant sGP alone or together with TNF-α and the death receptors TRAIL and FAS neither increased nor decreased apoptosis of Jurkat cells, a well-established human lymphocytic cell line. In addition, Jurkat cell adhesion to native or activated human umbilical vein endothelial cells was also found to be not altered by sGP.

PMID: 21987774 [PubMed - indexed for MEDLINE]

1125. J Infect Dis. 2011 Nov;204 Suppl 3:S941-6. doi: 10.1093/infdis/jir321.

Genomic RNA editing and its impact on Ebola virus adaptation during serial passages in cell culture and infection of guinea pigs.

Volchkova VA(1), Dolnik O, Martinez MJ, Reynard O, Volchkov VE.

Author information: (1)Filovirus Laboratory, INSERM U758, Human Virology Department, Université de Lyon, Claude Bernard Université Lyon-1, Ecole Normale Supérieure de Lyon, France.

Synthesis of the structural, surface glycoprotein (GP) of Ebola virus (EBOV) is dependent on transcriptional RNA editing phenomenon. Editing results in the insertion of an extra adenosine by viral polymerase at the editing site (7 consecutive template uridines) during transcription of GP gene of the wild-type virus (EBOV/7U). In this study, we demonstrate that passage of EBOV/7U in Vero E6 cells results in the appearance and rapid accumulation of a variant (EBOV/8U) containing an additional uridine at the editing site in the viral genome. EBOV/8U outgrows and eventually replaces the wild-type EBOV during 4-5 passages. On the contrary, infection of guinea pigs with EBOV/8U leads to the appearance and rapid predominance by EBOV/7U. These rapid conversions suggest that editing of the genomic RNA occurs at a higher frequency than previously thought. In addition, it indicates that the EBOV/7U phenotype has a selective advantage that is linked to controlled expression of GP and/or expression of secreted sGP, the primary gene product for wild-type EBOV. This study demonstrates the potential for insertion and deletion of uridines in the editing site of the EBOV genomic RNA, depending on environmental constraints.

PMID: 21987773 [PubMed - indexed for MEDLINE]

1126. J Infect Dis. 2011 Nov;204 Suppl 3:S934-40. doi: 10.1093/infdis/jir320.

Role of VP30 phosphorylation in the Ebola virus replication cycle.

Martinez MJ(1), Volchkova VA, Raoul H, Alazard-Dany N, Reynard O, Volchkov VE.

Author information: (1)INSERM U758, Human Virology Department, Université de Lyon, Claude Bernard University Lyon-1, Ecole Normale Supérieure de Lyon, Lyon, France.

Ebola virus (EBOV) transcription is dependent on the phosphoprotein VP30, a component of the viral nucleocapsid. VP30 is phosphorylated at 2 serine residue clusters located at the N-terminal part of the protein. In this report, we have investigated the role of VP30 phosphorylation in EBOV replication using a reverse genetics approach. In effect, recombinant EBOVs with the VP30 serine clusters substituted either by nonphosphorylatable alanines or phosphorylation-mimicking aspartates were generated and characterized. We show that in comparison to the wild-type EBOV the mutated viruses possess reduced infectivity. This difference is explained by alterations in the balance between the transcription and replication processes and appear to be associated with the state of VP30 phosphorylation. Here we propose a model in which dynamic phosphorylation of VP30 is an important mechanism to regulate the EBOV replication cycle.

PMID: 21987772 [PubMed - indexed for MEDLINE]

1127. J Infect Dis. 2011 Nov;204 Suppl 3:S919-26. doi: 10.1093/infdis/jir324.

Contribution of Sec61α to the life cycle of Ebola virus.

Iwasa A(1), Halfmann P, Noda T, Oyama M, Kozuka-Hata H, Watanabe S, Shimojima M, Watanabe T, Kawaoka Y.

Author information: (1)Division of Virology, Department of Microbiology and Immunology, University of Tokyo, Tokyo, Japan.

BACKGROUND: Similar to other viruses, the viral proteins of Ebola virus (EBOV) interact with a variety of host proteins for its replication. Of the 7 structural proteins encoded in the EBOV genome, VP24 is the smallest and is multifunctional. METHODS: To identify host factors that interact with VP24 and are required for EBOV replication, we transfected 293 cells with plasmid expressing FLAG- and HA-tagged VP24, immunoprecipitated the host proteins that bound to VP24, and analyzed the immunoprecipitants with use of mass spectrometry. RESULTS: Of the 68 candidate host proteins identified, we selected Sec61α because of its similar intracellular localization to that of VP24 (ie, perinuclear region), its involvement in various biological functions, and its roles in pathogenesis, such as type 2 diabetes and hepatosteatosis, and investigated its possible role in the EBOV life cycle. Our results suggest that Sec61α is not involved in EBOV entry, interferon antagonism by VP24, nucleocapsid formation, or budding. However, Sec61α colocalized with VP24 contributed to the ability of VP24 to inhibit EBOV genome transcription and reduced the polymerase activity of EBOV. CONCLUSIONS: The present study indicates that Sec61α is a host protein involved in EBOV replication, specifically in EBOV genome transcription and replication.

PMCID: PMC3189986 PMID: 21987770 [PubMed - indexed for MEDLINE]

1128. J Infect Dis. 2011 Nov;204 Suppl 3:S911-8. doi: 10.1093/infdis/jir343.

DRBP76 associates with Ebola virus VP35 and suppresses viral polymerase function.

Shabman RS(I), Leung DW, Johnson J, Glennon N, Gulcicek EE, Stone KL, Leung L, Hensley L, Amarasinghe GK, Basler CF.
Author information: (I)Department of Microbiology, Mount Sinai School of Medicine, New York, New York 10029, USA.

The Zaire Ebola virus (EBOV) protein VP35 is multifunctional; it inhibits IFN-α/β production and functions as a cofactor of the viral RNA polymerase. Mass spectrometry identified the double stranded RNA binding protein 76 (DRBP76/NFAR-I/NF90) as a cellular factor that associates with the VP35 C-terminal interferon inhibitory domain (IID). DRBP76 is described to regulate host cell protein synthesis and play an important role in host defense. The VP35-IID-DRBP76 interaction required the addition of exogenous dsRNA, but full-length VP35 associated with DRBP76 in the absence of exogenous dsRNA. Cells infected with a Newcastle disease virus (NDV)-expressing VP35 redistributed DRBP76 from the nucleus to the cytoplasm, the compartment in which EBOV replicates. Overexpression of DRBP76 did not alter the ability of VP35 to inhibit type I IFN production but did impair the function of the EBOV transcription/replication complex. These data suggest that DRBP76, via its association with VP35, exerts an anti-EBOV function.

PMCID: PMC3218669 PMID: 21987769 [PubMed - indexed for MEDLINE]
1129. J Infect Dis. 2011 Nov;204 Suppl 3:S904-10. doi: 10.1093/infdis/jir323.

The Ebola virus VP24 protein prevents hnRNP C1/C2 binding to karyopherin αl and partially alters its nuclear import.

Shabman RS(I), Gulcicek EE, Stone KL, Basler CF.
Author information: (I)Mount Sinai School of Medicine, New York, New York 10029, USA.

The Ebola virus (EBOV) protein VP24 inhibits type I and II interferon (IFN) signaling by binding to NPI-I subfamily karyopherin α (KPNA) nuclear import proteins, preventing their interaction with tyrosine-phosphorylated STATI (phospho-STATI). This inhibits phospho-STATI nuclear import. A biochemical screen now identifies heterogeneous nuclear ribonuclear protein complex CI/C2 (hnRNP CI/C2) nuclear import as an additional target of VP24. Co-immunoprecipitation studies demonstrate that hnRNP CI/C2 interacts with multiple KPNA family members, including KPNAI. Interaction with hnRNP CI/C2 occurs through the same KPNAI C-terminal region (amino acids 424-457) that binds VP24 and phospho-STATI. The ability of hnRNP CI/C2 to bind KPNAI is diminished in the presence of VP24, and cells transiently expressing VP24 redistribute hnRNP CI/C2 from the nucleus to the cytoplasm. These data further define the mechanism of hnRNP CI/C2 nuclear import and demonstrate that the impact of EBOV VP24 on nuclear import extends beyond STATI.

PMCID: PMC3189985 PMID: 21987768 [PubMed - indexed for MEDLINE]
1130. J Infect Dis. 2011 Nov;204 Suppl 3:S897-903. doi: 10.1093/infdis/jir313.

sGP serves as a structural protein in Ebola virus infection.

Iwasa A(I), Shimojima M, Kawaoka Y.
Author information: (I)Division of Virology, Department of Microbiology and Immunology, University of Tokyo, Japan.

BACKGROUND: sGP, which is perceived as nonstructural, secretory glycoprotein, shares 295 amino acids at its N-terminal with GP(I,2), which include the specific residue necessary to interact with GP(2). In the present study, we tested whether the sGP protein of Zaire ebolavirus (ZEBOV) could substitute for GP(I) and form a complex with GP(2), thus serving as a structural protein. METHODS: We expressed ZEBOV GP(I,2), VP40, and NP proteins, together with sGP protein, from expression plasmids and examined the resultant virus-like particles by using Western blot. Cells expressing GP(2) in combination with either GP(I) or sGP were analyzed by using flow cytometry with the KZ52 antibody, which recognizes a GP(I,2) conformational epitope. A VSV pseudotype, VSVΔG*, which expresses a GFP reporter gene instead of the G protein, was used to produce pseudotyped viruses encoding sGP and variants of GP to test the contribution of sGP to infectivity. RESULTS: Western blot and flow cytometric analyses suggested the existence of a covalently linked sGP-GP(2) molecule. VSVΔG*(sGP + GP(2)) and VSVΔG*(GP(I,2)) infected Vero E6 cells and were neutralized by the KZ52 antibody. Overexpression of sGP reduced the titer of VSVΔG*(GP(I,2)). CONCLUSIONS: ZEBOV sGP can substitute for GP(I), forming a sGP-GP(2) complex and conferring infectivity. Our studies suggest a novel role for sGP as a structural protein.

PMCID: PMC3218668 PMID: 21987767 [PubMed - indexed for MEDLINE]
1131. J Infect Dis. 2011 Nov;204 Suppl 3:S892-6. doi: 10.1093/infdis/jir311.

Knockdown of Ebola virus VP24 impairs viral nucleocapsid assembly and prevents virus replication.

Mateo M(I), Carbonnelle C, Martinez MJ, Reynard O, Page A, Volchkova VA, Volchkov VE.
Author information: (I)Filovirus Laboratory, INSERM U758, Human Virology Department, Université de Lyon, Ecole Normale Supérieure de Lyon, Lyon, France.

The structural protein VP24 of Ebola virus (EBOV) is a determinant of virulence in rodent models and possesses an interferon antagonist function. In this study, we investigate the role of VP24 in EBOV replication using RNA interference by small interfering RNA to knock down the expression of this protein in virus-infected cells. We reveal that VP24 is required for assembly of viral nucleocapsids and that silencing of VP24 expression prevents the release of EBOV.

PMID: 21987766 [PubMed - indexed for MEDLINE]
1132. J Infect Dis. 2011 Nov;204 Suppl 3:S884-91. doi: 10.1093/infdis/jir359.

Conserved proline-rich region of Ebola virus matrix protein VP40 is essential for plasma membrane targeting and virus-like particle release.

Reynard O(I), Nemirov K, Page A, Mateo M, Raoul H, Weissenhorn W, Volchkov VE.
Author information: (I)Filovirus Laboratory, INSERM U758, Human Virology Department, Claude Bernard Université Lyon I, Ecole Normale Supérieure de Lyon, Lyon, France.

The matrix protein VP40 is essential for Ebola virus (EBOV) and Marburg virus assembly and budding at the plasma membrane. In this study we have investigated the effect of single amino acid substitutions in a conserved proline-rich region of the EBOV VP40 located in the carboxy-terminal part of the protein. We demonstrate that substitutions within this region result in an alteration of intracellular VP40 localization and also cause a reduction or a complete block of virus-like particle budding, a benchmark of VP40 function. Furthermore, some mutated VP40s revealed an enhanced binding with cellular Sec24C, a part of the coat protein complex II (COPII) vesicular transport system. Analysis of the 3-dimensional structure of VP40 revealed the spatial proximity of the proline-rich region and an earlier identified site of interaction with Sec24C, thus allowing us to hypothesize that the altered intracellular localization of the VP40 mutants is a consequence of defects in their interaction with COPII-mediated vesicular transport.

PMID: 21987765 [PubMed - indexed for MEDLINE]

1133. J Infect Dis. 2011 Nov;204 Suppl 3:S878-83. doi: 10.1093/infdis/jir310.

The importance of the NP: VP35 ratio in Ebola virus nucleocapsid formation.

Noda T(1), Kolesnikova L, Becker S, Kawaoka Y.

Author information: (1)Department of Special Pathogens, International Research Center for Infectious Diseases, The Institute of Medical Science, The University of Tokyo, Japan. t-noda@ims.u-tokyo.ac.jp

Ebola virus VP35 is a cofactor of the viral RNA polymerase complex and, together with NP and VP24, is an essential component for nucleocapsid formation. In the present study, we examined the interactions between VP35 and NP and found that VP35 interacts with helical NP-RNA complexes through the C-terminus of NP. We also found that coexpression of excess VP35 with NP reduced the yields of NP-RNA complexes purified by CsCl gradient ultracentrifugation and inhibited the formation of the NP-induced inclusion bodies that typically form in Ebola virus-infected cells. These findings suggest that the NP to VP35 ratio is important in the Ebola virus replication cycle and advance our knowledge of nucleocapsid morphogenesis.

PMCID: PMC3189984 PMID: 21987764 [PubMed - indexed for MEDLINE]

1134. J Infect Dis. 2011 Nov;204 Suppl 3:S850-60. doi: 10.1093/infdis/jir378.

The Ebola virus glycoprotein and HIV-1 Vpu employ different strategies to counteract the antiviral factor tetherin.

Kühl A(1), Banning C, Marzi A, Votteler J, Steffen I, Bertram S, Glowacka I, Konrad A, Stürzl M, Guo JT, Schubert U, Feldmann H, Behrens G, Schindler M, Pöhlmann S.

Author information: (1)Institute of Virology, Hannover Medical School, Germany.

The antiviral protein tetherin/BST2/CD317/HM1.24 restricts cellular egress of human immunodeficiency virus (HIV) and of particles mimicking the Ebola virus (EBOV), a hemorrhagic fever virus. The HIV-1 viral protein U (Vpu) and the EBOV-glycoprotein (EBOV-GP) both inhibit tetherin. Here, we compared tetherin counteraction by EBOV-GP and Vpu. We found that EBOV-GP but not Vpu counteracted tetherin from different primate species, indicating that EBOV-GP and Vpu target tetherin differentially. Tetherin interacted with the GP2 subunit of EBOV-GP, which might encode the determinants for tetherin counteraction. Vpu reduced cell surface expression of tetherin while EBOV-GP did not, suggesting that both proteins employ different mechanisms to counteract tetherin. Finally, Marburg virus (MARV)-GP also inhibited tetherin and downregulated tetherin in a cell type-dependent fashion, indicating that tetherin antagonism depends on the cellular source of tetherin. Collectively, our results indicate that EBOV-GP counteracts tetherin by a novel mechanism and that tetherin inhibition is conserved between EBOV-GP and MARV-GP.

PMCID: PMC3189996 PMID: 21987761 [PubMed - indexed for MEDLINE]

1135. J Infect Dis. 2011 Nov;204 Suppl 3:S833-9. doi: 10.1093/infdis/jir305.

Unconventional secretion of Ebola virus matrix protein VP40.

Reynard O(1), Reid SP, Page A, Mateo M, Alazard-Dany N, Raoul H, Basler CF, Volchkov VE.

Author information: (1)Filovirus Laboratory, Inserm U758, Human Virology Department, Université de Lyon, Ecole Normale Supérieure de Lyon, Lyon, France.

The Ebola virus matrix protein VP40 plays an essential role in virus assembly and budding. In this study we reveal that transient VP40 expression results in the release into the culture medium of substantial amounts of soluble monomeric VP40 in addition to the release of virus-like particles containing an oligomeric form of this protein as previously described. We show that VP40 secretion is endoplasmic reticulum/Golgi-independent and is not associated with cell death. Soluble VP40 was observed during Ebola virus infection of cells and was also found in the serum of virus-infected animals albeit in lower amounts. Unconventional secretion of VP40 may therefore play a role in Ebola virus pathogenicity.

PMCID: PMC3189981 PMID: 21987759 [PubMed - indexed for MEDLINE]

1136. J Infect Dis. 2011 Nov;204 Suppl 3:S825-32. doi: 10.1093/infdis/jir295.

Impact of Ebola mucin-like domain on antiglycoprotein antibody responses induced by Ebola virus-like particles.

Martinez O(1), Tantral L, Mulherkar N, Chandran K, Basler CF.

Author information: (1)Department of Microbiology, Mount Sinai School of Medicine, New York, NY 10029, USA.

Ebola virus (EBOV) glycoprotein (GP), responsible for mediating host-cell attachment and membrane fusion, contains a heavily glycosylated mucin-like domain hypothesized to shield GP from neutralizing antibodies. To test whether the mucin-like domain inhibits the production and function of anti-GP antibodies, we vaccinated mice with Ebola virus-like particles (VLPs) that express vesicular stomatitis virus G, wild-type EBOV GP (EBGP), EBOV GP without its mucin-like domain (ΔMucGP), or EBOV GP with a Crimean-Congo hemorrhagic fever virus mucin-like domain substituted for the EBOV mucin-like domain (CMsubGP). EBGP-VLP immunized mice elicited significantly higher serum antibody titers toward EBGP or its mutants, as detected by western blot analysis, than did VLP-ΔMucGP. However, EBGP-, ΔMucGP- and CMsubGP-VLP immunized mouse sera contained antibodies that bound to cell surface-expressed GP at similar levels. Furthermore, low but similar neutralizing antibody titers, measured against a vesicular stomatitis virus (VSV) expressing EBGP or ΔMucGP, were present in EBGP, ΔMucGP, and CMsubGP sera, although a slightly higher neutralizing titer (2- to 2.5-fold) was detected in ΔMucGP sera. We conclude that the EBOV GP mucin-like domain can increase relative anti-GP titers, however these titers appear to be directed, at least partly, to denatured GP. Furthermore, removing the mucin-like domain from immunizing VLPs has modest impact on neutralizing antibody titers in serum.

PMCID: PMC3189980 PMID: 21987758 [PubMed - indexed for MEDLINE]

1137. J Infect Dis. 2011 Nov;204 Suppl 3:S817-24. doi: 10.1093/infdis/jir293.

Characterization of filovirus protein-protein interactions in mammalian cells using bimolecular complementation.

Liu Y(1), Stone S, Harty RN.

Author information: (1)Department of Pathobiology, School of Veterinary Medicine, University of Pennsylvania, Philadelphia, PA 19104, USA.

The virion protein 40 (VP40) and nucleoprotein (NP) of Ebola (EBOV) and Marburg viruses (MARV) play key roles during virion assembly and egress. The ability to detect interactions between VP40-VP40, VP40-NP, and NP-NP and follow these complexes as they traffic through mammalian cells would enhance our understanding of the molecular events leading to filovirus assembly and budding, and provide new insights into filovirus replication and pathogenesis. Here, we successfully employed a bimolecular complementation (BiMC) approach to visualize interactions between EBOV and MARV VP40-VP40, NP-NP, and VP40-NP proteins and localize these protein complexes in mammalian cells using confocal microscopy. We demonstrate that VP40-VP40 complexes localized predominantly at the plasma membrane, whereas VP40-NP and NP-NP complexes displayed a more dispersed pattern throughout the cytoplasm. As expected based on previous findings, efficient interactions between EBOV or MARV VP40-VP40 proteins were independent of L-domains PTAPPEY and PPPY, respectively. In contrast, the formation of EBOV or MARV VP40-VP40 complexes was dependent on the previously characterized LPLGVA and LPLGIM motifs of EBOV and MARV VP40 proteins, respectively, indicating that these motifs are important for VP40 oligomerization and subsequent budding. These results highlight the feasibility and usefulness of the BiMC approach as a strategy to further characterize both filovirus protein interactions as well as filovirus-host interactions in real time in the natural environment of the cell.

PMCID: PMC3189979 PMID: 21987757 [PubMed - indexed for MEDLINE]

1138. J Infect Dis. 2011 Nov;204 Suppl 3:S810-6. doi: 10.1093/infdis/jir299.

Basic clinical and laboratory features of filoviral hemorrhagic fever.

Kortepeter MG(1), Bausch DG, Bray M.

Author information: (1)Department of Preventive Medicine, Infectious Disease Clinical Research Program, Uniformed Services University of Health Sciences, Bethesda, Maryland 20814-5119, USA. mkortepeter@idcrp.org

The filoviruses Marburg and Ebola cause severe hemorrhagic fever (HF) in humans. Beginning with the 1967 Marburg outbreak, 30 epidemics, isolated cases, and accidental laboratory infections have been described in the medical literature. We reviewed those reports to determine the basic clinical and laboratory features of filoviral HF. The most detailed information was found in descriptions of patients treated in industrialized countries; except for the 2000 outbreak of Ebola Sudan HF in Uganda, reports of epidemics in central Africa provided little controlled or objective clinical data. Other than the case fatality rate, there were no clear differences in the features of the various filovirus infections. This compilation will be of value to medical workers responding to epidemics and to investigators attempting to develop animal models of filoviral HF. By identifying key unanswered questions and gaps in clinical data, it will help guide clinical research in future outbreaks.

PMID: 21987756 [PubMed - indexed for MEDLINE]

1139. J Infect Dis. 2011 Nov;204 Suppl 3:S804-9. doi: 10.1093/infdis/jir300.

Ebola Reston virus infection of pigs: clinical significance and transmission potential.

Marsh GA(1), Haining J, Robinson R, Foord A, Yamada M, Barr JA, Payne J, White J, Yu M, Bingham J, Rollin PE, Nichol ST, Wang LF, Middleton D.

Author information: (1)Australian Animal Health Laboratory, Livestock Industries, Commonwealth Scientific and Industrial Research Organisation (CSIRO), Geelong, Australia. glenn.marsh@csiro.au

In 2008, Reston ebolavirus (REBOV) was isolated from pigs during a disease investigation in the Philippines. Porcine reproductive and respiratory syndrome virus (PRRSV) and porcine circovirus type 2 (PCV-2) infections were also confirmed in affected herds and the contribution of REBOV to the disease outbreak remains uncertain. We have conducted experimental challenge studies in 5-week-old pigs, with exposure of animals to 10(6) TCID(50) of a 2008 swine isolate of REBOV via either the oronasal or subcutaneous route. Replication of virus in internal organs and viral shedding from the nasopharynx were documented in the absence of clinical signs of disease in infected pigs. These observations confirm not only that asymptomatic infection of pigs with REBOV occurs, but that animals so affected pose a transmission risk to farm, veterinary, and abattoir workers.

PMID: 21987755 [PubMed - indexed for MEDLINE]

1140. J Infect Dis. 2011 Nov;204 Suppl 3:S785-90. doi: 10.1093/infdis/jir298.

Management of accidental exposure to Ebola virus in the biosafety level 4 laboratory, Hamburg, Germany.

Günther S(1), Feldmann H, Geisbert TW, Hensley LE, Rollin PE, Nichol ST, Ströher U, Artsob H, Peters CJ, Ksiazek TG, Becker S, ter Meulen J, Olschläger S, Schmidt-Chanasit J, Sudeck H, Burchard GD, Schmiedel S.

Author information: (1)Department of Virology, Bernhard Nocht Institute for Tropical Medicine, Hamburg, Germany. guenther@bni.uni-hamburg.de

A needlestick injury occurred during an animal experiment in the biosafety level 4 laboratory in Hamburg, Germany, in March 2009. The syringe contained Zaire ebolavirus (ZEBOV) mixed with Freund's adjuvant. Neither an approved treatment nor a postexposure prophylaxis (PEP) exists for Ebola hemorrhagic fever. Following a risk-benefit assessment, it was recommended the exposed person take an experimental vaccine that had shown PEP efficacy in ZEBOV-infected nonhuman primates (NHPs) [12]. The vaccine, which had not been used previously in humans, was a live-attenuated recombinant vesicular stomatitis virus (recVSV) expressing the glycoprotein of ZEBOV. A single dose of 5 × 10(7) plaque-forming units was injected 48 hours after the accident. The vaccinee developed fever 12 hours later and recVSV viremia was detectable by polymerase chain reaction (PCR) for 2 days. Otherwise, the person remained healthy, and ZEBOV RNA, except for the glycoprotein gene expressed in the vaccine, was never detected in serum and peripheral blood mononuclear cells during the 3-week observation period.

PMID: 21987751 [PubMed - indexed for MEDLINE]
1141. J Infect Dis. 2011 Nov;204 Suppl 3:S776-84. doi: 10.1093/infdis/jir364.

Emergence of divergent Zaire ebola virus strains in Democratic Republic of the Congo in 2007 and 2008.

Grard G(1), Biek R, Tamfum JJ, Fair J, Wolfe N, Formenty P, Paweska J, Leroy E.

Author information: (1)Centre International de Recherches Médicales de Franceville, Gabon. gildagrard@gmail.com

BACKGROUND: Zaire ebolavirus was responsible for 2 outbreaks in Democratic Republic of the Congo (DRC), in 1976 and 1995. The virus reemerged in DRC 12 years later, causing 2 successive outbreaks in the Luebo region, Kasai Occidental province, in 2007 and 2008. METHODS: Viruses of each outbreak were isolated and the full-length genomes were characterized. Phylogenetic analysis was then undertaken to characterize the relationships with previously described viruses. RESULTS: The 2 Luebo viruses are nearly identical but are not related to lineage A viruses known in DRC or to descendants of the lineage B viruses encountered in the Gabon-Republic of the Congo area, with which they do, however, share a common ancestor. CONCLUSIONS: Our findings strongly suggest that the Luebo 2007 outbreak did not result from viral spread from previously identified foci but from an independent viral emergence. The previously identified epidemiological link with migratory bat species known to carry Zaire ebolavirus RNA support the hypothesis of viral spillover from this widely dispersed reservoir. The high level of similarity between the Luebo2007 and Luebo2008 viruses suggests that local wildlife populations (most likely bats) became infected and allowed local viral persistence and reemergence from year to year.

PMCID: PMC3218671 PMID: 21987750 [PubMed - indexed for MEDLINE]
1142. J Infect Dis. 2011 Nov;204 Suppl 3:S768-75. doi: 10.1093/infdis/jir344.

Risk factors for Zaire ebolavirus--specific IgG in rural Gabonese populations.

Nkoghe D(1), Padilla C, Becquart P, Wauquier N, Moussavou G, Akué JP, Ollomo B, Pourrut X, Souris M, Kazanji M, Gonzalez JP, Leroy E.

Author information: (1)Centre International de Recherches Médicales de Franceville, Franceville, Gabon. dnkoghe@hotmail.com

BACKGROUND: In Gabon, several Ebolavirus outbreaks have occurred exclusively in the northeastern region. We conducted a large serosurvey to identify areas and populations at risk and potential demographic, clinical, and behavioral risk factors. METHODS: Blood samples and clinical and sociodemographic data were collected from 4349 adults and 362 children in a random sample of 220 villages in the 9 provinces of Gabon. An enzyme-linked immunosorbent assay was used to detect Zaire ebolavirus (ZEBOV)-specific IgG, and thin blood smears were used to detect parasites. Logistic regression was implemented using Stata software (Stata), and a probability level of < .001) in forest areas. No sociodemographic risk factors were found, but the antibody prevalence increased linearly up to 20 years of age. Chronic arthralgia and amicrofilaremia were the only factors associated with ZEBOV seropositivity. CONCLUSIONS: These findings confirm the endemicity of ZEBOV in Gabon and its link to the ecosystem. Human antibody positivity would appear to be to the result of exposure to contaminated fruits.

PMID: 21987749 [PubMed - indexed for MEDLINE]
1143. J Infect Dis. 2011 Nov;204 Suppl 3:S761-7. doi: 10.1093/infdis/jir294.

Filovirus outbreak detection and surveillance: lessons from Bundibugyo.

MacNeil A(1), Farnon EC, Morgan OW, Gould P, Boehmer TK, Blaney DD, Wiersma P, Tappero JW, Nichol ST, Ksiazek TG, Rollin PE.

Author information: (1)Viral Special Pathogens Branch, The Centers for Disease Control and Prevention, Atlanta, Georgia 30333, USA. aho3@cdc.gov

The first outbreak of Ebola hemorrhagic fever (EHF) due to Bundibugyo ebolavirus occurred in Uganda from August to December 2007. During outbreak response and assessment, we identified 131 EHF cases (44 suspect, 31 probable, and 56 confirmed). Consistent with previous large filovirus outbreaks, a long temporal lag (approximately 3 months) occurred between initial EHF cases and the subsequent identification of Ebola virus and outbreak response, which allowed for prolonged person-to-person transmission of the virus. Although effective control measures for filovirus outbreaks, such as patient isolation and contact tracing, are well established, our observations from the Bundibugyo EHF outbreak demonstrate the need for improved filovirus surveillance, reporting, and diagnostics, in endemic locations in Africa.

PMID: 21987748 [PubMed - indexed for MEDLINE]
1144. J Infect Dis. 2011 Nov;204 Suppl 3:S757-60. doi: 10.1093/infdis/jir296.

Reston ebolavirus in humans and animals in the Philippines: a review.

Miranda ME(1), Miranda NL.

Author information: (1)Veterinary Public Health Consultants, Research Institute for Tropical Medicine, Muntinlupa City, Philippines. betsygmiranda@gmail.com

The 2008 Reston ebolavirus infection event in domestic pigs has triggered continuing epidemiologic investigations among Philippine health and veterinary agencies in collaboration with international filovirus experts. Prior to this, there were only 3 known and documented Reston ebolavirus outbreaks in nonhuman primates in the world, all traced back to a single geographic source in the Philippines in a monkey breeding/export facility. The first one in 1989 was the first-ever Ebola virus that emerged outside of Africa and was also the first known natural infection of Ebola virus in nonhuman primates. When it was first discovered among laboratory monkeys in the United States, the source was immediately traced back to the farm located in the Philippines. The second outbreak was in 1992-93. The third episode in 1996 was the last known outbreak before Reston ebolavirus reemerged in pigs in 2008. The isolated outbreaks involving 2 animal species bring forth issues requiring further investigations, and highlight the significance of intersectoral collaboration to effectively address zoonoses prevention and control/response in the interest of minimizing public health risk.

PMID: 21987747 [PubMed - indexed for MEDLINE]
1145. J Infect Dis. 2011 Nov;204 Suppl 3:S1090-7. doi: 10.1093/infdis/jir379.

Protective efficacy of a bivalent recombinant vesicular stomatitis virus vaccine in the Syrian hamster model of lethal Ebola virus infection.

Tsuda Y(1), Safronetz D, Brown K, LaCasse R, Marzi A, Ebihara H, Feldmann H.
Author information: (1)Laboratory of Virology, Division of Intramural Research, National Institute of Allergy and Infectious Diseases, National Institutes of Health, Hamilton, Montana, USA.

BACKGROUND: Outbreaks of filoviral hemorrhagic fever occur sporadically and unpredictably across wide regions in central Africa and overlap with the occurrence of other infectious diseases of public health importance. METHODS: As a proof of concept we developed a bivalent recombinant vaccine based on vesicular stomatitis virus (VSV) expressing the Zaire ebolavirus (ZEBOV) and Andes virus (ANDV) glycoproteins (VSVΔG/Dual) and evaluated its protective efficacy in the common lethal Syrian hamster model. Hamsters were vaccinated with VSVΔG/Dual and were lethally challenged with ZEBOV or ANDV. Time to immunity and postexposure treatment were evaluated by immunizing hamsters at different times prior to and post ZEBOV challenge. RESULTS: A single immunization with VSVΔG/Dual conferred complete and sterile protection against lethal ZEBOV and ANDV challenge. Complete protection was achieved with an immunization as close as 3 days prior to ZEBOV challenge, and 40% of the animals were even protected when treated with VSVΔG/Dual one day postchallenge. In comparison to the monovalent VSV vaccine, the bivalent vaccine has slightly reduced postexposure efficacy most likely due to its restricted lymphoid organ replication. CONCLUSIONS: Bivalent VSV vectors are a feasible approach to vaccination against multiple pathogens.
PMCID: PMC3189997 PMID: 21987746 [PubMed - indexed for MEDLINE]

1146. J Infect Dis. 2011 Nov;204 Suppl 3:S1082-9. doi: 10.1093/infdis/jir350.

Single immunization with a monovalent vesicular stomatitis virus-based vaccine protects nonhuman primates against heterologous challenge with Bundibugyo ebolavirus.

Falzarano D(1), Feldmann F, Grolla A, Leung A, Ebihara H, Strong JE, Marzi A, Takada A, Jones S, Gren J, Geisbert J, Jones SM, Geisbert TW, Feldmann H.
Author information: (1)Special Pathogens Program, National Microbiology Laboratory, Public Health Agency of Canada, Winnipeg, Canada.

The recombinant vesicular stomatitis virus (rVSV) vector-based monovalent vaccine platform expressing a filovirus glycoprotein has been demonstrated to provide protection from lethal challenge with Ebola (EBOV) and Marburg (MARV) viruses both prophylactically and after exposure. This platform provides protection between heterologous strains within a species; however, protection from lethal challenge between species has been largely unsuccessful. To determine whether the rVSV-EBOV vaccines have the potential to provide protection against a newly emerging, phylogenetically related species, cynomolgus macaques were vaccinated with an rVSV vaccine expressing either the glycoprotein of Zaire ebolavirus (ZEBOV) or Côte d'Ivoire ebolavirus (CIEBOV) and then challenged with Bundibugyo ebolavirus (BEBOV), which was recently proposed as a new EBOV species following an outbreak in Uganda in 2007. A single vaccination with the ZEBOV-specific vaccine provided cross-protection (75% survival) against subsequent BEBOV challenge, whereas vaccination with the CIEBOV-specific vaccine resulted in an outcome similar to mock-immunized animals (33% and 25% survival, respectively). This demonstrates that monovalent rVSV-based vaccines may be useful against a newly emerging species; however, heterologous protection across species remains challenging and may depend on enhancing the immune responses either through booster immunizations or through the inclusion of multiple immunogens.
PMCID: PMC3189995 PMID: 21987745 [PubMed - indexed for MEDLINE]

1147. J Infect Dis. 2011 Nov;204 Suppl 3:S1075-81. doi: 10.1093/infdis/jir349.

Recombinant vesicular stomatitis virus-based vaccines against Ebola and Marburg virus infections.

Geisbert TW(1), Feldmann H.
Author information: (1)Galveston National Laboratory, University of Texas Medical Branch, 301 University Blvd., Galveston, TX 77550-0610, USA.
tom.geisbert@utmb.edu

The filoviruses, Marburg virus and Ebola virus, cause severe hemorrhagic fever with a high mortality rate in humans and nonhuman primates. Among the most-promising filovirus vaccines under development is a system based on recombinant vesicular stomatitis virus (rVSV) that expresses a single filovirus glycoprotein (GP) in place of the VSV glycoprotein (G). Importantly, a single injection of blended rVSV-based filovirus vaccines was shown to completely protect nonhuman primates against Marburg virus and 3 different species of Ebola virus. These rVSV-based vaccines have also shown utility when administered as a postexposure treatment against filovirus infections, and a rVSV-based Ebola virus vaccine was recently used to treat a potential laboratory exposure. Here, we review the history of rVSV-based vaccines and pivotal animal studies showing their utility in combating Ebola and Marburg virus infections.
PMCID: PMC3218670 PMID: 21987744 [PubMed - indexed for MEDLINE]

1148. J Infect Dis. 2011 Nov;204 Suppl 3:S1066-74. doi: 10.1093/infdis/jir348.

Vesicular stomatitis virus-based Ebola vaccines with improved cross-protective efficacy.

Marzi A(1), Ebihara H, Callison J, Groseth A, Williams KJ, Geisbert TW, Feldmann H.
Author information: (1)Laboratory of Virology, Division of Intramural Research, National Institute of Allergy and Infectious Diseases, National Institute of Health, Hamilton, Montana 59840, USA.

For Ebola virus (EBOV), 4 different species are known: Zaire, Sudan, Côte d'Ivoire, and Reston ebolavirus. The newly discovered Bundibugyo ebolavirus has been proposed as a 5th species. So far, no cross-neutralization among EBOV species has been described, aggravating progress toward cross-species protective vaccines. With the use of recombinant vesicular stomatitis virus (rVSV)-based vaccines, guinea pigs could be protected against Zaire ebolavirus (ZEBOV) infection only when immunized with a vector expressing the homologous, but not a heterologous, EBOV glycoprotein (GP). However, infection of guinea pigs with nonadapted wild-type strains of the different species resulted in full protection of all animals against subsequent challenge with guinea pig-adapted ZEBOV, showing that cross-species protection is possible. New vectors were generated that contain EBOV viral protein 40 (VP40) or EBOV nucleoprotein (NP) as a second antigen expressed by the same rVSV vector that encodes the heterologous GP. After applying a 2-dose immunization approach, we observed an improved cross-protection rate, with 5 of 6 guinea pigs surviving the lethal ZEBOV challenge if vaccinated with rVSV-expressing SEBOV-GP and -VP40. Our data demonstrate that cross-protection between the EBOV species can be achieved, although EBOV-GP alone cannot induce the required immune response.

PMCID: PMC3203393 PMID: 21987743 [PubMed - indexed for MEDLINE]

1149. J Infect Dis. 2011 Nov;204 Suppl 3:S1060-5. doi: 10.1093/infdis/jir347.

Kunjin virus replicon-based vaccines expressing Ebola virus glycoprotein GP protect the guinea pig against lethal Ebola virus infection.

Reynard O(1), Mokhonov V, Mokhonova E, Leung J, Page A, Mateo M, Pyankova O, Georges-Courbot MC, Raoul H, Khromykh AA, Volchkov VE.

Author information: (1)Filovirus Laboratory, INSERM U758, Human Virology Department, Claude Bernard University Lyon-1, Université de Lyon, Ecole Normale Supérieure de Lyon, Lyon, France.

Pre- or postexposure treatments against the filoviral hemorrhagic fevers are currently not available for human use. We evaluated, in a guinea pig model, the immunogenic potential of Kunjin virus (KUN)-derived replicons as a vaccine candidate against Ebola virus (EBOV). Virus like particles (VLPs) containing KUN replicons expressing EBOV wild-type glycoprotein GP, membrane anchor-truncated GP (GP/Ctr), and mutated GP (D637L) with enhanced shedding capacity were generated and assayed for their protective efficacy. Immunization with KUN VLPs expressing full-length wild-type and D637L-mutated GPs but not membrane anchor-truncated GP induced dose-dependent protection against a challenge of a lethal dose of recombinant guinea pig-adapted EBOV. The surviving animals showed complete clearance of the virus. Our results demonstrate the potential for KUN replicon vectors as vaccine candidates against EBOV infection.

PMCID: PMC3189994 PMID: 21987742 [PubMed - indexed for MEDLINE]

1150. J Infect Dis. 2011 Nov;204 Suppl 3:S1053-9. doi: 10.1093/infdis/jir346.

Advances in virus-like particle vaccines for filoviruses.

Warfield KL(1), Aman MJ.

Author information: (1)Vaccine Development, Integrated Biotherapeutics, 21 Firstfield Rd, Ste 100, Gaithersburg, MD 20878, USA. kelly@integratedbiotherapeutics.com

Ebola virus (EBOV) and Marburg virus (MARV) are among the deadliest human pathogens, with no vaccines or therapeutics available. Multiple vaccine platforms have been tested for efficacy as prophylactic pretreatments or therapeutics for prevention of filovirus hemorrhagic fever. Most successful vaccines are based on a virus-vectored approach expressing the protective glycoprotein (GP); protein-based subunit and DNA vaccines have been tested with moderate success. Virus-like particle (VLP) vaccines have realized promising results when tested in both rodents and nonhuman primates. VLPs rely on the natural properties of the viral matrix protein (VP) 40 to drive budding of filamentous particles that can also incorporate ≥ 1 other filovirus protein, including GP, VP24, and nucleoprotein (NP). Filovirus VLP vaccines have used particles containing 2 or 3 (GP and VP40, with or without NP) viral proteins generated in either mammalian or insect cells. Early studies successfully demonstrated efficacy of bivalent VLP vaccines in rodents; more recent studies have shown the ability of the VLP vaccines containing GP, NP, and VP40 to confer complete homologous protection against Ebola virus and Marburg virus in a prophylactic setting against in macaques. This review will discuss published work to date regarding development of the VLP vaccines for prevention of lethal filovirus hemorrhagic fever.

PMCID: PMC3189993 PMID: 21987741 [PubMed - indexed for MEDLINE]

1151. J Infect Dis. 2011 Nov;204 Suppl 3:S1043-52. doi: 10.1093/infdis/jir345.

Therapeutics of Ebola hemorrhagic fever: whole-genome transcriptional analysis of successful disease mitigation.

Yen JY(1), Garamszegi S, Geisbert JB, Rubins KH, Geisbert TW, Honko A, Xia Y, Connor JH, Hensley LE.

Author information: (1)Department of Microbiology, Boston University School of Medicine, Boston, MA 02118, USA.

The mechanisms of Ebola (EBOV) pathogenesis are only partially understood, but the dysregulation of normal host immune responses (including destruction of lymphocytes, increases in circulating cytokine levels, and development of coagulation abnormalities) is thought to play a major role. Accumulating evidence suggests that much of the observed pathology is not the direct result of virus-induced structural damage but rather is due to the release of soluble immune mediators from EBOV-infected cells. It is therefore essential to understand how the candidate therapeutic may be interrupting the disease process and/or targeting the infectious agent. To identify genetic signatures that are correlates of protection, we used a DNA microarray-based approach to compare the host genome-wide responses of EBOV-infected nonhuman primates (NHPs) responding to candidate therapeutics. We observed that, although the overall circulating immune response was similar in the presence and absence of coagulation inhibitors, surviving NHPs clustered together. Noticeable differences in coagulation-associated genes appeared to correlate with survival, which revealed a subset of distinctly differentially expressed genes, including chemokine ligand 8 (CCL8/MCP-2), that may provide possible targets for early-stage diagnostics or future therapeutics. These analyses will assist us in understanding the pathogenic mechanisms of EBOV infection and in identifying improved therapeutic strategies.

PMID: 21987740 [PubMed - indexed for MEDLINE]

1152. J Infect Dis. 2011 Nov;204 Suppl 3:S1032-42. doi: 10.1093/infdis/jir332.

Impact of systemic or mucosal immunity to adenovirus on Ad-based Ebola virus vaccine efficacy in guinea pigs.

Richardson JS(1), Abou MC, Tran KN, Kumar A, Sahai BM, Kobinger GP.

Author information: (1)Special Pathogens Department, National Microbiology Laboratory, Public Health Agency of Canada, Winnipeg, Canada.

BACKGROUND: Approximately 35% of the North American population and an estimated 90% of the sub-Saharan African population have antibodies against adenovirus serotype 5 (AdHu5) that are capable of neutralizing AdHu5-based vaccines. In mice, intranasal delivery of AdHu5 expressing the Zaire ebolavirus glycoprotein human adenovirus serotype 5 (Ad) containing the genes for the Zaire ebolavirus glycoprotein (ZGP) under the expressional control of a cytomegalovirus immediate early promoter (CMV)) can bypass systemic preexisting immunity, resulting in protection against mouse-adapted Zaire ebolavirus (Mayinga 1976). METHODS: Guinea pigs administered an adenovirus-based Ebola virus vaccine either intramuscularly or intranasally in the presence of systemically or mucosally induced adenovirus immunity were challenged with a lethal dose of guinea pig-adapted Zaire ebolavirus (Mayinga 1976) (GA-ZEBOV). The humoral immune response was assayed to determine the effect of vaccine delivery route and preexisting immunity. RESULTS: Intramuscular or intranasal vaccination fully protected guinea pigs against a lethal GA-ZEBOV challenge. However, intramuscular vaccination in animals with systemically induced preexisting immunity resulted in low survival following challenge. Interestingly, intranasal vaccination protected guinea pigs with systemic preexisting immunity to AdHu5. Mucosal adenoviral immunity induced by intranasal administration of AdHu5 decreased protection following intranasal vaccination with the first-generation but not with the second-generation vaccine. CONCLUSIONS: Intranasal vaccination is an effective vaccine delivery route in the presence of systemic and, to a lower extent, mucosal preexisting immunity to the vaccine vector in guinea pigs.

PMID: 21987739 [PubMed - indexed for MEDLINE]

1153. J Infect Dis. 2011 Nov;204 Suppl 3:S1021-31. doi: 10.1093/infdis/jir339.

Pathogenesis of Marburg hemorrhagic fever in cynomolgus macaques.

Hensley LE(1), Alves DA, Geisbert JB, Fritz EA, Reed C, Larsen T, Geisbert TW.

Author information: (1)Virology Division, US Army Medical Research Institute of Infectious Diseases, Fort Detrick, Maryland, USA.

BACKGROUND: Marburg virus (MARV) infection causes a severe and often fatal hemorrhagic disease in primates; however, little is known about the development of MARV hemorrhagic fever. In this study we evaluated the progression of MARV infection in nonhuman primates. METHODS: Eighteen cynomolgus monkeys were infected with MARV; blood and tissues were examined sequentially over an 8-day period to investigate disease pathogenesis. RESULTS: Disease caused by MARV in cynomolgus macaques was very similar to disease previously described for Ebola virus-infected macaques. Monocytes, macrophages, Kupffer cells, and dendritic cells (DCs) were identified as the initial targets of MARV infection. Bystander lymphocyte apoptosis occurred at early stages in the disease course in intravascular and extravascular locations. The loss of splenic and lymph node DCs or downregulation of dendritic cell-specific intercellular adhesion molecule-3-grabbing non-integrin (DC-SIGN) on DCs as early as day 2 and continuing through day 8 after MARV infection was a prominent finding. Evidence of disseminated intravascular coagulation was noted; however, the degree of fibrin deposition in tissues was less prominent than was reported in Ebola-infected macaques. CONCLUSIONS: The sequence of pathogenic events identified in this study provides an understanding of the development of disease processes and also may provide new targets for rational prophylactic and chemotherapeutic interventions.

PMID: 21987738 [PubMed - indexed for MEDLINE]

1154. J Infect Dis. 2011 Nov;204 Suppl 3:S1011-20. doi: 10.1093/infdis/jir338.

VP24 is a molecular determinant of Ebola virus virulence in guinea pigs.

Mateo M(1), Carbonnelle C, Reynard O, Kolesnikova L, Nemirov K, Page A, Volchkova VA, Volchkov VE.

Author information: (1)Filovirus Laboratory, INSERM U758, Human Virology Department, Université de Lyon, Ecole Normale Supérieure de Lyon, Lyon, France.

In sharp contrast to human and nonhuman primates, guinea pigs and some other mammals resist Ebola virus (EBOV) replication and do not develop illness upon virus inoculation. However, serial passaging of EBOV in guinea pigs results in a selection of variants with high pathogenicity. In this report, using a reverse genetics approach, we demonstrate that this dramatic increase in EBOV pathogenicity is associated with amino acid substitutions in the structural protein VP24. We show that although replication of recombinant EBOV carrying wild-type VP24 is impaired in primary peritoneal guinea pig macrophages and in the liver of infected animals, the substitutions in VP24 allow EBOV to replicate in guinea pig macrophages and spread in the liver of infected animals. Furthermore, we demonstrate that both VP24/wild type and the guinea pig-adapted VP24/8mc are similar in their ability to block expression of interferon-induced host genes, suggesting that the increase in EBOV virulence for guinea pigs is not associated with VP24 interferon antagonist function. This study sheds light on the mechanism of resistance to EBOV infection and highlights the critical role of VP24 in EBOV pathogenesis.

PMID: 21987737 [PubMed - indexed for MEDLINE]

1155. J Infect Dis. 2011 Nov;204 Suppl 3:S1000-10. doi: 10.1093/infdis/jir337.

Real-time monitoring of cardiovascular function in rhesus macaques infected with Zaire ebolavirus.

Kortepeter MG(1), Lawler JV, Honko A, Bray M, Johnson JC, Purcell BK, Olinger GG, Rivard R, Hepburn MJ, Hensley LE.

Author information: (1)Department of Preventive Medicine, Infectious Disease Clinical Research Program, Uniformed Services University, Bethesda, MD 20814, USA. mkortepeter@idcrp.org

Nine rhesus macaques were implanted with multisensor telemetry devices and internal jugular vein catheters before being infected with Zaire ebolavirus. All animals developed viremia, fever, a hemorrhagic rash, and typical changes of Ebola hemorrhagic fever in clinical laboratory tests. Three macaques unexpectedly survived this usually lethal disease, making it possible to compare physiological parameters in lethally challenged animals and survivors. After the onset of fever, lethal illness was characterized by a decline in mean arterial blood pressure, an increase in pulse and respiratory rate, lactic acidosis, and renal failure. Survivors showed less pronounced change in these parameters. Four macaques were randomized to receive supplemental volumes of intravenous normal saline when they became hypotensive. Although those animals had less severe renal compromise, no apparent survival benefit was observed. This is the first report of continuous physiologic monitoring in filovirus-infected nonhuman primates and the first to attempt cardiovascular support with intravenous fluids.

PMID: 21987736 [PubMed - indexed for MEDLINE]

1156. J Virol. 2011 Nov;85(22):11709-24. doi: 10.1128/JVI.05040-11. Epub 2011 Sep 7.

Crystal structure of swine major histocompatibility complex class I SLA-1 0401 and identification of 2009 pandemic swine-origin influenza A H1N1 virus cytotoxic T lymphocyte epitope peptides.

Zhang N(1), Qi J, Feng S, Gao F, Liu J, Pan X, Chen R, Li Q, Chen Z, Li X, Xia C, Gao GF.

Author information: (1)Department of Microbiology and Immunology, College of Veterinary Medicine, China Agricultural University, Beijing 100094, China.

The presentation of viral epitopes to cytotoxic T lymphocytes (CTLs) by swine leukocyte antigen class I (SLA I) is crucial for swine immunity. To illustrate the structural basis of swine CTL epitope presentation, the first SLA crystal structures, SLA-1 0401, complexed with peptides derived from either 2009 pandemic H1N1 (pH1N1) swine-origin influenza A virus (S-OIV(NW9); NSDTVGWSW) or Ebola virus (Ebola(AY9); ATAAATEAY) were determined in this study. The overall peptide-SLA-1 0401 structures resemble, as expected, the general conformations of other structure-solved peptide major histocompatibility complexes (pMHC). The major distinction of SLA-1 0401 is that Arg(156) has a "one-ballot veto" function in peptide binding, due to its flexible side chain. S-OIV(NW9) and Ebola(AY9) bind SLA-1 0401 with similar conformations but employ different water molecules to stabilize their binding. The side chain of P7 residues in both peptides is exposed, indicating that the epitopes are "featured" peptides presented by this SLA. Further analyses showed that SLA-1 0401 and human leukocyte antigen (HLA) class I HLA-A 0101 can present the same peptides, but in different conformations, demonstrating cross-species epitope presentation. CTL epitope peptides derived from 2009 pandemic S-OIV were screened and evaluated by the in vitro refolding method. Three peptides were identified as potential cross-species influenza virus (IV) CTL epitopes. The binding motif of SLA-1 0401 was proposed, and thermostabilities of key peptide-SLA-1 0401 complexes were analyzed by circular dichroism spectra. Our results not only provide the structural basis of peptide presentation by SLA I but also identify some IV CTL epitope peptides. These results will benefit both vaccine development and swine organ-based xenotransplantation.

PMCID: PMC3209268 PMID: 21900158 [PubMed - indexed for MEDLINE]

1157. PLoS Negl Trop Dis. 2011 Nov;5(11):e1395. doi: 10.1371/journal.pntd.0001395. Epub 2011 Nov 15.

Ebola virus glycoprotein needs an additional trigger, beyond proteolytic priming for membrane fusion.

Bale S(1), Liu T, Li S, Wang Y, Abelson D, Fusco M, Woods VL Jr, Saphire EO.

Author information: (1)Department of Immunology and Microbial Science, The Scripps Research Institute, La Jolla, California, USA.

BACKGROUND: Ebolavirus belongs to the family filoviridae and causes severe hemorrhagic fever in humans with 50-90% lethality. Detailed understanding of how the viruses attach to and enter new host cells is critical to development of medical interventions. The virus displays a trimeric glycoprotein (GP(1,2)) on its surface that is solely responsible for membrane attachment, virus internalization and fusion. GP(1,2) is expressed as a single peptide and is cleaved by furin in the host cells to yield two disulphide-linked fragments termed GP1 and GP2 that remain associated in a GP(1,2) trimeric, viral surface spike. After entry into host endosomes, GP(1,2) is enzymatically cleaved by endosomal cathepsins B and L, a necessary step in infection. However, the functional effects of the cleavage on the glycoprotein are unknown. PRINCIPAL FINDINGS: We demonstrate by antibody binding and Hydrogen-Deuterium Exchange Mass Spectrometry (DXMS) of glycoproteins from two different ebolaviruses that although enzymatic priming of GP(1,2) is required for fusion, the priming itself does not initiate the required conformational changes in the ectodomain of GP(1,2). Further, ELISA binding data of primed GP(1,2) to conformational antibody KZ52 suggests that the low pH inside the endosomes also does not trigger dissociation of GP1 from GP2 to effect membrane fusion. SIGNIFICANCE: The results reveal that the ebolavirus GP(1,2) ectodomain remains in the prefusion conformation upon enzymatic cleavage in low pH and removal of the glycan cap. The results also suggest that an additional endosomal trigger is necessary to induce the conformational changes in GP(1,2) and effect fusion. Identification of this trigger will provide further mechanistic insights into ebolavirus infection.

PMCID: PMC3216919 PMID: 22102923 [PubMed - indexed for MEDLINE]

1158. PLoS Pathog. 2011 Nov;7(11):e1002332. doi: 10.1371/journal.ppat.1002332. Epub 2011 Nov 3.

BST2/Tetherin enhances entry of human cytomegalovirus.

Viswanathan K(1), Smith MS, Malouli D, Mansouri M, Nelson JA, Früh K.

Author information: (1)Vaccine and Gene Therapy Institute, Oregon Health and Science University, Beaverton, Oregon, United States of America.

Interferon-induced BST2/Tetherin prevents budding of vpu-deficient HIV-1 by tethering mature viral particles to the plasma membrane. BST2 also inhibits release of other enveloped viruses including Ebola virus and Kaposi's sarcoma associated herpesvirus (KSHV), indicating that BST2 is a broadly acting antiviral host protein. Unexpectedly however, recovery of human cytomegalovirus (HCMV) from supernatants of BST2-expressing human fibroblasts was increased rather than decreased. Furthermore, BST2 seemed to enhance viral entry into cells since more virion proteins were released into BST2-expressing cells and subsequent viral gene expression was elevated. A significant increase in viral entry was also observed upon induction of endogenous BST2 during differentiation of the pro-monocytic cell line THP-1. Moreover, treatment of primary human monocytes with siRNA to BST2 reduced HCMV infection, suggesting that BST2 facilitates entry of HCMV into cells expressing high levels of BST2 either constitutively or in response to exogenous stimuli. Since BST2 is present in HCMV particles we propose that HCMV entry is enhanced via a reverse-tethering mechanism with BST2 in the viral envelope interacting with BST2 in the target cell membrane. Our data suggest that HCMV not only counteracts the well-established function of BST2 as inhibitor of viral egress but also employs this antiviral protein to gain entry into BST2-expressing hematopoietic cells, a process that might play a role in hematogenous dissemination of HCMV.

PMCID: PMC3207899 PMID: 22072961 [PubMed - indexed for MEDLINE]

1159. Virology. 2011 Oct 25;419(2):72-83. doi: 10.1016/j.virol.2011.08.009. Epub 2011 Sep 9.

The Ebola virus glycoprotein mediates entry via a non-classical dynamin-dependent macropinocytic pathway.

Mulherkar N(1), Raaben M, de la Torre JC, Whelan SP, Chandran K.

Author information: (1)Department of Microbiology and Immunology, Albert Einstein College of Medicine, Bronx, NY 10461, USA.

Ebola virus (EBOV) has been reported to enter cultured cell lines via a dynamin-2-independent macropinocytic pathway or clathrin-mediated endocytosis. The route(s) of productive EBOV internalization into physiologically relevant cell types remain unexplored, and viral-host requirements for this process are incompletely understood. Here, we use electron microscopy and complementary chemical and genetic approaches to demonstrate that the viral glycoprotein, GP, induces macropinocytic uptake of viral particles into cells. GP's highly-glycosylated mucin domain is dispensable for virus-induced macropinocytosis, arguing that interactions between other sequences in GP and the host cell surface are responsible. Unexpectedly, we also found a requirement for the large GTPase dynamin-2, which is proposed to be dispensable for several types of macropinocytosis. Our results provide evidence that EBOV uses an atypical dynamin-dependent macropinocytosis-like entry pathway to enter Vero cells, adherent human peripheral blood-derived monocytes, and a mouse dendritic cell line.

PMCID: PMC3177976 PMID: 21907381 [PubMed - indexed for MEDLINE]
1160. J Bioterror Biodef. 2011 Oct 20;(S1). pii: 007.

Evaluation of Different Strategies for Post-Exposure Treatment of Ebola Virus Infection in Rodents.

Richardson JS(1), Wong G, Pillet S, Schindle S, Ennis J, Turner J, Strong JE, Kobinger GP.

Author information: (1)Special Pathogens Program, National Microbiology Laboratory, Public Health Agency of Canada, Winnipeg, Manitoba, Canada.

Zaire Ebola virus (ZEBOV) is a pathogen that causes severe hemorrhagic fever in humans and non-human primates. There are currently no licensed vaccines or approved treatments available against ZEBOV infections. The goal of this work was to evaluate different treatment strategies in conjunction with a replication deficient, recombinant human adenovirus serotype 5-based vaccine expressing the Zaire Ebola virus glycoprotein (Ad-CAGoptZGP) in Ebola infected mice and guinea pigs. Guinea pigs were treated with Ad-CAGoptZGP in combination with different treatment strategies after challenge with guinea pig adapted-ZEBOV (GA-ZEBOV). B10.BR mice were used to further characterize efficacy and immune responses following co-administration of Ad-CAGoptZGP with the most effective treatment: AdHu5 expressing recombinant IFN-α (hereafter termed DEF201) after challenge with a lethal dose of mouse adapted-ZEBOV (MA-ZEBOV). In mice, DEF201 treatment was able to elicit full protection against a lethal dose of MA-ZEBOV when administered 30 minutes after infection. In guinea pigs the Ad-CAGoptZGP and DEF201 combination therapy elicited full protection when treated 30 minutes post-exposure and were a superior treatment to Ad-CAGoptZGP supplemented with recombinant IFN-α protein. Further analysis of the immune response revealed that addition of DEF201 to Ad-CAGoptZGP enhances the resulting adaptive immune response against ZGP. The results highlight the importance of the innate immune response in the prevention of ZEBOV pathogenesis and support further development of the Ad-CAGoptZGP with DEF201 treatment combination for post-exposure therapy against ZEBOV infection.

PMCID: PMC3509938 PMID: 23205319 [PubMed]
1161. Virology. 2011 Oct 10;419(1):1-9. doi: 10.1016/j.virol.2011.07.018. Epub 2011 Aug 19

Differential requirements for clathrin endocytic pathway components in cellular entry by Ebola and Marburg glycoprotein pseudovirions.

Bhattacharyya S(1), Hope TJ, Young JA.

Author information: (1)Nomis Center for Immunobiology and Microbial Pathogenesis, The Salk Institute for Biological Studies, 10010 N. Torrey Pines Road, La Jolla, CA 92037, USA.

Clathrin-mediated endocytosis was previously implicated as one of the cellular pathways involved in filoviral glycoprotein mediated viral entry into target cells. Here we have further dissected the requirements for different components of this pathway in Ebola versus Marburg virus glycoprotein (GP) mediated viral infection. Although a number of these components were involved in both cases; Ebola GP-dependent viral entry specifically required the cargo recognition proteins Eps15 and DAB2 as well as the clathrin adaptor protein AP-2. In contrast, Marburg GP-mediated infection was independent of these three proteins and instead required beta-arrestin 1 (ARRB1). These findings have revealed an unexpected difference between the clathrin pathway requirements for Ebola GP versus Marburg GP pseudovirion infection. Anthrax toxin also uses a clathrin-, and ARRB1-dependent pathway for cellular entry, indicating that the mechanism used by Marburg GP pseudovirions may be more generally important for pathogen entry.

PMCID: PMC3210186 PMID: 21855102 [PubMed - indexed for MEDLINE]
1162. Biochim Biophys Acta. 2011 Oct;1808(10):2343-51. doi: 10.1016/j.bbamem.2011.06.017. Epub 2011 Jul 5.

The fusogenic tilted peptide (67-78) of α-synuclein is a cholesterol binding domain.

Fantini J(1), Carlus D, Yahi N.

Author information: (1)Universite Paul Cezanne, France. jacques.fantini@univ-cezanne.fr

Parkinson's disease-associated α-synuclein is an amyloidogenic protein not only expressed in the cytoplasm of neurons, but also secreted in the extracellular space and internalized into glial cells through a lipid raft-dependent process. We previously showed that α-synuclein interacts with raft glycosphingolipids through a structural motif common to various viral and amyloidogenic proteins. Here we report that α-synuclein also interacts with cholesterol, as assessed by surface pressure measurements of cholesterol-containing monolayers. Using a panel of recombinant fragments and synthetic peptides, we identified two distinct cholesterol-binding domains in α-synuclein. One of these domains, which corresponds to the tilted peptide of α-synuclein (67-78), bound cholesterol with high affinity and was toxic for cultured astrocytes. Molecular modeling suggested that cholesterol binds to this peptide with a tilt angle of 46°. α-synuclein also contains a cholesterol recognition consensus motif, which had a lower affinity for cholesterol and was devoid of toxicity. This motif is encased in the glycosphingolipid-binding domain (34-45) of α-synuclein. In raft-like model membranes containing both cholesterol and glycosphingolipids, the head groups of glycosphingolipids prevented the accessibility of cholesterol to exogenous ligands. Nevertheless, cholesterol appeared to 'signal' its presence by tuning glycosphingolipid conformation, thereby facilitating α-synuclein binding to raft-like membranes. We propose that the association of α-synuclein with lipid rafts involves both the binding of α-synuclein (34-45) to glycosphingolipids, and the interaction of the fusogenic tilted peptide (67-78) with cholesterol. Coincidentally, a similar mechanism is used by viruses (HIV-I, HTLV-I, Ebola) which display a tilted peptide and fuse with host cell membranes through a sphingolipid/cholesterol-dependent process.

PMID: 21756873 [PubMed - indexed for MEDLINE]

1163. Immunol Cell Biol. 2011 Oct;89(7):792-802. doi: 10.1038/icb.2010.169. Epub 2011 Jan 25.

Ebolavirus VP35 suppresses IFN production from conventional but not plasmacytoid dendritic cells.

Leung LW(1), Park MS, Martinez O, Valmas C, López CB, Basler CF.

Author information: (1)Department of Microbiology, Mount Sinai School of Medicine, One Gustave L Levy Place, New York, NY 10029, USA.

Ebolaviruses naturally infect a wide variety of cells including macrophages and dendritic cells (DCs), and the resulting cytokine and interferon-α/β (IFN) responses of infected cells are thought to influence viral pathogenesis. The VP35 protein impairs RIG-I-like receptor-dependent signaling to inhibit IFN production, and this function has been suggested to promote the ineffective host immune response characteristic of ebolavirus infection. To assess the impact of VP35 on innate immunity in biologically relevant primary cells, we used a recombinant Newcastle disease virus encoding VP35 (NDV/VP35) to infect macrophages and conventional DCs, which primarily respond to RNA virus infection via RIG-I-like pathways. VP35 suppressed not only IFN but also tumor necrosis factor (TNF)-α secretion, which are normally produced from these cells upon NDV infection. Additionally, in cells susceptible to the activity of VP35, IRF7 activation is impaired. In contrast, NDV/VP35 infection of plasmacytoid DCs, which activate IRF7 and produce IFN through TLR-dependent signaling, leads to robust IFN production. When plasmacytoid DCs deficient for TLR signaling were infected, NDV/VP35 was able to inhibit IFN production. Consistent with this, VP35 was less able to inhibit TLR-dependent versus RIG-I-dependent signaling in vitro. These data demonstrate that ebolavirus VP35 suppresses both IFN and cytokine production in multiple primary human cell types. However, cells that utilize the TLR pathway can circumvent this inhibition, suggesting that the presence of multiple viral sensors enables the host to overcome viral immune evasion mechanisms.

PMCID: PMC4148147 PMID: 21263462 [PubMed - indexed for MEDLINE]

1164. Infect Genet Evol. 2011 Oct;11(7):1514-9. doi: 10.1016/j.meegid.2011.06.017. Epub 2011 Jun 30.

Current perspectives on the phylogeny of Filoviridae.

Barrette RW(1), Xu L, Rowland JM, McIntosh MT.

Author information: (1)Foreign Animal Disease Diagnostic Laboratory, National Veterinary Services Laboratories, Animal and Plant Health Inspection Services, USA.

Sporadic fatal outbreaks of disease in humans and non-human primates caused by Ebola or Marburg viruses have driven research into the characterization of these viruses with the hopes of identifying host tropisms and potential reservoirs. Such an understanding of the relatedness of newly discovered filoviruses may help to predict risk factors for outbreaks of hemorrhagic disease in humans and/or non-human primates. Recent discoveries such as three distinct genotypes of Reston ebolavirus, unexpectedly discovered in domestic swine in the Philippines; as well as a new species, Bundibugyo ebolavirus; the recent discovery of Lloviu virus as a potential new genus, Cuevavirus, within Filoviridae; and germline integrations of filovirus-like sequences in some animal species bring new insights into the relatedness of filoviruses, their prevalence and potential for transmission to humans. These new findings reveal that filoviruses are more diverse and may have had a greater influence on the evolution of animals than previously thought. Herein we review these findings with regard to the implications for understanding the host range, prevalence and transmission of Filoviridae.

Published by Elsevier B.V.

PMID: 21742058 [PubMed - indexed for MEDLINE]

1165. J Virol. 2011 Oct;85(20):10605-16. doi: 10.1128/JVI.00558-11. Epub 2011 Aug 17.

Inactivated or live-attenuated bivalent vaccines that confer protection against rabies and Ebola viruses.

Blaney JE(1), Wirblich C, Papaneri AB, Johnson RF, Myers CJ, Juelich TL, Holbrook MR, Freiberg AN, Bernbaum JG, Jahrling PB, Paragas J, Schnell MJ.

Author information: (1)Emerging Viral Pathogens Section, National Institute of Allergy and Infectious Diseases, National Institutes of Health, Bethesda, Maryland 20892, USA. jblaney@niaid.nih.gov

Comment in Expert Rev Vaccines. 2012 Feb;11(2):163-6.

The search for a safe and efficacious vaccine for Ebola virus continues, as no current vaccine candidate is nearing licensure. We have developed (i) replication-competent, (ii) replication-deficient, and (iii) chemically inactivated rabies virus (RABV) vaccines expressing Zaire Ebola virus (ZEBOV) glycoprotein (GP) by a reverse genetics system based on the SAD B19 RABV wildlife vaccine. ZEBOV GP is efficiently expressed by these vaccine candidates and is incorporated into virions. The vaccine candidates were avirulent after inoculation of adult mice, and viruses with a deletion in the RABV glycoprotein had greatly reduced neurovirulence after intracerebral inoculation in suckling mice. Immunization with live or inactivated RABV vaccines expressing ZEBOV GP induced humoral immunity against each virus and conferred protection from both lethal RABV and EBOV challenge in mice. The bivalent RABV/ZEBOV vaccines described here have several distinct advantages that may speed the development of inactivated vaccines for use in humans and potentially live or inactivated vaccines for use in nonhuman primates at risk of EBOV infection in endemic areas.

PMCID: PMC3187516 PMID: 21849459 [PubMed - indexed for MEDLINE]

1166. J Virol Methods. 2011 Oct;177(1):123-7. doi: 10.1016/j.jviromet.2011.06.021. Epub 2011 Jul 5.

An alternative method of measuring aerosol survival using spiders' webs and its use for the filoviruses.

Smither SJ(1), Piercy TJ, Eastaugh L, Steward JA, Lever MS.

Author information: (1)Biomedical Sciences Department, Dstl, Porton Down, Wiltshire, SP4 0JQ, UK. sjsmither@dstl.gov.uk

Understanding the ability to survive in an aerosol leads to better understanding of the hazard posed by pathogenic organisms and can inform decisions related to the control and management of disease outbreaks. This basic survival information is sometimes lacking for high priority select agents such as the filoviruses which cause severe disease with high case fatality rates and can be acquired through the aerosol route. Microthreads in the form of spiders' webs were used to capture aerosolised filoviruses, and the decay rates of Zaire ebolavirus and Marburgvirus were determined. Results were compared to data obtained using a Goldberg drum to measure survival as a dynamic aerosol. The two methods of obtaining aerostability information are compared.

PMID: 21762730 [PubMed - indexed for MEDLINE]

1167. Microbes Infect. 2011 Oct;13(11):930-6. doi: 10.1016/j.micinf.2011.05.002. Epub 2011 May 25.

Aerosol exposure to Zaire ebolavirus in three nonhuman primate species: differences in disease course and clinical pathology.

Reed DS(1), Lackemeyer MG, Garza NL, Sullivan LJ, Nichols DK.

Author information: (1)U.S. Army Medical Research Institute of Infectious Diseases, Frederick, MD, USA. dsreed@cvr.pitt.edu

There is little known concerning the disease caused by Zaire ebolavirus (ZEBOV) when inhaled, the likely route of exposure in a biological attack. Cynomolgus macaques, rhesus macaques, and African green monkeys were exposed to aerosolized ZEBOV to determine which species might be the most relevant model of the human disease. A petechial rash was noted on cynomolgus and rhesus macaques after fever onset but not on African green monkeys. Fever duration was shortest in rhesus macaques (62.7 ± 16.3 h) and longest in cynomolgus macaques (82.7 ± 22.3h) and African green monkeys (88.4 ± 16.7h). Virus was first detectable in the blood 3 days after challenge; the level of viremia was comparable among all three species. Hematological changes were noted in all three species, including decreases in lymphocyte and platelet counts. Increased blood coagulation times were most pronounced in African green monkeys. Clinical signs and time to death in all three species were comparable to what has been reported previously for each species after parenteral inoculation with ZEBOV. These data will be useful in selection of an animal model for efficacy studies.

Published by Elsevier Masson SAS.

PMID: 21651988 [PubMed - indexed for MEDLINE]

1168. PLoS Negl Trop Dis. 2011 Oct;5(10):e1359. doi: 10.1371/journal.pntd.0001359. Epub 2011 Oct 18.

Ebola virion attachment and entry into human macrophages profoundly effects early cellular gene expression.

Wahl-Jensen V(1), Kurz S, Feldmann F, Buehler LK, Kindrachuk J, DeFilippis V, da Silva Correia J, Früh K, Kuhn JH, Burton DR, Feldmann H.

Author information: (1)Integrated Research Facility at Fort Detrick, Division of Clinical Research, National Institute of Allergy and Infectious Diseases, National Institutes of Health, Fort Detrick, Maryland, United States of America. victoriajensen@nih.gov

Zaire ebolavirus (ZEBOV) infections are associated with high lethality in primates. ZEBOV primarily targets mononuclear phagocytes, which are activated upon infection and secrete mediators believed to trigger initial stages of pathogenesis. The characterization of the responses of target cells to ZEBOV infection may therefore not only further understanding of pathogenesis but also suggest possible points of therapeutic intervention. Gene expression profiles of primary human macrophages exposed to ZEBOV were determined using DNA microarrays and quantitative PCR to gain insight into the cellular response immediately after cell entry. Significant changes in mRNA concentrations encoding for 88 cellular proteins were observed. Most of these proteins have not yet been implicated in ZEBOV infection. Some, however, are inflammatory mediators known to be elevated during the acute phase of disease in the blood of ZEBOV-infected humans. Interestingly, the cellular response occurred within the first hour of Ebola virion exposure, i.e. prior to virus gene expression. This observation supports the hypothesis that virion binding or entry mediated by the spike glycoprotein (GP(1,2)) is the primary stimulus for an initial response. Indeed, ZEBOV virions, LPS, and virus-like particles consisting of only the ZEBOV matrix protein VP40 and GP(1,2) (VLP(VP40-GP)) triggered comparable responses in macrophages, including pro-inflammatory and pro-apoptotic signals. In contrast, VLP(VP40) (particles lacking GP(1,2)) caused an aberrant response. This suggests that GP(1,2) binding to macrophages plays an important role in the immediate cellular response.

PMCID: PMC3196478 PMID: 22028943 [PubMed - indexed for MEDLINE]

1169. PLoS Pathog. 2011 Oct;7(10):e1002304. doi: 10.1371/journal.ppat.1002304. Epub 2011 Oct 20.

Discovery of an ebolavirus-like filovirus in europe.

Negredo A(1), Palacios G, Vázquez-Morón S, González F, Dopazo H, Molero F, Juste J, Quetglas J, Savji N, de la Cruz Martínez M, Herrera JE, Pizarro M, Hutchison SK, Echevarría JE, Lipkin WI, Tenorio A.

Author information: (1)National Center of Microbiology, (ISCIII), Madrid, Spain.

Filoviruses, amongst the most lethal of primate pathogens, have only been reported as natural infections in sub-Saharan Africa and the Philippines. Infections of bats with the ebolaviruses and marburgviruses do not appear to be associated with disease. Here we report identification in dead insectivorous bats of a genetically distinct filovirus, provisionally named Lloviu virus, after the site of detection, Cueva del Lloviu, in Spain.

PMCID: PMC3197594 PMID: 22039362 [PubMed - indexed for MEDLINE]

1170. Nat Rev Drug Discov. 2011 Sep 30;10(10):731. doi: 10.1038/nrd3568.

Achilles heel of Ebola viral entry.

Flemming A.

Comment on Nature. 2011 Sep 15;477(7364):340-3. Nature. 2011 Sep 15;477(7364):344-8.

PMID: 21959282 [PubMed]

1171. J Bioterror Biodef. 2011 Sep 25;S1(4). pii: 2157-2526-S1-004.

Vesicular Stomatitis Virus-Based Vaccines for Prophylaxis and Treatment of Filovirus Infections.

Marzi A(1), Feldmann H, Geisbert TW, Falzarano D.

Author information: (1)Laboratory of Virology, Division of Intramural Research, National Institute of Allergy and Infectious Diseases, National Institutes of Health, Hamilton, Montana, USA.

Ebola and Marburg viruses are emerging/re-emerging zoonotic pathogens that cause severe viral hemorrhagic fever with case-fatality rates up to 90% in humans. Over the last three decades numerous outbreaks, of increasing frequency, have been documented in endemic regions. Furthermore, as a result of increased international travel filovirus infections have been imported into South Africa, Europe and North America. Both viruses possess the potential of being used as bioterrorism agents and are classified as category A pathogens. Currently there is neither a licensed vaccine nor effective treatment available, despite substantial efforts being dedicated to understanding filovirus well as vaccine and drug development. One of the most promising vaccine platforms is based on replication competent recombinant vesicular stomatitis viruses (rVSV) that express a filovirus glycoprotein as the surface antigen. These rVSVs have been extensively studied in rodent and nonhuman primate models of filovirus disease and, in general, have been shown to be 100% protective in pre-exposure prophylaxis. In addition, rVSVs have demonstrated potential for post-exposure treatment, and thus would be particularly useful in the event of intentional release as well as accidental exposures in outbreak and laboratory settings.

PMCID: PMC3265573 PMID: 22288023 [PubMed]

1172. Angew Chem Int Ed Engl. 2011 Sep 5;50(37):A46-51.

Sensing carbohydrate-protein interactions at picomolar concentrations using cantilever arrays.

Gruber K(1), Hermann BA, Seeberger PH.

Author information: (1)Walther-Meissner-Institute, Ludwig-Maximilians University München, Garching, Germany. kathrin.gruber@wmi.badw.de

Carbohydrates are important mediators of many biological processes that underlie cellular communication and disease mechanisms. Therapeutic agents include carbohydrate-based vaccines and the potent anti-viral protein Cyanovirin-N (CV-N). CV-N acts by specifically binding the carbohydrate structures decorating the cell surface of deadly viruses including human immunodeficiency virus (HI-V) or Ebola. In search for new carbohydrate-binding proteins and the development of sensors that exploit carbohydrate-protein interactions the label-free cantilever array technique can provides a fast, parallel and low-cost approach.

PMID: 22022717 [PubMed - indexed for MEDLINE]

1173. Am J Infect Control. 2011 Sep;39(7):e30-8. doi: 10.1016/j.ajic.2010.10.036. Epub 2011 May 6.

Detection of viruses in used ventilation filters from two large public buildings.

Goyal SM(1), Anantharaman S, Ramakrishnan MA, Sajja S, Kim SW, Stanley NJ, Farnsworth JE, Kuehn TH, Raynor PC.

Author information: (1)Department of Veterinary Population Medicine, College of Veterinary Medicine, University of Minnesota, Saint Paul, 55108, USA. goyal001@umn.edu

Comment in Am J Infect Control. 2012 Feb;40(1):89.

BACKGROUND: Viral and bacterial pathogens may be present in the air after being released from infected individuals and animals. Filters are installed in the heating, ventilation, and air-conditioning (HVAC) systems of buildings to protect ventilation equipment and maintain healthy indoor air quality. These filters process enormous volumes of air. This study was undertaken to determine the utility of sampling used ventilation filters to assess the types and concentrations of virus aerosols present in buildings. METHODS: The HVAC filters from 2 large public buildings in Minneapolis and Seattle were sampled to determine the presence of human respiratory viruses and viruses with bioterrorism potential. Four air-handling units were selected from each building, and a total of 64 prefilters and final filters were tested for the presence of influenza A, influenza B, respiratory syncytial, corona, parainfluenza 1-3, adeno, orthopox, entero, Ebola, Marburg, Lassa fever, Machupo, eastern equine encephalitis, western equine encephalitis, and Venezuelan equine encephalitis viruses. Representative pieces of each filter were cut and eluted with a buffer solution. RESULTS: Attempts were made to detect viruses by inoculation of these eluates in cell cultures (Vero, MDCK, and RK-13) and specific pathogen-free embryonated chicken eggs. Two passages of eluates in cell cultures or these eggs did not reveal the presence of any live virus. The eluates were also examined by polymerase chain reaction or reverse-transcription polymerase chain reaction to detect the presence of viral DNA or RNA, respectively. Nine of the 64 filters tested were positive for influenza A virus, 2 filters were positive for influenza B virus, and 1 filter was positive for parainfluenza virus 1. CONCLUSION: These findings indicate that existing building HVAC filters may be used as a method of detection for airborne viruses. As integrated long-term bioaerosol sampling devices, they may yield valuable information on the epidemiology and aerobiology of viruses in air that can inform the development of methods to prevent airborne transmission of viruses and possible deterrents against the spread of bioterrorism agents.

PMID: 21549446 [PubMed - indexed for MEDLINE]

1174. Future Virol. 2011 Sep;6(9):1091-1106.

Clinical aspects of Marburg hemorrhagic fever.

Mehedi M(1), Groseth A, Feldmann H, Ebihara H.

Author information: (1)Department of Medical Microbiology, University of Manitoba, Winnipeg, Manitoba, Canada.

Marburg virus belongs to the genus Marburgvirus in the family Filoviridae and causes a severe hemorrhagic fever, known as Marburg hemorrhagic fever (MHF), in both humans and nonhuman primates. Similar to the more widely known Ebola hemorrhagic fever, MHF is characterized by systemic viral replication, immunosuppression and abnormal inflammatory responses. These pathological features of the disease contribute to a number of systemic dysfunctions

including hemorrhages, edema, coagulation abnormalities and, ultimately, multiorgan failure and shock, often resulting in death. A detailed understanding of the pathological processes that lead to this devastating disease remains elusive, a fact that contributes to the lack of licensed vaccines or effective therapeutics. This article will review the clinical aspects of MHF and discuss the pathogenesis and possible options for diagnosis, treatment and prevention.
PMCID: PMC3201746 PMID: 22046196 [PubMed]

1175. J Virol. 2011 Sep;85(17):9060-8. doi: 10.1128/JVI.00659-11. Epub 2011 Jul 6.

Functional genomics reveals the induction of inflammatory response and metalloproteinase gene expression during lethal Ebola virus infection.

Cilloniz C(1), Ebihara H, Ni C, Neumann G, Korth MJ, Kelly SM, Kawaoka Y, Feldmann H, Katze MG.

Author information: (1)Department of Microbiology, School of Medicine, University of Washington, Box 358070, Seattle, WA 98195-8070, USA.

Ebola virus is the etiologic agent of a lethal hemorrhagic fever in humans and nonhuman primates with mortality rates of up to 90%. Previous studies with Zaire Ebola virus (ZEBOV), mouse-adapted virus (MA-ZEBOV), and mutant viruses (ZEBOV-NP(ma), ZEBOV-VP24(ma), and ZEBOV-NP/VP24(ma)) allowed us to identify the mutations in viral protein 24 (VP24) and nucleoprotein (NP) responsible for acquisition of high virulence in mice. To elucidate specific molecular signatures associated with lethality, we compared global gene expression profiles in spleen samples from mice infected with these viruses and performed an extensive functional analysis. Our analysis showed that the lethal viruses (MA-ZEBOV and ZEBOV-NP/VP24(ma)) elicited a strong expression of genes 72 h after infection. In addition, we found that although the host transcriptional response to ZEBOV-VP24(ma) was nearly the same as that to ZEBOV-NP/VP24(ma), the contribution of a mutation in the NP gene was required for a lethal phenotype. Further analysis indicated that one of the most relevant biological functions differentially regulated by the lethal viruses was the inflammatory response, as was the induction of specific metalloproteinases, which were present in our newly identify functional network that was associated with Ebola virus lethality. Our results suggest that this dysregulated proinflammatory response increased the severity of disease. Consequently, the newly discovered molecular signature could be used as the starting point for the development of new drugs and therapeutics. To our knowledge, this is the first study that clearly defines unique molecular signatures associated with Ebola virus lethality.
PMCID: PMC3165855 PMID: 21734050 [PubMed - indexed for MEDLINE]

1176. J Virol. 2011 Sep;85(17):8502-13. doi: 10.1128/JVI.02600-10. Epub 2011 Jun 22.

Ebolavirus delta-peptide immunoadhesins inhibit marburgvirus and ebolavirus cell entry.

Radoshitzky SR(1), Warfield KL, Chi X, Dong L, Kota K, Bradfute SB, Gearhart JD, Retterer C, Kranzusch PJ, Misasi JN, Hogenbirk MA, Wahl-Jensen V, Volchkov VE, Cunningham JM, Jahrling PB, Aman MJ, Bavari S, Farzan M, Kuhn JH.

Author information: (1)U.S. Army Medical Research Institute of Infectious Diseases, Fort Detrick, Frederick, Maryland 21702, USA.

With the exception of Reston and Lloviu viruses, filoviruses (marburgviruses, ebolaviruses, and "cuevaviruses") cause severe viral hemorrhagic fevers in humans. Filoviruses use a class I fusion protein, GP(1,2), to bind to an unknown, but shared, cell surface receptor to initiate virus-cell fusion. In addition to GP(1,2), ebolaviruses and cuevaviruses, but not marburgviruses, express two secreted glycoproteins, soluble GP (sGP) and small soluble GP (ssGP). All three glycoproteins have identical N termini that include the receptor-binding region (RBR) but differ in their C termini. We evaluated the effect of the secreted ebolavirus glycoproteins on marburgvirus and ebolavirus cell entry, using Fc-tagged recombinant proteins. Neither sGP-Fc nor ssGP-Fc bound to filovirus-permissive cells or inhibited GP(1,2)-mediated cell entry of pseudotyped retroviruses. Surprisingly, several Fc-tagged Δ-peptides, which are small C-terminal cleavage products of sGP secreted by ebolavirus-infected cells, inhibited entry of retroviruses pseudotyped with Marburg virus GP(1,2), as well as Marburg virus and Ebola virus infection in a dose-dependent manner and at low molarity despite absence of sequence similarity to filovirus RBRs. Fc-tagged Δ-peptides from three ebolaviruses (Ebola virus, Sudan virus, and Taï Forest virus) inhibited GP(1,2)-mediated entry and infection of viruses comparably to or better than the Fc-tagged RBRs, whereas the Δ-peptide-Fc of an ebolavirus nonpathogenic for humans (Reston virus) and that of an ebolavirus with lower lethality for humans (Bundibugyo virus) had little effect. These data indicate that Δ-peptides are functional components of ebolavirus proteomes. They join cathepsins and integrins as novel modulators of filovirus cell entry, might play important roles in pathogenesis, and could be exploited for the synthesis of powerful new antivirals.
PMCID: PMC3165852 PMID: 21697477 [PubMed - indexed for MEDLINE]

1177. Mol Immunol. 2011 Sep;48(15-16):2027-37. doi: 10.1016/j.molimm.2011.06.437. Epub 2011 Jul 12.

Isolation and characterisation of Ebolavirus-specific recombinant antibody fragments from murine and shark immune libraries.

Goodchild SA(1), Dooley H, Schoepp RJ, Flajnik M, Lonsdale SG.

Author information: (1)Defence Science and Technology Laboratory, Porton Down, Salisbury SP4 0JQ, UK. sagoodchild@mail.dstl.gov.uk

Members of the genus Ebolavirus cause fulminating outbreaks of disease in human and non-human primate populations with a mortality rate up to 90%. To facilitate rapid detection of these pathogens in clinical and environmental samples, robust reagents capable of providing sensitive and specific detection are required. In this work recombinant antibody libraries were generated from murine (single chain variable domain fragment; scFv) and nurse shark, Ginglymostoma cirratum (IgNAR V) hosts immunised with Zaire ebolavirus. This provides the first recorded IgNAR V response against a particulate antigen in the nurse shark. Both murine scFv and shark IgNAR V libraries were panned by phage display technology to identify useful antibodies for the generation of immunological detection reagents. Two murine scFv were shown to have specificity to the Zaire ebolavirus viral matrix protein VP40. Two isolated IgNAR V were shown to bind to the viral nucleoprotein (NP) and to capture viable Zaire ebolavirus with a high degree of sensitivity. Assays developed with IgNAR V cross-reacted to Reston ebolavirus, Sudan ebolavirus and Bundibugyo ebolavirus. Despite this broad reactivity, neither of IgNAR V showed reactivity to Côte d'Ivoire ebolavirus. IgNAR V was substantially more resistant to irreversible thermal denaturation than murine scFv and monoclonal IgG in a comparative test. The demonstrable robustness of the IgNAR V domains may offer enhanced utility as immunological detection reagents in fieldable biosensor applications for use in tropical or subtropical countries where outbreaks of Ebolavirus haemorrhagic fever occur.

PMID: 21752470 [PubMed - indexed for MEDLINE]
1178. Plant Biotechnol J. 2011 Sep;9(7):807-16. doi: 10.1111/j.1467-7652.2011.00593.x. Epub 2011 Feb 1.

Expression of an immunogenic Ebola immune complex in Nicotiana benthamiana.

Phoolcharoen W(1), Bhoo SH, Lai H, Ma J, Arntzen CJ, Chen Q, Mason HS.

Author information: (1)Biodesign Institute and School of Life Sciences, Arizona State University, Tempe, Arizona, USA.

Filoviruses (Ebola and Marburg viruses) cause severe and often fatal haemorrhagic fever in humans and non-human primates. The US Centers for Disease Control identifies Ebola and Marburg viruses as 'category A' pathogens (defined as posing a risk to national security as bioterrorism agents), which has lead to a search for vaccines that could prevent the disease. Because the use of such vaccines would be in the service of public health, the cost of production is an important component of their development. The use of plant biotechnology is one possible way to cost-effectively produce subunit vaccines. In this work, a geminiviral replicon system was used to produce an Ebola immune complex (EIC) in Nicotiana benthamiana. Ebola glycoprotein (GP1) was fused at the C-terminus of the heavy chain of humanized 6D8 IgG monoclonal antibody, which specifically binds to a linear epitope on GP1. Co-expression of the GP1-heavy chain fusion and the 6D8 light chain using a geminiviral vector in leaves of N. benthamiana produced assembled immunoglobulin, which was purified by ammonium sulphate precipitation and protein G affinity chromatography. Immune complex formation was confirmed by assays to show that the recombinant protein bound the complement factor C1q. Size measurements of purified recombinant protein by dynamic light scattering and size-exclusion chromatography also indicated complex formation. Subcutaneous immunization of BALB/C mice with purified EIC resulted in anti-Ebola virus antibody production at levels comparable to those obtained with a GP1 virus-like particle. These results show excellent potential for a plant-expressed EIC as a human vaccine.

© 2011 The Authors. Plant Biotechnology Journal © 2011 Society for Experimental Biology, Association of Applied Biologists and Blackwell Publishing Ltd.
PMCID: PMC4022790 PMID: 21281425 [PubMed - indexed for MEDLINE]
1179. Protein Sci. 2011 Sep;20(9):1587-96. doi: 10.1002/pro.688. Epub 2011 Aug 3.

Designed protein mimics of the Ebola virus glycoprotein GP2 α-helical bundle: stability and pH effects.

Harrison JS(1), Higgins CD, Chandran K, Lai JR.

Author information: (1)Department of Biochemistry, Albert Einstein College of Medicine, Bronx, New York 10461, USA.

Ebola virus (EboV) belongs to the Filoviridae family of viruses that causes severe and fatal hemhorragic fever. Infection by EboV involves fusion between the virus and host cell membranes mediated by the envelope glycoprotein GP2 of the virus. Similar to the envelope glycoproteins of other viruses, the central feature of the GP2 ectodomain postfusion structure is a six-helix bundle formed by the protein's N- and C-heptad repeat regions (NHR and CHR, respectively). Folding of this six-helix bundle provides the energetic driving force for membrane fusion; in other viruses, designed agents that disrupt formation of the six-helix bundle act as potent fusion inhibitors. To interrogate determinants of EboV GP2-mediated membrane fusion, we designed model proteins that consist of the NHR and CHR segments linked by short protein linkers. Circular dichroism and gel filtration studies indicate that these proteins adopt stable α-helical folds consistent with design. Thermal denaturation indicated that the GP2 six-helix bundle is highly stable at pH 5.3 (melting temperature, $T(m)$, of 86.8 ± 2.0°C and van't Hoff enthalpy, $\Delta H(vH)$, of -28.2 ± 1.0 kcal/mol) and comparable in stability to other viral membrane fusion six-helix bundles. We found that the stability of our designed α-helical bundle proteins was dependent on buffering conditions with increasing stability at lower pH. Small pH differences (5.3-6.1) had dramatic effects ($\Delta T(m)$ = 37°C) suggesting a mechanism for conformational control that is dependent on environmental pH. These results suggest a role for low pH in stabilizing six-helix bundle formation during the process of GP2-mediated viral membrane fusion.

PMCID: PMC3190153 PMID: 21739501 [PubMed - indexed for MEDLINE]
1180. Vet Clin North Am Exot Anim Pract. 2011 Sep;14(3):421-6, v. doi: 10.1016/j.cvex.2011.05.007. Epub 2011 Jul 2.

One health: zoonoses in the exotic animal practice.

Souza MJ(1).

Author information: (1)Department of Comparative Medicine, University of Tennessee College of Veterinary Medicine, Knoxville, TN 37996, USA. msouza@utk.edu

Zoonoses make up approximately ¾ of today's emerging infectious diseases; many of these zoonoses come from exotic pets and wildlife. Recent outbreaks in humans associated with nondomestic animals include Sudden Acute Respiratory Syndrome, Ebola virus, salmonellosis, and monkeypox. Expanding human populations, increased exotic pet ownership and changes in climate may contribute to increased incidence of zoonoses. Education and preventive medicine practices can be applied by veterinarians and other health professionals to reduce the risk of contracting a zoonotic disease. The health of humans, animals, and the environment must be treated as a whole to prevent the transmission of zoonoses.

PMID: 21872779 [PubMed - indexed for MEDLINE]
1181. Viruses. 2011 Sep;3(9):1634-49. doi: 10.3390/v3091634. Epub 2011 Sep 7.

Filoviral immune evasion mechanisms.

Ramanan P(1), Shabman RS, Brown CS, Amarasinghe GK, Basler CF, Leung DW.

Author information: (1)Department of Biochemistry, Biophysics and Molecular Biology, Iowa State University, Ames, IA 50011, USA.

The Filoviridae family of viruses, which includes the genera Ebolavirus (EBOV) and Marburgvirus (MARV), causes severe and often times lethal hemorrhagic fever in humans. Filoviral infections are associated with ineffective innate antiviral responses as a result of virally encoded immune antagonists, which render the host incapable of mounting effective innate or adaptive immune responses. The Type I interferon (IFN) response is critical for establishing an antiviral state in the host cell and subsequent activation of the adaptive immune responses. Several filoviral encoded components target Type I IFN responses, and this innate

immune suppression is important for viral replication and pathogenesis. For example, EBOV VP35 inhibits the phosphorylation of IRF-3/7 by the TBK-1/IKKε kinases in addition to sequestering viral RNA from detection by RIG-I like receptors. MARV VP40 inhibits STAT1/2 phosphorylation by inhibiting the JAK family kinases. EBOV VP24 inhibits nuclear translocation of activated STAT1 by karyopherin-α. The examples also represent distinct mechanisms utilized by filoviral proteins in order to counter immune responses, which results in limited IFN-α/β production and downstream signaling.
PMCID: PMC3187693 PMID: 21994800 [PubMed - indexed for MEDLINE]
1182. Nature. 2011 Aug 24;477(7364):340-3. doi: 10.1038/nature10348.

Ebola virus entry requires the cholesterol transporter Niemann-Pick C1.
Carette JE(1), Raaben M, Wong AC, Herbert AS, Obernosterer G, Mulherkar N, Kuehne AI, Kranzusch PJ, Griffin AM, Ruthel G, Dal Cin P, Dye JM, Whelan SP, Chandran K, Brummelkamp TR.

Author information: (1)Whitehead Institute for Biomedical Research, Nine Cambridge Center, Cambridge, Massachusetts 02142, USA.
Comment in Nat Rev Drug Discov. 2011 Oct;10(10):731.

Infections by the Ebola and Marburg filoviruses cause a rapidly fatal haemorrhagic fever in humans for which no approved antivirals are available. Filovirus entry is mediated by the viral spike glycoprotein (GP), which attaches viral particles to the cell surface, delivers them to endosomes and catalyses fusion between viral and endosomal membranes. Additional host factors in the endosomal compartment are probably required for viral membrane fusion; however, despite considerable efforts, these critical host factors have defied molecular identification. Here we describe a genome-wide haploid genetic screen in human cells to identify host factors required for Ebola virus entry. Our screen uncovered 67 mutations disrupting all six members of the homotypic fusion and vacuole protein-sorting (HOPS) multisubunit tethering complex, which is involved in the fusion of endosomes to lysosomes, and 39 independent mutations that disrupt the endo/lysosomal cholesterol transporter protein Niemann-Pick C1 (NPC1). Cells defective for the HOPS complex or NPC1 function, including primary fibroblasts derived from human Niemann-Pick type C1 disease patients, are resistant to infection by Ebola virus and Marburg virus, but remain fully susceptible to a suite of unrelated viruses. We show that membrane fusion mediated by filovirus glycoproteins and viral escape from the vesicular compartment require the NPC1 protein, independent of its known function in cholesterol transport. Our findings uncover unique features of the entry pathway used by filoviruses and indicate potential antiviral strategies to combat these deadly agents.
PMCID: PMC3175325 PMID: 21866103 [PubMed - indexed for MEDLINE]
1183. Nature. 2011 Aug 24;477(7364):344-8. doi: 10.1038/nature10380.

Small molecule inhibitors reveal Niemann-Pick C1 is essential for Ebola virus infection.
Côté M(1), Misasi J, Ren T, Bruchez A, Lee K, Filone CM, Hensley L, Li Q, Ory D, Chandran K, Cunningham J.

Author information: (1)Division of Hematology, Department of Medicine, Brigham and Women's Hospital, Boston, Massachusetts 02115, USA.
Comment in Nat Rev Drug Discov. 2011 Oct;10(10):731.

Ebola virus (EboV) is a highly pathogenic enveloped virus that causes outbreaks of zoonotic infection in Africa. The clinical symptoms are manifestations of the massive production of pro-inflammatory cytokines in response to infection and in many outbreaks, mortality exceeds 75%. The unpredictable onset, ease of transmission, rapid progression of disease, high mortality and lack of effective vaccine or therapy have created a high level of public concern about EboV. Here we report the identification of a novel benzylpiperazine adamantane diamide-derived compound that inhibits EboV infection. Using mutant cell lines and informative derivatives of the lead compound, we show that the target of the inhibitor is the endosomal membrane protein Niemann-Pick C1 (NPC1). We find that NPC1 is essential for infection, that it binds to the virus glycoprotein (GP), and that antiviral compounds interfere with GP binding to NPC1. Combined with the results of previous studies of GP structure and function, our findings support a model of EboV infection in which cleavage of the GP1 subunit by endosomal cathepsin proteases removes heavily glycosylated domains to expose the amino-terminal domain, which is a ligand for NPC1 and regulates membrane fusion by the GP2 subunit. Thus, NPC1 is essential for EboV entry and a target for antiviral therapy.
PMCID: PMC3230319 PMID: 21866101 [PubMed - indexed for MEDLINE]
1184. Nat Med. 2011 Aug 21;17(9):1128-31. doi: 10.1038/nm.2447.

CD8+ cellular immunity mediates rAd5 vaccine protection against Ebola virus infection of nonhuman primates.
Sullivan NJ(1), Hensley L, Asiedu C, Geisbert TW, Stanley D, Johnson J, Honko A, Olinger G, Bailey M, Geisbert JB, Reimann KA, Bao S, Rao S, Roederer M, Jahrling PB, Koup RA, Nabel GJ.

Author information: (1)Vaccine Research Center, US National Institute of Allergy and Infectious Diseases, US National Institutes of Health, Bethesda, Maryland, USA. nsullivan@nih.gov
Vaccine-induced immunity to Ebola virus infection in nonhuman primates (NHPs) is marked by potent antigen-specific cellular and humoral immune responses; however, the immune mechanism of protection remains unknown. Here we define the immune basis of protection conferred by a highly protective recombinant adenovirus virus serotype 5 (rAd5) encoding Ebola virus glycoprotein (GP) in NHPs. Passive transfer of high-titer polyclonal antibodies from vaccinated Ebola virus-immune cynomolgus macaques to naive macaques failed to confer protection against disease, suggesting a limited role of humoral immunity. In contrast, depletion of CD3(+) T cells in vivo after vaccination and immediately before challenge eliminated immunity in two vaccinated macaques, indicating a crucial requirement for T cells in this setting. The protective effect was mediated largely by CD8(+) cells, as depletion of CD8(+) cells in vivo using the cM-T807 monoclonal antibody (mAb), which does not affect CD4(+) T cell or humoral immune responses, abrogated protection in four out of five subjects. These findings indicate that CD8(+) cells have a major role in rAd5-GP-induced immune protection against Ebola virus infection in NHPs. Understanding the immunologic mechanism of Ebola virus protection will facilitate the development of vaccines for Ebola and related hemorrhagic fever viruses in humans.
PMID: 21857654 [PubMed - indexed for MEDLINE]

1185. Antiviral Res. 2011 Aug;91(2):89-93. doi: 10.1016/j.antiviral.2011.05.006. Epub 2011 May 17.

Depletion of GTP pool is not the predominant mechanism by which ribavirin exerts its antiviral effect on Lassa virus.

Ölschläger S(1), Neyts J, Günther S.

Author information: (1)Department of Virology, Bernhard-Nocht-Institute for Tropical Medicine, Bernhard-Nocht-Str. 74, 20359 Hamburg, Germany. oelschlaeger@bni-hamburg.de

Ribavirin (1-β-d-ribofuranosyl-1,2,4-triazole-3-carboxamide) is the standard treatment for Lassa fever, though its mode of action is unknown. One possibility is depletion of the intracellular GTP pool via inhibition of the cellular enzyme inosine monophosphate dehydrogenase (IMPDH). This study compared the anti-arenaviral effect of ribavirin with that of two other IMPDH inhibitors, mycophenolic acid (MPA) and 5-ethynyl-1-β-d-ribofuranosylimidazole-4-carboxamide (EICAR). All three compounds were able to inhibit Lassa virus replication by ≥2 log units in cell culture. Restoring the intracellular GTP pool by exogenous addition of guanosine reversed the inhibitory effects of MPA and EICAR, while ribavirin remained fully active. Analogous experiments performed with Zaire Ebola virus showed that IMPDH inhibitors are also active against this virus, although to a lesser extent than against Lassa virus. In conclusion, the experiments with MPA and EICAR indicate that replication of Lassa and Ebola virus is sensitive to depletion of the GTP pool mediated via inhibition of IMPDH. However, this is not the predominant mechanism by which ribavirin exerts its in-vitro antiviral effect on Lassa virus.

PMID: 21616094 [PubMed - indexed for MEDLINE]

1186. Emerg Infect Dis. 2011 Aug;17(8):1559-60. doi: 10.3201/eid1708.101693.

Reston Ebolavirus antibodies in bats, the Philippines.

Taniguchi S, Watanabe S, Masangkay JS, Omatsu T, Ikegami T, Alviola P, Ueda N, Iha K, Fujii H, Ishii Y, Mizutani T, Fukushi S, Saijo M, Kurane I, Kyuwa S, Akashi H, Yoshikawa Y, Morikawa S.

PMCID: PMC3381561 PMID: 21801651 [PubMed - indexed for MEDLINE]

1187. PLoS Negl Trop Dis. 2011 Aug;5(8):e1275. doi: 10.1371/journal.pntd.0001275. Epub 2011 Aug 9.

A replicating cytomegalovirus-based vaccine encoding a single Ebola virus nucleoprotein CTL epitope confers protection against Ebola virus.

Tsuda Y(1), Caposio P, Parkins CJ, Botto S, Messaoudi I, Cicin-Sain L, Feldmann H, Jarvis MA.

Author information: (1)Laboratory of Virology, Division of Intramural Research, National Institute of Allergy and Infectious Diseases, National Institutes of Health, Hamilton, Montana, United States of America.

BACKGROUND: Human outbreaks of Ebola virus (EBOV) are a serious human health concern in Central Africa. Great apes (gorillas/chimpanzees) are an important source of EBOV transmission to humans due to increased hunting of wildlife including the 'bush-meat' trade. Cytomegalovirus (CMV) is an highly immunogenic virus that has shown recent utility as a vaccine platform. CMV-based vaccines also have the unique potential to re-infect and disseminate through target populations regardless of prior CMV immunity, which may be ideal for achieving high vaccine coverage in inaccessible populations such as great apes. METHODOLOGY/PRINCIPAL FINDINGS: We hypothesize that a vaccine strategy using CMV-based vectors expressing EBOV antigens may be ideally suited for use in inaccessible wildlife populations. To establish a 'proof-of-concept' for CMV-based vaccines against EBOV, we constructed a mouse CMV (MCMV) vector expressing a CD8+ T cell epitope from the nucleoprotein (NP) of Zaire ebolavirus (ZEBOV) (MCMV/ZEBOV-NP(CTL)). MCMV/ZEBOV-NP(CTL) induced high levels of long-lasting (>8 months) CD8+ T cells against ZEBOV NP in mice. Importantly, all vaccinated animals were protected against lethal ZEBOV challenge. Low levels of anti-ZEBOV antibodies were only sporadically detected in vaccinated animals prior to ZEBOV challenge suggesting a role, at least in part, for T cells in protection. CONCLUSIONS/SIGNIFICANCE: This study demonstrates the ability of a CMV-based vaccine approach to protect against an highly virulent human pathogen, and supports the potential for 'disseminating' CMV-based EBOV vaccines to prevent EBOV transmission in wildlife populations.

PMCID: PMC3153429 PMID: 21858240 [PubMed - indexed for MEDLINE]

1188. Trans R Soc Trop Med Hyg. 2011 Aug;105(8):466-72. doi: 10.1016/j.trstmh.2011.04.011. Epub 2011 May 24.

A limited outbreak of Ebola haemorrhagic fever in Etoumbi, Republic of Congo, 2005

Nkoghe D(1), Kone ML, Yada A, Leroy E.

Author information: (1)Centre International de Recherches Médicales de Franceville, BP 769, Franceville, Gabon. dnkoghe@hotmail.com

Ebolavirus has caused highly lethal outbreaks of haemorrhagic fever in the Congo basin. The 2005 outbreak in the Republic of Congo occurred in the Etoumbi district of Cuvette Ouest Department between April and May. The two index cases were infected while poaching. The sanitary response consisted of active surveillance and contact tracing, public awareness campaigns and community mobilization, case management and safe burial practices, and laboratory confirmation. Twelve cases and ten deaths were reported (lethality 83%). A transmission tree was constructed from a sample collected by a medical team. This outbreak was remarkable by its short duration and limited size. Increased awareness among these previously affected populations and the rapid response of the healthcare system probably contributed to its extinction.

PMID: 21605882 [PubMed - indexed for MEDLINE]

1189. Viruses. 2011 Aug;3(8):1501-31. doi: 10.3390/v3081501.

Intracellular events and cell fate in filovirus infection.

Olejnik J(1), Ryabchikova E, Corley RB, Mühlberger E.

Author information: (1)Department of Microbiology, School of Medicine, Boston University, Boston, MA 02118, USA. jolejnik@bu.edu

Marburg and Ebola viruses cause a severe hemorrhagic disease in humans with high fatality rates. Early target cells of filoviruses are monocytes, macrophages, and dendritic cells. The infection spreads to the liver, spleen and later other organs by blood and lymph flow. A hallmark of filovirus infection is the depletion of non-infected lymphocytes; however, the molecular mechanisms leading to the observed bystander lymphocyte apoptosis are poorly understood. Also, there is limited knowledge about the fate of infected cells in filovirus disease. In this review we will explore what is known about the intracellular events leading to virus amplification and cell damage in filovirus infection. Furthermore, we will discuss how cellular dysfunction and cell death may correlate with disease pathogenesis.

PMCID: PMC3172725 PMID: 21927676 [PubMed - indexed for MEDLINE]

1190. Lancet. 2011 Jul 30;378(9789):389.

USA focuses on Ebola vaccine but research gaps remain.

Burki TK.

Erratum in Lancet. 2011 Oct 8;378(9799):1296.

PMID: 21809495 [PubMed - indexed for MEDLINE]

1191. Bioconjug Chem. 2011 Jul 20;22(7):1354-65. doi: 10.1021/bc2000403. Epub 2011 Jun 20

Pseudosaccharide functionalized dendrimers as potent inhibitors of DC-SIGN dependent Ebola pseudotyped viral infection.

Luczkowiak J(1), Sattin S, Sutkevičiūtė I, Reina JJ, Sánchez-Navarro M, Thépaut M, Martínez-Prats L, Daghetti A, Fieschi F, Delgado R, Bernardi A, Rojo J.

Author information: (1)Laboratorio de Microbiologa Molecular, Instituto de Investigación Hospital 12 de Octubre (imas12), 28041 Madrid, Spain.

The development of compounds with strong affinity for the receptor DC-SIGN is a topic of remarkable interest due to the role that this lectin plays in several pathogen infection processes and in the modulation of the immune response. DC-SIGN recognizes mannosylated and fucosylated oligosaccharides in a multivalent manner. Therefore, multivalent carbohydrate systems are required to interact in an efficient manner with this receptor and compete with the natural ligands. We have previously demonstrated that linear pseudodi- and pseudotrisaccharides are adequate ligands for DC-SIGN. In this work, we show that multivalent presentations of these glycomimetics based on polyester dendrons and dendrimers lead to very potent inhibitors (in the nanomolar range) of cell infection by Ebola pseudotyped viral particles by blocking DC-SIGN receptor. Furthermore, SPR model experiments confirm that the described multivalent glycomimetic compounds compete in a very efficient manner with polymannosylated ligands for binding to DC-SIGN.

PMID: 21650462 [PubMed - indexed for MEDLINE]

1192. J Infect Dis. 2011 Jul 15;204(2):200-8. doi: 10.1093/infdis/jir077. Epub 2011 May 12

Replication, pathogenicity, shedding, and transmission of Zaire ebolavirus in pigs.

Kobinger GP(1), Leung A, Neufeld J, Richardson JS, Falzarano D, Smith G, Tierney K, Patel A, Weingartl HM.

Author information: (1)Special Pathogens Program, National Microbiology Laboratory, Public Health Agency of Canada. gary_kobinger@phac-aspc.gc.ca

Comment in J Infect Dis. 2011 Jul 15;204(2):179-81.

(See the editorial commentary by Bausch, on pages 179-81.)BACKGROUND: Reston ebolavirus was recently detected in pigs in the Philippines. Specific antibodies were found in pig farmers, indicating exposure to the virus. This important observation raises the possibility that pigs may be susceptible to Ebola virus infection, including from other species, such as Zaire ebolavirus (ZEBOV), and can transmit to other susceptible hosts. METHODS: This study investigated whether ZEBOV, a species commonly reemerging in central Africa, can replicate and induce disease in pigs and can be transmitted to naive animals. Domesticated Landrace pigs were challenged through mucosal exposure with a total of 1 ×10(6) plaque-forming units of ZEBOV and monitored for virus replication, shedding, and pathogenesis. Using similar conditions, virus transmission from infected to naive animals was evaluated in a second set of pigs. RESULTS: Following mucosal exposure, pigs replicated ZEBOV to high titers (reaching 10(7) median tissue culture infective doses/mL), mainly in the respiratory tract, and developed severe lung pathology. Shedding from the oronasal mucosa was detected for up to 14 days after infection, and transmission was confirmed in all naive pigs cohabiting with inoculated animals. CONCLUSIONS: These results shed light on the susceptibility of pigs to ZEBOV infection and identify an unexpected site of virus amplification and shedding linked to transmission of infectious virus.

PMID: 21571728 [PubMed - indexed for MEDLINE]

1193. J Infect Dis. 2011 Jul 15;204(2):179-81. doi: 10.1093/infdis/jir201. Epub 2011 May 12.

Ebola virus as a foodborne pathogen? Cause for consideration, but not panic.

Bausch DG.

Comment on J Infect Dis. 2011 Jul 15;204(2):200-8.

PMID: 21571727 [PubMed - indexed for MEDLINE]

1194. Proc Natl Acad Sci U S A. 2011 Jul 5;108(27):11211-6. doi: 10.1073/pnas.1104760108. Epub 2011 Jun 20.

Structure and function of the complete internal fusion loop from Ebolavirus glycoprotein 2.

Gregory SM(1), Harada E, Liang B, Delos SE, White JM, Tamm LK.

Author information: (1)Center for Membrane Biology, University of Virginia, Charlottesville, VA 22908, USA.

Ebolavirus (Ebov), an enveloped virus of the family Filoviridae, causes hemorrhagic fever in humans and nonhuman primates. The viral glycoprotein (GP) is solely responsible for virus-host membrane fusion, but how it does so remains elusive. Fusion occurs after virions reach an endosomal compartment where GP is proteolytically primed by cathepsins. Fusion by primed GP is governed by an internal fusion loop found in GP2, the fusion subunit. This fusion loop contains a stretch of hydrophobic residues, some of which have been shown to be critical for GP-mediated infection. Here we present liposome fusion data and NMR structures for a complete (54-residue) disulfide-bonded internal fusion loop (Ebov FL) in a membrane mimetic. The Ebov FL induced rapid fusion of liposomes of varying compositions at pH values at or below 5.5. Consistently, circular dichroism experiments indicated that the α-helical content of the Ebov FL in the presence of either lipid-mimetic micelles or small liposomes increases in samples exposed to pH $\leq$5.5. NMR structures in dodecylphosphocholine micelles at pH 7.0 and 5.5 revealed a conformational change from a relatively flat extended loop structure at pH 7.0 to a structure with an $\sim$90° bend at pH 5.5. Induction of the bend at low pH reorients and compacts the hydrophobic patch at the tip of the FL. We propose that these changes facilitate disruption of lipids at the site of virus-host cell membrane contact and, hence, initiate Ebov fusion.

PMCID: PMC3131375 PMID: 21690393 [PubMed - indexed for MEDLINE]

1195. Virology. 2011 Jul 5;415(2):83-94. doi: 10.1016/j.virol.2011.04.002. Epub 2011 May 6.

Tyrosine kinase receptor Axl enhances entry of Zaire ebolavirus without direct interactions with the viral glycoprotein.

Brindley MA(1), Hunt CL, Kondratowicz AS, Bowman J, Sinn PL, McCray PB Jr, Quinn K, Weller ML, Chiorini JA, Maury W.

Author information: (1)Department of Microbiology, University of Iowa, Iowa City, IA 52242, USA.

In a bioinformatics-based screen for cellular genes that enhance Zaire ebolavirus (ZEBOV) transduction, AXL mRNA expression strongly correlated with ZEBOV infection. A series of cell lines and primary cells were identified that require Axl for optimal ZEBOV entry. Using one of these cell lines, we identified ZEBOV entry events that are Axl-dependent. Interactions between ZEBOV-GP and the Axl ectodomain were not detected in immunoprecipitations and reduction of surface-expressed Axl by RNAi did not alter ZEBOV-GP binding, providing evidence that Axl does not serve as a receptor for the virus. However, RNAi knock down of Axl reduced ZEBOV pseudovirion internalization and α-Axl antisera inhibited pseudovirion fusion with cellular membranes. Consistent with the importance of Axl for ZEBOV transduction, Axl transiently co-localized on the surface of cells with ZEBOV virus particles and was internalized during virion transduction. In total, these findings indicate that endosomal uptake of filoviruses is facilitated by Axl.

Copyright © 2011 Elsevier Inc. All rights reserved.

PMCID: PMC3107944 PMID: 21529875 [PubMed - indexed for MEDLINE]

1196. Clin Microbiol Infect. 2011 Jul;17(7):964-76. doi: 10.1111/j.1469-0691.2011.03535.x.

Ebola and Marburg haemorrhagic fever viruses: major scientific advances, but a relatively minor public health threat for Africa.

Leroy EM(1), Gonzalez JP, Baize S.

Author information: (1)Centre International de Recherches Médicales de Franceville, Franceville, Gabon. eric.leroy@ird.fr

Ebola and Marburg viruses are the only members of the Filoviridae family (order Mononegavirales), a group of viruses characterized by a linear, non-segmented, single-strand negative RNA genome. They are among the most virulent pathogens for humans and great apes, causing acute haemorrhagic fever and death within a matter of days. Since their discovery 50 years ago, filoviruses have caused only a few outbreaks, with 2317 clinical cases and 1671 confirmed deaths, which is negligible compared with the devastation caused by malnutrition and other infectious diseases prevalent in Africa (malaria, cholera, AIDS, dengue, tuberculosis ...). Yet considerable human and financial resourses have been devoted to research on these viruses during the past two decades, partly because of their potential use as bioweapons. As a result, our understanding of the ecology, host interactions, and control of these viruses has improved considerably.

© 2011 The Authors. Clinical Microbiology and Infection © 2011 European Society of Clinical Microbiology and Infectious Diseases.

PMID: 21722250 [PubMed - indexed for MEDLINE]

1197. Viruses. 2011 Jul;3(7):982-1000. doi: 10.3390/v3070982. Epub 2011 Jun 27.

Correlates of immunity to filovirus infection.

Bradfute SB(1), Bavari S.

Author information: (1)United States Army Medical Research Institute of Infectious Diseases, 1425 Porter Street, Fort Detrick, Maryland, MD 21702, USA. steven.bradfute@us.army.mil

Filoviruses can cause severe, often fatal hemorrhagic fever in humans. Recent advances in vaccine and therapeutic drug development have provided encouraging data concerning treatment of these infections. However, relatively little is known about immune responses in fatal versus non-fatal filovirus infection. This review summarizes the published literature on correlates of immunity to filovirus infection, and highlights deficiencies in our knowledge on this topic. It is likely that there are several types of successful immune responses, depending on the type of filovirus, and the presence and timing of vaccination or drug treatment.

PMCID: PMC3185794 PMID: 21994766 [PubMed - indexed for MEDLINE]

1198. Curr Protoc Cell Biol. 2011 Jun;Chapter 26:Unit 26.12. doi: 10.1002/0471143030.cb2612s51.

An enzymatic assay for detection of viral entry.

Tscherne DM(1), García-Sastre A.

Author information: (1)Department of Microbiology, Mount Sinai School of Medicine, New York, New York, USA.

This unit describes a viral entry assay where a beta-lactamase reporter protein fused to the matrix protein of either influenza (BlaM1) or ebola virus (BlaVP40) is packaged as a structural component into virus-like particles (VLPs). The Bla reporter is released upon fusion with target cells and can be detected in live cells by flow cytometry, microscopy, or a fluorometric plate reader for utility in high-throughput screening approaches. The transfer of Bla to a target cell by BlaM1 or BlaVP40 VLPs requires the presence of influenza hemagglutinin (HA) and neuraminidase (NA) or EboV glycoprotein (GP), respectively. This straightforward assay has broad application for studying the entry steps of enveloped viruses, especially those that require high levels of biosafety containment.

© 2011 by John Wiley & Sons, Inc.

PMID: 21688257 [PubMed - indexed for MEDLINE]
1199. Glycobiology. 2011 Jun;21(6):806-12. doi: 10.1093/glycob/cwr008. Epub 2011 Jan 21

Mouse LSECtin as a model for a human Ebola virus receptor.

Pipirou Z(1), Powlesland AS, Steffen I, Pöhlmann S, Taylor ME, Drickamer K.

Author information: (1)Division of Molecular Biosciences, Department of Life Sciences, Imperial College, London, UK.

The biochemical properties of mouse LSECtin, a glycan-binding receptor that is a member of the C-type lectin family found on sinusoidal endothelial cells, have been investigated. The C-type carbohydrate-recognition domain of mouse LSECtin, expressed in bacteria, has been used in solid-phase binding assays, and a tetramerized form has been used to probe a glycan array. In spite of sequence differences near the glycan-binding sites, the mouse receptor closely mimics the properties of the human receptor, showing high affinity binding to glycans bearing terminal GlcNAcβ1-2Man motifs. Site-directed mutagenesis has been used to confirm that residues near the binding site that differ between the human and the mouse proteins do not affect this binding specificity. Mouse and human LSECtin have been shown to bind Ebola virus glycoprotein with equivalent affinities, and the GlcNAcβ1-2Man disaccharide has been demonstrated to be an effective inhibitor of this interaction. These studies provide a basis for using mouse LSECtin, and knockout mice lacking this receptor, to model the biological properties of the human receptor.

PMCID: PMC3091528 PMID: 21257728 [PubMed - indexed for MEDLINE]
1200. J Virol. 2011 Jun;85(11):5406-14. doi: 10.1128/JVI.02190-10. Epub 2011 Mar 16.

A new Ebola virus nonstructural glycoprotein expressed through RNA editing.

Mehedi M(1), Falzarano D, Seebach J, Hu X, Carpenter MS, Schnittler HJ, Feldmann H.

Author information: (1)Department of Medical Microbiology, University of Manitoba, Public Health Agency of Canada, Winnipeg, Manitoba, Canada.

Ebola virus (EBOV), an enveloped, single-stranded, negative-sense RNA virus, causes severe hemorrhagic fever in humans and nonhuman primates. The EBOV glycoprotein (GP) gene encodes the nonstructural soluble glycoprotein (sGP) but also produces the transmembrane glycoprotein ($GP_{1,2}$) through transcriptional editing. A third GP gene product, a small soluble glycoprotein (ssGP), has long been postulated to be produced also as a result of transcriptional editing. To identify and characterize the expression of this new EBOV protein, we first analyzed the relative ratio of GP gene-derived transcripts produced during infection in vitro (in Vero E6 cells or Huh7 cells) and in vivo (in mice). The average percentages of transcripts encoding sGP, $GP_{1,2}$, and ssGP were approximately 70, 25, and 5%, respectively, indicating that ssGP transcripts are indeed produced via transcriptional editing. N-terminal sequence similarity with sGP, the absence of distinguishing antibodies, and the abundance of sGP made it difficult to identify ssGP through conventional methodology. Optimized 2-dimensional (2D) gel electrophoresis analyses finally verified the expression and secretion of ssGP in tissue culture during EBOV infection. Biochemical analysis of recombinant ssGP characterized this protein as a disulfide-linked homodimer that was exclusively N glycosylated. In conclusion, we have identified and characterized a new EBOV nonstructural glycoprotein, which is expressed as a result of transcriptional editing of the GP gene. While ssGP appears to share similar structural properties with sGP, it does not appear to have the same anti-inflammatory function on endothelial cells as sGP.

PMCID: PMC3094950 PMID: 21411529 [PubMed - indexed for MEDLINE]
1201. J Virol Methods. 2011 Jun;174(1-2):99-109. doi: 10.1016/j.jviromet.2011.04.003. Epub 2011 Apr 13.

Development and characterization of rabbit and mouse antibodies against ebolavirus envelope glycoproteins.

Ou W(1), Delisle J, Konduru K, Bradfute S, Radoshitzky SR, Retterer C, Kota K, Bavari S, Kuhn JH, Jahrling PB, Kaplan G, Wilson CA.

Author information: (1)Division of Cellular and Gene Therapies, Center for Biologics Evaluation and Research, FDA, Bethesda, MD, USA.

Ebolaviruses are the etiologic agents of severe viral hemorrhagic fevers in primates, including humans, and could be misused for the development of biological weapons. The ability to rapidly detect and differentiate these viruses is therefore crucial. Antibodies that can detect reliably the ebolavirus surface envelope glycoprotein $GP_{1,2}$ or a truncated variant that is secreted from infected cells (sGP) are required for advanced development of diagnostic assays such as sandwich ELISAs or Western blots (WB). We used a $GP_{1,2}$ peptide conserved among Bundibugyo, Ebola, Reston, Sudan, and Taï Forest viruses and a mucin-like domain-deleted Sudan virus $GP_{1,2}$ (SudanGPΔMuc) to immunize mice or rabbits, and developed a panel of antibodies that either cross-react or are virus-specific. These antibodies detected full-length $GP_{1,2}$ and sGP in different assays such as ELISA, FACS, or WB. In addition, some of the antibodies were shown to have potential clinical relevance, as they detected ebolavirus-infected cells by immunofluorescence assay and gave a specific increase in signal by sandwich ELISA against sera from mouse-adapted Ebola virus-infected mice over uninfected mouse sera. Rabbit anti-SudanGPΔMuc polyclonal antibody neutralized gammaretroviral particles pseudotyped with Sudan virus $GP_{1,2}$, but not particles pseudotyped with other ebolavirus$GP_{1,2}$. Together, our results suggest that this panel of antibodies may prove useful for both in vitro analyses of ebolavirus $GP_{1,2}$, as well as analysis of clinically relevant samples.
Published by Elsevier B.V.

PMCID: PMC3106979 PMID: 21513741 [PubMed - indexed for MEDLINE]
1202. Osong Public Health Res Perspect. 2011 Jun;2(1):3-7. doi: 10.1016/j.phrp.2011.04.001. Epub 2011 Apr 12.

Incubation period of ebola hemorrhagic virus subtype zaire.

Eichner M(1), Dowell SF, Firese N.

Author information: (1)Department of Medical Biometry, University of Tübingen, Tübingen, Germany.

OBJECTIVES: Ebola hemorrhagic fever has killed over 1300 people, mostly in equatorial Africa. There is still uncertainty about the natural reservoir of the virus and about some of the factors involved in disease transmission. Until now, a maximum incubation period of 21 days has been assumed. METHODS: We analyzed data collected during the Ebola outbreak (subtype Zaire) in Kikwit, Democratic Republic of the Congo, in 1995 using maximum likelihood inference and assuming a log-normally distributed incubation period. RESULTS: The mean incubation period was estimated to be 12.7 days (standard deviation 4.31 days), indicating that about 4.1% of patients may have incubation periods longer than 21 days. CONCLUSION: If the risk of new cases is to be reduced to 1% then 25 days should be used when investigating the source of an outbreak, when determining the duration of surveillance for contacts, and when declaring the end of an outbreak. PMCID: PMC3766904 PMID: 24159443 [PubMed]

1203. PLoS Negl Trop Dis. 2011 Jun;5(6):e1175. doi: 10.1371/journal.pntd.0001175. Epub 2011 Jun 7.

Serologic cross-reactivity of human IgM and IgG antibodies to five species of Ebola virus.

Macneil A(1), Reed Z, Rollin PE.

Author information: (1)Viral Special Pathogens Branch, The Centers for Disease Control and Prevention, Atlanta, Georgia, USA. aho3@cdc.gov

Five species of Ebola virus (EBOV) have been identified, with nucleotide differences of 30-45% between species. Four of these species have been shown to cause Ebola hemorrhagic fever (EHF) in humans and a fifth species (Reston ebolavirus) is capable of causing a similar disease in non-human primates. While examining potential serologic cross-reactivity between EBOV species is important for diagnostic assays as well as putative vaccines, the nature of cross-reactive antibodies following EBOV infection has not been thoroughly characterized. In order to examine cross-reactivity of human serologic responses to EBOV, we developed antigen preparations for all five EBOV species, and compared serologic responses by IgM capture and IgG enzyme-linked immunosorbent assay (ELISA) in groups of convalescent diagnostic sera from outbreaks in Kikwit, Democratic Republic of Congo (n=24), Gulu, Uganda (n=20), Bundibugyo, Uganda (n=33), and the Philippines (n=18), which represent outbreaks due to four different EBOV species. For groups of samples from Kikwit, Gulu, and Bundibugyo, some limited IgM cross-reactivity was noted between heterologous sera-antigen pairs, however, IgM responses were largely stronger against autologous antigen. In some instances IgG responses were higher to autologous antigen than heterologous antigen, however, in contrast to IgM responses, we observed strong cross-reactive IgG antibody responses to heterologous antigens among all sets of samples. Finally, we examined autologous IgM and IgG antibody levels, relative to time following EHF onset, and observed early peaking and declining IgM antibody levels (by 80 days) and early development and persistence of IgG antibodies among all samples, implying a consistent pattern of antibody kinetics, regardless of EBOV species. Our findings demonstrate limited cross-reactivity of IgM antibodies to EBOV, however, the stronger tendency for cross-reactive IgG antibody responses can largely circumvent limitations in the utility of heterologous antigen for diagnostic assays and may assist in the development of antibody-mediated vaccines to EBOV. PMCID: PMC3110169 PMID: 21666792 [PubMed - indexed for MEDLINE]

1204. Virol Sin. 2011 Jun;26(3):156-70. doi: 10.1007/s12250-011-3194-9. Epub 2011 Jun 12

Characterization of the receptor-binding domain of Ebola glycoprotein in viral entry.

Wang J(1), Manicassamy B, Caffrey M, Rong L.

Author information: (1)Department of Microbiology and Immunology, College of Medicine, University of Illinois at Chicago, USA.

Ebola virus infection causes severe hemorrhagic fever in human and non-human primates with high mortality. Viral entry/infection is initiated by binding of glycoprotein GP protein on Ebola virion to host cells, followed by fusion of virus-cell membrane also mediated by GP. Using an human immunodeficiency virus (HIV)-based pseudotyping system, the roles of 41 Ebola GP1 residues in the receptor-binding domain in viral entry were studied by alanine scanning substitutions. We identified that four residues appear to be involved in protein folding/structure and four residues are important for viral entry. An improved entry interference assay was developed and used to study the role of these residues that are important for viral entry. It was found that R64 and K95 are involved in receptor binding. In contrast, some residues such as I170 are important for viral entry, but do not play a major role in receptor binding as indicated by entry interference assay and/or protein binding data, suggesting that these residues are involved in post-binding steps of viral entry. Furthermore, our results also suggested that Ebola and Marburg viruses share a common cellular molecule for entry. PMID: 21667336 [PubMed - indexed for MEDLINE]

1205. Wkly Epidemiol Rec. 2011 May 27;86(22):221.

Outbreak news.Ebola, Uganda.

[Article in English, French]

[No authors listed]

PMID: 21661270 [PubMed - indexed for MEDLINE]

1206. Proc Natl Acad Sci U S A. 2011 May 17;108(20):8426-31. doi: 10.1073/pnas.1019030108. Epub 2011 May 2.

T-cell immunoglobulin and mucin domain 1 (TIM-1) is a receptor for Zaire Ebolavirus and Lake Victoria Marburgvirus.

Kondratowicz AS(1), Lennemann NJ, Sinn PL, Davey RA, Hunt CL, Moller-Tank S, Meyerholz DK, Rennert P, Mullins RF, Brindley M, Sandersfeld LM, Quinn K, Weller M, McCray PB Jr, Chiorini J, Maury W.

Author information: (1)Department of Microbiology, Carver College of Medicine, University of Iowa, Iowa City, IA 52242, USA.

The glycoproteins (GP) of enveloped viruses facilitate entry into the host cell by interacting with specific cellular receptors. Despite extensive study, a cellular receptor for the deadly filoviruses Ebolavirus and Marburgvirus has yet to be identified and characterized. Here, we show that T-cell Ig and mucin domain 1 (TIM-1) binds to the receptor binding domain of the Zaire Ebola virus (EBOV) glycoprotein, and ectopic TIM-1 expression in poorly permissive cells enhances EBOV infection by 10- to 30-fold. Conversely, reduction of cell-surface expression of TIM-1 by RNAi decreased infection of highly permissive Vero cells. TIM-1 expression within the human body is broader than previously appreciated, with expression on mucosal epithelia from the trachea, cornea, and conjunctiva--tissues believed to be important during in vivo transmission of filoviruses. Recognition that TIM-1 serves as a receptor for filoviruses on these mucosal epithelial surfaces provides a mechanistic understanding of routes of entry into the human body via inhalation of aerosol particles or hand-to-eye contact. ARD5, a monoclonal antibody against the IgV domain of TIM-1, blocked EBOV binding and infection, suggesting that antibodies or small molecules directed against this cellular receptor may provide effective filovirus antivirals.

PMCID: PMC3100998 PMID: 21536871 [PubMed - indexed for MEDLINE]
1207. Rev Med Suisse. 2011 May 11;7(294):991-2, 994.

[Indications for PCR in travel medicine].

[Article in French]

Chappuis F(1).

Author information: (1)Service de médecine internationale et humanitaire, Département de médecine communautaire, de premier recours et des urgences HUG, 1211 Genève 14. francois.chappuis@hcuge.ch

The use of PCR-based molecular diagnosis in travel medicine remains limited to specific indications such as clinical suspicion of some of the viral hemorrhagic fevers (e.g. Ebola, Marburg), differential diagnosis between Entamoeba histolytica (pathogen) and E. dispar (non pathogen) in the stools, and parasitological diagnosis of cutaneous leishmaniasis. The scope of indications is likely to expand in the coming years with the development of techniques (e.g. multiplex PCR) able to identify several pathogens from a single sample. Simplification and cost-reduction of molecular techniques, which would allow for more equitable access to these diagnostic tools in countries where the targeted diseases are highly prevalent, pose major technological and ethical challenges.

PMID: 21692311 [PubMed - indexed for MEDLINE]
1208. J Biol Chem. 2011 May 6;286(18):15854-61. doi: 10.1074/jbc.M110.207084. Epub 2011 Mar 16.

Inhibition of Ebola virus entry by a C-peptide targeted to endosomes.

Miller EH(1), Harrison JS, Radoshitzky SR, Higgins CD, Chi X, Dong L, Kuhn JH, Bavari S, Lai JR, Chandran K.

Author information: (1)Department of Microbiology and Immunology, Albert Einstein College of Medicine, Bronx, New York 10461, USA.

Ebola virus (EboV) and Marburg virus (MarV) (filoviruses) are the causative agents of severe hemorrhagic fever. Infection begins with uptake of particles into cellular endosomes, where the viral envelope glycoprotein (GP) catalyzes fusion between the viral and host cell membranes. This fusion event is thought to involve conformational rearrangements of the transmembrane subunit (GP2) of the envelope spike that ultimately result in formation of a six-helix bundle by the N- and C-terminal heptad repeat (NHR and CHR, respectively) regions of GP2. Infection by other viruses employing similar viral entry mechanisms (such as HIV-1 and severe acute respiratory syndrome coronavirus) can be inhibited with synthetic peptides corresponding to the native CHR sequence ("C-peptides"). However, previously reported EboV C-peptides have shown weak or insignificant antiviral activity. To determine whether the activity of a C-peptide could be improved by increasing its intracellular concentration, we prepared an EboV C-peptide conjugated to the arginine-rich sequence from HIV-1 Tat, which is known to accumulate in endosomes. We found that this peptide specifically inhibited viral entry mediated by filovirus GP proteins and infection by authentic filoviruses. We determined that antiviral activity was dependent on both the Tat sequence and the native EboV CHR sequence. Mechanistic studies suggested that the peptide acts by blocking a membrane fusion intermediate.

PMCID: PMC3091195 PMID: 21454542 [PubMed - indexed for MEDLINE]
1209. J Vis Exp. 2011 May 2;(51). pii: 2444. doi: 10.3791/2444.

Protocol for recombinant RBD-based SARS vaccines: protein preparation, animal vaccination and neutralization detection.

Du L(1), Zhang X, Liu J, Jiang S.

Author information: (1)Lindsley F. Kimball Research Institute, New York Blood Center, USA.

Based on their safety profile and ability to induce potent immune responses against infections, subunit vaccines have been used as candidates for a wide variety of pathogens. Since the mammalian cell system is capable of post-translational modification, thus forming properly folded and glycosylated proteins, recombinant proteins expressed in mammalian cells have shown the greatest potential to maintain high antigenicity and immunogenicity. Although no new cases of SARS have been reported since 2004, future outbreaks are a constant threat; therefore, the development of vaccines against SARS-CoV is a prudent preventive step and should be carried out. The RBD of SARS-CoV S protein plays important roles in receptor binding and induction of specific neutralizing antibodies against virus infection. Therefore, in this protocol, we describe novel methods for developing a RBD-based subunit vaccine against SARS. Briefly, the recombinant RBD protein (rRBD) was expressed in culture supernatant of mammalian 293T cells to obtain a correctly folded protein with proper conformation and high immunogenicity. The transfection of the recombinant plasmid encoding RBD to the cells was then performed using a calcium phosphate transfection method with some modifications. Compared with the lipid transfection method, this modified calcium phosphate transfection method is cheaper, easier to handle, and has the potential to reach high efficacy once a transfection complex with suitable size and shape is formed. Finally, a SARS pseudovirus neutralization assay was introduced in the protocol and used to detect the neutralizing activity of sera of mice vaccinated with rRBD protein. This assay is relatively safe, does not involve an infectious SARS-CoV, and can be performed without the requirement of a biosafety-3 laboratory. The protocol described here can also be used to design and study recombinant subunit vaccines against other viruses with class I fusion proteins, for example, HIV, respiratory syncytial virus (RSV), Ebola virus, influenza virus, as well as Nipah and Handra viruses. In addition, the methods for generating a pseudovirus and subsequently establishing a pseudovirus neutralization assay can be applied to all these viruses.

PMCID: PMC3197098 PMID: 21587153 [PubMed - indexed for MEDLINE]
1210. J Virol. 2011 May;85(9):4222-33. doi: 10.1128/JVI.02407-10. Epub 2011 Feb 16.

Recombinant adenovirus serotype 26 (Ad26) and Ad35 vaccine vectors bypass immunity to Ad5 and protect nonhuman primates against ebolavirus challenge.

Geisbert TW(1), Bailey M, Hensley L, Asiedu C, Geisbert J, Stanley D, Honko A, Johnson J, Mulangu S, Pau MG, Custers J, Vellinga J, Hendriks J, Jahrling P, Roederer M, Goudsmit J, Koup R, Sullivan NJ.

Author information: (1)United States Army Medical Research Institute of Infectious Diseases, Fort Detrick, Maryland 21702-5011, USA.

The use of adenoviruses (Ad) as vaccine vectors against a variety of pathogens has demonstrated their capacity to elicit strong antibody and cell-mediated immune responses. Adenovirus serotype C vectors, such as Ad serotype 5 (Ad5), expressing Ebolavirus (EBOV) glycoprotein (GP), protect completely after a single inoculation at a dose of 10(10) viral particles. However, the clinical application of a vaccine based on Ad5 vectors may be hampered, since impairment of Ad5 vaccine efficacy has been demonstrated for humans and nonhuman primates with high levels of preexisting immunity to the vector. Ad26 and Ad35 segregate genetically from Ad5 and exhibit lower seroprevalence in humans, making them attractive vaccine vector alternatives. In the series of studies presented, we show that Ad26 and Ad35 vectors generate robust antigen-specific cell-mediated and humoral immune responses against EBOV GP and that Ad5 immune status does not affect the generation of GP-specific immune responses by these vaccines. We demonstrate partial protection against EBOV by a single-shot Ad26 vaccine and complete protection when this vaccine is boosted by Ad35 1 month later. Increases in efficacy are paralleled by substantial increases in T- and B-cell responses to EBOV GP. These results suggest that Ad26 and Ad35 vectors warrant further development as candidate vaccines for EBOV.

PMCID: PMC3126236 PMID: 21325402 [PubMed - indexed for MEDLINE]

1211. Pol Merkur Lekarski. 2011 May;30(179):359-61.

[Antiviral drugs].

[Article in Polish]

Denys A(1).

Author information: (1)Akademia Humanistyczno-Ekonomiczna w Łodzi. adenys@ahe.lodz.pl

It is 50 years since the first antiviral drug--JUDR for the local herpes keratitis was introduced and over 25 years since HIV/AIDS was isolated and the Noble Prize in Medicine and Physiology was given to its discovers. Now, there are 50 antiviral drugs, in which 25 are for HIV, the others are for herpes virus, shingles, cytomegalovirus, hepatitis virus and influenza A virus. Drugs for hemorrhagic fever Ebola and Marbourg as well as Denga fever are under way In the paper the current knowledge on chemotherapy and prophylaxis is presented in the following viral infections: HIV, HBV, HCV, CMV, HSV, shingles and other. The paper also demonstrates different groups of antiviral drugs, their use and efficacy. Mechanisms of infections and activity of antiviral drugs are analyzed.

PMID: 21675143 [PubMed - indexed for MEDLINE]

1212. Travel Med Infect Dis. 2011 May;9(3):126-34. doi: 10.1016/j.tmaid.2010.05.003. Epub 2010 Jun 26.

Filovirus emergence and vaccine development: a perspective for health care practitioners in travel medicine.

Sarwar UN(1), Sitar S, Ledgerwood JE.

Author information: (1)Vaccine Research Center, National Institute of Allergy and Infectious Diseases, National Institutes of Health, 40 Convent Drive, Bethesda, MD 20892-3017, USA.

Recent case reports of viral hemorrhagic fever in Europe and the United States have raised concerns about the possibility for increased importation of filoviruses to non-endemic areas. This emerging threat is concerning because of the increase in global air travel and the rise of tourism in central and eastern Africa and the greater dispersion of military troops to areas of infectious disease outbreaks. Marburg viruses (MARV) and Ebola viruses (EBOV) have been associated with outbreaks of severe hemorrhagic fever involving high mortality (25-90% case fatality rates). First recognized in 1967 and 1976 respectively, subtypes of MARV and EBOV are the only known viruses of the Filoviridae family, and are among the world's most virulent pathogens. This article focuses on information relevant for health care practitioners in travel medicine to include, the epidemiology and clinical features of filovirus infection and efforts toward development of a filovirus vaccine.

Published by Elsevier Ltd.

PMCID: PMC3116067 PMID: 21208830 [PubMed - indexed for MEDLINE]

1213. Viruses. 2011 May;3(5):613-9. doi: 10.3390/v3050613. Epub 2011 May 12.

Meta-analysis of high-throughput datasets reveals cellular responses following hemorrhagic fever virus infection.

Bowick GC(1), McAuley AJ.

Author information: (1)Department of Microbiology & Immunology, Institute for Human Infections & Immunity, University of Texas Medical Branch, Galveston, TX 77555, USA. gabowick@utmb.edu

The continuing use of high-throughput assays to investigate cellular responses to infection is providing a large repository of information. Due to the large number of differentially expressed transcripts, often running into the thousands, the majority of these data have not been thoroughly investigated. Advances in techniques for the downstream analysis of high-throughput datasets are providing additional methods for the generation of additional hypotheses for further investigation. The large number of experimental observations, combined with databases that correlate particular genes and proteins with canonical pathways, functions and diseases, allows for the bioinformatic exploration of functional networks that may be implicated in replication or pathogenesis. Herein, we provide an example of how analysis of published high-throughput datasets of cellular responses to hemorrhagic fever virus infection can generate additional functional data. We describe enrichment of genes involved in metabolism, post-translational modification and cardiac damage; potential roles for specific transcription factors and a conserved involvement of a pathway based around cyclooxygenase-2. We believe that these types of analyses can provide virologists with additional hypotheses for continued investigation.

PMCID: PMC3185756 PMID: 21994748 [PubMed - indexed for MEDLINE]

1214. Euro Surveill. 2011 Apr 21;16(16). pii: 19845.

European risk assessment guidance for infectious diseases transmitted on aircraft--the RAGIDA project.

Leitmeyer K(1).

Author information: (1)European Centre for Disease Prevention and Control, Stockholm, Sweden. katrin.leitmeyer@ecdc.europa.eu

In order to assist national public health authorities in the European Union to assess the risks associated with the transmission of infectious agents on board aircrafts, the European Centre for Disease Prevention and Control initiated in 2007 the RAGIDA project (Risk Assessment Guidance for Infectious Diseases transmitted on Aircraft). RAGIDA consists of two parts: the production of a systematic review and a series of disease-specific guidance documents. The systematic review covered over 3,700 peer-reviewed articles and grey literature for the following diseases: tuberculosis, influenza, severe acute respiratory syndrome (SARS), invasive meningococcal disease, measles, rubella, diphtheria, Ebola and Marburg haemorrhagic fevers, Lassa fever, smallpox and anthrax. In addition, general guidelines on risk assessment and management from international aviation boards and national and international public health agencies were systematically searched. Experts were interviewed on case-based events by standardised questionnaires. Disease-specific guidance documents on tuberculosis, SARS, meningococcal infections, measles, rubella, Ebola and Marburg haemorrhagic fevers, Lassa fever, smallpox and anthrax were the result of consultations of disease-specific expert panels. Factors that influence the risk assessment of infectious disease transmission on board aircrafts and decision making for contact tracing are outlined.

PMID: 21527131 [PubMed - indexed for MEDLINE]

1215. Vaccine. 2011 Apr 5;29(16):2968-77. doi: 10.1016/j.vaccine.2011.01.113. Epub 2011 Feb 15.

Ebola virus glycoprotein Fc fusion protein confers protection against lethal challenge in vaccinated mice.

Konduru K(1), Bradfute SB, Jacques J, Manangeeswaran M, Nakamura S, Morshed S, Wood SC, Bavari S, Kaplan GG.

Author information: (1)Center for Biologics Evaluation and Research, Food and Drug Administration, Bethesda, MD 20892, USA.

Ebola virus is a Filoviridae that causes hemorrhagic fever in humans and induces high morbidity and mortality rates. Filoviruses are classified as "Category A bioterrorism agents", and currently there are no licensed therapeutics or vaccines to treat and prevent infection. The Filovirus glycoprotein (GP) is sufficient to protect individuals against infection, and several vaccines based on GP are under development including recombinant adenovirus, parainfluenza virus, Venezuelan equine encephalitis virus, vesicular stomatitis virus (VSV) and virus-like particles. Here we describe the development of a GP Fc fusion protein as a vaccine candidate. We expressed the extracellular domain of the Zaire Ebola virus (ZEBOV) GP fused to the Fc fragment of human IgG1 (ZEBOVGP-Fc) in mammalian cells and showed that GP undergoes the complex furin cleavage and processing observed in the native membrane-bound GP. Mice immunized with ZEBOVGP-Fc developed T-cell immunity against ZEBOV GP and neutralizing antibodies against replication-competent VSV-G deleted recombinant VSV containing ZEBOV GP. The ZEBOVGP-Fc vaccinated mice were protected against challenge with a lethal dose of ZEBOV. These results show that vaccination with the ZEBOVGP-Fc fusion protein alone without the need of a viral vector or assembly into virus-like particles is sufficient to induce protective immunity against ZEBOV in mice. Our data suggested that Filovirus GP Fc fusion proteins could be developed as a simple, safe, efficacious, and cost effective vaccine against Filovirus infection for human use.

Published by Elsevier Ltd.

PMCID: PMC3070761 PMID: 21329775 [PubMed - indexed for MEDLINE]

1216. Appl Environ Microbiol. 2011 Apr;77(7):2366-73. doi: 10.1128/AEM.01840-09. Epub 2011 Jan 28.

Campylobacter troglodytis sp. nov., isolated from feces of human-habituated wild chimpanzees (Pan troglodytes schweinfurthii) in Tanzania.

Kaur T(1), Singh J, Huffman MA, Petrzelková KJ, Taylor NS, Xu S, Dewhirst FE, Paster BJ, Debruyne L, Vandamme P, Fox JG.

Author information: (1)Virginia-Maryland Regional College of Veterinary Medicine, Virginia Tech, Blacksburg, Virginia 24061, USA.

The transmission of simian immunodeficiency and Ebola viruses to humans in recent years has heightened awareness of the public health significance of zoonotic diseases of primate origin, particularly from chimpanzees. In this study, we analyzed 71 fecal samples collected from 2 different wild chimpanzee (Pan troglodytes) populations with different histories in relation to their proximity to humans. Campylobacter spp. were detected by culture in 19/56 (34%) group 1 (human habituated for research and tourism purposes at Mahale Mountains National Park) and 0/15 (0%) group 2 (not human habituated but propagated from an introduced population released from captivity over 30 years ago at Rubondo Island National Park) chimpanzees, respectively. Using 16S rRNA gene sequencing, all isolates were virtually identical (at most a single base difference), and the chimpanzee isolates were most closely related to Campylobacter helveticus and Campylobacter upsaliensis (94.7% and 95.9% similarity, respectively). Whole-cell protein profiling, amplified fragment length polymorphism analysis of genomic DNA, hsp60 sequence analysis, and determination of the mol% G+C content revealed two subgroups among the chimpanzee isolates. DNA-DNA hybridization experiments confirmed that both subgroups represented distinct genomic species. In the absence of differential biochemical characteristics and morphology and identical 16S rRNA gene sequences, we propose to classify all isolates into a single novel nomenspecies, Campylobacter troglodytis, with strain MIT 05-9149 as the type strain; strain MIT 05-9157 is suggested as the reference strain for the second C. troglodytis genomovar. Further studies are required to determine whether the organism is pathogenic to chimpanzees and whether this novel Campylobacter colonizes humans and causes enteric disease.

PMCID: PMC3067447 PMID: 21278267 [PubMed - indexed for MEDLINE]

1217. Biochem Biophys Res Commun. 2011 Apr 1;407(1):74-8. doi: 10.1016/j.bbrc.2011.02.110. Epub 2011 Mar 6.

Involvement of viral envelope GP2 in Ebola virus entry into cells expressing the macrophage galactose-type C-type lectin.

Usami K(1), Matsuno K, Igarashi M, Denda-Nagai K, Takada A, Irimura T.

Author information: (1)Laboratory of Cancer Biology and Molecular Immunology, Graduate School of Pharmaceutical Sciences, University of Tokyo, Tokyo 113-0033, Japan.

Ebola virus (EBOV) infection is initiated by the interaction of the viral surface envelope glycoprotein (GP) with the binding sites on target cells. Differences in the mortality among different species of the Ebola viruses, i.e., Zaire ebolavirus (ZEBOV) and Reston ebolavirus (REBOV), correspond to the in vitro infectivity of the pseudo-typed virus constructed with the GPs in cells expressing macrophage galactose-type calcium-type lectin (MGL/CD301). Through mutagenesis of GP2, the transmembrane-anchored subunit of GP, we found that residues 502-527 of the GP2 sequence determined the different infectivity between VSV-ZEBOV GP and -REBOV GP in MGL/CD301-expressing cells and a histidine residue at position 516 of ZEBOV GP2 appeared essential in the differential infectivity. These findings may provide a clue to clarify a molecular basis of different pathogenicity among EBOV species.

PMID: 21362405 [PubMed - indexed for MEDLINE]
1218. J Clin Ethics. 2011 Spring;22(1):3-16.

How can careproviders most help patients during a disaster?

Howe EG(1).

Author information: (1)Programs in Medical Ethics, Uniformed Services University of the Health Sciences, Bethesda, Maryland, USA.

This article reviews careproviders' most difficult emotional challenges during disasters and provides approaches for responding optimally to them. It describes key approaches that careproviders may pursue to best help patients and others during a catastrophe. It raises unanswered questions regarding when, if ever, careproviders should provide active euthanasia to patients who are incompetent, and when, if ever, careproviders should give their own food and water to patients or others who may otherwise soon die without them.

PMID: 21595349 [PubMed - indexed for MEDLINE]
1219. J Virol. 2011 Apr;85(8):4041-2. doi: 10.1128/JVI.00181-11. Epub 2011 Feb 9.

Evidence for Ebola virus superantigen activity.

Leroy EM, Becquart P, Wauquier N, Baize S.

PMCID: PMC3126126 PMID: 21307193 [PubMed - indexed for MEDLINE]
1220. J Virol. 2011 Apr;85(7):3106-19. doi: 10.1128/JVI.01456-10. Epub 2011 Jan 26.

Identification of a small-molecule entry inhibitor for filoviruses.

Basu A(1), Li B, Mills DM, Panchal RG, Cardinale SC, Butler MM, Peet NP, Majgier-Baranowska H, Williams JD, Patel I, Moir DT, Bavari S, Ray R, Farzan MR, Rong L, Bowlin TL.

Author information: (1)Microbiotix, Inc., One Innovation Drive, Worcester, MA 01605, USA. abasu@microbiotix.com

Ebola virus (EBOV) causes severe hemorrhagic fever, for which therapeutic options are not available. Preventing the entry of EBOV into host cells is an attractive antiviral strategy, which has been validated for HIV by the FDA approval of the anti-HIV drug enfuvirtide. To identify inhibitors of EBOV entry, the EBOV envelope glycoprotein (EBOV-GP) gene was used to generate pseudotype viruses for screening of chemical libraries. A benzodiazepine derivative (compound 7) was identified from a high-throughput screen (HTS) of small-molecule compound libraries utilizing the pseudotype virus. Compound 7 was validated as an inhibitor of infectious EBOV and Marburg virus (MARV) in cell-based assays, with 50% inhibitory concentrations (IC(50)s) of 10 μM and 12 μM, respectively. Time-of-addition and binding studies suggested that compound 7 binds to EBOV-GP at an early stage during EBOV infection. Preliminary Schrödinger SiteMap calculations, using a published EBOV-GP crystal structure in its prefusion conformation, suggested a hydrophobic pocket at or near the GP1 and GP2 interface as a suitable site for compound 7 binding. This prediction was supported by mutational analysis implying that residues Asn69, Leu70, Leu184, Ile185, Leu186, Lys190, and Lys191 are critical for the binding of compound 7 and its analogs with EBOV-GP. We hypothesize that compound 7 binds to this hydrophobic pocket and as a consequence inhibits EBOV infection of cells, but the details of the mechanism remain to be determined. In summary, we have identified a novel series of benzodiazepine compounds that are suitable for optimization as potential inhibitors of filoviral infection.

PMCID: PMC3067866 PMID: 21270170 [PubMed - indexed for MEDLINE]
1221. Med Trop (Mars). 2011 Apr;71(2):111-21.

[Ebola and Marburg hemorrhagic fever viruses: update on filoviruses].

[Article in French]

Leroy E(1), Baize S, Gonzalez JP.

Author information: (1)Centre International de Recherches Médicales de Franceville, Franceville, Gabon. eric.leroy@ird.fr

The Ebola and Marburg viruses are the sole members of the Filoviridae family of viruses. They are characterized by a long filamentous form that is unique in the viral world. Filoviruses are among the most virulent pathogens currently known to infect humans. They cause fulminating disease characterized by acute fever followed by generalized hemorrhagic syndrome that is associated with 90% mortality in the most severe forms. Epidemic outbreaks of Marburg and Ebola viruses have taken a heavy toll on human life in Central Africa and devastated large ape populations in Gabon and Republic of Congo. Since their discovery in 1967 (Marburg) and 1976 (Ebola), more than 2,300 cases and 1,670 deaths have been reported. These numbers pale in comparison with the burden caused by malnutrition or other infectious disease scourges in Africa such as malaria, cholera, AIDS, dengue or tuberculosis. However, due to their extremely high lethality, association with multifocal hemorrhaging and specificity to the African continent, these hemorrhagic fever viruses have given rise to great interest on the part not only of the international scientific community but also of the general public because of their perceived potential as biological weapons. Much research has been performed on these viruses and major progress has been made in knowledge of their ecology, epidemiology and physiopathology and in development of vaccine candidates and therapeutic schemes. The purpose of this review is to present the main developments in these particular fields in the last decade.

PMID: 21695865 [PubMed - indexed for MEDLINE]
1222. Proteins. 2011 Apr;79(4):1109-17. doi: 10.1002/prot.22947. Epub 2011 Jan 18.

Effect of flanking residues on the conformational sampling of the internal fusion peptide from Ebola virus.

Jaskierny AJ(1), Panahi A, Feig M.

Author information: (1)Department of Biochemistry and Molecular Biology, Michigan State University, East Lansing, Michigan 48824, USA.

Fusion peptides mediate viral and host-cell membrane fusion during viral entry. The monomeric form of the internal fusion peptide from Ebola virus was studied in membrane bilayer and water environments with computer simulations using replica exchange sampling and an implicit solvent description of the environment. Wild-type Ebola fusion peptide (EFP), the W8A mutant form, and an extended construct with flanking residues were examined. It was found that the monomeric form of wild-type EFP adopts coil-helix-coil structure with a short helix from residues 8 to 11 mostly sampling orientations parallel to the membrane surface. W8A mutation disrupts the helicity in the N-terminal region of the peptide and leads to a preference for slightly oblique orientation relative to the membrane surface. The addition of flanking residues also alters the fusion peptide conformation with either a helix-break-helix structure or extended N and C-termini and reduced membrane insertion. In water, the fusion peptide is found to adopt structures with low helicity.

PMCID: PMC3075865 PMID: 21246633 [PubMed - indexed for MEDLINE]
1223. Virol Sin. 2011 Apr;26(2):73-80. doi: 10.1007/s12250-011-3186-9. Epub 2011 Apr 7.

Laboratory detection and diagnosis of filoviruses.

Wang YP(1), Zhang XE, Wei HP.

Author information: (1)Wuhan Institute of Virology, Chinese Academy of Sciences, Wuhan 430071, China.

Ebola virus (EBOV) and Marburg virus (MARV), belonging to the Filoviridae family, emerged four decades ago and caused severe viral hemorrhagic fever in human and other primates. As high as 50-90% mortality, filoviruses can cause significant threats to public health. However, so far no specific and efficient vaccine has been available, nor have other treatment methods proved to be effective. It is of great importance to detect these pathogens specific, rapidly and sensitively in order to control future filovirus outbreaks. Here, recent progresses in the development of detection and diagnosis methods for EBOV and MARV are summarized.

PMID: 21468930 [PubMed - indexed for MEDLINE]
1224. J Med Chem. 2011 Mar 10;54(5):1157-69. doi: 10.1021/jm100938u. Epub 2011 Jan 25.

A chemotype that inhibits three unrelated pathogenic targets: the botulinum neurotoxin serotype A light chain, P. falciparum malaria, and the Ebola filovirus.

Opsenica I(1), Burnett JC, Gussio R, Opsenica D, Todorović N, Lanteri CA, Sciotti RJ, Gettayacamin M, Basilico N, Taramelli D, Nuss JE, Wanner L, Panchal RG, Solaja BA, Bavari S.

Author information: (1)Faculty of Chemistry, University of Belgrade, Studentski trg 16, PO Box 51, 11158 Belgrade, Serbia.

A 1,7-bis(alkylamino)diazachrysene-based small molecule was previously identified as an inhibitor of the botulinum neurotoxin serotype A light chain metalloprotease. Subsequently, a variety of derivatives of this chemotype were synthesized to develop structure-activity relationships, and all are inhibitors of the BoNT/A LC. Three-dimensional analyses indicated that half of the originally discovered 1,7-DAAC structure superimposed well with 4-amino-7-chloroquinoline-based antimalarial agents. This observation led to the discovery that several of the 1,7-DAAC derivatives are potent in vitro inhibitors of Plasmodium falciparum and, in general, are more efficacious against CQ-resistant strains than against CQ-susceptible strains. In addition, by inhibiting β-hematin formation, the most efficacious 1,7-DAAC-based antimalarials employ a mechanism of action analogous to that of 4,7-ACQ-based antimalarials and are well tolerated by normal cells. One candidate was also effective when administered orally in a rodent-based malaria model. Finally, the 1,7-DAAC-based derivatives were examined for Ebola filovirus inhibition in an assay employing Vero76 cells, and three provided promising antiviral activities and acceptably low toxicities.

PMCID: PMC3056319 PMID: 21265542 [PubMed - indexed for MEDLINE]
1225. Lancet. 2011 Mar 5;377(9768):849-62. doi: 10.1016/S0140-6736(10)60667-8.

Ebola haemorrhagic fever.

Feldmann H(1), Geisbert TW.

Author information: (1)Laboratory of Virology, Division of Intramural Research, National Institute of Allergy and Infectious Diseases, National Institutes of Health, Rocky Mountain Laboratories, Hamilton, MT, USA. feldmannh@niaid.nih.gov

Ebola viruses are the causative agents of a severe form of viral haemorrhagic fever in man, designated Ebola haemorrhagic fever, and are endemic in regions of central Africa. The exception is the species Reston Ebola virus, which has not been associated with human disease and is found in the Philippines. Ebola virus constitutes an important local public health threat in Africa, with a worldwide effect through imported infections and through the fear of misuse for biological terrorism. Ebola virus is thought to also have a detrimental effect on the great ape population in Africa. Case-fatality rates of the African species in man are as high as 90%, with no prophylaxis or treatment available. Ebola virus infections are characterised by immune suppression and a systemic inflammatory response that causes impairment of the vascular, coagulation, and immune systems, leading to multiorgan failure and shock, and thus, in some ways, resembling septic shock.

PMCID: PMC3406178 PMID: 21084112 [PubMed - indexed for MEDLINE]

1226. Arch Virol. 2011 Mar;156(3):489-94. doi: 10.1007/s00705-010-0847-1. Epub 2010 Nov 23

Sensitivity to ultraviolet radiation of Lassa, vaccinia, and Ebola viruses dried on surfaces.

Sagripanti JL(1), Lytle CD.

Author information: (1)Research and Technology Directorate, Edgewood Chemical Biological Center, U.S. Army, Aberdeen Proving Ground, MD, USA. joseluis.sagripanti@us.army.mil

Germicidal UV (also known as UVC) provides a means to decontaminate infected environments as well as a measure of viral sensitivity to sunlight. The present study determined UVC inactivation slopes (and derived D(37) values) of viruses dried onto nonporous (glass) surfaces. The data obtained indicate that the UV resistance of Lassa virus is higher than that of Ebola virus. The UV sensitivity of vaccinia virus (a surrogate for variola virus) appeared intermediate between that of the two virulent viruses studied. In addition, the three viruses dried on surfaces showed a relatively small but significant population of virions (from 3 to 10 % of virus in the inoculum) that appeared substantially more protected by their environment from the effect of UV than the majority of virions tested. The findings reported in this study should assist in estimating the threat posed by the persistence of virus in environments contaminated during epidemics or after an accidental or intentional release.

PMID: 21104283 [PubMed - indexed for MEDLINE]

1227. Expert Opin Drug Discov. 2011 Mar;6(3):233-50. doi: 10.1517/17460441.2011.554815.

Nonhuman primates as models for the discovery and development of ebolavirus therapeutics.

Shurtleff AC(1), Warren TK, Bavari S.

Author information: (1)US Army Medical Research Institute of Infectious Diseases, Integrated Toxicology Division, 1425 Porter Street, Fort Detrick, Frederick, MD 21702, USA +1 301 619 4246 ; +1 541 754 3545 ; sina.bavari@us.army.mil.

INTRODUCTION: Ebolaviruses are human pathogenic Category A priority pathogens for which no vaccines or therapeutics are currently licensed; however, several therapeutic agents have shown promising efficacy in nonhuman primate models of infection and are potential candidates for use in humans. Demonstration of efficacy in nonhuman primate models of ebolavirus infection will probably be central to the development and eventual licensure of ebolavirus medical countermeasures given the ethical and feasibility constraints of human efficacy assessments. AREAS COVERED: The authors describe ebolavirus hemorrhagic fever (EHF), with an emphasis on comparing human and nonhuman primate pathophysiology. Published data examining human and animal clinical disease parameters, histopathological findings, and immune responses in fatal and nonfatal cases are synthesized and evaluated. Importantly, the authors also introduce and describe the FDA Animal Efficacy Rule as well as recent advances in antiviral drug development strategies for the treatment of EHF. EXPERT OPINION: Well-characterized models of ebolavirus infection are currently under development and scrutiny as to their accuracy and utility for modeling fatal infection in humans. The advanced development and eventual licensure of therapeutic agents will require demonstration that mechanisms conferring protection in nonhuman primate models of infection are predictive of protective responses in humans.

PMID: 22647202 [PubMed]

1228. Hum Vaccin. 2011 Mar;7(3):331-8. Epub 2011 Mar 1.

Geminiviral vectors based on bean yellow dwarf virus for production of vaccine antigens and monoclonal antibodies in plants.

Chen Q(1), He J, Phoolcharoen W, Mason HS.

Author information: (1)The Biodesign Institute and School of Life Sciences, Arizona State University, Tempe, AZ, USA.

Expression of recombinant vaccine antigens and monoclonal antibodies using plant viral vectors has developed extensively during the past several years. The approach benefits from high yields of recombinant protein obtained within days after transient delivery of viral vectors to leaves of Nicotiana benthamiana, a tobacco relative. Modified viral genomes of both RNA and DNA viruses have been created. Geminiviruses such as bean yellow dwarf virus (BeYDV) have a small, single stranded DNA genome that replicates in the nucleus of an infected plant cell, using the cellular DNA synthesis apparatus and a virus-encoded replication initiator protein (Rep). BeYDV-derived expression vectors contain deletions of the viral genes encoding coat and movement proteins and insertion of an expression cassette for a protein of interest. Delivery of the geminiviral vector to leaf cells via Agrobacterium-mediated delivery produces very high levels of recombinant DNA that can act as a transcription template, yielding high levels of mRNA for the protein of interest. Several vaccine antigens, including Norwalk virus capsid protein and hepatitis B core antigen, were expressed using the BeYDV vector at levels up to 1 mg per g of leaf mass. BeYDV replicons can be stacked in the same vector molecule by linking them in tandem, which enables production of multi-subunit proteins like monoclonal antibody (mAb) heavy and light chains. The protective mAb 6D8 against Ebola virus was produced at 0.5 mg per g of leaf mass. Multi-replicon vectors could be conveniently used to produce protein complexes, e.g. virus-like particles that require two or more subunits.

PMCID: PMC3166492 PMID: 21358270 [PubMed - indexed for MEDLINE]

1229. J Virol. 2011 Mar;85(6):2512-23. doi: 10.1128/JVI.01160-10. Epub 2011 Jan 12.

Ebolavirus proteins suppress the effects of small interfering RNA by direct interaction with the mammalian RNA interference pathway.

Fabozzi G(1), Nabel CS, Dolan MA, Sullivan NJ.

Author information: (1)Biodefense Research Section, Vaccine Research Center, National Institutes of Health, Vaccine Research Center, 40 Convent Drive, Bldg. 40/2509, Bethesda, MD 20892, USA.

Cellular RNA interference (RNAi) provides a natural response against viral infection, but some viruses have evolved mechanisms to antagonize this form of antiviral immunity. To determine whether Ebolavirus (EBOV) counters RNAi by encoding suppressors of RNA silencing (SRSs), we screened all EBOV proteins using an RNAi assay initiated by exogenously delivered small interfering RNAs (siRNAs) against either an EBOV or a reporter gene. In addition to viral protein 35 (VP35), we found that VP30 and VP40 independently act as SRSs. Here, we present the molecular mechanisms of VP30 and VP35. VP30 interacts with Dicer

independently of siRNA and with one Dicer partner, TRBP, only in the presence of siRNA. VP35 directly interacts with Dicer partners TRBP and PACT in an siRNA-independent fashion and in the absence of effects on interferon (IFN). Taken together, our findings elucidate a new mechanism of RNAi suppression that extends beyond the role of SRSs in double-stranded RNA (dsRNA) binding and IFN antagonism. The presence of three suppressors highlights the relevance of host RNAi-dependent antiviral immunity in EBOV infection and illustrates the importance of RNAi in shaping the evolution of RNA viruses.
PMCID: PMC3067942 PMID: 21228243 [PubMed - indexed for MEDLINE]

1230. J Med Chem. 2011 Feb 10;54(3):765-81. doi: 10.1021/jm1008715. Epub 2011 Jan 4.

Discovery, synthesis, and biological evaluation of a novel group of selective inhibitors of filoviral entry.

Yermolina MV(1), Wang J, Caffrey M, Rong LL, Wardrop DJ.

Author information: (1)Department of Chemistry, University of Illinois, 845 West Taylor Street, Chicago, IL 60607, USA.

Herein, we report the development of an antifiloviral screening system, based on a pseudotyping strategy, and its application in the discovery of a novel group of small molecules that selectively inhibit the Ebola and Marburg glycoprotein (GP)-mediated infection of human cells. Using Ebola Zaire GP-pseudotyped HIV particles bearing a luciferase reporter gene and 293T cells, a library of 237 small molecules was screened for inhibition of GP-mediated viral entry. From this assay, lead compound 8a was identified as a selective inhibitor of filoviral entry with an IC(50) of 30 μM. To analyze functional group requirements for efficacy, a structure-activity relationship analysis of this 3,5-disubstituted isoxazole was then conducted with 56 isoxazole and triazole derivatives prepared using "click" chemistry. This study revealed that while the isoxazole ring can be replaced by a triazole system, the 5-(diethylamino)acetamido substituent found in 8a is required for inhibition of viral-cell entry. Variation of the 3-aryl substituent provided a number of more potent antiviral agents with IC(50) values ranging to 2.5 μM. Lead compound 8a and three of its derivatives were also found to block the Marburg glycoprotein (GP)-mediated infection of human cells.
PMCID: PMC3081529 PMID: 21204524 [PubMed - indexed for MEDLINE]

1231. Ugeskr Laeger. 2011 Feb 7;173(6):414-6.

[The past decade's infectious diseases].

[Article in Danish]

Mølbak K(1).

Author information: (1)Epidemiologisk Afdeling, Statens Serum Institut, 2300 København S, Denmark. krm@ssi.dk

The past decade saw emerging infections such as SARS, avian and pandemic influenza, food-borne infections and the bioterror threat. New vaccines became available and novel technologies for detection and typing of microorganisms were applied. In the years to come, control of antimicrobial drug resistance and nosocomial infections will continue to pose challenges in the light of an increasing number of senior citizens and individuals with chronic diseases. There will also be unknown challenges: We have not faced the last HIV, ebola, SARS or avian or swine flu epidemic.
PMID: 21299933 [PubMed - indexed for MEDLINE]

1232. Retrovirology. 2011 Jan 30;8:7. doi: 10.1186/1742-4690-8-7.

Interplay between HIV entry and transportin-SR2 dependency.

Thys W(1), De Houwer S, Demeulemeester J, Taltynov O, Vancraenenbroeck R, Gérard M, De Rijck J, Gijsbers R, Christ F, Debyser Z.

Author information: (1)Laboratory of Molecular Virology and Gene Therapy, Katholieke Universiteit Leuven, Kapucijnenvoer 33, VCTB+5, B-3000 Leuven, Flanders, Belgium.

BACKGROUND: Transportin-SR2 (TRN-SR2, TNPO3, transportin 3) was previously identified as an interaction partner of human immunodeficiency virus type 1 (HIV-1) integrase and functions as a nuclear import factor of HIV-1. A possible role of capsid in transportin-SR2-mediated nuclear import was recently suggested by the findings that a chimeric HIV virus, carrying the murine leukemia virus (MLV) capsid and matrix proteins, displayed a transportin-SR2 independent phenotype, and that the HIV-1 N74D capsid mutant proved insensitive to transportin-SR2 knockdown. RESULTS: Our present analysis of viral specificity reveals that TRN-SR2 is not used to the same extent by all lentiviruses. The DNA flap does not determine the TRN-SR2 requirement of HIV-1. We corroborate the TRN-SR2 independent phenotype of the chimeric HIV virus carrying the MLV capsid and matrix proteins. We reanalyzed the HIV-1 N74D capsid mutant in cells transiently or stably depleted of transportin-SR2 and confirm that the N74D capsid mutant is independent of TRN-SR2 when pseudotyped with the vesicular stomatitis virus glycoprotein (VSV-G). Remarkably, although somewhat less dependent on TRN-SR2 than wild type virus, the N74D capsid mutant carrying the wild type HIV-1 envelope required TRN-SR2 for efficient replication. By pseudotyping with envelopes that mediate pH-independent viral uptake including HIV-1, measles virus and amphotropic MLV envelopes, we demonstrate that HIV-1 N74D capsid mutant viruses retain partial dependency on TRN-SR2. However, this dependency on TRN-SR2 is lost when the HIV N74D capsid mutant is pseudotyped with envelopes mediating pH-dependent endocytosis, such as the VSV-G and Ebola virus envelopes. CONCLUSION: Here we discover a link between the viral entry of HIV and its interaction with TRN-SR2. Our data confirm the importance of TRN-SR2 in HIV-1 replication and argue for careful interpretation of experiments performed with VSV-G pseudotyped viruses in studies on early steps of HIV replication including the role of capsid therein.
PMCID: PMC3041740 PMID: 21276267 [PubMed - indexed for MEDLINE]

1233. Genome Med. 2011 Jan 27;3(1):5. doi: 10.1186/gm219.

Tackling Ebola: new insights into prophylactic and therapeutic intervention strategies.

de Wit E(1), Feldmann H, Munster VJ.

Author information: (1)Laboratory of Virology, Division of Intramural Research, National Institute of Allergy and Infectious Diseases, National Institutes of Health, Hamilton, 903 South 4th Street, MT 59840, USA. vincent.munster@nih.gov.

Since its discovery in 1976, Ebolavirus has caused periodic outbreaks of viral hemorrhagic fever associated with severe and often fatal disease. Ebolavirus is endemic in Central Africa and the Philippines. Although there is currently no approved treatment available, the past 10 years has seen remarkable progress in our understanding of the pathogenicity of Ebolavirus and the development of prophylactic and post-exposure therapies against it. In vitro and in vivo experiments have shown that Ebolavirus pathogenicity is multifactorial, including viral and host determinants. Besides their function in the virus replication cycle, the viral glycoprotein, nucleoprotein, minor matrix protein and polymerase cofactor are viral determinants of pathogenicity, with evasion of the host innate and adaptive immune responses as the main mechanism. Although no licensed Ebolavirus vaccines are currently available, vaccine research in non-human primates, the 'gold standard' animal model for Ebolavirus, has produced several promising candidates. A combination of DNA vaccination and a recombinant adenovirus serotype 5 boost resulted in cross-protective immunity in non-human primates. A recombinant vesicular stomatitis vaccine vector protected non-human primates in pre- and post-exposure challenge studies. Several antiviral therapies are currently under investigation, but only a few of these have been tested in non-human primate models. Antisense therapies, in which oligonucleotides inhibit viral replication, have shown promising results in non-human primates following post-exposure treatment. In light of the severity of Ebolavirus disease and the observed increase in Ebolavirus outbreaks over the past decade, the expedited translation of potential candidate therapeutics and vaccines from bench to bedside is currently the most challenging task for the field. Here, we review the current state of Ebolavirus research, with emphasis on prophylactic and therapeutic intervention strategies.
PMCID: PMC3092090 PMID: 21349211 [PubMed]

1234. J Immunol. 2011 Jan 15;186(2):1068-80. doi: 10.4049/jimmunol.1002212. Epub 2010 Dec 17.

Genome-based in silico identification of new Mycobacterium tuberculosis antigens activating polyfunctional CD8+ T cells in human tuberculosis.

Tang ST(1), van Meijgaarden KE, Caccamo N, Guggino G, Klein MR, van Weeren P, Kazi F, Stryhn A, Zaigler A, Sahin U, Buus S, Dieli F, Lund O, Ottenhoff TH.
Author information: (1)Center for Biological Sequence Analysis, Technical University of Denmark, 2800 Lyngby, Denmark.

Although CD8(+) T cells help control Mycobacterium tuberculosis infection, their M. tuberculosis Ag repertoire, in vivo frequency, and functionality in human tuberculosis (TB) remains largely undefined. We have performed genome-based bioinformatics searches to identify new M. tuberculosis epitopes presented by major HLA class I supertypes A2, A3, and B7 (covering 80% of the human population). A total of 432 M. tuberculosis peptides predicted to bind to HLA-A*0201, HLA-A*0301, and HLA-B*0702 (representing the above supertypes) were synthesized and HLA-binding affinities determined. Peptide-specific CD8(+) T cell proliferation assays (CFSE dilution) in 41 M. tuberculosis-responsive donors identified 70 new M. tuberculosis epitopes. Using HLA/peptide tetramers for the 18 most prominently recognized HLA-A*0201-binding M. tuberculosis peptides, recognition by cured TB patients' CD8(+) T cells was validated for all 18 epitopes. Intracellular cytokine staining for IFN-γ, IL-2, and TNF-α revealed mono-, dual-, as well as triple-positive CD8(+) T cells, indicating these M. tuberculosis peptide-specific CD8(+) T cells were (poly)functional. Moreover, these T cells were primed during natural infection, because they were absent from M. tuberculosis-noninfected individuals. Control CMV peptide/HLA-A*0201 tetramers stained CD8(+) T cells in M. tuberculosis-infected and noninfected individuals equally, whereas Ebola peptide/HLA-A*0201 tetramers were negative. In conclusion, the M. tuberculosis-epitope/Ag repertoire for human CD8(+) T cells is much broader than hitherto suspected, and the newly identified M. tuberculosis Ags are recognized by (poly)functional CD8(+) T cells during control of infection. These results impact on TB-vaccine design and biomarker identification.

PMID: 21169544 [PubMed - indexed for MEDLINE]

1235. J Infect Dis. 2011 Jan 15;203(2):175-9. doi: 10.1093/infdis/jiq025.

High-dose mannose-binding lectin therapy for Ebola virus infection.

Michelow IC(1), Lear C, Scully C, Prugar LI, Longley CB, Yantosca LM, Ji X, Karpel M, Brudner M, Takahashi K, Spear GT, Ezekowitz RA, Schmidt EV, Olinger GG.
Author information: (1)Program of Developmental Immunology, Department of Pediatrics, Massachusetts General Hospital, Harvard Medical School, Boston, Massachusetts, USA.

Mannose-binding lectin (MBL) targets diverse microorganisms for phagocytosis and complement-mediated lysis by binding specific surface glycans. Although recombinant human MBL (rhMBL) trials have focused on reconstitution therapy, safety studies have identified no barriers to its use at higher levels. Ebola viruses cause fatal hemorrhagic fevers for which no treatment exists and that are feared as potential biothreat agents. We found that mice whose rhMBL serum concentrations were increased ≥7-fold above average human levels survived otherwise fatal Ebola virus infections and became immune to virus rechallenge. Because Ebola glycoproteins potentially model other glycosylated viruses, rhMBL may offer a novel broad-spectrum antiviral approach.

PMCID: PMC3071052 PMID: 21288816 [PubMed - indexed for MEDLINE]

1236. PLoS One. 2011 Jan 13;6(1):e15756. doi: 10.1371/journal.pone.0015756.

Measuring the strength of interaction between the Ebola fusion peptide and lipid rafts: implications for membrane fusion and virus infection.

Freitas MS(1), Follmer C, Costa LT, Vilani C, Bianconi ML, Achete CA, Silva JL.
Author information: (1)Centro Nacional de Ressonância Magnética Nuclear Jiri Jonas, Instituto de Bioquímica Médica, Instituto de Ciências e Tecnologia de Biologia Estrutural e Bioimagem, Universidade Federal do Rio de Janeiro, Rio de Janeiro, Brazil.

Erratum in PLoS One. 2011;6(5). doi: 10.1371/annotation/6a5deee5-b766-49e5-a4ef-6079c2b25830.

The Ebola fusion peptide (EBO_{16}) is a hydrophobic domain that belongs to the GP2 membrane fusion protein of the Ebola virus. It adopts a helical structure in the presence of mimetic membranes that is stabilized by the presence of an aromatic-aromatic interaction established by Trp8 and Phe12. In spite of its infectious cycle becoming better understood recently, several steps still remain unclear, a lacuna that makes it difficult to develop strategies to block infection. In order to gain insight into the mechanism of membrane fusion, we probed the structure, function and energetics of EBO_{16} and its mutant W8A, in the absence or presence of different lipid membranes, including isolated domain-resistant membranes (DRM), a good experimental model for lipid rafts. The depletion of cholesterol from living mammalian cells reduced the ability of EBO_{16} to induce lipid mixing. On the other hand, EBO_{16} was structurally sensitive to interaction with lipid rafts (DRMs), but the same was not observed for W8A mutant. In agreement with these data, W8A showed a poor ability to promote membrane aggregation in comparison to EBO_{16}. Single molecule AFM experiments showed a high affinity force pattern for the interaction of EBO_{16} and DRM, which seems to be a complex energetic event as observed by the calorimetric profile. Our study is the first to show a strong correlation between the initial step of Ebola virus infection and cholesterol, thus providing a rationale for Ebola virus proteins being co-localized with lipid-raft domains. In all, the results show how small fusion peptide sequences have evolved to adopt highly specific and strong interactions with membrane domains. Such features suggest these processes are excellent targets for therapeutic and vaccine approaches to viral diseases.

PMCID: PMC3020948 PMID: 21249196 [PubMed - indexed for MEDLINE]

1237. Virol J. 2011 Jan 12;8:11. doi: 10.1186/1743-422X-8-11.

Full-length Ebola glycoprotein accumulates in the endoplasmic reticulum.

Bhattacharyya S(1), Hope TJ.

Author information: (1)Department of Cell and Molecular Biology, Feinberg School of Medicine, Northwestern University, 303 East Chicago Avenue, Chicago, Illinois 60611, USA.

The Filoviridae family comprises of Ebola and Marburg viruses, which are known to cause lethal hemorrhagic fever. However, there is no effective anti-viral therapy or licensed vaccines currently available for these human pathogens. The envelope glycoprotein (GP) of Ebola virus, which mediates entry into target cells, is cytotoxic and this effect maps to a highly glycosylated mucin-like region in the surface subunit of GP (GP1). However, the mechanism underlying this cytotoxic property of GP is unknown. To gain insight into the basis of this GP-induced cytotoxicity, HEK293T cells were transiently transfected with full-length and mucin-deleted (Δmucin) Ebola GP plasmids and GP localization was examined relative to the nucleus, endoplasmic reticulum (ER), Golgi, early and late endosomes using deconvolution fluorescent microscopy. Full-length Ebola GP was observed to accumulate in the ER. In contrast, GPΔmucin was uniformly expressed throughout the cell and did not localize in the ER. The Ebola major matrix protein VP40 was also co-expressed with GP to investigate its influence on GP localization. GP and VP40 co-expression did not alter GP localization to the ER. Also, when VP40 was co-expressed with the nucleoprotein (NP), it localized to the plasma membrane while NP accumulated in distinct cytoplasmic structures lined with vimentin. These latter structures are consistent with aggresomes and may serve as assembly sites for filoviral nucleocapsids. Collectively, these data suggest that full-length GP, but not GPΔmucin, accumulates in the ER in close proximity to the nuclear membrane, which may underscore its cytotoxic property.

PMCID: PMC3024955 PMID: 21223600 [PubMed - indexed for MEDLINE]

1238. J Antivir Antiretrovir. 2011 Jan 7;3:8-10.

Development of an Antiviral Screening Protocol: One-Stone-Two-Birds.

Rumschlag-Booms E(1), Zhang H, Soejarto DD, Fong HH, Rong L.

Author information: (1)Department of Microbiology and Immunology, University of Illinois at Chicago, Chicago, IL 60612.

As prophylactic therapies and vaccines against viral infections continue to improve, drug resistant strains are continuing to arise; therefore it is imperative to develop new therapeutics against these diseases. For highly pathogenic viruses, such as Ebola and H5N1 influenza virus, the need for antivirals is even more urgent due to limited therapeutics against these viruses. Furthermore, the high pathogenicity of such viruses often makes it difficult to work with such agents. In this report, we describe a protocol called One-stone-two-birds which provides a safe and efficient screening system to identify anti-flu (entry) and anti-HIV (replication) activities. Using plant extracts as an example, we demonstrate the utility of this protocol in antiviral screening.

PMCID: PMC3227027 PMID: 22140608 [PubMed]

1239. PLoS Pathog. 2011 Jan 6;7(1):e1001258. doi: 10.1371/journal.ppat.1001258.

Distinct patterns of IFITM-mediated restriction of filoviruses, SARS coronavirus, and influenza A virus.

Huang IC(1), Bailey CC, Weyer JL, Radoshitzky SR, Becker MM, Chiang JJ, Brass AL, Ahmed AA, Chi X, Dong L, Longobardi LE, Boltz D, Kuhn JH, Elledge SJ, Bavari S, Denison MR, Choe H, Farzan M.

Author information: (1)Department of Microbiology and Molecular Genetics, Harvard Medical School, New England Primate Research Center, Southborough, Massachusetts, United States of America. I-Chueh_Huang@hms.harvard.edu

Interferon-inducible transmembrane proteins 1, 2, and 3 (IFITM1, 2, and 3) are recently identified viral restriction factors that inhibit infection mediated by the influenza A virus (IAV) hemagglutinin (HA) protein. Here we show that IFITM proteins restricted infection mediated by the entry glycoproteins (GP(1,2)) of Marburg and Ebola filoviruses (MARV, EBOV). Consistent with these observations, interferon-β specifically restricted filovirus and IAV entry processes. IFITM proteins also inhibited replication of infectious MARV and EBOV. We observed distinct patterns of IFITM-mediated restriction: compared with IAV, the entry processes of MARV and EBOV were less restricted by IFITM3, but more restricted by IFITM1. Moreover, murine Ifitm5 and 6 did not restrict IAV, but efficiently inhibited filovirus entry. We further demonstrate that replication of infectious SARS coronavirus (SARS-CoV) and entry mediated by the SARS-CoV spike (S) protein are restricted by IFITM proteins. The profile of IFITM-mediated restriction of SARS-CoV was more similar to that of filoviruses than to IAV. Trypsin treatment of receptor-associated SARS-CoV pseudovirions, which bypasses their dependence on lysosomal cathepsin L, also bypassed IFITM-mediated restriction. However, IFITM proteins did not reduce cellular cathepsin activity or limit access of virions to acidic intracellular compartments. Our data indicate that IFITM-mediated restriction is localized to a late stage in the endocytic pathway. They further show that IFITM proteins differentially restrict the entry of a broad range of enveloped viruses, and modulate cellular tropism independently of viral receptor expression.

PMCID: PMC3017121 PMID: 21253575 [PubMed - indexed for MEDLINE]

1240. Adv Virol. 2011 Jan 1;2011. pii: 341816.

Bimolecular Complementation to Visualize Filovirus VP40-Host Complexes in Live Mammalian Cells: Toward the Identification of Budding Inhibitors.

Liu Y(1), Lee MS, Olson MA, Harty RN.
Author information: (1)Department of Pathobiology, School of Veterinary Medicine, University of Pennsylvania, 3800 Spruce Street, Philadelphia, PA 19104, USA.
Virus-host interactions play key roles in promoting efficient egress of many RNA viruses, including Ebola virus (EBOV or "e") and Marburg virus (MARV or "m"). Late- (L-) domains conserved in viral matrix proteins recruit specific host proteins, such as Tsg101 and Nedd4, to facilitate the budding process. These interactions serve as attractive targets for the development of broad-spectrum budding inhibitors. A major gap still exists in our understanding of the mechanism of filovirus budding due to the difficulty in detecting virus-host complexes and mapping their trafficking patterns in the natural environment of the cell. To address this gap, we used a bimolecular complementation (BiMC) approach to detect, localize, and follow the trafficking patterns of eVP40-Tsg101 complexes in live mammalian cells. In addition, we used the BiMC approach along with a VLP budding assay to test small molecule inhibitors identified by in silico screening for their ability to block eVP40 PTAP-mediated interactions with Tsg101 and subsequent budding of eVP40 VLPs. We demonstrated the potential broad spectrum activity of a lead candidate inhibitor by demonstrating its ability to block PTAP-dependent binding of HIV-1 Gag to Tsg101 and subsequent egress of HIV-1 Gag VLPs.

PMCID: PMC3217271 PMID: 22102845 [PubMed]

1241. Curr Med Chem. 2011;18(22):3431-6.

Quasi-life self-organizing systems: based on ensembles of succinylated derivatives of interferon-gamma.

Martynov A(1), Farber B, Farber S.
Author information: (1)American Medical Technologies, Inc., Noigel LLC, 1781 East 17th Street Suite D6, Brooklyn, NY 11229, USA.

Research has been conducted on the chemical and biological properties of combinatorial succinylated derivatives of interferon-γ with various levels of acylation, which create quasi-life, self-organizing ensembles. As a result of the research, it has been established that acylation by succinic anhydride of two lysines in the structure of interferon-γ (Gammaferon) leads to both an increase in its affinity to cell receptors and a decrease in the time of maximum effect from 48 hours to 15 minutes. Moreover, treatment of cells with these interferon ensembles led to the shielding of 100% of the cells after a 15-minute incubation period, whereas native interferon shielded no more than 80% of the cells after 48 hours. Other ensembles also protected cells from viral action, but this protective effect did not exceed two hours in duration. The ensemble of succinylated interferon- γ with two modified lysines may hold promise for the treatment of severe viral infections with fast courses, such as influenza and the diseases caused by the Ebola, Marburg, SARS, and other viruses.

PMID: 21728956 [PubMed - indexed for MEDLINE]

1242. Expert Rev Vaccines. 2011 Jan;10(1):63-77. doi: 10.1586/erv.10.152.

Progress in filovirus vaccine development: evaluating the potential for clinical use.

Falzarano D(1), Geisbert TW, Feldmann H.
Author information: (1)Laboratory of Virology, Rocky Mountain Laboratories, Division of Intramural Research, National Institute of Allergy and Infectious Disease, National Institutes of Health, 903 South 4th Street, Hamilton, MT 59840, USA.

Marburg and Ebola viruses cause severe hemorrhagic fever in humans and nonhuman primates. Currently, there are no effective treatments and no licensed vaccines; although a number of vaccine platforms have proven successful in animal models. The ideal filovirus vaccine candidate should be able to provide rapid protection following a single immunization, have the potential to work postexposure and be cross-reactive or multivalent against all Marburg virus strains and all relevant Ebola virus species and strains. Currently, there are multiple platforms that have provided prophylactic protection in nonhuman primates, including DNA, recombinant adenovirus serotype 5, recombinant human parainfluenza virus 3 and virus-like particles. In addition, a single platform, recombinant vesicular stomatitis virus, has demonstrated both prophylactic and postexposure protection in nonhuman primates. These results demonstrate that achieving a vaccine that is protective against filoviruses is possible; the challenge now is to prove its safety and efficacy in order to obtain a vaccine that is ready for human use.

PMCID: PMC3398800 PMID: 21162622 [PubMed - indexed for MEDLINE]

1243. J Biomed Biotechnol. 2011;2011:984241. doi: 10.1155/2011/984241. Epub 2011 Dec 28

Protective role of cytotoxic T lymphocytes in filovirus hemorrhagic fever.

Warfield KL(1), Olinger GG.
Author information: (1)Vaccine Development, Integrated Biotherapeutics, Inc., 21 Firstfield Road Suite 100, Gaithersburg, MD 20878, USA.
kelly@integratedbiotherapeutics.com

Infection with many emerging viruses, such as the hemorrhagic fever disease caused by the filoviruses, Marburg (MARV), and Ebola virus (EBOV), leaves the host with a short timeframe in which to mouse a protective immune response. In lethal cases, uncontrolled viral replication and virus-induced immune dysregulation are too severe to overcome, and mortality is generally associated with a lack of notable immune responses. Vaccination studies in animals have demonstrated an association of IgG and neutralizing antibody responses against the protective glycoprotein antigen with survival from lethal challenge. More recently, studies in animal models of filovirus hemorrhagic fever have established that induction of a strong filovirus-specific cytotoxic T lymphocyte (CTL) response can facilitate complete viral clearance. In this review, we describe assays used to discover CTL responses after vaccination or live filovirus infection in both animal models and human clinical trials. Unfortunately, little data regarding CTL responses have been collected from infected human survivors, primarily due to the low frequency of disease and the inability to perform these studies in the field. Advancements in assays and technologies may allow these studies to occur during future outbreaks.

PMCID: PMC3255346 PMID: 22253531 [PubMed - indexed for MEDLINE]

1244. J Virol. 2011 Jan;85(1):334-47. doi: 10.1128/JVI.01278-09. Epub 2010 Nov 3.

The Tyro3 receptor kinase Axl enhances macropinocytosis of Zaire ebolavirus.

Hunt CL(1), Kolokoltsov AA, Davey RA, Maury W.

Author information: (1)Dept. Microbiology, University of Iowa, Iowa City, IA 52242, USA.

Axl, a plasma membrane-associated Tyro3/Axl/Mer (TAM) family member, is necessary for optimal Zaire ebolavirus (ZEBOV) glycoprotein (GP)-dependent entry into some permissive cells but not others. To date, the role of Axl in virion entry is unknown. The focus of this study was to characterize entry pathways that are used for ZEBOV uptake in cells that require Axl for optimal transduction and to define the role of Axl in this process. Through the use of biochemical inhibitors, interfering RNA (RNAi), and dominant negative constructs, we demonstrate that ZEBOV-GP-dependent entry into these cells occurs through multiple uptake pathways, including both clathrin-dependent and caveola/lipid raft-mediated endocytosis. Other dynamin-dependent and -independent pathways such as macropinocytosis that mediate high-molecular-weight dextran uptake also stimulated ZEBOV-GP entry into these cells, and inhibitors that are known to block macropinocytosis inhibited both dextran uptake and ZEBOV infection. These findings provided strong evidence for the importance of this pathway in filovirus entry. Reduction of Axl expression by RNAi treatment resulted in decreased ZEBOV entry via macropinocytosis but had no effect on the clathrin-dependent or caveola/lipid raft-mediated endocytic mechanisms. Our findings demonstrate for the first time that Axl enhances macropinocytosis, thereby increasing productive ZEBOV entry.

PMCID: PMC3014168 PMID: 21047970 [PubMed - indexed for MEDLINE]

1245. J Virol Methods. 2011 Jan;171(1):310-3. doi: 10.1016/j.jviromet.2010.11.010. Epub 2010 Nov 17.

Detection of all known filovirus species by reverse transcription-polymerase chain reaction using a primer set specific for the viral nucleoprotein gene.

Ogawa H(1), Miyamoto H, Ebihara H, Ito K, Morikawa S, Feldmann H, Takada A.

Author information: (1)Hokudai Center for Zoonosis Control in Zambia, School of Veterinary Medicine, The University of Zambia, Lusaka, Zambia.

The filoviruses, Marburg virus (MARV) and Ebola virus (EBOV), are causative agents of severe hemorrhagic fever with high mortality rates in humans and non-human primates. Sporadic outbreaks of filovirus infection have occurred in Central Africa and parts of Asia. Identification of the natural reservoir animals that are unknown yet and epidemiological investigations are current challenges to forestall outbreaks of filovirus diseases. The filovirus species identified currently include one in the MARV group and five in the EBOV group, with large genetic variations found among the species. Therefore, it has been difficult to develop a single sensitive assay to detect all filovirus species, which would advance laboratory diagnosis greatly in endemic areas. In this study, a highly sensitive universal RT-PCR assay targeting the nucleoprotein (NP) gene of filoviruses was developed. The genomic RNAs of all known MARV and EBOV species were detected by using an NP-specific primer set. In addition, this RT-PCR procedure was verified further for its application to detect viral RNAs in tissue samples of animals infected experimentally and blood specimens of infected patients. This assay will be a useful method for diagnostics and epidemiological studies of filovirus infections.

PMCID: PMC3393132 PMID: 21093485 [PubMed - indexed for MEDLINE]

1246. Pan Afr Med J. 2011;9:43. Epub 2011 Aug 23.

Reporting epidemics: newspapers, information dissemination and the story of Ebola in the Ugandan district of Luweero.

Mwesiga A(1).

Author information: (1)Pan African Medical Journal, African Field Epidemiology Network, Kampala, Uganda.

When an outbreak occurs, the affected population needs timely information in order to make informed decisions on how best to deal with the situation. Most target populations rely on the media for their information and the authorities use the media to disseminate outbreak information. The media, particularly locally based media, is as a result, crucial to public health outcomes. Reports on outbreaks should be as easy to understand as possible. However, there is, at times, a mismatch between the ideal and the practice. In looking at an example of the practice, this opinion hopes to influence the negotiation for the ideal in outbreak reporting.

PMCID: PMC3215565 PMID: 22355441 [PubMed - indexed for MEDLINE]

1247. PLoS One. 2011;6(12):e29030. doi: 10.1371/journal.pone.0029030. Epub 2011 Dec 22.

Consequences of non-intervention for infectious disease in African great apes.

Ryan SJ(1), Walsh PD.

Author information: (1)Department of Environmental and Forest Biology, SUNY College of Environmental Science and Forestry, Syracuse, New York, USA. sjryan@esf.edu

Infectious disease has recently joined poaching and habitat loss as a major threat to African apes. Both "naturally" occurring pathogens, such as Ebola and Simian Immunodeficiency Virus (SIV), and respiratory pathogens transmitted from humans, have been confirmed as important sources of mortality in wild gorillas and chimpanzees. While awareness of the threat has increased, interventions such as vaccination and treatment remain controversial. Here we explore both the risk of disease to African apes, and the status of potential responses. Through synthesis of published data, we summarize prior disease impact on African apes. We then use a simple demographic model to illustrate the resilience of a well-known gorilla population to disease, modeled on prior documented outbreaks. We found that the predicted recovery time for this specific gorilla population from a single outbreak ranged from 5 years for a low mortality (4%) respiratory outbreak, to 131 years for an Ebola outbreak that killed 96% of the population. This shows that mortality rates comparable to those recently reported for disease outbreaks in wild populations are not sustainable. This is particularly troubling given the rising pathogen risk created by increasing habituation of wild apes for tourism, and the growth of human populations surrounding protected areas. We assess potential future disease spillover risk in terms of vaccination rates amongst humans that may come into contact with wild apes, and the availability of vaccines against potentially threatening diseases. We discuss and evaluate non-interventionist responses such as limiting tourist access to apes, community health programs, and safety, logistic, and cost issues that constrain the potential of vaccination.

© 2011 Ryan and Walsh.

PMCID: PMC3245243 PMID: 22216162 [PubMed - indexed for MEDLINE]

1248. PLoS One. 2011;6(10):e26040. doi: 10.1371/journal.pone.0026040. Epub 2011 Oct 24.

Rapid high yield production of different glycoforms of Ebola virus monoclonal antibody.

Castilho A(1), Bohorova N, Grass J, Bohorov O, Zeitlin L, Whaley K, Altmann F, Steinkellner H.

Author information: (1)Department of Applied Genetics and Cell Biology, University of Natural Resources and Life Sciences, Vienna, Austria.

BACKGROUND: Fc-glycosylation of monoclonal antibodies (mAbs) has profound implications on the Fc-mediated effector functions. Alteration of this glycosylation may affect the efficiency of an antibody. However, difficulties in the production of mAbs with homogeneous N-glycosylation profiles in sufficient amounts hamper investigations of the potential biological impact of different glycan residues. METHODOLOGY/PRINCIPAL FINDINGS: Here we set out to evaluate a transient plant viral based production system for the rapid generation of different glycoforms of a monoclonal antibody. Ebola virus mAb h-13F6 was generated using magnICON expression system in Nicotiana benthamiana, a plant species developed for commercial scale production of therapeutic proteins. h-13F6 was co-expressed with a series of modified mammalian enzymes involved in the processing of complex N-glycans. Using wild type (WT) plants and the glycosylation mutant ΔXTFT that synthesizes human like biantennary N-glycans with terminal N-acetylglucosamine on each branch (GnGn structures) as expression hosts we demonstrate the generation of h-13F6 complex N-glycans with (i) bisected structures, (ii) core α1,6 fucosylation and (iii) β1,4 galactosylated oligosaccharides. In addition we emphasize the significance of precise sub Golgi localization of enzymes for engineering of IgG Fc-glycosylation. CONCLUSION: The method described here allows the efficient generation of a series of different human-like glycoforms at large homogeneity of virtually any antibody within one week after cDNA delivery to plants. This accelerates follow up functional studies and thus may contribute to study the biological role of N-glycan residues on Fcs and maximizing the clinical efficacy of therapeutic antibodies.

PMCID: PMC3200319 PMID: 22039433 [PubMed - indexed for MEDLINE]

1249. PLoS One. 2011;6(10):e26180. doi: 10.1371/journal.pone.0026180. Epub 2011 Oct 12.

Infection of XC cells by MLVs and Ebola virus is endosome-dependent but acidification-independent.

Kamiyama H(1), Kakoki K, Yoshii H, Iwao M, Igawa T, Sakai H, Hayashi H, Matsuyama T, Yamamoto N, Kubo Y.

Author information: (1)Department of AIDS Research, Institute of Tropical Medicine, Global COE Program, Nagasaki University, Nagasaki, Japan.

Inhibitors of endosome acidification or cathepsin proteases attenuated infections mediated by envelope proteins of xenotropic murine leukemia virus-related virus (XMRV) and Ebola virus, as well as ecotropic, amphotropic, polytropic, and xenotropic murine leukemia viruses (MLVs), indicating that infections by these viruses occur through acidic endosomes and require cathepsin proteases in the susceptible cells such as TE671 cells. However, as previously shown, the endosome acidification inhibitors did not inhibit these viral infections in XC cells. It is generally accepted that the ecotropic MLV infection in XC cells occurs at the plasma membrane. Because cathepsin proteases are activated by low pH in acidic endosomes, the acidification inhibitors may inhibit the viral infections by suppressing cathepsin protease activation. The acidification inhibitors attenuated the activities of cathepsin proteases B and L in TE671 cells, but not in XC cells. Processing of cathepsin protease L was suppressed by the acidification inhibitor in NIH3T3 cells, but again not in XC cells. These results indicate that cathepsin proteases are activated without endosome acidification in XC cells. Treatment with an endocytosis inhibitor or knockdown of dynamin 2 expression by siRNAs suppressed MLV infections in all examined cells including XC cells. Furthermore, endosomal cathepsin proteases were required for these viral infections in XC cells as other susceptible cells. These results suggest that infections of XC cells by the MLVs and Ebola virus occur through endosomes and pH-independent cathepsin activation induces pH-independent infection in XC cells.

PMCID: PMC3192169 PMID: 22022555 [PubMed - indexed for MEDLINE]

1250. Viruses. 2011 Jan;3(1):26-31. doi: 10.3390/v3010026.

Un-"ESCRT"-ed budding.

Yondola M(1), Carter C.

Author information: (1)Department of Microbiology, Mount Sinai School of Medicine, New York, NY 10128, USA. mark.yondola@mssm.edu

In their recent publication, Rossman et al. describe how the inherent budding capability of its M2 protein allows influenza A virus to bypass recruitment of the cellular ESCRT machinery enlisted by several other enveloped RNA and DNA viruses, including HIV, Ebola, rabies, herpes simplex type I and hepatitis B. Studies from the same laboratory and other laboratories indicate that budding of plasmid-derived virus-like particles can be mediated by the influenza virus hemagglutinin and neuraminidase proteins in the absence of M2. These events are also independent of canonical ESCRT components. Understanding how intrinsic properties of these influenza virus proteins permit ESCRT-independent budding expands our understanding of the budding process itself.

PMCID: PMC3110670 PMID: 21666754 [PubMed - indexed for MEDLINE]

1251. Vopr Virusol. 2011 Jan-Feb;56(1):37-40.

[Study of the functional role of mutation in the guinea pig-adapted Ebola virus genome on a Drosophila melanogaster model].

[Article in Russian]

Shelemba-Chepurnova AA, Omel'ianchuk LV, Chepurnov AA.

Ebola virus virulence in guinea pigs, which appears through virus adaptation to this animal host, correlates with substitutions in the gene encoding vp24 protein. In particular, the substitution His-->Tyr186 was found when obtaining strain 8 ms. An attempt was made to clarify the functional role of this substitution in a transgenic fruit fly model. Using the drosophila transformation technique provided transgenic strains that contained genomic insertions of wild-type Ebola virus vp24 gene and the mutant gene with the His-->Tyr substitution at the above position. Thus, the drosophila strains carrying the sequences encoding for the vp24 proteins of Ebola virus Zaire and 8 ms in pUAST vector were obtained. This makes it possible to study the expression of transgenic constructs in various D. melanogaster organs and tissues.

PMID: 21427954 [PubMed - indexed for MEDLINE]

1252. Vaccine. 2010 Dec 16;29(2):304-13. doi: 10.1016/j.vaccine.2010.10.037. Epub 2010 Oct 27.

A replication defective recombinant Ad5 vaccine expressing Ebola virus GP is safe and immunogenic in healthy adults.

Ledgerwood JE(1), Costner P, Desai N, Holman L, Enama ME, Yamshchikov G, Mulangu S, Hu Z, Andrews CA, Sheets RA, Koup RA, Roederer M, Bailer R, Mascola JR, Pau MG, Sullivan NJ, Goudsmit J, Nabel GJ, Graham BS; VRC 205 Study Team.

Collaborators: Gordon I, Hubka S, Hendel CS, Novik L, Larkin B, Jones S, Johnson D, Sitar S, Casazza J, Goswami T, Cruz R, Gomez P, Decederfelt H, Starling J, Washington-Lewis R, Rhone K, Stanford L, Zaia P.

Author information: (1)Vaccine Research Center, National Institute of Allergy and Infectious Diseases, National Institutes of Health, 40 Convent Drive, Bethesda, MD 20892-3017, United States. Ledgerwood@mail.nih.gov

Ebola virus causes irregular outbreaks of severe hemorrhagic fever in equatorial Africa. Case mortality remains high; there is no effective treatment and outbreaks are sporadic and unpredictable. Studies of Ebola virus vaccine platforms in non-human primates have established that the induction of protective immunity is possible and safety and human immunogenicity has been demonstrated in a previous Phase I clinical trial of a 1st generation Ebola DNA vaccine. We now report the safety and immunogenicity of a recombinant adenovirus serotype 5 (rAd5) vaccine encoding the envelope glycoprotein (GP) from the Zaire and Sudan Ebola virus species, in a randomized, placebo-controlled, double-blinded, dose escalation, Phase I human study. Thirty-one healthy adults received vaccine at 2×10(9) (n=12), or 2×10(10) (n=11) viral particles or placebo (n=8) as an intramuscular injection. Antibody responses were assessed by ELISA and neutralizing assays; and T cell responses were assessed by ELISpot and intracellular cytokine staining assays. This recombinant Ebola virus vaccine was safe and subjects developed antigen specific humoral and cellular immune responses.

Published by Elsevier Ltd.

PMID: 21034824 [PubMed - indexed for MEDLINE]

1253. Vaccine. 2010 Dec 10;29(1):17-25. doi: 10.1016/j.vaccine.2010.10.024. Epub 2010 Oct 27.

Respiratory tract immunization of non-human primates with a Newcastle disease virus-vectored vaccine candidate against Ebola virus elicits a neutralizing antibody response.

DiNapoli JM(1), Yang L, Samal SK, Murphy BR, Collins PL, Bukreyev A.

Author information: (1)Laboratory of Infectious Diseases, National Institute of Allergy and Infectious Diseases, National Institutes of Health, Bethesda, MD 20892-MSC, USA.

We previously developed a respiratory tract vaccine candidate against Ebola virus (EBOV) based on human parainfluenza virus type 3 (HPIV3), a respiratory paramyxovirus, expressing the EBOV GP envelope protein (HPIV3/GP) from an added gene. Two doses of this vaccine candidate delivered by the intranasal and intratracheal route protected monkeys against intraperitoneal challenge with EBOV; however, concerns exist that the vaccine candidate may have reduced immunogenicity in the adult human population due to pre-existing immunity against HPIV3. Here we developed a new vaccine candidate (NDV/GP) based on Newcastle disease virus (NDV), an avian paramyxovirus that is antigenically distinct from human viral pathogens and is highly attenuated in monkeys. Following one intranasal and intratracheal inoculation of Rhesus monkeys with NDV/GP, titers of EBOV-specific antibodies in respiratory tract secretions and serum samples determined by ELISA, as well as serum EBOV-neutralizing antibodies, were undetectable or low compared to those induced by HPIV3/GP. A second immunization resulted in a substantial boost in serum IgG ELISA titers, yet the titers remained lower than those induced by a second dose of HPIV3/GP. In contrast, the ELISA IgA titers in respiratory tract secretions and, more importantly, the serum EBOV-neutralizing antibody titers were equal to those induced after the second dose of HPIV3/GP. These data suggest that NDV/GP can be effective for immunization against EBOV alone, or in combination with either HPIV3/GP or another vaccine platform in a heterologous prime-boost regimen.

Published by Elsevier Ltd.

PMCID: PMC3428043 PMID: 21034822 [PubMed - indexed for MEDLINE]

1254. Nano Lett. 2010 Dec 8;10(12):4962-9. doi: 10.1021/nl103025u. Epub 2010 Nov 5.

An optofluidic nanoplasmonic biosensor for direct detection of live viruses from biological media.

Yanik AA(1), Huang M, Kamohara O, Artar A, Geisbert TW, Connor JH, Altug H.

Author information: (1)Photonics Center.

Fast and sensitive virus detection techniques, which can be rapidly deployed at multiple sites, are essential to prevent and control future epidemics and bioterrorism threats. In this Letter, we demonstrate a label-free optofluidic nanoplasmonic sensor that can directly detect intact viruses from biological media at clinically relevant concentrations with little to no sample preparation. Our sensing platform is based on an extraordinary light transmission effect in plasmonic nanoholes and utilizes group-specific antibodies for highly divergent strains of rapidly evolving viruses. So far, the questions remain for the possible limitations of this technique for virus detection, as the penetration depths of the surface plasmon polaritons are comparable to the dimensions of the pathogens. Here, we demonstrate detection and recognition of small enveloped RNA viruses (vesicular stomatitis virus and pseudotyped Ebola) as well as large enveloped DNA viruses (vaccinia virus) within a dynamic range spanning 3 orders of magnitude. Our platform, by enabling high signal to noise measurements without any mechanical or optical isolation, opens up opportunities for detection of a broad range of pathogens in typical biology laboratory settings.

PMCID: PMC3123676 PMID: 21053965 [PubMed - indexed for MEDLINE]
1255. Arch Virol. 2010 Dec;155(12):2083-103. doi: 10.1007/s00705-010-0814-x. Epub 2010 Oct 30.

Proposal for a revised taxonomy of the family Filoviridae: classification, names of taxa and viruses, and virus abbreviations.

Kuhn JH(1), Becker S, Ebihara H, Geisbert TW, Johnson KM, Kawaoka Y, Lipkin WI, Negredo AI, Netesov SV, Nichol ST, Palacios G, Peters CJ, Tenorio A, Volchkov VE, Jahrling PB.

Author information: (1)Integrated Research Facility at Fort Detrick, Division of Clinical Research, National Institute of Allergy and Infectious Diseases, National Institutes of Health, National Interagency Biodefense Campus, B-8200 Research Plaza, Fort Detrick, Frederick, MD 21702, USA. kuhnjens@mail.nih.gov

The taxonomy of the family Filoviridae (marburgviruses and ebolaviruses) has changed several times since the discovery of its members, resulting in a plethora of species and virus names and abbreviations. The current taxonomy has only been partially accepted by most laboratory virologists. Confusion likely arose for several reasons: species names that consist of several words or which (should) contain diacritical marks, the current orthographic identity of species and virus names, and the similar pronunciation of several virus abbreviations in the absence of guidance for the correct use of vernacular names. To rectify this problem, we suggest (1) to retain the current species names Reston ebolavirus, Sudan ebolavirus, and Zaire ebolavirus, but to replace the name Cote d'Ivoire ebolavirus [sic] with Taï Forest ebolavirus and Lake Victoria marburgvirus with Marburg marburgvirus; (2) to revert the virus names of the type marburgviruses and ebolaviruses to those used for decades in the field (Marburg virus instead of Lake Victoria marburgvirus and Ebola virus instead of Zaire ebolavirus); (3) to introduce names for the remaining viruses reminiscent of jargon used by laboratory virologists but nevertheless different from species names (Reston virus, Sudan virus, Taï Forest virus), and (4) to introduce distinct abbreviations for the individual viruses (RESTV for Reston virus, SUDV for Sudan virus, and TAFV for Taï Forest virus), while retaining that for Marburg virus (MARV) and reintroducing that used over decades for Ebola virus (EBOV). Paying tribute to developments in the field, we propose (a) to create a new ebolavirus species (Bundibugyo ebolavirus) for one member virus (Bundibugyo virus, BDBV); (b) to assign a second virus to the species Marburg marburgvirus (Ravn virus, RAVV) for better reflection of now available high-resolution phylogeny; and (c) to create a new tentative genus (Cuevavirus) with one tentative species (Lloviu cuevavirus) for the recently discovered Lloviu virus (LLOV). Furthermore, we explain the etymological derivation of individual names, their pronunciation, and their correct use, and we elaborate on demarcation criteria for each taxon and virus.

PMCID: PMC3074192 PMID: 21046175 [PubMed - indexed for MEDLINE]
1256. Arch Virol. 2010 Dec;155(12):2035-9. doi: 10.1007/s00705-010-0791-0. Epub 2010 Sep 15.

Persistence in darkness of virulent alphaviruses, Ebola virus, and Lassa virus deposited on solid surfaces.

Sagripanti JL(1), Rom AM, Holland LE.

Author information: (1)Edgewood Chemical Biological Center, 5183 Blackhawk Road (RDCB-DR) Aberdeen Proving Ground, Maryland 21010-5424, USA. joseluis.sagripanti@us.army.mil

Ebola, Lassa, Venezuelan equine encephalitis, and Sindbis viruses were dried onto solid surfaces, incubated for various time periods under controlled conditions of temperature and relative humidity, and quantitatively eluted from surfaces, and viral titers in the recovered samples were determined. The viral inactivation kinetics that were obtained indicated that viral resistance to natural inactivation in the dark follows (in decreasing order of stability) alphavirus > Lassa virus > Ebola virus. The findings reported in this study on the natural decay in the dark should assist in understanding the biophysical properties of enveloped RNA viruses outside the host and in estimating the persistence of viruses in the environment during epidemics or after an accidental or intentional release.

PMID: 20842393 [PubMed - indexed for MEDLINE]
1257. Curr Protoc Pharmacol. 2010 Dec;Chapter 13:Unit 13B.3. doi: 10.1002/0471141755.ph13b03s51.

High-throughput screening of viral entry inhibitors using pseudotyped virus.

Basu A(1), Mills DM, Bowlin TL.

Author information: (1)Microbiotix, Worcester, Massachusetts, USA.

Virus entry into a host cell is an attractive target for therapy because propagation of virus can be blocked at an early stage, minimizing chances for the virus to acquire drug resistance. Anti-infective drug discovery for BSL-4 viruses like Ebola or Lassa hemorrhagic fever virus presents challenges due to the requirement for a BSL-4 laboratory containment facility. Pseudotyped viruses provide a surrogate model in which the native envelope glycoprotein of a BSL-2 level virus (e.g., vesicular stomatitis virus) is replaced with envelope glycoprotein of a foreign BSL-4 virus (e.g., Ebola virus). Because the envelope glycoprotein determines interaction of virus with its cellular receptors, pseudotyped viruses can mimic the viral entry process of the original virus. Moreover, they are competent for only a single cycle of infection, and therefore can be used in BSL-2 facilities. Pseudotyped viruses have been used in high-throughput screening of entry inhibitors for a number of BSL-4 level viruses. This unit includes protocols for preparing pseudotyped viruses using lentiviral vectors and use of pseudotyped viruses for high-throughput screening of viral entry inhibitors.

PMID: 21935898 [PubMed - indexed for MEDLINE]
1258. Emerg Infect Dis. 2010 Dec;16(12):1969-72. doi: 10.3201/eid1612.100627.

Proportion of deaths and clinical features in Bundibugyo Ebola virus infection, Uganda.

MacNeil A(1), Farnon EC, Wamala J, Okware S, Cannon DL, Reed Z, Towner JS, Tappero JW, Lutwama J, Downing R, Nichol ST, Ksiazek TG, Rollin PE.

Author information: (1)Centers for Disease Control and Prevention, Atlanta, Georgia 30333, USA. aho3@cdc.gov

The first known Ebola hemorrhagic fever (EHF) outbreak caused by Bundibugyo Ebola virus occurred in Bundibugyo District, Uganda, in 2007. Fifty-six cases of EHF were laboratory confirmed. Although signs and symptoms were largely nonspecific and similar to those of EHF outbreaks caused by Zaire and Sudan Ebola viruses, proportion of deaths among those infected was lower (≈40%).

PMCID: PMC3294552 PMID: 21122234 [PubMed - indexed for MEDLINE]

1259. Immunogenetics. 2010 Dec;62(11-12):767-71. doi: 10.1007/s00251-010-0480-x. Epub 2010 Sep 29.

Association of KIR2DS1 and KIR2DS3 with fatal outcome in Ebola virus infection.

Wauquier N(1), Padilla C, Becquart P, Leroy E, Vieillard V.

Author information: (1)Centre International de Recherches Médicales de Franceville, Franceville, Gabon. nadia.wauquier@gmail.com

Zaïre ebolavirus (ZEBOV) infection rapidly outruns the host's immunity and leads to death within a week. Fatal cases have been associated with an aberrant innate, proinflammatory immune response followed by a suppressed adaptive response leading to the rapid depletion of peripheral NK cells and lymphocytes. A critical role for NK cells has been suggested but not elucidated. In this genetic study, we investigated the association of KIR genotype with disease outcome by comparing genotypes of a Gabonese control population, IgG+ contacts, survivors, and fatalities of ZEBOV infection. We showed that the activating KIR2DS1 and KIR2DS3 genes associate with fatal outcome in Ebola virus infection. In addition, this study brings supplemental evidence in favor of the specificity of the IgG+ contact population. The outcome of fulminating Ebola virus infection could depend in part on the host's inherited KIR gene repertoire. This supports a key role for KIRs in disease susceptibility to infections.

PMCID: PMC2978320 PMID: 20878400 [PubMed - indexed for MEDLINE]

1260. J Virol. 2010 Dec;84(24):13004-18. doi: 10.1128/JVI.01255-10. Epub 2010 Oct 6.

Metagenomic analysis of the viromes of three North American bat species: viral diversity among different bat species that share a common habitat.

Donaldson EF(1), Haskew AN, Gates JE, Huynh J, Moore CJ, Frieman MB.

Author information: (1)Department of Epidemiology, University of North Carolina, Chapel Hill, NC 27599, USA. eric_donaldson@med.unc.edu

Effective prediction of future viral zoonoses requires an in-depth understanding of the heterologous viral population in key animal species that will likely serve as reservoir hosts or intermediates during the next viral epidemic. The importance of bats as natural hosts for several important viral zoonoses, including Ebola, Marburg, Nipah, Hendra, and rabies viruses and severe acute respiratory syndrome-coronavirus (SARS-CoV), has been established; however, the large viral population diversity (virome) of bats has been partially determined for only a few of the ~1,200 bat species. To assess the virome of North American bats, we collected fecal, oral, urine, and tissue samples from individual bats captured at an abandoned railroad tunnel in Maryland that is cohabitated by 7 to 10 different bat species. Here, we present preliminary characterization of the virome of three common North American bat species, including big brown bats (Eptesicus fuscus), tricolored bats (Perimyotis subflavus), and little brown myotis (Myotis lucifugus). In samples derived from these bats, we identified viral sequences that were similar to at least three novel group I CoVs, large numbers of insect and plant virus sequences, and nearly full-length genomic sequences of two novel bacteriophages. These observations suggest that bats encounter and disseminate a large assortment of viruses capable of infecting many different animals, insects, and plants in nature.

PMCID: PMC3004358 PMID: 20926577 [PubMed - indexed for MEDLINE]

1261. Mol Cell Probes. 2010 Dec;24(6):370-5. doi: 10.1016/j.mcp.2010.08.004. Epub 2010 Aug 21.

Cross-platform evaluation of commercial real-time reverse transcription PCR master mix kits using a quantitative 5'nuclease assay for Ebola virus.

Stephens KW(1), Hutchins RJ, Dauphin LA.

Author information: (1)Bioterrorism Rapid Response and Advanced Technology (BRRAT) Laboratory, Laboratory Preparedness and Response Branch (LPRB), Division of Preparedness and Emerging Infections (DPEI), Centers for Disease Control and Prevention (CDC), Mail Stop G-42, 1600 Clifton Road, Atlanta, GA 30333, USA.

Selection of optimal reaction master mix reagents is essential to obtain the best performance with diagnostic real-time reverse transcription polymerase chain reaction (RT-PCR) assays. Every year the number of commercially available master mix kits increases, so it is prudent to periodically evaluate kits on the market. In this study we evaluated five commercial real-time RT-PCR master mix kits, the RealMasterMix RT-PCR ROX kit, the AgPath-ID One-Step RT-PCR kit, the SuperScript III Platinum One-step Quantitative RT-PCR system, the QuantiTect Probe RT-PCR kit, and the LightCycler RNA HybProbe amplification kit, using a 5'nuclease assay for Ebola virus. The kits were evaluated using the manufacturer's recommended conditions, as well as conditions which have been used with the Ebola virus assay during outbreaks. When evaluated for use in Ebola virus RNA detection, the AgPath-ID kit resulted in the greatest sensitivity in comparison to the other four kits. The efficacy of the AgPath-ID kit was instrument-independent in the five real-time PCR platforms tested. This study demonstrated that Ebola virus RNA detection was not equivalent among the master mix reagents studied and, thus, that this variable can affect real-time RT-PCR assay sensitivity. Furthermore, this study rates the master mix reagents for their suitability, providing diagnostic laboratories the option to select from these kits to suit their specific laboratory needs for real-time RT-PCR.

Published by Elsevier Ltd.

PMID: 20732412 [PubMed - indexed for MEDLINE]

1262. Mol Cell Proteomics. 2010 Dec;9(12):2690-703. doi: 10.1074/mcp.M110.003418. Epub 2010 Aug 11.

Identification of essential filovirion-associated host factors by serial proteomic analysis and RNAi screen.

Spurgers KB(1), Alefantis T, Peyser BD, Ruthel GT, Bergeron AA, Costantino JA, Enterlein S, Kota KP, Boltz RC, Aman MJ, Delvecchio VG, Bavari S.

Author information: (1)The United States Army Medical Research Institute of Infectious Diseases, 1425 Porter Street, Fort Detrick, Frederick, MD 21702, USA.

An assessment of the total protein composition of filovirus (ebolavirus and marburgvirus) virions is currently lacking. In this study, liquid chromatography-linked tandem mass spectrometry of purified ebola and marburg virions was performed to identify associated cellular proteins. Host proteins involved in cell adhesion, cytoskeleton, cell signaling, intracellular trafficking, membrane organization, and chaperones were identified. Significant overlap exists between this data set and proteomic studies of disparate viruses, including HIV-1 and influenza A, generated in multiple cell types. However, the great majority of proteins identified here have not been previously described to be incorporated within filovirus particles. Host proteins identified by liquid chromatography-linked tandem mass spectrometry could lack biological relevance because they represent protein contaminants in the virus preparation, or because they are incorporated within virions by chance. These issues were addressed using siRNA library-mediated gene knockdown (targeting each identified virion-associated host protein), followed by filovirus infection. Knockdown of several host proteins (e.g. HSPA5 and RPL18) significantly interfered with ebolavirus and marburgvirus infection, suggesting specific and relevant virion incorporation. Notably, select siRNAs inhibited ebolavirus, but enhanced marburgvirus infection, suggesting important differences between the two viruses. The proteomic analysis presented here contributes to a greater understanding of filovirus biology and potentially identifies host factors that can be targeted for antiviral drug development.

PMCID: PMC3101857 PMID: 20702783 [PubMed - indexed for MEDLINE]

1263. PLoS One. 2010 Nov 30;5(11):e15091. doi: 10.1371/journal.pone.0015091.

Liposome-coupled peptides induce long-lived memory CD8 T cells without CD4 T cells.

Taneichi M(1), Tanaka Y, Kakiuchi T, Uchida T.

Author information: (1)Department of Safety Research on Blood and Biological Products, National Institute of Infectious Diseases, Tokyo, Japan.

CD8(+) T cells provide broad immunity to viruses, because they are able to recognize all types of viral proteins. Therefore, the development of vaccines capable of inducing long-lived memory CD8(+) T cells is desired to prevent diseases, especially those for which no vaccines currently exist. However, in designing CD8(+) T cell vaccines, the role of CD4(+) T cells in the induction and maintenance of memory CD8(+) T cells remains uncertain. In the present study, the necessity or not of CD4(+) T cells in the induction and maintenance of memory CD8(+) T cells was investigated in mice immunized with liposome-coupled CTL epitope peptides. When OVA-derived CTL epitope peptides were chemically coupled to the surfaces of liposomes and inoculated into mice, both primary and secondary CTL responses were successfully induced. The results were further confirmed in CD4(+) T cell-eliminated mice, suggesting that CD4(+) T cells were not required for the generation of memory CD8(+) T cells in the case of immunization with liposome-coupled peptides. Thus, surface-linked liposomal antigens, capable of inducing long-lived memory CD8(+) T cells without the contribution of CD4(+) T cells, might be applicable for the development of vaccines to prevent viral infection, especially for those viruses that evade humoral immunity by varying their surface proteins, such as influenza viruses, HIV, HCV, SARS coronaviruses, and Ebola viruses.

PMCID: PMC3020143 PMID: 21264321 [PubMed - indexed for MEDLINE]

1264. Virol J. 2010 Nov 9;7:306. doi: 10.1186/1743-422X-7-306.

Shedding of soluble glycoprotein 1 detected during acute Lassa virus infection in human subjects.

Branco LM(1), Grove JN, Moses LM, Goba A, Fullah M, Momoh M, Schoepp RJ, Bausch DG, Garry RF.

Author information: (1)Tulane University Health Sciences Center, New Orleans, LA, USA.

BACKGROUND: Lassa hemorrhagic fever (LHF) is a neglected tropical disease with significant impact on the health care system, society, and economy of Western and Central African nations where it is endemic. With a high rate of infection that may lead to morbidity and mortality, understanding how the virus interacts with the host's immune system is of great importance for generating vaccines and therapeutics. Previous work by our group identified a soluble isoform of the Lassa virus (LASV) GP1 (sGP1) in vitro resulting from the expression of the glycoprotein complex (GPC) gene [1, 2]. Though no work has directly been done to demonstrate the function of this soluble isoform in arenaviral infections, evidence points to immunomodulatory effects against the host's immune system mediated by a secreted glycoprotein component in filoviruses, another class of hemorrhagic fever-causing viruses. A significant fraction of shed glycoprotein isoforms during viral infection and biogenesis may attenuate the host's inflammatory response, thereby enhancing viral replication and tissue damage. Such shed glycoprotein mediated effects were previously reported for Ebola virus (EBOV), a filovirus that also causes hemorrhagic fever with nearly 90 percent fatality rates [3 - 5]. The identification of an analogous phenomenon in vivo could establish a new correlate of LHF infection leading to the development of sensitive diagnostics targeting the earliest molecular events of the disease. Additionally, the reversal of potentially untoward immunomodulatory functions mediated by sGP1 could potentiate the development of novel therapeutic intervention. To this end, we investigated the presence of sGP1 in the serum of suspected LASV patients admitted to the Kenema Government Hospital (KGH) Lassa Fever Ward (LFW), in Kenema, Sierra Leone that tested positive for viral antigen or displayed classical signs of Lassa fever. RESULTS: It is reasonable to expect that a narrow window exists for detection of sGP1 as the sole protein shed during early arenaviral biogenesis. This phenomenon was clearly distinguishable from virion-associated GP1 only prior to the emergence of de novo viral particles. Despite this restricted time frame, in 2/46 suspected cases in two studies performed in late 2009 and early 2010, soluble glycoprotein component shedding was identified. Differential detection of viral antigens GP1, GP2, and NP by western blot yielded five different scenarios: whole LASV virions (GP1, GP2, NP; i.e. active viremia), different combinations of these three proteins, sGP1 only, NP only, and absence of all three proteins. Four additional samples showed inconclusive evidence for sGP1 shedding due to lack of detection of GP2 and NP in western blot; however, a sensitive LASV NP antigen capture ELISA generated marginally positive signals. CONCLUSIONS: During a narrow window following active infection with LASV, soluble GP1 can be detected in patient sera. This phenomenon parallels other VHF infection profiles, with the actual role of a soluble viral glycoprotein component in vivo remaining largely speculative. The expenditure of energy and cellular resources toward secretion of a critical protein during viral biogenesis without apparent specific function requires further investigation. Future studies will be aimed at systematically identifying the role of LASV sGP1 in the infection process and outcome in vitro and in vivo.

PMCID: PMC2993672 PMID: 21062490 [PubMed - indexed for MEDLINE]
1265. Clin Vaccine Immunol. 2010 Nov;17(11):1723-8. doi: 10.1128/CVI.00170-10. Epub 2010 Sep 22.

Enzyme-linked immunosorbent assay for detection of filovirus species-specific antibodies.

Nakayama E(1), Yokoyama A, Miyamoto H, Igarashi M, Kishida N, Matsuno K, Marzi A, Feldmann H, Ito K, Saijo M, Takada A.

Author information: (1)Department of Global Epidemiology, Hokkaido University Research Center for Zoonosis Control, Kita-20, Nishi-10, Kita-ku, Sapporo 001-0020, Japan.

Several enzyme-linked immunosorbent assays (ELISAs) for the detection of filovirus-specific antibodies have been developed. However, diagnostic methods to distinguish antibodies specific to the respective species of filoviruses, which provide the basis for serological classification, are not readily available. We established an ELISA using His-tagged secreted forms of the transmembrane glycoproteins (GPs) of five different Ebola virus (EBOV) species and one Marburg virus (MARV) strain as antigens for the detection of filovirus species-specific antibodies. The GP-based ELISA was evaluated by testing antisera collected from mice immunized with virus-like particles as well as from humans and nonhuman primates infected with EBOV or MARV. In our ELISA, little cross-reactivity of IgG antibodies was observed in most of the mouse antisera. Although sera and plasma from some patients and monkeys showed notable cross-reactivity with the GPs from multiple filovirus species, the highest reactions of IgG were uniformly detected against the GP antigen homologous to the virus species that infected individuals. We further confirmed that MARV-specific IgM antibodies were specifically detected in specimens collected from patients during the acute phase of infection. These results demonstrate the usefulness of our ELISA for diagnostics as well as ecological and serosurvey studies.
PMCID: PMC2976089 PMID: 20861331 [PubMed - indexed for MEDLINE]
1266. J Appl Microbiol. 2010 Nov;109(5):1531-9. doi: 10.1111/j.1365-2672.2010.04778.x. Epub 2010 Jun 10.

The survival of filoviruses in liquids, on solid substrates and in a dynamic aerosol.

Piercy TJ(1), Smither SJ, Steward JA, Eastaugh L, Lever MS.

Author information: (1)Biomedical Sciences Department, Defence Science and Technology Laboratory, Salisbury, Wiltshire, UK.

AIMS: Filoviruses are associated with high morbidity and lethality rates in humans, are capable of human-to-human transmission, via infected material such as blood, and are believed to have low infectious doses for humans. Filoviruses are able to infect via the respiratory route and are lethal at very low doses in experimental animal models, but there is minimal information on how well the filoviruses survive within aerosol particles. There is also little known about how well filoviruses survive in liquids or on solid surfaces which is important in management of patients or samples that have been exposed to filoviruses. METHODS AND RESULTS: Filoviruses were tested for their ability to survive in different liquids and on different solid substrates at different temperatures. The decay rates of filoviruses in a dynamic aerosol were also determined. CONCLUSIONS: Our study has shown that Lake Victoria marburgvirus (MARV) and Zaire ebolavirus (ZEBOV) can survive for long periods in different liquid media and can also be recovered from plastic and glass surfaces at low temperatures for over 3 weeks. The decay rates of ZEBOV and Reston ebolavirus (REBOV) plus MARV within a dynamic aerosol were calculated. ZEBOV and MARV had similar decay rates, whilst REBOV showed significantly better survival within an aerosol. SIGNIFICANCE AND IMPACT OF THE STUDY: Data on the survival of two ebolaviruses are presented for the first time. Extended data on the survival of MARV are presented. Data from this study extend the knowledge on the survival of filoviruses under different conditions and provide a basis with which to inform risk assessments and manage exposure to filoviruses.
PMID: 20553340 [PubMed - indexed for MEDLINE]
1267. J Virol. 2010 Nov;84(21):11374-84. doi: 10.1128/JVI.01067-10. Epub 2010 Aug 11.

Endogenous CD317/Tetherin limits replication of HIV-1 and murine leukemia virus in rodent cells and is resistant to antagonists from primate viruses.

Goffinet C(1), Schmidt S, Kern C, Oberbremer L, Keppler OT.

Author information: (1)Department of Infectious Diseases, Virology, University of Heidelberg, Im Neuenheimer Feld 324, D-69120 Heidelberg, Germany.

Human CD317 (BST-2/tetherin) is an intrinsic immunity factor that blocks the release of retroviruses, filoviruses, herpesviruses, and arenaviruses. It is unclear whether CD317 expressed endogenously in rodent cells has the capacity to interfere with the replication of the retroviral rodent pathogen murine leukemia virus (MLV) or, in the context of small-animal model development, contributes to the well-established late-phase restriction of human immunodeficiency virus type 1 (HIV-1). Here, we show that small interfering RNA (siRNA)-mediated knockdown of CD317 relieved a virion release restriction and markedly enhanced the egress of HIV-1, HIV-2, and simian immunodeficiency virus (SIV) in rat cells, including primary macrophages. Moreover, rodent CD317 potently inhibited MLV release, and siRNA-mediated depletion of CD317 in a mouse T-cell line resulted in the accelerated spread of MLV. Several virus-encoded antagonists have recently been reported to overcome the restriction imposed by human or monkey CD317, including HIV-1 Vpu, envelope glycoproteins of HIV-2 and Ebola virus, Kaposi's sarcoma-associated herpesvirus K5, and SIV Nef. In contrast, both rat and mouse CD317 showed a high degree of resistance to these viral antagonists. These data suggest that CD317 is a broadly acting and conserved mediator of innate control of retroviral infection and pathogenesis that restricts the release of retroviruses and lentiviruses in rodents. The high degree of resistance of the rodent CD317 restriction factors to antagonists from primate viruses has implications for HIV-1 small-animal model development and may guide the design of novel antiviral interventions.
PMCID: PMC2953199 PMID: 20702620 [PubMed - indexed for MEDLINE]
1268. Mol Immunol. 2010 Nov-Dec;48(1-3):240-7. doi: 10.1016/j.molimm.2010.08.004. Epub 2010 Sep 15.

Myeloid cell death associated with Toll-like receptor 7/8-mediated inflammatory response. Implication of ASK1, HIF-1 alpha, IL-1 beta and TNF-alpha.

Nicholas SA(1), Oniku AE, Sumbayev VV.

Author information: (1)Medway School of Pharmacy, University of Kent, Kent, United Kingdom.

Programmed cell death or apoptosis is an important part of the host innate immune defence, especially against ssRNA viruses (influenza virus, HIV-1, ebola virus, hepatitis C virus and many others). Viral ssRNA is recognised by endosomal Toll-like receptors 7 and 8 (TLR7/8) which induce further stages of immune defence against these pathogens. Some of the immune cells die because of inflammatory stress allowing for the selection of those cells which are resistant to stress-induced apoptosis and which are used in further stages of the host immune response. On the other hand, apoptosis could be used as an instrument to suppress the function of activated inflammatory cells. However, the mechanisms underlying death of the inflammatory cells associated with stress induced by ligands of TLR7/8 remain unclear. In this study we have found that programmed death of human myeloid cells from different cell lines associated with ligand-induced TLR7/8-mediated inflammatory stress depends on activation of apoptosis signal-regulating kinase 1 (ASK1). This enzyme is, however, not required for the production of pro-inflammatory cytokines - TNF-α and IL-1β. We have found that released IL-1β and TNF-α are involved in apoptosis of myeloid cells associated with TLR7/8-mediated inflammatory stress. The pro-apoptotic effect of released TNF-α in this case is much lower compared to that of IL-1β.

Copyright © 2010 Elsevier Ltd. All rights reserved.

PMID: 20828827 [PubMed - indexed for MEDLINE]

1269. Pharm Unserer Zeit. 2010 Nov;39(6):427-8. doi: 10.1002/pauz.201090092.

[Treatment of Ebola infection with siRNA.].

[Article in German]

Winckler T.

PMID: 20967928 [PubMed - indexed for MEDLINE]

1270. Rev Med Virol. 2010 Nov;20(6):344-57. doi: 10.1002/rmv.661.

Prospects for immunisation against Marburg and Ebola viruses.

Geisbert TW(1), Bausch DG, Feldmann H.

Author information: (1)Galveston National Laboratory1 and Department of Microbiology and Immunology2, University of Texas Medical Branch, 301 University Blvd., Galveston, TX, USA. twgeisbe@utmb.edu

For more than 30 years the filoviruses, Marburg virus and Ebola virus, have been associated with periodic outbreaks of hemorrhagic fever that produce severe and often fatal disease. The filoviruses are endemic primarily in resource-poor regions in Central Africa and are also potential agents of bioterrorism. Although no vaccines or antiviral drugs for Marburg or Ebola are currently available, remarkable progress has been made over the last decade in developing candidate preventive vaccines against filoviruses in nonhuman primate models. Due to the generally remote locations of filovirus outbreaks, a single-injection vaccine is desirable. Among the prospective vaccines that have shown efficacy in nonhuman primate models of filoviral hemorrhagic fever, two candidates, one based on a replication-defective adenovirus serotype 5 and the other on a recombinant VSV (rVSV), were shown to provide complete protection to nonhuman primates when administered as a single injection. The rVSV-based vaccine has also shown utility when administered for postexposure prophylaxis against filovirus infections. A VSV-based Ebola vaccine was recently used to manage a potential laboratory exposure.

2010 John Wiley & Sons, Ltd.

PMCID: PMC3394174 PMID: 20658513 [PubMed - indexed for MEDLINE]

1271. Virulence. 2010 Nov-Dec;1(6):526-31. Epub 2010 Nov 1.

Ebolavirus VP35 is a multifunctional virulence factor.

Leung DW(1), Prins KC, Basler CF, Amarasinghe GK.

Author information: (1)Department of Biochemistry, Biophysics and Molecular Biology, Iowa State University, Ames, IA, USA.

Ebola virus (EBOV) is a member of the filoviridae family that causes severe hemorrhagic fever during sporadic outbreaks, and no approved treatments are currently available. The multifunctional EBOV VP35 protein facilitates immune evasion by antagonizing antiviral signaling pathways and is important for viral RNA synthesis. In order to elucidate regulatory mechanisms and to develop countermeasures, we recently solved the structures of the Zaire and Reston EBOV VP35 interferon inhibitory domain (IID) in the free form and of the Zaire EBOV VP35 IID bound to dsRNA. Together with biochemical, cell biological, and virological studies, our structural work revealed that distinct regions within EBOV VP35 IID contribute to virulence through host immune evasion and viral RNA synthesis. Here we summarize our recent structural and functional studies and discuss the potential of multifunctional Ebola VP35 as a therapeutic target.

PMCID: PMC3061251 PMID: 21178490 [PubMed - indexed for MEDLINE]

1272. Vopr Virusol. 2010 Nov-Dec;55(6):35-8.

[Antigenic differences in wild-type and guinea pig-adapted Ebola virus strains].

[Article in Russian]

Razumov IA, Kazachinskaia EI, Chepurnov AA.

The splenocytes isolated from the mice immunized with wild-type or guinea pig-adapted Ebola virus strains were used to obtain hybridoma collections. Investigation of the monoclonal antibodies (mAb) obtained to one of the strains to another revealed antigenic interstrain differences in nucleoprotein and VP40. It is interesting that the differences were found in the hydridoma collection obtained against the wild-type strain. The mAbs produced by hydridomas to the adapted strain were found to equally well the antigens of both strains.

PMID: 21381339 [PubMed - indexed for MEDLINE]

1273. PLoS Negl Trop Dis. 2010 Oct 5;4(10). pii: e837. doi: 10.1371/journal.pntd.0000837.

Human fatal zaire ebola virus infection is associated with an aberrant innate immunity and with massive lymphocyte apoptosis.

Wauquier N(1), Becquart P, Padilla C, Baize S, Leroy EM.
Author information: (1)Unité des Maladies Virales Émergentes, Centre International de Recherches Médicales de Franceville, Franceville, Gabon.
BACKGROUND: Ebolavirus species Zaire (ZEBOV) causes highly lethal hemorrhagic fever, resulting in the death of 90% of patients within days. Most information on immune responses to ZEBOV comes from in vitro studies and animal models. The paucity of data on human immune responses to this virus is mainly due to the fact that most outbreaks occur in remote areas. Published studies in this setting, based on small numbers of samples and limited panels of immunological markers, have given somewhat different results. METHODOLOGY/PRINCIPAL FINDINGS: Here, we studied a unique collection of 56 blood samples from 42 nonsurvivors and 14 survivors, obtained during the five outbreaks that occurred between 1996 and 2003 in Gabon and Republic of Congo. Using Luminex technology, we assayed 50 cytokines in all 56 samples and performed phenotypic analyses by flow cytometry. We found that fatal outcome was associated with hypersecretion of numerous proinflammatory cytokines (IL-1β, IL-IRA, IL-6, IL-8, IL-15 and IL-16), chemokines and growth factors (MIP-Iα, MIP-Iβ, MCP-I, M-CSF, MIF, IP-IO, GRO-α and eotaxin). Interestingly, no increase of IFNα2 was detected in patients. Furthermore, nonsurvivors were also characterized by very low levels of circulating cytokines produced by T lymphocytes (IL-2, IL-3, IL-4, IL-5, IL-9, IL-13) and by a significant drop of CD3+CD4+ and CD3+CD8+ peripheral cells as well as a high increase in CD95 expression on T lymphocytes. CONCLUSIONS/SIGNIFICANCE: This work, the largest study to be conducted to date in humans, showed that fatal outcome is associated with aberrant innate immune responses and with global suppression of adaptive immunity. The innate immune reaction was characterized by a "cytokine storm," with hypersecretion of numerous proinflammatory cytokines, chemokines and growth factors, and by the noteworthy absence of antiviral IFNα2. Immunosuppression was characterized by very low levels of circulating cytokines produced by T lymphocytes and by massive loss of peripheral CD4 and CD8 lymphocytes, probably through Fas/FasL-mediated apoptosis.
PMCID: PMC2950153 PMID: 20957152 [PubMed - indexed for MEDLINE]

1274. Future Microbiol. 2010 Oct;5(10):1469-73. doi: 10.2217/fmb.10.117.

Towards broad protection against Ebolaviruses.

Baize S(1).
Author information: (1)Unité de Biologie des Infections Virales Emergentes, Institut Pasteur, IFR128 Biosciences Gerland, Lyon Sud, 21 av. Tony Garnier, 69365 Lyon cedex 7, France. sylvain.baize@inserm.fr
Comment on PLoS Pathog. 2010 May;6(5):e1000904.

The Ebola and Marburg viruses (from the filovirus family) induce deadly hemorrhagic fevers for which there is currently no licensed vaccine or treatment. Frequent outbreaks have occurred in sub-Saharan Africa, in humans and nonhuman primates over the last 15 years or so and constitute a major public health problem. Of particular concern, a new species of Ebolavirus recently emerged in Uganda, highlighting the high potential of these viruses to evolve and the need to develop 'broad-spectrum' vaccines against filoviruses. Hensley et al. used their well studied vaccine platform based on DNA vectors and recombinant, replication-defective, adenoviruses producing Ebolavirus glycoproteins to protect cynomolgus monkeys against a heterologous challenge with the new species. Further developments are required before this experimental approach could be adapted for field use in humans, but this study nevertheless constitutes a proof-of-concept for broad protection against Ebolaviruses.
PMID: 21073307 [PubMed]

1275. J Virol. 2010 Oct;84(20):10569-80. doi: 10.1128/JVI.00103-10. Epub 2010 Aug 4.

Infectious Lassa virus, but not filoviruses, is restricted by BST-2/tetherin.

Radoshitzky SR(1), Dong L, Chi X, Clester JC, Retterer C, Spurgers K, Kuhn JH, Sandwick S, Ruthel G, Kota K, Boltz D, Warren T, Kranzusch PJ, Whelan SP, Bavari S.
Author information: (1)U.S. Army Medical Research Institute of Infectious Diseases, 1425 Porter St., Fort Detrick, Frederick, MD 21702, USA.
Bone marrow stromal antigen 2 (BST-2/tetherin) is a cellular membrane protein that inhibits the release of HIV-1. We show for the first time, using infectious viruses, that BST-2 also inhibits egress of arenaviruses but has no effect on filovirus replication and spread. Specifically, infectious Lassa virus (LASV) release significantly decreased or increased in human cells in which BST-2 was either stably expressed or knocked down, respectively. In contrast, replication and spread of infectious Zaire ebolavirus (ZEBOV) and Lake Victoria marburgvirus (MARV) were not affected by these conditions. Replication of infectious Rift Valley fever virus (RVFV) and cowpox virus (CPXV) was also not affected by BST-2 expression. Elevated cellular levels of human or murine BST-2 inhibited the release of virus-like particles (VLPs) consisting of the matrix proteins of multiple highly virulent NIAID Priority Pathogens, including arenaviruses (LASV and Machupo virus [MACV]), filoviruses (ZEBOV and MARV), and paramyxoviruses (Nipah virus). Although the glycoproteins of filoviruses counteracted the antiviral activity of BST-2 in the context of VLPs, they could not rescue arenaviral (LASV and MACV) VLP release upon BST-2 overexpression. Furthermore, we did not observe colocalization of filoviral glycoproteins with BST-2 during infection with authentic viruses. None of the arenavirus-encoded proteins rescued budding of VLPs in the presence of BST-2. Our results demonstrate that BST-2 might be a broad antiviral factor with the ability to restrict release of a wide variety of human pathogens. However, at least filoviruses, RVFV, and CPXV are immune to its inhibitory effect.
PMCID: PMC2950602 PMID: 20686043 [PubMed - indexed for MEDLINE]

1276. J Virol. 2010 Oct;84(20):10581-91. doi: 10.1128/JVI.00925-10. Epub 2010 Aug 4.

Basic residues within the ebolavirus VP35 protein are required for its viral polymerase cofactor function.

Prins KC(1), Binning JM, Shabman RS, Leung DW, Amarasinghe GK, Basler CF.
Author information: (1)Department of Microbiology, Mount Sinai School of Medicine, Box 1124, 1 Gustave L. Levy Place, New York, NY 10029, USA.
The ebolavirus (EBOV) VP35 protein binds to double-stranded RNA (dsRNA), inhibits host alpha/beta interferon (IFN-α/β) production, and is an essential component of the viral polymerase complex. Structural studies of the VP35 C-terminal IFN inhibitory domain (IID) identified specific structural features,

including a central basic patch and a hydrophobic pocket, that are important for dsRNA binding and IFN inhibition. Several other conserved basic residues bordering the central basic patch and a separate cluster of basic residues, called the first basic patch, were also identified. Functional analysis of alanine substitution mutants indicates that basic residues outside the central basic patch are not required for dsRNA binding or for IFN inhibition. However, minigenome assays, which assess viral RNA polymerase complex function, identified these other basic residues to be critical for viral RNA synthesis. Of these, a subset located within the first basic patch is important for VP35-nucleoprotein (NP) interaction, as evidenced by the inability of alanine substitution mutants to coimmunoprecipitate with NP. Therefore, first basic patch residues are likely critical for replication complex formation through interactions with NP. Coimmunoprecipitation studies further demonstrate that the VP35 IID is sufficient to interact with NP and that dsRNA can modulate VP35 IID interactions with NP. Other basic residue mutations that disrupt the VP35 polymerase cofactor function do not affect interaction with NP or with the amino terminus of the viral polymerase. Collectively, these results highlight the importance of conserved basic residues from the EBOV VP35 C-terminal IID and validate the VP35 IID as a potential therapeutic target.

PMCID: PMC2950600 PMID: 20686031 [PubMed - indexed for MEDLINE]

1277. Virus Res. 2010 Oct;153(1):121-33. doi: 10.1016/j.virusres.2010.07.015. Epub 2010 Jul 21.

Genetic factors of Ebola virus virulence in guinea pigs.

Subbotina E(1), Dadaeva A, Kachko A, Chepurnov A.

Author information: (1)Department of Molecular Virology, State Research Center of Virology and Biotechnology Vector, Koltsovo, 630559, Russia. Subbotina@ngs.ru

Zaire ebolavirus (ZEBOV) causes severe hemorrhagic fever in primates, whereas in guinea pigs it induces a nonlethal infection with a mild fever and subsequent recovery. We performed 7 selective passages in guinea pigs resulted in obtaining of guinea pig-adapted strain (GPA-P7) strain. By the 7th passage, the infection with EBOV induced a lethal disease in animals accompanied by the characteristic hematological changes: leukocytosis (primarily due to neutrophilia) as well as pronounced deficiencies in platelets, lymphocytes, monocytes and significant decrease of blood neutrophils phagocytic capacity. Increasing of virulence correlated with appearance of several nucleotide substitutions: in the genes NP, A2166G (N566S), VP24, U10784C (L147P), G10557A (M711), G10805U (R154L), and L, G12286A (V2361). It has been theoretically calculated that the mutations associated with an increase in EBOV virulence can confer characteristic secondary structure on the proteins NP (C-terminal region) and full-sized VP24.

PMID: 20654661 [PubMed - indexed for MEDLINE]

1278. Wien Klin Wochenschr. 2010 Oct;122 Suppl 3:19-30. doi: 10.1007/s00508-010-1434-x.

[Bats and other reservoir hosts of Filoviridae. Danger of epidemic on the African continent?--a deductive literature analysis].

[Article in German]

Laminger F(1), Prinz A.

Author information: (1)Abteilung für Allgemein- und Familienmedizin am Zentrum für Public Health, Unit Ethnomedizin und International Health der Medizinischen Universität Wien, Wien, Österreich. n0542217@students.meduniwien.ac.at

Ebola and Marburg virus, forming the Filoviridae family, cause hemorrhagic fever in countries of sub-Saharan Africa. These viral diseases are characterized by a sudden epidemic occurrence as well as a high lethality. Even though a reservoir host has not been approved yet, literature indicates the order of bats (Chiroptera) as a potential reservoir host. Significant references lead to a delineation of a hypothetical ecosystem of Filoviridae including Chiroptera. IgG-specific Ebola-Zaire antibodies were detected in Hammer-headed Bats (Hypsignathus monstrosus), Epauletted Fruit Bats (Epomops franqueti), and Little Collared Fruit Bats (Myonycteris torquata) during Ebola outbreaks between 2001 and 2005 in Gabon and the Republic of the Congo. The discovery of IgG-specific-Marburg virus antibodies and virus-specific ribonucleic acid in Egyptian Fruit Bats (Rousettus aegyptiacus) provided further indication for the exploration of the reservoir host. In 2007, the Marburg virus isolation could for the first time be accomplished directly from apparently healthy and naturally infected Egyptian Fruit Bats (Rousettus aegyptiacus) in Kitaka Mine (Uganda). Risk groups can be defined through chronological reprocessing and interpretation of existing epidemic-outbreaks on the African continent and the search for infection reasons of the index cases. The following risk factors for an infection with Ebola or Marburg virus must be put into consideration: Contact with and consumption of wild animal carcasses, sightseeing in caves as well as work in mines. The focus of this review is the demonstration of risk profiles and their exposure to Chiroptera and other potential reservoir hosts.

PMID: 20924703 [PubMed - indexed for MEDLINE]

1279. PLoS Pathog. 2010 Sep 23;6(9):e1001121. doi: 10.1371/journal.ppat.1001121.

Ebolavirus is internalized into host cells via macropinocytosis in a viral glycoprotein-dependent manner.

Nanbo A(1), Imai M, Watanabe S, Noda T, Takahashi K, Neumann G, Halfmann P, Kawaoka Y.

Author information: (1)Influenza Research Institute, Department of Pathological Sciences, School of Veterinary Medicine, University of Wisconsin-Madison, Madison, Wisconsin, United States of America.

Ebolavirus (EBOV) is an enveloped, single-stranded, negative-sense RNA virus that causes severe hemorrhagic fever with mortality rates of up to 90% in humans and nonhuman primates. Previous studies suggest roles for clathrin- or caveolae-mediated endocytosis in EBOV entry; however, ebolavirus virions are long, filamentous particles that are larger than the plasma membrane invaginations that characterize clathrin- or caveolae-mediated endocytosis. The mechanism of EBOV entry remains, therefore, poorly understood. To better understand Ebolavirus entry, we carried out internalization studies with fluorescently labeled, biologically contained Ebolavirus and Ebolavirus-like particles (Ebola VLPs), both of which resemble authentic Ebolavirus in their morphology. We examined the mechanism of Ebolavirus internalization by real-time analysis of these fluorescently labeled Ebolavirus particles and found that

their internalization was independent of clathrin- or caveolae-mediated endocytosis, but that they co-localized with sorting nexin (SNX) 5, a marker of macropinocytosis-specific endosomes (macropinosomes). Moreover, the internalization of Ebolavirus virions accelerated the uptake of a macropinocytosis-specific cargo, was associated with plasma membrane ruffling, and was dependent on cellular GTPases and kinases involved in macropinocytosis. A pseudotyped vesicular stomatitis virus possessing the Ebolavirus glycoprotein (GP) also co-localized with SNX5 and its internalization and infectivity were affected by macropinocytosis inhibitors. Taken together, our data suggest that Ebolavirus is internalized into cells by stimulating macropinocytosis in a GP-dependent manner. These findings provide new insights into the lifecycle of Ebolavirus and may aid in the development of therapeutics for Ebolavirus infection.
PMCID: PMC2944813 PMID: 20886108 [PubMed - indexed for MEDLINE]

1280. Proc Natl Acad Sci U S A. 2010 Sep 21;107(38):16637-42. doi: 10.1073/pnas.1008509107. Epub 2010 Sep 3.

Cell adhesion-dependent membrane trafficking of a binding partner for the ebolavirus glycoprotein is a determinant of viral entry.

Dube D(1), Schornberg KL, Shoemaker CJ, Delos SE, Stantchev TS, Clouse KA, Broder CC, White JM.

Author information: (1)Department of Microbiology, University of Virginia, Charlottesville, VA 22908, USA.

Ebolavirus is a hemorrhagic fever virus associated with high mortality. Although much has been learned about the viral lifecycle and pathogenesis, many questions remain about virus entry. We recently showed that binding of the receptor binding region (RBR) of the ebolavirus glycoprotein (GP) and infection by GP pseudovirions increase on cell adhesion independently of mRNA or protein synthesis. One model to explain these observations is that, on cell adhesion, an RBR binding partner translocates from an intracellular vesicle to the cell surface. Here, we provide evidence for this model by showing that suspension 293F cells contain an RBR binding site within a membrane-bound compartment associated with the trans-Golgi network and microtubule-organizing center. Consistently, trafficking of the RBR binding partner to the cell surface depends on microtubules, and the RBR binding partner is internalized when adherent cells are placed in suspension. Based on these observations, we reexamined the claim that lymphocytes, which are critical for ebolavirus pathogenesis, are refractory to infection because they lack an RBR binding partner. We found that both cultured and primary human lymphocytes (in suspension) contain an intracellular pool of an RBR binding partner. Moreover, we identified two adherent primate lymphocytic cell lines that bind RBR at their surface and strikingly, support GP-mediated entry and infection. In summary, our results reveal a mode of determining viral entry by a membrane-trafficking event that translocates an RBR binding partner to the cell surface, and they suggest that this process may be operative in cells important for ebolavirus pathogenesis (e.g., lymphocytes and macrophages).
PMCID: PMC2944755 PMID: 20817853 [PubMed - indexed for MEDLINE]

1281. PLoS Pathog. 2010 Sep 16;6(9):e1001110. doi: 10.1371/journal.ppat.1001110.

Cellular entry of ebola virus involves uptake by a macropinocytosis-like mechanism and subsequent trafficking through early and late endosomes.

Saeed MF(1), Kolokoltsov AA, Albrecht T, Davey RA.

Author information: (1)Department of Microbiology & Immunology, The University of Texas Medical Branch, Galveston, Texas, United States of America.

Zaire ebolavirus (ZEBOV), a highly pathogenic zoonotic virus, poses serious public health, ecological and potential bioterrorism threats. Currently no specific therapy or vaccine is available. Virus entry is an attractive target for therapeutic intervention. However, current knowledge of the ZEBOV entry mechanism is limited. While it is known that ZEBOV enters cells through endocytosis, which of the cellular endocytic mechanisms used remains unclear. Previous studies have produced differing outcomes, indicating potential involvement of multiple routes but many of these studies were performed using noninfectious surrogate systems such as pseudotyped retroviral particles, which may not accurately recapitulate the entry characteristics of the morphologically distinct wild type virus. Here we used replication-competent infectious ZEBOV as well as morphologically similar virus-like particles in specific infection and entry assays to demonstrate that in HEK293T and Vero cells internalization of ZEBOV is independent of clathrin, caveolae, and dynamin. Instead the uptake mechanism has features of macropinocytosis. The binding of virus to cells appears to directly stimulate fluid phase uptake as well as localized actin polymerization. Inhibition of key regulators of macropinocytosis including Pak1 and CtBP/BARS as well as treatment with the drug EIPA, which affects macropinosome formation, resulted in significant reduction in ZEBOV entry and infection. It is also shown that following internalization, the virus enters the endolysosomal pathway and is trafficked through early and late endosomes, but the exact site of membrane fusion and nucleocapsid penetration in the cytoplasm remains unclear. This study identifies the route for ZEBOV entry and identifies the key cellular factors required for the uptake of this filamentous virus. The findings greatly expand our understanding of the ZEBOV entry mechanism that can be applied to development of new therapeutics as well as provide potential insight into the trafficking and entry mechanism of other filoviruses.
PMCID: PMC2940741 PMID: 20862315 [PubMed - indexed for MEDLINE]

1282. PLoS Pathog. 2010 Sep 9;6(9):e1001098. doi: 10.1371/journal.ppat.1001098.

Steric shielding of surface epitopes and impaired immune recognition induced by the ebola virus glycoprotein.

Francica JR(1), Varela-Rohena A, Medvec A, Plesa G, Riley JL, Bates P.

Author information: (1)Department of Microbiology, University of Pennsylvania School of Medicine, Philadelphia, Pennsylvania, United States of America.

Many viruses alter expression of proteins on the surface of infected cells including molecules important for immune recognition, such as the major histocompatibility complex (MHC) class I and II molecules. Virus-induced downregulation of surface proteins has been observed to occur by a variety of mechanisms including impaired transcription, blocks to synthesis, and increased turnover. Viral infection or transient expression of the Ebola virus (EBOV) glycoprotein (GP) was previously shown to result in loss of staining of various host cell surface proteins including MHCI and β1 integrin; however, the mechanism responsible for this effect has not been delineated. In the present study we demonstrate that EBOV GP does not decrease surface levels of β1 integrin or MHCI, but rather impedes recognition by steric occlusion of these proteins on the cell surface. Furthermore, steric occlusion also occurs for epitopes on the EBOV glycoprotein itself. The occluded epitopes in host proteins and EBOV GP can be revealed by removal of the surface subunit of GP or by removal of surface N- and O- linked glycans, resulting in increased surface staining by flow cytometry. Importantly, expression of EBOV GP impairs CD8 T-cell recognition of MHCI on antigen presenting cells. Glycan-mediated steric shielding of host cell surface proteins by EBOV GP represents a novel mechanism for a virus to affect host cell function, thereby escaping immune detection.

PMCID: PMC2936550 PMID: 20844579 [PubMed - indexed for MEDLINE]

1283. J Virol Methods. 2010 Sep;168(1-2):248-50. doi: 10.1016/j.jviromet.2010.04.025. Epub 2010 May 4.

Anti-Ebola MAb 17A3 reacts with bovine and human alpha-2-macroglobulin proteins.

Yu JS(1), Ma BJ, Scearce RM, Liao HX, Haynes BF.

Author information: (1)Departments of Medicine, Human Vaccine Institute, Duke University Medical Center, Durham, NC 27710, USA. yu000022@mc.duke.edu

Monoclonal antibodies (MAbs) were developed against soluble Ebola virus (EBOV) envelope glycoprotein (GP) for the study of the diversity of EBOV envelope and development of diagnostic reagents. Of the three anti-EBOV GP mouse MAbs produced, MAb 15H10 recognized all human EBOV GP species tested (Zaire, Sudan, Ivory Coast), and as well as reacted with the Reston nonhuman primate EBOV GPs. A second MAb, 6D11 recognized EBOV GP species of Sudan and Sudan-Gulu. The third MAb, 17A3, was reported originally in the same article to be EBOV GP specific has now been found to be specific for bovine and human alpha-2-macroglobulin (alpha-2M) proteins which were contaminants in the Ebola envelope protein preparation. Thus, while MAbs 15H10 and 6D11 are indeed EBOV GP specific, MAb 17A3 is an alpha-2-macroglobulin MAb.

Copyright 2010 Elsevier B.V. All rights reserved.

PMCID: PMC2910138 PMID: 20447422 [PubMed - indexed for MEDLINE]

1284. Nat Med. 2010 Sep;16(9):991-4. doi: 10.1038/nm.2202. Epub 2010 Aug 22.

Advanced antisense therapies for postexposure protection against lethal filovirus infections.

Warren TK(1), Warfield KL, Wells J, Swenson DL, Donner KS, Van Tongeren SA, Garza NL, Dong L, Mourich DV, Crumley S, Nichols DK, Iversen PL, Bavari S.

Author information: (1)United States Army Medical Research Institute of Infectious Diseases, Fort Detrick, Maryland, USA.

Comment in Nat Rev Drug Discov. 2010 Oct;9(10):764-5.

Currently, no vaccines or therapeutics are licensed to counter Ebola or Marburg viruses, highly pathogenic filoviruses that are causative agents of viral hemorrhagic fever. Here we show that administration of positively charged phosphorodiamidate morpholino oligomers (PMOplus), delivered by various dosing strategies initiated 30-60 min after infection, protects>60% of rhesus monkeys against lethal Zaire Ebola virus (ZEBOV) and 100% of cynomolgus monkeys against Lake Victoria Marburg virus (MARV) infection. PMOplus may be useful for treating these and other highly pathogenic viruses in humans.

PMID: 20729866 [PubMed - indexed for MEDLINE]

1285. PLoS Negl Trop Dis. 2010 Aug 24;4(8):e802. doi: 10.1371/journal.pntd.0000802.

Establishment of fruit bat cells (Rousettus aegyptiacus) as a model system for the investigation of filoviral infection.

Krähling V(1), Dolnik O, Kolesnikova L, Schmidt-Chanasit J, Jordan I, Sandig V, Günther S, Becker S.

Author information: (1)Institut für Virologie, Philipps-Universität Marburg, Marburg, Germany.

BACKGROUND: The fruit bat species Rousettus aegyptiacus was identified as a potential reservoir for the highly pathogenic filovirus Marburg virus. To establish a basis for a molecular understanding of the biology of filoviruses in the reservoir host, we have adapted a set of molecular tools for investigation of filovirus replication in a recently developed cell line, R06E, derived from the species Rousettus aegyptiacus. METHODOLOGY/PRINCIPAL FINDINGS: Upon infection with Ebola or Marburg viruses, R06E cells produced viral titers comparable to VeroE6 cells, as shown by TCID(50) analysis. Electron microscopic analysis of infected cells revealed morphological signs of filovirus infection as described for human- and monkey-derived cell lines. Using R06E cells, we detected an unusually high amount of intracellular viral proteins, which correlated with the accumulation of high numbers of filoviral nucleocapsids in the cytoplasm. We established protocols to produce Marburg infectious virus-like particles from R06E cells, which were then used to infect naïve target cells to investigate primary transcription. This was not possible with other cell lines previously tested. Moreover, we established protocols to reliably rescue recombinant Marburg viruses from R06E cells. CONCLUSION/SIGNIFICANCE: These data indicated that R06E cells are highly suitable to investigate the biology of filoviruses in cells derived from their presumed reservoir.

PMCID: PMC2927428 PMID: 20808767 [PubMed - indexed for MEDLINE]

1286. J Biol Chem. 2010 Aug 6;285(32):24729-39. doi: 10.1074/jbc.M110.106260. Epub 2010 Jun 1.

A novel L-ficolin/mannose-binding lectin chimeric molecule with enhanced activity against Ebola virus.

Michelow IC(1), Dong M, Mungall BA, Yantosca LM, Lear C, Ji X, Karpel M, Rootes CL, Brudner M, Houen G, Eisen DP, Kinane TB, Takahashi K, Stahl GL, Olinger GG, Spear GT, Ezekowitz RA, Schmidt EV.

Author information: (1)From the Program of Developmental Immunology, Department of Pediatrics, Massachusetts General Hospital, Harvard Medical School, Boston, Massachusetts 2114

Ebola viruses constitute a newly emerging public threat because they cause rapidly fatal hemorrhagic fevers for which no treatment exists, and they can be manipulated as bioweapons. We targeted conserved N-glycosylated carbohydrate ligands on viral envelope surfaces using novel immune therapies. Mannose-binding lectin (MBL) and L-ficolin (L-FCN) were selected because they function as opsonins and activate complement. Given that MBL has a complex quaternary structure unsuitable for large scale cost-effective production, we sought to develop a less complex chimeric fusion protein with similar ligand recognition and enhanced effector functions. We tested recombinant human MBL and three L-FCN/MBL variants that contained the MBL carbohydrate recognition domain and varying lengths of the L-FCN collagenous domain. Non-reduced chimeric proteins formed predominantly nona- and dodecameric oligomers, whereas recombinant human MBL formed octadecameric and larger oligomers. Surface plasmon resonance revealed that L-FCN/MBL76 had the highest binding affinities for N-acetylglucosamine-bovine serum albumin and mannan. The same chimeric protein displayed superior complement C4 cleavage and binding to calreticulin (cClqR), a putative receptor for MBL. L-FCN/MBL76 reduced infection by wild type Ebola virus Zaire significantly greater than the other molecules. Tapping mode atomic force microscopy revealed that L-FCN/MBL76 was significantly less tall than the other molecules despite similar polypeptide lengths. We propose that alterations in the quaternary structure of L-FCN/MBL76 resulted in greater flexibility in the collagenous or neck region. Similarly, a more pliable molecule might enhance cooperativity between the carbohydrate recognition domains and their cognate ligands, complement activation, and calreticulin binding dynamics. L-FCN/MBL chimeric proteins should be considered as potential novel therapeutics.

PMCID: PMC2915709 PMID: 20516066 [PubMed - indexed for MEDLINE]

1287. PLoS One. 2010 Aug 4;5(8):e11978. doi: 10.1371/journal.pone.0011978.

Long-term survival of an urban fruit bat seropositive for Ebola and Lagos bat viruses.

Hayman DT(1), Emmerich P, Yu M, Wang LF, Suu-Ire R, Fooks AR, Cunningham AA, Wood JL.

Author information: (1)Cambridge Infectious Diseases Consortium, University of Cambridge, Cambridge, UK. dtsh2@cam.ac.uk

Ebolaviruses (EBOV) (family Filoviridae) cause viral hemorrhagic fevers in humans and non-human primates when they spill over from their wildlife reservoir hosts with case fatality rates of up to 90%. Fruit bats may act as reservoirs of the Filoviridae. The migratory fruit bat, Eidolon helvum, is common across sub-Saharan Africa and lives in large colonies, often situated in cities. We screened sera from 262 E. helvum using indirect fluorescent tests for antibodies against EBOV subtype Zaire. We detected a seropositive bat from Accra, Ghana, and confirmed this using western blot analysis. The bat was also seropositive for Lagos bat virus, a Lyssavirus, by virus neutralization test. The bat was fitted with a radio transmitter and was last detected in Accra 13 months after release post-sampling, demonstrating long-term survival. Antibodies to filoviruses have not been previously demonstrated in E. helvum. Radio-telemetry data demonstrates long-term survival of an individual bat following exposure to viruses of families that can be highly pathogenic to other mammal species. Because E. helvum typically lives in large urban colonies and is a source of bushmeat in some regions, further studies should determine if this species forms a reservoir for EBOV from which spillover infections into the human population may occur.

PMCID: PMC2915915 PMID: 20694141 [PubMed - indexed for MEDLINE]

1288. Antiviral Res. 2010 Aug;87(2):187-94. doi: 10.1016/j.antiviral.2010.04.015. Epub 2010 May 7.

Inhibition of heat-shock protein 90 reduces Ebola virus replication.

Smith DR(1), McCarthy S, Chrovian A, Olinger G, Stossel A, Geisbert TW, Hensley LE, Connor JH.

Author information: (1)U.S. Army Medical Research Institute of Infectious Diseases, Virology Division, Fort Detrick, MD, United States.

Ebola virus (EBOV), a negative-sense RNA virus in the family Filoviridae, is known to cause severe hemorrhagic fever in humans and other primates. Infection with EBOV causes a high mortality rate and currently there is no FDA-licensed vaccine or therapeutic treatment available. Recently, heat-shock protein 90 (Hsp90), a molecular chaperone, was shown to be an important host factor for the replication of several negative-strand viruses. We tested the effect of several different Hsp90 inhibitors including geldanamycin, radicicol, and 17-allylamino-17-demethoxygeldanamycin (17-AAG; a geldanamycin analog) on the replication of Zaire EBOV. Our results showed that inhibition of Hsp90 significantly reduced the replication of EBOV. Classic Hsp90 inhibitors reduced viral replication with an effective concentration at 50% (EC(50)) in the high nanomolar to low micromolar range, while drugs from a new class of Hsp90 inhibitors showed markedly more potent inhibition. These compounds blocked EBOV replication with an EC(50) in the low nanomolar range and showed significant potency in blocking replication in primary human monocytes. These results validated that Hsp90 is an important host factor for the replication of filoviruses and suggest that Hsp90 inhibitors may be therapeutically effective in treating EBOV infection.

PMCID: PMC2907434 PMID: 20452380 [PubMed - indexed for MEDLINE]

1289. J Biomol Screen. 2010 Aug;15(7):755-65. doi: 10.1177/1087057110374357. Epub 2010 Jul 16.

Development of high-content imaging assays for lethal viral pathogens.

Panchal RG(1), Kota KP, Spurgers KB, Ruthel G, Tran JP, Boltz RC, Bavari S.

Author information: (1)United States Army Medical Research Institute of Infectious Diseases, Fort Detrick, Frederick, MD, USA. rekha.panchal@amedd.army.mil

Filoviruses such as Ebola (EBOV) and Marburg (MARV) are single-stranded negative sense RNA viruses that cause acute hemorrhagic fever with high mortality rates. Currently, there are no licensed vaccines or therapeutics to counter filovirus infections in humans. The development of higher throughput/high-content primary screening assays followed by validation using the low-throughput traditional plaque or real-time PCR assays will greatly aid efforts toward the discovery of novel antiviral therapeutics. Specifically, high-content imaging technology is increasingly being applied for primary drug screening. In this study, the authors describe the challenges encountered when optimizing bioassays based on image acquisition and analyses for the highly pathogenic filoviruses Ebola and Marburg. A number of biological and imaging-related variables such as plating density, multiplicity of infection, the number of fields scanned per well, fluorescence intensity, and the cell number analyzed were evaluated during the development of these assays. Furthermore, the authors demonstrate the benefits related to the statistical analyses of single-cell data to account for heterogeneity in the subcellular localization and whole-cell integrated intensity of the viral antigen staining pattern. In conclusion, they show that image-based methods represent powerful screening tools for identifying antiviral compounds for highly pathogenic viruses.

PMID: 20639507 [PubMed - indexed for MEDLINE]

1290. Mol Pharmacol. 2010 Aug;78(2):319-24. doi: 10.1124/mol.110.064261. Epub 2010 May 13

A small-molecule oxocarbazate inhibitor of human cathepsin L blocks severe acute respiratory syndrome and ebola pseudotype virus infection into human embryonic kidney 293T cells.

Shah PP(1), Wang T, Kaletsky RL, Myers MC, Purvis JE, Jing H, Huryn DM, Greenbaum DC, Smith AB 3rd, Bates P, Diamond SL.

Author information: (1)Department of Chemical and Biomolecular Engineering, Penn Center for Molecular Discovery, Institute for Medicine and Engineering, University of Pennsylvania, Philadelphia, Pennsylvania 19104-6383, USA.

A tetrahydroquinoline oxocarbazate (PubChem CID 23631927) was tested as an inhibitor of human cathepsin L (EC 3.4.22.15) and as an entry blocker of severe acute respiratory syndrome (SARS) coronavirus and Ebola pseudotype virus. In the cathepsin L inhibition assay, the oxocarbazate caused a time-dependent 17-fold drop in IC(50) from 6.9 nM (no preincubation) to 0.4 nM (4-h preincubation). Slowly reversible inhibition was demonstrated in a dilution assay. A transient kinetic analysis using a single-step competitive inhibition model provided rate constants of k(on) = 153,000 M(-1)s(-1) and k(off) = 4.40 x 10(-5) s(-1) (K(i) = 0.29 nM). The compound also displayed cathepsin L/B selectivity of >700-fold and was nontoxic to human aortic endothelial cells at 100 muM. The oxocarbazate and a related thiocarbazate (PubChem CID 16725315) were tested in a SARS coronavirus (CoV) and Ebola virus-pseudotype infection assay with the oxocarbazate but not the thiocarbazate, demonstrating activity in blocking both SARS-CoV (IC(50) = 273 +/- 49 nM) and Ebola virus (IC(50) = 193 +/- 39 nM) entry into human embryonic kidney 293T cells. To trace the intracellular action of the inhibitors with intracellular cathepsin L, the activity-based probe biotin-Lys-C5 alkyl linker-Tyr-Leu-epoxide (DCG-04) was used to label the active site of cysteine proteases in 293T lysates. The reduction in active cathepsin L in inhibitor-treated cells correlated well with the observed potency of inhibitors observed in the virus pseudotype infection assay. Overall, the oxocarbazate CID 23631927 was a subnanomolar, slow-binding, reversible inhibitor of human cathepsin L that blocked SARS-CoV and Ebola pseudotype virus entry in human cells.
PMCID: PMC2917856 PMID: 20466822 [PubMed - indexed for MEDLINE]
1291. Protein Cell. 2010 Aug;1(8):752-9. doi: 10.1007/s13238-010-0096-9. Epub 2010 Aug 28

Analyses of SELEX-derived ZAP-binding RNA aptamers suggest that the binding specificity is determined by both structure and sequence of the RNA.

Huang Z(1), Wang X, Gao G.

Author information: (1)Key Laboratory of Infection and Immunity, Institute of Biophysics, Chinese Academy of Sciences, Beijing 100101, China.

The zinc-finger antiviral protein (ZAP) is a host factor that specifically inhibits the replication of certain viruses, including murine leukemia virus, Sindbis virus and Ebola virus, by targeting the viral mRNAs for degradation. ZAP directly binds to the target viral mRNA and recruits the cellular RNA degradation machinery to degrade the RNA. No significant sequence similarity or obvious common motifs have been found in the so far identified target viral mRNAs. The minimum length of the target sequence is about 500 nt long. Short workable ZAP-binding RNAs should facilitate further studies on the ZAP-RNA interaction and characterization of such RNAs may provide some insights into the underlying mechanism. In this study, we used the SELEX method to isolate ZAP-binding RNA aptamers. After 21 rounds of selection, ZAP-binding aptamers were isolated. Sequence analysis revealed that they are G-rich RNAs with predicted stem-loop structures containing conserved "GGGUGG" and "GAGGG" motifs in the loop region. Insertion of the aptamer sequence into a luciferase reporter failed to render the reporter sensitive to ZAP. However, overexpression of the aptamers modestly but significantly reduced ZAP's antiviral activity. Substitution of the conserved motifs of the aptamers significantly impaired their ZAP-binding ability and ZAP-antagonizing activity, suggesting that the RNA sequence is important for specific interaction between ZAP and the target RNA. The aptamers identified in this report should provide useful tools to further investigate the details of the interaction between ZAP and the target RNAs.
PMID: 21203916 [PubMed - indexed for MEDLINE]
1292. PLoS Pathog. 2010 Jul 29;6(7):e1001030. doi: 10.1371/journal.ppat.1001030.

Unexpected inheritance: multiple integrations of ancient bornavirus and ebolavirus/marburgvirus sequences in vertebrate genomes.

Belyi VA(1), Levine AJ, Skalka AM.

Author information: (1)Simons Center for Systems Biology, Institute for Advanced Study, Princeton, New Jersey, USA.

Vertebrate genomes contain numerous copies of retroviral sequences, acquired over the course of evolution. Until recently they were thought to be the only type of RNA viruses to be so represented, because integration of a DNA copy of their genome is required for their replication. In this study, an extensive sequence comparison was conducted in which 5,666 viral genes from all known non-retroviral families with single-stranded RNA genomes were matched against the germline genomes of 48 vertebrate species, to determine if such viruses could also contribute to the vertebrate genetic heritage. In 19 of the tested vertebrate species, we discovered as many as 80 high-confidence examples of genomic DNA sequences that appear to be derived, as long ago as 40 million years, from ancestral members of 4 currently circulating virus families with single strand RNA genomes. Surprisingly, almost all of the sequences are related to only two families in the Order Mononegavirales: the Bornaviruses and the Filoviruses, which cause lethal neurological disease and hemorrhagic fevers, respectively. Based on signature landmarks some, and perhaps all, of the endogenous virus-like DNA sequences appear to be LINE element-facilitated integrations derived from viral mRNAs. The integrations represent genes that encode viral nucleocapsid, RNA-dependent-RNA-polymerase, matrix and, possibly, glycoproteins. Integrations are generally limited to one or very few copies of a related viral gene per species, suggesting that once the initial germline integration was obtained (or selected), later integrations failed or provided little advantage to the host. The conservation of relatively long open reading frames for several of the endogenous sequences, the virus-like protein regions represented, and a potential correlation between their presence and a species' resistance to the diseases caused by these pathogens, are consistent with the notion that their products provide some important biological advantage to the species. In addition, the viruses could also benefit, as some resistant species (e.g. bats) may serve as natural reservoirs for their persistence and transmission. Given the stringent limitations imposed in this informatics search, the examples described here should be considered a low estimate of the number of such integration events that have persisted over evolutionary time scales. Clearly, the sources of genetic information in vertebrate genomes are much more diverse than previously suspected.
PMCID: PMC2912400 PMID: 20686665 [PubMed - indexed for MEDLINE]

1293. Virology. 2010 Jul 20;403(1):56-66. doi: 10.1016/j.virol.2010.04.002. Epub 2010 May 4.

Both matrix proteins of Ebola virus contribute to the regulation of viral genome replication and transcription.

Hoenen T(1), Jung S, Herwig A, Groseth A, Becker S.

Author information: (1)Institute for Virology, Philipps University Marburg, Marburg, Germany.

Ebola virus (EBOV) causes severe hemorrhagic fevers in humans and non-human primates. While the role of the EBOV major matrix protein VP40 in morphogenesis is well understood, nothing is known about its contributions to the regulation of viral genome replication and/or transcription. Similarly, while it was reported that the minor matrix protein VP24 impairs viral genome replication, it remains unclear whether it also regulates transcription, since all common experimental systems measure the combined products of replication and transcription. We have developed systems that allow the independent monitoring of viral transcription and replication, based on qRT-PCR and a replication-deficient minigenome. Using these systems we show that VP24 regulates not only viral genome replication, but also transcription. Further, we show for the first time that VP40 is also involved in regulating these processes. These functions are conserved among EBOV species and, in the case of VP40, independent of its budding or RNA-binding functions.

Copyright 2010 Elsevier Inc. All rights reserved.

PMID: 20444481 [PubMed - indexed for MEDLINE]

1294. JAMA. 2010 Jul 7;304(1):31. doi: 10.1001/jama.2010.868.

Experimental RNA therapy shows promise against Ebola virus in monkey studies.

Mitka M.

PMID: 20606143 [PubMed - indexed for MEDLINE]

1295. Antimicrob Agents Chemother. 2010 Jul;54(7):3007-10. doi: 10.1128/AAC.00138-10. Epub 2010 Apr 26.

Minigenome-based reporter system suitable for high-throughput screening of compounds able to inhibit Ebolavirus replication and/or transcription.

Jasenosky LD(1), Neumann G, Kawaoka Y.

Author information: (1)Department of Pathobiological Sciences, School of Veterinary Medicine, University of Wisconsin-Madison, 2015 Linden Drive, Madison, WI 53706, USA.

We describe an Ebolavirus minigenome-based system that is suitable for high-throughput screening of compounds able to impair Ebolavirus virus replication and/or transcription. The assay is robust (Z' factor, >0.6) and can be carried out in low-biosafety containment. Results from a pilot screen of 960 compounds are presented.

PMCID: PMC2897319 PMID: 20421407 [PubMed - indexed for MEDLINE]

1296. Bull World Health Organ. 2010 Jul 1;88(7):488-9. doi: 10.2471/BLT.10.030710.

Time to put Ebola in context. Interview with Dr Melissa Leach.

Leach M.

Viruses that cause haemorrhagic fevers have been popularized by the media as fierce predators that threaten to devastate global populations. Professor Melissa Leach says there is much to learn from combining local and scientific knowledge in dealing with these deadly pathogens.

PMCID: PMC2897993 PMID: 20616966 [PubMed - indexed for MEDLINE]

1297. Emerg Infect Dis. 2010 Jul;16(7):1087-92. doi: 10.3201/eid1607.091525.

Ebola hemorrhagic fever associated with novel virus strain, Uganda, 2007-2008.

Wamala JF(1), Lukwago L, Malimbo M, Nguku P, Yoti Z, Musenero M, Amone J, Mbabazi W, Nanyunja M, Zaramba S, Opio A, Lutwama JJ, Talisuna AO, Okware SI.
Author information: (1)Ministry of Heath, Kampala, Uganda. j_wamala@yahoo.com

During August 2007-February 2008, the novel Bundibugyo ebolavirus species was identified during an outbreak of Ebola viral hemorrhagic fever in Bundibugyo district, western Uganda. To characterize the outbreak as a requisite for determining response, we instituted a case-series investigation. We identified 192 suspected cases, of which 42 (22%) were laboratory positive for the novel species; 74 (38%) were probable, and 77 (40%) were negative. Laboratory confirmation lagged behind outbreak verification by 3 months. Bundibugyo ebolavirus was less fatal (case-fatality rate 34%) than Ebola viruses that had caused previous outbreaks in the region, and most transmission was associated with handling of dead persons without appropriate protection (adjusted odds ratio 3.83, 95% confidence interval 1.78-8.23). Our study highlights the need for maintaining a high index of suspicion for viral hemorrhagic fevers among healthcare workers, building local capacity for laboratory confirmation of viral hemorrhagic fevers, and institutionalizing standard precautions.

PMCID: PMC3321896 PMID: 20587179 [PubMed - indexed for MEDLINE]

1298. Future Virol. 2010 Jul 1;5(4):481-491.

Viral and host proteins that modulate filovirus budding.

Liu Y(1), Harty RN.

Author information: (1)Department of Pathobiology, School of Veterinary Medicine, University of Pennsylvania, 3800 Spruce St., Philadelphia, PA 19104, USA.

The filoviruses, Ebola and Marburg, utilize a multifaceted mechanism for assembly and budding of infectious virions from mammalian cells. Growing evidence not only demonstrates the importance of multiple viral proteins for efficient assembly and budding, but also the exploitation of various host proteins/pathways by the virus during this late stage of filovirus replication, including endocytic compartments, vacuolar protein sorting pathways, ubiquitination machinery, lipid rafts and cytoskeletal components. Continued elucidation of these complex and orchestrated virus-host interactions will provide a fundamental understanding of the molecular mechanisms of filovirus assembly/budding and ultimately lead to the development of novel viral- and/or host-oriented therapeutics to inhibit filovirus egress and spread. This article will focus on the most recent studies on host interactions and modulation of filovirus budding and summarize the key findings from these investigations.

PMCID: PMC2922766 PMID: 20730024 [PubMed]

1299. J Clin Microbiol. 2010 Jul;48(7):2330-6. doi: 10.1128/JCM.01224-09. Epub 2010 Apr 26

Development and evaluation of a simple assay for Marburg virus detection using a reverse transcription-loop-mediated isothermal amplification method.

Kurosaki Y(1), Grolla A, Fukuma A, Feldmann H, Yasuda J.

Author information: (1)National Research Institute of Police Science, Kashiwa, Japan.

Marburg virus (MARV) causes a severe hemorrhagic fever in humans with a high mortality rate. The rapid and accurate identification of the virus is required to appropriately provide infection control and outbreak management. Here, we developed and evaluated a one-step reverse transcription-loop-mediated isothermal amplification (RT-LAMP) assay for the rapid and simple detection of MARV. By combining two sets of primers specific for the Musoke and Ravn genetic lineages, a multiple RT-LAMP assay detected MARV strains of both lineages, and no cross-reactivity with other hemorrhagic fever viruses (Ebola virus and Lassa virus) was observed. The assay could detect 10(2) copies of the viral RNA per tube within 40 min by real-time monitoring of the turbidities of the reaction mixtures. The assay was further evaluated using viral RNA extracted from clinical specimens collected in the 2005 Marburg hemorrhagic fever outbreak in Angola and yielded positive results for samples containing MARV at greater than 10(4) 50% tissue culture infective doses/ml, exhibiting 78% (14 of 18 samples positive) consistency with the results of a reverse transcription-PCR assay carried out in the field laboratory. The results obtained by both agarose gel electrophoresis and naked-eye judgment indicated that the RT-LAMP assay developed in this study is an effective tool for the molecular detection of MARV. Furthermore, it seems suitable for use for field diagnostics or in laboratories in areas where MARV is endemic.

PMCID: PMC2897471 PMID: 20421440 [PubMed - indexed for MEDLINE]

1300. J Virol. 2010 Jul;84(14):7053-63. doi: 10.1128/JVI.00737-10. Epub 2010 May 12.

Oligomerization of Ebola virus VP40 is essential for particle morphogenesis and regulation of viral transcription.

Hoenen T(1), Biedenkopf N, Zielecki F, Jung S, Groseth A, Feldmann H, Becker S.

Author information: (1)Institut für Virologie, Hans-Meerwein-Str. 2, 35043 Marburg, Germany.

The morphogenesis and budding of virus particles represent an important stage in the life cycle of viruses. For Ebola virus, this process is driven by its major matrix protein, VP40. Like the matrix proteins of many other nonsegmented, negative-strand RNA viruses, VP40 has been demonstrated to oligomerize and to occur in at least two distinct oligomeric states: hexamers and octamers, which are composed of antiparallel dimers. While it has been shown that VP40 oligomers are essential for the viral life cycle, their function is completely unknown. Here we have identified two amino acids essential for oligomerization of VP40, the mutation of which blocked virus-like particle production. Consistent with this observation, oligomerization-deficient VP40 also showed impaired intracellular transport to budding sites and reduced binding to cellular membranes. However, other biological functions, such as the interaction of VP40 with the nucleoprotein, NP, remained undisturbed. Furthermore, both wild-type VP40 and oligomerization-deficient VP40 were found to negatively regulate viral genome replication, a novel function of VP40, which we have recently reported. Interestingly, while wild-type VP40 was also able to negatively regulate viral genome transcription, oligomerization-deficient VP40 was no longer able to fulfill this function, indicating that regulation of viral replication and transcription by VP40 are mechanistically distinct processes. These data indicate that VP40 oligomerization not only is a prerequisite for intracellular transport of VP40 and efficient membrane binding, and as a consequence virion morphogenesis, but also plays a critical role in the regulation of viral transcription by VP40.

PMCID: PMC2898221 PMID: 20463076 [PubMed - indexed for MEDLINE]

1301. J Virol. 2010 Jul;84(14):7243-55. doi: 10.1128/JVI.02636-09. Epub 2010 May 5.

Ebola virus glycoprotein counteracts BST-2/Tetherin restriction in a sequence-independent manner that does not require tetherin surface removal.

Lopez LA(1), Yang SJ, Hauser H, Exline CM, Haworth KG, Oldenburg J, Cannon PM.

Author information: (1)Department of Molecular Microbiology and Immunology, USC Keck School of Medicine, 2011 Zonal Ave., HMR502, Los Angeles, CA 90033, USA.

BST-2/tetherin is an interferon-inducible protein that restricts the release of enveloped viruses from the surface of infected cells by physically linking viral and cellular membranes. It is present at both the cell surface and in a perinuclear region, and viral anti-tetherin factors including HIV-1 Vpu and HIV-2 Env have been shown to decrease the cell surface population. To map the domains of human tetherin necessary for both virus restriction and sensitivity to viral anti-tetherin factors, we constructed a series of tetherin derivatives and assayed their activity. We found that the cytoplasmic tail (CT) and transmembrane (TM) domains of tetherin alone produced its characteristic cellular distribution, while the ectodomain of the protein, which includes a glycosylphosphatidylinositol (GPI) anchor, was sufficient to restrict virus release when presented by the CT/TM regions of a different type II membrane protein. To counteract tetherin restriction and remove it from the cell surface, HIV-1 Vpu required the specific sequence present in the TM domain of human tetherin. In contrast, the HIV-2 Env required only the ectodomain of the protein and was sensitive to a point mutation in this region. Strikingly, the anti-tetherin factor, Ebola virus GP, was able to overcome restriction conferred by both tetherin and a series of functional tetherin derivatives, including a wholly artificial tetherin molecule. Moreover, GP overcame restriction without significantly removing tetherin from the cell surface. These findings suggest that Ebola virus GP uses a novel mechanism to circumvent tetherin restriction.

PMCID: PMC2898217 PMID: 20444895 [PubMed - indexed for MEDLINE]

1302. PLoS Pathog. 2010 Jul 1;6:e1000972. doi: 10.1371/journal.ppat.1000972.

Identification of GBV-D, a novel GB-like flavivirus from old world frugivorous bats (Pteropus giganteus) in Bangladesh.

Epstein JH(1), Quan PL, Briese T, Street C, Jabado O, Conlan S, Ali Khan S, Verdugo D, Hossain MJ, Hutchison SK, Egholm M, Luby SP, Daszak P, Lipkin WI.

Author information: (1)Conservation Medicine Program, Wildlife Trust, New York, New York, United States of America.

Bats are reservoirs for a wide range of zoonotic agents including lyssa-, henipah-, SARS-like corona-, Marburg-, Ebola-, and astroviruses. In an effort to survey for the presence of other infectious agents, known and unknown, we screened sera from 16 Pteropus giganteus bats from Faridpur, Bangladesh, using high-throughput pyrosequencing. Sequence analyses indicated the presence of a previously undescribed virus that has approximately 50% identity at the amino acid level to GB virus A and C (GBV-A and -C). Viral nucleic acid was present in 5 of 98 sera (5%) from a single colony of free-ranging bats. Infection was not associated with evidence of hepatitis or hepatic dysfunction. Phylogenetic analysis indicates that this first GBV-like flavivirus reported in bats constitutes a distinct species within the Flaviviridae family and is ancestral to the GBV-A and -C virus clades.

PMCID: PMC2895649 PMID: 20617167 [PubMed - indexed for MEDLINE]

1303. Vopr Virusol. 2010 Jul-Aug;55(4):33-8.

[Evaluation of Ebola virus reproduction in adult ICR white mice].

[Article in Russian]

Chepurnov AA, Sizikova LP, Shalemba-Chepurnova AA, Shestopalova LV.

The investigators studied the ability of adult ICR mice (a laboratory model that was most approximated to the wildtype populations of mice) to maintain Ebola virus (EV) reproduction in the organism. The adult ICR mice inoculated with EV during 23 passages were shown to maintain viral reproduction in the liver. The elevated levels of platelets and the early generation of fibrin and fibrinogen degradation products suggested there were hemostatic changes that did not, however, progress to severe coagulopathy. The animals were in appearance apparently, other than adynamia observed on days 5-7. Thus, the susceptibility of the adult ICR mice to EV is characterized by their ability to maintain virus reproduction in the liver without evident signs of the infection. This pattern of susceptibility in the mice shows a possible role of this rodent species in the transmissive cycle of EV.

PMID: 20886711 [PubMed - indexed for MEDLINE]

1304. BMC Evol Biol. 2010 Jun 22;10:193. doi: 10.1186/1471-2148-10-193.

Filoviruses are ancient and integrated into mammalian genomes.

Taylor DJ(1), Leach RW, Bruenn J.

Author information: (1)Department of Biological Sciences, The State University of New York at Buffalo, Buffalo, NY 14260, USA. djtaylor@buffalo.edu

BACKGROUND: Hemorrhagic diseases from Ebolavirus and Marburgvirus (Filoviridae) infections can be dangerous to humans because of high fatality rates and a lack of effective treatments or vaccine. Although there is evidence that wild mammals are infected by filoviruses, the biology of host-filovirus systems is notoriously poorly understood. Specifically, identifying potential reservoir species with the expected long-term coevolutionary history of filovirus infections has been intractable. Integrated elements of filoviruses could indicate a coevolutionary history with a mammalian reservoir, but integration of nonretroviral RNA viruses is thought to be nonexistent or rare for mammalian viruses (such as filoviruses) that lack reverse transcriptase and replication inside the nucleus. Here, we provide direct evidence of integrated filovirus-like elements in mammalian genomes by sequencing across host-virus gene boundaries and carrying out phylogenetic analyses. Further we test for an association between candidate reservoir status and the integration of filoviral elements and assess the previous age estimate for filoviruses of less than 10,000 years. RESULTS: Phylogenetic and sequencing evidence from gene boundaries was consistent with integration of filoviruses in mammalian genomes. We detected integrated filovirus-like elements in the genomes of bats, rodents, shrews, tenrecs and marsupials. Moreover, some filovirus-like elements were transcribed and the detected mammalian elements were homologous to a fragment of the filovirus genome whose expression is known to interfere with the assembly of Ebolavirus. The phylogenetic evidence strongly indicated that the direction of transfer was from virus to mammal. Eutherians other than bats, rodents, and insectivores (i.e., the candidate reservoir taxa for filoviruses) were significantly underrepresented in the taxa with detected integrated filovirus-like elements. The existence of orthologous filovirus-like elements shared among mammalian genera whose divergence dates have been estimated suggests that filoviruses are at least tens of millions of years old. CONCLUSIONS: Our findings indicate that filovirus infections have been recorded as paleoviral elements in the genomes of small mammals despite extranuclear replication and a requirement for cooption of reverse transcriptase. Our results show that the mammal-filovirus association is ancient and has resulted in candidates for functional gene products (RNA or protein).

PMCID: PMC2906475 PMID: 20569424 [PubMed - indexed for MEDLINE]

1305. Virology. 2010 Jun 20;402(1):203-8. doi: 10.1016/j.virol.2010.03.024. Epub 2010 Apr 14.

Reduced virus replication, proinflammatory cytokine production, and delayed macrophage cell death in human PBMCs infected with the newly discovered Bundibugyo ebolavirus relative to Zaire ebolavirus.

Gupta M(1), Goldsmith CS, Metcalfe MG, Spiropoulou CF, Rollin PE.

Author information: (1)Special Pathogens Branch, DVRD, Centers for Disease Control and Prevention, Atlanta, GA, USA. mgupta@cdc.gov

Erratum in Virology. 2010 Oct 10;406(1):165. Spipopoulou, Christina F [corrected to Spiropoulou, Christina F].

Bundibugyo ebolavirus is a newly identified Ebolavirus species. The virus was responsible for a recent hemorrhagic fever outbreak in Uganda with an approximate 30% case fatality rate. In this study, we compared the pathogenesis of Bundibugyo with highly lethal Zaire Ebolavirus by using in vitro human PBMCs. We found that PBMCs infected with Bundibugyo ebolaviruses resulted in 1 to 2 log lower virus yields compared to Zaire ebolavirus and produced 2- to 10-fold lower levels of TNF-alpha, MCP-1, IL-1beta, MIP1-alpha and IL-10 than PBMCs infected with Zaire ebolavirus. In addition, flow cytometric studies have shown lower levels and delay of the macrophage cell death in Bundibugyo ebolavirus compared to Zaire ebolavirus infection. The findings of slower Bundibugyo ebolavirus replication, lower production of proinflammatory cytokines and delay in macrophage cell death provide insight into the basis of the lower case fatality observed with Bundibugyo ebolavirus.

Published by Elsevier Inc.

PMID: 20394957 [PubMed - indexed for MEDLINE]

1306. J Mol Biol. 2010 Jun 11;399(3):347-57. doi: 10.1016/j.jmb.2010.04.022. Epub 2010 Apr 24.

Structural and functional characterization of Reston Ebola virus VP35 interferon inhibitory domain.

Leung DW(1), Shabman RS, Farahbakhsh M, Prins KC, Borek DM, Wang T, Mühlberger E, Basler CF, Amarasinghe GK.

Author information: (1)Department of Biochemistry, Biophysics, and Molecular Biology, Iowa State University, Ames, IA 50011, USA.

Ebolaviruses are causative agents of lethal hemorrhagic fever in humans and nonhuman primates. Among the filoviruses characterized thus far, Reston Ebola virus (REBOV) is the only Ebola virus that is nonpathogenic to humans despite the fact that REBOV can cause lethal disease in nonhuman primates. Previous studies also suggest that REBOV is less effective at inhibiting host innate immune responses than Zaire Ebola virus (ZEBOV) or Marburg virus. Virally encoded VP35 protein is critical for immune suppression, but an understanding of the relative contributions of VP35 proteins from REBOV and other filoviruses is currently lacking. In order to address this question, we characterized the REBOV VP35 interferon inhibitory domain (IID) using structural, biochemical, and virological studies. These studies reveal differences in double-stranded RNA binding and interferon inhibition between the two species. These observed differences are likely due to increased stability and loss of flexibility in REBOV VP35 IID, as demonstrated by thermal shift stability assays. Consistent with this finding, the 1.71-A crystal structure of REBOV VP35 IID reveals that it is highly similar to that of ZEBOV VP35 IID, with an overall backbone r.m.s.d. of 0.64 A, but contains an additional helical element at the linker between the two subdomains of VP35 IID. Mutations near the linker, including swapping sequences between REBOV and ZEBOV, reveal that the linker sequence has limited tolerance for variability. Together with the previously solved ligand-free and double-stranded-RNA-bound forms of ZEBOV VP35 IID structures, our current studies on REBOV VP35 IID reinforce the importance of VP35 in immune suppression. Functional differences observed between REBOV and ZEBOV VP35 proteins may contribute to observed differences in pathogenicity, but these are unlikely to be the major determinant. However, the high level of similarity in structure and the low tolerance for sequence variability, coupled with the multiple critical roles played by Ebola virus VP35 proteins, highlight the viability of VP35 as a potential target for therapeutic development.

Copyright 2010 Elsevier Ltd. All rights reserved.

PMCID: PMC2917615 PMID: 20399790 [PubMed - indexed for MEDLINE]

1307. Virology. 2010 Jun 5;401(2):228-35. doi: 10.1016/j.virol.2010.02.029. Epub 2010 Mar 20.

Antibody-mediated neutralization of Ebola virus can occur by two distinct mechanisms.

Shedlock DJ(1), Bailey MA, Popernack PM, Cunningham JM, Burton DR, Sullivan NJ.

Author information: (1)Biodefense Research Section, Vaccine Research Center, National Institute for Allergy and Infectious Disease, National Institutes of Health, 40 Convent Drive, MSC 3005, Bethesda, MD 20814, USA. shedlock@mail.med.upenn.edu

Human Ebola virus causes severe hemorrhagic fever disease with high mortality and there is no vaccine or treatment. Antibodies in survivors occur early, are sustained, and can delay infection when transferred into nonhuman primates. Monoclonal antibodies (mAbs) from survivors exhibit potent neutralizing activity in vitro and are protective in rodents. To better understand targets and mechanisms of neutralization, we investigated a panel of mAbs shown previously to react with the envelope glycoprotein (GP). While one non-neutralizing mAb recognized a GP epitope in the nonessential mucin-like domain, the rest were specific for GP1, were neutralizing, and could be further distinguished by reactivity with secreted GP. We show that survivor antibodies, human KZ52 and monkey JP3K11, were specific for conformation-dependent epitopes comprising residues in GP1 and GP2 and that neutralization occurred by two distinct mechanisms; KZ52 inhibited cathepsin cleavage of GP whereas JP3K11 recognized the cleaved, fusion-active form of GP.

Published by Elsevier Inc.

PMCID: PMC3351102 PMID: 20304456 [PubMed - indexed for MEDLINE]

1308. Acta Crystallogr Sect F Struct Biol Cryst Commun. 2010 Jun 1;66(Pt 6):689-92. doi: 10.1107/S1744309110013266. Epub 2010 May 27.

Crystallization and preliminary X-ray analysis of Ebola VP35 interferon inhibitory domain mutant proteins.

Leung DW(1), Borek D, Farahbakhsh M, Ramanan P, Nix JC, Wang T, Prins KC, Otwinowski Z, Honzatko RB, Helgeson LA, Basler CF, Amarasinghe GK.

Author information: (1)Department of Biochemistry, Biophysics and Molecular Biology, Iowa State University, Ames, IA 50011, USA.

VP35 is one of seven structural proteins encoded by the Ebola viral genome and mediates viral replication, nucleocapsid formation and host immune suppression. The C-terminal interferon inhibitory domain (IID) of VP35 is critical for dsRNA binding and interferon inhibition. The wild-type VP35 IID structure revealed several conserved residues that are important for dsRNA binding and interferon antagonism. Here, the expression, purification and crystallization of recombinant Zaire Ebola VP35 IID mutants R312A, K319A/R322A and K339A in space groups P6(1)22, P2(1)2(1)2(1) and P2(1), respectively, are described. Diffraction data were collected using synchrotron sources at the Advanced Light Source and the Advanced Photon Source.

PMCID: PMC2882771 PMID: 20516601 [PubMed - indexed for MEDLINE]

1309. Hum Vaccin. 2010 Jun;6(6):439-49. Epub 2010 Jun 1.

Recent advances in Ebolavirus vaccine development.

Richardson JS(1), Dekker JD, Croyle MA, Kobinger GP.

Author information: (1)Special Pathogens Program, National Microbiology Laboratory, Public Health Agency of Canada, Winnipeg, MB, Canada.

Ebolavirus is a highly infectious pathogen with a case fatality rate as high as 90%. Currently there is a lack of licensed Ebolavirus vaccines as well as pre- and post-exposure treatments. Recent increases in the frequency of natural human Ebolavirus infections and its potential use as a bioterrorism agent makes

vaccine development a priority for many nations. Significant progress has been made in understanding the pathogenesis of Ebolavirus infection and several promising vaccine candidates were shown to be successful in protecting NHPs against lethal infection. These include replication-deficient adenovirus vectors, replication-competent VSV, HPIV-3 vectors and virus-like particle preparations. Recent advances in the generation of effective post-exposure immunization strategies highlight the possibility of developing a single dose vaccine that will confer full protection in humans following Ebolavirus exposure. Post-exposure protection is particularly important in outbreak and biodefense settings, as well as clinical and laboratory settings in the case of accidental exposure.
PMID: 20671437 [PubMed - indexed for MEDLINE]

1310. J Gen Virol. 2010 Jun;91(Pt 6):1478-83. doi: 10.1099/vir.0.019794-0. Epub 2010 Feb 17.

Characterization of the Ebola virus nucleoprotein-RNA complex.

Noda T(1), Hagiwara K, Sagara H, Kawaoka Y.

Author information: (1)International Research Center for Infectious Diseases, Institute of Medical Science, University of Tokyo, Shirokanedai, Minato-ku, Tokyo 108-8639, Japan.

When Ebola virus nucleoprotein (NP) is expressed in mammalian cells, it assembles into helical structures. Here, the recombinant NP helix purified from cells expressing NP was characterized biochemically and morphologically. We found that the recombinant NP helix is associated with non-viral RNA, which is not protected from RNase digestion and that the morphology of the helix changes depending on the environmental salt concentration. The N-terminal 450 aa residues of NP are sufficient for these properties. However, digestion of the NP-associated RNA eliminates the plasticity of the helix, suggesting that this RNA is an essential structural component of the helix, binding to individual NP molecules via the N-terminal 450 aa. These findings enhance our knowledge of Ebola virus assembly and understanding of the Ebola virus life cycle.
PMCID: PMC2878588 PMID: 20164259 [PubMed - indexed for MEDLINE]

1311. J Gen Virol. 2010 Jun;91(Pt 6):1464-72. doi: 10.1099/vir.0.018523-0. Epub 2010 Feb 3.

Measles virus M protein-driven particle production does not involve the endosomal sorting complex required for transport (ESCRT) system.

Salditt A(1), Koethe S, Pohl C, Harms H, Kolesnikova L, Becker S, Schneider-Schaulies S.

Author information: (1)Institute for Virology and Immunobiology, University of Wuerzburg, Versbacher Str. 7, D-97078 Wuerzburg, Germany.

Assembly and budding of enveloped RNA viruses rely on viral matrix (M) proteins and host proteins involved in sorting and vesiculation of cellular cargoes, such as the endosomal sorting complex required for transport (ESCRT). The measles virus (MV) M protein promotes virus-like particle (VLP) production, and we now show that it shares association with detergent-resistant or tetraspanin-enriched membrane microdomains with ebolavirus VP40 protein, yet accumulates less efficiently at the plasma membrane. Unlike VP40, which recruits ESCRT components via its N-terminal late (L) domain and exploits them for particle production, the M protein does this independently of this pathway, as (i) ablation of motifs bearing similarity to canonical L domains did not affect VLP production, (ii) it did not redistribute Tsg101, AIP-1 or Vps4A to the plasma membrane, and (iii) neither VLP nor infectious virus production was sensitive to inhibition by dominant-negative Vps4A. Importantly, transfer of the VP40 L domain into the MV M protein did not cause recruitment of ESCRT proteins or confer sensitivity of VLP release to Vps4A, indicating that MV particle production occurs independently of and cannot be routed into an ESCRT-dependent pathway.
PMID: 20130136 [PubMed - indexed for MEDLINE]

1312. J Virol. 2010 Jun;84(11):5687-94. doi: 10.1128/JVI.02583-09. Epub 2010 Mar 24.

Studies of the "chain reversal regions" of the avian sarcoma/leukosis virus (ASLV) and ebolavirus fusion proteins: analogous residues are important, and a His residue unique to EnvA affects the pH dependence of ASLV entry.

Delos SE(1), La B, Gilmartin A, White JM.

Author information: (1)Department of Cell Biology, University of Virginia, Charlottesville, Virginia 22908, USA. sed7a@virginia.edu

Most class I fusion proteins exist as trimers of dimers composed of a receptor binding and a fusion subunit. In their postfusion forms, the three fusion subunits form trimers of hairpins consisting of a central coiled coil (formed by the N-terminal helices), an intervening sequence, and a region containing the C helix (and flanking strands) that runs antiparallel to and packs in the grooves of the N-terminal coiled coil. For filoviruses and most retroviruses, the intervening sequence includes a "chain reversal region" consisting of a short stretch of hydrophobic residues, a Gly-Gly pair, a CX(6)CC motif, and a bulky hydrophobic residue. Maerz and coworkers (A. L. Maerz, R. J. Center, B. E. Kemp, B. Kobe, and P. Poumbourios, J. Virol. 74:6614-6621, 2000) proposed a model for this region of human T-cell leukemia virus type I (HTLV-I) Env in which expulsion of the final bulky hydrophobic residue is important for early conformational changes and specific residues in the chain reversal region are important for forming the final, stable trimer of hairpins. Here, we used mutagenesis and pseudovirus entry assays to test this model for the avian retrovirus avian sarcoma/leukosis virus (ASLV) and the filovirus ebolavirus Zaire. Our results are generally consistent with the model proposed for HTLV-I Env. In addition, we show with ASLV EnvA that the bulky hydrophobic residue following the CX(6)CC motif is required for the step of prehairpin target membrane insertion, whereas other residues are required for the foldback step of fusion. We further found that a His residue that is unique to the chain reversal region of ASLV EnvA controls the pH at which ASLV entry occurs.
PMCID: PMC2876614 PMID: 20335266 [PubMed - indexed for MEDLINE]

1313. Sci Am. 2010 Jun;302(6):21.

Bad wraps on viruses.

Roeher B.

Erratum in Sci Am. 2010 Oct;303(4):12.
PMID: 20521472 [PubMed - indexed for MEDLINE]

1314. Lancet. 2010 May 29;375(9729):1896-905. doi: 10.1016/S0140-6736(10)60357-1.

Postexposure protection of non-human primates against a lethal Ebola virus challenge with RNA interference: a proof-of-concept study.

Geisbert TW(1), Lee AC, Robbins M, Geisbert JB, Honko AN, Sood V, Johnson JC, de Jong S, Tavakoli I, Judge A, Hensley LE, Maclachlan I.

Author information: (1)National Emerging Infectious Diseases Laboratories Institute, Boston University School of Medicine, Boston, MA 02118, USA. geisbert@bu.edu

Comment in Lancet. 2010 May 29;375(9729):1850-2.

BACKGROUND: We previously showed that small interfering RNAs (siRNAs) targeting the Zaire Ebola virus (ZEBOV) RNA polymerase L protein formulated in stable nucleic acid-lipid particles (SNALPs) completely protected guineapigs when administered shortly after a lethal ZEBOV challenge. Although rodent models of ZEBOV infection are useful for screening prospective countermeasures, they are frequently not useful for prediction of efficacy in the more stringent non-human primate models. We therefore assessed the efficacy of modified non-immunostimulatory siRNAs in a uniformly lethal non-human primate model of ZEBOV haemorrhagic fever. METHODS: A combination of modified siRNAs targeting the ZEBOV L polymerase (EK-1 mod), viral protein (VP) 24 (VP24-1160 mod), and VP35 (VP35-855 mod) were formulated in SNALPs. A group of macaques (n=3) was given these pooled anti-ZEBOV siRNAs (2 mg/kg per dose, bolus intravenous infusion) after 30 min, and on days 1, 3, and 5 after challenge with ZEBOV. A second group of macaques (n=4) was given the pooled anti-ZEBOV siRNAs after 30 min, and on days 1, 2, 3, 4, 5, and 6 after challenge with ZEBOV. FINDINGS: Two (66%) of three rhesus monkeys given four postexposure treatments of the pooled anti-ZEBOV siRNAs were protected from lethal ZEBOV infection, whereas all macaques given seven postexposure treatments were protected. The treatment regimen in the second study was well tolerated with minor changes in liver enzymes that might have been related to viral infection. INTERPRETATION: This complete postexposure protection against ZEBOV in non-human primates provides a model for the treatment of ZEBOV-induced haemorrhagic fever. These data show the potential of RNA interference as an effective postexposure treatment strategy for people infected with Ebola virus, and suggest that this strategy might also be useful for treatment of other emerging viral infections. FUNDING: Defense Threat Reduction Agency.

PMID: 20511019 [PubMed - indexed for MEDLINE]

1315. Lancet. 2010 May 29;375(9729):1850-2. doi: 10.1016/S0140-6736(10)60597-1.

Are we any closer to combating Ebola infections?

Feldmann H(1).

Author information: (1)Rocky Mountain Laboratories, Hamilton, MT 59840, USA. feldmannh@niaid.nih.gov

Comment on Lancet. 2010 May 29;375(9729):1896-905.

PMCID: PMC3398603 PMID: 20511001 [PubMed - indexed for MEDLINE]

1316. Proc Natl Acad Sci U S A. 2010 May 25;107(21):9556-61. doi: 10.1073/pnas.0915002107. Epub 2010 May 10.

Effects of the USA PATRIOT Act and the 2002 Bioterrorism Preparedness Act on select agent research in the United States.

Dias MB(1), Reyes-Gonzalez L, Veloso FM, Casman EA.

Author information: (1)Department of Engineering and Public Policy, Carnegie Mellon University, Pittsburgh, PA 15213, USA.

A bibliometric analysis of the Bacillus anthracis and Ebola virus archival literature was conducted to determine whether negative consequences of the Uniting and Strengthening America by Providing Appropriate Tools Required to Intercept and Obstruct Terrorism" (USA PATRIOT) Act and the 2002 Bioterrorism Preparedness Act on US select agent research could be discerned. Indicators of the health of the field, such as number of papers published per year, number of researchers authoring papers, and influx rate of new authors, indicated an overall stimulus to the field after 2002. As measured by interorganizational coauthorships, both B. anthracis and Ebola virus research networks expanded after 2002 in terms of the number of organizations and the degree of collaboration. Coauthorship between US and non US scientists also grew for Ebola virus but contracted for the subset of B. anthracis research that did not involve possession of viable, virulent bacteria. Some non-US institutions were dropped, and collaborations with others intensified. Contrary to expectations, research did not become centralized around a few gatekeeper institutions. Two negative effects were detected. There was an increased turnover rate of authors in the select agent community that was not observed in the control organism (Klebsiella pneumoniae) research community. However, the most striking effect observed was not associated with individual authors or institutions; it was a loss of efficiency, with an approximate 2- to 5-fold increase in the cost of doing select agent research as measured by the number of research papers published per millions of US research dollars awarded.

PMCID: PMC2906869 PMID: 20457912 [PubMed - indexed for MEDLINE]

1317. Virology. 2010 May 25;401(1):18-28. doi: 10.1016/j.virol.2010.02.015. Epub 2010 Mar 3.

Ebola virus uses clathrin-mediated endocytosis as an entry pathway.

Bhattacharyya S(1), Warfield KL, Ruthel G, Bavari S, Aman MJ, Hope TJ.

Author information: (1)Department of Cell and Molecular Biology, Feinberg School of Medicine, Northwestern University, 303 East Chicago Avenue, Chicago, IL 60611, USA.

Ebola virus (EBOV) infects several cell types and while viral entry is known to be pH-dependent, the exact entry pathway(s) remains unknown. To gain insights into EBOV entry, the role of several inhibitors of clathrin-mediated endocytosis in blocking infection mediated by HIV pseudotyped with the EBOV envelope glycoprotein (EbGP) was examined. Wild type HIV and envelope-minus HIV pseudotyped with Vesicular Stomatitis Virus glycoprotein (VSVg) were used as controls to assess cell viability after inhibiting clathrin pathway. Inhibition of clathrin pathway using dominant-negative Eps15, siRNA-mediated knockdown of clathrin heavy chain, chlorpromazine and sucrose blocked EbGP pseudotyped HIV infection. Also, both chlorpromazine and Bafilomycin A1 inhibited entry of infectious EBOV. Sensitivity of EbGP pseudotyped HIV as well as infectious EBOV to inhibitors of clathrin suggests that EBOV uses clathrin-mediated endocytosis as an entry pathway. Furthermore, since chlorpromazine inhibits EBOV infection, novel therapeutic modalities could be designed based on this lead compound.

PMCID: PMC3732189 PMID: 20202662 [PubMed - indexed for MEDLINE]

1318. PLoS Pathog. 2010 May 20;6(5):e1000904. doi: 10.1371/journal.ppat.1000904.

Demonstration of cross-protective vaccine immunity against an emerging pathogenic Ebolavirus Species.

Hensley LE(1), Mulangu S, Asiedu C, Johnson J, Honko AN, Stanley D, Fabozzi G, Nichol ST, Ksiazek TG, Rollin PE, Wahl-Jensen V, Bailey M, Jahrling PB, Roederer M, Koup RA, Sullivan NJ.

Author information: (1)Virology Division, United States Army Medical Research Institute of Infectious Diseases, Fort Detrick, Maryland, USA.

Comment in Future Microbiol. 2010 Oct;5(10):1469-73.

A major challenge in developing vaccines for emerging pathogens is their continued evolution and ability to escape human immunity. Therefore, an important goal of vaccine research is to advance vaccine candidates with sufficient breadth to respond to new outbreaks of previously undetected viruses. Ebolavirus (EBOV) vaccines have demonstrated protection against EBOV infection in nonhuman primates (NHP) and show promise in human clinical trials but immune protection occurs only with vaccines whose antigens are matched to the infectious challenge species. A 2007 hemorrhagic fever outbreak in Uganda demonstrated the existence of a new EBOV species, Bundibugyo (BEBOV), that differed from viruses covered by current vaccine candidates by up to 43% in genome sequence. To address the question of whether cross-protective immunity can be generated against this novel species, cynomolgus macaques were immunized with DNA/rAd5 vaccines expressing ZEBOV and SEBOV glycoprotein (GP) prior to lethal challenge with BEBOV. Vaccinated subjects developed robust, antigen-specific humoral and cellular immune responses against the GP from ZEBOV as well as cellular immunity against BEBOV GP, and immunized macaques were uniformly protected against lethal challenge with BEBOV. This report provides the first demonstration of vaccine-induced protective immunity against challenge with a heterologous EBOV species, and shows that Ebola vaccines capable of eliciting potent cellular immunity may provide the best strategy for eliciting cross-protection against newly emerging heterologous EBOV species.

PMCID: PMC2873919 PMID: 20502688 [PubMed - indexed for MEDLINE]

1319. PLoS Pathog. 2010 May 13;6(5):e1000913. doi: 10.1371/journal.ppat.1000913.

The great escape: viral strategies to counter BST-2/tetherin.

Douglas JL(1), Gustin JK, Viswanathan K, Mansouri M, Moses AV, Früh K.

Author information: (1)Vaccine and Gene Therapy Institute, Oregon Health & Science University, Beaverton, Oregon, United States of America.

The interferon-induced BST-2 protein has the unique ability to restrict the egress of HIV-1, Kaposi's sarcoma-associated herpesvirus (KSHV), Ebola virus, and other enveloped viruses. The observation that virions remain attached to the surface of BST-2-expressing cells led to the renaming of BST-2 as "tetherin". However, viral proteins such as HIV-1 Vpu, simian immunodeficiency virus Nef, and KSHV K5 counteract BST-2, thereby allowing mature virions to readily escape from infected cells. Since the anti-viral function of BST-2 was discovered, there has been an explosion of research into several aspects of this intriguing interplay between host and virus. This review focuses on recent work addressing the molecular mechanisms involved in BST-2 restriction of viral egress and the species-specific countermeasures employed by various viruses.

PMCID: PMC2869331 PMID: 20485522 [PubMed - indexed for MEDLINE]

1320. Am J Emerg Med. 2010 May;28(4):515-8. doi: 10.1016/j.ajem.2009.03.024. Epub 2010 Feb 25.

Bioterrorism: what might be walking into the ED?

Goffman TE(1).

Author information: (1)Cancer Intelligence and Research, PC, Virginia Beach, VA 23455, USA. tetomtg@yahoo.com

PMID: 20466236 [PubMed - indexed for MEDLINE]

1321. Am J Trop Med Hyg. 2010 May;82(5):954-60. doi: 10.4269/ajtmh.2010.09-0636.

Comprehensive panel of real-time TaqMan polymerase chain reaction assays for detection and absolute quantification of filoviruses, arenaviruses, and New World hantaviruses.

Trombley AR(1), Wachter L, Garrison J, Buckley-Beason VA, Jahrling J, Hensley LE, Schoepp RJ, Norwood DA, Goba A, Fair JN, Kulesh DA.

Author information: (1)Diagnostic Systems Division, and Virology Division, United States Army Medical Research Institute of Infectious Diseases, Fort Detrick, MD 21701-5011, USA.

Viral hemorrhagic fever is caused by a diverse group of single-stranded, negative-sense or positive-sense RNA viruses belonging to the families Filoviridae (Ebola and Marburg), Arenaviridae (Lassa, Junin, Machupo, Sabia, and Guanarito), and Bunyaviridae (hantavirus). Disease characteristics in these families mark each with the potential to be used as a biological threat agent. Because other diseases have similar clinical symptoms, specific laboratory diagnostic tests are necessary to provide the differential diagnosis during outbreaks and for instituting acceptable quarantine procedures. We designed 48 TaqMan-based polymerase chain reaction (PCR) assays for specific and absolute quantitative detection of multiple hemorrhagic fever viruses. Forty-six assays were determined to be virus-specific, and two were designated as pan assays for Marburg virus. The limit of detection for the assays ranged from 10 to 0.001 plaque-forming units (PFU)/PCR. Although these real-time hemorrhagic fever virus assays are qualitative (presence of target), they are also quantitative (measure a single DNA/RNA target sequence in an unknown sample and express the final results as an absolute value (e.g., viral load, PFUs, or copies/mL) on the basis of concentration of standard samples and can be used in viral load, vaccine, and antiviral drug studies.

PMCID: PMC2861391 PMID: 20439981 [PubMed - indexed for MEDLINE]

1322. Antimicrob Agents Chemother. 2010 May;54(5):2152-9. doi: 10.1128/AAC.01315-09. Epub 2010 Mar 8.

Antiviral activity of a small-molecule inhibitor of filovirus infection.

Warren TK(1), Warfield KL, Wells J, Enterlein S, Smith M, Ruthel G, Yunus AS, Kinch MS, Goldblatt M, Aman MJ, Bavari S.

Author information: (1)US Army Medical Research Institute of Infectious Diseases, Fort Detrick, Frederick, Maryland, USA.

There exists an urgent need to develop licensed drugs and vaccines for the treatment or prevention of filovirus infections. FGI-103 is a low-molecular-weight compound that was discovered through an in vitro screening assay utilizing a variant of Zaire ebolavirus (ZEBOV) that expresses green fluorescent protein. In vitro analyses demonstrated that FGI-103 also exhibits antiviral activity against wild-type ZEBOV and Sudan ebolavirus, as well as Marburgvirus (MARV) strains Ci67 and Ravn. In vivo administration of FGI-103 as a single intraperitoneal dose of 10 mg/kg delivered 24 h after infection is sufficient to completely protect mice against a lethal challenge with a mouse-adapted strain of either ZEBOV or MARV-Ravn. In a murine model of ZEBOV infection, delivery of FGI-103 reduces viremia and the viral burden in kidney, liver, and spleen tissues and is associated with subdued and delayed proinflammatory cytokine responses and tissue pathology. Taken together, these results identify a promising antiviral therapeutic candidate for the treatment of filovirus infections.

PMCID: PMC2863630 PMID: 20211898 [PubMed - indexed for MEDLINE]

1323. Biotechnol Bioeng. 2010 May 1;106(1):9-17. doi: 10.1002/bit.22652.

High-level rapid production of full-size monoclonal antibodies in plants by a single-vector DNA replicon system.

Huang Z(1), Phoolcharoen W, Lai H, Piensook K, Cardineau G, Zeitlin L, Whaley KJ, Arntzen CJ, Mason HS, Chen Q.

Author information: (1)The Biodesign Institute and School of Life Sciences, Arizona State University, Tempe, Arizona 85287-4501, USA.

Plant viral vectors have great potential in rapid production of important pharmaceutical proteins. However, high-yield production of hetero-oligomeric proteins that require the expression and assembly of two or more protein subunits often suffers problems due to the "competing" nature of viral vectors derived from the same virus. Previously we reported that a bean yellow dwarf virus (BeYDV)-derived, three-component DNA replicon system allows rapid production of single recombinant proteins in plants (Huang et al., 2009. Biotechnol Bioeng 103: 706-714). In this article, we report further development of this expression system for its application in high-yield production of oligomeric protein complexes including monoclonal antibodies (mAbs) in plants. We showed that the BeYDV replicon system permits simultaneous efficient replication of two DNA replicons and thus, high-level accumulation of two recombinant proteins in the same plant cell. We also demonstrated that a single vector that contains multiple replicon cassettes was as efficient as the three-component system in driving the expression of two distinct proteins. Using either the non-competing, three-vector system or the multi-replicon single vector, we produced both the heavy and light chain subunits of a protective IgG mAb 6D8 against Ebola virus GP1 (Wilson et al., 2000. Science 287: 1664-1666) at 0.5 mg of mAb per gram leaf fresh weight within 4 days post-infiltration of Nicotiana benthamiana leaves. We further demonstrated that full-size tetrameric IgG complex containing two heavy and two light chains was efficiently assembled and readily purified, and retained its functionality in specific binding to inactivated Ebola virus. Thus, our single-vector replicon system provides high-yield production capacity for hetero-oligomeric proteins, yet eliminates the difficult task of identifying non-competing virus and the need for co-infection of multiple expression modules. The multi-replicon vector represents a significant advance in transient expression technology for antibody production in plants.

PMCID: PMC2905544 PMID: 20047189 [PubMed - indexed for MEDLINE]

1324. J Virol. 2010 May;84(9):4816-20. doi: 10.1128/JVI.00010-10. Epub 2010 Feb 17.

Role of the GTPase Rab1b in ebolavirus particle formation.

Yamayoshi S(1), Neumann G, Kawaoka Y.

Author information: (1)Division of Virology, Department of Microbiology and Immunology, Institute of Medical Science, University of Tokyo, Shirokanedai, Minato-ku, Tokyo 108-8639, Japan.

The Ebolavirus matrix protein VP40 is essential for virion assembly and egress. Recently, we reported that the coat protein complex II (COPII) transport system plays an important role in the transport of VP40 to the plasma membrane. Here, we show that dominant-negative mutants of the GTPase Rab1b interfere with VP40-mediated particle formation. Rab1b activates GBF1 (Golgi-specific BFA [brefeldin A] resistance factor 1), a critical factor in the assembly of COPI vesicles. Activated GBF1 stimulates ARF1 (ADP ribosylation factor 1), which recruits coat protein to cellular membranes for the assembly of COPI vesicles. Here, we demonstrate that GBF1 and ARF1 are involved in Ebolavirus virion formation, suggesting that both the COPII and COPI transport systems play a role in Ebolavirus VP40-mediated particle formation. These findings provide new insights into the cellular pathways employed for Ebolavirus virion formation.

PMCID: PMC2863720 PMID: 20164217 [PubMed - indexed for MEDLINE]

1325. PLoS Pathog. 2010 Apr 29;6(4):e1000875. doi: 10.1371/journal.ppat.1000875.

Electron tomography reveals the steps in filovirus budding.

Welsch S(1), Kolesnikova L, Krähling V, Riches JD, Becker S, Briggs JA.

Author information: (1)Structural and Computational Biology Unit, European Molecular Biology Laboratory, Heidelberg, Germany.

The filoviruses, Marburg and Ebola, are non-segmented negative-strand RNA viruses causing severe hemorrhagic fever with high mortality rates in humans and nonhuman primates. The sequence of events that leads to release of filovirus particles from cells is poorly understood. Two contrasting mechanisms have been proposed, one proceeding via a "submarine-like" budding with the helical nucleocapsid emerging parallel to the plasma membrane, and the other via perpendicular rocket-like protrusion. Here we have infected cells with Marburg virus under BSL-4 containment conditions, and reconstructed the sequence of steps in the budding process in three dimensions using electron tomography of plastic-embedded cells. We find that highly infectious filamentous particles are released at early stages in infection. Budding proceeds via lateral association of intracellular nucleocapsid along its whole length with the plasma membrane, followed by rapid envelopment initiated at one end of the nucleocapsid, leading to a protruding intermediate. Scission results in local membrane instability at the rear of the virus. After prolonged infection, increased vesiculation of the plasma membrane correlates with changes in shape and infectivity of released viruses. Our observations demonstrate a cellular determinant of virus shape. They reconcile the contrasting models of filovirus budding and allow us to describe the sequence of events taking place during budding and release of Marburg virus. We propose that this represents a general sequence of events also followed by other filamentous and rod-shaped viruses.

PMCID: PMC2861712 PMID: 20442788 [PubMed - indexed for MEDLINE]

1326. Virology. 2010 Apr 10;399(2):290-8. doi: 10.1016/j.virol.2010.01.015. Epub 2010 Feb 2.

Mucosal parainfluenza virus-vectored vaccine against Ebola virus replicates in the respiratory tract of vector-immune monkeys and is immunogenic.

Bukreyev AA(1), Dinapoli JM, Yang L, Murphy BR, Collins PL.

Author information: (1)Laboratory of Infectious Diseases, National Institute of Allergy and Infectious Diseases, National Institutes of Health, Bethesda, MD 20892, USA. abukreyev@niaid.nih.gov

We previously used human parainfluenza virus type 3 (HPIV3) as a vector to express the Ebola virus (EBOV) GP glycoprotein. The resulting HPIV3/EboGP vaccine was immunogenic and protective against EBOV challenge in a non-human primate model. However, it remained unclear whether the vaccine would be effective in adults due to preexisting immunity to HPIV3. Here, the immunogenicity of HPIV3/EboGP was compared in HPIV3-naive and HPIV3-immune Rhesus monkeys. After a single dose of HPIV3/EboGP, the titers of EBOV-specific serum ELISA or neutralization antibodies were substantially less in HPIV3-immune animals compared to HPIV3-naive animals. However, after two doses, which were previously determined to be required for complete protection against EBOV challenge, the antibody titers were indistinguishable between the two groups. The vaccine virus appeared to replicate, at a reduced level, in the respiratory tract despite the preexisting immunity. This may reflect the known ability of HPIV3 to re-infect and may also reflect the presence of EBOV GP in the vector virion, which confers resistance to neutralization in vitro by HPIV3-specific antibodies. These data suggest that HPIV3/EboGP will be immunogenic in adults as well as children.

Published by Elsevier Inc.

PMCID: PMC2842940 PMID: 20129638 [PubMed - indexed for MEDLINE]

1327. Arch Virol. 2010 Apr;155(4):507-14. doi: 10.1007/s00705-010-0612-5. Epub 2010 Mar 10

Identification of SARS-like coronaviruses in horseshoe bats (Rhinolophus hipposideros) in Slovenia.

Rihtaric D(1), Hostnik P, Steyer A, Grom J, Toplak I.

Author information: (1)Virology Unit, Veterinary Faculty, Institute of Microbiology and Parasitology, University of Ljubljana, Gerbiceva 60, 1115 Ljubljana, Slovenia.

Bats have been identified as a natural reservoir for an increasing number of emerging zoonotic viruses, such as Hendra virus, Nipah virus, Ebola virus, Marburg virus, rabies and other lyssaviruses. Recently, a large number of viruses closely related to members of the genus Coronavirus have been associated with severe acute respiratory syndrome (SARS) and detected in bat species. In this study, samples were collected from 106 live bats of seven different bat species from 27 different locations in Slovenia. Coronaviruses were detected by RT-PCR in 14 out of 36 horseshoe bat (Rhinolophus hipposideros) fecal samples, with 38.8% virus prevalence. Sequence analysis of a 405-nucleotide region of the highly conserved RNA polymerase gene (pol) showed that all coronaviruses detected in this study are genetically closely related, with 99.5-100% nucleotide identity, and belong to group 2 of the coronaviruses. The most closely related virus sequence in GenBank was SARS bat isolate Rp3/2004 (DQ071615) within the SARS-like CoV cluster, sharing 85% nucleotide identity and 95.6% amino acid identity. The potential risk of a new group of bat coronaviruses as a reservoir for human infections is highly suspected, and further molecular epidemiologic studies of these bat coronaviruses are needed.

PMID: 20217155 [PubMed - indexed for MEDLINE]

1328. Clin Vaccine Immunol. 2010 Apr;17(4):572-81. doi: 10.1128/CVI.00467-09. Epub 2010 Feb 24.

Protection of nonhuman primates against two species of Ebola virus infection with a single complex adenovirus vector.

Pratt WD(1), Wang D, Nichols DK, Luo M, Woraratanadharm J, Dye JM, Holman DH, Dong JY.

Author information: (1)U.S. Army Medical Research Institute of Infectious Diseases, 1425 Porter St., Fort Detrick, MD 21702-5011, USA. williamd.pratt@us.army.mil

Ebola viruses are highly pathogenic viruses that cause outbreaks of hemorrhagic fever in humans and other primates. To meet the need for a vaccine against the several types of Ebola viruses that cause human diseases, we developed a multivalent vaccine candidate (EBO7) that expresses the glycoproteins of Zaire ebolavirus (ZEBOV) and Sudan ebolavirus (SEBOV) in a single complex adenovirus-based vector (CAdVax). We evaluated our vaccine in nonhuman primates against the parenteral and aerosol routes of lethal challenge. EBO7 vaccine provided protection against both Ebola viruses by either route of infection. Significantly, protection against SEBOV given as an aerosol challenge, which has not previously been shown, could be achieved with a boosting vaccination. These results demonstrate the feasibility of creating a robust, multivalent Ebola virus vaccine that would be effective in the event of a natural virus outbreak or biological threat.

PMCID: PMC2849326 PMID: 20181765 [PubMed - indexed for MEDLINE]

1329. Rapid Commun Mass Spectrom. 2010 Mar 15;24(5):571-85. doi: 10.1002/rcm.4410.

Identification of N-glycans from Ebola virus glycoproteins by matrix-assisted laser desorption/ionisation time-of-flight and negative ion electrospray tandem mass spectrometry.

Ritchie G(1), Harvey DJ, Stroeher U, Feldmann F, Feldmann H, Wahl-Jensen V, Royle L, Dwek RA, Rudd PM.

Author information: (1)Oxford Glycobiology Institute, Department of Biochemistry, University of Oxford, Oxford, UK.

The larger fragment of the transmembrane glycoprotein (GP1) and the soluble glycoprotein (sGP) of Ebola virus were expressed in human embryonic kidney cells and the secreted products were purified from the supernatant for carbohydrate analysis. The N-glycans were released with PNGase F from within sodium dodecyl sulphate/polyacrylamide gel electrophoresis (SDS-PAGE) gels. Identification of the glycans was made with normal-phase high-performance liquid chromatography (HPLC), matrix-assisted laser desorption/ionisation mass spectrometry, negative ion electrospray ionisation fragmentation mass spectrometry and exoglycosidase digestion. Most glycans were complex bi-, tri- and tetra-antennary compounds with reduced amounts of galactose. No bisected compounds were detected. Triantennary glycans were branched on the 6-antenna; fucose was attached to the core GlcNAc residue. Sialylated glycans were present on sGP but were largely absent from GP1, the larger fragment of the transmembrane glycoprotein. Consistent with this was the generally higher level of processing of carbohydrates found on sGP as evidenced by a higher percentage of galactose and lower levels of high-mannose glycans than were found on GP1. These results confirm and expand previous findings on partial characterisation of the Ebola virus transmembrane glycoprotein. They represent the first detailed data on carbohydrate structures of the Ebola virus sGP.

PMCID: PMC3399782 PMID: 20131323 [PubMed - indexed for MEDLINE]
1330. Clin Lab Med. 2010 Mar;30(1):161-77. doi: 10.1016/j.cll.2009.12.001.

Ebola and marburg hemorrhagic fever.

Hartman AL(1), Towner JS, Nichol ST.

Author information: (1)University of Pittsburgh, Center for Vaccine Research, PA 15261, USA. hartman2@pitt.edu

Ebola and Marburg viruses cause a severe viral hemorrhagic fever disease mainly in Sub-Saharan Africa. Although outbreaks are sporadic, there is the potential for filoviruses to spread to other continents unintentionally because of air travel or intentionally because of bioterrorism. This article discusses the natural history, epidemiology, and clinical presentation of patients infected with Ebola and Marburg viruses. Clinicians in the United States should be aware of the symptoms of these viral infections in humans and know the appropriate procedures for contacting local, state, and national reference laboratories in the event of a suspected case of filoviral hemorrhagic fever.

PMID: 20513546 [PubMed - indexed for MEDLINE]
1331. East Afr J Public Health. 2010 Mar;7(1):30-6.

Lessons learned during active epidemiological surveillance of Ebola and Marburg viral hemorrhagic fever epidemics in Africa.

Allaranga Y(1), Kone ML, Formenty P, Libama F, Boumandouki P, Woodfill CJ, Snw I, Duale S, Alemu W, Yada A.

Author information: (1)WHO, Regional office for Africa, Brazzaville, Congo. allarangary@gw.afro.who.int

OBJECTIVE: To review epidemiological surveillance approaches used during Ebola and Marburg hemorrhagic fever epidemics in Africa in the past fifteen years. Overall, 26 hemorrhagic epidemic outbreaks have been registered in 12 countries; 18 caused by the Ebola virus and eight by the Marburg virus. About 2551 cases have been reported, among which 268 were health workers (9,3%). METHODS: Based on articles and epidemic management reports, this review analyses surveillance approaches, route of introduction of the virus into the population (urban and rural), the collaboration between the human health sector and the wildlife sector and factors that have affected epidemic management. FINDINGS: Several factors affecting the epidemiological surveillance during Ebola and Marburg viruses hemorrhagic epidemics have been observed. During epidemics in rural settings, outbreak investigations have shown multiple introductions of the virus into the human population through wildlife. In contrast, during epidemics in urban settings a single introduction of the virus in the community was responsible for the epidemic. Active surveillance is key to containing outbreaks of Ebola and Marburg viruses CONCLUSIONS: Collaboration with those in charge of the conservation of wildlife is essential for the early detection of viral hemorrhagic fever epidemics. Hemorrhagic fever epidemics caused by Ebola and Marburg viruses are occurring more and more frequently in Sub-Saharan Africa and only an adapted epidemiological surveillance system will allow for early detection and effective response.

PMID: 21413569 [PubMed - indexed for MEDLINE]
1332. East Afr J Public Health. 2010 Mar;7(1):20-9.

Trends of major disease outbreaks in the African region, 2003-2007.

Kebede S(1), Duales S, Yokouide A, Alemu W.

Author information: (1)International Health Consultancy, Altanta, Georgia, USA. kebed4@sph.emory.edu

BACKGROUND: Communicable disease outbreaks cause millions of deaths throughout Sub-Saharan Africa each year. Most of the diseases causing epidemics in the region have been nearly eradicated or brought under control in other parts of the world. In recent years, considerable effort has been directed toward public health initiatives and strategies with a potential for significant impact in the fight against infectious diseases. In 1998, the World Health Organization African Regional Office (WHO/AFRO) launched the Integrated Disease Surveillance and Response (IDSR) strategy aimed at mitigating the impact of communicable diseases, including epidemic-prone diseases, through improving surveillance, laboratory confirmation and appropriate and timely public health interventions. Over the past decade, WHO and its partners have been providing technical and financial resources to African countries to strengthen epidemic preparedness and response (EPR) activities. METHODS: This review examined the major epidemics reported to WHO/AFRO from 2003 to 2007. we conduct a review of documents and reports obtained from WHO/AFRO, WHO inter-country team, and partners and held meeting and discussions with key stakeholders to elicit the experiences of local, regional and international efforts against these epidemics to evaluate the lessons learned and to stimulate discussion on the future course for enhancing EPR. RESULTS: The most commonly reported epidemic outbreaks in Africa include: cholera, dysentery, malaria and hemorrhagic fevers (e.g. Ebola, Rift Valley fever, Crimean-Congo fever and yellow fever). The cyclic meningococcal meningitis outbreak that affects countries along the "meningitis belt" (spanning Sub-Saharan Africa from Senegal and The Gambia to Kenya and Ethiopia) accounts for other major epidemics in the region. The reporting of disease outbreaks to WHO/AFRO has improved since the launch of the IDSR strategy in 1998. Although the epidemic trends for cholera showed a

decline in case fatality rate (CFR) suggesting improvement in detection and quality of response by the health sector, the number of countries affected has increased. Major epidemic diseases continue to occur in most countries in the region. Among the major challenges to overcome are: poor coordination of EPR, weak public health infrastructure, lack of trained workers and inconsistent supply of diagnostic, treatment and prevention commodities. CONCLUSIONS: To successfully reduce the levels of morbidity and mortality resulting from epidemic outbreaks, urgent and long-term investments are needed to strengthen capacities for early detection and timely and effective response. Effective advocacy, collaboration and resource mobilization efforts involving local health officials, governments and the international community are critically needed to reduce the heavy burden of disease outbreaks on African populations.
PMID: 21413568 [PubMed - indexed for MEDLINE]

1333. J Virol. 2010 Mar;84(6):3004-15. doi: 10.1128/JVI.02459-09. Epub 2010 Jan 13.

Mutations abrogating VP35 interaction with double-stranded RNA render Ebola virus avirulent in guinea pigs.

Prins KC(1), Delpeut S, Leung DW, Reynard O, Volchkova VA, Reid SP, Ramanan P, Cárdenas WB, Amarasinghe GK, Volchkov VE, Basler CF.

Author information: (1)Department of Microbiology, Mount Sinai School of Medicine, New York, New York 10029, USA.

Ebola virus (EBOV) protein VP35 is a double-stranded RNA (dsRNA) binding inhibitor of host interferon (IFN)-alpha/beta responses that also functions as a viral polymerase cofactor. Recent structural studies identified key features, including a central basic patch, required for VP35 dsRNA binding activity. To address the functional significance of these VP35 structural features for EBOV replication and pathogenesis, two point mutations, K319A/R322A, that abrogate VP35 dsRNA binding activity and severely impair its suppression of IFN-alpha/beta production were identified. Solution nuclear magnetic resonance (NMR) spectroscopy and X-ray crystallography reveal minimal structural perturbations in the K319A/R322A VP35 double mutant and suggest that loss of basic charge leads to altered function. Recombinant EBOVs encoding the mutant VP35 exhibit, relative to wild-type VP35 viruses, minimal growth attenuation in IFN-defective Vero cells but severe impairment in IFN-competent cells. In guinea pigs, the VP35 mutant virus revealed a complete loss of virulence. Strikingly, the VP35 mutant virus effectively immunized animals against subsequent wild-type EBOV challenge. These in vivo studies, using recombinant EBOV viruses, combined with the accompanying biochemical and structural analyses directly correlate VP35 dsRNA binding and IFN inhibition functions with viral pathogenesis. Moreover, these studies provide a framework for the development of antivirals targeting this critical EBOV virulence factor.
PMCID: PMC2826052 PMID: 20071589 [PubMed - indexed for MEDLINE]

1334. J Virol. 2010 Mar;84(6):2972-82. doi: 10.1128/JVI.02151-09. Epub 2010 Jan 6.

Biochemical and structural characterization of cathepsin L-processed Ebola virus glycoprotein: implications for viral entry and immunogenicity.

Hood CL(1), Abraham J, Boyington JC, Leung K, Kwong PD, Nabel GJ.

Author information: (1)Vaccine Research Center, National Institute of Allergy and Infectious Diseases, National Institutes of Health,Room 4502, Building 40, MSC-3005, 40 Convent Drive, Bethesda, Maryland 20892-3005, USA.

Ebola virus (EBOV) cellular attachment and entry is initiated by the envelope glycoprotein (GP) on the virion surface. Entry of this virus is pH dependent and associated with the cleavage of GP by proteases, including cathepsin L (CatL) and/or CatB, in the endosome or cell membrane. Here, we characterize the product of CatL cleavage of Zaire EBOV GP (ZEBOV-GP) and evaluate its relevance to entry. A stabilized recombinant form of the EBOV GP trimer was generated using a trimerization domain linked to a cleavable histidine tag. This trimer was purified to homogeneity and cleaved with CatL. Characterization of the trimeric product by N-terminal sequencing and mass spectrometry revealed three cleavage fragments, with masses of 23, 19, and 4 kDa. Structure-assisted modeling of the cathepsin L-cleaved ZEBOV-GP revealed that cleavage removes a glycosylated glycan cap and mucin-like domain (MUC domain) and exposes the conserved core residues implicated in receptor binding. The CatL-cleaved ZEBOV-GP intermediate bound with high affinity to a neutralizing antibody, KZ52, and also elicited neutralizing antibodies, supporting the notion that the processed intermediate is required for viral entry. Together, these data suggest that CatL cleavage of EBOV GP exposes its receptor-binding domain, thereby facilitating access to a putative cellular receptor in steps that lead to membrane fusion.
PMCID: PMC2826059 PMID: 20053739 [PubMed - indexed for MEDLINE]

1335. J Virol. 2010 Mar;84(5):2294-303. doi: 10.1128/JVI.02034-09. Epub 2009 Dec 23.

Conserved motifs within Ebola and Marburg virus VP40 proteins are important for stability, localization, and subsequent budding of virus-like particles.

Liu Y(1), Cocka L, Okumura A, Zhang YA, Sunyer JO, Harty RN.

Author information: (1)Laboratory 412, Department of Pathobiology, School of Veterinary Medicine, University of Pennsylvania, Philadelphia, Pennsylvania 19104, USA.

The filovirus VP40 protein is capable of budding from mammalian cells in the form of virus-like particles (VLPs) that are morphologically indistinguishable from infectious virions. Ebola virus VP40 (eVP40) contains well-characterized overlapping L domains, which play a key role in mediating efficient virus egress. L domains represent only one component required for efficient budding and, therefore, there is a need to identify and characterize additional domains important for VP40 function. We demonstrate here that the (96)LPLGVA(101) sequence of eVP40 and the corresponding (84)LPLGIM(89) sequence of Marburg virus VP40 (mVP40) are critical for efficient release of VP40 VLPs. Indeed, deletion of these motifs essentially abolished the ability of eVP40 and mVP40 to bud as VLPs. To address the mechanism by which the (96)LPLGVA(101) motif of eVP40 contributes to egress, a series of point mutations were introduced into this motif. These mutants were then compared to the eVP40 wild type in a VLP budding assay to assess budding competency. Confocal microscopy and gel filtration analyses were performed to assess their pattern of intracellular localization and ability to oligomerize, respectively. Our results show that mutations disrupting the (96)LPLGVA(101) motif resulted in both altered patterns of intracellular localization and self-assembly compared to wild-type controls. Interestingly, coexpression of either Ebola virus GP-WT or mVP40-WT with eVP40-DeltaLPLGVA failed to rescue the budding defective eVP40-DeltaLPLGVA mutant into VLPs;

however, coexpression of eVP40-WT with mVP40-DeltaLPLGIM successfully rescued budding of mVP40-DeltaLPLGIM into VLPs at mVP40-WT levels. In sum, our findings implicate the LPLGVA and LPLGIM motifs of eVP40 and mVP40, respectively, as being important for VP40 structure/stability and budding.

PMCID: PMC2820906 PMID: 20032189 [PubMed - indexed for MEDLINE]

1336. Proc Natl Acad Sci U S A. 2010 Feb 23;107(8):3463-8. doi: 10.1073/pnas.0913083107. Epub 2010 Feb 8.

Histidine-mediated RNA transfer to GDP for unique mRNA capping by vesicular stomatitis virus RNA polymerase.

Ogino T(1), Yadav SP, Banerjee AK.

Author information: (1)Department of Molecular Genetics, Lerner Research Institute, Cleveland Clinic, Cleveland, OH 44195, USA.

Comment in Proc Natl Acad Sci U S A. 2010 Feb 23;107(8):3283-4.

The RNA-dependent RNA polymerase L protein of vesicular stomatitis virus, a prototype of nonsegmented negative-strand (NNS) RNA viruses, forms a covalent complex with a 5'-phosphorylated viral mRNA-start sequence (L-pRNA), a putative intermediate in the unconventional mRNA capping reaction catalyzed by the RNA:GDP polyribonucleotidyltransferase (PRNTase) activity. Here, we directly demonstrate that the purified L-pRNA complex transfers pRNA to GDP to produce the capped RNA (Gpp-pRNA), indicating that the complex is a bona fide intermediate in the RNA transfer reaction. To locate the active site of the PRNTase domain in the L protein, the covalent RNA attachment site was mapped. We found that the 5'-monophosphate end of the RNA is linked to the histidine residue at position 1,227 (H1227) of the L protein through a phosphoamide bond. Interestingly, H1227 is part of the histidine-arginine (HR) motif, which is conserved within the L proteins of the NNS RNA viruses including rabies, measles, Ebola, and Borna disease viruses. Mutagenesis analyses revealed that the HR motif is required for the PRNTase activity at the step of the enzyme-pRNA intermediate formation. Thus, our findings suggest that an ancient NNS RNA viral polymerase has acquired the PRNTase domain independently of the eukaryotic mRNA capping enzyme during evolution and PRNTase becomes a rational target for designing antiviral agents.

PMCID: PMC2840475 PMID: 20142503 [PubMed - indexed for MEDLINE]

1337. Proc Natl Acad Sci U S A. 2010 Feb 16;107(7):3157-62. doi: 10.1073/pnas.0909587107. Epub 2010 Jan 28.

A broad-spectrum antiviral targeting entry of enveloped viruses.

Wolf MC(1), Freiberg AN, Zhang T, Akyol-Ataman Z, Grock A, Hong PW, Li J, Watson NF, Fang AQ, Aguilar HC, Porotto M, Honko AN, Damoiseaux R, Miller JP, Woodson SE, Chantasirivisal S, Fontanes V, Negrete OA, Krogstad P, Dasgupta A, Moscona A, Hensley LE, Whelan SP, Faull KF, Holbrook MR, Jung ME, Lee B.

Author information: (1)Department of Microbiology, Immunology, and Molecular Genetics, University of California, Los Angeles, CA 90025, USA.

Comment in Expert Rev Anti Infect Ther. 2010 Jun;8(6):635-8.

We describe an antiviral small molecule, LJ001, effective against numerous enveloped viruses including Influenza A, filoviruses, poxviruses, arenaviruses, bunyaviruses, paramyxoviruses, flaviviruses, and HIV-1. In sharp contrast, the compound had no effect on the infection of nonenveloped viruses. In vitro and in vivo assays showed no overt toxicity. LJ001 specifically intercalated into viral membranes, irreversibly inactivated virions while leaving functionally intact envelope proteins, and inhibited viral entry at a step after virus binding but before virus-cell fusion. LJ001 pretreatment also prevented virus-induced mortality from Ebola and Rift Valley fever viruses. Structure-activity relationship analyses of LJ001, a rhodanine derivative, implicated both the polar and nonpolar ends of LJ001 in its antiviral activity. LJ001 specifically inhibited virus-cell but not cell-cell fusion, and further studies with lipid biosynthesis inhibitors indicated that LJ001 exploits the therapeutic window that exists between static viral membranes and biogenic cellular membranes with reparative capacity. In sum, our data reveal a class of broad-spectrum antivirals effective against enveloped viruses that target the viral lipid membrane and compromises its ability to mediate virus-cell fusion.

PMCID: PMC2840368 PMID: 20133606 [PubMed - indexed for MEDLINE]

1338. PLoS One. 2010 Feb 9;5(2):e9126. doi: 10.1371/journal.pone.0009126.

High prevalence of both humoral and cellular immunity to Zaire ebolavirus among rural populations in Gabon.

Becquart P(1), Wauquier N, Mahlakõiv T, Nkoghe D, Padilla C, Souris M, Ollomo B, Gonzalez JP, De Lamballerie X, Kazanji M, Leroy EM.

Author information: (1)Unité des Maladies Virales Emergentes, Centre International de Recherches Médicales de Franceville, Franceville, Gabon.

Erratum in PLoS One. 2010;5(2) doi: 10.1371/annotation/9bc62f9e-8386-4e9b-951c-1eeba930a41c.

To better understand Zaire ebolavirus (ZEBOV) circulation and transmission to humans, we conducted a large serological survey of rural populations in Gabon, a country characterized by both epidemic and non epidemic regions. The survey lasted three years and covered 4,349 individuals from 220 randomly selected villages, representing 10.7% of all villages in Gabon. Using a sensitive and specific ELISA method, we found a ZEBOV-specific IgG seroprevalence of 15.3% overall, the highest ever reported. The seroprevalence rate was significantly higher in forested areas (19.4%) than in other ecosystems, namely grassland (12.4%), savannah (10.5%), and lakeland (2.7%). No other risk factors for seropositivity were found. The specificity of anti-ZEBOV IgG was confirmed by Western blot in 138 individuals, and CD8 T cells from seven IgG+ individuals were shown to produce IFN-gamma after ZEBOV stimulation. Together, these findings show that a large fraction of the human population living in forested areas of Gabon has both humoral and cellular immunity to ZEBOV. In the absence of identified risk factors, the high prevalence of "immune" persons suggests a common source of human exposure such as fruits contaminated by bat saliva. These findings provide significant new insights into ZEBOV circulation and human exposure, and raise important questions as to the human pathogenicity of ZEBOV and the existence of natural protective immunization.

PMCID: PMC2817732 PMID: 20161740 [PubMed - indexed for MEDLINE]

1339. Cell Microbiol. 2010 Feb;12(2):148-57. doi: 10.1111/j.1462-5822.2009.01385.x. Epub 2009 Sep 22.

Zaire Ebola virus entry into human dendritic cells is insensitive to cathepsin L inhibition.

Martinez O(1), Johnson J, Manicassamy B, Rong L, Olinger GG, Hensley LE, Basler CF.

Author information: (1)Department of Microbiology, Mount Sinai School of Medicine, New York, NY 10029, USA.

Cathepsins B and L contribute to Ebola virus (EBOV) entry into Vero cells and mouse embryonic fibroblasts. However, the role of cathepsins in EBOV-infection of human dendritic cells (DCs), important targets of infection in vivo, remains undefined. Here, EBOV-like particles containing a beta-lactamase-VP40 fusion reporter and Ebola virus were used to demonstrate the cathepsin dependence of EBOV entry into human monocyte-derived DCs. However, while DC infection is blocked by cathepsin B inhibitor, it is insensitive to cathepsin L inhibitor. Furthermore, DCs pre-treated for 48 h with TNFalpha were generally less susceptible to entry and infection by EBOV. This decrease in infection was associated with a decrease in cathepsin B activity. Thus, cathepsin L plays a minimal, if any, role in EBOV infection in human DCs. The inflammatory cytokine TNFalpha modulates cathepsin B activity and affects EBOV entry into and infection of human DCs.

PMCID: PMC2996272 PMID: 19775255 [PubMed - indexed for MEDLINE]

1340. J Gen Virol. 2010 Feb;91(Pt 2):352-61. doi: 10.1099/vir.0.017343-0. Epub 2009 Oct 14

The VP35 protein of Ebola virus impairs dendritic cell maturation induced by virus and lipopolysaccharide.

Jin H(1), Yan Z, Prabhakar BS, Feng Z, Ma Y, Verpooten D, Ganesh B, He B.

Author information: (1)Department of Microbiology and Immunology, College of Medicine, University of Illinois, Chicago, IL 60612, USA.

Ebola virus causes rapidly progressive haemorrhagic fever, which is associated with severe immuosuppression. In infected dendritic cells (DCs), Ebola virus replicates efficiently and inhibits DC maturation without inducing cytokine expression, leading to impaired T-cell proliferation. However, the underlying mechanism remains unclear. In this study, we report that Ebola virus VP35 impairs the maturation of mouse DCs. When expressed in mouse immature DCs, Ebola virus VP35 prevents virus-stimulated expression of CD40, CD80, CD86 and major histocompatibility complex class II. Further, it suppresses the induction of cytokines such as interleukin (IL)-6, IL-12, tumour necrosis factor alpha and alpha/beta interferon (IFN-alpha/beta). Notably, Ebola VP35 attenuates the ability of DCs to stimulate the activation of CD4(+) T cells. Addition of type I IFN to mouse DCs only partially reverses the inhibitory effects of VP35. Moreover, VP35 perturbs mouse DC functions induced by lipopolysaccharide, an agonist of Toll-like receptor 4. Deletion of the amino terminus abolishes its activity, whereas a mutation in the RNA binding motif has no effect. Our work highlights a critical role of VP35 in viral interference in DC function with resultant deficiency in T-cell function, which may contribute to the profound virulence of Ebola virus infection.

PMCID: PMC2831215 PMID: 19828757 [PubMed - indexed for MEDLINE]

1341. J Virol Methods. 2010 Feb;163(2):336-43. doi: 10.1016/j.jviromet.2009.10.020. Epub 2009 Oct 29.

An enzymatic virus-like particle assay for sensitive detection of virus entry.

Tscherne DM(1), Manicassamy B, García-Sastre A.

Author information: (1)Department of Microbiology, Mount Sinai School of Medicine, 1 Gustave L. Levy Place, New York, NY 10029, USA.

A viral entry assay where a beta-lactamase reporter protein fused to the influenza matrix protein-1 (BlaM1) is packaged as a structural component into influenza virus-like particles (VLPs) is described. The Bla reporter is released upon fusion with target cells and can be detected in live cells by flow cytometry, microscopy, or fluorometric plate reader for utility in high-throughput screening approaches. The production of BlaM1 VLPs and subsequent transfer of Bla activity to target cells requires the presence of influenza hemagglutinin (HA) and neuraminidase (NA). In addition, transfer of Bla by the VLPs can be blocked by an influenza neutralizing antibody, is impeded by a chemical inhibitor of influenza virus entry, and requires HA that is cleaved by a protease specific for its cleavage site. An analogous VLP system also was developed for Ebola (EBOV) and Marburg (MARV) viruses, demonstrating that this straightforward assay has broad application for studying the entry steps of enveloped viruses, especially those that require high levels of biosafety containment.

PMCID: PMC2814992 PMID: 19879300 [PubMed - indexed for MEDLINE]

1342. Nat Struct Mol Biol. 2010 Feb;17(2):165-72. doi: 10.1038/nsmb.1765. Epub 2010 Jan 17

Structural basis for dsRNA recognition and interferon antagonism by Ebola VP35.

Leung DW(1), Prins KC, Borek DM, Farahbakhsh M, Tufariello JM, Ramanan P, Nix JC, Helgeson LA, Otwinowski Z, Honzatko RB, Basler CF, Amarasinghe GK.

Author information: (1)Department of Biochemistry, Biophysics and Molecular Biology, Iowa State University, Ames, Iowa, USA.

Ebola viral protein 35 (VP35), encoded by the highly pathogenic Ebola virus, facilitates host immune evasion by antagonizing antiviral signaling pathways, including those initiated by RIG-I-like receptors. Here we report the crystal structure of the Ebola VP35 interferon inhibitory domain (IID) bound to short double-stranded RNA (dsRNA), which together with in vivo results reveals how VP35-dsRNA interactions contribute to immune evasion. Conserved basic residues in VP35 IID recognize the dsRNA backbone, whereas the dsRNA blunt ends are 'end-capped' by a pocket of hydrophobic residues that mimic RIG-I-like receptor recognition of blunt-end dsRNA. Residues critical for RNA binding are also important for interferon inhibition in vivo but not for viral polymerase cofactor function of VP35. These results suggest that simultaneous recognition of dsRNA backbone and blunt ends provides a mechanism by which Ebola VP35 antagonizes host dsRNA sensors and immune responses.

PMCID: PMC2872155 PMID: 20081868 [PubMed - indexed for MEDLINE]

1343. PLoS Pathog. 2010 Jan 15;6(1):e1000721. doi: 10.1371/journal.ppat.1000721.

Marburg virus evades interferon responses by a mechanism distinct from ebola virus.

Valmas C(1), Grosch MN, Schümann M, Olejnik J, Martinez O, Best SM, Krähling V, Basler CF, Mühlberger E.

Author information: (1)Department of Microbiology, Mount Sinai School of Medicine, New York, New York, USA.

Previous studies have demonstrated that Marburg viruses (MARV) and Ebola viruses (EBOV) inhibit interferon (IFN)-alpha/beta signaling but utilize different mechanisms. EBOV inhibits IFN signaling via its VP24 protein which blocks the nuclear accumulation of tyrosine phosphorylated STAT1. In contrast, MARV infection inhibits IFNalpha/beta induced tyrosine phosphorylation of STAT1 and STAT2. MARV infection is now demonstrated to inhibit not only IFNalpha/beta but also IFNgamma-induced STAT phosphorylation and to inhibit the IFNalpha/beta and IFNgamma-induced tyrosine phosphorylation of upstream Janus (Jak) family kinases. Surprisingly, the MARV matrix protein VP40, not the MARV VP24 protein, has been identified to antagonize Jak and STAT tyrosine phosphorylation, to inhibit IFNalpha/beta or IFNgamma-induced gene expression and to inhibit the induction of an antiviral state by IFNalpha/beta. Global loss of STAT and Jak tyrosine phosphorylation in response to both IFNalpha/beta and IFNgamma is reminiscent of the phenotype seen in Jak1-null cells. Consistent with this model, MARV infection and MARV VP40 expression also inhibit the Jak1-dependent, IL-6-induced tyrosine phosphorylation of STAT1 and STAT3. Finally, expression of MARV VP40 is able to prevent the tyrosine phosphorylation of Jak1, STAT1, STAT2 or STAT3 which occurs following over-expression of the Jak1 kinase. In contrast, MARV VP40 does not detectably inhibit the tyrosine phosphorylation of STAT2 or Tyk2 when Tyk2 is over-expressed. Mutation of the VP40 late domain, essential for efficient VP40 budding, has no detectable impact on inhibition of IFN signaling. This study shows that MARV inhibits IFN signaling by a mechanism different from that employed by the related EBOV. It identifies a novel function for the MARV VP40 protein and suggests that MARV may globally inhibit Jak1-dependent cytokine signaling.

PMCID: PMC2799553 PMID: 20084112 [PubMed - indexed for MEDLINE]

1344. Proc Natl Acad Sci U S A. 2010 Jan 5;107(1):314-9. doi: 10.1073/pnas.0910547107. Epub 2009 Dec 14.

Ebolavirus VP35 uses a bimodal strategy to bind dsRNA for innate immune suppression.

Kimberlin CR(1), Bornholdt ZA, Li S, Woods VL Jr, MacRae IJ, Saphire EO.

Author information: (1)Department of Immunology and Microbial Science, The Scripps Research Institute, La Jolla, CA 92037, USA.

Ebolavirus causes a severe hemorrhagic fever and is divided into five distinct species, of which Reston ebolavirus is uniquely nonpathogenic to humans. Disease caused by ebolavirus is marked by early immunosuppression of innate immune signaling events, involving silencing and sequestration of double-stranded RNA (dsRNA) by the viral protein VP35. Here we present unbound and dsRNA-bound crystal structures of the dsRNA-binding domain of Reston ebolavirus VP35. The structures show that VP35 forms an unusual, asymmetric dimer on dsRNA binding, with each of the monomers binding dsRNA in a different way: one binds the backbone whereas the other caps the terminus. Additional SAXS, DXMS, and dsRNA-binding experiments presented here support a model of cooperative dsRNA recognition in which binding of the first monomer assists binding of the next monomer of the oligomeric VP35 protein. This work illustrates how ebolavirus VP35 could mask key recognition sites of molecules such as RIG-I, MDA-5, and Dicer to silence viral dsRNA in infection.

PMCID: PMC2806767 PMID: 20018665 [PubMed - indexed for MEDLINE]

1345. Virology. 2010 Jan 5;396(1):135-42. doi: 10.1016/j.virol.2009.10.028. Epub 2009 Nov 10.

Phenylalanines at positions 88 and 159 of Ebolavirus envelope glycoprotein differentially impact envelope function.

Ou W(1), King H, Delisle J, Shi D, Wilson CA.

Author information: (1)Division of Cellular and Gene Therapies, Center for Biologics Evaluation and Research, FDA, Bethesda, MD 20892, USA.

The envelope glycoprotein (GP) of Ebolavirus (EBOV) mediates viral entry into host cells. Through mutagenesis, we and other groups reported that two phenylalanines at positions 88 and 159 of GP are critical for viral entry. However, it remains elusive which steps of viral entry are impaired by F88 or F159 mutations and how. In this study, we further characterized these two phenylalanines through mutagenesis and examined the impact on GP expression, function, and structure. Our data suggest that F159 plays an indirect role in viral entry by maintaining EBOV GP's overall structure. In contrast, we did not detect any evidence for conformational differences in GP with F88 mutations. The data suggest that F88 influences viral entry during a step after cathepsin processing, presumably impacting viral fusion.

PMID: 19906395 [PubMed - indexed for MEDLINE]

1346. Br Med Bull. 2010;95:193-225. doi: 10.1093/bmb/ldq022. Epub 2010 Aug 3.

Viral haemorrhagic fevers imported into non-endemic countries: risk assessment and management.

Bannister B(1).

Author information: (1)Department of Infectious Diseases, Royal Free Hospital, Hampstead, London NW3 2QG, UK. barbara.bannister@royalfree.nhs.uk

BACKGROUND: Viral haemorrhagic fevers (VHFs) are severe infections capable of causing haemorrhagic disease and fatal multi-organ failure. Crimean-Congo, Marburg, Ebola and Lassa viruses cause both sporadic cases and large epidemics over wide endemic areas. SOURCES OF DATA: Original articles and reviews identified by PubMed search and personal reading; European and United States national guidance and legislation. World Health Organization information, documents and reports. VHFs cause significant morbidity and mortality in their endemic areas; they can cause healthcare-related infections, and their broad diversity and range are increasingly recognized. AREAS OF CONTROVERSY: There is uncertainty about the risks presented by VHFs in non-endemic countries, particularly in healthcare environments. Consensus on the best modes of care and infection control are only slowly emerging. GROWING POINTS: With increasing commerce in rural and low-income areas, VHF outbreaks increasingly expand, causing social and economic damage. AREAS TIMELY FOR DEVELOPING RESEARCH: New ecologies, viral strains and clinical syndromes are being discovered. There is a great need for rapid diagnostic tests and effective antiviral treatments. Vaccine development programmes are challenged by multiple viral strains and the need for trials in rural communities.

PMID: 20682627 [PubMed - indexed for MEDLINE]

1347. Emerg Health Threats J. 2010;3:e7. doi: 10.3134/ehtj.10.163. Epub 2010 Jun 3.

Emerging viral threats in Gabon: health capacities and response to the risk of emerging zoonotic diseases in Central Africa.

Bourgarel M(1), Wauquier N, Gonzalez JP.

Author information: (1)Centre de Coopération Internationale en Recherche Agronomique pour le Développement (CIRAD), UPR AGIRs, Campus International de Baillarguet, Montpellier cedex 5, France.

Emerging infectious diseases (EID) are currently the major threat to public health worldwide and most EID events have involved zoonotic infectious agents. Central Africa in general and Gabon in particular are privileged areas for the emergence of zoonotic EIDs. Indeed, human incursions in Gabonese forests for exploitation purposes lead to intensified contacts between humans and wildlife thus generating an increased risk of emergence of zoonotic diseases. In Gabon, 51 endemic or potential endemic viral infectious diseases have been reported. Among them, 22 are of zoonotic origin and involve 12 families of viruses. The most notorious are dengue, yellow fever, ebola, marburg, Rift Valley fever and chikungunya viruses. Potential EID due to wildlife in Gabon are thereby plentiful and need to be inventoried. The Gabonese Public Health system covers geographically most of the country allowing a good access to sanitary information and efficient monitoring of emerging diseases. However, access to treatment and prevention is better in urban areas where medical structures are more developed and financial means are concentrated even though the population is equally distributed between urban and rural areas. In spite of this, Gabon could be a good field for investigating the emergence or re-emergence of zoonotic EID. Indeed Gabonese health research structures such as CIRMF, advantageously located, offer high quality researchers and facilities that study pathogens and wildlife ecology, aiming toward a better understanding of the contact and transmission mechanisms of new pathogens from wildlife to human, the emergence of zoonotic EID and the breaking of species barriers by pathogens.
PMCID: PMC3167654 PMID: 22460397 [PubMed]

1348. Front Biosci (Schol Ed). 2010 Jan 1;2:527-46.

Role of surfactant protein A and D (SP-A and SP-D) in human antiviral host defense.

Hartshorn KL(1).

Author information: (1)Department of Medicine, Boston University School of Medicine, Boston, MA 02118, USA. khartsho@bu.edu

SP-A and SP-D contribute to host defense against respiratory viral infection. The most extensive body of evidence relates to influenza A viruses (IAV), and evidence from gene-deleted mice also indicate a role for surfactant collectins in defense against respiratory syncytial virus (RSV) and adenovirus. Some important respiratory pathogens including rhinovirus and metapneumovirus have not yet been examined. Viral pathogens that enter the body via the respiratory tract (e.g., Ebola virus), replicate in the lung (e.g., human immunodeficiency virus or HIV) or infect the lung in immuno-compromised hosts (e.g., herpes simplex virus or HSV) are inhibited by collectins. SP-A and SP-D are expressed in other mucosal surfaces (e.g., the eye or genitourinary tract) where they may play roles in antiviral defense. In addition to direct antiviral activities, the SP-A and SP-D modulate innate and adaptive immunity and inflammation associated with infection. The relative importance of antiviral vs anti-inflammatory effects of SP-A and SP-D in viral infections and the potential use of these collectins as therapeutics for viral infections are under investigation.
PMID: 20036966 [PubMed - indexed for MEDLINE]

1349. J Gen Virol. 2010 Jan;91(Pt 1):228-34. doi: 10.1099/vir.0.015495-0. Epub 2009 Oct 7

Regulation of Marburg virus (MARV) budding by Nedd4.1: a different WW domain of Nedd4.1 is critical for binding to MARV and Ebola virus VP40.

Urata S(1), Yasuda J.

Author information: (1)First Department of Forensic Science, National Research Institute of Police Science, Kashiwa 277-0882, Japan.

The VP40 matrix protein of Marburg virus (MARV) has been shown to be the driving force behind MARV budding, a process in which the PPPY L-domain motif of VP40 plays a critical role. Here, we report that Vps4B and Nedd4.1 play critical roles in MARV VP40-mediated budding. We showed that unidentified activities of the Nedd4.1 HECT domain, along with its E3 ubiquitin ligase activity, may be required for MARV budding. Moreover, we showed that the first WW domain of Nedd4.1, WW1, is critical for binding to MARV VP40, indicating that MARV VP40 and Ebola virus VP40 are recognized by a different WW domain of Nedd4.1. This is the first report showing that the viral L-domains containing PPxY have specificities for binding to WW domains. Our findings provide new insights into MARV budding, which may contribute to the development of novel anti-MARV therapeutic strategies.
PMID: 19812267 [PubMed - indexed for MEDLINE]

1350. J Immunol. 2010 Jan 1;184(1):327-35. doi: 10.4049/jimmunol.0901231.

Mechanisms and consequences of ebolavirus-induced lymphocyte apoptosis.

Bradfute SB(1), Swanson PE, Smith MA, Watanabe E, McDunn JE, Hotchkiss RS, Bavari S.

Author information: (1)United States Army Medical Research Institute of Infectious Diseases, Fort Detrick, MD 21702, USA.

Ebolavirus (EBOV) is a member of the filovirus family and causes severe hemorrhagic fever, resulting in death in up to 90% of infected humans. EBOV infection induces massive bystander lymphocyte apoptosis; however, neither the cellular apoptotic pathway(s) nor the systemic implications of lymphocyte apoptosis in EBOV infection are known. In this study, we show data suggesting that EBOV-induced lymphocyte apoptosis in vivo occurs via both the death receptor (extrinsic) and mitochondrial (intrinsic) pathways, as both Fas-associated death domain dominant negative transgenic mice and mice overexpressing bcl-2 were resistant to EBOV-induced lymphocyte apoptosis. Surprisingly, inhibiting lymphocyte apoptosis during EBOV infection did not result in improved animal survival. Furthermore, we show for the first time that hepatocyte apoptosis likely occurs in EBOV infection, and that mice lacking the proapoptotic genes Bim and Bid had reduced hepatocyte apoptosis and liver enzyme levels postinfection. Collectively, these data suggest that EBOV induces multiple proapoptotic stimuli and that blocking lymphocyte apoptosis is not sufficient to improve survival in EBOV infection. These data suggest that hepatocyte apoptosis may play a role in the pathogenesis of EBOV infection, whereas lymphocyte apoptosis appears to be nonessential for EBOV disease progression.
PMID: 20028660 [PubMed - indexed for MEDLINE]

1351. J Virol. 2010 Jan;84(2):1169-75. doi: 10.1128/JVI.01372-09. Epub 2009 Nov 4.

Ebolavirus VP24 binding to karyopherins is required for inhibition of interferon signaling.

Mateo M(1), Reid SP, Leung LW, Basler CF, Volchkov VE.

Author information: (1)Laboratoire des Filovirus, INSERM U758, University Claude Bernard Lyon-1, 21 Av. Tony Garnier, 69365 Lyon Cedex 07, France.

The Ebolavirus VP24 protein counteracts alpha/beta interferon (IFN-alpha/beta) and IFN-gamma signaling by blocking the nuclear accumulation of tyrosine-phosphorylated STAT1 (PY-STAT1). According to the proposed model, VP24 binding to members of the NP1-1 subfamily of karyopherin alpha (KPNalpha) nuclear localization signal receptors prevents their binding to PY-STAT1, thereby preventing PY-STAT1 nuclear accumulation. This study now identifies two domains of VP24 required for inhibition of IFN-beta-induced gene expression and PY-STAT1 nuclear accumulation. We demonstrate that loss of function correlates with loss of binding to KPNalpha proteins. Thus, the VP24 IFN antagonist function requires the ability of VP24 to interact with KPNalpha.
PMCID: PMC2798383 PMID: 19889762 [PubMed - indexed for MEDLINE]

1352. J Virol. 2010 Jan;84(1):163-75. doi: 10.1128/JVI.01832-09.

A forward genetic strategy reveals destabilizing mutations in the Ebolavirus glycoprotein that alter its protease dependence during cell entry.

Wong AC(1), Sandesara RG, Mulherkar N, Whelan SP, Chandran K.

Author information: (1)Department of Microbiology and Immunology, Albert Einstein College of Medicine, Bronx, NY 10461, USA.

Ebolavirus (EBOV) entry into cells requires proteolytic disassembly of the viral glycoprotein, GP. This proteolytic processing, unusually extensive for an enveloped virus entry protein, is mediated by cysteine cathepsins, a family of endosomal/lysosomal proteases. Previous work has shown that cleavage of GP by cathepsin B (CatB) is specifically required to generate a critical entry intermediate. The functions of this intermediate are not well understood. We used a forward genetic strategy to investigate this CatB-dependent step. Specifically, we generated a replication-competent recombinant vesicular stomatitis virus bearing EBOV GP as its sole entry glycoprotein and used it to select viral mutants resistant to a CatB inhibitor. We obtained mutations at six amino acid positions in GP that independently confer complete resistance. All of the mutations reside at or near the GP1-GP2 intersubunit interface in the membrane-proximal base of the prefusion GP trimer. This region forms a part of the "clamp" that holds the fusion subunit GP2 in its metastable prefusion conformation. Biochemical studies suggest that most of the mutations confer CatB independence not by altering specific cleavage sites in GP but rather by inducing conformational rearrangements in the prefusion GP trimer that dramatically enhance its susceptibility to proteolysis. The remaining mutants did not show the preceding behavior, indicating the existence of multiple mechanisms for acquiring CatB independence during entry. Altogether, our findings suggest that CatB cleavage is required to facilitate the triggering of viral membrane fusion by destabilizing the prefusion conformation of EBOV GP.
PMCID: PMC2798398 PMID: 19846533 [PubMed - indexed for MEDLINE]

1353. J Virol. 2010 Jan;84(1):27-33. doi: 10.1128/JVI.01462-09.

Interaction between Ebola virus glycoprotein and host toll-like receptor 4 leads to induction of proinflammatory cytokines and SOCS1.

Okumura A(1), Pitha PM, Yoshimura A, Harty RN.

Author information: (1)Department of Pathobiology, University of Pennsylvania, Philadelphia, PA 19104, USA.

Ebola virus initially targets monocytes and macrophages, which can lead to the release of proinflammatory cytokines and chemokines. These inflammatory cytokines are thought to contribute to the development of circulatory shock seen in fatal Ebola virus infections. Here we report that host Toll-like receptor 4 (TLR4) is a sensor for Ebola virus glycoprotein (GP) on virus-like particles (VLPs) and that resultant TLR4 signaling pathways lead to the production of proinflammatory cytokines and suppressor of cytokine signaling 1 (SOCS1) in a human monocytic cell line and in HEK293-TLR4/MD2 cells stably expressing the TLR4/MD2 complex. Ebola virus GP was found to interact with TLR4 by immunoprecipitation/Western blot analyses, and Ebola virus GP on VLPs was able to stimulate expression of NF-kappaB in a TLR4-dependent manner. Interestingly, we found that budding of Ebola virus VLPs was more pronounced in TLR4-stimulated cells than in unstimulated control cells. In sum, these findings identify the host innate immune protein TLR4 as a sensor for Ebola virus GP which may play an important role in the immunopathogenesis of Ebola virus infection.
PMCID: PMC2798428 PMID: 19846529 [PubMed - indexed for MEDLINE]

1354. Mol Ther. 2010 Jan;18(1):143-50. doi: 10.1038/mt.2009.190. Epub 2009 Sep 1.

Activation of transgene-specific T cells following lentivirus-mediated gene delivery to mouse lung.

Limberis MP(1), Bell CL, Heath J, Wilson JM.

Author information: (1)Gene Therapy Program, Department of Pathology and Laboratory Medicine, University of Pennsylvania, Philadelphia, Pennsylvania 19104-3403, USA.

Integrating lentiviral vectors based on the human immunodeficiency virus type-1 (HIV-1) can transduce quiescent cells, which in lung account for almost 95% of the epithelial cell population. Pseudotyping lentiviral vectors with the envelope glycoprotein from the Ebola Zaire virus, the lymphocytic choriomeningitis virus (LCMV), the Mokola virus, and the vesicular stomatitis virus (VSV-G) resulted in transduction of mouse alveolar epithelium, but gene expression in the lung of C57BL/6 and BALB/c mice waned within 90 days of vector injection. Intratracheal delivery of the four pseudotyped lentiviral vectors resulted in transgene-specific T-cell activation in both mouse strains, albeit lower than that achieved by intramuscular injection of the vectors. We performed an adoptive transfer of luciferase-specific T cells, isolated from spleen or lung of donor mice injected with VSV-G-pseudotyped lentivirus vector expressing luciferase into the muscle or lung, respectively, into recipient recombination-activating gene (RAG)-deficient mice transduced in lung with adenovirus expressing firefly luciferase (ffluc2). Gene expression declined within 7 days of adoptive transfer approaching background levels by day 36. Taken together, our results suggest that the loss of transduced cells in lung is due to VSV-G.HIV vector-mediated activation of transgene-specific T cells rather than as result of normal turnover of airway cells.
PMCID: PMC2839217 PMID: 19724265 [PubMed - indexed for MEDLINE]

1355. Trans R Soc Trop Med Hyg. 2010 Jan;104(1):48-50. doi: 10.1016/j.trstmh.2009.07.011. Epub 2009 Sep 23.

Infection control during filoviral hemorrhagic fever outbreaks: preferences of community members and health workers in Masindi, Uganda.

Raabe VN(1), Mutyaba I, Roddy P, Lutwama JJ, Geissler W, Borchert M.

Author information: (1)London School of Hygiene and Tropical Medicine, Keppel Street, London WC1E 7HT, UK. raab0016@umn.edu

Interviews were conducted with health workers and community members in Masindi, Uganda on improving the acceptability of infection control measures used during an Ebola outbreak. Measures that promote cultural sensitivity and transparency of control activities were preferred and should be employed in future control efforts. We suggest assessing the practicality of body bags with viewing windows, and face shields with or without chin protectors, in future outbreaks.

PMID: 19783269 [PubMed - indexed for MEDLINE]

1356. Viruses. 2010 Jan;2(1):262-82. doi: 10.3390/v2010262. Epub 2010 Jan 21.

Evasion of the interferon-mediated antiviral response by filoviruses.

Cárdenas WB(1).

Author information: (1)Laboratorio de Biomedicina, FIMCM, Escuela Superior Politécnica del Litoral (ESPOL), Campus Gustavo Galindo, Km 30.5 via Perimetral, Apartado 09-01-5863, Guayaquil, Ecuador; E-Mail: wbcarden@espol.edu.ec ; Tel.: +5934 226 9589;

The members of the filoviruses are recognized as some of the most lethal viruses affecting human and non-human primates. The only two genera of the Filoviridae family, Marburg virus (MARV) and Ebola virus (EBOV), comprise the main etiologic agents of severe hemorrhagic fever outbreaks in central Africa, with case fatality rates ranging from 25 to 90%. Fatal outcomes have been associated with a late and dysregulated immune response to infection, very likely due to the virus targeting key host immune cells, such as macrophages and dendritic cells (DCs) that are necessary to mediate effective innate and adaptive immune responses. Despite major progress in the development of vaccine candidates for filovirus infections, a licensed vaccine or therapy for human use is still not available. During the last ten years, important progress has been made in understanding the molecular mechanisms of filovirus pathogenesis. Several lines of evidence implicate the impairment of the host interferon (IFN) antiviral innate immune response by MARV or EBOV as an important determinant of virulence. In vitro and in vivo experimental infections with recombinant Zaire Ebola virus (ZEBOV), the best characterized filovirus, demonstrated that the viral protein VP35 plays a key role in inhibiting the production of IFN-α/β. Further, the action of VP35 is synergized by the inhibition of cellular responses to IFN-α/β by the minor matrix viral protein VP24. The dual action of these viral proteins may contribute to an efficient initial virus replication and dissemination in the host. Noticeably, the analogous function of these viral proteins in MARV has not been reported. Because the IFN response is a major component of the innate immune response to virus infection, this chapter reviews recent findings on the molecular mechanisms of IFN-mediated antiviral evasion by filovirus infection.

PMCID: PMC3185555 PMID: 21994610 [PubMed]

1357. Vopr Virusol. 2010 Jan-Feb;55(1):45-8.

[Stabilization of peroxidase conjugates used in enzyme immunoassay systems to detect Ebola and Marburg virus antigens].

[Article in Russian]

Pirozhkov AP, Borisevich IV, Snetkova Olu, Androshchuk IA, Syromiatnikova SI, Khmelev AL, Shatokhina IV, Kudrin VIu, Timofeev MA, Pantiukhov VB, Borisevich SV, Markov VI, Bondarev VP.

The time course of changes in the activity of solutions of horseradish peroxidase conjugates with immunoglobulins against Ebola and Marburg fevers was studied in the presence of different components. The series of the conjugates of ELISA kits for the detection of Ebola and Marburg virus antigens, which were prepared on the basis of the designed stabilizing solution, preserved at less than 90% of its baseline activity during 10 months at a storage temperature of 2 to 8 degrees C.

PMID: 20364672 [PubMed - indexed for MEDLINE]

1358. BMC Syst Biol. 2009 Dec 30;3:121. doi: 10.1186/1752-0509-3-121.

Metabolic investigation of host/pathogen interaction using MS2-infected Escherichia coli.

Jain R(1), Srivastava R.

Author information: (1)Department of Chemical, Materials and Biomolecular Engineering, University of Connecticut, Storrs, CT 06269, USA. jainr@ornl.gov

BACKGROUND: RNA viruses are responsible for a variety of illnesses among people, including but not limited to the common cold, the flu, HIV, and ebola. Developing new drugs and new strategies for treating diseases caused by these viruses can be an expensive and time-consuming process. Mathematical modeling may be used to elucidate host-pathogen interactions and highlight potential targets for drug development, as well providing the basis for optimizing patient treatment strategies. The purpose of this work was to determine whether a genome-scale modeling approach could be used to understand how metabolism is impacted by the host-pathogen interaction during a viral infection. Escherichia coli/MS2 was used as the host-pathogen model system as MS2 is easy to work with, harmless to humans, but shares many features with eukaryotic viruses. In addition, the genome-scale metabolic model of E. coli is the most comprehensive model at this time. RESULTS: Employing a metabolic modeling strategy known as "flux balance analysis" coupled with experimental studies, we were able to predict how viral infection would alter bacterial metabolism. Based on our simulations, we predicted that cell growth and biosynthesis of the cell wall would be halted. Furthermore, we predicted a substantial increase in metabolic activity of the pentose phosphate pathway as a means to enhance viral biosynthesis, while a break down in the citric acid cycle was predicted. Also, no changes were predicted in the glycolytic pathway. CONCLUSIONS: Through our approach, we have developed a technique of modeling virus-infected host metabolism and have investigated the metabolic effects of viral infection. These studies may provide insight into how to design better drugs. They also illustrate the potential of extending such metabolic analysis to higher order organisms, including humans.

PMCID: PMC2813233 PMID: 20042079 [PubMed - indexed for MEDLINE]

1359. PLoS One. 2009 Dec 18;4(12):e8375. doi: 10.1371/journal.pone.0008375.

How Ebola impacts genetics of Western lowland gorilla populations.

Le Gouar PJ(1), Vallet D, David L, Bermejo M, Gatti S, Levréro F, Petit EJ, Ménard N.
Author information: (1)UMR 6553 Ecobio, Université RennesI/CNRS, Paimpont, France. pascalinelegouar@free.fr

BACKGROUND: Emerging infectious diseases in wildlife are major threats for both human health and biodiversity conservation. Infectious diseases can have serious consequences for the genetic diversity of populations, which could enhance the species' extinction probability. The Ebola epizootic in western and central Africa induced more than 90% mortality in Western lowland gorilla population. Although mortality rates are very high, the impacts of Ebola on genetic diversity of Western lowland gorilla have never been assessed. METHODOLOGY/PRINCIPAL FINDINGS: We carried out long term studies of three populations of Western lowland gorilla in the Republic of the Congo (Odzala-Kokoua National Park, Lossi gorilla sanctuary both affected by Ebola and Lossi's periphery not affected). Using 17 microsatellite loci, we compared genetic diversity and structure of the populations and estimate their effective size before and after Ebola outbreaks. Despite the effective size decline in both populations, we did not detect loss in genetic diversity after the epizootic. We revealed temporal changes in allele frequencies in the smallest population. CONCLUSIONS/SIGNIFICANCE: Immigration and short time elapsed since outbreaks could explain the conservation of genetic diversity after the demographic crash. Temporal changes in allele frequencies could not be explained by genetic drift or random sampling. Immigration from genetically differentiated populations and a non random mortality induced by Ebola, i.e., selective pressure and cost of sociality, are alternative hypotheses. Understanding the influence of Ebola on gorilla genetic dynamics is of paramount importance for human health, primate evolution and conservation biology.
PMCID: PMC2791222 PMID: 20020045 [PubMed - indexed for MEDLINE]

1360. PLoS One. 2009 Dec 11;4(12):e8266. doi: 10.1371/journal.pone.0008266.
Establishment, immortalisation and characterisation of pteropid bat cell lines.
Crameri G(1), Todd S, Grimley S, McEachern JA, Marsh GA, Smith C, Tachedjian M, De Jong C, Virtue ER, Yu M, Bulach D, Liu JP, Michalski WP, Middleton D, Field HE, Wang LF.
Author information: (1)CSIRO Livestock Industries, Australian Animal Health Laboratory, Geelong, Australia.

BACKGROUND: Bats are the suspected natural reservoir hosts for a number of new and emerging zoonotic viruses including Nipah virus, Hendra virus, severe acute respiratory syndrome coronavirus and Ebola virus. Since the discovery of SARS-like coronaviruses in Chinese horseshoe bats, attempts to isolate a SL-CoV from bats have failed and attempts to isolate other bat-borne viruses in various mammalian cell lines have been similarly unsuccessful. New stable bat cell lines are needed to help with these investigations and as tools to assist in the study of bat immunology and virus-host interactions. METHODOLOGY/FINDINGS: Black flying foxes (Pteropus alecto) were captured from the wild and transported live to the laboratory for primary cell culture preparation using a variety of different methods and culture media. Primary cells were successfully cultured from 20 different organs. Cell immortalisation can occur spontaneously, however we used a retroviral system to immortalise cells via the transfer and stable production of the Simian virus 40 Large T antigen and the human telomerase reverse transcriptase protein. Initial infection experiments with both cloned and uncloned cell lines using Hendra and Nipah viruses demonstrated varying degrees of infection efficiency between the different cell lines, although it was possible to infect cells in all tissue types. CONCLUSIONS/SIGNIFICANCE: The approaches developed and optimised in this study should be applicable to bats of other species. We are in the process of generating further cell lines from a number of different bat species using the methodology established in this study.
PMCID: PMC2788226 PMID: 20011515 [PubMed - indexed for MEDLINE]

1361. AIDS Res Hum Retroviruses. 2009 Dec;25(12):1197-210. doi: 10.1089/aid.2009.0253.
Antiviral activity of the interferon-induced cellular protein BST-2/tetherin.
Tokarev A(1), Skasko M, Fitzpatrick K, Guatelli J.
Author information: (1)Department of Medicine, University of California San Diego, California 92093-0679, USA.

Pathogenic microorganisms encode proteins that antagonize specific aspects of innate or adaptive immunity. Just as the study of the HIV-1 accessory protein Vif led to the identification of cellular cytidine deaminases as host defense proteins, the study of HIV-1 Vpu recently led to the discovery of the interferon-induced transmembrane protein BST-2 (CD317; tetherin) as a novel component of the innate defense against enveloped viruses. BST-2 is an unusually structured protein that restricts the release of fully formed progeny virions from infected cells, presumably by a direct retention mechanism that is independent of any viral protein target. Its spectrum of activity includes at least four virus families: retroviruses, filoviruses, arenaviruses, and herpesviruses. Viral antagonists of BST-2 include HIV-1 Vpu, HIV-2 and SIV Env, SIV Nef, the Ebola envelope glycoprotein, and the K5 protein of KSHV. The mechanisms of antagonism are diverse and currently include viral cooption of cellular endosomal trafficking and protein degradation pathways, including those mediated by ubiquitination. Orthologs of human BST-2 are present in mammals. Primate BST-2 proteins are differentially sensitive to antagonism by lentiviral Vpu and Nef proteins, suggesting that BST-2 has subjected lentiviruses to evolutionary pressure and presents barriers to cross-species transmission. BST-2 functions not only as an effector of the interferon-induced antiviral response but also as a negative feedback regulator of interferon production by plasmacytoid dendritic cells. Future work will focus on the role and regulation of BST-2 during the innate response to viral infection, on the mechanisms of restriction and of antagonism by viral gene products, and on the role of BST-2 in primate lentiviral evolution. The augmentation of BST-2 activity and the inhibition of virally encoded antagonists, in particular Vpu, represent new approaches to the prevention and treatment of HIV-1 infection.
PMCID: PMC2858902 PMID: 19929170 [PubMed - indexed for MEDLINE]

1362. Ecohealth. 2009 Dec;6(4):496-508. doi: 10.1007/s10393-010-0284-3. Epub 2010 Mar 16
Cross-species pathogen transmission and disease emergence in primates.
Pedersen AB(1), Davies TJ.

Author information: (1)Centre for Immunity, Infection and Evolution, Institutes of Evolutionary Biology, Immunology and Infection Research, School of Biological Sciences, University of Edinburgh, Ashworth Labs, Edinburgh EH93JT, UK. amy.pedersen@ed.ac.uk

Many of the most virulent emerging infectious diseases in humans, e.g., AIDS and Ebola, are zoonotic, having shifted from wildlife populations. Critical questions for predicting disease emergence are: (1) what determines when and where a disease will first cross from one species to another, and (2) which factors facilitate emergence after a successful host shift. In wild primates, infectious diseases most often are shared between species that are closely related and inhabit the same geographic region. Therefore, humans may be most vulnerable to diseases from the great apes, which include chimpanzees and gorillas, because these species represent our closest relatives. Geographic overlap may provide the opportunity for cross-species transmission, but successful infection and establishment will be determined by the biology of both the host and pathogen. We extrapolate the evolutionary relationship between pathogen sharing and divergence time between primate species to generate "hotspot" maps, highlighting regions where the risk of disease transfer between wild primates and from wild primates to humans is greatest. We find that central Africa and Amazonia are hotspots for cross-species transmission events between wild primates, due to a high diversity of closely related primate species. Hotspots of host shifts to humans will be most likely in the forests of central and west Africa, where humans come into frequent contact with their wild primate relatives. These areas also are likely to sustain a novel epidemic due to their rapidly growing human populations, close proximity to apes, and population centers with high density and contact rates among individuals.
PMID: 20232229 [PubMed - indexed for MEDLINE]

1363. Expert Rev Vaccines. 2009 Dec;8(12):1739-54. doi: 10.1586/erv.09.132.

DNA vaccines for biodefense.

Dupuy LC(1), Schmaljohn CS.

Author information: (1)Heaadquauarters, Unnited Staates Army Medical Research Institute of Infectious Diseases, Fort Detrick, MD 21702, USA. lesley.dupuy@amedd.army.mil

An ideal biodefense vaccine platform would allow for the quick formulation of novel vaccines in response to emerging or engineered pathogens. The resultant vaccine should elicit protective immune responses in one to three doses and be unaffected by pre-existing immunity to vaccine components. In addition, it should be amenable to combination and multi-agent formulation, and should be safe for all populations and the environment. DNA vaccines can potentially meet all of these requirements; thus, this platform is being tested with several biodefense threats. Here, we provide a review of the current status of the development efforts for DNA vaccines against several relevant biodefense pathogens: Bacillus anthracis, Ebola and Marburg viruses, smallpox virus, and Venezuelan equine encephalitis virus.
PMID: 19943766 [PubMed - indexed for MEDLINE]

1364. Public Health. 2009 Dec;123(12):814-6. doi: 10.1016/j.puhe.2009.10.013.

When Nature turns cook: an epidemiological feast: report of the John Snow Society Pumphandle Lecture 2009, delivered by Dr David Heymann.

Stanwell-Smith R(1).

Author information: (1)London School of Hygiene and Tropical Medicine, Keppel Street, London, WC1E 7HT, UK. r.stanwellsmith@btinternet.com
PMID: 19958919 [PubMed - indexed for MEDLINE]

1365. Vector Borne Zoonotic Dis. 2009 Dec;9(6):723-8. doi: 10.1089/vbz.2008.0167.

Human Ebola outbreak resulting from direct exposure to fruit bats in Luebo, Democratic Republic of Congo, 2007.

Leroy EM(1), Epelboin A, Mondonge V, Pourrut X, Gonzalez JP, Muyembe-Tamfum JJ, Formenty P.

Author information: (1)Centre International de Recherches Médicales de Franceville (CIRMF), Franceville, Gabon. eric.leroy@ird.fr

Twelve years after the Kikwit Ebola outbreak in 1995, Ebola virus reemerged in the Occidental Kasaï province of the Democratic Republic of Congo (DRC) between May and November 2007, affecting more than 260 humans and causing 186 deaths. During this latter outbreak we conducted several epidemiological investigations to identify the underlying ecological conditions and animal sources. Qualitative social and environmental data were collected through interviews with villagers and by direct observation. The local populations reported no unusual morbidity or mortality among wild or domestic animals, but they described a massive annual fruit bat migration toward the southeast, up the Lulua River. Migrating bats settled in the outbreak area for several weeks, between April and May, nestling in the numerous fruit trees in Ndongo and Koumelele islands as well as in palm trees of a largely abandoned plantation. They were massively hunted by villagers, for whom they represented a major source of protein. By tracing back the initial human-human transmission events, we were able to show that, in May, the putative first human victim bought freshly killed bats from hunters to eat. We were able to reconstruct the likely initial human-human transmission events that preceded the outbreak. This study provides the most likely sequence of events linking a human Ebola outbreak to exposure to fruit bats, a putative virus reservoir. These findings support the suspected role of bats in the natural cycle of Ebola virus and indicate that the massive seasonal fruit bat migrations should be taken into account in operational Ebola risk maps and seasonal alerts in the DRC.
PMID: 19323614 [PubMed - indexed for MEDLINE]

1366. Acta Crystallogr D Biol Crystallogr. 2009 Nov;65(Pt 11):1162-80. doi: 10.1107/S0907444909032314. Epub 2009 Oct 22.

Techniques and tactics used in determining the structure of the trimeric ebolavirus glycoprotein.

Lee JE(1), Fusco ML, Abelson DM, Hessell AJ, Burton DR, Saphire EO.

Author information: (1)Department of Immunology and Microbial Science, The Scripps Research Institute, La Jolla, CA 92037, USA.

The trimeric membrane-anchored ebolavirus envelope glycoprotein (GP) is responsible for viral attachment, fusion and entry. Knowledge of its structure is important both for understanding ebolavirus entry and for the development of medical interventions. Crystal structures of viral glycoproteins, especially those in their metastable prefusion oligomeric states, can be difficult to achieve given the challenges in production, purification, crystallization and diffraction that are inherent in the heavily glycosylated flexible nature of these types of proteins. The crystal structure of ebolavirus GP in its trimeric prefusion conformation in complex with a human antibody derived from a survivor of the 1995 Kikwit outbreak has now been determined [Lee et al. (2008), Nature (London), 454, 177-182]. Here, the techniques, tactics and strategies used to overcome a series of technical roadblocks in crystallization and phasing are described. Glycoproteins were produced in human embryonic kidney 293T cells, which allowed rapid screening of constructs and expression of protein in milligram quantities. Complexes of GP with an antibody fragment (Fab) promoted crystallization and a series of deglycosylation strategies, including sugar mutants, enzymatic deglycosylation, insect-cell expression and glycan anabolic pathway inhibitors, were attempted to improve the weakly diffracting glycoprotein crystals. The signal-to-noise ratio of the search model for molecular replacement was improved by determining the structure of the uncomplexed Fab. Phase combination with Fab model phases and a selenium anomalous signal, followed by NCS-averaged density modification, resulted in a clear interpretable electron-density map. Model building was assisted by the use of B-value-sharpened electron-density maps and the proper sequence register was confirmed by building alternate sequences using N-linked glycan sites as anchors and secondary-structural predictions.

PMCID: PMC2777170 PMID: 19923712 [PubMed - indexed for MEDLINE]

1367. Prehosp Disaster Med. 2009 Nov-Dec;24(6):525-8.

Personal protection during resuscitation of casualties contaminated with chemical or biological warfare agents--a survey of medical first responders.

Brinker A(1), Prior K, Schumacher J.

Author information: (1)Departmnet of Anaesthetics, Guy's and St Thomas' NHS Foundation Trust, London, UK.

INTRODUCTION: The threat of mass casualties caused by an unconventional terrorist attack is a challenge for the public health system, with special implications for emergency medicine, anesthesia, and intensive care. Advanced life support of patients injured by chemical or biological warfare agents requires an adequate level of personal protection. The aim of this study was to evaluate the personal protection knowledge of emergency physicians and anesthetists who would be at the frontline of the initial health response to a chemical/biological warfare agent incident. METHODS: After institutional review board approval, knowledge of personal protection measures among emergency medicine (n = 28) and anesthetics (n = 47) specialty registrars in the South Thames Region of the United Kingdom was surveyed using a standardized questionnaire. Participants were asked for the recommended level of personal protection if a chemical/biological warfare agent(s) casualty required advanced life support in the designated hospital resuscitation area. RESULTS: The best awareness within both groups was regarding severe acute respiratory syndrome, and fair knowledge was found regarding anthrax, plague, Ebola, and smallpox. In both groups, knowledge about personal protection requirements against chemical warfare agents was limited. Knowledge about personal protection measures for biological agents was acceptable, but was limited for chemical warfare agents. CONCLUSIONS: The results highlight the need to improve training and education regarding personal protection measures for medical first receivers.

PMID: 20301071 [PubMed - indexed for MEDLINE]

1368. Cell. 2009 Oct 30;139(3):499-511. doi: 10.1016/j.cell.2009.08.039.

Tetherin inhibits HIV-1 release by directly tethering virions to cells.

Perez-Caballero D(1), Zang T, Ebrahimi A, McNatt MW, Gregory DA, Johnson MC, Bieniasz PD.

Author information: (1)Aaron Diamond AIDS Research Center, The Rockefeller University, New York, NY 10016, USA.

Comment in Cell. 2009 Oct 30;139(3):456-7.

Tetherin is an interferon-induced protein whose expression blocks the release of HIV-1 and other enveloped viral particles. The underlying mechanism by which tetherin functions and whether it directly or indirectly causes virion retention are unknown. Here, we elucidate the mechanism by which tetherin exerts its antiviral activity. We demonstrate, through mutational analyses and domain replacement experiments, that tetherin configuration rather than primary sequence is critical for antiviral activity. These findings allowed the design of a completely artificial protein, lacking sequence homology with native tetherin, that nevertheless mimicked its antiviral activity. We further show that tetherin is incorporated into HIV-1 particles as a parallel homodimer using either of its two membrane anchors. These results indicate that tetherin functions autonomously and directly and that infiltration of virion envelopes by one or both of tetherin's membrane anchors is necessary, and likely sufficient, to tether enveloped virus particles that bud through the plasma membrane.

PMCID: PMC2844890 PMID: 19879838 [PubMed - indexed for MEDLINE]

1369. Biosystems. 2009 Oct;98(1):43-50. doi: 10.1016/j.biosystems.2009.05.006. Epub 2009 May 21.

Optimal treatment of an SIR epidemic model with time delay.

Zaman G(1), Kang YH, Jung IH.

Author information: (1)Centre for Advanced Mathematics and Physics, National University of Sciences and Technology, Rawalpindi 46000, Pakistan. zaman@pusan.ac.kr

In this paper the optimal control strategies of an SIR (susceptible-infected-recovered) epidemic model with time delay are introduced. In order to do this, we consider an optimally controlled SIR epidemic model with time delay where a control means treatment for infectious hosts. We use optimal control approach to minimize the probability that the infected individuals spread and to maximize the total number of susceptible and recovered individuals. We first derive the basic reproduction number and investigate the dynamical behavior of the controlled SIR epidemic model. We also show the existence of an optimal control for the control system and present numerical simulations on real data regarding the course of Ebola virus in Congo. Our results indicate that a small contact rate(probability of infection) is suitable for eradication of the disease (Ebola virus) and this is one way of optimal treatment strategies for infectious hosts.

PMID: 19464340 [PubMed - indexed for MEDLINE]

1370. J Virol. 2009 Oct;83(19):10176-86. doi: 10.1128/JVI.00422-09. Epub 2009 Jul 22.

Rho GTPases modulate entry of Ebola virus and vesicular stomatitis virus pseudotyped vectors.

Quinn K(1), Brindley MA, Weller ML, Kaludov N, Kondratowicz A, Hunt CL, Sinn PL, McCray PB Jr, Stein CS, Davidson BL, Flick R, Mandell R, Staplin W, Maury W, Chiorini JA.

Author information: (1)Molecular Physiology and Therapeutics Branch, National Institute of Dental and Craniofacial Research, National Institutes of Health, Bethesda, Maryland 20892, USA.

To explore mechanisms of entry for Ebola virus (EBOV) glycoprotein (GP) pseudotyped virions, we used comparative gene analysis to identify genes whose expression correlated with viral transduction. Candidate genes were identified by using EBOV GP pseudotyped virions to transduce human tumor cell lines that had previously been characterized by cDNA microarray. Transduction profiles for each of these cell lines were generated, and a significant positive correlation was observed between RhoC expression and permissivity for EBOV vector transduction. This correlation was not specific for EBOV vector alone as RhoC also correlated highly with transduction of vesicular stomatitis virus GP (VSVG) pseudotyped vector. Levels of RhoC protein in EBOV and VSV permissive and nonpermissive cells were consistent with the cDNA gene array findings. Additionally, vector transduction was elevated in cells that expressed high levels of endogenous RhoC but not RhoA. RhoB and RhoC overexpression significantly increased EBOV GP and VSVG pseudotyped vector transduction but had minimal effect on human immunodeficiency virus (HIV) GP pseudotyped HIV or adeno-associated virus 2 vector entry, indicating that not all virus uptake was enhanced by expression of these molecules. RhoB and RhoC overexpression also significantly enhanced VSV infection. Similarly, overexpression of RhoC led to a significant increase in fusion of EBOV virus-like particles. Finally, ectopic expression of RhoC resulted in increased nonspecific endocytosis of fluorescent dextran and in formation of increased actin stress fibers compared to RhoA-transfected cells, suggesting that RhoC is enhancing macropinocytosis. In total, our studies implicate RhoB and RhoC in enhanced productive entry of some pseudovirions and suggest the involvement of actin-mediated macropinocytosis as a mechanism of uptake of EBOV GP and VSVG pseudotyped viral particles.

PMCID: PMC2747995 PMID: 19625394 [PubMed - indexed for MEDLINE]

1371. New Microbiol. 2009 Oct;32(4):359-67.

Case definition for Ebola and Marburg haemorrhagic fevers: a complex challenge for epidemiologists and clinicians.

Pittalis S(1), Fusco FM, Lanini S, Nisii C, Puro V, Lauria FN, Ippolito G.

Author information: (1)Epidemiological and Pre-clinical Research Department, National Institute for Infectious Diseases (INMI) "L. Spallanzani", Rome, Italy. pittalis@inmi.it

Viral haemorrhagic fevers (VHFs) represent a challenge for public health because of their epidemic potential, and their possible use as bioterrorism agents poses particular concern. In 1999 the World Health Organization (WHO) proposed a case definition for VHFs, subsequently adopted by other international institutions with the aim of early detection of initial cases/outbreaks in western countries. We applied this case definition to reports of Ebola and Marburg virus infections to estimate its sensitivity to detect cases of the disease. We analyzed clinical descriptions of 795 reported cases of Ebola haemorrhagic fever: only 58.5% of patients met the proposed case definition. A similar figure was obtained reviewing 169 cases of Marburg diseases, of which only 64.5% were in accordance with the case definition. In conclusion, the WHO case definition for hemorrhagic fevers is too specific and has poor sensitivity both for case finding during Ebola or Marburg outbreaks, and for early detection of suspected cases in western countries. It can lead to a hazardous number of false negatives and its use should be discouraged for early detection of cases.

PMID: 20128442 [PubMed - indexed for MEDLINE]

1372. BMC Infect Dis. 2009 Sep 28;9:159. doi: 10.1186/1471-2334-9-159.

Large serological survey showing cocirculation of Ebola and Marburg viruses in Gabonese bat populations, and a high seroprevalence of both viruses in Rousettus aegyptiacus.

Pourrut X(1), Souris M, Towner JS, Rollin PE, Nichol ST, Gonzalez JP, Leroy E.

Author information: (1)Institut de Recherche pour le Développement, UR 178, Marseille, France. xavier.pourrut@ird.fr

BACKGROUND: Ebola and Marburg viruses cause highly lethal hemorrhagic fevers in humans. Recently, bats of multiple species have been identified as possible natural hosts of Zaire ebolavirus (ZEBOV) in Gabon and Republic of Congo, and also of marburgvirus (MARV) in Gabon and Democratic Republic of Congo. METHODS: We tested 2147 bats belonging to at least nine species sampled between 2003 and 2008 in three regions of Gabon and in the Ebola epidemic region of north Congo for IgG antibodies specific for ZEBOV and MARV. RESULTS: Overall, IgG antibodies to ZEBOV and MARV were found in 4% and 1% of bats, respectively. ZEBOV-specific antibodies were found in six bat species (Epomops franqueti, Hypsignathus monstrosus, Myonycteris torquata, Micropteropus pusillus, Mops condylurus and Rousettus aegyptiacus), while MARV-specific antibodies were only found in Rousettus aegyptiacus and Hypsignathus monstrosus. The prevalence of MARV-specific IgG was significantly higher in R. aegyptiacus members captured inside caves than elsewhere. No significant difference in prevalence was found according to age or gender. A higher prevalence of ZEBOV-specific IgG was found in pregnant females than in non pregnant females. CONCLUSION: These findings confirm that ZEBOV and MARV co-circulate in Gabon, the only country where bats infected by each virus have been found. IgG antibodies to both viruses were detected only in Rousettus aegyptiacus, suggesting that this bat species may be involved in the natural cycle of both Marburg and Ebola viruses. The presence of MARV in Gabon indicates a potential risk for a first human outbreak. Disease surveillance should be enhanced in areas near caves.

PMCID: PMC2761397 PMID: 19785757 [PubMed - indexed for MEDLINE]

1373. Virology. 2009 Sep 15;392(1):11-5. doi: 10.1016/j.virol.2009.06.032. Epub 2009 Jul 23.

RIG-I activation inhibits ebolavirus replication.

Spiropoulou CF(1), Ranjan P, Pearce MB, Sealy TK, Albariño CG, Gangappa S, Fujita T, Rollin PE, Nichol ST, Ksiazek TG, Sambhara S.

Author information: (1)Special Pathogens Branch, Division of Viral and Rickettsial Diseases, Centers for Disease Control and Prevention, Atlanta, GA, USA. ccs8@cdc.gov

Hemorrhagic fever viruses are associated with rapidly progressing severe disease with high case fatality, making them of public health and biothreat importance. Effective antivirals are not available for most of the members of this diverse group of viruses. A broad spectrum strategy for antiviral development would be very advantageous. Perhaps the most challenging target would be the highly immunosuppressive filoviruses, ebolavirus and marburgvirus, associated with aerosol infectivity and case fatalities in the 80-90% range. Here we report that activation of evolutionarily conserved cytosolic viral nucleic acid sensor, RIG-I can cause severe inhibition of ebolavirus replication. These findings indicate that RIG-I-based therapies may provide an attractive approach for antivirals against Ebola hemorrhagic fever, and possibly other HF viruses.

PMID: 19628240 [PubMed - indexed for MEDLINE]

1374. Science. 2009 Sep 4;325(5945):1200. doi: 10.1126/science.325_1200a.

American Chemical Society fall meeting, 16-20 August, Washington, D.C. Sugary Achilles' heel raises hope for broad-acting antiviral drugs.

Service RF.

PMID: 19729635 [PubMed - indexed for MEDLINE]

1375. Ann N Y Acad Sci. 2009 Sep;1171 Suppl 1:E6-11. doi: 10.1111/j.1749-6632.2009.05056.x.

Diagnostics and discovery in viral hemorrhagic fevers.

Lipkin WI(1), Palacios G, Briese T.

Author information: (1)Center for Infection and Immunity, Mailman School of Public Health of Columbia University, New York, New York, USA. wil2001@columbia.edu

The rate of discovery of new microbes and of new associations of microbes with health and disease is accelerating. Many factors contribute to this phenomenon including those that favor the true emergence of new pathogens as well as new technologies and paradigms that enable their detection and characterization. This chapter reviews recent progress in the field of pathogen surveillance and discovery with a focus on viral hemorrhagic fevers.

PMCID: PMC4109264 PMID: 19751404 [PubMed - indexed for MEDLINE]

1376. Antiviral Res. 2009 Sep;83(3):245-51. doi: 10.1016/j.antiviral.2009.06.001. Epub 2009 Jun 10.

Development of a broad-spectrum antiviral with activity against Ebola virus.

Aman MJ(1), Kinch MS, Warfield K, Warren T, Yunus A, Enterlein S, Stavale E, Wang P, Chang S, Tang Q, Porter K, Goldblatt M, Bavari S.

Author information: (1)United States Army Medical Research Institute for Infectious Diseases, Fort Detrick, MD 21702, USA. mkinch@functional-genetics.com

We report herein the identification of a small molecule therapeutic, FGI-106, which displays potent and broad-spectrum inhibition of lethal viral hemorrhagic fevers pathogens, including Ebola, Rift Valley and Dengue Fever viruses, in cell-based assays. Using mouse models of Ebola virus, we further demonstrate that FGI-106 can protect animals from an otherwise lethal infection when used either in a prophylactic or therapeutic setting. A single treatment, administered 1 day after infection, is sufficient to protect animals from lethal Ebola virus challenge. Cell-based assays also identified inhibitory activity against divergent virus families, which supports a hypothesis that FGI-106 interferes with a common pathway utilized by different viruses. These findings suggest FGI-106 may provide an opportunity for targeting viral diseases.

PMID: 19523489 [PubMed - indexed for MEDLINE]

1377. J Interferon Cytokine Res. 2009 Sep;29(9):511-20. doi: 10.1089/jir.2009.0076.

Evasion of interferon responses by Ebola and Marburg viruses.

Basler CF(1), Amarasinghe GK.

Author information: (1)Department of Microbiology, Mount Sinai School of Medicine, New York, New York 10029, USA. chris.basler@mssm.edu

The filoviruses, Ebola virus (EBOV) and Marburg virus (MARV), cause frequently lethal viral hemorrhagic fever. These infections induce potent cytokine production, yet these host responses fail to prevent systemic virus replication. Consistent with this, filoviruses have been found to encode proteins VP35 and VP24 that block host interferon (IFN)-alpha/beta production and inhibit signaling downstream of the IFN-alpha/beta and the IFN-gamma receptors, respectively. VP35, which is a component of the viral nucleocapsid complex and plays an essential role in viral RNA synthesis, acts as a pseudosubstrate for the cellular kinases IKK-epsilon and TBK-1, which phosphorylate and activate interferon regulatory factor 3 (IRF-3) and interferon regulatory factor 7 (IRF-7). VP35 also promotes SUMOylation of IRF-7, repressing IFN gene transcription. In addition, VP35 is a dsRNA-binding protein, and mutations that disrupt dsRNA binding impair VP35 IFN-antagonist activity while leaving its RNA replication functions intact. The phenotypes of recombinant EBOV bearing mutant VP35s unable to inhibit IFN-alpha/beta demonstrate that VP35 IFN-antagonist activity is critical for full virulence of these lethal pathogens. The structure of the VP35 dsRNA-binding domain, which has recently become available, is expected to provide insight into how VP35 IFN-antagonist and dsRNA-binding functions are related. The EBOV VP24 protein inhibits IFN signaling through an interaction with select host cell karyopherin-alpha proteins, preventing the nuclear import of otherwise activated STAT1. It remains to be determined to what extent VP24 may also modulate the nuclear import of other host cell factors and to what extent this may influence the outcome of infection. Notably, the Marburg virus VP24 protein does not detectably block STAT1 nuclear import, and, unlike EBOV, MARV infection inhibits STAT1 and STAT2 phosphorylation. Thus, despite their similarities, there are fundamental differences by which these deadly viruses counteract the IFN system. It will be of interest to determine how these differences influence pathogenesis.

PMCID: PMC2988466 PMID: 19694547 [PubMed - indexed for MEDLINE]

1378. J Virol. 2009 Sep;83(18):9596-601. doi: 10.1128/JVI.00784-09. Epub 2009 Jul 8.

Ebolavirus glycoprotein GP masks both its own epitopes and the presence of cellular surface proteins.

Reynard O(1), Borowiak M, Volchkova VA, Delpeut S, Mateo M, Volchkov VE.

Author information: (1)INSERM, Laboratoire des Filovirus, Lyon, France.

Ebolavirus (EBOV) is the etiological agent of a severe hemorrhagic fever with a high mortality rate. The spike glycoprotein (GP) is believed to be one of the major determinants of virus pathogenicity. In this study, we demonstrated the molecular mechanism responsible for the downregulation of surface markers caused by EBOV GP expression. We showed that expression of mature GP on the plasma membrane results in the masking of cellular surface proteins, including major histocompatibility complex class I. Overexpression of GP also results in the masking of certain antigenic epitopes on GP itself, causing an illusory effect of disappearance from the plasma membrane.

PMCID: PMC2738224 PMID: 19587051 [PubMed - indexed for MEDLINE]

1379. J Virol. 2009 Sep;83(17):8993-7. doi: 10.1128/JVI.00523-09. Epub 2009 Jun 10.

Ebola virus VP35 antagonizes PKR activity through its C-terminal interferon inhibitory domain.

Schümann M(1), Gantke T, Mühlberger E.

Author information: (1)Department of Virology, Philipps University Marburg, 35043 Marburg, Germany.

Ebola virus VP35 contains a C-terminal cluster of basic amino acids required for double-stranded RNA (dsRNA) binding and inhibition of interferon regulatory factor 3 (IRF3). VP35 also blocks protein kinase R (PKR) activation; however, the responsible domain has remained undefined. Here we show that the IRF inhibitory domain of VP35 mediates the inhibition of PKR and enhances the synthesis of coexpressed proteins. In contrast to dsRNA binding and IRF inhibition, alanine substitutions of at least two basic amino acids are required to abrogate PKR inhibition and enhanced protein expression. Moreover, we show that PKR activation is not only blocked but reversed by Ebola virus infection.

PMCID: PMC2738155 PMID: 19515768 [PubMed - indexed for MEDLINE]

1380. J Virol. 2009 Sep;83(17):8575-86. doi: 10.1128/JVI.00526-09. Epub 2009 Jun 10.

A charged second-site mutation in the fusion peptide rescues replication of a mutant avian sarcoma and leukosis virus lacking critical cysteine residues flanking the internal fusion domain.

Melder DC(1), Yin X, Delos SE, Federspiel MJ.

Author information: (1)Department of Molecular Medicine, Mayo Clinic, 200 First Street, SW, Rochester, MN 55905, USA.

The entry process of the avian sarcoma and leukosis virus (ASLV) family of retroviruses requires first a specific interaction between the viral surface (SU) glycoproteins and a receptor on the cell surface at a neutral pH, triggering conformational changes in the viral SU and transmembrane (TM) glycoproteins, followed by exposure to low pH to complete fusion. The ASLV TM glycoprotein has been proposed to adopt a structure similar to that of the Ebola virus GP2 protein: each contains an internal fusion peptide flanked by cysteine residues predicted to be in a disulfide bond. In a previous study, we concluded that the cysteines flanking the internal fusion peptide in ASLV TM are critical for efficient function of the ASLV viral glycoproteins in mediating entry. In this study, replication-competent ASLV mutant subgroup A [ASLV(A)] variants with these cysteine residues mutated were constructed and genetically selected for improved replication capacity in chicken fibroblasts. Viruses with single cysteine-to-serine mutations reverted to the wild-type sequence. However, viruses with both C9S and C45S (C9,45S) mutations retained both mutations and acquired a second-site mutation that significantly improved the infectivity of the genetically selected virus population. A charged-amino-acid second-site substitution in the TM internal fusion peptide at position 30 is preferred to rescue the C9,45S mutant ASLV(A). ASLV(A) envelope glycoproteins that contain the C9,45S and G30R mutations bind the Tva receptor at wild-type levels and have improved abilities to trigger conformational changes and to form stable TM oligomers compared to those of the C9,45S mutant glycoprotein.

PMCID: PMC2738199 PMID: 19515762 [PubMed - indexed for MEDLINE]

1381. Sci Am. 2009 Sep;301(3):15.

Swine Ebola.

Borrell B.

PMID: 19708514 [PubMed - indexed for MEDLINE]

1382. Virus Res. 2009 Sep;144(1-2):1-7. doi: 10.1016/j.virusres.2009.02.005. Epub 2009 Feb 21.

Characterization of Ebolavirus regulatory genomic regions.

Neumann G(1), Watanabe S, Kawaoka Y.

Author information: (1)Department of Pathobiological Sciences, School of Veterinary Medicine, University of Wisconsin-Madison, Madison, WI 53706, USA.

For filoviruses, such as Ebolavirus and the closely related Marburgvirus, transcriptional regulation is poorly understood. The open reading frames (ORFs) that encode the viral proteins are separated by regulatory regions composed of the 3' nontranslated region (NTR) of the upstream gene, highly conserved transcription stop and start signals, and the 5'NTR of the downstream gene. The conserved transcription stop and start signals either overlap, or they are separated by intergenic regions (IGRs) of different lengths. To assess the contribution of the regulatory regions to transcription, we established bicistronic minireplicons in which these regions were flanked by upstream and downstream ORFs, the Ebolavirus leader and trailer regions, and by T7 RNA polymerase promoter and ribozyme sequences. We found that the individual viral regulatory regions differ in their ability to direct protein synthesis from the upstream or downstream ORFs. Deletion or modification of the NTRs, IGRs, or transcription stop and start signals affected protein expression levels to various extents; for example, 5'NTRs appear to affect efficient protein expression from the downstream ORF, whereas 3'NTRs seem to attenuate protein expression from the upstream ORF. Overall, our data suggest that the regulation of Ebolavirus protein levels is complex.

PMCID: PMC2845284 PMID: 19481829 [PubMed - indexed for MEDLINE]

1383. Cell Host Microbe. 2009 Aug 20;6(2):162-73. doi: 10.1016/j.chom.2009.07.003.

Reduced levels of protein tyrosine phosphatase CD45 protect mice from the lethal effects of Ebola virus infection.

Panchal RG(1), Bradfute SB, Peyser BD, Warfield KL, Ruthel G, Lane D, Kenny TA, Anderson AO, Raschke WC, Bavari S.

Author information: (1)United States Army Medical Research Institute of Infectious Diseases, 1425 Porter Street, Fort Detrick, Frederick, MD 21702-5011, USA. rekha.panchal@amedd.army.mil

Ebola virus (EBOV) infection of humans is a lethal but accidental dead-end event. Understanding resistance to EBOV in other species may help establish the basis of susceptibility differences among its hosts. Although rodents are resistant to EBOV, a murine-adapted variant is lethal when injected intraperitoneally into mice. We find that mice expressing reduced levels of the tyrosine phosphatase CD45 are protected against EBOV, whereas wild-type, CD45-deficient, or enzymatically inactive CD45-expressing mice succumbed to infection. Protection was dependent on CD8(+) T cells and interferon gamma. Reduced CD45-expressing mice retained greater control of gene expression and immune cell proliferation following EBOV infection, which contributed to reduced apoptosis, enhanced viral clearance, and increased protection against the virus. Together, these findings suggest that host susceptibility to EBOV is dependent on the delicate balance of immune homeostasis, which, as demonstrated here, can be determined by the levels of a single regulator.

PMID: 19683682 [PubMed - indexed for MEDLINE]

1384. PLoS One. 2009 Aug 11;4(8):e6569. doi: 10.1371/journal.pone.0006569.

Testing and validation of high density resequencing microarray for broad range biothreat agents detection.

Leski TA(1), Lin B, Malanoski AP, Wang Z, Long NC, Meador CE, Barrows B, Ibrahim S, Hardick JP, Aitichou M, Schnur JM, Tibbetts C, Stenger DA.

Author information: (1)Center for Bio/Molecular Science and Engineering, Code 6900, Naval Research Laboratory, Washington, DC, USA.

Rapid and effective detection and identification of emerging microbiological threats and potential biowarfare agents is very challenging when using traditional culture-based methods. Contemporary molecular techniques, relying upon reverse transcription and/or polymerase chain reaction (RT-PCR/PCR) provide a rapid and effective alternative, however, such assays are generally designed and optimized to detect only a limited number of targets, and seldom are capable of differentiation among variants of detected targets. To meet these challenges, we have designed a broad-range resequencing pathogen microarray (RPM) for detection of tropical and emerging infectious agents (TEI) including biothreat agents: RPM-TEI v 1.0 (RPM-TEI). The scope of the RPM-TEI assay enables detection and differential identification of 84 types of pathogens and 13 toxin genes, including most of the class A, B and C select agents as defined by the Centers for Disease Control and Prevention (CDC, Atlanta, GA). Due to the high risks associated with handling these particular target pathogens, the sensitivity validation of the RPM-TEI has been performed using an innovative approach, in which synthetic DNA fragments are used as templates for testing the assay's limit of detection (LOD). Assay specificity and sensitivity was subsequently confirmed by testing with full-length genomic nucleic acids of selected agents. The LOD for a majority of the agents detected by RPM-TEI was determined to be at least 10(4) copies per test. Our results also show that the RPM-TEI assay not only detects and identifies agents, but is also able to differentiate near neighbors of the same agent types, such as closely related strains of filoviruses of the Ebola Zaire group, or the Machupo and Lassa arenaviruses. Furthermore, each RPM-TEI assay results in specimen-specific agent gene sequence information that can be used to assess pathogenicity, mutations, and virulence markers, results that are not generally available from multiplexed RT-PCR/PCR-based detection assays.

PMCID: PMC2719057 PMID: 19668365 [PubMed - indexed for MEDLINE]

1385. Curr Opin Struct Biol. 2009 Aug;19(4):408-17. doi: 10.1016/j.sbi.2009.05.004. Epub 2009 Jun 24.

Neutralizing ebolavirus: structural insights into the envelope glycoprotein and antibodies targeted against it.

Lee JE(1), Saphire EO.

Author information: (1)Department of Immunology and Microbial Science, The Scripps Research Institute, 10550 North Torrey Pines Road, La Jolla, CA 92037, USA.

The ebolavirus (EBOV) envelope glycoprotein (GP) is solely responsible for viral attachment to, fusion with, and entry of new host cells, and consequently is a major target of vaccine design efforts. Recently determined crystal structures of key antibodies in complex with their EBOV epitopes have provided insights into the molecular architecture of GP and defined likely hotspots for viral neutralization. In this review, we discuss the structural basis for antibody-mediated neutralization of ebolavirus and its implications for novel therapeutic or vaccine strategies.

PMCID: PMC2759674 PMID: 19559599 [PubMed - indexed for MEDLINE]

1386. J Struct Biol. 2009 Aug;167(2):136-44. doi: 10.1016/j.jsb.2009.05.001. Epub 2009 May 15.

Fold prediction of VP24 protein of Ebola and Marburg viruses using de novo fragment assembly.

Lee MS(1), Lebeda FJ, Olson MA.

Author information: (1)Computational Sciences and Engineering Branch, US Army Research Laboratory, Aberdeen, MD 21005, USA. michael.lee@amedd.army.mil

Virus particle 24 (VP24) is the smallest protein of the Ebola and Marburg virus genomes. Recent experiments show that Ebola VP24 blocks binding of tyrosine-phosphorylated STAT-1 homodimer (PY-STAT1) to the NPI-1 subfamily of importin alpha, thereby preventing nuclear accumulation of this interferon-promoting transcription factor which, in turn, reduces the innate immune response of the host target. Lacking an experimental structure for VP24, we applied de novo protein structure prediction using the fragment assembly-based Rosetta method to classify its fold topology and better understand its biological function. Filtering and ranking of models were performed with the DFIRE all-atom statistical potential and the CHARMM22 force field with a generalized Born solvent model. From 40,000 Rosetta-generated structures and selective comparisons with the SCOP database, a structural match to two of our top 10-ranking models was the Armadillo repeat fold topology. Specific members of this fold family include importin alpha, importin beta, and exportin. We propose that, unlike the nuclear import of host cargo, VP24 lacks a classical nuclear localization signal (NLS) and targets importin alpha in a similar manner to the observed heterodimeric complex with exportin, thereby interfering with the auto-inhibitory NLS on importin alpha and blocking peripheral docking sites for PY-STAT1 assembly.

PMID: 19447180 [PubMed - indexed for MEDLINE]
1387. Zoonoses Public Health. 2009 Aug;56(6-7):407-28. doi: 10.1111/j.1863-2378.2009.01255.x.

Emerging infections: a tribute to the one medicine, one health concept.

Kahn RE(1), Clouser DF, Richt JA.

Author information: (1)Avian Flu Action, Warrington, Cheshire, UK.

Events in the last decade have taught us that we are now, more than ever, vulnerable to fatal zoonotic diseases such as those caused by haemorrhagic fever viruses, influenza, rabies and BSE/vCJD. Future research activities should focus on solutions to these problems arising at the interface between animals and humans. A 4-fold classification of emerging zoonoses was proposed: Type 1: from wild animals to humans (Hanta); Type 1 plus: from wild animals to humans with further human-to-human transmission (AIDS); Type 2: from wild animals to domestic animals to humans (Avian flu) and Type 2 plus: from wild animals to domestic animals to humans, with further human-to-human transmission (Severe Acute Respiratory Syndrome, SARS). The resulting holistic approach to emerging infections links microbiology, veterinary medicine, human medicine, ecology, public health and epidemiology. As emerging 'new' respiratory viruses are identified in many wild and domestic animals, issues of interspecies transmission have become of increasing concern. The development of safe and effective human and veterinary vaccines is a priority. For example, the spread of different influenza viruses has stimulated influenza vaccine development, just as the spread of Ebola and Marburg viruses has led to new approaches to filovirus vaccines. Interdisciplinary collaboration has become essential because of the convergence of human disease, animal disease and a common approach to biosecurity. High containment pathogens pose a significant threat to public health systems, as well as a major research challenge, because of limited experience in case management, lack of appropriate resources in affected areas and a limited number of animal research facilities in developed countries. Animal models that mimic certain diseases are key elements for understanding the underlying mechanisms of disease pathogenesis, as well as for the development and efficacy testing of therapeutics and vaccines. An updated veterinary curriculum is essential to empower future graduates to work in an international environment, applying international standards for disease surveillance, veterinary public health, food safety and animal welfare.

PMID: 19486315 [PubMed - indexed for MEDLINE]
1388. Science. 2009 Jul 10;325(5937):204-6. doi: 10.1126/science.1172705.

Discovery of swine as a host for the Reston ebolavirus.

Barrette RW(1), Metwally SA, Rowland JM, Xu L, Zaki SR, Nichol ST, Rollin PE, Towner JS, Shieh WJ, Batten B, Sealy TK, Carrillo C, Moran KE, Bracht AJ, Mayr GA, Sirios-Cruz M, Catbagan DP, Lautner EA, Ksiazek TG, White WR, McIntosh MT.

Author information: (1)Foreign Animal Disease Diagnostic Laboratory, National Veterinary Services Laboratories, Animal and Plant Health Inspection Services, United States Department of Agriculture, Plum Island Animal Disease Center, New York, NY 11944, USA.

Since the discovery of the Marburg and Ebola species of filovirus, seemingly random, sporadic fatal outbreaks of disease in humans and nonhuman primates have given impetus to identification of host tropisms and potential reservoirs. Domestic swine in the Philippines, experiencing unusually severe outbreaks of porcine reproductive and respiratory disease syndrome, have now been discovered to host Reston ebolavirus (REBOV). Although REBOV is the only member of Filoviridae that has not been associated with disease in humans, its emergence in the human food chain is of concern. REBOV isolates were found to be more divergent from each other than from the original virus isolated in 1989, indicating polyphyletic origins and that REBOV has been circulating since, and possibly before, the initial discovery of REBOV in monkeys.

PMID: 19590002 [PubMed - indexed for MEDLINE]
1389. Antiviral Res. 2009 Jul;83(1):10-20. doi: 10.1016/j.antiviral.2009.04.004. Epub 2009 Apr 16.

Applications of high-throughput genomics to antiviral research: evasion of antiviral responses and activation of inflammation during fulminant RNA virus infection.

Kash JC(1).

Author information: (1)Viral Pathogenesis and Evolution Section, Laboratory of Infectious Diseases, National Institute of Allergy and Infectious Diseases (NIAID), National Institutes of Health (NIH), Bethesda, MD 20892-3203, USA. kashj@niaid.nih.gov

Host responses can contribute to the severity of viral infection, through the failure of innate antiviral mechanisms to recognize and restrict the pathogen, the development of intense systemic inflammation leading to circulatory failure or through tissue injury resulting from overly exuberant cell-mediated immune responses. High-throughput genomics methods are now being used to identify the biochemical pathways underlying ineffective or damaging host responses in a number of acute and chronic viral infections. This article reviews recent gene expression studies of 1918 H1N1 influenza and Ebola hemorrhagic fever in cell culture and animal models, focusing on how genomics experiments can be used to increase our understanding of the mechanisms that permit those viruses to cause rapidly overwhelming infection. Particular attention is paid to how evasion of type I IFN responses in infected cells might contribute to over-activation of inflammatory responses. Reviewing recent research and describing how future studies might be tailored to understand the relationship between the infected cell and its environment, this article discusses how the rapidly growing field of high-throughput genomics can contribute to a more complete understanding of severe, acute viral infections and identify novel targets for therapeutic intervention.

PMCID: PMC3457704 PMID: 19375457 [PubMed - indexed for MEDLINE]
1390. Emerg Infect Dis. 2009 Jul;15(7):1136-7. doi: 10.3201/eid1507.090402.

Immunoglobulin G in Ebola outbreak survivors, Gabon.

Wauquier N, Becquart P, Gasquet C, Leroy EM.
PMCID: PMC2744259 PMID: 19624943 [PubMed - indexed for MEDLINE]

1391. J Virol. 2009 Jul;83(13):6952-6. doi: 10.1128/JVI.00480-09. Epub 2009 Apr 29.

Ebolavirus VP35 interacts with the cytoplasmic dynein light chain 8.

Kubota T(1), Matsuoka M, Chang TH, Bray M, Jones S, Tashiro M, Kato A, Ozato K.

Author information: (1)Department of Virology III, National Institute of Infectious Diseases, Gakuen 4-7-1, Musashi-Murayama, Tokyo 208-0011, Japan. kubota@nih.go.jp

The viral protein VP35 of ebolavirus (EBOV) is implicated to have diverse roles in the viral life cycle. We employed a yeast two-hybrid screen to search for VP35 binding partners and identified the cytoplasmic dynein light chain (DLC8) as a protein that interacts with VP35. Mapping analysis unraveled a consensus motif, SQTQT, within VP35 through which VP35 binds to DLC8. The disruption of DLC8 binding does not affect the ability of VP35 to inhibit type I IFN production. Given that VP35 from various EBOV species interacts with DLC8, this interaction may have a role in regulating the EBOV life cycle.

PMCID: PMC2698516 PMID: 19403681 [PubMed - indexed for MEDLINE]

1392. J Virol. 2009 Jul;83(14):7296-304. doi: 10.1128/JVI.00561-09. Epub 2009 Apr 22.

Single-injection vaccine protects nonhuman primates against infection with marburg virus and three species of ebola virus.

Geisbert TW(1), Geisbert JB, Leung A, Daddario-DiCaprio KM, Hensley LE, Grolla A, Feldmann H.

Author information: (1)Department of Microbiology, National Emerging Infectious Diseases Laboratories Institute, Boston University School of Medicine, Boston, Massachusetts 02118, USA. geisbert@bu.edu

The filoviruses Marburg virus and Ebola virus cause severe hemorrhagic fever with high mortality in humans and nonhuman primates. Among the most promising filovirus vaccines under development is a system based on recombinant vesicular stomatitis virus (VSV) that expresses a single filovirus glycoprotein (GP) in place of the VSV glycoprotein (G). Here, we performed a proof-of-concept study in order to determine the potential of having one single-injection vaccine capable of protecting nonhuman primates against Sudan ebolavirus (SEBOV), Zaire ebolavirus (ZEBOV), Cote d'Ivoire ebolavirus (CIEBOV), and Marburgvirus (MARV). In this study, 11 cynomolgus monkeys were vaccinated with a blended vaccine consisting of equal parts of the vaccine vectors VSVDeltaG/SEBOVGP, VSVDeltaG/ZEBOVGP, and VSVDeltaG/MARVGP. Four weeks later, three of these animals were challenged with MARV, three with CIEBOV, three with ZEBOV, and two with SEBOV. Three control animals were vaccinated with VSV vectors encoding a nonfilovirus GP and challenged with SEBOV, ZEBOV, and MARV, respectively, and five unvaccinated control animals were challenged with CIEBOV. Importantly, none of the macaques vaccinated with the blended vaccine succumbed to a filovirus challenge. As expected, an experimental control animal vaccinated with VSVDeltaG/ZEBOVGP and challenged with SEBOV succumbed, as did the positive controls challenged with SEBOV, ZEBOV, and MARV, respectively. All five control animals challenged with CIEBOV became severely ill, and three of the animals succumbed on days 12, 12, and 14, respectively. The two animals that survived CIEBOV infection were protected from subsequent challenge with either SEBOV or ZEBOV, suggesting that immunity to CIEBOV may be protective against other species of Ebola virus. In conclusion, we developed an immunization scheme based on a single-injection vaccine that protects nonhuman primates against lethal challenge with representative strains of all human pathogenic filovirus species.

PMCID: PMC2704787 PMID: 19386702 [PubMed - indexed for MEDLINE]

1393. J Virol. 2009 Jul;83(13):6404-15. doi: 10.1128/JVI.00126-09. Epub 2009 Apr 15.

Development and characterization of a mouse model for Marburg hemorrhagic fever.

Warfield KL(1), Bradfute SB, Wells J, Lofts L, Cooper MT, Alves DA, Reed DK, VanTongeren SA, Mech CA, Bavari S.

Author information: (1)United States Army Medical Research Institute of Infectious Diseases, Fort Detrick, Maryland 21702, USA. kelly@integratedbiotherapeutics.com

The lack of a mouse model has hampered an understanding of the pathogenesis and immunity of Marburg hemorrhagic fever (MHF), the disease caused by marburgvirus (MARV), and has created a bottleneck in the development of antiviral therapeutics. Primary isolates of the filoviruses, i.e., ebolavirus (EBOV) and MARV, are not lethal to immunocompetent adult mice. Previously, pathological, virologic, and immunologic evaluation of a mouse-adapted EBOV, developed by sequential passages in suckling mice, identified many similarities between this model and EBOV infections in nonhuman primates. We recently demonstrated that serially passaging virus recovered from the liver homogenates of MARV-infected immunodeficient (SCID) mice was highly successful in reducing the time to death in these mice from 50 to 70 days to 7 to 10 days after challenge with the isolate MARV-Ci67, -Musoke, or -Ravn. In this study, we extended our findings to show that further sequential passages of MARV-Ravn in immunocompetent mice caused the MARV to kill BALB/c mice. Serial sampling studies to characterize the pathology of mouse-adapted MARV-Ravn revealed that this model is similar to the guinea pig and nonhuman primate MHF models. Infection of BALB/c mice with mouse-adapted MARV-Ravn caused uncontrolled viremia and high viral titers in the liver, spleen, lymph node, and other organs; profound lymphopenia; destruction of lymphocytes within the spleen and lymph nodes; and marked liver damage and thrombocytopenia. Sequencing the mouse-adapted MARV-Ravn strain revealed differences in 16 predicted amino acids from the progenitor virus, although the exact changes required for adaptation are unclear at this time. This mouse-adapted MARV strain can now be used to develop and evaluate novel vaccines and therapeutics and may also help to provide a better understanding of the virulence factors associated with MARV.

PMCID: PMC2698517 PMID: 19369350 [PubMed - indexed for MEDLINE]

1394. J Virol Methods. 2009 Jul;159(1):29-33. doi: 10.1016/j.jviromet.2009.02.021. Epub 2009 Mar 3.

Non-infectious plasmid engineered to simulate multiple viral threat agents.

Carrera M(1), Sagripanti JL.

Author information: (1)Laboratory of the Association of Biochemists and Pharmacists (COFYB, Argentina), Buenos Aires CP 1184, Argentina.

The aim of this study was to design and construct a non-virulent simulant to replace several pathogenic viruses in the development of detection and identification methods in biodefense. A non-infectious simulant was designed and engineered to include the nucleic acid signature of VEEV (Venezuelan Equine Encephalitis virus), Influenza virus, Rift Valley Fever virus, Machupo virus, Lassa virus, Yellow Fever virus, Ebola virus, Eastern Equine Encephalitis virus, Junin virus, Marburg virus, Dengue virus, and Crimean-Congo virus, all in a single construct. The nucleic acid sequences of all isolates available for each virus species were aligned using ClustalW software in order to obtain conserved regions of the viral genomes. Specific primers were designed to permit the identification and differentiation between viral threat agents. A chimera of 3143 base pairs was engineered to produce 13 PCR amplicons of different sizes. PCR amplification of the simulant with virus-specific primers revealed products of the predicted length, in bands of similar intensity, and without detectable unspecific products by electrophoresis analysis. The simulant described could reduce the need to use infectious viruses in the development of detection and diagnostic methods, and could also be useful as a non-virulent positive control in nucleic acid-based tests against biological threat agents.

PMID: 19442841 [PubMed - indexed for MEDLINE]

1395. Nat Nanotechnol. 2009 Jul;4(7):430-6. doi: 10.1038/nnano.2009.93. Epub 2009 May 3

Multifunctional nanoarchitectures from DNA-based ABC monomers.

Lee JB(1), Roh YH, Um SH, Funabashi H, Cheng W, Cha JJ, Kiatwuthinon P, Muller DA, Luo D.

Author information: (1)Department of Biological and Environmental Engineering, Cornell University, Ithaca, New York 14850, USA.

The ability to attach different functional moieties to a molecular building block could lead to applications in nanoelectronics, nanophotonics, intelligent sensing and drug delivery. The building unit needs to be both multivalent and anisotropic, and although many anisotropic building blocks have been created, these have not been universally applicable. Recently, DNA has been used to generate various nanostructures or hybrid systems, and as a generic building block for various applications. Here, we report the creation of anisotropic, branched and crosslinkable building blocks (ABC monomers) from which multifunctional nanoarchitectures have been assembled. In particular, we demonstrate a target-driven polymerization process in which polymers are generated only in the presence of a specific DNA molecule, leading to highly sensitive pathogen detection. Using this monomer system, we have also designed a biocompatible nanovector that delivers both drugs and tracers simultaneously. Our approach provides a general yet versatile route towards the creation of a range of multifunctional nanoarchitectures.

PMID: 19581895 [PubMed - indexed for MEDLINE]

1396. Protein Expr Purif. 2009 Jul;66(1):113-9. doi: 10.1016/j.pep.2009.02.008. Epub 2009 Feb 20.

Purification and functional characterization of the full length recombinant Ebola virus VP35 protein expressed in E. coli.

Zinzula L(1), Esposito F, Mühlberger E, Trunschke M, Conrad D, Piano D, Tramontano E.

Author information: (1)Department of Applied Sciences in Biosystems, University of Cagliari, Cittadella di Monserrato SS554, Monserrato, Cagliari, Italy.

In this work is presented, for the first time, the expression and purification in a prokaryotic system of the functionally active, recombinant full length VP35 protein of Ebola virus (EBOV). EBOV is an enveloped non-segmented negative-stranded RNA virus belonging to the filovirus family which causes a severe hemorrhagic fever in humans with mortality rates as high as 90%. Several lines of evidence suggest that EBOV interferes with host interferon responses and that the lack of these responses allows its rapidly progressive, overwhelming infection. Recently, the EBOV-encoded VP35 protein, essential cofactor of the viral RNA polymerase complex, has been shown to play an important role as interferon antagonist and the structure of his C-terminal IFN inhibitory domain has been solved. Although it is clearly important to better understand VP35 biochemical functions and its interplay with viral and cellular factors, the attempts to obtain full length E. coli recombinant VP35 (rVP35) have, until now, failed. In this study, we expressed the full length EBOV VP35 in E. coli as a soluble N-terminal His(6)-tag fusion protein and purified it to >95% homogeneity. In order to compare native and rVP35 functions, we characterized the rVP35 for its homo-oligomeric status and its RNA binding capacity showing that bacterially expressed rVP35 has the same properties as VP35 expressed in eukaryotic cells and that, therefore, rVP35 can be used as a valid model for functional studies and the validation of biochemical assays aimed to identify antiviral inhibitors which can interfere with the EBOV replication cycle.

PMID: 19233284 [PubMed - indexed for MEDLINE]

1397. Theor Biol Med Model. 2009 Jun 29;6:11. doi: 10.1186/1742-4682-6-11.

Models of epidemics: when contact repetition and clustering should be included.

Smieszek T(1), Fiebig L, Scholz RW.

Author information: (1)Institute for Environmental Decisions, Natural and Social Science Interface, ETH Zurich, Universitaetsstrasse 22, 8092 Zurich, Switzerland. timo.smieszek@env.ethz.ch

BACKGROUND: The spread of infectious disease is determined by biological factors, e.g. the duration of the infectious period, and social factors, e.g. the arrangement of potentially contagious contacts. Repetitiveness and clustering of contacts are known to be relevant factors influencing the transmission of droplet or contact transmitted diseases. However, we do not yet completely know under what conditions repetitiveness and clustering should be included for realistically modelling disease spread. METHODS: We compare two different types of individual-based models: One assumes random mixing without repetition of contacts, whereas the other assumes that the same contacts repeat day-by-day. The latter exists in two variants, with and without clustering. We systematically test and compare how the total size of an outbreak differs between these model types depending on the key parameters transmission probability, number of contacts per day, duration of the infectious period, different levels of clustering and varying proportions of repetitive contacts. RESULTS: The simulation runs under different parameter constellations provide the following results: The difference between both model types is highest for low numbers of contacts per day and low transmission probabilities. The number of contacts and the transmission probability have a higher influence on this difference than the duration of the infectious period. Even when only minor parts of the daily contacts are repetitive and clustered can there be relevant

293

differences compared to a purely random mixing model. CONCLUSION: We show that random mixing models provide acceptable estimates of the total outbreak size if the number of contacts per day is high or if the per-contact transmission probability is high, as seen in typical childhood diseases such as measles. In the case of very short infectious periods, for instance, as in Norovirus, models assuming repeating contacts will also behave similarly as random mixing models. If the number of daily contacts or the transmission probability is low, as assumed for MRSA or Ebola, particular consideration should be given to the actual structure of potentially contagious contacts when designing the model.
PMCID: PMC2709892 PMID: 19563624 [PubMed - indexed for MEDLINE]

1398. Virol J. 2009 Jun 8;6:75. doi: 10.1186/1743-422X-6-75.

Expression of Ebolavirus glycoprotein on the target cells enhances viral entry.

Manicassamy B(1), Rong L.

Author information: (1)Department of Microbiology and Immunology, College of Medicine, University of Illinois at Chicago, Chicago, Illinois, USA. balaji.manicassamy@mssm.edu

BACKGROUND: Entry of Ebolavirus to the target cells is mediated by the viral glycoprotein GP. The native GP exists as a homotrimer on the virions and contains two subunits, a surface subunit (GP1) that is involved in receptor binding and a transmembrane subunit (GP2) that mediates the virus-host membrane fusion. Previously we showed that over-expression of GP on the target cells blocks GP-mediated viral entry, which is mostly likely due to receptor interference by GP1. RESULTS: In this study, using a tetracycline inducible system, we report that low levels of GP expression on the target cells, instead of interfering, specifically enhance GP mediated viral entry. Detailed mapping analysis strongly suggests that the fusion subunit GP2 is primarily responsible for this novel phenomenon, here referred to as trans enhancement. CONCLUSION: Our data suggests that GP2 mediated trans enhancement of virus fusion occurs via a mechanism analogous to eukaryotic membrane fusion processes involving specific trans oligomerization and cooperative interaction of fusion mediators. These findings have important implications in our current understanding of virus entry and superinfection interference.
PMCID: PMC2699336 PMID: 19505320 [PubMed - indexed for MEDLINE]

1399. Biosecur Bioterror. 2009 Jun;7(2):227-33. doi: 10.1089/bsp.2009.0023.

Report of the International Conference on Risk Communication Strategies for BSL-4 laboratories, Tokyo, October 3-5, 2007.

Dickmann P(1), Keith K, Comer C, Abraham G, Gopal R, Marui E.

Author information: (1)Frankfurt University Hospital, Department of Infectious Diseases, Germany. pdickmann@dickmann-drc.com

Working with highly pathogenic agents such as Ebola or Marburg virus in the context of infection control or biodefense research requires high-biocontainment laboratories of the Biosafety Level 4 (BSL-4) to protect researchers and laboratory staff from infection and to prevent the unintentional release of harmful agents. The public perception of research on highly pathogenic agents and the operation of high-containment facilities is often ambivalent: while the output of the biomedical research is highly valued, the existence of a BSL-4 lab is often viewed with concern. Biomedical research perspectives and public perceptions often differ and can lead to tensions that could have negative effects on research, society, and politics. Therefore, risk communication plays a crucial role in siting, building, and operating a high-containment facility. The Japanese government invited risk communication experts and scientists from Canada, the U.S., Europe, and Australia to discuss their risk communication strategies for BSL-4 labs. This article describes the international perspective on risk communication and gives recommendations for successful strategies.
PMID: 19635008 [PubMed - indexed for MEDLINE]

1400. Drug Dev Res. 2009 Jun 1;70(4):255-265.

Identification of novel cellular targets for therapeutic intervention against Ebola virus infection by siRNA screening.

Kolokoltsov AA(1), Saeed MF, Freiberg AN, Holbrook MR, Davey RA.

Author information: (1)Dept. of Microbiology & Immunology.

While much progress has been made in developing drugs against a few prominent viruses such as HIV, few examples exist for emerging infectious agents. In some cases broad spectrum anti-viral drugs, such as ribavirin, are effective, but for some groups of viruses, these show little efficacy in animal models. Traditional methods focus on screening small molecule libraries to identify drugs that target virus factors, with the intention that side-effects to the host can be minimized. However, this greatly limits potential drug targets and virus genes can rapidly mutate to avoid drug action. Recent advances in siRNA gene targeting technologies have provided a powerful tool to specifically target and suppress the expression of cell genes. Since viruses are completely dependent upon host cell proteins for propagation, siRNA screening promises to reveal novel cell proteins and signaling pathways that may be viable targets for drug therapy regimens. Here we used an siRNA screening approach to identify gene products that play critical roles in Ebola virus infection. By gene cluster analysis, proteins in phosphatidylinositol-3-kinase and calcium/calmodulin kinase related networks were identified as important for Zaire Ebola virus infection and prioritized for further evaluation. Key roles of each were confirmed by testing available drugs specific for members of each pathway. Interestingly, both sets of proteins are also important in cancer and subject to intense investigation. Thus development of new drugs against these cancer targets may also prove useful in combating Ebola virus.
PMCID: PMC2949974 PMID: 20930947 [PubMed]

1401. Dtsch Med Wochenschr. 2009 Jun;134(25-26):1343-8. doi: 10.1055/s-0029-1225288. Epub 2009 Jun 10.

[Infectiology and tropical medicine 2009].

[Article in German]

Löscher T(1), Bogner JR.

Author information: (1)Abteilung für Infektions- und Tropenmedizin, Klinikum der Ludwig-Maximilians-Universität München. loescher@lrz.uni-muenchen.de

PMID: 19517328 [PubMed - indexed for MEDLINE]
1402. PLoS Pathog. 2009 Jun;5(6):e1000493. doi: 10.1371/journal.ppat.1000493. Epub 2009 Jun 26.

Ebola Zaire virus blocks type I interferon production by exploiting the host SUMO modification machinery.

Chang TH(1), Kubota T, Matsuoka M, Jones S, Bradfute SB, Bray M, Ozato K.

Author information: (1)Program in Genomics of Differentiation, Eunice Kennedy Shriver National Institute of Child Health and Human Development, National Institutes of Health, Bethesda, Maryland, United States of America.

Ebola Zaire virus is highly pathogenic for humans, with case fatality rates approaching 90% in large outbreaks in Africa. The virus replicates in macrophages and dendritic cells (DCs), suppressing production of type I interferons (IFNs) while inducing the release of large quantities of proinflammatory cytokines. Although the viral VP35 protein has been shown to inhibit IFN responses, the mechanism by which it blocks IFN production has not been fully elucidated. We expressed VP35 from a mouse-adapted variant of Ebola Zaire virus in murine DCs by retroviral gene transfer, and tested for IFN transcription upon Newcastle Disease virus (NDV) infection and toll-like receptor signaling. We found that VP35 inhibited IFN transcription in DCs following these stimuli by disabling the activity of IRF7, a transcription factor required for IFN transcription. By yeast two-hybrid screens and coimmunoprecipitation assays, we found that VP35 interacted with IRF7, Ubc9 and PIAS1. The latter two are the host SUMO E2 enzyme and E3 ligase, respectively. VP35, while not itself a SUMO ligase, increased PIAS1-mediated SUMOylation of IRF7, and repressed Ifn transcription. In contrast, VP35 did not interfere with the activation of NF-kappaB, which is required for induction of many proinflammatory cytokines. Our findings indicate that Ebola Zaire virus exploits the cellular SUMOylation machinery for its advantage and help to explain how the virus overcomes host innate defenses, causing rapidly overwhelming infection to produce a syndrome resembling fulminant septic shock.

PMCID: PMC2696038 PMID: 19557165 [PubMed - indexed for MEDLINE]
1403. Uirusu. 2009 Jun;59(1):99-106.

[Electron microscopic analysis of viral assembly and budding].

[Article in Japanese]

Noda T(1).

Author information: (1)Department of Special Pathogens, International Research Center for Infectious Diseases, Institute of Medical Science, University of Tokyo, Japan. t-noda@ims.u-tokyo.ac.jp

Viruses show ultrastructural changes during viral assembly and budding processes in which viral genome and proteins are systemically assembled. Electron microscopy is the only way that enables us to observe such ultrastructural changes. We have investigated the mechanisms of Ebola and influenza virion formation by electron microscopy. We have elucidated the roles of each Ebola virus protein in viral assembly and budding as well as the mechanisms of genome packaging of influenza A viruses.

PMID: 19927994 [PubMed - indexed for MEDLINE]
1404. Proc Natl Acad Sci U S A. 2009 May 12;106(19):8003-8. doi: 10.1073/pnas.0807578106. Epub 2009 Apr 28.

Alpha5beta1-integrin controls ebolavirus entry by regulating endosomal cathepsins.

Schornberg KL(1), Shoemaker CJ, Dube D, Abshire MY, Delos SE, Bouton AH, White JM.

Author information: (1)Department of Microbiology, University of Virginia, Charlottesville, VA 22908-0734, USA.

Integrins are involved in the binding and internalization of both enveloped and nonenveloped viruses. By using 3 distinct cell systems-CHO cells lacking expression of alpha(5)beta(1)-integrin, HeLa cells treated with siRNA to alpha(5)-integrin, and mouse beta(1)-integrin knockout fibroblasts, we show that alpha(5)beta(1)-integrin is required for efficient infection by pseudovirions bearing the ebolavirus glycoprotein (GP). These integrins are necessary for viral entry but not for binding or internalization. Given the need for endosomal cathepsins B and L (CatB and CatL) to prime GPs for fusion, we investigated the status of CatB and CatL in integrin-positive and integrin-negative cell lines. Alpha(5)beta(1)-Integrin-deficient cells lacked the double-chain (DC) forms of CatB and CatL, and this correlated with decreased CatL activity in integrin-negative CHO cells. These data indicate that alpha(5)beta(1)-integrin-negative cells may be refractory to infection by GP pseudovirions because they lack the necessary priming machinery (the double-chain forms of CatB and CatL). In support of this model, we show that GP pseudovirions that have been preprimed in vitro to generate the 19-kDa form of GP overcome the requirement for alpha(5)beta(1)-integrin for infection. These results provide further support for the requirement for endosomal cathepsins for ebolavirus infection, identify the DC forms of these cathepsins as previously unrecognized factors that contribute to cell tropism of this virus, and reveal a previously undescribed role for integrins during viral entry as regulators of endosomal cathepsins, which are required to prime the entry proteins of ebolavirus and other pathogenic viruses.

PMCID: PMC2683081 PMID: 19416892 [PubMed - indexed for MEDLINE]
1405. Antimicrob Agents Chemother. 2009 May;53(5):2089-99. doi: 10.1128/AAC.00936-08. Epub 2009 Feb 17.

Chemical modifications of antisense morpholino oligomers enhance their efficacy against Ebola virus infection.

Swenson DL(1), Warfield KL, Warren TK, Lovejoy C, Hassinger JN, Ruthel G, Blouch RE, Moulton HM, Weller DD, Iversen PL, Bavari S.

Author information: (1)U.S. Army Medical Research Institute of Infectious Diseases, 1425 Porter Street, Fort Detrick, MD 21702, USA.

Phosphorodiamidate morpholino oligomers (PMOs) are uncharged nucleic acid-like molecules designed to inactivate the expression of specific genes via the antisense-based steric hindrance of mRNA translation. PMOs have been successful at knocking out viral gene expression and replication in the case of acute viral infections in animal models and have been well tolerated in human clinical trials. We propose that antisense PMOs represent a promising class of therapeutic agents that may be useful for combating filoviral infections. We have previously shown that mice treated with a PMO whose sequence is complementary to a region spanning the start codon of VP24 mRNA were protected against lethal Ebola virus challenge. In the present study, we report on the abilities of two additional VP24-specific PMOs to reduce the cell-free translation of a VP24 reporter, to inhibit the in vitro replication of Ebola virus, and to protect mice against lethal challenge when the PMOs are delivered prior to infection. Additionally, structure-activity relationship evaluations were conducted to assess the enhancement of antiviral efficacy associated with PMO chemical modifications that included conjugation with peptides of various lengths and compositions, positioning of conjugated peptides to either the 5' or the 3' terminus, and the conferring of charge modifications by the addition of piperazine moieties. Conjugation with arginine-rich peptides greatly enhanced the antiviral efficacy of VP24-specific PMOs in infected cells and mice during lethal Ebola virus challenge.

PMCID: PMC2681561 PMID: 19223614 [PubMed - indexed for MEDLINE]

1406. Expert Rev Anti Infect Ther. 2009 May;7(4):423-35. doi: 10.1586/eri.09.13.

Fibroblastic reticular cells and their role in viral hemorrhagic fevers.

Steele KE(1), Anderson AO, Mohamadzadeh M.

Author information: (1)Division of Pathology, US Army Medical Research Institute of Infectious Diseases, 1425 Porter Street, Frederick, MD 21702, USA. keith.steele1@us.army.mil

Viral hemorrhagic fevers (VHFs) caused by Ebola, Marburg and Lassa viruses often manifest as multiple organ dysfunction and hemorrhagic shock with high mortality. These viruses target numerous cell types, including monocytes and dendritic cells, which are primary early targets that mediate critical pathogenetic processes. This review focuses on fibroblastic reticular cells (FRCs), another prevalent infected cell type that is known as a key regulator of circulatory and immune functions. Viral infection of FRCs could have debilitating effects in secondary lymphoid organs and various other tissues. FRCs may also contribute to the spread of these deadly viruses throughout the body. Here, we review the salient features of these VHFs and the biology of FRCs, emphasizing the potential role of these cells in VHFs and the rapid deterioration of immune and hemovascular sytems that are characteristic of such acute infections.

PMID: 19400762 [PubMed - indexed for MEDLINE]

1407. J Virol. 2009 May;83(9):4508-19. doi: 10.1128/JVI.02429-08. Epub 2009 Feb 18.

The marburg virus 3' noncoding region structurally and functionally differs from that of ebola virus.

Enterlein S(1), Schmidt KM, Schümann M, Conrad D, Krähling V, Olejnik J, Mühlberger E.

Author information: (1)Institute of Virology, Philipps University Marburg, Marburg, Germany.

We have previously shown that the first transcription start signal (TSS) of Zaire Ebola virus (ZEBOV) is involved in formation of an RNA secondary structure regulating VP30-dependent transcription activation. Interestingly, transcription of Marburg virus (MARV) minigenomes occurs independently of VP30. In this study, we analyzed the structure of the MARV 3' noncoding region and its influence on VP30 necessity. Secondary structure formation of the TSS of the first gene was experimentally determined and showed substantial differences from the structure formed by the ZEBOV TSS. Chimeric MARV minigenomes mimicking the ZEBOV-specific RNA secondary structure were neither transcribed nor replicated. Mapping of the MARV genomic replication promoter revealed that the region homologous to the sequence involved in formation of the regulatory ZEBOV RNA structure is part of the MARV promoter. The MARV promoter is contained within the first 70 nucleotides of the genome and consists of two elements separated by a spacer region, comprising the TSS of the first gene. Mutations within the spacer abolished transcription activity and led to increased replication, indicating competitive transcription and replication initiation. The second promoter element is located within the nontranslated region of the first gene and consists of a stretch of three UN(5) hexamers. Recombinant full-length MARV clones, in which the three conserved U residues were substituted, could not be rescued, underlining the importance of the UN(5) hexamers for replication activity. Our data suggest that differences in the structure of the genomic replication promoters might account for the different transcription strategies of Marburg and Ebola viruses.

PMCID: PMC2668471 PMID: 19225002 [PubMed - indexed for MEDLINE]

1408. Nat Rev Microbiol. 2009 May;7(5):393-400. doi: 10.1038/nrmicro2129.

Correlates of protective immunity for Ebola vaccines: implications for regulatory approval by the animal rule.

Sullivan NJ(1), Martin JE, Graham BS, Nabel GJ.

Author information: (1)Biodefense Research Section, Bethesda, Maryland 20892, USA. nsullivan@nih.gov

Erratum in Nat Rev Microbiol. 2009 Sep;7(9):684.

Ebola virus infection is a highly lethal disease for which there are no effective therapeutic or preventive treatments. Several vaccines have provided immune protection in laboratory animals, but because outbreaks occur unpredictably and sporadically, vaccine efficacy cannot be proven in human trials, which is required for traditional regulatory approval. The Food and Drug Administration has introduced the 'animal rule', to allow laboratory animal data to be used to show efficacy when human trials are not logistically feasible. In this Review, we describe immune correlates of vaccine protection against Ebola virus in animals. This research provides a basis for bridging the gap from basic research to human vaccine responses in support of the licensing of vaccines through the animal rule.

PMID: 19369954 [PubMed - indexed for MEDLINE]

1409. Infect Disord Drug Targets. 2009 Apr;9(2):191-200.

Drug targets in infections with Ebola and Marburg viruses.

Gene OG(1), Julia BE, Vanessa MR, Victoria WJ, Thomas GW, Lisa HE.

Author information: (1)United States Army Medical Research Institute of Infectious Diseases, Division of Virology, Frederick, Maryland 21702-5011, USA.

The development of antiviral drugs for Ebola and Marburg viruses has been slow. To date, beyond supportive care, no effective treatments, prophylactic measures, therapies, or vaccines are approved to treat or prevent filovirus infections. In this review, we examine the current treatments available to administer care for filovirus infection, the potential therapeutic targets that can be used for filovirus drug development, and the various drug targeting techniques used against filoviruses.

PMID: 19275706 [PubMed - indexed for MEDLINE]

1410. J Vet Med Sci. 2009 Apr;71(4):505-7.

Generation of vero cells expressing ebola virus glycoprotein.

Makino A(1), Kawaoka Y.

Author information: (1)Division of Virology, Department of Microbiology and Immunology, Institute of Medical Science, The University of Tokyo, Japan.

To establish replication-incompetent Ebola virus (EBOV) lacking its glycoprotein (GP), we attempted to generate a Vero cell line that constitutively expressed GP. We used a retroviral vector to transduce Vero cells with the EBOV GP gene, resulting in a high expression level of GP on the cell surface. The Vero cells expressing EBOV GP complemented the replication cycle of vesicular stomatitis virus, which lacks the essential viral glycoprotein. This cell line might be useful for basic research on EBOV GP as well as for vaccine production.

PMID: 19420858 [PubMed - indexed for MEDLINE]

1411. J Virol. 2009 Apr;83(8):3810-5. doi: 10.1128/JVI.00074-09. Epub 2009 Feb 11.

Replication-deficient ebolavirus as a vaccine candidate.

Halfmann P(1), Ebihara H, Marzi A, Hatta Y, Watanabe S, Suresh M, Neumann G, Feldmann H, Kawaoka Y.

Author information: (1)Department of Pathobiological Sciences, School of Veterinary Medicine, University of Wisconsin-Madison, Madison, Wisconsin 53706, USA.
Ebolavirus causes severe hemorrhagic fever, with case fatality rates as high as 90%. Currently, no licensed vaccine is available against Ebolavirus. We previously generated a replication-deficient, biologically contained Ebolavirus, EbolaDeltaVP30, which lacks the essential VP30 gene, grows only in cells stably expressing this gene product, and is genetically stable. Here, we evaluated the vaccine potential of EbolaDeltaVP30. First, we demonstrated its safety in STAT-1-knockout mice, a susceptible animal model for Ebolavirus infection. We then tested its protective efficacy in two animal models, mice and guinea pigs. Mice immunized twice with EbolaDeltaVP30 were protected from a lethal infection of mouse-adapted Ebolavirus. Virus titers in the serum of vaccinated mice were significantly lower than those in nonvaccinated mice. Protection of mice immunized with EbolaDeltaVP30 was associated with a high antibody response to the Ebolavirus glycoprotein and the generation of an Ebolavirus NP-specific CD8(+) T-cell response. Guinea pigs immunized twice with EbolaDeltaVP30 were also protected from a lethal infection of guinea pig-adapted Ebolavirus. Our study demonstrates the potential of the EbolaDeltaVP30 virus as a new vaccine platform.

PMCID: PMC2663241 PMID: 19211761 [PubMed - indexed for MEDLINE]

1412. J Virol. 2009 Apr;83(7):3069-77. doi: 10.1128/JVI.01875-08. Epub 2009 Jan 19.

Ebola virus protein VP35 impairs the function of interferon regulatory factor-activating kinases IKKepsilon and TBK-1.

Prins KC(1), Cárdenas WB, Basler CF.

Author information: (1)Department of Microbiology, Mount Sinai School of Medicine, New York, New York 10029, USA.

The Ebola virus (EBOV) VP35 protein antagonizes the early antiviral alpha/beta interferon (IFN-alpha/beta) response. We previously demonstrated that VP35 inhibits the virus-induced activation of the IFN-beta promoter by blocking the phosphorylation of IFN-regulatory factor 3 (IRF-3), a transcription factor that is crucial for the induction of IFN-alpha/beta expression. Furthermore, VP35 blocks IFN-beta promoter activation induced by any of several components of the retinoic acid-inducible gene I (RIG-I)/melanoma differentiation-associated gene 5 (MDA-5)-activated signaling pathways including RIG-I, IFN-beta promoter stimulator I (IPS-I), TANK-binding kinase I (TBK-1), and IkappaB kinase epsilon (IKKepsilon). These results suggested that VP35 may target the IRF kinases TBK-1 and IKKepsilon. Coimmunoprecipitation experiments now demonstrate physical interactions of VP35 with IKKepsilon and TBK-1, and the use of an IKKepsilon deletion construct further demonstrates that the amino-terminal kinase domain of IKKepsilon is sufficient for interactions with either IRF-3 or VP35. In vitro, either IKKepsilon or TBK-1 phosphorylates not only IRF-3 but also VP35. Moreover, VP35 overexpression impairs IKKepsilon-IRF-3, IKKepsilon-IRF-7, and IKKepsilon-IPS-I interactions. Finally, lysates from cells overexpressing IKKepsilon contain kinase activity that can phosphorylate IRF-3 in vitro. When VP35 is expressed in the IKKepsilon-expressing cells, this kinase activity is suppressed. These data suggest that VP35 exerts its IFN-antagonist function, at least in part, by blocking necessary interactions between the kinases IKKepsilon and TBK-1 and their normal interaction partners, including their substrates, IRF-3 and IRF-7.

PMCID: PMC2655579 PMID: 19153231 [PubMed - indexed for MEDLINE]

1413. J Virol. 2009 Apr;83(7):2883-91. doi: 10.1128/JVI.01956-08. Epub 2009 Jan 14.

The primed ebolavirus glycoprotein (19-kilodalton GP1,2): sequence and residues critical for host cell binding.

Dube D(1), Brecher MB, Delos SE, Rose SC, Park EW, Schornberg KL, Kuhn JH, White JM.

Author information: (1)Department of Cell Biology, University of Virginia, Charlottesville, Virginia 22908-0732, USA.

Entry of ebolavirus (EBOV) into cells is mediated by its glycoprotein (GP(1,2)), a class I fusion protein whose structure was recently determined (J. E. Lee et al., Nature 454:177-182, 2008). Here we confirmed two major predictions of the structural analysis, namely, the residues in GP(1) and GP(2) that remain after GP(1,2) is proteolytically primed by endosomal cathepsins for fusion and residues in GP(1) that are critical for binding to host cells. Mass spectroscopic analysis indicated that primed GP(1,2) contains residues 33 to 190 of GP(1) and all residues of GP(2). The location of the receptor binding site was determined by a two-pronged approach. We identified a small receptor binding region (RBR), residues 90 to 149 of GP(1), by comparing the cell binding abilities of four RBR proteins

produced in high yield. We characterized the binding properties of the optimal RBR (containing GP(1) residues 57 to 149) and then conducted a mutational analysis to identify critical binding residues. Substitutions at four lysines (K95, K114, K115, and K140) decreased binding and the ability of RBR proteins to inhibit GP(1,2)-mediated infection. K114, K115, and K140 lie in a small region modeled to be located on the top surface of the chalice following proteolytic priming; K95 lies deeper in the chalice bowl. Combined with those of Lee et al., our findings provide structural insight into how GP(1,2) is primed for fusion and define the core of the EBOV RBR (residues 90 to 149 of GP(1)) as a highly conserved region containing a two-stranded beta-sheet, the two intra-GP(1) disulfide bonds, and four critical Lys residues.
PMCID: PMC2655554 PMID: 19144707 [PubMed - indexed for MEDLINE]
1414. Virol Sin. 2009 Apr;24(2):121-135.

The Role of the Charged Residues of the GP2 Helical Regions in Ebola Entry().

Jiang H(1), Wang J, Manicassamy B, Manicassamy S, Caffrey M, Rong L.

Author information: (1)Department of Microbiology and Immunology, College of Medicine, University of Illinois at Chicag.

The glycoprotein (GP) of Ebola is the sole structural protein that forms the spikes on the viral envelope. The GP contains two subunits, GP1 and GP2, linked by a disulfide bond, which are responsible for receptor binding and membrane fusion, respectively. In this study, the full length of GP gene of Ebola Zaire species, 2028 base pairs in length, was synthesized using 38 overlapping oligonucleotides by multiple rounds of polymerase chain reaction (PCR). The synthesized GP gene was shown to be efficiently expressed in mammalian cells. Furthermore, an efficient HIV-based pseudotyping system was developed using the synthetic GP gene, providing a safe approach to dissecting the entry mechanism of Ebola viruses. Using this pseudotyping system and mutational analysis, the role of the charged residues in the GP2 helical regions was examined. It was found that substitutions of the most charged residues in the regions did not adversely affect GP expression, processing, or viral incorporation, however, most of the mutations greatly impaired the ability of GP to mediate efficient viral infection. These results demonstrate that these charged residues of GP2 play an important role in GP-mediated Ebola entry into its host cells. We propose that these charged residues are involved in forming the intermediate conformation(s) of GP in membrane fusion and Ebola entry.
PMCID: PMC3516429 PMID: 23227032 [PubMed]
1415. BMJ. 2009 Mar 23;338:b1223. doi: 10.1136/bmj.b1223.

Experimental vaccine may have saved Hamburg scientist from Ebola fever.

Tuffs A.

PMID: 19307268 [PubMed - indexed for MEDLINE]
1416. Structure. 2009 Mar 11;17(3):427-37. doi: 10.1016/j.str.2008.12.020.

Three-dimensional structure of AAA ATPase Vps4: advancing structural insights into the mechanisms of endosomal sorting and enveloped virus budding.

Landsberg MJ(1), Vajjhala PR, Rothnagel R, Munn AL, Hankamer B.

Author information: (1)Institute for Molecular Bioscience, The University of Queensland, St. Lucia QLD 4072, Australia.

Vps4 is a AAA ATPase that mediates endosomal membrane protein sorting. It is also a host factor hijacked by a diverse set of clinically important viruses, including HIV and Ebola, to facilitate viral budding. Here we present the three-dimensional structure of the hydrolysis-defective Vps4p(E233Q) mutant. Single-particle analysis, multiangle laser light scattering, and the docking of independently determined atomic models of Vps4 monomers reveal a complex with C6 point symmetry, distinguishing between a range of previously suggested oligomeric states (8-14 subunits). The 3D reconstruction also reveals a tail-to-tail subunit organization between the two rings of the complex and identifies the location of domains critical to complex assembly and interaction with partner proteins. Our refined Vps4 structure is better supported by independent lines of evidence than those previously proposed, and provides insights into the mechanism of endosomal membrane protein sorting and viral envelope budding.
PMID: 19278657 [PubMed - indexed for MEDLINE]
1417. Proc Natl Acad Sci U S A. 2009 Mar 10;106(10):3710-5. doi: 10.1073/pnas.0808101106. Epub 2009 Feb 23.

Crystal structure of the Borna disease virus matrix protein (BDV-M) reveals ssRNA binding properties.

Neumann P(1), Lieber D, Meyer S, Dautel P, Kerth A, Kraus I, Garten W, Stubbs MT.

Author information: (1)Institut für Biochemie und Biotechnologie, Martin-Luther-Universität Halle-Wittenberg, Kurt-Mothes-Strasse 3, D-06120 Halle (Saale), Germany.

Borna disease virus (BDV) is a neurotropic enveloped RNA virus that causes a noncytolytic, persistent infection of the central nervous system in mammals. BDV belongs to the order Mononegavirales, which also includes the negative-strand RNA viruses (NSVs) Ebola, Marburg, vesicular stomatitis, rabies, mumps, and measles. BDV-M, the matrix protein (M-protein) of BDV, is the smallest M-protein (16.2 kDa) among the NSVs. M-proteins play a critical role in virus assembly and budding, mediating the interaction between the viral capsid, envelope, and glycoprotein spikes, and are as such responsible for the structural stability and individual form of virus particles. Here, we report the 3D structure of BDV-M, a full-length M-protein structure from a nonsegmented RNA NSV. The BDV-M monomer exhibits structural similarity to the N-terminal domain of the Ebola M-protein (VP40), while the surface charge of the tetramer provides clues to the membrane association of BDV-M. Additional electron density in the crystal reveals the presence of bound nucleic acid, interpreted as cytidine-5'-monophosphate. The heterologously expressed BDV-M copurifies with and protects ssRNA oligonucleotides of a median length of 16 nt taken up from the expression host. The results presented here show that BDV-M would be able to bind RNA and lipid membranes simultaneously, expanding the repertoire of M-protein functionalities.
PMCID: PMC2656145 PMID: 19237566 [PubMed - indexed for MEDLINE]

1418. Antiviral Res. 2009 Mar;81(3):189-97. doi: 10.1016/j.antiviral.2008.12.003. Epub 2008 Dec 27.

No exit: targeting the budding process to inhibit filovirus replication.

Harty RN(1).

Author information: (1)Department of Pathobiology, School of Veterinary Medicine, University of Pennsylvania, 3800 Spruce Street, Philadelphia, PA 19104, USA. rharty@vet.upenn.edu

The filoviruses, Ebola and Marburg, cause severe hemorrhagic fever in humans and nonhuman primates, with high mortality rates. Although the filovirus replication pathway is now understood in considerable detail, no antiviral drugs have yet been developed that directly inhibit steps in the replication cycle. One potential target is the filovirus VP40 matrix protein, the key viral protein that drives the budding process, in part by mediating specific virus-host interactions to facilitate the efficient release of virions from the infected cell. This review will summarize current knowledge of key structural and functional domains of VP40 believed to be necessary for efficient budding of virions and virus-like particles. A better understanding of the structure and function of these key regions of VP40 will be crucial, as they may represent novel and rational targets for inhibitors of filovirus egress.

PMCID: PMC2666966 PMID: 19114059 [PubMed - indexed for MEDLINE]

1419. Curr Mol Med. 2009 Mar;9(2):174-85.

Potential factors induced by filoviruses that lead to immune supression.

Mohamadzadeh M(1).

Author information: (1)Northwestern University, School of Medicine, Chicago, IL 60611, USA. m.zadeh@northwestern.edu

The filoviruses, Ebola (EBOV) and Marburg (MARV), are among the deadliest of human pathogens, causing acute diseases typified by rapidly fatal hemorrhagic fevers. Upon filoviral infection, innate immune cells become paralyzed and lose the capacity to properly co-stimulate and activate filovirus-specific, T-cell responses. Deleterious inflammation and upregulation of co-inhibitory molecules expressed by monocytic lineage cells (e.g., dendritic cells) and their co-inhibitory receptors on T- and B-cells may lead to incomplete humoral and T-cell immunity, anergy, exhaustion, apoptosis, and subsequent immune subversion. Hence, the dysregulation of inflammatory and co-inhibitory molecules may be exploited by filoviruses to further deteriorate host immune responses, ultimately leading to fulminant infections in susceptible species. Thus, in light of accumulating scientific observations, the challenge is now to characterize the molecular mechanisms that may result in rational strategies leading to new therapeutics and vaccines.

PMID: 19275625 [PubMed - indexed for MEDLINE]

1420. Immunotherapy. 2009 Mar;1(2):187-97. doi: 10.2217/1750743X.1.2.187.

Fibroblastic reticular cell infection by hemorrhagic fever viruses.

Steele KE(1), Anderson AO, Mohamadzadeh M.

Author information: (1)Division of Pathology, US Army Medical Research Institute of Infectious Diseases, 1425 Porter Street, Frederick, MD 21702, USA. keith.steele1@us.army.mil

Viral hemorrhagic fevers (VHFs) often cause high mortality with high infectivity, multiorgan failure, shock and hemorrhagic diathesis. Fibroblastic reticular cells (FRCs) within secondary lymphoid organs provide a supporting scaffold to T-lymphocyte areas. These cells regulate the movement of various immune cells and soluble molecules that promote T-lymphocyte homeostasis. We previously reported Ebola virus infection of FRCs, but ascribed little significance to this finding. Here, we studied infection of FRCs by Ebola, Marburg and Lassa viruses. We demonstrate that FRCs, or the extracellular 'conduit' of the fibroblastic reticulum of nonhuman primates, are targets of Ebola, Marburg and Lassa viruses. Furthermore, we observed that FRC damage correlates temporally and spatially with lymphocyte damage and that FRCs serve as nidi of fibrin deposition. In addition, we show that nonhuman primate FRCs express p75 NGF receptor and tissue transglutaminase. Our data suggest that viral infection of FRCs may be crucial to the immunological dysfunction and coagulopathy characteristic of VHFs. We further propose that p75 NGF receptor and tissue transglutaminase may be involved in FRC-associated dysfunction during the course of infection.

PMID: 20635940 [PubMed - indexed for MEDLINE]

1421. Virus Res. 2009 Mar;140(1-2):8-14. doi: 10.1016/j.virusres.2008.10.017. Epub 2008 Dec 16.

The Ebola virus ribonucleoprotein complex: a novel VP30-L interaction identified.

Groseth A(1), Charton JE, Sauerborn M, Feldmann F, Jones SM, Hoenen T, Feldmann H.

Author information: (1)National Laboratory for Zoonotic Diseases and Special Pathogens, National Microbiology Laboratory, Public Health Agency of Canada, 1015 Arlington Street, Winnipeg R3E 3R2, Canada. groseth@staff.uni-marburg.de

The ribonucleoprotein (RNP) complex of Ebola virus (EBOV) is known to be a multiprotein/RNA structure, however, knowledge is rather limited regarding the actual protein-protein interactions involved in its formation. Here we show that singularly expressed VP35 and VP30 are present throughout the cytoplasm, while NP forms prominent cytoplasmic inclusions and L forms smaller perinuclear inclusions. We could demonstrate the existence of NP-VP35, NP-VP30 and VP35-L interactions, similar to those described for Marburg virus (MARV) based on the redistribution of protein partners into NP and L inclusion bodies. Significantly, a novel VP30-L interaction was also identified and found to form as part of an NP-VP30-L bridge structure, similar to that formed by VP35. The identification of these interactions allows a preliminary model of the EBOV RNP complex structure to be proposed, and may provide insight into filovirus transcriptional regulation.

PMCID: PMC3398801 PMID: 19041915 [PubMed - indexed for MEDLINE]

1422. Proc Natl Acad Sci U S A. 2009 Feb 24;106(8):2886-91. doi: 10.1073/pnas.0811014106. Epub 2009 Jan 28.

Tetherin-mediated restriction of filovirus budding is antagonized by the Ebola glycoprotein.

Kaletsky RL(1), Francica JR, Agrawal-Gamse C, Bates P.

Author information: (1)Department of Microbiology, School of Medicine, University of Pennsylvania, 225 Johnson Pavilion, 3610 Hamilton Walk, Philadelphia, PA 19104-6076, USA.

Mammalian cells employ numerous innate cellular mechanisms to inhibit viral replication and spread. Tetherin, also known as Bst-2 or CD317, is a recently identified, IFN-induced, cellular response factor that blocks release of HIV-1 and other retroviruses from infected cells. The means by which tetherin retains retroviruses on the cell surface, as well as the mechanism used by the HIV-1 accessory protein Vpu to antagonize tetherin function and promote HIV-1 release, are unknown. Here, we document that tetherin functions as a broadly acting antiviral factor by demonstrating that both human and murine tetherin potently inhibit the release of the filovirus, Ebola, from the surface of cells. Expression of the Ebola glycoprotein (GP) antagonized the antiviral effect of human and murine tetherin and facilitated budding of Ebola particles, as did the HIV-1 Vpu protein. Conversely, Ebola GP could substitute for Vpu to promote HIV-1 virion release from tetherin-expressing cells, demonstrating a common cellular target for these divergent viral proteins. Ebola GP efficiently coimmunoprecipitated with tetherin, suggesting that the viral glycoprotein directly interferes with this host antiviral factor. These results demonstrate that tetherin is a cellular antiviral factor that restricts budding of structurally diverse enveloped viruses. Additionally, Ebola has evolved a highly effective strategy to combat this antiviral response elicited in the host during infection.

PMCID: PMC2650360 PMID: 19179289 [PubMed - indexed for MEDLINE]

1423. Wkly Epidemiol Rec. 2009 Feb 13;84(7):49-50.

Outbreak news. Ebola Reston in pigs and humans, Philippines.

[Article in English, French]

[No authors listed]

PMID: 19219963 [PubMed - indexed for MEDLINE]

1424. Acta Crystallogr Sect F Struct Biol Cryst Commun. 2009 Feb 1;65(Pt 2):163-5. doi: 10.1107/S1744309108044187. Epub 2009 Jan 31.

Expression, purification, crystallization and preliminary X-ray studies of the Ebola VP35 interferon inhibitory domain.

Leung DW(1), Ginder ND, Nix JC, Basler CF, Honzatko RB, Amarasinghe GK.

Author information: (1)Department of Biochemistry, Biophysics and Molecular Biology, Iowa State University, Ames, IA 50011, USA.

Ebola VP35 is a multifunctional protein that is important for host immune suppression and pathogenesis. VP35 contains an N-terminal oligomerization domain and a C-terminal interferon inhibitory domain (IID). Mutations within the VP35 IID result in loss of host immune suppression. Here, efforts to crystallize recombinantly overexpressed VP35 IID that was purified from Escherichia coli are described. Native and selenomethionine-labeled crystals belonging to the orthorhombic space group P2(1)2(1)2(1) were obtained by the hanging-drop vapor-diffusion method and diffraction data were collected at the ALS synchrotron.

PMCID: PMC2635856 PMID: 19194011 [PubMed - indexed for MEDLINE]

1425. J Virol. 2009 Feb;83(4):1837-44. doi: 10.1128/JVI.02211-08. Epub 2008 Nov 26.

Broad-spectrum inhibition of retroviral and filoviral particle release by tetherin.

Jouvenet N(1), Neil SJ, Zhadina M, Zang T, Kratovac Z, Lee Y, McNatt M, Hatziioannou T, Bieniasz PD.

Author information: (1)Aaron Diamond AIDS Research Center, Rockefeller University, New York, New York, USA.

The expression of many putative antiviral genes is upregulated when cells encounter type I interferon (IFN), but the actual mechanisms by which many IFN-induced gene products inhibit virus replication are poorly understood. A recently identified IFN-induced antiretroviral protein, termed tetherin (previously known as BST-2 or CD317), blocks the release of nascent human immunodeficiency virus type 1 (HIV-1) particles from infected cells, and an HIV-1 accessory protein, Vpu, acts as a viral antagonist of tetherin. Here, we show that tetherin is capable of blocking not only the release of HIV-1 particles but also the release of particles assembled using the major structural proteins of a variety of prototype retroviruses, including members of the alpharetrovirus, betaretrovirus, deltaretrovirus, lentivirus, and spumaretrovirus families. Moreover, we show that the release of particles assembled using filovirus matrix proteins from Marburg virus and Ebola virus is also sensitive to inhibition by tetherin. These findings indicate that tetherin is a broadly specific inhibitor of enveloped particle release, and therefore, inhibition is unlikely to require specific interactions with viral proteins. Nonetheless, tetherin colocalized with nascent virus-like particles generated by several retroviral and filoviral structural proteins, indicating that it is present at, or recruited to, sites of particle assembly. Overall, tetherin is potentially active against many enveloped viruses and likely to be an important component of the antiviral innate immune defense.

PMCID: PMC2643743 PMID: 19036818 [PubMed - indexed for MEDLINE]

1426. Euro Surveill. 2009 Jan 29;14(4). pii: 19105.

Ebola Reston virus detected pigs in the Philippines.

Editorial team.

PMID: 19215709 [PubMed - indexed for MEDLINE]

1427. Science. 2009 Jan 23;323(5913):451. doi: 10.1126/science.323.5913.451a.

Emerging infectious diseases. Scientists puzzle over Ebola-Reston virus in pigs.

Normile D.

PMID: 19164717 [PubMed - indexed for MEDLINE]

1428. Nature. 2009 Jan 22;457(7228):364-5. doi: 10.1038/457364b.

Ebola outbreak has experts rooting for answers.

Cyranoski D.

PMID: 19158753 [PubMed - indexed for MEDLINE]

1429. Virology. 2009 Jan 20;383(2):237-47. doi: 10.1016/j.virol.2008.10.029. Epub 2008 Nov 14.

Requirements for cell rounding and surface protein down-regulation by Ebola virus glycoprotein.

Francica JR(1), Matukonis MK, Bates P.

Author information: (1)Department of Microbiology, University of Pennsylvania School of Medicine, Philadelphia, 19104-6076, USA.

Ebola virus causes an acute hemorrhagic fever that is associated with high morbidity and mortality. The viral glycoprotein is thought to contribute to pathogenesis, though precise mechanisms are unknown. Cellular pathogenesis can be modeled in vitro by expression of the Ebola viral glycoprotein (GP) in cells, which causes dramatic morphological changes, including cell rounding and surface protein down-regulation. These effects are known to be dependent on the presence of a highly glycosylated region of the glycoprotein, the mucin domain. Here we show that the mucin domain from the highly pathogenic Zaire subtype of Ebola virus is sufficient to cause characteristic cytopathology when expressed in the context of a foreign glycoprotein. Similarly to full length Ebola GP, expression of the mucin domain causes rounding, detachment from the extracellular matrix, and the down-regulation of cell surface levels of beta1 integrin and major histocompatibility complex class I. These effects were not seen when the mucin domain was expressed in the context of a glycophosphatidylinositol-anchored isoform of the foreign glycoprotein. In contrast to earlier analysis of full length Ebola glycoproteins, chimeras carrying the mucin domains from the Zaire and Reston strains appear to cause similar levels of down-modulation and cell detachment. Cytopathology associated with Ebola glycoprotein expression does not occur when GP expression is restricted to the endoplasmic reticulum. In contrast to a previously published report, our results demonstrate that GP-induced surface protein down-regulation is not mediated through a dynamin-dependent pathway. Overall, these results support a model in which the mucin domain of Ebola GP acts at the cell surface to induce protein down modulation and cytopathic effects.

PMCID: PMC2654768 PMID: 19013626 [PubMed - indexed for MEDLINE]

1430. Virology. 2009 Jan 20;383(2):348-61. doi: 10.1016/j.virol.2008.09.030. Epub 2008 Nov 17.

Chimeric human parainfluenza virus bearing the Ebola virus glycoprotein as the sole surface protein is immunogenic and highly protective against Ebola virus challenge.

Bukreyev A(1), Marzi A, Feldmann F, Zhang L, Yang L, Ward JM, Dorward DW, Pickles RJ, Murphy BR, Feldmann H, Collins PL.

Author information: (1)National Institute of Allergy and Infectious Diseases, Building 50, Room 6505, NIAID, National Institutes of Health, 50 South Dr. MSC 8007, Bethesda, MD 20892-8007, USA. abukreyev@nih.gov

We generated a new live-attenuated vaccine against Ebola virus (EBOV) based on a chimeric virus HPIV3/DeltaF-HN/EboGP that contains the EBOV glycoprotein (GP) as the sole transmembrane envelope protein combined with the internal proteins of human parainfluenza virus type 3 (HPIV3). Electron microscopy analysis of the virus particles showed that they have an envelope and surface spikes resembling those of EBOV and a particle size and shape resembling those of HPIV3. When HPIV3/DeltaF-HN/EboGP was inoculated via apical surface of an in vitro model of human ciliated airway epithelium, the virus was released from the apical surface; when applied to basolateral surface, the virus infected basolateral cells but did not spread through the tissue. Following intranasal (IN) inoculation of guinea pigs, scattered infected cells were detected in the lungs by immunohistochemistry, but infectious HPIV3/DeltaF-HN/EboGP could not be recovered from the lungs, blood, or other tissues. Despite the attenuation, the virus was highly immunogenic, and a single IN dose completely protected the animals against a highly lethal intraperitoneal challenge of guinea pig-adapted EBOV.

PMCID: PMC2649782 PMID: 19010509 [PubMed - indexed for MEDLINE]

1431. Proc Natl Acad Sci U S A. 2009 Jan 13;106(2):411-6. doi: 10.1073/pnas.0807854106. Epub 2009 Jan 2.

Structure of the Ebola VP35 interferon inhibitory domain.

Leung DW(1), Ginder ND, Fulton DB, Nix J, Basler CF, Honzatko RB, Amarasinghe GK.

Author information: (1)Department of Biochemistry, Biophysics and Molecular Biology, Iowa State University, Ames, IA 50011, USA.

Ebola viruses (EBOVs) cause rare but highly fatal outbreaks of viral hemorrhagic fever in humans, and approved treatments for these infections are currently lacking. The Ebola VP35 protein is multifunctional, acting as a component of the viral RNA polymerase complex, a viral assembly factor, and an inhibitor of host interferon (IFN) production. Mutation of select basic residues within the C-terminal half of VP35 abrogates its dsRNA-binding activity, impairs VP35-mediated IFN antagonism, and attenuates EBOV growth in vitro and in vivo. Because VP35 contributes to viral escape from host innate immunity and is required for EBOV virulence, understanding the structural basis for VP35 dsRNA binding, which correlates with suppression of IFN activity, is of high importance. Here, we report the structure of the C-terminal VP35 IFN inhibitory domain (IID) solved to a resolution of 1.4 A and show that VP35 IID forms a unique fold. In the structure, we identify 2 basic residue clusters, one of which is important for dsRNA binding. The dsRNA binding cluster is centered on Arg-312, a highly conserved residue required for IFN inhibition. Mutation of residues within this cluster significantly changes the surface electrostatic potential and diminishes dsRNA binding activity. The high-resolution structure and the identification of the conserved dsRNA binding residue cluster provide opportunities for antiviral therapeutic design. Our results suggest a structure-based model for dsRNA-mediated innate immune antagonism by Ebola VP35 and other similarly constructed viral antagonists.

PMCID: PMC2626716 PMID: 19122151 [PubMed - indexed for MEDLINE]

1432. Am J Transl Res. 2009 Jan 5;1(1):87-98.

FGI-104: a broad-spectrum small molecule inhibitor of viral infection.

Kinch MS, Yunus AS, Lear C, Mao H, Chen H, Fesseha Z, Luo G, Nelson EA, Li L, Huang Z, Murray M, Ellis WY, Hensley L, Christopher-Hennings J, Olinger GG, Goldblatt M.

The treatment of viral diseases remains an intractable problem facing the medical community. Conventional antivirals focus upon selective targeting of virus-encoded targets. However, the plasticity of viral nucleic acid mutation, coupled with the large number of progeny that can emerge from a single infected cells, often conspire to render conventional antivirals ineffective as resistant variants emerge. Compounding this, new viral pathogens are increasingly recognized and it is highly improbable that conventional approaches could address emerging pathogens in a timely manner. Our laboratories have adopted an orthogonal approach to combat viral disease: Target the host to deny the pathogen the ability to cause disease. The advantages of this novel approach are many-fold, including the potential to identify host pathways that are applicable to a broad-spectrum of pathogens. The acquisition of drug resistance might also be minimized since selective pressure is not directly placed upon the viral pathogen. Herein, we utilized this strategy of host-oriented therapeutics to screen small molecules for their abilities to block infection by multiple, unrelated virus types and identified FGI-104. FGI-104 demonstrates broad-spectrum inhibition of multiple blood-borne pathogens (HCV, HBV, HIV) as well as emerging biothreats (Ebola, VEE, Cowpox, PRRSV infection). We also demonstrate that FGI-104 displays an ability to prevent lethality from Ebola in vivo. Altogether, these findings reinforce the concept of host-oriented therapeutics and present a much-needed opportunity to identify antiviral drugs that are broad-spectrum and durable in their application.

PMCID: PMC2776286 PMID: 19966942 [PubMed]

1433. Virology. 2009 Jan 5;383(1):12-21. doi: 10.1016/j.virol.2008.09.020. Epub 2008 Nov 4.

Protection against lethal challenge by Ebola virus-like particles produced in insect cells.

Sun Y(1), Carrion R Jr, Ye L, Wen Z, Ro YT, Brasky K, Ticer AE, Schwegler EE, Patterson JL, Compans RW, Yang C.

Author information: (1)Department of Microbiology and Immunology and Emory Vaccine Center, Emory University School of Medicine, 1510 Clifton Road, Room 3086 Rollins Research Center, Atlanta, GA 30322, USA.

Erratum in Virology. 2010 Mar 30;399(1):186.

Ebola virus-like particles (VLPs) were produced in insect cells using a recombinant baculovirus expression system and their efficacy for protection against Ebola virus infection was investigated. Two immunizations with 50 microg Ebola VLPs (high dose) induced a high level of antibodies against Ebola GP that exhibited strong neutralizing activity against GP-mediated virus infection and conferred complete protection of vaccinated mice against lethal challenge by a high dose of mouse-adapted Ebola virus. In contrast, two immunizations with 10 microg Ebola VLPs (low dose) induced 5-fold lower levels of antibodies against GP and these mice were not protected against lethal Ebola virus challenge, similar to control mice that were immunized with 50 microg SIV Gag VLPs. However, the antibody responses against GP were boosted significantly after a third immunization with 10 microg Ebola VLPs to similar levels as those induced by two immunizations with 50 microg Ebola VLPs, and vaccinated mice were also effectively protected against lethal Ebola virus challenge. Furthermore, serum viremia levels in protected mice were either below the level of detection or significantly lower compared to the viremia levels in control mice. These results show that effective protection can be achieved by immunization with Ebola VLPs produced in insect cells, which give high production yields, and lend further support to their development as an effective vaccine strategy against Ebola virus.

PMCID: PMC2657000 PMID: 18986663 [PubMed - indexed for MEDLINE]

1434. Bull Mem Acad R Med Belg. 2009;164(1-2):7-15; discussion 15-6.

[Viruses and bats: rabies and Lyssavirus].

[Article in French]

Tordo N(1), Marianneau MP.

Author information: (1)Institut Pasteur de Paris, France.

Recent emerging zoonoses (hemorrhagic fevers due to Ebola or Marburg virus, encephalitis due to Nipah virus, severe acute respiratory syndrome due to SRAS virus...) outline the potential of bats as vectors for transmission of infectious disease to humans. Such a potential is already known for rabies encephalitis since seven out of the eight genotypes of Lyssavirus are transmitted by bats. In addition, phylogenetic reconstructions indicate that Lyssavirus have evolved in chiropters before their emergence in carnivores. Nevertheless, carnivores remain the most critical vectors for public health, in particular dogs that are originating 55.000 rabies deaths per year, essentially in developing countries. Rabies control in carnivores by parenteral (dog) or oral (wild carnivores) vaccination is efficacious and campaigns start to be more widely applied. On the other hand, rabies control in bat still remains non realistic, particularly as the pathogenicity of bat Lyssavirus for bats is still under debate, suggesting that a "diplomatic relationship" between partners would have arisen from a long term cohabitation. While comparing the interactions that humans and bats establish with Lyssavirus, scientists try to understand the molecular basis ofpathogenicity in man, a indispensable prerequisite to identify antiviral targets in a perspective of therapy.

PMID: 19718950 [PubMed - indexed for MEDLINE]

1435. Dis Model Mech. 2009 Jan-Feb;2(1-2):12-7. doi: 10.1242/dmm.000471.

Disease modeling for Ebola and Marburg viruses.

Bente D(1), Gren J, Strong JE, Feldmann H.

Author information: (1)Laboratory for Zoonotic Diseases and Special Pathogens, National Microbiology Laboratory, Public Health Agency of Canada, Winnipeg, Manitoba, Canada.

The filoviruses Ebola and Marburg are zoonotic agents that are classified as both biosafety level 4 and category A list pathogens. These viruses are pathogenic in humans and cause isolated infections or epidemics of viral hemorrhagic fever, mainly in Central Africa. Their natural reservoir has not been definitely identified, but certain species of African bat have been associated with Ebola and Marburg infections. Currently, there are no licensed options available for either treatment or prophylaxis. Different animal models have been developed for filoviruses including mouse, guinea pig and nonhuman primates. The 'gold standard' animal models for pathogenesis, treatment and vaccine studies are rhesus and cynomolgus macaques. This article provides a brief overview of the clinical picture and the pathology/pathogenesis of human filovirus infections. The current animal model options are discussed and compared with regard to their value in different applications. In general, the small animal models, in particular the mouse, are the most feasible for high biocontainment facilities and they offer the most options for research owing to the greater availability of immunologic and genetic tools. However, their mimicry of the human diseases as well as their predictive value for therapeutic efficacy in primates is limited, thereby making them, at best, valuable initial screening tools for pathophysiology, treatment and vaccine studies.

PMCID: PMC2615158 PMID: 19132113 [PubMed - indexed for MEDLINE]

1436. Future Virol. 2009;4(6):621-635.

Ebolavirus glycoprotein structure and mechanism of entry.

Lee JE(1), Saphire EO.

Author information: (1)Department of Immunology & Microbial Science, The Scripps Research Institute, 10550 North Torrey Pines Road, La Jolla, CA 92037, USA, Tel.: +1 858 784 7976.

Ebolavirus (EBOV) is a highly virulent pathogen capable of causing a severe hemorrhagic fever with 50-90% lethality. The EBOV glycoprotein (GP) is the only virally expressed protein on the virion surface and is critical for attachment to host cells and catalysis of membrane fusion. Hence, the EBOV GP is a critical component of vaccines as well as a target of neutralizing antibodies and inhibitors of attachment and fusion. The crystal structure of the Zaire ebolavirus GP in its trimeric, prefusion conformation (3 GP(1) plus 3 GP(2)) in complex with a neutralizing antibody fragment, derived from a human survivor of the 1995 Kikwit outbreak, was recently determined. This is the first near-complete structure of any filovirus glycoprotein. The overall molecular architecture of the Zaire ebolavirus GP and its role in viral entry and membrane fusion are discussed in this article.

PMCID: PMC2829775 PMID: 20198110 [PubMed]

1437. Hepatology. 2009 Jan;49(1):287-96. doi: 10.1002/hep.22678.

The pathogen receptor liver and lymph node sinusoidal endotelial cell C-type lectin is expressed in human Kupffer cells and regulated by PU.1.

Domínguez-Soto A(1), Aragoneses-Fenoll L, Gómez-Aguado F, Corcuera MT, Cláría J, García-Monzón C, Bustos M, Corbí AL.

Author information: (1)Centro de Investigaciones Biológicas, CSIC, Madrid, Spain.

Human LSECtin (liver and lymph node sinusoidal endothelial cell C-type lectin, CLEC4G) is a C-type lectin encoded within the L-SIGN/DC-SIGN/CD23 gene cluster. LSECtin acts as a pathogen attachment factor for Ebolavirus and the SARS coronavirus, and its expression can be induced by interleukin-4 on monocytes and macrophages. Although reported as a liver and lymph node sinusoidal endothelial cell-specific molecule, LSECtin could be detected in the MUTZ-3 dendritic-like cell line at the messenger RNA (mRNA) and protein level, and immunohistochemistry analysis on human liver revealed its presence in Kupffer cells coexpressing the myeloid marker CD68. The expression of LSECtin in myeloid cells was further corroborated through the analysis of the proximal regulatory region of the human LSECtin gene, whose activity was maximal in LSECtin+ myeloid cells, and which contains a highly conserved PU.1-binding site. PU.1 transactivated the LSECtin regulatory region in collaboration with hematopoietic-restricted transcription factors (Myb, RUNX3), and was found to bind constitutively to the LSECtin proximal promoter. Moreover, knockdown of PU.1 through the use of small interfering RNA led to a decrease in LSECtin mRNA levels in THP-1 and monocyte-derived dendritic cells, thus confirming the involvement of PU.1 in the myeloid expression of the lectin. CONCLUSION: LSECtin is expressed by liver myeloid cells, and its expression is dependent on the PU.1 transcription factor.

PMID: 19111020 [PubMed - indexed for MEDLINE]

1438. J Clin Virol. 2009 Jan;44(1):39-42. doi: 10.1016/j.jcv.2008.09.003. Epub 2008 Nov 1

Detection of viral RNA from paraffin-embedded tissues after prolonged formalin fixation.

McKinney MD(1), Moon SJ, Kulesh DA, Larsen T, Schoepp RJ.

Author information: (1)GEO-CENTERS, Inc., United States Army Medical Research Institute of Infectious Diseases, Fort Detrick, Frederick, MD 21702-5011, United States.

BACKGROUND: Isolating amplifiable RNA from formalin-fixed, paraffin-embedded (FFPE) tissues is more difficult than isolating DNA because of RNases, chemical modification of the RNA, and cross-linking of nucleic acids and proteins. Tissues containing infectious disease agents that require biosafety level (BSL)-3 and -4 necessitate fixation times of 21 and 30 days, respectively. OBJECTIVE: To improve procedures for extracting RNA from these FFPE tissues and detect the RNA with the more sensitive TaqManbased reverse transcriptase (RT)-PCR. STUDY DESIGN: Through a single modification of a commercially available kit, we were able to extract amplifiable RNA and detect West Nile virus (WNV), Marburg virus (MARV), and Ebola virus (EBOV)-infected tissues using TaqMan assays. RESULTS: Formalin fixation results in an approximately 2log(10) reduction in detection limit when compared to fresh tissues. Increasing proteinase K digestion (24h) improved extraction of amplifiable RNA from FFPE tissues. The TaqMan results were comparable to more traditional detection results such as virus isolation. CONCLUSION: This improved extraction procedure for obtaining RNA combined with the TaqMan RT-PCR assays permit retrospective and prospective studies on FFPE tissues infected with BSL-3 and -4 pathogens.

PMID: 18977691 [PubMed - indexed for MEDLINE]

1439. PLoS One. 2009;4(5):e5547. doi: 10.1371/journal.pone.0005547. Epub 2009 May 14.

Mucosal immunization of cynomolgus macaques with the VSVDeltaG/ZEBOVGP vaccine stimulates strong ebola GP-specific immune responses.

Qiu X(1), Fernando L, Alimonti JB, Melito PL, Feldmann F, Dick D, Ströher U, Feldmann H, Jones SM.

Author information: (1)Special Pathogens Program, National Microbiology Laboratory, Public Health Agency of Canada, Winnipeg, Manitoba, Canada.

BACKGROUND: Zaire ebolavirus (ZEBOV) produces a lethal viral hemorrhagic fever in humans and non-human primates. METHODOLOGY/PRINCIPAL FINDINGS: We demonstrate that the VSVDeltaG/ZEBOVGP vaccine given 28 days pre-challenge either intranasally (IN), orally (OR), or intramuscularly (IM) protects non-human primates against a lethal systemic challenge of ZEBOV, and induces cellular and humoral immune responses. We demonstrated that ZEBOVGP-specific T-cell and humoral responses induced in the IN and OR groups, following an immunization and challenge, produced the most IFN-gamma and IL-2 secreting cells, and long term memory responses. CONCLUSIONS/SIGNIFICANCE: We have shown conclusively that mucosal immunization can protect from systemic ZEBOV challenge and that mucosal delivery, particularly IN immunization, seems to be more potent than IM injection in the immune parameters we have tested. Mucosal immunization would be a huge benefit in any emergency mass vaccination campaign during a natural outbreak, or following intentional release, or for mucosal immunization of great apes in the wild.

PMCID: PMC2678264 PMID: 19440245 [PubMed - indexed for MEDLINE]

1440. PLoS One. 2009;4(4):e5308. doi: 10.1371/journal.pone.0005308. Epub 2009 Apr 23.

Enhanced protection against Ebola virus mediated by an improved adenovirus-based vaccine.

Richardson JS(1), Yao MK, Tran KN, Croyle MA, Strong JE, Feldmann H, Kobinger GP.

Author information: (1)Special Pathogens Program, National Microbiology Laboratory, Public Health Agency of Canada, Winnipeg, Manitoba, Canada.

BACKGROUND: The Ebola virus is transmitted by direct contact with bodily fluids of infected individuals, eliciting death rates as high as 90% among infected humans. Currently, replication defective adenovirus-based Ebola vaccine is being studied in a phase I clinical trial. Another Ebola vaccine, based on an attenuated vesicular stomatitis virus has shown efficacy in post-exposure treatment of nonhuman primates to Ebola infection. In this report, we modified the common recombinant adenovirus serotype 5-based Ebola vaccine expressing the wild-type ZEBOV glycoprotein sequence from a CMV promoter (Ad-CMVZGP). The immune response elicited by this improved expression cassette vector (Ad-CAGoptZGP) and its ability to afford protection against lethal ZEBOV challenge in mice was compared to the standard Ad-CMVZGP vector. METHODOLOGY/PRINCIPAL FINDINGS: Ad-CMVZGP was previously shown to protect mice, guinea pigs and nonhuman primates from an otherwise lethal challenge of Zaire ebolavirus. The antigenic expression cassette of this vector was improved through codon optimization, inclusion of a consensus Kozak sequence and reconfiguration of a CAG promoter (Ad-CAGoptZGP). Expression of GP from Ad-CAGoptZGP was substantially higher than from Ad-CMVZGP. Ad-CAGoptZGP significantly improved T and B cell responses at doses 10 to 100-fold lower than that needed with Ad-CMVZGP. Additionally, Ad-CAGoptZGP afforded full protections in mice against lethal challenge at a dose 100 times lower than the dose required for Ad-CMVZGP. Finally, Ad-CAGoptZGP induced full protection to mice when given 30 minutes post-challenge. CONCLUSIONS/SIGNIFICANCE: We describe an improved adenovirus-based Ebola vaccine capable of affording post-exposure protection against lethal challenge in mice. The molecular modifications of the new improved vaccine also translated in the induction of significantly enhanced immune responses and complete protection at a dose 100 times lower than with the previous generation adenovirus-based Ebola vaccine. Understanding and improving the molecular components of adenovirus-based vaccines can produce potent, optimized product, useful for vaccination and post-exposure therapy.

PMCID: PMC2669164 PMID: 19390586 [PubMed - indexed for MEDLINE]

1441. Viruses. 2009;1(3):441-459.

Simultaneous Detection of CDC Category "A" DNA and RNA Bioterrorism Agents by Use of Multiplex PCR & RT-PCR Enzyme Hybridization Assays.

He J(1), Kraft AJ, Fan J, Van Dyke M, Wang L, Bose ME, Khanna M, Metallo JA, Henrickson KJ.

Author information: (1)Department of Pediatric, Medical College of Wisconsin, Milwaukee, WI 53226, USA; jhe@mcw.edu (J.H.); akraft@mcw.edu (A.J.K.); jfan@mcw.edu (J.F.); mvandyke@mcw.edu (M.V.D.); lwang@mcw.edu (L.W.); mbose@mcw.edu (M.E.B.); jmetallo@mcw.edu (J.A.M.).

Assays to simultaneously detect multiple potential agents of bioterrorism are limited. Two multiplex PCR and RT-PCR enzyme hybridization assays (mPCR-EHA, mRT-PCR-EHA) were developed to simultaneously detect many of the CDC category "A" bioterrorism agents. The "Bio T" DNA assay was developed to detect: Variola major (VM), Bacillus anthracis (BA), Yersinia pestis (YP), Francisella tularensis (FT) and Varicella zoster virus (VZV). The "Bio T" RNA assay (mRT-PCR-EHA) was developed to detect: Ebola virus (Ebola), Lassa fever virus (Lassa), Rift Valley fever (RVF), Hantavirus Sin Nombre species (HSN) and dengue virus (serotypes 1-4). Sensitivity and specificity of the 2 assays were tested by using genomic DNA, recombinant plasmid positive controls, RNA transcripts controls, surrogate (spiked) clinical samples and common respiratory pathogens. The analytical sensitivity (limit of detection (LOD)) of the DNA asssay for genomic DNA was $1\times10(0)\sim1\times10(2)$ copies/mL for BA, FT and YP. The LOD for VZV whole organism was $1\times10(-2)$ TCID(50)/mL. The LOD for recombinant controls ranged from $1\times10(2)\sim1\times10(3)$copies/mL for BA, FT, YP and VM. The RNA assay demonstrated LOD for RNA transcript controls of $1\times10(4)\sim1\times10(6)$ copies/mL without extraction and $1\times10(5)\sim1\times10(6)$ copies/mL with extraction for Ebola, RVF, Lassa and HSN. The LOD for dengue whole organisms was $\sim1\times10(-4)$ dilution for dengue 1 and 2, $1\times10(4)$ LD(50)/mL and $1\times10(2)$ LD(50)/mL for dengue 3 and 4. The LOD without extraction for recombinant plasmid DNA controls was $\sim1\times10(3)$ copies/mL (1.5 input copies/reaction) for Ebola, RVF, Lassa and HSN. No cross-reactivity of primers and probes used in both assays was detected with common respiratory pathogens or between targeted analytes. Clinical sensitivity was estimated using 264 surrogate clinical samples tested with the BioT DNA assay and 549 samples tested with the BioT RNA assay. The clinical specificity is 99.6% and 99.8% for BioT DNA assay and BioT RNA assay, respectively. The surrogate sensitivities of these two assays were 100% (95%CI 83-100) for FT, BA (pXO2), YP, VM, VZV, dengue 2,3,4 and 95% (95%CI 75-100) for BA (pXO1) and dengue 1 using spiked clinical specimens. The specificity of both BioT multiplex assays on spiked specimens was 100% (95% CI 99-100). Compared to other available assays (culture, serology, PCR, etc.) both the BioT DNA mPCR-EHA and BioT RNA mRT-PCR-EHA are rapid, sensitive and specific assays for detecting many category "A" Bioterrorism agents using a standard thermocycler.

PMCID: PMC2836126 PMID: 20224751 [PubMed]

1442. Vaccine. 2008 Dec 9;26(52):6894-900. doi: 10.1016/j.vaccine.2008.09.082. Epub 2008 Oct 18.

Vesicular stomatitis virus-based vaccines protect nonhuman primates against aerosol challenge with Ebola and Marburg viruses.

Geisbert TW(1), Daddario-Dicaprio KM, Geisbert JB, Reed DS, Feldmann F, Grolla A, Ströher U, Fritz EA, Hensley LE, Jones SM, Feldmann H.

Author information: (1)National Emerging Infectious Diseases Laboratories Institute, Boston University School of Medicine, Boston, MA, USA. geisbert@bu.edu

Considerable progress has been made over the last decade in developing candidate preventive vaccines that can protect nonhuman primates against Ebola and Marburg viruses. A vaccine based on recombinant vesicular stomatitis virus (VSV) seems to be particularly robust as it can also confer protection when

administered as a postexposure treatment. While filoviruses are not thought to be transmitted by aerosol in nature the inhalation route is among the most likely portals of entry in the setting of a bioterrorist event. At present, all candidate filoviral vaccines have been evaluated against parenteral challenges but none have been tested against an aerosol exposure. Here, we evaluated our recombinant VSV-based Zaire ebolavirus (ZEBOV) and Marburg virus (MARV) vaccines against aerosol challenge in cynomolgus macaques. All monkeys vaccinated with a VSV vector expressing the glycoprotein of ZEBOV were completely protected against an aerosol exposure of ZEBOV. Likewise, all monkeys vaccinated with a VSV vector expressing the glycoprotein of MARV were completely protected against an aerosol exposure of MARV. All control animals challenged by the aerosol route with either ZEBOV or MARV succumbed. Interestingly, disease in control animals appeared to progress slower than previously seen in macaques exposed to comparable doses by intramuscular injection.
PMCID: PMC3398796 PMID: 18930776 [PubMed - indexed for MEDLINE]

1443. J Virol. 2008 Dec;82(24):12569-73. doi: 10.1128/JVI.01395-08. Epub 2008 Oct 1.

Role of Ebola virus VP30 in transcription reinitiation.

Martínez MJ(1), Biedenkopf N, Volchkova V, Hartlieb B, Alazard-Dany N, Reynard O, Becker S, Volchkov V.

Author information: (1)INSERM, U758, Filovirus Laboratory, 21 Av. Tony Garnier, 69365 Lyon, Cedex 07, France.

VP30 is a phosphoprotein essential for the initiation of Ebola virus transcription. In this work, we have studied the effect of mutations in VP30 phosphorylation sites on the ebolavirus replication cycle by using a reverse genetics system. We demonstrate that VP30 is involved in reinitiation of gene transcription and that this activity is affected by mutations at the phosphorylation sites.
PMCID: PMC2593317 PMID: 18829754 [PubMed - indexed for MEDLINE]

1444. J Virol. 2008 Dec;82(23):11628-36. doi: 10.1128/JVI.01344-08. Epub 2008 Sep 24.

Crystal structure and carbohydrate analysis of Nipah virus attachment glycoprotein: a template for antiviral and vaccine design.

Bowden TA(1), Crispin M, Harvey DJ, Aricescu AR, Grimes JM, Jones EY, Stuart DI.

Author information: (1)Division of Structural Biology, University of Oxford, Henry Wellcome Building of Genomic Medicine, Roosevelt Drive, Oxford OX3 7BN, United Kingdom.

Two members of the paramyxovirus family, Nipah virus (NiV) and Hendra virus (HeV), are recent additions to a growing number of agents of emergent diseases which use bats as a natural host. Identification of ephrin-B2 and ephrin-B3 as cellular receptors for these viruses has enabled the development of immunotherapeutic reagents which prevent virus attachment and subsequent fusion. Here we present the structural analysis of the protein and carbohydrate components of the unbound viral attachment glycoprotein of NiV glycoprotein (NiV-G) at a 2.2-A resolution. Comparison with its ephrin-B2-bound form reveals that conformational changes within the envelope glycoprotein are required to achieve viral attachment. Structural differences are particularly pronounced in the 579-590 loop, a major component of the ephrin binding surface. In addition, the 236-245 loop is rather disordered in the unbound structure. We extend our structural characterization of NiV-G with mass spectrometric analysis of the carbohydrate moieties. We demonstrate that NiV-G is largely devoid of the oligomannose-type glycans that in viruses such as human immunodeficiency virus type 1 and Ebola virus influence viral tropism and the host immune response. Nevertheless, we find putative ligands for the endothelial cell lectin, LSECtin. Finally, by mapping structural conservation and glycosylation site positions from other members of the paramyxovirus family, we suggest the molecular surface involved in oligomerization. These results suggest possible pathways of virus-host interaction and strategies for the optimization of recombinant vaccines.
PMCID: PMC2583688 PMID: 18815311 [PubMed - indexed for MEDLINE]

1445. Ugeskr Laeger. 2008 Nov 24;170(48):3949-52.

[Ebola--haemorrhagic fever].

[Article in Danish]

Fabiansen C(1), Kronborg G, Thybo S, Nielsen JO.

Author information: (1)Paediatrisk Klinik, Juliane Marie Centeret, Rigshospitalet, DK-2100 København Ø. fabiansen@dadlnet.dk

This review presents the latest findings on ebola. Ebola presents one of the highest case-fatality rates of all infectious diseases, and in 2007 outbreaks were observed first in the Democratic Republic of Congo and later in Uganda with a new subtype. Accumulating evidence suggests that fruit bats are a likely reservoir for the ebola virus. The frequency of filovirus outbreaks in Central Africa is increasing and the potential for introduction and patient care in Denmark is evaluated.
PMID: 19087734 [PubMed - indexed for MEDLINE]

1446. Proc Natl Acad Sci U S A. 2008 Nov 18;105(46):17982-7. doi: 10.1073/pnas.0809698105. Epub 2008 Nov 3.

Stimulation of Ebola virus production from persistent infection through activation of the Ras/MAPK pathway.

Strong JE(1), Wong G, Jones SE, Grolla A, Theriault S, Kobinger GP, Feldmann H.

Author information: (1)Special Pathogens Program, National Microbiology Laboratory, Public Health Agency of Canada, Winnipeg, MB,Canada R3E 3R2. jim_strong@phac-aspc.gc.ca

Human infections with Ebola virus (EBOV) result in a deadly viral disease known as Ebola hemorrhagic fever. Up to 90% of infected patients die, and there is no available treatment or vaccine. The sporadic human outbreaks are believed to result when EBOV "jumps" from an infected animal to a person and is subsequently transmitted between persons by direct contact with infected blood or body fluids. This study was undertaken to investigate the mechanism by which EBOV can persistently infect and then escape from model cell and animal reservoir systems. We report a model system in which infection of mouse and bat cell lines with EBOV leads to persistence, which can be broken with low levels of lipopolysaccharide or phorbol-12-myristate-13-acetate (PMA). This reactivation depends on the Ras/MAPK pathway through inhibition of RNA-dependent protein kinase and eukaryotic initiation factor 2alpha phosphorylation and

occurs at the level of protein synthesis. EBOV also can be evoked from mice 7 days after infection by PMA treatment, indicating that a similar mechanism occurs in vivo. Our findings suggest that EBOV may persist in nature through subclinical infection of a reservoir species, such as bats, and that appropriate physiological stimulation may result in increased replication and transmission to new hosts. Identification of a presumptive mechanism responsible for EBOV emergence from its reservoir underscores the "hit-and-run" nature of the initiation of human and/or nonhuman primate EBOV outbreaks and may provide insight into possible countermeasures to interfere with transmission.
PMCID: PMC2577702 PMID: 18981410 [PubMed - indexed for MEDLINE]
1447. Bioorg Med Chem Lett. 2008 Nov 15;18(22):5871-4. doi: 10.1016/j.bmcl.2008.07.064. Epub 2008 Jul 18.

Sensitive and selective viral DNA detection assay via microbead-based rolling circle amplification.

Schopf E(1), Fischer NO, Chen Y, Tok JB.

Author information: (1)BioSecurity and NanoSciences Laboratory, Lawrence Livermore National Laboratory, 7000 East Avenue, Livermore, CA 94551, USA.
We report a sensitive and efficient magnetic bead-based assay for viral DNA identification using isothermal amplification of a reporting probe.
PMID: 18694640 [PubMed - indexed for MEDLINE]
1448. Virol J. 2008 Nov 10;5:137. doi: 10.1186/1743-422X-5-137.

The YPLGVG sequence of the Nipah virus matrix protein is required for budding.

Patch JR(1), Han Z, McCarthy SE, Yan L, Wang LF, Harty RN, Broder CC.

Author information: (1)Department of Microbiology and Immunology, Uniformed Services University, Bethesda, Maryland 20814, USA.
Jared.Patch@ARS.USDA.GOV

BACKGROUND: Nipah virus (NiV) is a recently emerged paramyxovirus capable of causing fatal disease in a broad range of mammalian hosts, including humans. Together with Hendra virus (HeV), they comprise the genus Henipavirus in the family Paramyxoviridae. Recombinant expression systems have played a crucial role in studying the cell biology of these Biosafety Level-4 restricted viruses. Henipavirus assembly and budding occurs at the plasma membrane, although the details of this process remain poorly understood. Multivesicular body (MVB) proteins have been found to play a role in the budding of several enveloped viruses, including some paramyxoviruses, and the recruitment of MVB proteins by viral proteins possessing late budding domains (L-domains) has become an important concept in the viral budding process. Previously we developed a system for producing NiV virus-like particles (VLPs) and demonstrated that the matrix (M) protein possessed an intrinsic budding ability and played a major role in assembly. Here, we have used this system to further explore the budding process by analyzing elements within the M protein that are critical for particle release. RESULTS: Using rationally targeted site-directed mutagenesis we show that a NiV M sequence YPLGVG is required for M budding and that mutation or deletion of the sequence abrogates budding ability. Replacement of the native and overlapping Ebola VP40 L-domains with the NiV sequence failed to rescue VP40 budding; however, it did induce the cellular morphology of extensive filamentous projection consistent with wild-type VP40-expressing cells. Cells expressing wild-type NiV M also displayed this morphology, which was dependent on the YPLGVG sequence, and deletion of the sequence also resulted in nuclear localization of M. Dominant-negative VPS4 proteins had no effect on NiV M budding, suggesting that unlike other viruses such as Ebola, NiV M accomplishes budding independent of MVB cellular proteins. CONCLUSION: These data indicate that the YPLGVG motif within the NiV M protein plays an important role in M budding; however, involvement of any specific components of the cellular MVB sorting pathway in henipavirus budding remains to be demonstrated. Further investigation of henipavirus assembly and budding may yet reveal a novel mechanism(s) of viral assembly and release that could be applicable to other enveloped viruses or have therapeutic implications.
PMCID: PMC2625347 PMID: 19000317 [PubMed - indexed for MEDLINE]
1449. J Theor Biol. 2008 Nov 7;255(1):69-80. doi: 10.1016/j.jtbi.2008.08.007. Epub 2008 Aug 13.

Adaptive modeling of viral diseases in bats with a focus on rabies.

Dimitrov DT(1), Hallam TG, Rupprecht CE, McCracken GF.

Author information: (1)Department of Ecology and Evolutionary Biology, University of Tennessee, 569 Dabney Hall, 1416 Circle Drive, Knoxville, TN 37996-1610, USA. dobromir@scharp.org

Many emerging and reemerging viruses, such as rabies, SARS, Marburg, and Ebola have bat populations as disease reservoirs. Understanding the spillover from bats to humans and other animals, and the associated health risks requires an analysis of the disease dynamics in bat populations. Traditional compartmental epizootic models, which are relatively easy to implement and analyze, usually impose unrealistic aggregation assumptions about disease-related structure and depend on parameters that frequently are not measurable in field conditions. We propose a novel combination of computational and adaptive modeling approaches that address the maintenance of emerging diseases in bat colonies through individual (intra-host) models of the response of the host to a viral challenge. The dynamics of the individual models are used to define survival, susceptibility and transmission conditions relevant to epizootics as well as to develop and parametrize models of the disease evolution into uniform and diverse populations. Applications of the proposed approach to modeling the effects of immunological heterogeneity on the dynamics of bat rabies are presented.
PMID: 18761020 [PubMed - indexed for MEDLINE]
1450. Mol Biol (Mosk). 2008 Nov-Dec;42(6):1093-6.

[An approach the quantitative determination of the area of glycoprotein spikes at the surface of enveloped viruses].

[Article in Russian]

Ksenofontov AL, Badun GA, Fedorova NV, Kordiukova LV.
The density of distribution of glycoproteins on virion surface seriously influences the virus infectivity and pathogenicity. In the present work a method of quantitative determination of the area occupied by the surface glycoprotein spikes is proposed for influenza virus (strain A/PR/8/34) based on data of tritium

bombardment and dynamic light scattering (DLS). The method of DLS was used for measuring the diameter of the intact virions and the subviral particles (influenza virions lacking glycoprotein spikes after bromelain digestion). The intact virions and the subviral particles were bombarded by the hot tritium atom flux followed by the analysis of the specific radioactivity of the matrix MI protein. It was shown that the tritium label was incorporated into the amino acid residues of a thin exposed protein layer and partially penetrated through the lipid bilayer of the viral envelope. As a result, the matrix MI protein which is located under the lipid bilayer became labeled. The tritium label distribution among different amino acid residues was the same for the MI protein isolated from the subviral particles and the one isolated from the intact virions. This testifies that the MI protein spatial structure remains unchanged during proteolysis of the glycoprotein spikes. The difference between the specific radioactivity of the MI protein isolated from the intact virions and that of the MI protein isolated from the subviral particles allowed us to calculate the portion of the viral surface which is free of the glycoprotein spikes. If approximate the influenza virion as as here the area occupied by the surface glycoproteins could be calculated. It appeared to be equal to approximately 1.4 yen 10 nm that is about 40% of the total viral surface. This is consistent with the cryoelectron tomography data published for the influenza virus (strain A/X-31). The developed approach could be applied for other enveloped high pathogenic viruses such as HIV and Ebola.
PMID: 19140331 [PubMed - indexed for MEDLINE]

1451. PLoS Pathog. 2008 Nov;4(11):e1000225. doi: 10.1371/journal.ppat.1000225. Epub 2008 Nov 28.

Vesicular stomatitis virus-based ebola vaccine is well-tolerated and protects immunocompromised nonhuman primates.

Geisbert TW(1), Daddario-Dicaprio KM, Lewis MG, Geisbert JB, Grolla A, Leung A, Paragas J, Matthias L, Smith MA, Jones SM, Hensley LE, Feldmann H, Jahrling PB.
Author information: (1)National Emerging Infectious Diseases Laboratories Institute, Boston, Massachusetts, USA. geisbert@bu.edu

Ebola virus (EBOV) is a significant human pathogen that presents a public health concern as an emerging/re-emerging virus and as a potential biological weapon. Substantial progress has been made over the last decade in developing candidate preventive vaccines that can protect nonhuman primates against EBOV. Among these prospects, a vaccine based on recombinant vesicular stomatitis virus (VSV) is particularly robust, as it can also confer protection when administered as a postexposure treatment. A concern that has been raised regarding the replication-competent VSV vectors that express EBOV glycoproteins is how these vectors would be tolerated by individuals with altered or compromised immune systems such as patients infected with HIV. This is especially important as all EBOV outbreaks to date have occurred in areas of Central and Western Africa with high HIV incidence rates in the population. In order to address this concern, we evaluated the safety of the recombinant VSV vector expressing the Zaire ebolavirus glycoprotein (VSVDeltaG/ZEBOVGP) in six rhesus macaques infected with simian-human immunodeficiency virus (SHIV). All six animals showed no evidence of illness associated with the VSVDeltaG/ZEBOVGP vaccine, suggesting that this vaccine may be safe in immunocompromised populations. While one goal of the study was to evaluate the safety of the candidate vaccine platform, it was also of interest to determine if altered immune status would affect vaccine efficacy. The vaccine protected 4 of 6 SHIV-infected macaques from death following ZEBOV challenge. Evaluation of CD4+ T cells in all animals showed that the animals that succumbed to lethal ZEBOV challenge had the lowest CD4+ counts, suggesting that CD4+ T cells may play a role in mediating protection against ZEBOV.
PMCID: PMC2582959 PMID: 19043556 [PubMed - indexed for MEDLINE]

1452. PLoS Pathog. 2008 Nov;4(11):e1000212. doi: 10.1371/journal.ppat.1000212. Epub 2008 Nov 21.

Newly discovered ebola virus associated with hemorrhagic fever outbreak in Uganda.

Towner JS(1), Sealy TK, Khristova ML, Albariño CG, Conlan S, Reeder SA, Quan PL, Lipkin WI, Downing R, Tappero JW, Okware S, Lutwama J, Bakamutumaho B, Kayiwa J, Comer JA, Rollin PE, Ksiazek TG, Nichol ST.
Author information: (1)Special Pathogens Branch, Centers for Disease Control and Prevention, Atlanta, Georgia, United States of America.

Over the past 30 years, Zaire and Sudan ebolaviruses have been responsible for large hemorrhagic fever (HF) outbreaks with case fatalities ranging from 53% to 90%, while a third species, Côte d'Ivoire ebolavirus, caused a single non-fatal HF case. In November 2007, HF cases were reported in Bundibugyo District, Western Uganda. Laboratory investigation of the initial 29 suspect-case blood specimens by classic methods (antigen capture, IgM and IgG ELISA) and a recently developed random-primed pyrosequencing approach quickly identified this to be an Ebola HF outbreak associated with a newly discovered ebolavirus species (Bundibugyo ebolavirus) distantly related to the Côte d'Ivoire ebolavirus found in western Africa. Due to the sequence divergence of this new virus relative to all previously recognized ebolaviruses, these findings have important implications for design of future diagnostic assays to monitor Ebola HF disease in humans and animals, and ongoing efforts to develop effective antivirals and vaccines.
PMCID: PMC2581435 PMID: 19023410 [PubMed - indexed for MEDLINE]

1453. Biol Chem. 2008 Oct;389(10):1273-82. doi: 10.1515/BC.2008.145.

RNA viruses and the mitogenic Raf/MEK/ERK signal transduction cascade.

Pleschka S(1).
Author information: (1)Institute for Medical Virology, Justus Liebig University, Frankfurter Str. 107, D-35392 Giessen, Germany. stephan.pleschka@mikro.bio.uni-giessen.de

The Raf/MEK/ERK signal transduction cascade belongs to the mitogen-activated protein kinase (MAPK) cascades. Raf/MEK/ERK signaling leads to stimulus-specific changes in gene expression, alterations in cell metabolism or induction of programmed cell death (apoptosis), and thus controls cell differentiation and proliferation. It is induced by extracellular agents, including pathogens such as RNA viruses. Many DNA viruses are known to induce cellular signaling via this pathway. As these pathogens partly use the DNA synthesis machinery for their replication, they aim to drive cells into a proliferative state. In contrast, the consequences of RNA virus-induced Raf/MEK/ERK signaling were less clear for a long time, but since the turn of the century the number of publications on this topic has rapidly increased. Research on this virus/host-interaction will broaden our understanding of its relevance in viral replication. This important control center of cellular responses is differently employed to support the replication of several important human pathogenic RNA viruses including influenza, Ebola, hepatitis C and SARS corona viruses.

PMID: 18713014 [PubMed - indexed for MEDLINE]

1454. Immunol Rev. 2008 Oct;225:9-26. doi: 10.1111/j.1600-065X.2008.00677.x.

Emerging and reemerging diseases: a historical perspective.

Snowden FM(1).

Author information: (1)Department of History, Yale University, New Haven, CT 06520-8324, USA.

SUMMARY: Between mid-century and 1992, there was a consensus that the battle against infectious diseases had been won, and the Surgeon General announced that it was time to close the book. Experience with human immunodeficiency virus/acquired immunodeficiency syndrome, the return of cholera to the Americas in 1991, the plague outbreak in India in 1994, and the emergence of Ebola in Zaire in 1995 created awareness of a new vulnerability to epidemics due to population growth, unplanned urbanization, antimicrobial resistance, poverty, societal change, and rapid mass movement of people. The increasing virulence of dengue fever with dengue hemorrhagic fever and dengue shock syndrome disproved the theory of the evolution toward commensalism, and the discovery of the microbial origins of peptic ulcer demonstrated the reach of infectious diseases. The Institute of Medicine coined the term 'emerging and reemerging diseases' to explain that the world had entered an era in which the vulnerability to epidemics in the United States and globally was greater than ever. The United States and the World Health Organization took devised rapid response systems to monitor and contain disease outbreaks and to develop new weapons against microbes. These mechanisms were tested by severe acute respiratory syndrome in 2003, and a series of practical and conceptual blind spots in preparedness were revealed.

PMID: 18837773 [PubMed - indexed for MEDLINE]

1455. Biochem Biophys Res Commun. 2008 Sep 5;373(4):561-6. doi: 10.1016/j.bbrc.2008.06.078. Epub 2008 Jun 30.

DC-SIGN mediates avian H5N1 influenza virus infection in cis and in trans.

Wang SF(1), Huang JC, Lee YM, Liu SJ, Chan YJ, Chau YP, Chong P, Chen YM.

Author information: (1)Department of Biotechnology and Laboratory Science in Medicine, School of Medicine, National Yang-Ming University, Taipei 112, Taiwan. DC-SIGN, a C-type lectin receptor expressed in dendritic cells (DCs), has been identified as a receptor for human immunodeficiency virus type 1, hepatitis C virus, Ebola virus, cytomegalovirus, dengue virus, and the SARS coronavirus. We used H5N1 pseudotyped and reverse-genetics (RG) virus particles to study their ability to bind with DC-SIGN. Electronic microscopy and functional assay results indicate that pseudotyped viruses containing both HA and NA proteins express hemagglutination and are capable of infecting cells expressing alpha-2,3-linked sialic acid receptors. Results from a capture assay show that DC-SIGN-expressing cells (including B-THP-1/DC-SIGN and T-THP-1/DC-SIGN) and peripheral blood dendritic cells are capable of transferring H5N1 pseudotyped and RG virus particles to target cells; this action can be blocked by anti-DC-SIGN monoclonal antibodies. In summary, (a) DC-SIGN acts as a capture or attachment molecule for avian H5N1 virus, and (b) DC-SIGN mediates infections in cis and in trans.

PMID: 18593570 [PubMed - indexed for MEDLINE]

1456. Gen Hosp Psychiatry. 2008 Sep-Oct;30(5):446-52. doi: 10.1016/j.genhosppsych.2008.05.003. Epub 2008 Jul 23.

The 1995 Kikwit Ebola outbreak: lessons hospitals and physicians can apply to future viral epidemics.

Hall RC(1), Hall RC, Chapman MJ.

Author information: (1)Case Western Reserve University, Cleveland, OH 44106, USA. rcwh@att.net

OBJECTIVE: This article looks at lessons learned from the 1995 Kikwit Ebola outbreak and suggests how modern hospitals should apply these lessons to the next lethal viral epidemic that occurs. METHOD: The 1995 Kikwit Ebola outbreak in the Democratic Republic of the Congo (formally Zaire) is one of the most well studied epidemics to have occurred to date. Many of the lessons learned from identifying, containing and treating that epidemic are applicable to future viral outbreaks, natural disasters and bioterrorist attacks. This is due to Ebola's highly contagious nature and high mortality rate. RESULTS: When an outbreak occurs, it often produces fear in the community and causes the basic practice of medicine to be altered. Changes seen at Kikwit included limited physical examinations, hesitance to give intravenous medications and closure of supporting hospital facilities. The Kikwit Ebola outbreak also provided beneficial psychological insight into how patients, staff and the general community respond to a biological crisis and how this will affect physicians working in an epidemic. CONCLUSIONS: General lessons from the outbreak include the importance of having simple, well-defined triage procedures; staff who are flexible and able to adapt to situations with unknowns; and the need to protect staff physically and emotionally to ensure a sustained effort to provide care.

PMID: 18774428 [PubMed - indexed for MEDLINE]

1457. Hum Vaccin. 2008 Sep-Oct;4(5):344-6. Epub 2008 Sep 2.

Next generation of human vaccines: what does the future hold?

Awasthi S(1).

Author information: (1)Infectious Disease Division, Department of Medicine, School of Medicine, University of Pennsylvania, Philadelphia, Pennsylvania 19104, USA. sawasthi@mail.med.upenn.edu

The World Vaccine Congress was held in Arlington, VA April 21st-24th, 2008. Tevi Troy, the deputy secretary of the US Department of Health and Human Services, set the tone of the meeting during his keynote address. He discussed the government's plan to deliver a strategic outlook and follow a road map for vaccine development. He also emphasized the importance of ongoing cooperation between industry and the government's many departments. In an electrifying keynote address Gregory Poland, Professor of Medicine and Infectious Diseases at the Mayo Clinic in Rochester, MN discussed the role of recent advancements in the fields of Immunology, Genetics, Molecular Biology, Bioinformatics and the completion of the Human Genome Project. Poland described the recent emergence of the field of Vaccinomics and laid out his vision for an era of personalized medicine. Next-generation vaccine approaches targeting cervical cancer, meningitis, childhood diarrhea and renal cell carcinoma were presented by leaders in the field. Preclinical and early-stage clinical successes of vaccines against Malaria, TB and Ebola were discussed along with a road map for HIV, TB and Malaria vaccine development. The importance of collaborations among government departments, academic institutions, industries and philanthropic foundations was a common theme stressed throughout the conference.

PMID: 18849649 [PubMed - indexed for MEDLINE]

1458. J Virol. 2008 Sep;82(18):9107-14. doi: 10.1128/JVI.00857-08. Epub 2008 Jun 11.

Novel astroviruses in insectivorous bats.

Chu DK(1), Poon LL, Guan Y, Peiris JS.

Author information: (1)Department of Microbiology, The University of Hong Kong, Hong Kong SAR, China.

Bats are increasingly recognized to harbor a wide range of viruses, and in most instances these viruses appear to establish long-term persistence in these animals. They are the reservoir of a number of human zoonotic diseases including Nipah, Ebola, and severe acute respiratory syndrome. We report the identification of novel groups of astroviruses in apparently healthy insectivorous bats found in Hong Kong, in particular, bats belonging to the genera Miniopterus and Myotis. Astroviruses are important causes of diarrhea in many animal species, including humans. Many of the bat astroviruses form distinct phylogenetic clusters in the genus Mamastrovirus within the family Astroviridae. Virus detection rates of 36% to 100% and 50% to 70% were found in Miniopterus magnater and Miniopterus pusillus bats, respectively, captured within a single bat habitat during four consecutive visits spanning 1 year. There was high genetic diversity of viruses in bats found within this single habitat. Some bat astroviruses may be phylogenetically related to human astroviruses, and further studies with a wider range of bat species in different geographic locations are warranted. These findings are likely to provide new insights into the ecology and evolution of astroviruses and reinforce the role of bats as a reservoir of viruses with potential to pose a zoonotic threat to human health.

PMCID: PMC2546893 PMID: 18550669 [PubMed - indexed for MEDLINE]

1459. PLoS Pathog. 2008 Aug 29;4(8):e1000141. doi: 10.1371/journal.ppat.1000141.

Phosphoinositide-3 kinase-Akt pathway controls cellular entry of Ebola virus.

Saeed MF(1), Kolokoltsov AA, Freiberg AN, Holbrook MR, Davey RA.

Author information: (1)Department of Microbiology and Immunology, University of Texas Medical Branch, Galveston, Texas, United States of America.

The phosphoinositide-3 kinase (PI3K) pathway regulates diverse cellular activities related to cell growth, migration, survival, and vesicular trafficking. It is known that Ebola virus requires endocytosis to establish an infection. However, the cellular signals that mediate this uptake were unknown for Ebola virus as well as many other viruses. Here, the involvement of PI3K in Ebola virus entry was studied. A novel and critical role of the PI3K signaling pathway was demonstrated in cell entry of Zaire Ebola virus (ZEBOV). Inhibitors of PI3K and Akt significantly reduced infection by ZEBOV at an early step during the replication cycle. Furthermore, phosphorylation of Akt-1 was induced shortly after exposure of cells to radiation-inactivated ZEBOV, indicating that the virus actively induces the PI3K pathway and that replication was not required for this induction. Subsequent use of pseudotyped Ebola virus and/or Ebola virus-like particles, in a novel virus entry assay, provided evidence that activity of PI3K/Akt is required at the virus entry step. Class IA PI3Ks appear to play a predominant role in regulating ZEBOV entry, and Rac1 is a key downstream effector in this regulatory cascade. Confocal imaging of fluorescently labeled ZEBOV indicated that inhibition of PI3K, Akt, or Rac1 disrupted normal uptake of virus particles into cells and resulted in aberrant accumulation of virus into a cytosolic compartment that was non-permissive for membrane fusion. We conclude that PI3K-mediated signaling plays an important role in regulating vesicular trafficking of ZEBOV necessary for cell entry. Disruption of this signaling leads to inappropriate trafficking within the cell and a block in steps leading to membrane fusion. These findings extend our current understanding of Ebola virus entry mechanism and may help in devising useful new strategies for treatment of Ebola virus infection.

PMCID: PMC2516934 PMID: 18769720 [PubMed - indexed for MEDLINE]

1460. Cell Host Microbe. 2008 Aug 14;4(2):87-9. doi: 10.1016/j.chom.2008.07.011.

Ebola images emerge from the cave.

Diamond MS(1), Fremont DH.

Author information: (1)Department of Medicine, Washington University School of Medicine, 660 South Euclid Avenue, St. Louis, MO 63110, USA. diamond@borcim.wustl.edu

Ebola virus causes a lethal hemorrhagic disease for which no therapy or vaccine is currently approved. Recently, the crystal structure of the Ebola virus glycoprotein in complex with a human neutralizing antibody was illuminated, providing a path from the shadows toward understanding cellular attachment, viral fusion, and immune evasion.

PMID: 18692765 [PubMed - indexed for MEDLINE]

1461. Org Biomol Chem. 2008 Aug 7;6(15):2743-54. doi: 10.1039/b802144a. Epub 2008 Jun 5

Docking, synthesis, and NMR studies of mannosyl trisaccharide ligands for DC-SIGN lectin.

Reina JJ(1), Díaz I, Nieto PM, Campillo NE, Páez JA, Tabarani G, Fieschi F, Rojo J.

Author information: (1)Grupo de Carbohidratos, Instituto de Investigaciones Químicas, CSIC, Universidad de Sevilla, Américo Vespucio 49, Seville, Spain.

DC-SIGN, a lectin, which presents at the surface of immature dendritic cells, constitutes nowadays a promising target for the design of new antiviral drugs. This lectin recognizes highly glycosylated proteins present at the surface of several pathogens such as HIV, Ebola virus, Candida albicans, Mycobacterium tuberculosis, etc. Understanding the binding mode of this lectin is a topic of tremendous interest and will permit a rational design of new and more selective ligands. Here, we present computational and experimental tools to study the interaction of di- and trisaccharides with DC-SIGN. Docking analysis of complexes involving mannosyl di- and trisaccharides and the carbohydrate recognition domain (CRD) of DC-SIGN have been performed. Trisaccharides Manalphal,2[Manalphal,6]Man 1 and Manalphal,3[Manalphal,6]Man 2 were synthesized from an orthogonally protected mannose as a common intermediate. Using these ligands and the soluble extracellular domain (ECD) of DC-SIGN, NMR experiments based on STD and transfer-NOE were performed providing additional information. Conformational analysis of the mannosyl ligands in the free and bound states was done. These studies have demonstrated that terminal mannoses at positions 2 or 3 in the trisaccharides are the most important moiety and present the strongest contact with the binding site of the lectin. Multiple binding modes could be proposed and therefore should be considered in the design of new ligands.

PMID: 18633532 [PubMed - indexed for MEDLINE]

1462. Am J Bioeth. 2008 Aug;8(8):37-8. doi: 10.1080/15265160802318014.

Remembering the "pan" in "pandemic": considering the impact of global resource disparity on a duty to treat.

Reiheld A(1).

Author information: (1)35 East Holmes Hall, Lyman Briggs College, Michigan State University, East Lansing, MI 48825-1107, USA. reiheld@msu.edu

Comment on Am J Bioeth. 2008 Aug;8(8):4-19.

PMID: 18802860 [PubMed - indexed for MEDLINE]

1463. Med Hypotheses. 2008 Aug;71(2):298-301. doi: 10.1016/j.mehy.2008.03.019. Epub 2008 Apr 29.

What caused lymphopenia in SARS and how reliable is the lymphokine status in glucocorticoid-treated patients?

Panesar NS(1).

Author information: (1)Department of Chemical Pathology, The Chinese University of Hong Kong, Shatin, New Territories, Hong Kong. nspanesar@chuk.edu.hk

Severe Acute Respiratory Syndrome (SARS) outbreak in 2002-03 caused morbidity in over 8000 individuals and mortality in 744 in 29 countries. Lymphopenia along with neutrophilia was a feature of SARS, as it is in respiratory syncytial virus (RSV) and Ebola infections, to name a few. Direct infestation of lymphocytes, neutrophils and macrophages by SARS coronavirus (CoV) has been debated as a cause of lymphopenia, but there is no convincing data. Lymphopenia can be caused by glucocorticoids, and thus any debilitating condition has the potential to induce lymphopenia via stress mechanism involving the hypothalamic-pituitary-adrenal axis. Cortisol levels are elevated in patients with RSV and Ebola, and cortisol was higher in SARS patients with lymphopenia before any steroid therapy. Glucocorticoids also down-regulate the production of proinflammatory lymphokines. Because of the insidious presentation, SARS was treated with antibacterial, antiviral and supra-physiological doses of glucocorticoids. Treatment with glucocorticoids complicated the issue regarding lymphopenia, and certainly calls into question the status of lymphokines and their prognostic implications in SARS.

PMID: 18448259 [PubMed - indexed for MEDLINE]

1464. Virology. 2008 Aug 1;377(2):255-64. doi: 10.1016/j.virol.2008.04.029.

A paramyxovirus-vectored intranasal vaccine against Ebola virus is immunogenic in vector-immune animals.

Yang L(1), Sanchez A, Ward JM, Murphy BR, Collins PL, Bukreyev A.

Author information: (1)Laboratory of Infectious Disease, National Institute of Allergy and Infectious Diseases, National Institutes of Health, 50 South Drive, Rm. 6505, Bethesda, Maryland 20892-8007, USA.

Ebola virus (EBOV) causes outbreaks of a highly lethal hemorrhagic fever in humans. The virus can be transmitted by direct contact as well as by aerosol and is considered a potential bioweapon. Because direct immunization of the respiratory tract should be particularly effective against infection of mucosal surfaces, we previously developed an intranasal vaccine based on replication-competent human parainfluenza virus type 3 (HPIV3) expressing EBOV glycoprotein GP (HPIV3/EboGP) and showed that it is immunogenic and protective against a high dose parenteral EBOV challenge. However, because the adult human population has considerable immunity to HPIV3, which is a common human pathogen, replication and immunogenicity of the vaccine in this population might be greatly restricted. Indeed, in the present study, replication of the vaccine in the respiratory tract of HPIV3-immune guinea pigs was found to be restricted to undetectable levels. This restriction appeared to be based on both neutralizing antibodies and cellular or other components of the immunity to HPIV3. Surprisingly, even though replication of HPIV3/EboGP was highly restricted in HPIV3-immune animals, it induced a high level of EBOV-specific antibodies that nearly equaled that obtained in HPIV3-naive animals. We also show that the previously demonstrated presence of functional GP in the vector particle was not associated with increased replication in the respiratory tract nor with spread beyond the respiratory tract of HPIV3-naive guinea pigs, indicating that expression and functional incorporation of the attachment/penetration glycoprotein of this systemic virus did not mediate a change in tissue tropism.

PMCID: PMC2519172 PMID: 18570964 [PubMed - indexed for MEDLINE]

1465. Nature. 2008 Jul 10;454(7201):177-82. doi: 10.1038/nature07082.

Structure of the Ebola virus glycoprotein bound to an antibody from a human survivor.

Lee JE(1), Fusco ML, Hessell AJ, Oswald WB, Burton DR, Saphire EO.

Author information: (1)Department of Immunology and Microbial Science, The Scripps Research Institute, 10550 North Torrey Pines Road, Mail Drop IMM-2, La Jolla, California 92037, USA.

Ebola virus (EBOV) entry requires the surface glycoprotein (GP) to initiate attachment and fusion of viral and host membranes. Here we report the crystal structure of EBOV GP in its trimeric, pre-fusion conformation (GP1+GP2) bound to a neutralizing antibody, KZ52, derived from a human survivor of the 1995 Kikwit outbreak. Three GP1 viral attachment subunits assemble to form a chalice, cradled by the GP2 fusion subunits, while a novel glycan cap and projected mucin-like domain restrict access to the conserved receptor-binding site sequestered in the chalice bowl. The glycocalyx surrounding GP is likely central to immune evasion and may explain why survivors have insignificant neutralizing antibody titres. KZ52 recognizes a protein epitope at the chalice base where it clamps several regions of the pre-fusion GP2 to the amino terminus of GP1. This structure provides a template for unravelling the mechanism of EBOV GP-mediated fusion and for future immunotherapeutic development.

PMCID: PMC2700032 PMID: 18615077 [PubMed - indexed for MEDLINE]

1466. Nature. 2008 Jul 10;454(7201):159. doi: 10.1038/454159a.

Action needed to prevent extinctions caused by disease.

Hoffmann M, Hawkins CE, Walsh PD.

PMID: 18615062 [PubMed - indexed for MEDLINE]

1467. PLoS Pathog. 2008 Jul 4;4(7):e1000097. doi: 10.1371/journal.ppat.1000097.

Molecular ecology and natural history of simian foamy virus infection in wild-living chimpanzees.

Liu W(1), Worobey M, Li Y, Keele BF, Bibollet-Ruche F, Guo Y, Goepfert PA, Santiago ML, Ndjango JB, Neel C, Clifford SL, Sanz C, Kamenya S, Wilson ML, Pusey AE, Gross-Camp N, Boesch C, Smith V, Zamma K, Huffman MA, Mitani JC, Watts DP, Peeters M, Shaw GM, Switzer WM, Sharp PM, Hahn BH.

Author information: (1)Department of Medicine, University of Alabama at Birmingham, Birmingham, Alabama, United States of America.

Identifying microbial pathogens with zoonotic potential in wild-living primates can be important to human health, as evidenced by human immunodeficiency viruses types 1 and 2 (HIV-1 and HIV-2) and Ebola virus. Simian foamy viruses (SFVs) are ancient retroviruses that infect Old and New World monkeys and apes. Although not known to cause disease, these viruses are of public health interest because they have the potential to infect humans and thus provide a more general indication of zoonotic exposure risks. Surprisingly, no information exists concerning the prevalence, geographic distribution, and genetic diversity of SFVs in wild-living monkeys and apes. Here, we report the first comprehensive survey of SFVcpz infection in free-ranging chimpanzees (Pan troglodytes) using newly developed, fecal-based assays. Chimpanzee fecal samples (n = 724) were collected at 25 field sites throughout equatorial Africa and tested for SFVcpz-specific antibodies (n = 706) or viral nucleic acids (n = 392). SFVcpz infection was documented at all field sites, with prevalence rates ranging from 44% to 100%. In two habituated communities, adult chimpanzees had significantly higher SFVcpz infection rates than infants and juveniles, indicating predominantly horizontal rather than vertical transmission routes. Some chimpanzees were co-infected with simian immunodeficiency virus (SIVcpz); however, there was no evidence that SFVcpz and SIVcpz were epidemiologically linked. SFVcpz nucleic acids were recovered from 177 fecal samples, all of which contained SFVcpz RNA and not DNA. Phylogenetic analysis of partial gag (616 bp), pol-RT (717 bp), and pol-IN (425 bp) sequences identified a diverse group of viruses, which could be subdivided into four distinct SFVcpz lineages according to their chimpanzee subspecies of origin. Within these lineages, there was evidence of frequent superinfection and viral recombination. One chimpanzee was infected by a foamy virus from a Cercopithecus monkey species, indicating cross-species transmission of SFVs in the wild. These data indicate that SFVcpz (i) is widely distributed among all chimpanzee subspecies; (ii) is shed in fecal samples as viral RNA; (iii) is transmitted predominantly by horizontal routes; (iv) is prone to superinfection and recombination; (v) has co-evolved with its natural host; and (vi) represents a sensitive marker of population structure that may be useful for chimpanzee taxonomy and conservation strategies.

PMCID: PMC2435277 PMID: 18604273 [PubMed - indexed for MEDLINE]

1468. J Immunotoxicol. 2008 Jul;5(3):315-35. doi: 10.1080/15376510802312464.

Biodistribution and toxicological safety of adenovirus type 5 and type 35 vectored vaccines against human immunodeficiency virus-1 (HIV-1), Ebola, or Marburg are similar despite differing adenovirus serotype vector, manufacturer's construct, or gene inserts.

Sheets RL(1), Stein J, Bailer RT, Koup RA, Andrews C, Nason M, He B, Koo E, Trotter H, Duffy C, Manetz TS, Gomez P.

Author information: (1)Vaccine Research Center, NIH/NIAID, Bethesda, Maryland 20892-7628, USA. rsheets@niaid.nih.gov

The Vaccine Research Center has developed vaccine candidates for different diseases/infectious agents (including HIV-1, Ebola, and Marburg viruses) built on an adenovirus vector platform, based on adenovirus type 5 or 35. To support clinical development of each vaccine candidate, pre-clinical studies were performed in rabbits to determine where in the body they biodistribute and how rapidly they clear, and to screen for potential toxicities (intrinsic and immunotoxicities). The vaccines biodistribute only to spleen, liver (Ad5 only), and/or iliac lymph node (Ad35 only) and otherwise remain in the site of injection muscle and overlying subcutis. Though approximately 10(11) viral particles were inoculated, already by Day 9, all but 10(3) to 10(5) genome copies per mu g of DNA had cleared from the injection site muscle. By three months, the adenovector was cleared with, at most, a few animals retaining a small number of copies in the injection site, spleen (Ad5), or iliac lymph node (Ad35). This pattern of limited biodistribution and extensive clearance is consistent regardless of differences in adenovector type (Ad5 or 35), manufacturer's construct and production methods, or gene-insert. Repeated dose toxicology studies identified treatment-related toxicities confined primarily to the sites of injection, in certain clinical pathology parameters, and in body temperatures (Ad5 vectors) and food consumption immediately post-inoculation. Systemic reactogenicity and reactogenicity at the sites of injection demonstrated reversibility. These data demonstrate the safety and suitability for investigational human use of Ad5 or Ad35 adenovector-based vaccine candidates at doses of up to 2 x 10(11) given intramuscularly to prevent various infectious diseases.

PMCID: PMC2777703 PMID: 18830892 [PubMed - indexed for MEDLINE]

1469. J Prev Med Public Health. 2008 Jul;41(4):209-13. doi: 10.3961/jpmph.2008.41.4.209.

[The strategic plan for preparedness and response to bioterrorism in Korea].

[Article in Korean]

Hwang HS(1).

Author information: (1)Korea Centers for Disease Control and Prevention, Ministry for Health, Welfare and Family Affairs. hyunsoon@mw.go.kr

Following the Anthrax bioterrorism attacks in the US in 2001, the Korean government established comprehensive countermeasures against bioterrorism. These measures included the government assuming management of all infectious agents that cause diseases, including smallpox, anthrax, plaque, botulism, and the causative agents of viral hemorrhagic fevers (ebola fever, marburg fever, and lassa fever) for national security. In addition, the Korean government is reinforcing the ability to prepare and respond to bioterrorism. Some of the measures being implemented include revising the laws and guidelines that apply to the use of infectious agents, the construction and operation of dual surveillance systems for bioterrorism, stockpiling and managing products necessary to respond to an emergency (smallpox vaccine, antibiotics, etc.) and vigorously training emergency room staff and heath workers to ensure they can respond appropriately. In addition, the government's measures include improved public relations, building and maintaining international cooperation, and developing new vaccines and drugs for treatments of infectious agents used to create bioweapons.

PMID: 18664725 [PubMed - indexed for MEDLINE]

1470. J Virol. 2008 Jul;82(14):7238-42. doi: 10.1128/JVI.00425-08. Epub 2008 Apr 30.

Cell adhesion promotes Ebola virus envelope glycoprotein-mediated binding and infection.

Dube D(1), Schornberg KL, Stantchev TS, Bonaparte MI, Delos SE, Bouton AH, Broder CC, White JM.

Author information: (1)Department of Microbiology, University of Virginia, 1300 Jefferson Park Ave., Charlottesville, Virginia 22908-0734, USA.

Ebola virus infects a wide variety of adherent cell types, while nonadherent cells are found to be refractory. To explore this correlation, we compared the ability of pairs of related adherent and nonadherent cells to bind a recombinant Ebola virus receptor binding domain (EboV RBD) and to be infected with Ebola virus glycoprotein (GP)-pseudotyped particles. Both human 293F and THP-1 cells can be propagated as adherent or nonadherent cultures, and in both cases adherent cells were found to be significantly more susceptible to both EboV RBD binding and GP-pseudotyped virus infection than their nonadherent counterparts. Furthermore, with 293F cells the acquisition of EboV RBD binding paralleled cell spreading and did not require new mRNA or protein synthesis.

PMCID: PMC2446962 PMID: 18448524 [PubMed - indexed for MEDLINE]

1471. J Virol. 2008 Jul;82(13):6190-9. doi: 10.1128/JVI.02731-07. Epub 2008 Apr 16.

A filovirus-unique region of Ebola virus nucleoprotein confers aberrant migration and mediates its incorporation into virions.

Shi W(1), Huang Y, Sutton-Smith M, Tissot B, Panico M, Morris HR, Dell A, Haslam SM, Boyington J, Graham BS, Yang ZY, Nabel GJ.

Author information: (1)Vaccine Research Center, NIAID, National Institutes of Health, Bldg. 40, Rm. 4502, MSC-3005, 40 Convent Dr., Bethesda, MD 20892-3005, USA.

The Ebola virus nucleoprotein (NP) is an essential component of the nucleocapsid, required for filovirus particle formation and replication. Together with virion protein 35 (VP35) and VP24, this gene product gives rise to the filamentous nucleocapsid within transfected cells. Ebola virus NP migrates aberrantly, with an apparent molecular mass of 115 kDa, although it is predicted to encode an approximately 85-kDa protein. In this report, we show that two domains of this protein determine this aberrant migration and that this region mediates its incorporation into virions. These regions, amino acids 439 to 492 and amino acids 589 to 739, alter the mobility of Ebola virus NP by sodium dodecyl sulfate-polyacrylamide gel electrophoresis by 5 and 15 kDa, respectively, and confer similar effects on a heterologous protein, LacZ, in a position-independent fashion. Furthermore, when coexpressed with VP40, VP35, and VP24, this region mediated incorporation of NP into released viruslike particles. When fused to chimeric paramyxovirus NPs derived from measles or respiratory syncytial virus, this domain directed these proteins into the viruslike particle. The COOH-terminal NP domain comprises a conserved highly acidic region of NP with predicted disorder, distinguishing Ebola virus NPs from paramyxovirus NPs. The acidic character of this domain is likely responsible for its aberrant biochemical properties. These findings demonstrate that this region is essential for the assembly of the filamentous nucleocapsids that give rise to filoviruses.

PMCID: PMC2447054 PMID: 18417588 [PubMed - indexed for MEDLINE]

1472. J Virol Methods. 2008 Jul;151(1):126-31. doi: 10.1016/j.jviromet.2008.03.005. Epub 2008 Apr 28.

Rapid bio-barcode assay for multiplex DNA detection based on capillary DNA Analyzer.

He M(1), Li K, Xiao J, Zhou Y.

Author information: (1)Institute of Bioengineering, College of Biochemistry and Molecular Biology, East China University of Science and Technology, Shanghai 200237, China.

The detection of virus at low copy number is important for clinical diagnosis. In this study, a rapid bio-barcode assay was developed and it could detect short sequences of four types of virus DNA simultaneously at the concentration as low as 5p mol/L in 40 min with capillary 3730 DNA Analyzer. The background of the assay using high salt concentration prepared nanogold particle probes was five times less than that of the assay using conventionally prepared probes. With further optimization, the specificity of the complementary strands to the noncomplementary strands observed in the assay approached 140:1. Compared with the conventional bio-barcode assay, the current assay provides an alternative enzyme and labor-free selection of timesaving, better sensitivity and specificity, as well as higher throughput.

PMID: 18440653 [PubMed - indexed for MEDLINE]

1473. Curr Opin Mol Ther. 2008 Jun;10(3):285-93.

A DNA vaccine for the prevention of Ebola virus infection.

Dery M(1), Bausch DG.

Author information: (1)Tulane University Health Sciences Center, Department of Medicine, Infectious Diseases Section, 1430 Tulane Ave SL-87, New Orleans, LA 70112-2699, USA. madery@tulane.edu

The NIH and Vical Inc are developing an intramuscular needle-free DNA vaccine containing plasmids encoding the envelope glycoprotein of Ebola virus (EBOV) from the Sudan and Zaire strains, and the nucleoprotein of EBOV Zaire strain. A phase I clinical trial demonstrated a good safety profile, with most adverse events limited to the site of injection and largely attributable to the delivery.

PMID: 18535936 [PubMed - indexed for MEDLINE]

1474. Emerg Infect Dis. 2008 Jun;14(6):881-7. doi: 10.3201/eid1406.071489.

Managing potential laboratory exposure to ebola virus by using a patient biocontainment care unit.

Kortepeter MG(1), Martin JW, Rusnak JM, Cieslak TJ, Warfield KL, Anderson EL, Ranadive MV.

Author information: (1)US Army Medical Research Institute of Infectious Diseases, Fort Detrick, Maryland, USA. mark.kortepeter@na.amedd.army.mil

In 2004, a scientist from the US Army Medical Research Institute of Infectious Diseases (USAMRIID) was potentially exposed to a mouse-adapted variant of the Zaire species of Ebola virus. The circumstances surrounding the case are presented, in addition to an update on historical admissions to the medical containment suite at USAMRIID. Research facilities contemplating work with pathogens requiring Biosafety Level 4 laboratory precautions should be mindful of the occupational health issues highlighted in this article.

PMCID: PMC2600302 PMID: 18507897 [PubMed - indexed for MEDLINE]

1475. J Virol. 2008 Jun;82(11):5664-8. doi: 10.1128/JVI.00456-08. Epub 2008 Apr 2.

Recombinant vesicular stomatitis virus vector mediates postexposure protection against Sudan Ebola hemorrhagic fever in nonhuman primates.

Geisbert TW(1), Daddario-DiCaprio KM, Williams KJ, Geisbert JB, Leung A, Feldmann F, Hensley LE, Feldmann H, Jones SM.

Author information: (1)National Emerging Infectious Diseases Laboratories Institute, Boston, Massachusetts, USA. geisbert@bu.edu

Recombinant vesicular stomatitis virus (VSV) vectors expressing homologous filoviral glycoproteins can completely protect rhesus monkeys against Marburg virus when administered after exposure and can partially protect macaques after challenge with Zaire ebolavirus. Here, we administered a VSV vector expressing the Sudan ebolavirus (SEBOV) glycoprotein to four rhesus macaques shortly after exposure to SEBOV. All four animals survived SEBOV challenge, while a control animal that received a nonspecific vector developed fulminant SEBOV hemorrhagic fever and succumbed. This is the first demonstration of complete postexposure protection against an Ebola virus in nonhuman primates and provides further evidence that postexposure vaccination may have utility in treating exposures to filoviruses.

PMCID: PMC2395203 PMID: 18385248 [PubMed - indexed for MEDLINE]

1476. J Virol. 2008 Jun;82(11):5348-58. doi: 10.1128/JVI.00215-08. Epub 2008 Mar 19.

Whole-genome expression profiling reveals that inhibition of host innate immune response pathways by Ebola virus can be reversed by a single amino acid change in the VP35 protein.

Hartman AL(1), Ling L, Nichol ST, Hibberd ML.

Author information: (1)Centers for Disease Control and Prevention, Special Pathogens Branch, Atlanta, Georgia 30329, USA.

Ebola hemorrhagic fever is a rapidly progressing acute febrile illness characterized by high virus replication, severe immunosuppression, and case fatalities of ca. 80%. Inhibition of phosphorylation of interferon regulatory factor 3 (IRF-3) by the Ebola VP35 protein may block the host innate immune response and play an important role in the severity of disease. We used two precisely defined reverse genetics-generated Ebola viruses to investigate global host cell responses resulting from the inhibition of IRF-3 phosphorylation. The two viruses encoded either wild-type (WT) VP35 protein (recEbo-VP35/WT) or VP35 with an arginine (R)-to-alanine (A) amino acid substitution at position 312 (recEbo-VP35/R312A) within a previously defined IRF-3 inhibitory domain. When sucrose-gradient purified virus was used for infection, host cell whole-genome expression profiling revealed striking differences in human liver cell responses to these viruses differing by a single amino acid. The inhibition of host innate immune responses by WT Ebola virus was so potent that little difference in interferon and antiviral gene expression could be discerned between cells infected with purified WT, inactivated virus, or mock-infected cells. However, infection with recEbo-VP35/R312A virus resulted in a strong innate immune response including increased expression of MDA-5, RIG-I, RANTES, MCP-1, ISG-15, ISG-54, ISG-56, ISG-60, STAT1, IRF-9, OAS, and Mx1. The clear gene expression differences were obscured if unpurified virus stocks were used to initiate infection, presumably due to soluble factors present in virus-infected cell supernatant preparations. Ebola virus VP35 protein clearly plays a pivotal role in the potent inhibition of the host innate immune responses, and the present study indicates that VP35 has a wider effect on host cell responses than previously shown. The ability to eliminate this inhibitory effect with a single amino acid change in VP35 demonstrates the critical role this protein must play in the severe aspects this highly fatal disease.

PMCID: PMC2395193 PMID: 18353943 [PubMed - indexed for MEDLINE]

1477. Mol Aspects Med. 2008 Jun;29(3):151-85. Epub 2007 Oct 22.

Ebolavirus and Marburgvirus: insight the Filoviridae family.

Ascenzi P(1), Bocedi A, Heptonstall J, Capobianchi MR, Di Caro A, Mastrangelo E, Bolognesi M, Ippolito G.

Author information: (1)National Institute for Infectious Diseases IRCCS Lazzaro Spallanzani, Via Portuense 292, I-00149 Roma, Italy.

Ebolavirus and Marburgvirus (belonging to the Filoviridae family) emerged four decades ago and cause epidemics of haemorrhagic fever with high case-fatality rates. The genome of filoviruses encodes seven proteins. No significant homology is observed between filovirus proteins and any known macromolecule. Moreover, Marburgvirus and Ebolavirus show significant differences in protein homology. The natural maintenance cycle of filoviruses is unknown, the natural reservoir, the mode of transmission, the epidemic disease generation, and temporal dynamics are unclear. Lastly, Ebolavirus and Marburgvirus are considered as potential biological weapons. Vaccine appears the unique therapeutic frontier. Here, molecular and clinical aspects of filoviral haemorrhagic fevers are summarized.

PMID: 18063023 [PubMed - indexed for MEDLINE]

1478. Cell Host Microbe. 2008 May 15;3(5):285-92. doi: 10.1016/j.chom.2008.04.004.

HIV-1 assembly: viral glycoproteins segregate quantally to lipid rafts that associate individually with HIV-1 capsids and virions.

Leung K(1), Kim JO, Ganesh L, Kabat J, Schwartz O, Nabel GJ.

Author information: (1)Vaccine Research Center, NIAID, National Institutes of Health, Bethesda, MD 20892-0485, USA.
HIV-1 assembly depends on its structural protein, Gag, which after synthesis on ribosomes, traffics to the late endosome/plasma membrane, associates with HIV Env glycoprotein, and forms infectious virions. While Env and Gag migrate to lipid microdomains, their stoichiometry and specificity of interaction are unknown. Pseudotyped viral particles can be made with one viral core surrounded by heterologous envelope proteins. Taking advantage of this property, we analyzed the association of HIV Env and Ebola glycoprotein (GP), with HIV-1 Gag coexpressed in the same cell. Though both viral glycoproteins were expressed, each associated independently with Gag, giving rise to distinct virion populations, each with a single glycoprotein type. Confocal imaging demonstrated that Env and GP localized to distinct lipid raft microdomains within the same cell where they associated with different virions. Thus, a single Gag particle associates "quantally" with one lipid raft, containing homogeneous trimeric viral envelope proteins, to assemble functional virions.
PMCID: PMC2998762 PMID: 18474355 [PubMed - indexed for MEDLINE]
1479. CMAJ. 2008 May 6;178(10):1266-7. doi: 10.1503/cmaj.080524.

The strains of Ebola.

Mason C.
PMCID: PMC2335200 PMID: 18458253 [PubMed - indexed for MEDLINE]
1480. Am J Primatol. 2008 May;70(5):439-51. doi: 10.1002/ajp.20514. Epub 2008 Jan 4.

Comparing ape densities and habitats in northern Congo: surveys of sympatric gorillas and chimpanzees in the Odzala and Ndoki regions.

Devos C(1), Sanz C, Morgan D, Onononga JR, Laporte N, Huynen MC.
Author information: (1)Department of Behavioral Ecology, University of Liège, Liège, Belgium. vt638276@versateladsl.be
The conservation status of western lowland gorillas and central chimpanzees in western equatorial Africa remains largely speculative because many remote areas have never been surveyed and the impact of emergent diseases in the region has not been well documented. In this study, we compared ape densities and habitats in the Lokoué study area in Odzala National Park and the Goualougo Triangle in Nouabalé-Ndoki National Park in northern Republic of Congo. Both of these sites have long been considered strongholds for the conservation of chimpanzees and gorillas, but supposedly differ in vegetative composition and relative ape abundance. We compared habitats between these sites using conventional ground surveys and classified Landsat-7 ETM+ satellite images. We present density estimates via both standing-crop and marked-nest methods for the first time for sympatric apes of the Congo Basin. The marked-nest method was effective in depicting chimpanzee densities, but underestimated gorilla densities at both sites. Marked-nest surveys also revealed a dramatic decline in the ape population of Lokoué which coincided with a local Ebola epidemic. Normal baseline fluctuations in ape nest encounter rates during the repeated passages of marked-nest surveys were clearly distinguishable from a 80% decline in ape nest encounter rates at Lokoué. Our results showed that ape densities, habitat composition, and population dynamics differed between these populations in northern Congo. We emphasize the importance of intensifying monitoring efforts and further refinement of ape survey methods, as our results indicated that even the largest remaining ape populations in intact and protected forests are susceptible to sudden and dramatic declines.
© 2008 Wiley-Liss, Inc.
PMID: 18176937 [PubMed - indexed for MEDLINE]
1481. Cuad Bioet. 2008 May-Aug;19(66):321-53.

[Vaccines, biotechnology and their connection with induced abortion].

[Article in Spanish]
Redondo Calderón JL(1).
Author information: (1)Alminares del Genil, 18006 Granada. redondojoseluis@telefonica.net
Diploid cells (WI-38, MRC-5) vaccines have their origin in induced abortions. Among these vaccines we find the following: rubella, measles, mumps, rabies, polio, smallpox, hepatitis A, chickenpox, and herpes zoster. Nowadays, other abortion tainted vaccines cultivated on transformed cells (293, PER.C6) are in the pipeline: flu, Respiratory Syncytial and parainfluenza viruses, HIV, West Nile virus, Ebola, Marburg and Lassa, hepatitis B and C, foot and mouth disease, Japanese encephalitis, dengue, tuberculosis, anthrax, plague, tetanus and malaria. The same method is used for the production of monoclonal antibodies and other proteins, gene therapy and genomics. Technology enables us to develop the aforementioned products without resorting to induced abortion. Full disclosure of the cell origin in the labelling of vaccines and other products must be supported. There are vaccines from non-objectionable sources which should be made available to the public. When no alternative vaccines exist, ethical research must be promoted. Non-objectionable sources in the production of monoclonal antibodies, gene therapy and genomics must be encouraged. It is not be consistent to abstain from products originated in embryonic stem cells and at the same time approve of products obtained from induced abortions. It is of paramount importance to avoid that induced abortion technology seeps into every field of Medicine.
PMID: 18611078 [PubMed - indexed for MEDLINE]
1482. PLoS One. 2008 Apr 30;3(4):e2032. doi: 10.1371/journal.pone.0002032.

Processing of genome 5' termini as a strategy of negative-strand RNA viruses to avoid RIG-I-dependent interferon induction.

Habjan M(1), Andersson I, Klingström J, Schümann M, Martin A, Zimmermann P, Wagner V, Pichlmair A, Schneider U, Mühlberger E, Mirazimi A, Weber F.
Author information: (1)Department of Virology, University of Freiburg, Freiburg, Germany.
Innate immunity is critically dependent on the rapid production of interferon in response to intruding viruses. The intracellular pathogen recognition receptors RIG-I and MDA5 are essential for interferon induction by viral RNAs containing 5' triphosphates or double-stranded structures, respectively. Viruses with a negative-stranded RNA genome are an important group of pathogens causing emerging and re-emerging diseases. We investigated the ability of genomic RNAs

from substantial representatives of this virus group to induce interferon via RIG-I or MDA5. RNAs isolated from particles of Ebola virus, Nipah virus, Lassa virus, and Rift Valley fever virus strongly activated the interferon-beta promoter. Knockdown experiments demonstrated that interferon induction depended on RIG-I, but not MDA5, and phosphatase treatment revealed a requirement for the RNA 5' triphosphate group. In contrast, genomic RNAs of Hantaan virus, Crimean-Congo hemorrhagic fever virus and Borna disease virus did not trigger interferon induction. Sensitivity of these RNAs to a 5' monophosphate-specific exonuclease indicates that the RIG-I-activating 5' triphosphate group was removed post-transcriptionally by a viral function. Consequently, RIG-I is unable to bind the RNAs of Hantaan virus, Crimean-Congo hemorrhagic fever virus and Borna disease virus. These results establish RIG-I as a major intracellular recognition receptor for the genome of most negative-strand RNA viruses and define the cleavage of triphosphates at the RNA 5' end as a strategy of viruses to evade the innate immune response.

PMCID: PMC2323571 PMID: 18446221 [PubMed - indexed for MEDLINE]

1483. J Biol Chem. 2008 Apr 4;283(14):8783-7. doi: 10.1074/jbc.C800030200. Epub 2008 Feb 20.

ISG15 inhibits Nedd4 ubiquitin E3 activity and enhances the innate antiviral response.

Malakhova OA(1), Zhang DE.

Author information: (1)Department of Molecular and Experimental Medicine, The Scripps Research Institute, La Jolla, CA 92037, USA.

Interferons regulate diverse immune functions through the transcriptional activation of hundreds of genes involved in anti-viral responses. The interferon-inducible ubiquitin-like protein ISG15 is expressed in cells in response to a variety of stress conditions like viral or bacterial infection and is present in its free form or is conjugated to cellular proteins. In addition, protein ubiquitination plays a regulatory role in the immune system. Many viruses modulate the ubiquitin (Ub) pathway to alter cellular signaling and the antiviral response. Ubiquitination of retroviral group-specific antigen precursors and matrix proteins of the Ebola, vesicular stomatitis, and rabies viruses by Nedd4 family HECT domain E3 ligases is an important step in facilitating viral release. We found that Nedd4 is negatively regulated by ISG15. Free ISG15 specifically bound to Nedd4 and blocked its interaction with Ub-E2 molecules, thus preventing further Ub transfer from E2 to E3. Furthermore, overexpression of ISG15 diminished the ability of Nedd4 to ubiquitinate viral matrix proteins and led to a decrease in the release of Ebola VP40 virus-like particles from the cells. These results point to a mechanistically novel function of ISG15 in the enhancement of the innate anti-viral response through specific inhibition of Nedd4 Ub-E3 activity. To our knowledge, this is the first example of a Ub-like protein with the ability to interfere with Ub-E2 and E3 interaction to inhibit protein ubiquitination.

PMCID: PMC2276364 PMID: 18287095 [PubMed - indexed for MEDLINE]

1484. Antiviral Res. 2008 Apr;78(1):150-61. doi: 10.1016/j.antiviral.2008.01.152. Epub 2008 Feb 26.

Treatment of Marburg and Ebola hemorrhagic fevers: a strategy for testing new drugs and vaccines under outbreak conditions.

Bausch DG(1), Sprecher AG, Jeffs B, Boumandouki P.

Author information: (1)Tulane University Health Sciences Center, New Orleans, LA, United States. dbausch@tulane.edu

The filoviruses, Marburg and Ebola, have the dubious distinction of being associated with some of the highest case-fatality rates of any known infectious disease--approaching 90% in many outbreaks. In recent years, laboratory research on the filoviruses has produced treatments and vaccines that are effective in laboratory animals and that could potentially drastically reduce case-fatality rates and curtail outbreaks in humans. However, there are significant challenges in clinical testing of these products and eventual delivery to populations in need. Most cases of filovirus infection are recognized only in the setting of large outbreaks, often in the most remote and resource-poor areas of sub-Saharan Africa, with little infrastructure and few personnel experienced in clinical research. Significant political, legal, and socio-cultural barriers also exist. Here, we review the present research priorities and environment for field study of the filovirus hemorrhagic fevers and outline a strategy for future prospective clinical research on treatment and vaccine prevention.

PMID: 18336927 [PubMed - indexed for MEDLINE]

1485. Antiviral Res. 2008 Apr;78(1):51-9. Epub 2007 Nov 9.

NIAID resources for developing new therapies for severe viral infections.

Greenstone H(1), Spinelli B, Tseng C, Peacock S, Taylor K, Laughlin C.

Author information: (1)Division of Microbiology and Infectious Diseases, National Institute of Allergy and Infectious Diseases, National Institutes of Health, Bethesda, MD 20892, United States.

Severe viral infections, including hemorrhagic fever and encephalitis, occur throughout the world, but are most prevalent in developing areas that are most vulnerable to infectious diseases. Some of these can also infect related species as illustrated by the threatened extinction of gorillas by Ebola infection in west and central Africa. There are no safe and effective treatments available for these serious infections. In addition to the logistical difficulties inherent in developing a drug for infections that are sporadic and occur mainly in the third world, there is the overwhelming barrier of no hope for return on investment to encourage the pharmaceutical industry to address these unmet medical needs. Therefore, the National Institute of Allergy and infectious Disease (NIAID) has developed and supported a variety of programs and resources to provide assistance and lower the barrier for those who undertake these difficult challenges. The primary programs relevant to the development of therapies for severe viral infections are described and three case studies illustrate how they have been used. In addition, contact information for accessing these resources is supplied.

PMID: 18061283 [PubMed - indexed for MEDLINE]

1486. Expert Rev Vaccines. 2008 Apr;7(3):333-44. doi: 10.1586/14760584.7.3.333.

Protection against filovirus infection: virus-like particle vaccines.

Yang C(1), Ye L, Compans RW.

Author information: (1)Department of Microbiology and Immunology and Emory Vaccine Center, Emory University School of Medicine, 1510 Clifton Road, Atlanta, GA 30322, USA. chyang@emory.edu

Significant progress has been made in vaccine development against infection by Ebola and Marburg viruses, members of the Filoviridae, which cause severe hemorrhagic fevers in humans with no effective treatment and a mortality rate of up to 90%. Several vaccine strategies have been shown to effectively protect immunized animals against filovirus infection. Among these candidate vaccine strategies, virus-like particles represent a promising approach and have been shown to protect small laboratory animals as well as nonhuman primates against lethal challenge by Ebola and/or Marburg viruses. This review briefly summarizes filovirus epidemiology and pathogenesis, and focuses on the discussion of recent advances in filovirus vaccine development and the current understanding of protective immune responses against filovirus infection with an emphasis on the progress and challenge of filovirus virus-like particle vaccine development.

PMID: 18393603 [PubMed - indexed for MEDLINE]

1487. Virology. 2008 Mar 30;373(1):189-201. Epub 2008 Feb 20.

Interactions of LSECtin and DC-SIGN/DC-SIGNR with viral ligands: Differential pH dependence, internalization and virion binding.

Gramberg T(1), Soilleux E, Fisch T, Lalor PF, Hofmann H, Wheeldon S, Cotterill A, Wegele A, Winkler T, Adams DH, Pöhlmann S.

Author information: (1)Institute of Virology, University Hospital Erlangen, 91054 Erlangen, Germany.

The calcium-dependent lectins DC-SIGN and DC-SIGNR (collectively termed DC-SIGN/R) bind to high-mannose carbohydrates on a variety of viruses. In contrast, the related lectin LSECtin does not recognize mannose-rich glycans and interacts with a more restricted spectrum of viruses. Here, we analyzed whether these lectins differ in their mode of ligand engagement. LSECtin and DC-SIGNR, which we found to be co-expressed by liver, lymph node and bone marrow sinusoidal endothelial cells, bound to soluble Ebola virus glycoprotein (EBOV-GP) with comparable affinities. Similarly, LSECtin, DC-SIGN and the Langerhans cell-specific lectin Langerin readily bound to soluble human immunodeficiency virus type-1 (HIV-1) GP. However, only DC-SIGN captured HIV-1 particles, indicating that binding to soluble GP is not necessarily predictive of binding to virion-associated GP. Capture of EBOV-GP by LSECtin triggered ligand internalization, suggesting that LSECtin like DC-SIGN might function as an antigen uptake receptor. However, the intracellular fate of lectin-ligand complexes might differ. Thus, exposure to low-pH medium, which mimics the acidic luminal environment in endosomes/lysosomes, released ligand bound to DC-SIGN/R but had no effect on LSECtin interactions with ligand. Our results reveal important differences between pathogen capture by DC-SIGN/R and LSECtin and hint towards different biological functions of these lectins.

PMID: 18083206 [PubMed - indexed for MEDLINE]

1488. J Immunol. 2008 Mar 15;180(6):4058-66.

Functional CD8+ T cell responses in lethal Ebola virus infection.

Bradfute SB(1), Warfield KL, Bavari S.

Author information: (1)United States Army Medical Research Institute of Infectious Diseases, Fort Detrick, MD 21702, USA.

Ebola virus (EBOV) causes highly lethal hemorrhagic fever that leads to death in up to 90% of infected humans. Like many other infections, EBOV induces massive lymphocyte apoptosis, which is thought to prevent the development of a functional adaptive immune response. In a lethal mouse model of EBOV infection, we show that there is an increase in expression of the activation/maturation marker CD44 in CD4(+) and CD8(+) T cells late in infection, preceding a dramatic rebound of lymphocyte numbers in the blood. Furthermore, we observed both lymphoblasts and apoptotic lymphocytes in spleen late in infection, suggesting that there is lymphocyte activation despite substantial bystander apoptosis. To test whether these activated lymphocytes were functional, we performed adoptive transfer studies. Whole splenocytes from moribund day 7 EBOV-infected animals protected naive animals from EBOV, but not Marburgvirus, challenge. In addition, we observed EBOV-specific CD8(+) T cell IFN-gamma responses in moribund day 7 EBOV-infected mice, and adoptive transfer of CD8(+) T cells alone from day 7 mice could confer protection to EBOV-challenged naive mice. Furthermore, CD8(+) cells from day 7, but not day 0, mice proliferated after transfer to infected recipients. Therefore, despite significant lymphocyte apoptosis, a functional and specific, albeit insufficient, adaptive immune response is made in lethal EBOV infection and is protective upon transfer to naive infected recipients. These findings should cause a change in the current view of the 'impaired' immune response to EBOV challenge and may help spark new therapeutic strategies to control lethal filovirus disease.

PMID: 18322215 [PubMed - indexed for MEDLINE]

1489. Cell Host Microbe. 2008 Mar 13;3(3):168-77. doi: 10.1016/j.chom.2008.02.001.

Ebola virus matrix protein VP40 uses the COPII transport system for its intracellular transport.

Yamayoshi S(1), Noda T, Ebihara H, Goto H, Morikawa Y, Lukashevich IS, Neumann G, Feldmann H, Kawaoka Y.

Author information: (1)Division of Virology, Department of Microbiology and Immunology, Institute of Medical Science, University of Tokyo, Shirokanedai, Tokyo 108-8639, Japan.

The Ebola virus matrix protein VP40 plays an important role in virion formation and viral egress from cells. However, the host cell proteins and mechanisms responsible for intracellular transport of VP40 prior to its contribution to virion formation remain to be elucidated. Therefore we used coimmunoprecipitation and mass spectrometric analyses to identify host proteins interacting with VP40. We found that Sec24C, a component of the host COPII vesicular transport system, interacts specifically with VP40 via VP40 amino acids 303 to 307. Coimmunoprecipitation and dominant-negative mutant studies indicated that the COPII transport system plays a critical role in VP40 intracellular transport to the plasma membrane. Marburg virus VP40 was also shown to use the COPII transport system for intracellular transport. These findings identify a conserved intersection between a host pathway and filovirus replication, an intersection that can be targeted in the development of new antiviral drugs.

PMCID: PMC2330329 PMID: 18329616 [PubMed - indexed for MEDLINE]

1490. Proc Natl Acad Sci U S A. 2008 Mar 11;105(10):3974-9. doi: 10.1073/pnas.0710629105. Epub 2008 Feb 27.

ISG15 inhibits Ebola VP40 VLP budding in an L-domain-dependent manner by blocking Nedd4 ligase activity.

Okumura A(1), Pitha PM, Harty RN.

Author information: (1)Department of Pathobiology, School of Veterinary Medicine, University of Pennsylvania, Philadelphia, PA 19104, USA.

Ebola virus budding is mediated by the VP40 matrix protein. VP40 can bud from mammalian cells independent of other viral proteins, and efficient release of VP40 virus-like particles (VLPs) requires interactions with host proteins such as tsg101 and Nedd4, an E3 ubiquitin ligase. Ubiquitin itself is thought to be exploited by Ebola virus to facilitate efficient virus egress. Disruption of VP40 function and thus virus budding remains an attractive target for the development of novel antiviral therapies. Here, we investigate the effect of ISG15 protein on the release of Ebola VP40 VLPs. ISG15 is an IFN-inducible, ubiquitin-like protein expressed after bacterial or viral infection. Our results show that expression of free ISG15, or the ISGylation system (UbEIL and UbcH8), inhibits budding of Ebola virus VP40 VLPs. Addressing the molecular mechanism of this inhibition, we show that ISG15 interacts with Nedd4 ubiquitin ligase and inhibits ubiquitination of VP40. Furthermore, the L-domain deletion mutant of VP40 (DeltaPT/PY), which does not interact with Nedd4, was insensitive to ISG15-mediated inhibition of VLP release. These data provide evidence of antiviral activity of ISG15 against Ebola virus and suggest a mechanism of action involving disruption of Nedd4 function and subsequent ubiquitination of VP40.

PMCID: PMC2268823 PMID: 18305167 [PubMed - indexed for MEDLINE]

1491. Wkly Epidemiol Rec. 2008 Mar 7;83(10):89-90.

Outbreak news. Ebola haemorrhagic fever, Uganda--end of the outbreak.

[Article in English, French]

[No authors listed]

PMID: 18326109 [PubMed - indexed for MEDLINE]

1492. Cell Mol Life Sci. 2008 Mar;65(5):756-76.

Filoviruses: Interactions with the host cell.

Dolnik O(1), Kolesnikova L, Becker S.

Author information: (1)Philipps-Universität Marburg, Institut für Virologie, Marburg, Germany.

The highly pathogenic filoviruses, Marburg and Ebola virus, are difficult to handle and knowledge of the interactions between filoviruses and their host cells remained enigmatic for many years. Two developments were crucial for the presented advances in our understanding of the cell biology of filoviruses, which is still fragmentary. On the one hand, the number of high containment laboratories increased where handling of the highly pathogenic filoviruses is possible. On the other hand, molecular biological tools have been developed that allow investigation of certain aspects of filoviral replication under normal laboratory conditions which considerably accelerated research on filoviruses. This review describes advances in understanding the interactions between host cells and filoviruses during viral attachment, entry, transcription, assembly and budding.

PMID: 18158582 [PubMed - indexed for MEDLINE]

1493. Clin Vaccine Immunol. 2008 Mar;15(3):460-7. doi: 10.1128/CVI.00431-07. Epub 2008 Jan 23.

Vaccine to confer to nonhuman primates complete protection against multistrain Ebola and Marburg virus infections.

Swenson DL(1), Wang D, Luo M, Warfield KL, Woraratanadharm J, Holman DH, Dong JY, Pratt WD.

Author information: (1)U.S. Army Medical Research Institute of Infectious Diseases, 1425 Porter St., Fort Detrick, Frederick, Maryland 21702-5011, USA.

Filoviruses (Ebola and Marburg viruses) are among the deadliest viruses known to mankind, with mortality rates nearing 90%. These pathogens are highly infectious through contact with infected body fluids and can be easily aerosolized. Additionally, there are currently no licensed vaccines available to prevent filovirus outbreaks. Their high mortality rates and infectious capabilities when aerosolized and the lack of licensed vaccines available to prevent such infectious make Ebola and Marburg viruses serious bioterrorism threats, placing them both on the category A list of bioterrorism agents. Here we describe a panfilovirus vaccine based on a complex adenovirus (CAdVax) technology that expresses multiple antigens from five different filoviruses de novo. Vaccination of nonhuman primates demonstrated 100% protection against infection by two species of Ebola virus and three Marburg virus subtypes, each administered at 1,000 times the lethal dose. This study indicates the feasibility of vaccination against all current filovirus threats in the event of natural hemorrhagic fever outbreak or biological attack.

PMCID: PMC2268273 PMID: 18216185 [PubMed - indexed for MEDLINE]

1494. J Virol. 2008 Mar;82(6):2699-704. doi: 10.1128/JVI.02344-07. Epub 2008 Jan 16.

Inhibition of IRF-3 activation by VP35 is critical for the high level of virulence of ebola virus.

Hartman AL(1), Bird BH, Towner JS, Antoniadou ZA, Zaki SR, Nichol ST.

Author information: (1)Centers for Disease Control and Prevention, 1600 Clifton Rd., MS G-14, Atlanta, GA 30329, USA.

Zaire ebolavirus causes a rapidly progressing hemorrhagic disease with high mortality. Identification of the viral virulence factors that contribute to the severity of disease induced by Ebola virus is critical for the design of therapeutics and vaccines against the disease. Given the rapidity of disease progression, virus interaction with the innate immune system early in the course of infection likely plays an important role in determining the outcome of the disease. The Ebola virus VP35 protein inhibits the activation of IRF-3, a critical transcription factor for the induction of early antiviral immunity. Previous studies revealed that a single amino acid change (R312A) in VP35 renders the protein unable to inhibit IRF-3 activation. A reverse-genetics-generated, mouse-adapted, recombinant Ebola virus that encodes the R312A mutation in VP35 was produced. We found that relative to the case for wild-type virus containing the authentic VP35 sequence, this single amino acid change in VP35 renders the virus completely attenuated in mice. Given that these viruses differ by only a single amino acid in the IRF-3 inhibitory domain of VP35, the level of alteration of virulence is remarkable and highlights the importance of VP35 for the pathogenesis of Ebola virus.

PMCID: PMC2259001 PMID: 18199658 [PubMed - indexed for MEDLINE]

1495. J Virol. 2008 Mar;82(6):3131-4. doi: 10.1128/JVI.02266-07. Epub 2008 Jan 9.

Cysteines flanking the internal fusion peptide are required for the avian sarcoma/leukosis virus glycoprotein to mediate the lipid mixing stage of fusion with high efficiency.

Delos SE(1), Brecher MB, Chen Z, Melder DC, Federspiel MJ, White JM.

Author information: (1)Department of Cell Biology, UVA Health System, School of Medicine, P.O. Box 800732, Charlottesville, VA 22908-0732, USA. sed7a@virginia.edu

We previously showed that the cysteines flanking the internal fusion peptide of the avian sarcoma/leukosis virus subtype A (ASLV-A) Env (EnvA) are important for infectivity and cell-cell fusion. Here we define the stage of fusion at which the cysteines are required. The flanking cysteines are dispensable for receptor-triggered membrane association but are required for the lipid mixing step of fusion, which, interestingly, displays a high pH onset and a biphasic profile. Second-site mutations that partially restore infection partially restore lipid mixing. These findings indicate that the cysteines flanking the internal fusion peptide of EnvA (and perhaps by analogy Ebola virus glycoprotein) are important for the foldback stage of the conformational changes that lead to membrane merger.

PMCID: PMC2259008 PMID: 18184714 [PubMed - indexed for MEDLINE]

1496. J Virol Methods. 2008 Mar;148(1-2):237-43. doi: 10.1016/j.jviromet.2007.12.004. Epub 2008 Feb 1.

The creation of stable cell lines expressing Ebola virus glycoproteins and the matrix protein VP40 and generating Ebola virus-like particles utilizing an ecdysone inducible mammalian expression system.

Melito PL(1), Qiu X, Fernando LM, deVarennes SL, Beniac DR, Booth TF, Jones SM.

Author information: (1)Special Pathogens Program, National Microbiology Laboratory, Public Health Agency of Canada, 1015 Arlington Street, Winnipeg Manitoba, R3E 3R2 Canada. pasquale_melito@phac-aspc.gc.ca

Ebola virus is a filovirus that causes hemorrhagic fever in humans and is associated with case fatality rates of up to 90%. The lack of therapeutic interventions in combination with the threat of weaponizing this organism has enhanced research investigations. The expression of key viral proteins and the production of virus-like particles in mammalian systems are often pursued for characterization and functional studies. Common practice is to express these proteins through transient transfection of mammalian cells. Unfortunately the transfection reagents are expensive and the process is time consuming and labour intensive. This work describes utilizing an ecdysone inducible mammalian expression system to create stable cell lines that express the Ebola virus transmembrane glycoprotein (GP), the soluble glycoprotein (sGP) and the matrix protein (VP40) individually as well as GP and VP40 simultaneously (for the production of virus like particles). These products were the same as those expressed by the transient system, by Western blot analysis and electron microscopy. The inducible system proved to be an improvement of the current technology by enhancing the cost effectiveness and simplifying the process.

PMID: 18242720 [PubMed - indexed for MEDLINE]

1497. Nature. 2008 Feb 21;451(7181):990-3. doi: 10.1038/nature06536.

Global trends in emerging infectious diseases.

Jones KE(1), Patel NG, Levy MA, Storeygard A, Balk D, Gittleman JL, Daszak P.

Author information: (1)Institute of Zoology, Zoological Society of London, Regents Park, London NW1 4RY, UK.

Comment in Nature. 2008 Feb 21;451(7181):898-9. Nature. 2008 Mar 20;452(7185):282.

Emerging infectious diseases (EIDs) are a significant burden on global economies and public health. Their emergence is thought to be driven largely by socio-economic, environmental and ecological factors, but no comparative study has explicitly analysed these linkages to understand global temporal and spatial patterns of EIDs. Here we analyse a database of 335 EID 'events' (origins of EIDs) between 1940 and 2004, and demonstrate non-random global patterns. EID events have risen significantly over time after controlling for reporting bias, with their peak incidence (in the 1980s) concomitant with the HIV pandemic. EID events are dominated by zoonoses (60.3% of EIDs): the majority of these (71.8%) originate in wildlife (for example, severe acute respiratory virus, Ebola virus), and are increasing significantly over time. We find that 54.3% of EID events are caused by bacteria or rickettsia, reflecting a large number of drug-resistant microbes in our database. Our results confirm that EID origins are significantly correlated with socio-economic, environmental and ecological factors, and provide a basis for identifying regions where new EIDs are most likely to originate (emerging disease 'hotspots'). They also reveal a substantial risk of wildlife zoonotic and vector-borne EIDs originating at lower latitudes where reporting effort is low. We conclude that global resources to counter disease emergence are poorly allocated, with the majority of the scientific and surveillance effort focused on countries from where the next important EID is least likely to originate.

PMID: 18288193 [PubMed - indexed for MEDLINE]

1498. Hamostaseologie. 2008 Feb;28(1-2):77-84.

Viral haemorrhagic fever and vascular alterations.

Aleksandrowicz P(1), Wolf K, Falzarano D, Feldmann H, Seebach J, Schnittler H.

Author information: (1)Institut für Physiologie, Technische Universität, Medizinische Fakultät, Fetcherstrasse 74, 01307 Dresden, Germany.

Pathogenesis of viral haemorrhagic fever (VHF) is closely associated with alterations of the vascular system. Among the virus families causing VHF, filoviruses (Marburg and Ebola) are the most fatal, and will be focused on here. After entering the body, Ebola primarily targets monocytes/macrophages and dendritic cells. Infected dendritic cells are largely impaired in their activation potency, likely contributing to the immune suppression that occurs during filovirus infection. Monocytes/macrophages, however, immediately activate after viral contact and release reasonable amounts of cytokines that target the vascular system, particularly the endothelial cells. Some underlying molecular mechanisms such as alteration of the vascular endothelial cadherin/catenin complex, tyrosine phosphorylation, expression of cell adhesion molecules, tissue factor and the effect of soluble viral proteins released from infected cells to the blood stream will be discussed.

PMID: 18278167 [PubMed - indexed for MEDLINE]

1499. Proc Natl Acad Sci U S A. 2008 Jan 29;105(4):1129-33. doi: 10.1073/pnas.0708057105. Epub 2008 Jan 22.

Generation of biologically contained Ebola viruses.

Halfmann P(1), Kim JH, Ebihara H, Noda T, Neumann G, Feldmann H, Kawaoka Y.

Author information: (1)Department of Pathobiological Sciences, School of Veterinary Medicine, University of Wisconsin, Madison, WI 53706, USA.

Ebola virus (EBOV), a public health concern in Africa and a potential biological weapon, is classified as a biosafety level-4 agent because of its high mortality rate and the lack of approved vaccines and antivirals. Basic research into the mechanisms of EBOV pathogenicity and the development of effective countermeasures are restricted by the current biosafety classification of EBOVs. We therefore developed biologically contained EBOV that express a reporter gene instead of the VP30 gene, which encodes an essential transcription factor. A Vero cell line that stably expresses VP30 provides this essential protein in trans and biologically confines the virus to its complete replication cycle in this cell line. This complementation approach is highly efficient because biologically contained EBOVs lacking the VP30 gene grow to titers similar to those obtained with wild-type virus. Moreover, EBOVs lacking the VP30 gene are indistinguishable in their morphology from wild-type virus and are genetically stable, as determined by sequence analysis after seven serial passages in VP30-expressing Vero cells. We propose that this system provides a safe means to handle EBOV outside a biosafety level-4 facility and will stimulate critical studies on the EBOV life cycle as well as large-scale screening efforts for compounds with activity against this lethal virus.

PMCID: PMC2234103 PMID: 18212124 [PubMed - indexed for MEDLINE]

1500. BMC Genomics. 2008 Jan 7;9:5. doi: 10.1186/1471-2164-9-5.

Viral genome sequencing by random priming methods.

Djikeng A(1), Halpin R, Kuzmickas R, Depasse J, Feldblyum J, Sengamalay N, Afonso C, Zhang X, Anderson NG, Ghedin E, Spiro DJ.

Author information: (1)Viral Genomics Group, J, Craig Venter Institute, Rockville, MD 20850, USA. adjikeng@jcvi.org

BACKGROUND: Most emerging health threats are of zoonotic origin. For the overwhelming majority, their causative agents are RNA viruses which include but are not limited to HIV, Influenza, SARS, Ebola, Dengue, and Hantavirus. Of increasing importance therefore is a better understanding of global viral diversity to enable better surveillance and prediction of pandemic threats; this will require rapid and flexible methods for complete viral genome sequencing. RESULTS: We have adapted the SISPA methodology 123 to genome sequencing of RNA and DNA viruses. We have demonstrated the utility of the method on various types and sources of viruses, obtaining near complete genome sequence of viruses ranging in size from 3,000-15,000 kb with a median depth of coverage of 14.33. We used this technique to generate full viral genome sequence in the presence of host contaminants, using viral preparations from cell culture supernatant, allantoic fluid and fecal matter. CONCLUSION: The method described is of great utility in generating whole genome assemblies for viruses with little or no available sequence information, viruses from greatly divergent families, previously uncharacterized viruses, or to more fully describe mixed viral infections.

PMCID: PMC2254600 PMID: 18179705 [PubMed - indexed for MEDLINE]

1501. J Biol Chem. 2008 Jan 4;283(1):593-602. Epub 2007 Nov 5.

A novel mechanism for LSECtin binding to Ebola virus surface glycoprotein through truncated glycans.

Powlesland AS(1), Fisch T, Taylor ME, Smith DF, Tissot B, Dell A, Pöhlmann S, Drickamer K.

Author information: (1)Division of Molecular Biosciences, Imperial College, London, United Kingdom.

LSECtin is a member of the C-type lectin family of glycan-binding receptors that is expressed on sinusoidal endothelial cells of the liver and lymph nodes. To compare the sugar and pathogen binding properties of LSECtin with those of related but more extensively characterized receptors, such as DC-SIGN, a soluble fragment of LSECtin consisting of the C-terminal carbohydrate-recognition domain has been expressed in bacteria. A biotin-tagged version of the protein was also generated and complexed with streptavidin to create tetramers. These forms of the carbohydrate-recognition domain were used to probe a glycan array and to characterize binding to oligosaccharide and glycoprotein ligands. LSECtin binds with high selectivity to glycoproteins terminating in GlcNAcbetal-2Man. The inhibition constant for this disaccharide is 3.5 microm, making it one of the best low molecular weight ligands known for any C-type lectin. As a result of the selective binding of this disaccharide unit, the receptor recognizes glycoproteins with a truncated complex and hybrid N-linked glycans on glycoproteins. Glycan analysis of the surface glycoprotein of Ebola virus reveals the presence of such truncated glycans, explaining the ability of LSECtin to facilitate infection by Ebola virus. High mannose glycans are also present on the viral glycoprotein, which explains why DC-SIGN also binds to this virus. Thus, multiple receptors interact with surface glycoproteins of enveloped viruses that bear different types of relatively poorly processed glycans.

PMCID: PMC2275798 PMID: 17984090 [PubMed - indexed for MEDLINE]

1502. J Mol Biol. 2008 Jan 4;375(1):202-16. Epub 2007 Oct 16.

Complex of a protective antibody with its Ebola virus GP peptide epitope: unusual features of a V lambda x light chain.

Lee JE(1), Kuehne A, Abelson DM, Fusco ML, Hart MK, Saphire EO.

Author information: (1)Department of Immunology, The Scripps Research Institute, 10550 North Torrey Pines Road, La Jolla, CA 92037, USA.

13F6-1-2 is a murine monoclonal antibody that recognizes the heavily glycosylated mucin-like domain of the Ebola virus virion-attached glycoprotein (GP) and protects animals against lethal viral challenge. Here we present the crystal structure, at 2.0 A, of 13F6-1-2 in complex with its Ebola virus GP peptide epitope.

The GP peptide binds in an extended conformation, anchored primarily by interactions with the heavy chain. Two GP residues, Gln P406 and Arg P409, make extensive side-chain hydrogen bond and electrostatic interactions with the antibody and are likely critical for recognition and affinity. The 13F6-1-2 antibody utilizes a rare V lambda(x) light chain. The three light-chain complementarity-determining regions do not adopt canonical conformations and represent new classes of structures distinct from V kappa and other V lambda light chains. In addition, although V lambda(x) had been thought to confer specificity, all light-chain contacts are mediated through germ-line-encoded residues. This structure of an antibody that protects against the Ebola virus now provides a framework for humanization and development of a postexposure immunotherapeutic.
PMCID: PMC2173910 PMID: 18005986 [PubMed - indexed for MEDLINE]

1503. Chemotherapy. 2008;54(3):176-80. doi: 10.1159/000140361. Epub 2008 Jun 18.

Potent in vitro activity of the albumin fusion type I interferons (albumin-interferon-alpha and albumin-interferon-beta) against RNA viral agents of bioterrorism and the severe acute respiratory syndrome (SARS) virus.

Subramanian GM(1), Moore PA, Gowen BB, Olsen AL, Barnard DL, Paragas J, Hogan RJ, Sidwell RW.

Author information: (1)Human Genome Sciences, Inc., Rockville, MD 20850, USA. Mani_Subramanian@hgsi.com

BACKGROUND: The type I interferons (INF-alpha and INF-beta) are potent antiviral agents. Albumin-INF-alpha and albumin-INF-beta are novel recombinant proteins consisting of IFN-alpha or IFN-beta genetically fused to human albumin. METHODS: The in vitro antiviral activity of albumin-IFN-alpha was evaluated against representative bioterrorism viral agents and the severe acute respiratory syndrome virus. Antiviral activity was assessed using inhibition of cytopathic effect and neutral red staining. RESULTS: EC(50) values for albumin-IFN-alpha ranged from

(c) 2008 S. Karger AG, Basel.
PMID: 18560223 [PubMed - indexed for MEDLINE]

1504. Curr Pharm Des. 2008;14(25):2619-34.

Inhibition of RNA virus infections with peptide-conjugated morpholino oligomers.

Stein DA(1).

Author information: (1)Department of Microbiology, Oregon State University, Corvallis, OR 97331, USA. dave.stein@comcast.net

RNA virus infections cause immense human disease burdens globally, and few effective antiviral drugs are available for their treatment. Peptide-conjugated phosphorodiamidate morpholino oligomers (PPMO) are nuclease resistant and water-soluble single-stranded-DNA-analogues that can enter cells readily and act as steric-blocking antisense agents through stable duplex formation with complementary RNA. Recently there have been a number of publications documenting sequence-specific and dose-dependent inhibition of non-retroviral RNA virus infections by PPMO in both cell culture and murine experimental systems. PPMO have suppressed viral titers by several orders of magnitude in cell cultures, and have reduced viral replication in and/or increased survivorship of mice experimentally infected with poliovirus, coxsackievirus B3, dengue virus, West Nile virus, Venezuelan Equine encephalitis virus, respiratory syncytial virus, Ebola virus and influenza A virus. Along with evaluating PPMO efficacy and toxicity, these studies also explored PPMO mechanism of action, pharmacologic properties and the generation and characterization of resistant virus. Effective PPMO target sites in viral RNA have included regions of highly conserved sequence thought to be important in the pre-initiation or initiation of translation, or in long-range RNA-RNA interactions involved in viral RNA synthesis. These studies provide guidance for the design of steric-blocking antisense agents against RNA viruses, insights into viral molecular biology and novel strategies for the development of antiviral therapeutics. The purpose of this review is to summarize notable findings from the reports documenting antiviral activity by PPMO, with a focus on the specific regions of viral RNA that provided the most effective targets for PPMO-based inhibition of viral replication.
PMID: 18991679 [PubMed - indexed for MEDLINE]

1505. ILAR J. 2008;49(2):145-56.

Nonhuman primate quarantine: its evolution and practice.

Roberts JA(1), Andrews K.

Author information: (1)Valley Biosystems, 1265 Triangle Court, West Sacramento, CA 95605, USA. j.roberts@valleybiosystems.com

Nonhuman primates (NHPs) are imported to the United States for use in research, domestic breeding, and propagation of endangered populations in zoological gardens. During the past 60 years, individuals responsible for NHP importation programs have observed morbidity and mortality typically associated with infectious disease outbreaks. These outbreaks have included infectious agents such as tuberculosis, Herpesvirus sp., simian hemorrhagic fever, and filovirus infections such as the Ebola and Marburg viruses. Some outbreaks have affected both animal and human populations. These epizootics are attributable to a variety of factors, including increased population density, exposure of naïve populations to new infectious agents, and stress. The practice of quarantining animals arriving in the United States was first applied by individual research programs to improve animal health and ensure the quality of animals entering research programs. The development of government regulations for nonhuman primate quarantine accompanied the recognition that imported NHPs could pose a risk to public health. This article briefly reviews the history of US NHP importation and the factors behind the development of NHP quarantine regulations. The focus is on regulations concerned with infectious disease, public health, and the health of domestic primate colonies. These regulations have had the dual benefit of protecting public health as well as reducing animal morbidity and mortality during importation and quarantine. We review current practices and facilities for nonhuman primate quarantine and identify challenges for the future.
PMID: 18323577 [PubMed - indexed for MEDLINE]

1506. J Mater Res. 2008;23(12):3161-3168.

Design and synthesis of an antigenic mimic of the Ebola glycoprotein.

Rutledge RD(1), Huffman BJ, Cliffel DE, Wright DW.
Author information: (1)Vanderbilt University, Department of Chemistry, Nashville, Tennessee 37235.

An antigenic mimic of the Ebola glycoprotein was synthesized and tested for its ability to be recognized by an anti-Ebola glycoprotein antibody. Epitope-mapping procedures yielded a suitable epitope that, when presented on the surface of a nanoparticle, forms a structure that is recognized by an antibody specific for the native protein. This mimic-antibody interaction has been quantitated through ELISA and QCM-based methods and yielded an affinity (K(d) = 12 × 10(-6) M) within two orders of magnitude of the reported affinity of the native Ebola glycoprotein for the same antibody. These results suggest that the rational design approach described herein is a suitable method for the further development of protein-based antigenic mimics with potential applications in vaccine development and sensor technology.

PMCID: PMC2711029 PMID: 19609372 [PubMed]

1507. PLoS One. 2008;3(10):e3548. doi: 10.1371/journal.pone.0003548. Epub 2008 Oct 29.

Nasal delivery of an adenovirus-based vaccine bypasses pre-existing immunity to the vaccine carrier and improves the immune response in mice.

Croyle MA(1), Patel A, Tran KN, Gray M, Zhang Y, Strong JE, Feldmann H, Kobinger GP.
Author information: (1)Division of Pharmaceutics, College of Pharmacy, The University of Texas at Austin, Austin, Texas, USA.

Pre-existing immunity to human adenovirus serotype 5 (Ad5) is common in the general population. Bypassing pre-existing immunity could maximize Ad5 vaccine efficacy. Vaccination by the intramuscular (I.M.), nasal (I.N.) or oral (P.O.) route with Ad5 expressing Ebola Zaire glycoprotein (Ad5-ZGP) fully protected naïve mice against lethal challenge with Ebola. In the presence of pre-existing immunity, only mice vaccinated I.N. survived. The frequency of IFN-gamma+ CD8+ T cells was reduced by 80% and by 15% in animals vaccinated by the I.M. and P.O. routes respectively. Neutralizing antibodies could not be detected in serum from either treatment group. Pre-existing immunity did not compromise the frequency of IFN-gamma+ CD8+ T cells (3.9+/-1% naïve vs. 3.6+/-1% pre-existing immunity, PEI) nor anti-Ebola neutralizing antibody (NAB, 40+/-10 reciprocal dilution, both groups). The number of INF-gamma+ CD8+ cells detected in bronchioalveolar lavage fluid (BAL) after I.N. immunization was not compromised by pre-existing immunity to Ad5 (146+/-14, naïve vs. 120+/-16 SFC/million MNCs, PEI). However, pre-existing immunity reduced NAB levels in BAL by approximately 25% in this group. To improve the immune response after oral vaccination, the Ad5-based vaccine was PEGylated. Mice given the modified vaccine did not survive challenge and had reduced levels of IFN-gamma+ CD8+ T cells 10 days after administration (0.3+/-0.3% PEG vs. 1.7+/-0.5% unmodified). PEGylation did increase NAB levels 2-fold. These results provide some insight about the degree of T and B cell mediated immunity necessary for protection against Ebola virus and suggest that modification of the virus capsid can influence the type of immune response elicited by an Ad5-based vaccine.

PMCID: PMC2569416 PMID: 18958172 [PubMed - indexed for MEDLINE]

1508. Lancet. 2007 Dec 22;370(9605):2085.

Ebola outbreak in Uganda "atypical", say experts.

Alsop Z.

PMID: 18161067 [PubMed - indexed for MEDLINE]

1509. J Virol. 2007 Dec;81(24):13378-84. Epub 2007 Oct 10.

Proteolysis of the Ebola virus glycoproteins enhances virus binding and infectivity.

Kaletsky RL(1), Simmons G, Bates P.
Author information: (1)Department of Microbiology, University of Pennsylvania School of Medicine, 225 Johnson Pavilion, 3610 Hamilton Walk, Philadelphia, PA 19104-6076, USA.

Cellular cathepsins are required for Ebola virus infection and are believed to proteolytically process the Ebola virus glycoprotein (GP) during entry. However, the significance of cathepsin cleavage during infection remains unclear. Here we demonstrate a role for cathepsin L (CatL) cleavage of Ebola virus GP in the generation of a stable 18-kDa GP1 viral intermediate that exhibits increased binding to and infectivity for susceptible cell targets. Cell binding to a lymphocyte line was increased when CatL-proteolysed pseudovirions were used, but lymphocytes remained resistant to Ebola virus GP-mediated infection. Genetic removal of the highly glycosylated mucin domain in Ebola virus GP resulted in cell binding similar to that observed with CatL-treated full-length GP, and no overall enhancement of binding or infectivity was observed when mucin-deleted virions were treated with CatL. These results suggest that cathepsin cleavage of Ebola virus GP facilitates an interaction with a cellular receptor(s) and that removal of the mucin domain may facilitate receptor binding. The influence of CatL in Ebola virus GP receptor binding should be useful in future studies characterizing the mechanism of Ebola virus entry.

PMCID: PMC2168880 PMID: 17928356 [PubMed - indexed for MEDLINE]

1510. J Virol. 2007 Dec;81(24):13469-77. Epub 2007 Oct 10.

Ebola virus VP24 proteins inhibit the interaction of NPI-1 subfamily karyopherin alpha proteins with activated STAT1.

Reid SP(1), Valmas C, Martinez O, Sanchez FM, Basler CF.
Author information: (1)Department of Microbiology, Box 1124, Mount Sinai School of Medicine, 1 Gustave L. Levy Place, New York, NY 10029, USA.

The Zaire ebolavirus protein VP24 was previously demonstrated to inhibit alpha/beta interferon (IFN-alpha/beta)- and IFN-gamma-induced nuclear accumulation of tyrosine-phosphorylated STAT1 (PY-STAT1) and to inhibit IFN-alpha/beta- and IFN-gamma-induced gene expression. These properties correlated with the ability of VP24 to interact with the nuclear localization signal receptor for PY-STAT1, karyopherin alpha1. Here, VP24 is demonstrated to interact not only with overexpressed but also with endogenous karyopherin alpha1. Mutational analysis demonstrated that VP24 binds within the PY-STAT1 binding region located in the C terminus of karyopherin alpha1. In addition, VP24 was found to inhibit PY-STAT1 binding to both overexpressed and endogenous karyopherin alpha1. We assessed the binding of both PY-STAT1 and the VP24 proteins from Zaire, mouse-adapted Zaire, and Reston Ebola viruses for interaction with all six members of the human karyopherin alpha family. We found, in contrast to previous studies, that PY-STAT1 can interact not only with karyopherin alpha1 but also with karyopherins alpha5 and alpha6, which together comprise the NPI-1 subfamily of karyopherin alphaS. Similarly, all three VP24s bound and inhibited PY-STAT1 interaction with karyopherins alpha1, alpha5, and alpha6. Consistent with their ability to inhibit the karyopherin-PY-STAT1 interaction, Zaire, mouse-adapted Zaire, and Reston Ebola virus VP24s displayed similar capacities to inhibit IFN-beta-induced gene expression in human and mouse cells. These findings suggest that VP24 inhibits interaction of PY-STAT1 with karyopherins alpha1, alpha5, or alpha6 by binding within the PY-STAT1 binding region of the karyopherins and that this function is conserved among the VP24 proteins of different Ebola virus species.

PMCID: PMC2168840 PMID: 17928350 [PubMed - indexed for MEDLINE]

1511. Virus Genes. 2007 Dec;35(3):511-20. Epub 2007 Jun 15.

Influence of calcium/calmodulin on budding of Ebola VLPs: implications for the involvement of the Ras/Raf/MEK/ERK pathway.

Han Z(1), Harty RN.

Author information: (1)Department of Pathobiology, School of Veterinary Medicine, University of Pennsylvania, 3800 Spruce St., Philadelphia, PA 19104-6049, USA.

The VP40 matrix protein of Ebola virus is able to bud from mammalian cells as a virus-like particle (VLP). Interactions between L-domain motifs of VP40 and host proteins such as Tsg101 and Nedd4 serve to facilitate budding of VP40 VLPs. Since intracellular levels of calcium are known to influence localization and function of host proteins involved in virus budding, we sought to determine, whether alterations of calcium or calmodulin levels in cells would affect budding of VP40 VLPs. VP40 VLP release was assessed in cells treated with BAPTA/AM, a calcium ion chelator, or with ionomycin, a calcium ionophore. In addition, VLP budding was assessed in cells treated with W7, W13, or TFP; all calmodulin antagonists. Results from these experiments indicated that: (i) budding of VP40 VLPs was reduced in a dose-dependent manner in the presence of BAPTA/AM, and slightly enhanced in the presence of ionomycin, (ii) VP40 VLP budding was reduced in a dose-dependent manner in the presence of W7, whereas VP40 VLP budding was unaffected in the presence of cyclosporine-A, (iii) budding of VSV-WT and a VSV recombinant (M40 virus) possessing the L-domains of Ebola VP40 was inhibited in the presence of W7, W13, or TFP, (iv) inhibition of virus budding by W7, W13, and TFP appears to be L-domain independent, and (v) the mechanism of calcium/calmodulin-mediated inhibition of Ebola VLP budding may involve the Ras/Raf/MEK/ERK signaling pathway.

PMID: 17570046 [PubMed - indexed for MEDLINE]

1512. J Infect Dis. 2007 Nov 15;196 Suppl 2:S438-43.

Filovirus research: knowledge expands to meet a growing threat.

Bray M(1), Murphy FA.

Author information: (1)Integrated Research Facility, National Institute of Allergy and Infectious Diseases, National Institutes of Health, Bethesda, MD 20892, USA. mbray@niaid.nih.gov

PMID: 17940981 [PubMed - indexed for MEDLINE]

1513. J Infect Dis. 2007 Nov 15;196 Suppl 2:S430-7.

Ebola virus-like particle-based vaccine protects nonhuman primates against lethal Ebola virus challenge.

Warfield KL(1), Swenson DL, Olinger GG, Kalina WV, Aman MJ, Bavari S.

Author information: (1)US Army Medical Research Institute of Infectious Diseases, Fort Detrick, MD 21702, USA.

BACKGROUND: Currently, there are no licensed vaccines or therapeutics for the prevention or treatment of infection by the highly lethal filoviruses, Ebola virus (EBOV) and Marburg virus (MARV), in humans. We previously had demonstrated the protective efficacy of virus-like particle (VLP)-based vaccines against EBOV and MARV infection in rodents. METHODS: To determine the efficacy of vaccination with Ebola VLPs (eVLPs) in nonhuman primates, we vaccinated cynomolgus macaques with eVLPs containing EBOV glycoprotein (GP), nucleoprotein (NP), and VP40 matrix protein and challenged the macaques with 1000 pfu of EBOV. RESULTS: Serum samples from the eVLP-vaccinated nonhuman primates demonstrated EBOV-specific antibody titers, as measured by enzyme-linked immunosorbent assay, complement-mediated lysis assay, and antibody-dependent cell-mediated cytotoxicity assay. CD44+ T cells from eVLP-vaccinated macaques but not from a naive macaque responded with vigorous production of tumor necrosis factor- alpha after EBOV-peptide stimulation. All 5 eVLP-vaccinated monkeys survived challenge without clinical or laboratory signs of EBOV infection, whereas the control animal died of infection. CONCLUSION: On the basis of safety and efficacy, eVLPs represent a promising filovirus vaccine for use in humans.

PMID: 17940980 [PubMed - indexed for MEDLINE]

1514. J Infect Dis. 2007 Nov 15;196 Suppl 2:S421-9.

Filovirus-like particles produced in insect cells: immunogenicity and protection in rodents.

Warfield KL(1), Posten NA, Swenson DL, Olinger GG, Esposito D, Gillette WK, Hopkins RF, Costantino J, Panchal RG, Hartley JL, Aman MJ, Bavari S.

Author information: (1)US Army Medical Research Institute of Infectious Diseases, Fort Detrick, MD 21702, USA.

BACKGROUND: Virus-like particles (VLPs) of Ebola virus (EBOV) and Marburg virus (MARV) produced in human 293T embryonic kidney cells have been shown to be effective vaccines against filoviral infection. In this study, we explored alternative strategies for production of filovirus-like particle-based vaccines, to accelerate the development process. The goal of this work was to increase the yield of VLPs, while retaining their immunogenic properties. METHODS: Ebola and Marburg VLPs (eVLPs and mVLPs, respectively) were generated by use of recombinant baculovirus constructs expressing glycoprotein, VP40 matrix protein, and nucleoprotein from coinfected insect cells. The baculovirus-derived eVLPs and mVLPs were characterized biochemically, and then the immune responses produced by the eVLPs in insect cells were studied further. RESULTS: The baculovirus-derived eVLPs elicited maturation of human myeloid dendritic cells (DCs), indicating their immunogenic properties. Mice vaccinated with insect cell-derived eVLPs generated antibody and cellular responses equivalent to those vaccinated with mammalian 293T cell-derived eVLPs and were protected from EBOV challenge in a dose-dependent manner. CONCLUSION: Together, these data suggest that filovirus-like particles produced by baculovirus expression systems, which are amenable to large-scale production, are highly immunogenic and are suitable as safe and effective vaccines for the prevention of filoviral infection.

PMID: 17940979 [PubMed - indexed for MEDLINE]

1515. J Infect Dis. 2007 Nov 15;196 Suppl 2:S413-20.

Mucosal delivery of adenovirus-based vaccine protects against Ebola virus infection in mice.

Patel A(1), Zhang Y, Croyle M, Tran K, Gray M, Strong J, Feldmann H, Wilson JM, Kobinger GP.

Author information: (1)Special Pathogens Program, National Microbiology Laboratory, Public Health Agency of Canada, Canada.

BACKGROUND: Mucosal vaccination can offer several advantages over conventional intramuscular immunization to protect against Ebola virus (EBOV) infection, such as immune protection at sites of viral entry into susceptible individuals, and can be administered using needle-free devices. METHODS: The present study evaluated oral and nasal vaccination of mice with human adenovirus serotype 5 (Ad) expressing the Zaire ebolavirus glycoprotein (Ad-ZGP) in terms of their protection against and underlying immune responses to EBOV. RESULTS: Similar to intramuscular administration, oral or nasal vaccination of mice with Ad-ZGP fully protected the mice against a lethal challenge with mouse-adapted EBOV. Both T and B cell responses developed in mice receiving oral or nasal vaccination in different body compartments, indicating qualitative improvement of the immune response after mucosal immunization, compared with intramuscular vaccination. CONCLUSIONS: Overall, the breadth of the immune response noted after nasal or oral immunization, including stimulation of CD8+ T cells or effector memory T cells from the gastrointestinal tract or the lungs, was superior to that noted after intramuscular administration of the vaccine. The present study showed that adenovirus-based vaccine is effective against EBOV infection in mice after oral and nasal immunization.

PMID: 17940978 [PubMed - indexed for MEDLINE]

1516. J Infect Dis. 2007 Nov 15;196 Suppl 2:S404-12.

Assessment of a vesicular stomatitis virus-based vaccine by use of the mouse model of Ebola virus hemorrhagic fever.

Jones SM(1), Stroher U, Fernando L, Qiu X, Alimonti J, Melito P, Bray M, Klenk HD, Feldmann H.

Author information: (1)Special Pathogens Program, National Microbiology Laboratory, Public Health Agency of Canada, Canada. Steven_jones@phac-aspc.gc.ca

BACKGROUND: In humans and nonhuman primates, Ebola virus causes a virulent viral hemorrhagic fever for which no licensed vaccines or therapeutic drugs exist. In the present study, we used the mouse model for Ebola hemorrhagic fever to assess the safety and efficacy of a vaccine based on a live attenuated vesicular stomatitis virus expressing the Zaire ebolavirus (ZEBOV) glycoprotein. METHODS: Healthy mice were given the vaccine in various doses, decreasing from 2 x 10(4) to 2 plaque-forming units (pfu), with both systemic and mucosal vaccination routes used. Mice were challenged with 10(3) to 10(6) lethal doses of mouse-adapted ZEBOV. Severely immunocompromised mice were injected with 2 x 10(5) pfu, which is 10 times greater than the immunization dose normally used, to test vaccine safety. RESULTS: Two plaque-forming units of the vaccine protected against lethal challenge, and mucosal immunization was found to be as protective as systemic injection. The replicating vaccine was never detected in the immunized animals, nor were there clinical signs after immunization. Immunization of severely immunocompromised mice with 200,000 pfu of vaccine resulted in no clinical symptoms. CONCLUSIONS: Our data suggest that the vaccine is highly potent and safe and that it very rapidly induces "sterile" immunity in mice. The potential for mucosal delivery, if confirmed in nonhuman primates, makes it an excellent candidate for mass immunization during outbreaks or in the event of intentional release.

PMID: 17940977 [PubMed - indexed for MEDLINE]

1517. J Infect Dis. 2007 Nov 15;196 Suppl 2:S400-3.

Ebola hemorrhagic fever: evaluation of passive immunotherapy in nonhuman primates.

Jahrling PB(1), Geisbert JB, Swearengen JR, Larsen T, Geisbert TW.

Author information: (1)Integrated Research Facility at Fort Detrick, National Institute of Allergy and Infectious Diseases, National Institutes of Health, Fort Detrick, MD, USA. jahrlingp@niaid.nih.gov

The survival of 7 of 8 patients with Ebola virus (EBOV) infection after transfusions of convalescent-phase blood during a 1995 outbreak of EBOV infection is frequently cited as evidence that passive immunotherapy is a viable treatment option. To test whether whole-blood transfusions were more efficacious than passively administered immunoglobulins or monoclonal antibodies, we transfused convalescent-phase blood from EBOV-immune monkeys into naive animals shortly after challenge with EBOV. Although passively acquired antibody titers comparable to those associated with effective vaccination were obtained, all monkeys that had received transfusions succumbed to infection concurrently with control monkeys. These data cast further doubt on the value of passive immunotherapy for the treatment of EBOV infection.

PMID: 17940976 [PubMed - indexed for MEDLINE]

1518. J Infect Dis. 2007 Nov 15;196 Suppl 2:S390-9.

Recombinant human activated protein C for the postexposure treatment of Ebola hemorrhagic fever.

Hensley LE(1), Stevens EL, Yan SB, Geisbert JB, Macias WL, Larsen T, Daddario-DiCaprio KM, Cassell GH, Jahrling PB, Geisbert TW.

Author information: (1)Virology Division, US Army Medical Research Institute of Infectious Diseases, Fort Detrick, MD, USA.

BACKGROUND: Infection of primates with Zaire ebolavirus (ZEBOV) leads to hypotension, coagulation disorders, and an impaired immune response and, in many ways, resembles severe sepsis. Rapid decreases in plasma levels of protein C are a prominent feature of severe sepsis and ZEBOV hemorrhagic fever (ZHF). Currently, recombinant human activated protein C (rhAPC [Xigris; Eli Lilly]) is licensed for treating human patients with severe sepsis who are at high risk of death. The aim of this study was to test the efficacy of rhAPC as a potential treatment for ZHF. METHODS: Fourteen rhesus macaques were challenged with a uniformly lethal dose of ZEBOV; 11 of these monkeys were treated by intravenous infusion with rhAPC beginning 30-60 min after challenge and continuing for 7 days. Three control monkeys received sterile saline in parallel. RESULTS: All 3 control monkeys died on day 8, whereas 2 of the 11 rhAPC-treated monkeys survived. The mean time to death for the rhAPC-treated monkeys that did not survive ZEBOV challenge was 12.6 days. The difference in survival was significant when the rhAPC-treated monkeys were compared with historical controls. CONCLUSIONS: The experimental findings provide evidence that ZHF and severe sepsis share underlying mechanisms and may respond to the same therapies.

PMID: 17940975 [PubMed - indexed for MEDLINE]

1519. J Infect Dis. 2007 Nov 15;196 Suppl 2:S382-9.

In vitro evaluation of antisense RNA efficacy against filovirus infection, by use of reverse genetics.

Groseth A(1), Hoenen T, Alimonti JB, Zielecki F, Ebihara H, Theriault S, Ströher U, Becker S, Feldmann H.

Author information: (1)National Laboratory for Zoonotic Diseases and Special Pathogens, National Microbiology Laboratory, Public Health Agency of Canada. BACKGROUND: Recent reports indicate the possibility of using small interfering RNAs (siRNAs) to treat filovirus infections; however, they also show that the effectiveness of this approach is highly dependent on target site selection. Therefore, we explored the application of minigenomes as screening tools to identify functional siRNA targets under biosafety level 2 conditions. METHODS: siRNA candidates were screened using the minigenome system to identify those with potential antiviral activity, compared with controls with poor predicted function on the basis of design guidelines, or those that were noncomplementary to Zaire ebolavirus (ZEBOV). These findings were then validated in cell culture by use of a previously developed ZEBOV expressing green fluorescent protein (ZEBOV-GFP), which allowed siRNA function to be easily assessed via flow cytometry or focus formation. RESULTS: The most promising siRNA based on minigenome screening, targeting the nucleoprotein (NP) mRNA (ZNP1), also reduced protein expression and decreased viral titers after infection with ZEBOV-GFP to an extent similar to that reported for an siRNA recently shown to be therapeutic in guinea pigs. CONCLUSIONS: Minigenome screening appears to be an effective and convenient method of evaluating the therapeutic potential of siRNA targets, and findings suggest that its use would increase success rates in later stages of siRNA testing.

PMID: 17940974 [PubMed - indexed for MEDLINE]

1520. J Infect Dis. 2007 Nov 15;196 Suppl 2:S372-81.

Marburg virus Angola infection of rhesus macaques: pathogenesis and treatment with recombinant nematode anticoagulant protein c2.

Geisbert TW(1), Daddario-DiCaprio KM, Geisbert JB, Young HA, Formenty P, Fritz EA, Larsen T, Hensley LE.

Author information: (1)Integrated Research Facility at Fort Detrick, National Institute of Allergy and Infectious Diseases, National Institutes of Health, Fort Detrick, MD, USA. tgeisbert@bu.edu

BACKGROUND: The procoagulant tissue factor (TF) is thought to play a role in the coagulation disorders that characterize filoviral infections. In this study, we evaluated the pathogenesis of lethal infection with the Angola strain of Marburg virus (MARV-Ang) in rhesus macaques and tested the efficacy of recombinant nematode anticoagulant protein c2 (rNAPc2), an inhibitor of TF/factor VIIa, as a potential treatment. METHODS: Twelve rhesus macaques were challenged with a high dose (1000 pfu) of MARV-Ang. Six macaques were treated with rNAPc2, and 6 macaques served as control animals. RESULTS: All 6 control animals succumbed to MARV-Ang challenge by day 8 (mean, 7.3 days), whereas 5 of 6 rNAPc2-treated animals died on day 9 and 1 rNAPc2-treated animal survived. The disease course for MARV-Ang infection appeared to progress more rapidly in rhesus macaques than has been previously reported for other strains of MARV. In contrast to Ebola virus (EBOV) infection in macaques, up-regulation of TF was not as striking, and deposition of fibrin was a less prominent pathologic feature of disease in these animals. CONCLUSIONS: These data show that the pathogenicity of MARV-Ang infection appears to be consistent with the apparent increased human virulence attributed to this strain. The apparent reduced efficacy of rNAPc2 against MARV-Ang infection, compared with its efficacy against EBOV infection, appears to be associated with differences in TF induction and fibrin deposition.

PMID: 17940973 [PubMed - indexed for MEDLINE]

1521. J Infect Dis. 2007 Nov 15;196 Suppl 2:S364-71.

Blood chemistry measurements and D-Dimer levels associated with fatal and nonfatal outcomes in humans infected with Sudan Ebola virus.

Rollin PE(1), Bausch DG, Sanchez A.

Author information: (1)Special Pathogens Branch, Division of Viral and Rickettsial Diseases, National Center for Infectious Diseases, Centers for Disease Control and Prevention, Atlanta, GA 30333, USA.

Blood samples from patients infected with the Sudan species of Ebola virus (EBOV), obtained during an outbreak of disease in Uganda in 2000, were tested for a panel of analytes to evaluate their clinical condition and to compare values obtained for patients with fatal and nonfatal cases and for uninfected (hospitalized control) patients. Liver function tests showed higher levels of aspartate aminotransferase (AST) in blood samples from patients with fatal cases than in samples from patients with nonfatal cases, whereas alanine aminotransferase levels were comparable and only slightly increased in all patients, suggesting that increased blood AST levels are due to a greater degree of injury in tissues other than the liver. Significantly higher levels of amylase, urea nitrogen, and creatinine suggest that acute pancreatitis and renal dysfunction develop in fatal cases, whereas reduced albumin and calcium levels may be linked to these conditions or to liver damage. d-Dimer levels in blood specimens were drastically increased in patients with fatal and nonfatal infections but were 4 times higher in patients with fatal cases than in patients who survived (180,000 vs. 44,000 ng/mL), during the most acute period of the infection (6-8 days after onset). These results indicate that disseminated intravascular coagulation is an early and important component of EBOV disease. This study has identified levels of analytes with prognostic value, which can also be used to target therapeutic interventions, and expands on the findings of prior blood tests conducted on this group of patients.

PMID: 17940972 [PubMed - indexed for MEDLINE]

1522. J Infect Dis. 2007 Nov 15;196 Suppl 2:S357-63.

Cytokine and chemokine expression in humans infected with Sudan Ebola virus.

Hutchinson KL(1), Rollin PE.

Author information: (1)Special Pathogens Branch, Centers for Disease Control and Prevention, Atlanta, GA 30333, USA. kbh6@cdc.gov

The size and duration of the 2000 outbreak of Sudan Ebola virus (SEBOV) infection in Uganda made it possible to collect serial serum samples from 87 patients (53 survivors and 34 nonsurvivors). Surprisingly, the levels of tumor necrosis factor- alpha and interferon (IFN)- gamma , which had been found to be increased in patients with fatal Zaire Ebola virus infection, were not increased in any of the patients with SEBOV infection. The levels of interleukin (IL)-1 beta , IFN- gamma -inducible protein-10, and RANTES (regulated on activation, normally T cell-expressed and -secreted) were higher in samples from all patients with SEBOV infection than in control samples from healthy hospital staff members, but their levels did not differ between those who survived and those who did not. The levels of IFN- alpha were significantly higher in surviving patients with SEBOV infection, whereas the levels of IL-6, IL-8, IL-10, and macrophage inflammatory protein-1 beta were higher in patients with fatal SEBOV infections.

PMID: 17940971 [PubMed - indexed for MEDLINE]

1523. J Infect Dis. 2007 Nov 15;196 Suppl 2:S347-56.

Epitopes required for antibody-dependent enhancement of Ebola virus infection.

Takada A(1), Ebihara H, Feldmann H, Geisbert TW, Kawaoka Y.

Author information: (1)Department of Global Epidemiology, Research Center for Zoonosis Control, Hokkaido University, Sapporo 060-0818, Japan. atakada@czc.hokudai.ac.jp

We have shown that antibody-dependent enhancement (ADE) of infection with Zaire Ebola virus (ZEBOV) is mediated by interaction of virus-specific antibodies with Fc receptors or complement component C1q and its receptors in vitro. ADE activities of the antisera to the viral glycoprotein (GP) were virus species specific and were primarily correlated with immunoglobulin (Ig) G2a and IgM levels but not with IgG1 levels. Interestingly, compared with ZEBOV, Reston Ebola virus (REBOV) had substantially weaker potential to induce ADE antibodies. Using monoclonal antibodies, we identified ZEBOV-specific ADE epitopes. To confirm epitope specificity, we constructed a chimeric ZEBOV GP, the ADE epitopes of which were replaced with the corresponding regions of REBOV GP. We found that mouse antisera to the chimeric ZEBOV GP showed less potential to induce ADE activity than did mouse antisera to wild-type ZEBOV GP, although they retained neutralizing activity. These data suggest that GP lacking the ADE-inducing epitopes may increase the potential of GP as a vaccine antigen.

PMID: 17940970 [PubMed - indexed for MEDLINE]

1524. J Infect Dis. 2007 Nov 15;196 Suppl 2:S329-36.

Sequence-based human leukocyte antigen-B typing of patients infected with Ebola virus in Uganda in 2000: identification of alleles associated with fatal and nonfatal disease outcomes.

Sanchez A(1), Wagoner KE, Rollin PE.

Author information: (1)Special Pathogens Branch, Division of Viral and Rickettsial Diseases, National Center for Infectious Diseases, Centers for Disease Control and Prevention, Atlanta, GA 30333, USA. ans1@cdc.gov

The Sudan species of Ebola virus (SEBOV) causes severe, often fatal infection in approximately 50% of infected humans. We sought to determine whether the human leukocyte antigen-B (HLA-B) locus has a role in the outcome of SEBOV disease by typing 77 cases from an outbreak in northern Uganda in 2000-2001. Sequence-based HLA-B typing was performed using leukocytes isolated from 77 patients. Statistical analysis and a predictive discriminant analysis (PDA) were applied to typing data. Epitope prediction software was also applied to SEBOV sequences. Statistically significant associations were found between certain sets of alleles and either fatal or nonfatal disease outcomes. Alleles B*67 and B*15 were associated with fatal outcomes, whereas B*07 and B*14 were associated with nonfatal outcomes. The PDA-derived functions that were produced were 81.8% accurate in classifying patients into their correct outcome group. Several epitopes predicted to bind strongly to HLA-B*07 molecules were identified in the viral polymerase, nucleoprotein, and VP35 protein. HLA-B alleles associated with either fatal or nonfatal outcomes of SEBOV disease were identified and can be used in a predictive model. Studies of HLA-B-restricted epitopes could contribute to characterization of protective host responses and to vaccine development.

PMID: 17940968 [PubMed - indexed for MEDLINE]

1525. J Infect Dis. 2007 Nov 15;196 Suppl 2:S323-8.

Pathologic findings associated with delayed death in nonhuman primates experimentally infected with Zaire Ebola virus.

Larsen T(1), Stevens EL, Davis KJ, Geisbert JB, Daddario-DiCaprio KM, Jahrling PB, Hensley LE, Geisbert TW.

Author information: (1)Pathology Division, US Army Medical Research Institute of Infectious Diseases, Fort Detrick, MD, USA.

Zaire Ebola virus infection in macaques causes a fatal disease with a pathogenesis similar to that in humans. During several independent therapy studies, we noted altered tissue tropism in 6 rhesus macaques that survived longer than those with a typical disease course. The mean time to death for these 6 macaques was 21.7 days, which is significantly longer than the average mean time to death of 8.3 days for 20 untreated historical control animals. In addition to living significantly longer, these 6 animals exhibited a variety of deteriorating clinical signs with pathologic findings that were not seen in the untreated control animals, as well as the presence of viral antigen in the brain, eye, pancreas, thyroid, and lung. We suggest that treatment extended the time course of the disease and permitted the virus to infect tissues not usually affected in the typical model.

PMID: 17940967 [PubMed - indexed for MEDLINE]

1526. J Infect Dis. 2007 Nov 15;196 Suppl 2:S313-22.

In vitro and in vivo characterization of recombinant Ebola viruses expressing enhanced green fluorescent protein.

Ebihara H(1), Theriault S, Neumann G, Alimonti JB, Geisbert JB, Hensley LE, Groseth A, Jones SM, Geisbert TW, Kawaoka Y, Feldmann H.

Author information: (1)Department of Special Pathogens, International Research Center for Infectious Diseases, University of Tokyo, Tokyo, Japan. Hideki_Ebihara@phac-aspc.gc.ca

To facilitate an understanding of the molecular aspects of the pathogenesis of Zaire ebolavirus (ZEBOV) infection, we generated 2 different recombinant viruses expressing enhanced green fluorescent protein (eGFP) from additional transcription units inserted at different positions in the virus genome. These viruses showed in vitro phenotypes similar to that of wild-type ZEBOV (wt-ZEBOV) and were stable over multiple passages. Infection with one of the viruses expressing eGFP produced only mild disease in rhesus macaques, demonstrating a marked attenuation in this animal model. However, in mice lacking signal transducer and activator of transcription 1, both viruses expressing eGFP caused lethal cases of disease that were moderately attenuated, compared with that caused by wt-ZEBOV. In mice, viral replication could be easily tracked by the detection of eGFP-positive cells in tissues, by use of flow cytometry. These findings demonstrate that the incorporation of a foreign gene will attenuate ZEBOV in vivo but that these viruses still have potential for in vitro and in vivo research applications.

PMID: 17940966 [PubMed - indexed for MEDLINE]

1527. J Infect Dis. 2007 Nov 15;196 Suppl 2:S296-304.

Lymphocyte death in a mouse model of Ebola virus infection.

Bradfute SB(1), Braun DR, Shamblin JD, Geisbert JB, Paragas J, Garrison A, Hensley LE, Geisbert TW.

Author information: (1)Virology Division, US Army Medical Research Institute of Infectious Diseases, Fort Detrick, MD, USA.

BACKGROUND: A striking feature of Zaire Ebola virus (ZEBOV) infection in nonhuman primates is the rapid depletion of T and NK lymphocytes by apoptosis. In a mouse model of ZEBOV infection, lymphocyte death is a prominent finding; however, the mechanism of death and the lymphocyte subsets that are targeted remain unknown. METHODS: We extended the characterization of lymphocyte death in a mouse model of ZEBOV infection by evaluating lymphocytes during the course of disease, using flow cytometry, electron microscopy, and terminal deoxynucleotidyl transferase-mediated deoxyuridine triphosphate nick-end labeling (TUNEL). RESULTS: B cell, CD4+ and CD8+ T cell, and NK cell counts all dropped dramatically in the blood of infected BALB/c mice, and lymphocyte death was observed in the spleen by means of TUNEL staining and in the blood by means of electron microscopy. Morphologically, lymphocyte death occurred by both classic apoptosis and apoptosis-like programmed cell death. CONCLUSIONS: The early and severe loss of peripheral blood NK and CD8+ lymphocytes in ZEBOV-infected mice is similar to that seen in macaques. The morphological basis of lymphocyte death in ZEBOV-infected mice appears to be both classic apoptosis and apoptosis-like programmed cell death, although lymphocyte apoptosis in ZEBOV-infected nonhuman primates seems to occur primarily via classic apoptosis. The mouse model of ZEBOV infection may be useful for the screening of therapeutics directed against limiting lymphocyte death.

PMID: 17940964 [PubMed - indexed for MEDLINE]

1528. J Infect Dis. 2007 Nov 15;196 Suppl 2:S291-5.

Mapping of a region of Ebola virus VP40 that is important in the production of virus-like particles.

Yamayoshi S(1), Kawaoka Y.

Author information: (1)Division of Virology, Department of Microbiology and Immunology, University of Tokyo, Tokyo 108-8639, Japan.

Ebola virus VP40 contains 2 overlapping late domains (7-PTAP-10 and 10-PPEY-13) that are essential for its interaction with Tsg101 and Nedd4 in the promotion of viral egress. Deletion of the late domains inhibits VP40-induced virus-like particles (VLPs). However, a truncated form of VP40, which lacks a late domain because of the deletion of amino acids 1-30, is released into supernatant as a VLP, indicating that the remaining portion of VP40 contains the structural elements required for VLP release. Thus, the purpose of this study was to identify the VP40 sequence essential for VLP budding, through the generation of deletion and alanine-scanning mutants. We found that the amino acid sequence around the proline at position 53 plays a critical role in VLP production and intracellular transport. These data also may suggest that a novel host factor(s) is involved in virus budding.

PMID: 17940963 [PubMed - indexed for MEDLINE]

1529. J Infect Dis. 2007 Nov 15;196 Suppl 2:S284-90.

Ebola virus (EBOV) VP24 inhibits transcription and replication of the EBOV genome.

Watanabe S(1), Noda T, Halfmann P, Jasenosky L, Kawaoka Y.

Author information: (1)Department of Pathobiological Sciences, School of Veterinary Medicine, University of Wisconsin, Madison, WI, USA.

The roles of Ebola virus (EBOV) VP24 in nucleocapsid (NC) formation and the effect of VP24 on transcription and replication of the viral genome during NC formation remain unknown. We therefore examined the effect of VP24 on the expression of a reporter gene (luciferase), viral RNA, and messenger RNA from the EBOV minigenome. VP24 inhibited the expression of luciferase and both RNAs in a dose-dependent manner, suggesting that VP24 inhibits transcription and replication of the EBOV genome. By contrast, FLAG-tagged VP24, which cannot support NC-like structure formation, did not appreciably decrease luciferase expression, indicating that association of VP24 with the ribonucleoprotein complex is required for inhibition. Glycoprotein and VP40 did not affect VP24-mediated inhibition of transcription and replication. Together, these results suggest that VP24 reduces transcription and replication of the EBOV genome by direct association with the ribonucleoprotein complex in virus-infected cells.

PMID: 17940962 [PubMed - indexed for MEDLINE]

1530. J Infect Dis. 2007 Nov 15;196 Suppl 2:S276-83.

Ebola virus inactivation with preservation of antigenic and structural integrity by a photoinducible alkylating agent.

Warfield KL(1), Swenson DL, Olinger GG, Kalina WV, Viard M, Aitichou M, Chi X, Ibrahim S, Blumenthal R, Raviv Y, Bavari S, Aman MJ.

Author information: (1)US Army Medical Research Institute of Infectious Diseases, Fort Detrick, MD, USA.

Current methods for inactivating filoviruses are limited to high doses of irradiation or formalin treatment, which may cause structural perturbations that are reflected by poor immunogenicity. In this report, we describe a novel inactivation technique for Zaire Ebola virus (ZEBOV) that uses the photoinduced alkylating probe 1,5-iodonaphthylazide (INA). INA is incorporated into lipid bilayers and, when activated by ultraviolet irradiation, alkylates the proteins therein. INA treatment of ZEBOV resulted in the complete loss of infectivity in cells. Results of electron microscopy and virus-capture assays suggested the preservation of conformational surface epitopes. Challenge with 50,000 pfu of INA-inactivated, mouse-adapted ZEBOV did not cause disease or death in mice. A single vaccination with INA-inactivated ZEBOV (equivalent to 5 x 10(4) pfu) protected mice against lethal challenge with 1000 pfu of ZEBOV. INA-inactivated virus induced a protective response in 100% of mice when administered 3 days before challenge. Thus, INA may have significant potential for the development of vaccines and immunotherapeutics for filoviruses and other enveloped viruses.
PMID: 17940961 [PubMed - indexed for MEDLINE]
1531. J Infect Dis. 2007 Nov 15;196 Suppl 2:S271-5.

Blockage of filoviral glycoprotein processing by use of a protein-based inhibitor.

Ströher U(1), Willihnganz L, Jean F, Feldmann H.

Author information: (1)Special Pathogens Program, National Microbiology Laboratory, Public Health Agency of Canada, Manitoba, Canada R3E 3R2. Ute_Stroeher@phac-aspc.gc.ca

Cleavage of the glycoproteins of many virus species by furin and other host cell proteases is required for virus infectivity and, hence, determines viral pathogenicity. Proteolytic processing of Marburg virus and Ebola virus glycoproteins is also mediated by furin; however, for Ebola virus, in contrast to other viruses, glycoprotein cleavage is dispensable for replication in vitro, as has been shown in previous studies. In the present study, by use of a highly potent and selective furin inhibitor, we demonstrate that glycoprotein cleavage inhibition results in a minimal reduction in the virus titer that is insufficient to block filoviral replication. Thus, furin inhibitors are unlikely to be effective in the treatment of filoviral infections.
PMID: 17940960 [PubMed - indexed for MEDLINE]
1532. J Infect Dis. 2007 Nov 15;196 Suppl 2:S264-70.

Involvement of vacuolar protein sorting pathway in Ebola virus release independent of TSG101 interaction.

Silvestri LS(1), Ruthel G, Kallstrom G, Warfield KL, Swenson DL, Nelle T, Iversen PL, Bavari S, Aman MJ.

Author information: (1)United States Army Medical Research Institute of Infectious Diseases, Fort Detrick, MD 21704, USA.

Budding of Ebola virus (EBOV) particles from the plasma membrane of infected cells requires viral and host proteins. EBOV virus matrix protein VP40 recruits TSG101, an ESCRT-I (host cell endosomal sorting complex required for transport-I) complex protein in the vacuolar protein sorting (vps) pathway, to the plasma membrane during budding. Involvement of other vps proteins in EBOV budding has not been established. Therefore, we used VP40 deletion analysis, virus-like particle-release assays, and confocal microscopy to investigate the potential role of ESCRT-I proteins VPS4, VPS28, and VPS37B in EBOV budding. We found that VP40 could redirect each protein from endosomes to the cell surface independently of TSG101 interaction. A lack of VPS4 adenosine triphosphatase activity reduced budding by up to 80%. Inhibition of VPS4 gene expression by use of phosphorodiamidite morpholino antisense oligonucleotides protected mice from lethal EBOV infection. These data show that EBOV can use vps proteins independently of TSG101 for budding and reveal VPS4 as a potential target for filovirus therapeutics.
PMID: 17940959 [PubMed - indexed for MEDLINE]
1533. J Infect Dis. 2007 Nov 15;196 Suppl 2:S259-63.

The mechanism of Axl-mediated Ebola virus infection.

Shimojima M(1), Ikeda Y, Kawaoka Y.

Author information: (1)Division of Virology, Department of Microbiology and Immunology, University of Tokyo, Tokyo 108-8639, Japan.

We previously reported that expression of the receptor-type tyrosine kinase Axl, which regulates cell survival and activation, enhances both pseudotype and live Ebola virus (EBOV) infection. To clarify the mechanistic basis of this enhancement, we created a series of Axl mutants and identified amino acids/domains necessary for this function, by using a pseudotype virus carrying the EBOV glycoprotein (GP). Analyses of the Axl mutants showed the importance of extracellular and intracellular regions for Axl functions, including ligand binding and signal transduction, in EBOV GP-mediated infection. These data suggest that EBOV uses the physiological functions of Axl to enter cells.
PMID: 17940958 [PubMed - indexed for MEDLINE]
1534. J Infect Dis. 2007 Nov 15;196 Suppl 2:S251-8.

Analysis of filovirus entry into vero e6 cells, using inhibitors of endocytosis, endosomal acidification, structural integrity, and cathepsin (B and L) activity.

Sanchez A(1).

Author information: (1)Special Pathogens Branch, Division of Viral and Rickettsial Diseases, National Center for Infectious Diseases, Centers for Disease Control and Prevention, Atlanta, GA 30333, USA. ans1@cdc.gov

Ebola and Marburg viruses are believed to enter host cells by receptor-mediated endocytosis. The process has been studied through the use of inhibitors that affect host cell properties and recombinant pseudotyping systems in which filovirus structural glycoproteins mediate entry of foreign virus particles. The aim of the present study was to determine the effects of such treatments on the entry of wild-type filoviruses. Vero E6 cells were exposed to various inhibitors before, during, and after infection with filoviruses. Infected cultures were harvested early (18-24 h) and late (72 h) after infection, and effects of treatment on entry were measured by fluorescent antibody staining of cells or by antigen capture immunoassays, respectively. These preliminary results suggest that filoviruses enter host cells through receptor-mediated endocytosis via clathrin-coated pits and caveolae, that actin filaments and microtubules are important in the entry process, and that proteolytic digestion of glycoprotein 1 by endosomal proteases facilitates entry. These observations obtained using wild-type viruses confirm the results of studies utilizing recombinant systems and offer additional insights into filovirus entry.

PMID: 17940957 [PubMed - indexed for MEDLINE]

1535. J Infect Dis. 2007 Nov 15;196 Suppl 2:S247-50.

Regions in Ebola virus VP24 that are important for nucleocapsid formation.

Noda T(1), Halfmann P, Sagara H, Kawaoka Y.

Author information: (1)International Research Center for Infectious Diseases, Institute of Medical Science, University of Tokyo, Tokyo 108-8639, Japan. t-noda@ims.u-tokyo.ac.jp

Ebola virus (EBOV) VP24, together with nucleoprotein and VP35, is an essential component of viral RNA-protein complexes called "nucleocapsids." In this study, using a series of deletion mutants of VP24, we identified regions within VP24 that are important for the formation of nucleocapsid-like structures and determined that both termini of VP24 are essential for nucleocapsid formation. This finding advances our knowledge of both EBOV morphogenesis and the nature of VP24 molecules in nucleocapsid formation, which will be useful for the development of antiviral compounds.

PMID: 17940956 [PubMed - indexed for MEDLINE]

1536. J Infect Dis. 2007 Nov 15;196 Suppl 2:S237-46.

Analysis of the interaction of Ebola virus glycoprotein with DC-SIGN (dendritic cell-specific intercellular adhesion molecule 3-grabbing nonintegrin) and its homologue DC-SIGNR.

Marzi A(1), Möller P, Hanna SL, Harrer T, Eisemann J, Steinkasserer A, Becker S, Baribaud F, Pöhlmann S.

Author information: (1)Institute of Virology, Nikolaus-Fiebiger-Center for Molecular Medicine, Erlangen, Germany.

BACKGROUND: The lectin DC-SIGN (dendritic cell-specific intercellular adhesion molecule 3-grabbing nonintegrin) augments Ebola virus (EBOV) infection. However, it its unclear whether DC-SIGN promotes only EBOV attachment (attachment factor function, nonessential) or actively facilitates EBOV entry (receptor function, essential). METHODS: We investigated whether DC-SIGN on B cell lines and dendritic cells acts as an EBOV attachment factor or receptor. RESULTS: Engineered DC-SIGN expression rendered some B cell lines susceptible to EBOV glycoprotein (EBOV GP)-driven infection, whereas others remained refractory, suggesting that cellular factors other than DC-SIGN are also required for susceptibility to EBOV infection. Augmentation of entry was independent of efficient DC-SIGN internalization and might not involve lectin-mediated endocytic uptake of virions. Therefore, DC-SIGN is unlikely to function as an EBOV receptor on B cell lines; instead, it might concentrate virions onto cells, thereby allowing entry into cell lines expressing low levels of endogenous receptor(s). Indeed, artificial concentration of virions onto cells mirrored DC-SIGN expression, confirming that optimization of viral attachment is sufficient for EBOV GP-driven entry into some B cell lines. Finally, EBOV infection of dendritic cells was only partially dependent on mannose-specific lectins, such as DC-SIGN, suggesting an important contribution of other factors. CONCLUSIONS: Our results indicate that DC-SIGN is not an EBOV receptor but, rather, is an attachment-promoting factor that boosts entry into B cell lines susceptible to low levels of EBOV GP-mediated infection.

PMID: 17940955 [PubMed - indexed for MEDLINE]

1537. J Infect Dis. 2007 Nov 15;196 Suppl 2:S220-31.

Secreted glycoprotein from Live Zaire ebolavirus-infected cultures: preparation, structural and biophysical characterization, and thermodynamic stability.

Barrientos LG(1), Martin AM, Wohlhueter RM, Rollin PE.

Author information: (1)Special Pathogens Branch, Division of Viral and Rickettsial Diseases, National Center for Zoonotic, Vector-Borne, and Enteric Diseases, Centers for Disease Control and Prevention, Atlanta, GA 30333, USA. LBarrientos1@cdc.gov

Milligram quantities of Zaire ebolavirus nonstructural, secreted glycoprotein (sGP) were purified to homogeneity, and this preparation was characterized by an array of biophysical and biochemical experiments. Mass-spectrometry analysis revealed sGP posttranslational modifications and regions susceptible to limited proteolysis. In solution, sGP has an absolute molar mass of 103 kDa, is monodisperse, and folds into a predominantly beta -sheet conformation with a distinct tertiary structure. sGP appears to have a unique free-energy landscape that facilitates reversible folding and a strong propensity for disulfide-linked dimeric quaternary structure under a wide range of conditions; the low apparent free energy of conformation transition of sGP (Delta G=1.7+/-0.1 kcal/mol) suggests that the molecule is well suited as a thermodynamically facile switch, which would allow it to report on relatively subtle changes in milieu. In addition, a conformational transition at 37 degrees C was detected in thermal denaturing experiments. On the basis of biophysical and biochemical considerations alone, we propose that the property of being a thermodynamically facile switch is an important clue to reveal sGP functionality.

PMID: 17940953 [PubMed - indexed for MEDLINE]

1538. J Infect Dis. 2007 Nov 15;196 Suppl 2:S213-9.

Rapid assembly of sensitive antigen-capture assays for Marburg virus, using in vitro selection of llama single-domain antibodies, at biosafety level 4.

Sherwood LJ(1), Osborn LE, Carrion R Jr, Patterson JL, Hayhurst A.

Author information: (1)Department of Virology and Immunology, Southwest Foundation for Biomedical Research, San Antonio, TX 78245, USA.

There is a pressing need for rapid and reliable approaches to the delivery of sensitive yet rugged diagnostic assays specific for emerging viruses, to hasten containment of outbreaks when and wherever they occur. Within 3 weeks, we delivered an antigen-capture assay for Marburg virus (MARV) that was based on llama single-domain antibodies (sdAbs) selected at biosafety level 4. Four unique sdAbs were capable of independently detecting MARV variants Musoke, Ravn, and Angola without cross-reactivity with the 4 Ebola virus species. The unoptimized assays could be performed in

PMID: 17940952 [PubMed - indexed for MEDLINE]

1539. J Infect Dis. 2007 Nov 15;196 Suppl 2:S205-12.

High-throughput molecular detection of hemorrhagic fever virus threats with applications for outbreak settings.

Towner JS(1), Sealy TK, Ksiazek TG, Nichol ST.

Author information: (1)Special Pathogens Branch, National Center for Zoonotic, Vector-Borne, and Enteric Diseases, Centers for Disease Control and Prevention, Atlanta, GA 30333, USA.

Within the past dozen years, outbreaks of filoviral hemorrhagic fever within the human population have been occurring with increasing frequency, with an average of 1 epidemic now occurring every 1-2 years. Many of the outbreaks have been large (involving >150 cases), necessitating rapid responses from the international community to help implement infection control and surveillance. This increased activity, combined with today's climate of bioterrorism threats, has heightened the need for high-throughput methodologies for specific detection of these high-hazard viruses in sophisticated laboratory setups and mobile field laboratory situations. Using Zaire Ebola virus as an example, we describe here the development of a high-throughput protocol for RNA extraction and quantitative reverse-transcription polymerase chain reaction analysis that is safe, fast, and reliable. Furthermore, the applicability of this method to an outbreak setting was demonstrated by correct analysis of >500 specimens at a field laboratory established during a recent outbreak of Marburg hemorrhagic fever in Angola.

PMID: 17940951 [PubMed - indexed for MEDLINE]

1540. J Infect Dis. 2007 Nov 15;196 Suppl 2:S199-204.

Diagnostic reverse-transcription polymerase chain reaction kit for filoviruses based on the strain collections of all European biosafety level 4 laboratories.

Panning M(1), Laue T, Olschlager S, Eickmann M, Becker S, Raith S, Courbot MC, Nilsson M, Gopal R, Lundkvist A, Caro Ad, Brown D, Meyer H, Lloyd G, Kummerer BM, Gunther S, Drosten C.

Author information: (1)Bernhard-Nocht Institute for Tropical Medicine, Hamburg 20359, Germany.

A network of European biosafety level 4 laboratories has designed the first industry-standard molecular assay for all filoviruses species, based on the strain collections of all participants. It uses 5 optimized L gene primers and 3 probes, as well as an internal control with a separate detection probe. Detection limits (probit analysis, 95% detection chance) were as follows: Zaire ebolavirus, 487 copies/mL of plasma; Sudan ebolavirus Maleo, 586 copies/mL; Sudan ebolavirus Gulu, 1128 copies/mL; Cote d'Ivoire ebolavirus, 537 copies/mL; Reston ebolavirus, 4546 copies/mL; Lake Victoria marburgvirus Musoke, 860 copies/mL; and Lake Victoria marburgvirus Ravn, 1551 copies/mL. The assay facilitates reliable detection or exclusion screening of filovirus infections.

PMID: 17940950 [PubMed - indexed for MEDLINE]

1541. J Infect Dis. 2007 Nov 15;196 Suppl 2:S193-8.

Laboratory diagnosis of Ebola hemorrhagic fever during an outbreak in Yambio, Sudan, 2004.

Onyango CO(1), Opoka ML, Ksiazek TG, Formenty P, Ahmed A, Tukei PM, Sang RC, Ofula VO, Konongoi SL, Coldren RL, Grein T, Legros D, Bell M, De Cock KM, Bellini WJ, Towner JS, Nichol ST, Rollin PE.

Author information: (1)World Health Organization Collaborating Center for Arbovirus and Viral Hemorrhagic Fever Reference and Research, Nairobi, Kenya. conyango@mrc.gm

Between the months of April and June 2004, an Ebola hemorrhagic fever (EHF) outbreak was reported in Yambio county, southern Sudan. Blood samples were collected from a total of 36 patients with suspected EHF and were tested by enzyme-linked immunosorbent assay (ELISA) for immunoglobulin G and M antibodies, antigen ELISA, and reverse-transcription polymerase chain reaction (PCR) of a segment of the Ebolavirus (EBOV) polymerase gene. A total of 13 patients were confirmed to be infected with EBOV. In addition, 4 fatal cases were classified as probable cases, because no samples were collected. Another 12 patients were confirmed to have acute measles infection during the same period that EBOV was circulating. Genetic analysis of PCR-positive samples indicated that the virus was similar to but distinct from Sudan EBOV Maleo 1979. In response, case management, social mobilization, and follow-up of contacts were set up as means of surveillance. The outbreak was declared to be over on 7 August 2004.

PMID: 17940949 [PubMed - indexed for MEDLINE]

1542. J Infect Dis. 2007 Nov 15;196 Suppl 2:S184-92.

Development of an immunofiltration-based antigen-detection assay for rapid diagnosis of Ebola virus infection.

Lucht A(1), Formenty P, Feldmann H, Gotz M, Leroy E, Bataboukila P, Grolla A, Feldmann F, Wittmann T, Campbell P, Atsangandoko C, Boumandoki P, Finke EJ, Miethe P, Becker S, Grunow R.

Author information: (1)Bundeswehr Institute of Microbiology, Munich, Germany. andreaslu@gmx.de

Ebola virus (EBOV) has caused outbreaks of severe viral hemorrhagic fever in regions of Central Africa where medical facilities are ill equipped and diagnostic capabilities are limited. To obtain a reliable test that can be implemented easily under these conditions, monoclonal antibodies to the EBOV matrix protein (VP40), which previously had been found to work in a conventional enzyme-linked immunosorbent assay, were used to develop an immunofiltration assay for the detection of EBOV antigen in chemically inactivated clinical specimens. The assay was evaluated by use of defined virus stocks and specimens from experimentally infected animals. Its field application was tested during an outbreak of Ebola hemorrhagic fever in 2003. Although the original goal was to develop an assay that would detect all EBOV species, only the Zaire and Sudan species were detected in practice. The assay represents a first-generation rapid field test for the detection of EBOV antigen that can be performed in 30 min without electrical power or expensive or sensitive equipment.

PMID: 17940948 [PubMed - indexed for MEDLINE]

1543. J Infect Dis. 2007 Nov 15;196 Suppl 2:S176-83.

Spatial and temporal patterns of Zaire ebolavirus antibody prevalence in the possible reservoir bat species.

Pourrut X(1), Délicat A, Rollin PE, Ksiazek TG, Gonzalez JP, Leroy EM.

Author information: (1)Institut de Recherche pour le Développement, UR178, Franceville, Gabon. xavier.pourrut@ird.fr

To characterize the distribution of Zaire ebolavirus (ZEBOV) infection within the 3 bat species (Epomops franqueti, Hypsignathus monstrosus, and Myonycteris torquata) that are possible reservoirs, we collected 1390 bats during 2003-2006 in Gabon and the Republic of the Congo. Detection of ZEBOV immunoglobulin G (IgG) in 40 specimens supports the role of these bat species as the ZEBOV reservoirs. ZEBOV IgG prevalence rates (5%) were homogeneous across epidemic and nonepidemic regions during outbreaks, indicating that infected bats may well be present in nonepidemic regions of central Africa. ZEBOV IgG prevalence decreased, significantly, to 1% after the outbreaks, suggesting that the percentage of IgG-positive bats is associated with virus transmission to other animal species and outbreak appearance. The large number of ZEBOV IgG-positive adult bats and pregnant H. monstrosus females suggests virus transmission within bat populations through fighting and sexual contact. Our study, thus, helps to describe Ebola virus circulation in bats and offers some insight into the appearance of outbreaks.

PMID: 17940947 [PubMed - indexed for MEDLINE]

1544. J Infect Dis. 2007 Nov 15;196 Suppl 2:S142-7.

Assessment of the risk of Ebola virus transmission from bodily fluids and fomites.

Bausch DG(1), Towner JS, Dowell SF, Kaducu F, Lukwiya M, Sanchez A, Nichol ST, Ksiazek TG, Rollin PE.

Author information: (1)Tulane School of Public Health and Tropical Medicine, New Orleans, LA 70112, USA. dbausch@tulane.edu

Although Ebola virus (EBOV) is transmitted by unprotected physical contact with infected persons, few data exist on which specific bodily fluids are infected or on the risk of fomite transmission. Therefore, we tested various clinical specimens from 26 laboratory-confirmed cases of Ebola hemorrhagic fever, as well as environmental specimens collected from an isolation ward, for the presence of EBOV. Virus was detected by culture and/or reverse-transcription polymerase chain reaction in 16 of 54 clinical specimens (including saliva, stool, semen, breast milk, tears, nasal blood, and a skin swab) and in 2 of 33 environmental specimens. We conclude that EBOV is shed in a wide variety of bodily fluids during the acute period of illness but that the risk of transmission from fomites in an isolation ward and from convalescent patients is low when currently recommended infection control guidelines for the viral hemorrhagic fevers are followed.

PMID: 17940942 [PubMed - indexed for MEDLINE]

1545. J Infect Dis. 2007 Nov 15;196 Suppl 2:S136-41.

Outbreaks of filovirus hemorrhagic fever: time to refocus on the patient.

Bausch DG(1), Feldmann H, Geisbert TW, Bray M, Sprecher AG, Boumandouki P, Rollin PE, Roth C; Winnipeg Filovirus Clinical Working Group.

Author information: (1)Tulane School of Public Health and Tropical Medicine, New Orleans, LA 70112, USA. dbausch@tulane.edu

In the 40 years since the recognition of filoviruses as agents of lethal human disease, there have been no specific advances in antiviral therapies or vaccines and few clinical studies on the efficacy of supportive care. On 20 September 2006, experts from 14 countries representing 68 institutions integrally involved in the response to outbreaks of filovirus hemorrhagic fever gathered at the National Microbiology Laboratory of the Public Health Agency of Canada in Winnipeg to discuss possible remedies for this grim situation, in a unique workshop entitled "Marburg and Ebola Hemorrhagic Fever: Feasibility of Prophylaxis and Therapy." A summary of the opportunities for and challenges to improving treatment of filovirus hemorrhagic fevers is presented here.

PMID: 17940941 [PubMed - indexed for MEDLINE]

1546. Virology. 2007 Nov 10;368(1):83-90. Epub 2007 Jul 20.

Ebola sGP--the first viral glycoprotein shown to be C-mannosylated.

Falzarano D(1), Krokhin O, Van Domselaar G, Wolf K, Seebach J, Schnittler HJ, Feldmann H.

Author information: (1)Department of Medical Microbiology, University of Manitoba, Winnipeg, Manitoba, Canada R3E 0W3.

Mass spectrometry analysis of the Ebola virus soluble glycoprotein sGP identified a rare post-translation modification, C-mannosylation, which was found on tryptophan (W) 288. This modification has not been described for any other viral protein; however, many viral transmembrane glycoproteins contain one or more of the recognition motifs (W-x-x-W). Elimination of the C-mannose on sGP did not significantly alter protein biosynthesis, processing or structure. Furthermore, the protective effect of sGP on endothelial barrier function, currently the only known activity of sGP, was unaltered. It is possible that C-mannosylation may be a common post-translational modification of viral transmembrane glycoproteins where it could play a role in particle maturation and/or entry by stabilizing the structure of these proteins. In this regard, C-mannosylation of sGP may be an anomaly resulting from the unique manner in which this protein is generated as the product of unedited transcripts from the glycoprotein gene of Ebola.

PMID: 17659315 [PubMed - indexed for MEDLINE]

1547. Bioorg Khim. 2007 Nov-Dec;33(6):598-605.

[Recombinant full-size human antibody to Ebola virus].

[Article in Russian]

Shingarova LN, Tikunova NV, Iun TE, Chepurnov AA, Aliev TK, Batanova TA, Boldyreva EF, Nekrasova OV, Toporova VA, Panina AA, Kirpichnikov MP, Sandakhchiev LS.

A full-size human antibody to Ebola virus was constructed by joining genes encoding the constant domains of the heavy and light chains of human immunoglobulin with the corresponding DNA fragments encoding variable domains of the single-chain antibody 4DI specific to Ebola virus, which was chosen from a combinatorial phage display library of single-strand human antibodies. Two expression plasmids. pCHI and pCLI, containing the artificial genes encoding the light and heavy chains of human immunoglobulin, respectively, were constructed. Their cotransfection into the human embryonic kidney cell line HEK293T provided the production of a full-size recombinant human antibody. The affinity constant for the antibody was estimated by solid-phase enzyme-linked immunoassay to be $7.7 \times 10(7) +/- 1.5 \times 10(7)$ M(-I). Like the parent single-chain antibody 4DI, the resulting antibody bound the nucleoprotein of Ebola virus and did not interact with the proteins of Marburg virus.
PMID: 18173122 [PubMed - indexed for MEDLINE]

1548. J Mol Diagn. 2007 Nov;9(5):639-44.

Development of a novel one-tube isothermal reverse transcription thermophilic helicase-dependent amplification platform for rapid RNA detection.

Goldmeyer J(I), Kong H, Tang W.

Author information: (1)BioHelix Corporation, 32 Tozer Road, Beverly, MA 01915, USA.

The high complexity and cost of polymerase chain reaction-based molecular diagnostics sometimes limits their use in the clinical diagnostics setting. A new helicase-based isothermal amplification method offers an alternative to standard polymerase chain reaction, allowing amplification and detection of specific DNA sequences at a constant reaction temperature without thermocycling equipment. Herein, we describe the development of a novel one-tube isothermal reverse transcription-thermophilic helicase-dependent amplification (RT-tHDA) platform for RNA target detection based on the already established tHDA system. The RT-tHDA platform is highly sensitive and specific for a variety of RNA targets tested, including purified RNA molecules, armored RNA particles, and RNA virus. Moreover, rapid one-step RT-tHDA can be achieved by inclusion of an extreme thermostable single-stranded DNA binding protein in the reaction, resulting in one millionfold amplification of Ebola virus-armored RNA in less than 10 minutes. This RT-tHDA method expands on the known methods to amplify specific RNA targets and results in an easily prepared and contained platform.
PMCID: PMC2049050 PMID: 17975029 [PubMed - indexed for MEDLINE]

1549. Nat Immunol. 2007 Nov;8(11):1159-64.

Immunopathology of highly virulent pathogens: insights from Ebola virus.

Zampieri CA(I), Sullivan NJ, Nabel GJ.

Author information: (1)Vaccine Research Center, National Institute of Allergy and Infectious Diseases, National Institutes of Health, Bethesda, Maryland 20892-3005, USA.

Ebola virus is a highly virulent pathogen capable of inducing a frequently lethal hemorrhagic fever syndrome. Accumulating evidence indicates that the virus actively subverts both innate and adaptive immune responses and triggers harmful inflammatory responses as it inflicts direct tissue damage. The host immune system is ultimately overwhelmed by a combination of inflammatory factors and virus-induced cell damage, particularly in the liver and vasculature, often leading to death from septic shock. We summarize the mechanisms of immune dysregulation and virus-mediated cell damage in Ebola virus-infected patients. Future approaches to prevention and treatment of infection will be guided by answers to unresolved questions about interspecies transmission, molecular mechanisms of pathogenesis, and protective adaptive and innate immune responses to Ebola virus.
PMID: 17952040 [PubMed - indexed for MEDLINE]

1550. Virol J. 2007 Oct 25;4:108.

Development of a model for marburgvirus based on severe-combined immunodeficiency mice.

Warfield KL(I), Alves DA, Bradfute SB, Reed DK, VanTongeren S, Kalina WV, Olinger GG, Bavari S.

Author information: (1)United States Army Medical Research Institute of Infectious Diseases, Fort Detrick, Maryland, USA. kelly.warfield@us.army.mil

The filoviruses, Ebola (EBOV) and Marburg (MARV), cause a lethal hemorrhagic fever. Human isolates of MARV are not lethal to immmunocompetent adult mice and, to date, there are no reports of a mouse-adapted MARV model. Previously, a uniformly lethal EBOV-Zaire mouse-adapted virus was developed by performing 9 sequential passages in progressively older mice (suckling to adult). Evaluation of this model identified many similarities between infection in mice and nonhuman primates, including viral tropism for antigen-presenting cells, high viral titers in the spleen and liver, and an equivalent mean time to death. Existence of the EBOV mouse model has increased our understanding of host responses to filovirus infections and likely has accelerated the development of countermeasures, as it is one of the only hemorrhagic fever viruses that has multiple candidate vaccines and therapeutics. Here, we demonstrate that serially passaging liver homogenates from MARV-infected severe combined immunodeficient (scid) mice was highly successful in reducing the time to death in scid mice from 50-70 days to 7-10 days after MARV-Ci67, -Musoke, or -Ravn challenge. We performed serial sampling studies to characterize the pathology of these scid mouse-adapted MARV strains. These scid mouse-adapted MARV models appear to have many similar properties as the MARV models previously developed in guinea pigs and nonhuman primates. Also, as shown here, the scid-adapted MARV mouse models can be used to evaluate the efficacy of candidate antiviral therapeutic molecules, such as phosphorodiamidate morpholino oligomers or antibodies.
PMCID: PMC2164958 PMID: 17961252 [PubMed - indexed for MEDLINE]

1551. Proc Natl Acad Sci U S A. 2007 Oct 23;104(43):17123-7. Epub 2007 Oct 17.

Isolates of Zaire ebolavirus from wild apes reveal genetic lineage and recombinants.

Wittmann TJ(I), Biek R, Hassanin A, Rouquet P, Reed P, Yaba P, Pourrut X, Real LA, Gonzalez JP, Leroy EM.

Author information: (1)Centre International de Recherches Médicales de Franceville, BP 769 Franceville, Gabon.

Erratum in Proc Natl Acad Sci U S A. 2007 Dec 4;104(49):19656.

Over the last 30 years, Zaire ebolavirus (ZEBOV), a virus highly pathogenic for humans and wild apes, has emerged repeatedly in Central Africa. Thus far, only a few virus isolates have been characterized genetically, all belonging to a single genetic lineage and originating exclusively from infected human patients. Here, we describe the first ZEBOV sequences isolated from great ape carcasses in the Gabon/Congo region that belong to a previously unrecognized genetic lineage. According to our estimates, this lineage, which we also encountered in the two most recent human outbreaks in the Republic of the Congo in 2003 and 2005, diverged from the previously known viruses around the time of the first documented human outbreak in 1976. These results suggest that virus spillover from the reservoir has occurred more than once, as predicted by the multiple emergence hypothesis. However, the young age of both ZEBOV lineages and the spatial and temporal sequence of outbreaks remain at odds with the idea that the virus simply emerged from a long-established and widespread reservoir population. Based on data from two ZEBOV genes, we also demonstrate, within the family Filoviridae, recombination between the two lineages. According to our estimates, this event took place between 1996 and 2001 and gave rise to a group of recombinant viruses that were responsible for a series of outbreaks in 2001-2003. The potential for recombination adds an additional level of complexity to unraveling and potentially controlling the emergence of ZEBOV in humans and wildlife species.

PMCID: PMC2040453 PMID: 17942693 [PubMed - indexed for MEDLINE]

1552. Rev Med Suisse. 2007 Oct 10;3(128):2273-4, 2276-7.

[Bad bats?].

[Article in French]

Genné D(1).

Author information: (1)Service de médecine interne, Hôpital de la ville, 2300 La Chaux-de-Fonds. daniel.genne@ne.ch

For many centuries, man is fascinated by bats, the only flying mammals. Probably because of their particular immune system, bats can be considered an important reservoir for new emerging viral diseases like SARS-Coronavirus, Marburg fever, Ebola fever and Nipah virus encephalitis. During closer contact, they can transmit rabies and probably other nonviral infectious diseases. Bats get closer to man due to ecological modifications like deforestation, so that transmission of new infectious agents might provoke dramatic epidemics.

PMID: 17985603 [PubMed - indexed for MEDLINE]

1553. Wkly Epidemiol Rec. 2007 Oct 5;82(40):345-6.

Outbreak news. Ebola virus haemorrhagic fever, Democratic Republic of the Congo--update.

[Article in English, French]

[No authors listed]

PMID: 17918654 [PubMed - indexed for MEDLINE]

1554. J Virol. 2007 Oct;81(20):11452-60. Epub 2007 Aug 15.

Role for amino acids 212KLR214 of Ebola virus VP40 in assembly and budding.

McCarthy SE(1), Johnson RF, Zhang YA, Sunyer JO, Harty RN.

Author information: (1)Department of Pathobiology, School of Veterinary Medicine, University of Pennsylvania, 3800 Spruce Street, Philadelphia, PA 19104, USA. Ebola virus VP40 is able to produce virus-like particles (VLPs) in the absence of other viral proteins. At least three domains within VP40 are thought to be required for efficient VLP release: the late domain (L-domain), membrane association domain (M-domain), and self-interaction domain (I-domain). While the L-domain of Ebola VP40 has been well characterized, the exact mechanism by which VP40 mediates budding through the M- and I-domains remains unclear. To identify additional domains important for VP40 assembly/budding, amino acids (212)KLR(214) were targeted for mutagenesis based on the published crystal structure of VP40. These residues are part of a loop connecting two beta sheets in the C-terminal region and thus are potentially important for overall structure and/or oligomerization of VP40. A series of alanine substitutions were generated in the KLR region of VP40, and these mutants were examined for VLP budding, intracellular localization, and oligomerization. Our results indicated that (i) (212)KLR(214) residues of VP40 are important for efficient release of VP40 VLPs, with Leu213 being the most critical; (ii) VP40 KLR mutants displayed altered patterns of cellular localization compared to that of wild-type VP40 (VP40-WT); and (iii) self-assembly of VP40 KLR mutants into oligomers was altered compared to that of VP40-WT. These results suggest that (12)KLR(214) residues of VP40 are important for proper assembly/oligomerization of VP40 which subsequently leads to efficient budding of VLPs.

PMCID: PMC2045517 PMID: 17699576 [PubMed - indexed for MEDLINE]

1555. Med Trop (Mars). 2007 Oct;67(5):447-57.

[Medicine and health in the Democratic Republic of Congo: from Independence to the Third Republic].

[Article in French]

Wembonyama S(1), Mpaka S, Tshilolo L.

Author information: (1)Hôpital Général de Référence Provincial Jackson Sendwe. The birth and mortality rates in the Democratic Republic of Congo (DRC), a former Belgian colony, are high, i.e., 48.9/1000 and 17/1000 respectively. The DRC also has one of the highest maternal death rates in the world, i.e., 1289/100,000 live births. Health conditions have not improved since independence. Access to drinking water is limited, living conditions are poor, and food availability in households is low. The mean health services utilization rate in the DRC is estimated to be 0.15 visits/inhabitant/year. The incidence of transmissible diseases is rising. This increase is observed even for illnesses that were under control before independence such as sleeping sickness, onchocerciasis, leprosy, and tuberculosis. One the main causes of mortality and morbidity in the population is malaria that is responsible for the deaths of 150,000 to 250,000 children under the age of 5 every year. The HIV prevalence rate is 4.5% with 1.19 million persons with AIDS and 930,000 orphans whose parents died of AIDS. Other potentially epidemic diseases including bubonic plague and Ebola hemorrhagic fever are serious threats. Non-transmissible diseases are also on the rise including diabetes, systemic arterial hypertension, cancer and neglected diseases such as sickle cell anemia. To meet these challenges, the country's health authorities have established a program called the Strategy for Reinforcement of the Health System (SRHS). One goal of the SRHS is to develop health zones in order to improve access to quality health care for the whole population.

PMID: 18225727 [PubMed - indexed for MEDLINE]

1556. Wkly Epidemiol Rec. 2007 Sep 21;82(38):329.

Outbreak news. Ebola virus haemorrhagic fever, Democratic Republic of the Congo.

[Article in English, French]

[No authors listed]

Erratum in Wkly Epidemiol Rec. 2007 Sep 28;82(39):344.

PMID: 17886402 [PubMed - indexed for MEDLINE]

1557. J Biol Chem. 2007 Sep 14;282(37):27306-14. Epub 2007 Jun 1.

Structure of the Ebola fusion peptide in a membrane-mimetic environment and the interaction with lipid rafts.

Freitas MS(1), Gaspar LP, Lorenzoni M, Almeida FC, Tinoco LW, Almeida MS, Maia LF, Degrève L, Valente AP, Silva JL.

Author information: (1)Programa de Biologia Estrutural, Instituto de Bioquímica Médica, Centro Nacional de Ressonância Magnética Nuclear Jiri Jonas, Universidade Federal do Rio de Janeiro, 21941-590 Rio de Janeiro, RJ, Brazil.

The fusion peptide EBO(16) (GAAIGLAWIPYFGPAA) comprises the fusion domain of an internal sequence located in the envelope fusion glycoprotein (GP2) of the Ebola virus. This region interacts with the cellular membrane of the host and leads to membrane fusion. To gain insight into the mechanism of the peptide-membrane interaction and fusion, insertion of the peptide was modeled by experiments in which the tryptophan fluorescence and (1)H NMR were monitored in the presence of sodium dodecyl sulfate micelles or in the presence of detergent-resistant membrane fractions. In the presence of SDS micelles, EBO(16) undergoes a random coil-helix transition, showing a tendency to self-associate. The three-dimensional structure displays a 3(10)-helix in the central part of molecule, similar to the fusion peptides of many known membrane fusion proteins. Our results also reveal that EBO(16) can interact with detergent-resistant membrane fractions and strongly suggest that Trp-8 and Phe-12 are important for structure maintenance within the membrane bilayer. Replacement of tryptophan 8 with alanine (W8A) resulted in dramatic loss of helical structure, proving the importance of the aromatic ring in stabilizing the helix. Molecular dynamics studies of the interaction between the peptide and the target membrane also corroborated the crucial participation of these aromatic residues. The aromatic-aromatic interaction may provide a mechanism for the free energy coupling between random coil-helical transition and membrane anchoring. Our data shed light on the structural "domains" of fusion peptides and provide a clue for the development of a drug that might block the early steps of viral infection.

PMID: 17545161 [PubMed - indexed for MEDLINE]

1558. Science. 2007 Sep 14;317(5844):1484.

Conservation. Scientists say Ebola has pushed western gorillas to the brink.

Vogel G.

PMID: 17872416 [PubMed - indexed for MEDLINE]

1559. Cell Host Microbe. 2007 Sep 13;2(3):193-203.

An interferon-alpha-induced tethering mechanism inhibits HIV-1 and Ebola virus particle release but is counteracted by the HIV-1 Vpu protein.

Neil SJ(1), Sandrin V, Sundquist WI, Bieniasz PD.

Author information: (1)Aaron Diamond AIDS Research Center and the Laboratory of Retrovirology, The Rockefeller University, 455 First Avenue, New York, NY 10016, USA.

Type I interferon (IFN) inhibits the release of HIV-1 virus particles via poorly defined mechanisms. Here, we show that IFNalpha induces retention of viral particles on the surface of fibroblasts, T cells, or primary lymphocytes infected with HIV-1 lacking the Vpu protein. Retained particles are tethered to cell surfaces, can be endocytosed, appear fully assembled, exhibit mature morphology, and can be detached by protease. Strikingly, expression of the HIV-1 Vpu protein attenuates the ability of human cells to adhere to, and thereby retain, nascent HIV-1 particles upon IFNalpha treatment. Vpu also counteracts the IFNalpha-induced retention of virus-like particles assembled from the Ebola virus matrix protein. Furthermore, levels of IFNalpha that suppress replication of Vpu-defective HIV-1 have little effect on wild-type HIV-1. Thus, we propose that HIV-1 expresses Vpu to counteract an IFNalpha-induced, general host defense that inhibits dissemination of enveloped virions from the surface of infected cells.

PMCID: PMC3793644 PMID: 18005734 [PubMed - indexed for MEDLINE]

1560. Nature. 2007 Sep 13;449(7159):127.

Gorillas on the list.

Hopkin M.

PMID: 17851485 [PubMed - indexed for MEDLINE]

1561. Am J Disaster Med. 2007 Sep-Oct;2(5):270-6.

The 1995 Kikwit Ebola outbreak--model of virus properties on system capacity and function: a lesson for future viral epidemics.

Hall RC(1), Hall RC.

Author information: (1)Case Western Reserve, Cleveland, Ohio, USA.
The 1995 Kikwit Ebola outbreak in the Democratic Republic of the Congo is one of the first Ebola outbreaks to be treated in a hospital setting and is one of the most well-studied Ebola epidemics to have occurred to date. Many of the lessons learned from identifying, containing, and treating the epidemic are applicable to future viral outbreaks. This article looks at the characteristics of the Ebola virus and health system issues, which affected the healthcare providers' ability to contain and treat the virus. It specifically examines factors such as the disease characteristics, surge capacity, supply issues, press involvement, and the involvement of voluntary organizations.

PMID: 18491842 [PubMed - indexed for MEDLINE]

1562. Comp Immunol Microbiol Infect Dis. 2007 Sep;30(5-6):391-8. Epub 2007 Jul 3.

Current knowledge on lower virulence of Reston Ebola virus (in French: Connaissances actuelles sur la moindre virulence du virus Ebola Reston).

Morikawa S(1), Saijo M, Kurane I.

Author information: (1)Department of Virology 1, National Institute of Infectious Diseases, 4-7-1 Gakuen, Musashimurayama, Tokyo 208-0011, Japan. morikawa@nih.go.jp

Ebola viruses (EBOV) and Marburg virus belong to the family Filoviridae, order Mononegavirales. The genus Ebolavirus consists of four species: Zaire ebolavirus (ZEBOV), Sudan ebolavirus (SEBOV), Ivory Coast ebolavirus (ICEBOV) and Reston ebolavirus (REBOV). Three species of ebolaviruses, ZEBOV, SEBOV, ICEBOV, and Marburg virus are known to be extremely pathogenic in primates and humans and cause severe hemorrhagic fever leading up to case fatality rate of some 90%, while REBOV is thought to be pathogenic in Asian monkeys but not in African monkeys and humans. Recent studies indicated several factors involved in different virulence between African EBOV and REBOV. This article reviews the history, epidemiology, and virulence of REBOV.

PMID: 17610952 [PubMed - indexed for MEDLINE]

1563. J Virol. 2007 Sep;81(17):8967-76. Epub 2007 Jun 13.

Ebola virus VP30 is an RNA binding protein.

John SP(1), Wang T, Steffen S, Longhi S, Schmaljohn CS, Jonsson CB.

Author information: (1)Graduate Program in Biochemistry and Molecular Genetics, University of Alabama at Birmingham, Birmingham, Alabama 35294, USA.
The Ebola virus (EBOV) genome encodes for several proteins that are necessary and sufficient for replication and transcription of the viral RNAs in vitro; NP, VP30, VP35, and L. VP30 acts in trans with an RNA secondary structure upstream of the first transcriptional start site to modulate transcription. Using a bioinformatics approach, we identified a region within the N terminus of VP30 with sequence features that typify intrinsically disordered regions and a putative RNA binding site. To experimentally assess the ability of VP30 to directly interact with the viral RNA, we purified recombinant EBOV VP30 to >90% homogeneity and assessed RNA binding by UV cross-linking and filter-binding assays. VP30 is a strongly acidophilic protein; RNA binding became stronger as pH was decreased. $Zn(2+)$, but not $Mg(2+)$, enhanced activity. Enhancement of transcription by VP30 requires a RNA stem-loop located within nucleotides 54 to 80 of the leader region. VP30 showed low binding affinity to the predicted stem-loop alone or to double-stranded RNA but showed a good binding affinity for the stem-loop when placed in the context of upstream and downstream sequences. To map the region responsible for interacting with RNA, we constructed, purified, and assayed a series of N-terminal deletion mutations of VP30 for RNA binding. The key amino acids supporting RNA binding activity map to residues 26 to 40, a region rich in arginine. Thus, we show for the first time the direct interaction of EBOV VP30 with RNA and the importance of the N-terminal region for binding RNA.

PMCID: PMC1951390 PMID: 17567691 [PubMed - indexed for MEDLINE]

1564. Trends Microbiol. 2007 Sep;15(9):408-16. Epub 2007 Aug 15.

The ecology of Ebola virus.

Groseth A(1), Feldmann H, Strong JE.

Author information: (1)Special Pathogens Program, National Laboratory for Zoonotic Diseases and Special Pathogens, National Microbiology Laboratory, Public Health Agency of Canada, 1015 Arlington St., Winnipeg, MB R3E 3R2, Canada.
Since Ebola virus was first identified more than 30 years ago, tremendous progress has been made in understanding the molecular biology and pathogenesis of this virus. However, the means by which Ebola virus is maintained and transmitted in nature remains unclear despite dedicated efforts to answer these questions. Recent work has provided new evidence that fruit bats might have a role as a reservoir species, but it is not clear whether other species are also involved or how transmission to humans or apes takes place. Two opposing hypotheses for Ebola emergence have surfaced; one of long-term local persistence in a cryptic and infrequently contacted reservoir, versus another of a more recent introduction of the virus and directional spread through susceptible populations. Nevertheless, with the increasing frequency of human filovirus outbreaks and the tremendous impact of infection on the already threatened great ape populations, there is an urgent need to better understand the ecology of Ebola virus in nature.

PMID: 17698361 [PubMed - indexed for MEDLINE]

1565. PLoS One. 2007 Aug 22;2(8):e764.

Marburg virus infection detected in a common African bat.

Towner JS(1), Pourrut X, Albariño CG, Nkogue CN, Bird BH, Grard G, Ksiazek TG, Gonzalez JP, Nichol ST, Leroy EM.

Author information: (1)Centers for Disease Control and Prevention, Special Pathogens Branch, Atlanta, Georgia, United States of America.
Marburg and Ebola viruses can cause large hemorrhagic fever (HF) outbreaks with high case fatality (80-90%) in human and great apes. Identification of the natural reservoir of these viruses is one of the most important topics in this field and a fundamental key to understanding their natural history. Despite the discovery of this virus family almost 40 years ago, the search for the natural reservoir of these lethal pathogens remains an enigma despite numerous

ecological studies. Here, we report the discovery of Marburg virus in a common species of fruit bat (Rousettus aegyptiacus) in Gabon as shown by finding virus-specific RNA and IgG antibody in individual bats. These Marburg virus positive bats represent the first naturally infected non-primate animals identified. Furthermore, this is the first report of Marburg virus being present in this area of Africa, thus extending the known range of the virus. These data imply that more areas are at risk for MHF outbreaks than previously realized and correspond well with a recently published report in which three species of fruit bats were demonstrated to be likely reservoirs for Ebola virus.

PMCID: PMC1942080 PMID: 17712412 [PubMed - indexed for MEDLINE]

1566. Virology. 2007 Aug 1;364(2):342-54. Epub 2007 Apr 16.

Ebola virus-like particle-induced activation of NF-kappaB and Erk signaling in human dendritic cells requires the glycoprotein mucin domain.

Martinez O(1), Valmas C, Basler CF.

Author information: (1)Department of Microbiology, Box 1124, Mount Sinai School of Medicine, 1 Gustave L Levy Place, New York, NY 10029, USA.

Dendritic cells (DCs), important early targets of Ebola virus (EBOV) infection in vivo, are activated by Ebola virus-like particles (VLPs). To better understand this phenomenon, we have systematically assessed the response of DCs to VLPs of different compositions. VLPs containing the viral matrix protein (VP40) and the viral glycoprotein (GP), were found to induce a proinflammatory response highly similar to a prototypical DC activator, LPS. This response included the production of several proinflammatory cytokines, activation of numerous transcription factors including NF-kappaB, the functional importance of which was demonstrated by employing inhibitors of NF-kappaB activation, and activation of ERK1/2 MAP kinase. In contrast, VLPs constituted with a mutant GP lacking the heavily glycosylated mucin domain showed impaired NF-kappaB and Erk activation and induced less DC cytokine production. We conclude that the GP mucin domain is required for VLPs to stimulate human dendritic cells through NF-kappaB and MAPK signaling pathways.

PMCID: PMC2034500 PMID: 17434557 [PubMed - indexed for MEDLINE]

1567. Virology. 2007 Jul 20;364(1):45-54. Epub 2007 Mar 27.

Ebola virus infection of human PBMCs causes massive death of macrophages, CD4 and CD8 T cell sub-populations in vitro.

Gupta M(1), Spiropoulou C, Rollin PE.

Author information: (1)Special Pathogens Branch, DVRD, Centers for Disease Control and Prevention, Mailstop G14, 1600 Clifton Road, Atlanta, GA 30333, USA. mgupta@cdc.gov

Ebola virus causes an often fatal disease characterized by poor immune response and high inflammatory reaction in the patients. One of the causes for poor immunity is virus-mediated apoptosis of lymphocytes in the host. In this study, we infected human PBMCs with Ebola Zaire virus and study apoptosis of different cell types using flow cytometry. We have shown that Ebola virus causes bystander death of CD4 and CD8 T cells. Cells infected with virus had 30-40% active caspase 3(+), annexin-V(+) and Bcl2(low) phenotype by day 8 PI as compared to inactivated virus-treated cells. 60-70% of the macrophages were also dead by day 8 PI and had similar phenotype. Our data also showed that virus may induce death signals in Fas(+)/FasL(+) T lymphocytes and macrophages but did not upregulate Fas/FasL expression in these cells. Lastly, CD4, CD8 and CD14 cells were purified after infection and were studied for death signals by RNAse protection assay. We found an upregulation of TRAIL mRNA in CD4 and CD8 T cells on day 7 PI. A two-fold increase in CD4 T cells and three-fold increase in CD8 T cells were observed in TRAIL mRNA levels as compared to uninfected controls and inactive virus-treated cells. Surprisingly, we did not find any difference in TRAIL mRNA levels between infected macrophages and uninfected controls. These data suggest that Ebola virus evades the immune response by causing massive lymphocyte death. In addition, they may give an explanation on why the host is unable to produce a good antibody response in the absence of CD4 T cells.

PMID: 17391724 [PubMed - indexed for MEDLINE]

1568. ChemMedChem. 2007 Jul;2(7):1030-6.

1,2-Mannobioside mimic: synthesis, DC-SIGN interaction by NMR and docking, and antiviral activity.

Reina JJ(1), Sattin S, Invernizzi D, Mari S, Martínez-Prats L, Tabarani G, Fieschi F, Delgado R, Nieto PM, Rojo J, Bernardi A.

Author information: (1)Departamento de Química Bioorgánica, Instituto de Investigaciones Químicas, CSIC, Américo Vespucio 49, 41092 Sevilla, Spain.

The design and preparation of carbohydrate ligands for DC-SIGN is a topic of high interest because of the role played by this C-type lectin in immunity and infection processes. The low chemical stability of carbohydrates against enzymatic hydrolysis by glycosylases has stimulated the search for new alternatives more stable in vivo. Herein, we present a good alternative for a DC-SIGN ligand based on a mannobioside mimic with a higher enzymatic stability than the corresponding disaccharide. NMR and docking studies have been performed to study the interaction of this mimic with DC-SIGN in solution demonstrating that this pseudomannobioside is a good ligand for this lectin. In vitro studies using an infection model with Ebola pseudotyped virus demonstrates that this compound presents an antiviral activity even better than the corresponding disaccharide and could be an interesting ligand to prepare multivalent systems with higher affinities for DC-SIGN with potential biomedical applications.

PMID: 17508368 [PubMed - indexed for MEDLINE]

1569. J Virol. 2007 Jul;81(14):7702-9. Epub 2007 May 2.

Ebola virus glycoprotein 1: identification of residues important for binding and postbinding events.

Brindley MA(1), Hughes L, Ruiz A, McCray PB Jr, Sanchez A, Sanders DA, Maury W.

Author information: (1)Department of Microbiology, Carver College of Medicine, University of Iowa, Iowa City, IA 52242, USA.

The filoviruses Ebola virus (EBOV) and Marburg virus (MARV) are responsible for devastating hemorrhagic fever outbreaks. No therapies are available against these viruses. An understanding of filoviral glycoprotein 1 (GP1) residues involved in entry events would facilitate the development of antivirals. Towards this end, we performed alanine scanning mutagenesis on selected residues in the amino terminus of GP1. Mutant GPs were evaluated for their incorporation onto feline immunodeficiency virus (FIV) particles, transduction efficiency, receptor binding, and ability to be cleaved by cathepsins L and B. FIV virions bearing 39 out of 63 mutant glycoproteins transduced cells efficiently, whereas virions bearing the other 24 had reduced levels of transduction. Virions pseudotyped with 23 of the poorly transducing GPs were characterized for their block in entry. Ten mutant GPs were very poorly incorporated onto viral particles. Nine additional mutant GPs (G87A/F88A, K114A/K115A, K140A, G143A, P146A/C147A, F153A/H154A, F159A, F160A, and Y162A) competed poorly with wild-type GP for binding to permissive cells. Four of these nine mutants (P146A/C147A, F153A/H154A, F159A, and F160A) were also inefficiently cleaved by cathepsins. An additional four mutant GPs (K84A, R134A, D150A, and E305/E306A) that were partially defective in transduction were found to compete effectively for receptor binding and were readily cleaved by cathepsins. This finding suggested that this latter group of mutants might be defective at a postbinding, cathepsin cleavage-independent step. In total, our study confirms the role of some GP1 residues in EBOV entry that had previously been recognized and identifies for the first time other residues that are important for productive entry.

PMCID: PMC1933332 PMID: 17475648 [PubMed - indexed for MEDLINE]

1570. J Virol Methods. 2007 Jul;143(1):29-37. Epub 2007 Mar 19.

Production and characterization of monoclonal antibodies against different epitopes of Ebola virus antigens.

Shahhosseini S(1), Das D, Qiu X, Feldmann H, Jones SM, Suresh MR.

Author information: (1)Faculty of Pharmacy and Pharmaceutical Sciences, University of Alberta, Edmonton, AB, Canada.

Ebola virus (EBOV) causes hemorrhagic fever in humans and nonhuman primates with up to 90% mortality rate. In this study, Ebola virus like particles (EVLPs) and the aglycosyl subfragment of glycoprotein (GP(1) subfragment D) were used to generate monoclonal antibodies (MAbs) against different epitopes of the viral antigens. Such MAbs could be useful in diagnostics and potential therapeutics of viral infection and its hemorrhagic symptoms. Hybridoma cell fusion technology was used for production of MAbs. The MAbs were characterized using ELISA and Western blot analysis. Furthermore, five recombinant sub-domains of GP(1) subfragment D were produced, which were used as antigen in Western blot analysis for epitope mapping. Seventeen MAbs of different epitope specificities against EBOV antigens [virion protein (VP40), secreted glycoprotein (sGP), and GP(1) subfragment D] were developed. Based on epitope mapping studies, the anti-GP MAbs were categorized into six groups. The binding of the three anti-sGP MAbs with different epitope specificities were mostly between aa 157 and 221. The two anti-VP40 MAbs with the same or overlapping epitopes are potentially good candidates for developing antigen detection assays for early diagnosis of EBOV infection. The anti-GP MAbs with different epitope specificities as an oligoclonal cocktail could be tested for therapy.

PMID: 17368819 [PubMed - indexed for MEDLINE]

1571. Nat Rev Immunol. 2007 Jul;7(7):556-67.

How Ebola and Marburg viruses battle the immune system.

Mohamadzadeh M(1), Chen L, Schmaljohn AL.

Author information: (1)US Army Medical Research Institute for Infectious Diseases, Frederick, Maryland, USA. Mansour.mohamadzadeh@amedd.army.mil

The filoviruses Ebola and Marburg have emerged in the past decade from relative obscurity to serve now as archetypes for some of the more intriguing and daunting challenges posed by such agents. Public imagination is captured by deadly outbreaks of these viruses and reinforced by the specter of bioterrorism. As research on these agents has accelerated, it has been found increasingly that filoviruses use a combination of familiar and apparently new ways to baffle and battle the immune system. Filoviruses have provided thereby a new lens through which to examine the immune system itself.

PMID: 17589545 [PubMed - indexed for MEDLINE]

1572. Protein Expr Purif. 2007 Jul;54(1):117-25. Epub 2007 Feb 15.

Differential expression of the Ebola virus GP(1,2) protein and its fragments in E. coli.

Das D(1), Jacobs F, Feldmann H, Jones SM, Suresh MR.

Author information: (1)University of Alberta, Edmonton, Alta., Canada T6G 2N8.

Bacterial expression platforms are frequently used for the expression and production of different recombinant proteins. The full length Ebola virus (EBOV) GP(1,2) gene and subfragments of the GP(1) gene were cloned in a bacterial expression vector as a C-terminal His(6) fusion protein. Surprisingly, the full length EBOV GP(1,2) gene could not be expressed in Escherichia coli. The subfragments of GP(1) were only expressed in small amounts with the exception of one small fragment (subfragment D) which was expressed at very high levels as inclusion bodies. This was seen even in the in vitro translation system with no expression of full length GP(1,2), GP(1) subfragments A and C and low level expression of subfragment B. Only the subfragment D showed high level of expression. In E. coli (Top10), the recombinant GP(1) subfragment D protein was expressed exclusively as an insoluble approximately 25 kDa His(6) fusion protein, which is the expected size for a non-glycosylated recombinant protein. The IMAC purified and refolded non-glycosylated protein was used to immunize mice for the development of monoclonal anti-EBOV antibodies which successfully yielded several monoclonal antibodies with different specificities. The monoclonal and polyclonal antiserum derived from the animals immunized with this recombinant GP(1) subfragment D protein was found to specifically recognize the full length glycosylated EBOV GP(1,2) protein expressed in mammalian 293T cells, thus, demonstrating the immunogenicity of the recombinant subfragment.

PMID: 17383893 [PubMed - indexed for MEDLINE]

1573. US Army Med Dep J. 2007 Jul-Sep:28-37.

Challenges in biodefense research and the role of US Army veterinary pathologists.

Steele KE(1), Alves DA, Chapman JL.

Author information: (1)Division of Pathology, US Army Medical Research Institute of Infectious Diseases, Fort Detrick, Maryland, USA.

For years the nation's development of medical countermeasures to biowarfare agents has primarily existed as the domain of the United States military, but it has taken on increased urgency in the last few years. The realization that the civilian population is also at risk from biological agents has resulted in the institution of new biodefense programs at a variety of nonmilitary organizations. USAMRIID, a long-time leader in the nation's biodefense effort, will soon be joined by other US government agencies as part of a planned National Interagency Biodefense Campus at Fort Detrick Maryland. US Army veterinary pathologists at USAMRIID have played an important role in the nation's biodefense effort, along with our veterinary colleagues representing other specialties, our military colleagues in other Army Medical Department corps, and our civilian colleagues. Together, we will continue to strive to develop the diagnostics, vaccines, therapeutic agents, and operational practices that are required to meet the great demands posed by the threat of biowarfare agents.

PMID: 20088227 [PubMed - indexed for MEDLINE]

1574. Blood. 2007 Jun 15;109(12):5337-45. Epub 2007 Mar 5.

The DC-SIGN-related lectin LSECtin mediates antigen capture and pathogen binding by human myeloid cells.

Dominguez-Soto A(1), Aragoneses-Fenoll L, Martin-Gayo E, Martinez-Prats L, Colmenares M, Naranjo-Gomez M, Borras FE, Munoz P, Zubiaur M, Toribio ML, Delgado R, Corbi AL.

Author information: (1)Centro de Investigaciones Biológicas, Consejo Superior de Investigaciones Científicas (CSIC), Madrid, Spain.

Liver and lymph node sinusoidal endothelial cell C-type lectin (LSECtin [CLEC4G]) is a C-type lectin encoded within the liver/lymph node-specific intercellular adhesion molecule-3-grabbing nonintegrin (L-SIGN)/dendritic cell-specific intercellular adhesion molecule-3-grabbing nonintegrin (DC-SIGN)/CD23 gene cluster. LSECtin expression has been previously described as restricted to sinusoidal endothelial cells of the liver and lymph node. We now report LSECtin expression in human peripheral blood and thymic dendritic cells isolated ex vivo. LSECtin is also detected in monocyte-derived macrophages and dendritic cells at the RNA and protein level. In vitro, interleukin-4 (IL-4) induces the expression of 3 LSECtin alternatively spliced isoforms, including a potentially soluble form (Delta 2 isoform) and a shorter version of the prototypic molecule (Delta3/4 isoform). LSECtin functions as a pathogen receptor, because its expression confers Ebola virus-binding capacity to leukemic cells. Sugar-binding studies indicate that LSECtin specifically recognizes N-acetyl-glucosamine, whereas no LSECtin binding to Mannan- or N-acetyl-galactosamine-containing matrices are observed. Antibody or ligand-mediated engagement triggers a rapid internalization of LSECtin,which is dependent on tyrosine and diglutamic-containing motifs within the cytoplasmic tail. Therefore, LSECtin is a pathogen-associated molecular pattern receptor in human myeloid cells. In addition, our results suggest that LSECtin participates in antigen uptake and internalization, and might be a suitable target molecule in vaccination strategies.

PMID: 17339424 [PubMed - indexed for MEDLINE]

1575. J Virol. 2007 Jun;81(12):6379-88. Epub 2007 Apr 11.

Successful topical respiratory tract immunization of primates against Ebola virus.

Bukreyev A(1), Rollin PE, Tate MK, Yang L, Zaki SR, Shieh WJ, Murphy BR, Collins PL, Sanchez A.

Author information: (1)Laboratory of Infectious Disease, National Institute of Allergy and Infectious Diseases, National Institutes of Health, Bethesda, MD 20892-8007, USA. AB176v@nih.gov

Ebola virus causes outbreaks of severe viral hemorrhagic fever with high mortality in humans. The virus is highly contagious and can be transmitted by contact and by the aerosol route. These features make Ebola virus a potential weapon for bioterrorism and biological warfare. Therefore, a vaccine that induces both systemic and local immune responses in the respiratory tract would be highly beneficial. We evaluated a common pediatric respiratory pathogen, human parainfluenza virus type 3 (HPIV3), as a vaccine vector against Ebola virus. HPIV3 recombinants expressing the Ebola virus (Zaire species) surface glycoprotein (GP) alone or in combination with the nucleocapsid protein NP or with the cytokine adjuvant granulocyte-macrophage colony-stimulating factor were administered by the respiratory route to rhesus monkeys--in which HPIV3 infection is mild and asymptomatic--and were evaluated for immunogenicity and protective efficacy against a highly lethal intraperitoneal challenge with Ebola virus. A single immunization with any construct expressing GP was moderately immunogenic against Ebola virus and protected 88% of the animals against severe hemorrhagic fever and death caused by Ebola virus. Two doses were highly immunogenic, and all of the animals survived challenge and were free of signs of disease and of detectable Ebola virus challenge virus. These data illustrate the feasibility of immunization via the respiratory tract against the hemorrhagic fever caused by Ebola virus. To our knowledge, this is the first study in which topical immunization through respiratory tract achieved prevention of a viral hemorrhagic fever infection in a primate model.

PMCID: PMC1900097 PMID: 17428868 [PubMed - indexed for MEDLINE]

1576. Med Trop (Mars). 2007 Jun;67(3):291-300.

[Risk of nosocomial infection in intertropical Africa--part 3: health care workers].

[Article in French]

Rebaudet S(1), Kraemer P, Savini H, De Pina JJ, Rapp C, Demortiere F, Simon F.

Author information: (1)Service de pathologie infectieuse et tropicale, Hôpital d'instruction des armées Laveran, 13998 Marseille Armées.

Parts of the nosocomial infections issue are the professionally-acquired infections of health care workers. This problem is widely neglected in sub-Saharan Africa, and little is known on the subject, in spite of the high prevalence of blood-borne infections such as HIV or hepatitis B and C, and air-borne diseases like tuberculosis. Besides, unsafe practices and accidents like blood exposures are more frequent than in western countries. This is due to the lack of political concern, of safer equipment and of specific teachings. Most of this severe infections' treatments are long, difficult or unavailable in Subsaharan Africa. The loss of contaminated health care workers can then become devastating for their family and the fragile health care structures of those developing countries. Finally, one should not underestimate the risk of infection transmission from health care provider to patient, like in several past outbreaks of Ebola hemorrhagic fever.

PMID: 17784685 [PubMed - indexed for MEDLINE]

1577. PLoS Pathog. 2007 Jun;3(6):e86.

The Ebola virus VP35 protein is a suppressor of RNA silencing.

Haasnoot J(1), de Vries W, Geutjes EJ, Prins M, de Haan P, Berkhout B.

Author information: (1)Laboratory of Experimental Virology, Department of Medical Microbiology, Center of Infection and Immunity Amsterdam, Academic Medical Center of the University of Amsterdam, Amsterdam, The Netherlands.

RNA silencing or interference (RNAi) is a gene regulation mechanism in eukaryotes that controls cell differentiation and developmental processes via expression of microRNAs. RNAi also serves as an innate antiviral defence response in plants, nematodes, and insects. This antiviral response is triggered by virus-specific double-stranded RNA molecules (dsRNAs) that are produced during infection. To overcome antiviral RNAi responses, many plant and insect viruses encode RNA silencing suppressors (RSSs) that enable them to replicate at higher titers. Recently, several human viruses were shown to encode RSSs, suggesting that RNAi also serves as an innate defence response in mammals. Here, we demonstrate that the Ebola virus VP35 protein is a suppressor of RNAi in mammalian cells and that its RSS activity is functionally equivalent to that of the HIV-I Tat protein. We show that VP35 can replace HIV-I Tat and thereby support the replication of a Tat-minus HIV-I variant. The VP35 dsRNA-binding domain is required for this RSS activity. Vaccinia virus E3L protein and influenza A virus NSI protein are also capable of replacing the HIV-I Tat RSS function. These findings support the hypothesis that RNAi is part of the innate antiviral response in mammalian cells. Moreover, the results indicate that RSSs play a critical role in mammalian virus replication.

PMCID: PMCI894824 PMID: 17590081 [PubMed - indexed for MEDLINE]

1578. Uirusu. 2007 Jun;57(1):75-82.

[Feline immunodeficiency virus tropism].

[Article in Japanese]

Shimojima M(1).

Author information: (1)Division of Virology, Department of Microbiology and Immunology, Institute of Medical Science, University of Tokyo, 4-6-I Shirokendai, Minato-ku, Tokyo 108-8639, Japan. shimoji-@ims.u-tokyo.ac.jp

Feline immunodeficiency virus (FIV) induces a disease similar to acquired immunodeficiency syndrome (AIDS) in cats, yet in contrast to human immunodeficiency virus (HIV), CD4 is not the viral receptor. We identified a primary receptor for FIV as CD134 (OX40), a T cell activation antigen and costimulatory molecule. CD134 expression promotes viral binding and renders cells permissive for viral entry, productive infection, and syncytium formation. Infection is CXCR4-dependent, analogous to infection with X4 strains of HIV. Thus, despite the evolutionary divergence of the feline and human lentiviruses, both viruses use receptors that target the virus to a subset of cells that are pivotal to the acquired immune response. Further, we applied the new method for FIV receptor to Ebola virus entry factors with some modifications, and identified receptor-type tyrosine kinases, Axl and Dtk (members of Tyro3 family). Distribution of the molecules matches well with the Ebola virus tropism.

PMID: 18040157 [PubMed - indexed for MEDLINE]

1579. Virus Genes. 2007 Jun;34(3):273-81. Epub 2006 Aug 22.

Permeabilization of the plasma membrane by Ebola virus GP2.

Han Z(1), Licata JM, Paragas J, Harty RN.

Author information: (1)Department of Pathobiology, School of Veterinary Medicine, University of Pennsylvania, 3800 Spruce St., Philadelphia, PA 19104-6049, USA.

The glycoprotein (GP) of Ebola virus (EBOV) is a multifunctional protein known to play a role in virus attachment and entry, cell rounding and cytotoxicity, down-regulation of host surface proteins, and enhancement of virus assembly and budding. EBOV GP is synthesized as a precursor which is subsequently cleaved to yield two disulfide-linked subunits: GP1 (surface-exposed [SU] subunit) and GP2 (membrane-anchored [TM] subunit). We sought to determine the effect of membrane-anchored GP2 protein expression on the integrity of host cell lipid membranes. Our findings indicated that: (i) expression of GP2 enhanced membrane permeability to hygromycin-B (hyg-B), (ii) the transmembrane (TM) domain of GP2 was essential for enhanced membrane permeability, (iii) amino acids (aa) 667ALF669 within the TM region of GP2 were important for enhanced membrane permeability, and (iv) EBOV infected cells were more permeable to hyg-B than mock infected cells. Together, these data suggest that the TM region of GP2 modifies the permeability of the plasma membrane. These findings may have important implications for GP-induced cell damage and pathogenesis of EBOV infection.

PMID: 16927113 [PubMed - indexed for MEDLINE]

1580. Time. 2007 May 7;169(19):73.

A deadly mystery. A savage outbreak of Ebola virus is killing gorillas and chimps. Epidemiologists have just figured out why.

Lemonick MD.

PMID: 17511316 [PubMed - indexed for MEDLINE]

1581. Am Nat. 2007 May;169(5):684-9. Epub 2007 Mar 21.

Potential for Ebola transmission between gorilla and chimpanzee social groups.

Walsh PD(1), Breuer T, Sanz C, Morgan D, Doran-Sheehy D.

Author information: (1)Max Planck Institute for Evolutionary Anthropology, Deutscher Platz 6, 04103 Leipzig, Germany. walsh@eva.mpg.de

Over the past decade Ebola hemorrhagic fever has emerged repeatedly in Gabon and Congo, causing numerous human outbreaks and massive die-offs of gorillas and chimpanzees. Why Ebola has emerged so explosively remains poorly understood. Previous studies have tended to focus on exogenous factors such as habitat disturbance and climate change as drivers of Ebola emergence while downplaying the contribution of transmission between gorilla or chimpanzee social groups. Here we report recent observations on behaviors that pose a risk of transmission among gorilla groups and between gorillas and chimpanzees. These observations support a reassessment of ape-to-ape transmission as an amplifier of Ebola outbreaks.

PMID: 17427138 [PubMed - indexed for MEDLINE]

1582. Anaesthesist. 2007 May;56(5):482-4.

[New reflections on inflammation and coagulation].

[Article in German]

Zacharowski K(1).

Author information: (1)Dept. of Anaesthesia, BHI, Bristol Royal Infirmary, BS2 8HW, Bristol, United Kingdom. kai.zacharowski@bristol.ac.uk

Inflammation is the host's defense mechanism to infection or injury, including surgical procedures. In the clinical setting non-infectious inflammation, activation of the coagulation cascade and deterioration of endothelial function play an important role in cardiology (e.g. percutaneous transluminal coronary angioplasty, PTCA), intensive care medicine (e.g. polytrauma), cardiac (e.g. extracorporal circulation) and vascular surgery (e.g. reperfusion injury). Imbalances in the inflammatory response are mainly responsible for the often fatal course in conditions such as myocardial infarction, sepsis, hemorrhagic fever (ebola, dengue), graft rejection and autoimmune diseases. Great efforts are being undertaken worldwide to understand the regulation of inflammation in order to develop new drugs which can modulate the pathologic inflammation reaction.

PMID: 17364187 [PubMed - indexed for MEDLINE]

1583. Anal Biochem. 2007 May 1;364(1):19-29. Epub 2007 Jan 17.

Identification of inhibitors using a cell-based assay for monitoring Golgi-resident protease activity.

Coppola JM(1), Hamilton CA, Bhojani MS, Larsen MJ, Ross BD, Rehemtulla A.

Author information: (1)Department of Biological Chemistry, University of Michigan Medical School, Ann Arbor, MI 48109, USA.

Noninvasive real-time quantification of cellular protease activity allows monitoring of enzymatic activity and identification of activity modulators within the protease's natural milieu. We developed a protease activity assay based on differential localization of a recombinant reporter consisting of a Golgi retention signal and a protease cleavage sequence fused to alkaline phosphatase (AP). When expressed in mammalian cells, this protein localizes to Golgi bodies and, on protease-mediated cleavage, AP translocates to the extracellular medium where its activity is measured. We used this system to monitor the Golgi-associated protease furin, a pluripotent enzyme with a key role in tumorigenesis, viral propagation of avian influenza, ebola, and HIV as well as in activation of anthrax, pseudomonas, and diphtheria toxins. This technology was adapted for high-throughput screening of 39,000-compound small molecule libraries, leading to identification of furin inhibitors. Furthermore, this strategy was used to identify inhibitors of another Golgi protease, the beta-site amyloid precursor protein (APP)-cleaving enzyme (BACE). BACE cleavage of the APP leads to formation of the Abeta peptide, a key event that leads to Alzheimer's disease. In conclusion, we describe a customizable noninvasive technology for real-time assessment of Golgi protease activity used to identify inhibitors of furin and BACE.

PMCID: PMC1995463 PMID: 17316541 [PubMed - indexed for MEDLINE]

1584. Epidemiol Infect. 2007 May;135(4):610-21. Epub 2006 Sep 26.

Understanding the dynamics of Ebola epidemics.

Legrand J(1), Grais RF, Boelle PY, Valleron AJ, Flahault A.

Author information: (1)INSERM, UMR-S 707, Paris, France. legrand@u707.jussieu.fr

Ebola is a highly lethal virus, which has caused at least 14 confirmed outbreaks in Africa between 1976 and 2006. Using data from two epidemics [in Democratic Republic of Congo (DRC) in 1995 and in Uganda in 2000], we built a mathematical model for the spread of Ebola haemorrhagic fever epidemics taking into account transmission in different epidemiological settings. We estimated the basic reproduction number (R0) to be 2.7 (95% CI 1.9-2.8) for the 1995 epidemic in DRC, and 2.7 (95% CI 2.5-4.1) for the 2000 epidemic in Uganda. For each epidemic, we quantified transmission in different settings (illness in the community, hospitalization, and traditional burial) and simulated various epidemic scenarios to explore the impact of control interventions on a potential epidemic. A key parameter was the rapid institution of control measures. For both epidemic profiles identified, increasing hospitalization rate reduced the predicted epidemic size.

PMCID: PMC2870608 PMID: 16999875 [PubMed - indexed for MEDLINE]

1585. Hum Gene Ther. 2007 May;18(5):413-22.

Human immunodeficiency viral vector pseudotyped with the spike envelope of severe acute respiratory syndrome coronavirus transduces human airway epithelial cells and dendritic cells.

Kobinger GP(1), Limberis MP, Somanathan S, Schumer G, Bell P, Wilson JM.

Author information: (1)Special Pathogens Program, National Microbiology Laboratory, Public Health Agency of Canada, Winnipeg, MB, Canada R3E 3R2.

The human severe acute respiratory syndrome coronavirus (SARS-CoV) is a highly infectious virus that causes severe respiratory infections in humans. The spike envelope glycoprotein of SARS-CoV, the main determinant of SARS-CoV tropism, was isolated and used to pseudotype a human immunodeficiency virus (HIV)-based vector. Spike-pseudotyped HIV vector was generated and evaluated in vitro on well-differentiated human airway epithelial cells and bronchial explants and in vivo in murine airways. The spike envelope was less efficient at promoting HIV vector transduction of murine airway epithelium than an optimized deletion mutant of the Zaire ebolavirus envelope glycoprotein (NTDGL), which was used as a benchmark. However, spike-pseudotyped HIV vector was substantially more efficient than NTDGL-pseudotyped vector on human airway epithelium as demonstrated by lacZ gene transfer in primary cultures of epithelial cells and bronchial explants. In addition, this study shows that spike-pseudotyped HIV -based vector can efficiently transduce human dendritic cells and epithelial cells of the esophagus, which may have implications in investigating mechanisms of SARS-CoV pathogenesis. Spike-pseudotyped HIV-based vector is a novel lung-directed gene transfer vehicle that holds promise for the treatment of genetic lung diseases such as cystic fibrosis or alpha(1)-antitrypsin deficiency.

PMID: 17518614 [PubMed - indexed for MEDLINE]

1586. J Virol. 2007 May;81(9):4895-9. Epub 2007 Feb 14.

Interaction of Tsg101 with Marburg virus VP40 depends on the PPPY motif, but not the PT/SAP motif as in the case of Ebola virus, and Tsg101 plays a critical role in the budding of Marburg virus-like particles induced by VP40, NP, and GP.

Urata S(1), Noda T, Kawaoka Y, Morikawa S, Yokosawa H, Yasuda J.

Author information: (1)First Department of Forensic Science, National Research Institute of Police Science, Kashiwa 277-0882, Japan.

Marburg virus (MARV) VP40 is a matrix protein that can be released from mammalian cells in the form of virus-like particles (VLPs) and contains the PPPY sequence, which is an L-domain motif. Here, we demonstrate that the PPPY motif is important for VP40-induced VLP budding and that VLP production is significantly enhanced by coexpression of NP and GP. We show that Tsg101 interacts with VP40 depending on the presence of the PPPY motif, but not the PT/SAP motif as in the case of Ebola virus, and plays an important role in VLP budding. These findings provide new insights into the mechanism of MARV budding.

PMCID: PMC1900181 PMID: 17301151 [PubMed - indexed for MEDLINE]

1587. Vopr Virusol. 2007 May-Jun;52(3):41-3.

[Development of a method for rapid detection of Ebola virus antibodies and antigen].

[Article in Russian]

Chepurnov AA, Fedosova NI, Egoricheva IN, Poltavchenko AG, Elgh F.

Despite the wide spectrum of reliable methods for identifying Ebola virus, their performance requires highly-skilled personnel, specialized laboratories, complicated equipment, and much time. Therefore, there is a need for a method that allows a physician or a medical attendant to identify the causative agent in field or bedside tests without special equipment as soon as possible. The immunoassay involving nitrocellulose membrane immuno-filtration, by using a fixed antigen (antibodies) or their immunosols, is a tried-and-true method. The time of the analysis is 7-15 min.

PMID: 17601052 [PubMed - indexed for MEDLINE]

1588. Virology. 2007 Apr 10;360(2):257-63. Epub 2006 Nov 22.

Computational prediction and identification of HLA-A2.1-specific Ebola virus CTL epitopes.

Sundar K(1), Boesen A, Coico R.

Author information: (1)Department of Microbiology and Immunology, City University of New York Medical School, New York, NY 10031, USA.

Ebola virus (EBOV) is known to cause a severe hemorrhagic fever resulting in high mortality. Although the precise host defense mechanism(s) that afford protection against EBOV is not completely understood, T cell-mediated immune responses is believed to play a pivotal role in controlling virus replication and EBOV infection. There have been no reports on mapping of MHC Class I-binding CTL epitopes for EBOV till to date. In this study, we identified five HLA-A2-binding 9-mer peptides of EBOV nucleoprotein (NP) using computer-assisted algorithm. The peptides were synthesized and examined for their ability to bind to MHC class I molecules using a flow cytometry based MHC stabilization assay. Three of the EBOV-NP peptides tested (FLSFASLFL, RLMRTNFLI and KLTEAITAA) stabilized HLA-A2. The ability of the HLA-A2-binding EBOV-NP peptides to generate peptide-specific CTLs was evaluated in HLA-A2.1 transgenic mice. Epitope-specific CTL responses were confirmed by cytotoxic assays against peptide-pulsed target cells and interferon-gamma ELISPOT assay. Each of the EBOV-NP peptides induced CTL responses in HLA-A2-transgenic mice. Interestingly, all the three peptides were conserved in three different strains of Ebola (Zaire and Reston and Sudan). Taken together, these findings provide direct evidence for the existence of EBOV-derived NP epitopes that may be useful in the development of protective immunogens for this hemorrhagic virus.

PMID: 17123567 [PubMed - indexed for MEDLINE]

1589. Cell Microbiol. 2007 Apr;9(4):962-76.

NKp30-dependent cytolysis of filovirus-infected human dendritic cells.

Fuller CL(1), Ruthel G, Warfield KL, Swenson DL, Bosio CM, Aman MJ, Bavari S.

Author information: (1)United States Army Medical Research Institute of Infectious Diseases, Frederick, MD 21702, USA.

Understanding how protective innate immune responses are generated is crucial to defeating highly lethal emerging pathogens. Accumulating evidence suggests that potent innate immune responses are tightly linked to control of Ebola and Marburg filoviral infections. Here, we report that unlike authentic or inactivated Ebola and Marburg, filovirus-derived virus-like particles directly activated human natural killer (NK) cells in vitro, evidenced by pro-inflammatory cytokine production and enhanced cytolysis of permissive target cells. Further, we observed perforin- and CD95L-mediated cytolysis of filovirus-infected human dendritic cells (DCs), primary targets of filovirus infection, by autologous NK cells. Gene expression knock-down studies directly linked NK cell lysis of infected DCs to upregulation of the natural cytotoxicity receptor, NKp30. These results are the first to propose a role for NK cells in the clearance of infected DCs and the potential involvement of NKp30-mediated cytolysis in control of viral infection in vivo. Further elucidation of the biology of NK cell activation, specifically natural cytotoxicity receptors like NKp30 and NKp46, promises to aid our understanding of microbial pathology.

PMID: 17381429 [PubMed - indexed for MEDLINE]

1590. Gene Ther. 2007 Apr;14(8):648-56. Epub 2007 Feb 1.

Gene transfer in human skin with different pseudotyped HIV-based vectors.

Hachiya A(1), Sriwiriyanont P, Patel A, Saito N, Ohuchi A, Kitahara T, Takema Y, Tsuboi R, Boissy RE, Visscher MO, Wilson JM, Kobinger GP.

Author information: (1)Kao Biological Science Laboratories, Haga, Tochigi, Japan. hachiya.akira@kao.co.jp
Erratum in Gene Ther. 2007 Apr;14(8):709. James, W M [corrected to Wilson, J M].

Pseudotyping lentiviral vector with other viral surface proteins could be applied for treating genetic anomalies in human skin. In this study, the modification of HIV vector tropism by pseudotyping with the envelope glycoprotein from vesicular stomatitis virus (VSV), the Zaire Ebola (EboZ) virus, murine leukemia virus (MuLV), lymphocytic choriomeningitis virus (LCMV), Rabies or the rabies-related Mokola virus encoding LacZ as a reporter gene was evaluated qualitatively and quantitatively in human skin xenografts. High transgene expression was detected in dermal fibroblasts transduced with VSV-G-, EboZ- or MuLV-pseudotyped HIV vector with tissue irregularities in the dermal compartments following repeated injections of EboZ- or LCMV-pseudotyped vectors. Four weeks after transduction, double-labeling immunofluorescence of beta-galactosidase and involucrin or integrin beta1 demonstrated that VSV-G-, EboZ- or MuLV-pseudotyped HIV vector effectively targeted quiescent epidermal stem cells which underwent terminal differentiation resulting in transgene expression in their progenies. Among the six different pseudotyped HIV-based vectors evaluated, VSV-G-pseudotyped vector was found to be the most efficient viral glycoprotein for cutaneous transduction as demonstrated by the highest level of beta-galactosidase expression and genome copy number evaluated by TaqMan PCR.
PMID: 17268532 [PubMed - indexed for MEDLINE]
1591. J Virol. 2007 Apr;81(7):3554-62. Epub 2007 Jan 17.

Mapping of the VP40-binding regions of the nucleoprotein of Ebola virus.

Noda T(1), Watanabe S, Sagara H, Kawaoka Y.

Author information: (1)Department of Pathobiological Sciences, School of Veterinary Medicine, University of Wisconsin-Madison, 2015 Linden Drive, Madison, WI 53706, USA.

Expression of Ebola virus nucleoprotein (NP) in mammalian cells leads to the formation of helical structures, which serve as a scaffold for the nucleocapsid. We recently found that NP binding with the matrix protein VP40 is important for nucleocapsid incorporation into virions (T. Noda, H. Ebihara, Y. Muramoto, K. Fujii, A. Takada, H. Sagara, J. H. Kim, H. Kida, H. Feldmann, and Y. Kawaoka, PLoS Pathog. 2:e99, 2006). To identify the region(s) on the NP molecule required for VP40 binding, we examined the interaction of a series of NP deletion mutants with VP40 biochemically and ultrastructurally. We found that both termini of NP (amino acids 2 to 150 and 601 to 739) are essential for its interaction with VP40 and for its incorporation into virus-like particles (VLPs). We also found that the C terminus of NP is important for nucleocapsid incorporation into virions. Of interest is that the formation of NP helices, which involves the N-terminal 450 amino acids of NP, is dispensable for NP incorporation into VLPs. These findings enhance our understanding of Ebola virus assembly and in so doing move us closer to the identification of targets for the development of antiviral compounds to combat Ebola virus infection.
PMCID: PMC1866061 PMID: 17229682 [PubMed - indexed for MEDLINE]
1592. J Virol Methods. 2007 Apr;141(1):78-83. Epub 2006 Dec 27.

Rapid and simple detection of Ebola virus by reverse transcription-loop-mediated isothermal amplification.

Kurosaki Y(1), Takada A, Ebihara H, Grolla A, Kamo N, Feldmann H, Kawaoka Y, Yasuda J.

Author information: (1)National Research Institute of Police Science, Kashiwa 277-0882, Japan.

Ebola virus (EBOV) causes severe hemorrhagic fever in humans and nonhuman primates with high mortality rates. Rapid identification of the virus is required to prevent spread of the infection. In this study, we developed and evaluated a one-step simple reverse transcription-loop mediated isothermal amplification (RT-LAMP) assay for the rapid detection of Zaire ebolavirus (ZEBOV), the most virulent species of EBOV, targeting the trailer region of the viral genome. The assay could detect 20 copies of the artificial ZEBOV RNA in 26 min with a real time-monitoring detection, and also detect 10(-3) FFU of the cell-culture propagated viruses. The reaction time needed to detect 10(4) FFU of ZEBOV was only 20 min. In addition, the assay was highly specific for ZEBOV. The RT-LAMP assay developed in this study is rapid, simple, highly specific, and sensitive for the detection of ZEBOV, and so may be an effective diagnostic tool. Furthermore, as this technique does not require sophisticated instrumentation, it seems very suitable for diagnosis in the field or laboratories in Ebola outbreak areas such as Central Africa.
PMID: 17194485 [PubMed - indexed for MEDLINE]
1593. Nihon Rinsho. 2007 Mar 28;65 Suppl 3:25-9.

[Ebola hemorrhagic fever].

[Article in Japanese]

Sata T(1).

Author information: (1)Department of Pathology, National Institute of Infectious Diseases.
PMID: 17491360 [PubMed - indexed for MEDLINE]
1594. Clin Dermatol. 2007 Mar-Apr;25(2):212-20.

Viral exanthems in the tropics.

Carneiro SC(1), Cestari T, Allen SH, Ramos e-Silva M.

Author information: (1)Sector of Dermatology, School of Medicine and HUCFF-UFRJ, Federal University of Rio de Janeiro, Rio de Janeiro, Brazil. sueli@hucff.ufrj.br

Viral exanthems are a common problem in tropical regions, particularly affecting children. Most exanthems are transient and harmless, but some are potentially very dangerous. Pregnant women and malnourished or immunocompromised infants carry the greatest risk of adverse outcome. In this article, parvovirus B19; dengue and yellow fever; West Nile, Barmah Forest, Marburg, and Ebola viruses, and human herpesviruses; asymmetric periflexural exanthema of childhood; measles; rubella; enteroviruses; Lassa fever; and South American hemorrhagic fevers will be discussed.

PMID: 17350501 [PubMed - indexed for MEDLINE]
1595. Future Virol. 2007 Mar;2(2):205-215.

Filovirus replication and transcription.

Mühlberger E(1).

Author information: (1)Philipps University of Marburg, Institute of Virology, Hans-Meerwein-Street 2, 35043 Marburg, Germany Tel.: +49 6421 2864 525; ; muehlber@staff.unimarburg.de.

The highly pathogenic filoviruses, Marburg and Ebola virus, belong to the nonsegmented negative-sense RNA viruses of the order Mononegavirales. The mode of replication and transcription is similar for these viruses. On one hand, the negative-sense RNA genome serves as a template for replication, to generate progeny genomes, and, on the other hand, for transcription, to produce mRNAs. Despite the similarities in the replication/transcription strategy, filoviruses have evolved structural and functional properties that are unique among the nonsegmented negative-sense RNA viruses. Moreover, there are also striking differences in the replication and transcription mechanisms of Marburg and Ebola virus. This includes nucleocapsid formation, the structure of the genomic replication promoter, the protein requirement for transcription and the use of mRNA editing. In this article, the current knowledge of the replication and transcription strategy of Marburg and Ebola virus is reviewed, with focus on the observed differences.

PMCID: PMC3787895 PMID: 24093048 [PubMed]
1596. J Virol. 2007 Mar;81(6):2995-8. Epub 2007 Jan 17.

Proteolytic processing of the Ebola virus glycoprotein is not critical for Ebola virus replication in nonhuman primates.

Neumann G(1), Geisbert TW, Ebihara H, Geisbert JB, Daddario-DiCaprio KM, Feldmann H, Kawaoka Y.

Author information: (1)Department of Pathobiological Sciences, School of Veterinary Medicine, University of Wisconsin-Madison, 2015 Linden Drive, Madison, WI 53706, USA.

Enveloped viruses often require cleavage of a surface glycoprotein by a cellular endoprotease such as furin for infectivity and virulence. Previously, we showed that Ebola virus glycoprotein does not require the furin cleavage motif for virus replication in cell culture. Here, we show that there are no appreciable differences in disease progression, hematology, serum biochemistry, virus titers, or lethality in nonhuman primates infected with an Ebola virus lacking the furin recognition sequence compared to those infected with wild-type virus. We conclude that glycoprotein cleavage by subtilisin-like endoproteases is not critical for Ebola virus infectivity and virulence in nonhuman primates.

PMCID: PMC1866002 PMID: 17229700 [PubMed - indexed for MEDLINE]
1597. J Virol. 2007 Mar;81(5):2391-400. Epub 2006 Dec 20.

Inhibition of filovirus replication by the zinc finger antiviral protein.

Müller S(1), Möller P, Bick MJ, Wurr S, Becker S, Günther S, Kümmerer BM.

Author information: (1)Department of Virology, Bernhard-Nocht-Strasse 74, Bernhard-Nocht-Institute for Tropical Medicine, 20359 Hamburg, Germany.

The zinc finger antiviral protein (ZAP) was recently shown to inhibit Moloney murine leukemia virus and Sindbis virus replication. We tested whether ZAP also acts against Ebola virus (EBOV) and Marburg virus (MARV). Antiviral effects were observed after infection of cells expressing the N-terminal part of ZAP fused to the product of the zeocin resistance gene (NZAP-Zeo) as well as after infection of cells inducibly expressing full-length ZAP. EBOV was inhibited by up to 4 log units, whereas MARV was inhibited between 1 to 2 log units. The activity of ZAP was dependent on the integrity of the second and fourth zinc finger motif, as tested with cell lines expressing NZAP-Zeo mutants. Heterologous expression of EBOV- and MARV-specific sequences fused to a reporter gene suggest that ZAP specifically targets L gene sequences. The activity of NZAP-Zeo in this assay was also dependent on the integrity of the second and fourth zinc finger motif. Time-course experiments with infectious EBOV showed that ZAP reduces the level of L mRNA before the level of genomic or antigenomic RNA is affected. Transient expression of ZAP decreased the activity of an EBOV replicon system by up to 95%. This inhibitory effect could be partially compensated for by overexpression of L protein. In conclusion, the data demonstrate that ZAP exhibits antiviral activity against filoviruses, presumably by decreasing the level of viral mRNA.

PMCID: PMC1865956 PMID: 17182693 [PubMed - indexed for MEDLINE]
1598. Rev Med Virol. 2007 Mar-Apr;17(2):67-91.

Bats as a continuing source of emerging infections in humans.

Wong S(1), Lau S, Woo P, Yuen KY.

Author information: (1)Department of Microbiology, Research Centre of Infection and Immunology, The University of Hong Kong, 4/F University Pathology Building, Queen Mary Hospital, 102 Pokfulam Road, Hong Kong.

Amongst the 60 viral species reported to be associated with bats, 59 are RNA viruses, which are potentially important in the generation of emerging and re-emerging infections in humans. The prime examples of these are the lyssaviruses and Henipavirus. The transmission of Nipah, Hendra and perhaps SARS coronavirus and Ebola virus to humans may involve intermediate amplification hosts such as pigs, horses, civets and primates, respectively. Understanding of the natural reservoir or introductory host, the amplifying host, the epidemic centre and at-risk human populations are crucial in the control of emerging zoonosis. The association between the bat coronaviruses and certain lyssaviruses with particular bat species implies co-evolution between specific viruses and bat hosts. Cross-infection between the huge number of bat species may generate new viruses which are able to jump the trans-mammalian species barrier more efficiently. The currently known viruses that have been found in bats are reviewed and the risks of transmission to humans are highlighted. Certain families of bats including the Pteropodidae, Molossidae, Phyllostomidae, and Vespertilionidae are most frequently associated with known human pathogens. A systematic survey of bats is warranted to better understand the ecology of these viruses.

PMID: 17042030 [PubMed - indexed for MEDLINE]
1599. Vaccine. 2007 Mar 1;25(11):1923-34. Epub 2006 Nov 29.

Status and challenges of filovirus vaccines.

Reed DS(1), Mohamadzadeh M.

Author information: (1)Center for Aerobiological Sciences, U.S. Army Medical Research Institute of Infectious Diseases, 1425 Porter Street, Fort Detrick, Frederick, MD 21702-5011, USA. doug.reed@det.amedd.army.mil

Vaccines that could protect humans against the highly lethal Marburg and Ebola viruses have eluded scientists for decades. Classical approaches have been generally unsuccessful for Marburg and Ebola viruses and pose enormous safety concerns as well. Modern approaches, in particular those using vector-based approaches have met with success in nonhuman primate models although success against Ebola has been more difficult to achieve than Marburg. Despite these successes, more work remains to be done. For the vector-based vaccines, safety in humans and potency in the face of pre-existing anti-vector immunity may be critical thresholds for licensure. The immunological mechanism(s) by which these vaccines protect has not yet been convincingly determined. Licensure of these vaccines for natural outbreaks may be possible through clinical trials although this will be very difficult; licensure may also be possible by pivotal efficacy studies in animal models with an appropriate challenge. Nevertheless, nonhuman primate studies have shown that protection against Marburg and Ebola is possible and there is hope that one day a vaccine will be licensed for human use.

PMID: 17241710 [PubMed - indexed for MEDLINE]
1600. Virology. 2007 Feb 5;358(1):79-88. Epub 2006 Sep 20.

Characterization of Marburg virus glycoprotein in viral entry.

Manicassamy B(1), Wang J, Rumschlag E, Tymen S, Volchkova V, Volchkov V, Rong L.

Author information: (1)Department of Microbiology and Immunology, College of Medicine Research Building, University of Illinois at Chicago, 8133 COMRB, 909 S. Wolcott Ave., Chicago, IL 60612, USA.

One major determinant of host tropism for filoviruses is viral glycoprotein (GP), which is involved in receptor binding and viral entry. Compared to Ebola GP (EGP), Marburg GP (MGP) is less well characterized in viral entry. In this study, using a human immunodeficiency virus-based pseudotyped virus as a surrogate system, we have characterized the role of MGP in viral entry. We have shown that like EGP, the mucin-like region of MGP (289-501) is not essential for virus entry. We have developed a viral entry interference assay for filoviruses, and using this assay, we have demonstrated that transfection of EGP or MGP in target cells can interfere with EGP/HIV and MGP/HIV pseudotyped virus entry in a dose-dependent manner. These results are consistent with the notion that Ebola and Marburg viruses use the same or a related host molecule(s) for viral entry. Substitutions of the non-conserved residues in MGP1 did not impair MGP-mediated viral entry. Unlike that of EGP1, individual substitutions of many conserved residues of MGP1 exerted severe defects in MGP expression, incorporation to HIV virions, and thus its ability to mediate viral entry. These results indicate that MGP is more sensitive to substitutions of the conserved residues, suggesting that MGP may fold differently from EGP.

PMID: 16989883 [PubMed - indexed for MEDLINE]
1601. Virology. 2007 Feb 5;358(1):1-9. Epub 2006 Sep 18.

Release of cellular proteases into the acidic extracellular milieu exacerbates Ebola virus-induced cell damage.

Barrientos LG(1), Rollin PE.

Author information: (1)Special Pathogens Branch, MS G-14, Division of Viral and Rickettsial Diseases, National Center for Infectious Diseases, Centers for Disease Control and Prevention, 1600 Clifton Road N.E., Atlanta, GA 30333, USA. LBarrientosl@cdc.gov

Ebola virus is highly cytopathic through mechanisms that are largely unknown. We present evidence that progressive acidification of the extracellular milieu by Ebola virus-infected cells combined with reduced levels of natural cysteine protease inhibitor makes the cells vulnerable to uncontrolled proteolysis of extracellular matrix components by released active endosomal cathepsins, thereby exacerbating Ebola virus-induced cell destruction. The cell surface microenvironment was shown to be crucial in aiding this activity. Blocking the proteolytic activity with the cathepsin inhibitor E64 resulted in remarkable improvements with respect to viral cytopathicity and cell survival despite an overwhelmingly high viral load. We propose that the observed enzymatic matrix degradation, enhanced by an associated protease/inhibitor imbalance and metabolic acidosis, represents an effective viral strategy to boost infection and underlies, in part, the remarkable pathogenesis caused by Ebola virus. Further in vitro and in vivo research will establish whether a cellular protease with hemorrhagic activity is the leading cause of vascular leakage-the hallmark of Ebola virus hemorrhagic fever-and help understand the Ebola virus caused cell death.

PMID: 16982079 [PubMed - indexed for MEDLINE]
1602. MMWR Morb Mortal Wkly Rep. 2007 Feb 2;56(4):73-6.

Rift Valley fever outbreak--Kenya, November 2006-January 2007.

Centers for Disease Control and Prevention (CDC).

In mid-December 2006, several unexplained fatalities associated with fever and generalized bleeding were reported to the Kenya Ministry of Health (KMOH) from Garissa District in North Eastern Province (NEP). By December 20, a total of 11 deaths had been reported. Of serum samples collected from the first 19 patients, Rift Valley fever (RVF) virus RNA or immunoglobulin M (IgM) antibodies against RVF virus were found in samples from 10 patients; all serum specimens were negative for yellow fever, Ebola, Crimean-Congo hemorrhagic fever, and dengue viruses. The outbreak was confirmed by isolation of RVF virus from six of the specimens. Humans can be infected with RVF virus from bites of mosquitoes or other arthropod vectors that have fed on animals infected with RVF virus, or through contact with viremic animals, particularly livestock. Reports of livestock deaths and unexplained animal abortions in NEP provided further evidence of an RVF outbreak. On December 20, an investigation was launched by KMOH, the Kenya Field Epidemiology and Laboratory Training Program (FELTP), the Kenya Medical Research Institute (KEMRI), the Walter Reed Project of the U.S. Army Medical Research Unit, CDC-Kenya's Global Disease Detection Center, and other partners, including the World Health Organization (WHO) and Médecins Sans Frontières (MSF). This report describes the findings from that initial investigation and the control measures taken in response to the RVF outbreak, which spread to multiple additional provinces and districts, resulting in 404 cases with 118 deaths as of January 25, 2007.

PMID: 17268404 [PubMed - indexed for MEDLINE]

1603. Emerg Infect Dis. 2007 Feb;13(2):191-8.

Prevention of immune cell apoptosis as potential therapeutic strategy for severe infections.

Parrino J(1), Hotchkiss RS, Bray M.

Author information: (1)National Institutes of Health, Bethesda, Maryland 20892, USA.

Some labile cell types whose numbers are normally controlled through programmed cell death are subject to markedly increased destruction during some severe infections. Lymphocytes, in particular, undergo massive and apparently unregulated apoptosis in human patients and laboratory animals with sepsis, potentially playing a major role in the severe immunosuppression that characterizes the terminal phase of fatal illness. Extensive lymphocyte apoptosis has also occurred in humans and animals infected with several exotic agents, including Bacillus anthracis, the cause of anthrax; Yersinia pestis, the cause of plague; and Ebola virus. Prevention of lymphocyte apoptosis, through either genetic modification of the host or treatment with specific inhibitors, markedly improves survival in murine sepsis models. These findings suggest that interventions aimed at reducing the extent of immune cell apoptosis could improve outcomes for a variety of severe human infections, including those caused by emerging pathogens and bioterrorism agents.

PMCID: PMC2725847 PMID: 17479879 [PubMed - indexed for MEDLINE]

1604. Expert Rev Vaccines. 2007 Feb;6(1):57-74.

Development of vaccines for Marburg hemorrhagic fever.

Bausch DG(1), Geisbert TW.

Author information: (1)Department of Tropical Medicine, SL-17, Tulane School of Public Health and Tropical Medicine, 1430 Tulane Avenue, New Orleans, LA 70112, USA. dbausch@tulane.edu

Comment in Expert Rev Vaccines. 2007 Feb;6(1):1-3.

Marburg (MARV) and Ebola viruses (EBOV) emerged from the rainforests of Central Africa more than 30 years ago causing outbreaks of severe and, usually, fatal hemorrhagic fever. EBOV has garnered the lion's share of the attention, fueled by the higher frequency of EBOV outbreaks, high mortality rates and importation into the USA, documented in such popular works as the best-selling novel 'The Hot Zone'. However, recent large outbreaks of hundreds of cases of MARV infection in the Democratic Republic of the Congo and Angola with case fatalities approaching 90% dramatically highlight its lethal potential. Although no vaccines or antiviral drugs for MARV are currently available, remarkable progress has been made over the last few years in developing potential countermeasures against MARV in nonhuman primate models. In particular, a vaccine based on attenuated recombinant vesicular stomatitis virus was recently shown to have both preventive and postexposure efficacy.

PMID: 17280479 [PubMed - indexed for MEDLINE]

1605. J Virol. 2007 Feb;81(4):1821-37. Epub 2006 Dec 6.

Influences of glycosylation on antigenicity, immunogenicity, and protective efficacy of ebola virus GP DNA vaccines.

Dowling W(1), Thompson E, Badger C, Mellquist JL, Garrison AR, Smith JM, Paragas J, Hogan RJ, Schmaljohn C.

Author information: (1)U.S. Army Medical Research Institute of Infectious Diseases, 1425 Porter St., Fort Detrick, MD 21702, USA.

The Ebola virus (EBOV) envelope glycoprotein (GP) is the primary target of protective immunity. Mature GP consists of two disulfide-linked subunits, GP1 and membrane-bound GP2. GP is highly glycosylated with both N- and O-linked carbohydrates. We measured the influences of GP glycosylation on antigenicity, immunogenicity, and protection by testing DNA vaccines comprised of GP genes with deleted N-linked glycosylation sites or with deletions in the central hypervariable mucin region. We showed that mutation of one of the two N-linked GP2 glycosylation sites was highly detrimental to the antigenicity and immunogenicity of GP. Our data indicate that this is likely due to the inability of GP2 and GP1 to dimerize at the cell surface and suggest that glycosylation at this site is required for achieving the conformational integrity of GP2 and GP1. In contrast, mutation of two N-linked sites on GP1, which flank previously defined protective antibody epitopes on GP, may enhance immunogenicity, possibly by unmasking epitopes. We further showed that although deleting the mucin region apparently had no effect on antigenicity in vitro, it negatively impacted the elicitation of protective immunity in mice. In addition, we confirmed the presence of previously identified B-cell and T-cell epitopes in GP but show that when analyzed individually none of them were neither absolutely required nor sufficient for protective immunity to EBOV. Finally, we identified other potential regions of GP that may contain relevant antibody or T-cell epitopes.

PMCID: PMC1797596 PMID: 17151111 [PubMed - indexed for MEDLINE]

1606. J Virol. 2007 Feb;81(3):1230-40. Epub 2006 Nov 15.

The ERK mitogen-activated protein kinase pathway contributes to Ebola virus glycoprotein-induced cytotoxicity.

Zampieri CA(1), Fortin JF, Nolan GP, Nabel GJ.

Author information: (1)Vaccine Research Center, NIAID, National Institutes of Health, Room 4502, Bldg. 40, MSC-3005, 40 Convent Drive, Bethesda, MD 20892-3005, USA.

Ebola virus is a highly lethal pathogen that causes hemorrhagic fever in humans and nonhuman primates. Among the seven known viral gene products, the envelope glycoprotein (GP) alone induces cell rounding and detachment that ultimately leads to cell death. Cellular cytoxicity is not seen with comparable levels of expression of a mutant form of GP lacking a mucin-like domain (GPDeltamuc). GP-induced cell death is nonapoptotic and is preceded by downmodulation of cell surface molecules involved in signaling pathways, including certain integrins and epidermal growth factor receptor. To investigate the mechanism of GP-induced cellular toxicity, we analyzed the activation of several signal transduction pathways involved in cell growth and survival. The active form of extracellular signal-regulated kinases types 1 and 2 (ERK1/2), phospho-ERK1/2, was reduced in cells expressing GP compared to those expressing GPDeltamuc as determined by flow cytometry, in contrast to the case for several other signaling proteins. Subsequent analysis of the activation states and kinase activities of related kinases revealed a more pronounced effect on the ERK2 kinase isoform. Disruption of ERK2 activity by a dominant negative ERK or by small interfering RNA-mediated ERK2 knockdown potentiated the decrease in alphaV integrin expression associated with toxicity. Conversely, activation of the pathway through the expression of a constitutively active form of ERK2 significantly protected against this effect. These results indicate that the ERK signaling cascade mediates GP-mediated cytotoxicity and plays a role in pathogenicity induced by this gene product.
PMCID: PMC1797502 PMID: 17108034 [PubMed - indexed for MEDLINE]

1607. PLoS Pathog. 2007 Feb;3(2):e25.

Mechanism of ad5 vaccine immunity and toxicity: fiber shaft targeting of dendritic cells.

Cheng C(1), Gall JG, Kong WP, Sheets RL, Gomez PL, King CR, Nabel GJ.

Author information: (1)Vaccine Research Center, National Institute of Allergy and Infectious Diseases, National Institutes of Health, Bethesda, Maryland, United States of America.

Recombinant adenoviral (rAd) vectors elicit potent cellular and humoral immune responses and show promise as vaccines for HIV-1, Ebola virus, tuberculosis, malaria, and other infections. These vectors are now widely used and have been generally well tolerated in vaccine and gene therapy clinical trials, with many thousands of people exposed. At the same time, dose-limiting adverse responses have been observed, including transient low-grade fevers and a prior human gene therapy fatality, after systemic high-dose recombinant adenovirus serotype 5 (rAd5) vector administration in a human gene therapy trial. The mechanism responsible for these effects is poorly understood. Here, we define the mechanism by which Ad5 targets immune cells that stimulate adaptive immunity. rAd5 tropism for dendritic cells (DCs) was independent of the coxsackievirus and adenovirus receptor (CAR), its primary receptor or the secondary integrin RGD receptor, and was mediated instead by a heparin-sensitive receptor recognized by a distinct segment of the Ad5 fiber, the shaft. rAd vectors with CAR and RGD mutations did not infect a variety of epithelial and fibroblast cell types but retained their ability to transfect several DC types and stimulated adaptive immune responses in mice. Notably, the pyrogenic response to the administration of rAd5 also localized to the shaft region, suggesting that this interaction elicits both protective immunity and vector-induced fevers. The ability of replication-defective rAd5 viruses to elicit potent immune responses is mediated by a heparin-sensitive receptor that interacts with the Ad5 fiber shaft. Mutant CAR and RGD rAd vectors target several DC and mononuclear subsets and induce both adaptive immunity and toxicity. Understanding of these interactions facilitates the development of vectors that target DCs through alternative receptors that can improve safety while retaining the immunogenicity of rAd vaccines.
PMCID: PMC1803013 PMID: 17319743 [PubMed - indexed for MEDLINE]

1608. Vaccine. 2007 Jan 22;25(6):993-9. Epub 2006 Oct 10.

Protective efficacy of neutralizing antibodies against Ebola virus infection.

Takada A(1), Ebihara H, Jones S, Feldmann H, Kawaoka Y.

Author information: (1)Department of Global Epidemiology, Hokkaido University Research Center for Zoonosis Control, Sapporo 060-0818, Japan. atakada@czc.hokudai.ac.jp

Ebola virus causes lethal hemorrhagic fever in humans and nonhuman primates, but no effective antiviral compounds are available for the treatment of this infection. The surface glycoprotein (GP) of Ebola virus is an important target of neutralizing antibodies. Although passive transfer of GP-specific antibodies has been evaluated in mouse and guinea pig models, protection was achieved only by treatment shortly before or after virus challenge. Using these animal models, we evaluated the protective efficacy of two monoclonal antibodies whose epitopes are distinct from those of the antibodies tested by others. Treatment of mice with these antibodies 2 days after challenge completely protected most of the animals; even treatment 3 or 4 days after challenge was partially effective. Although antibody treatment in the guinea pig model was not as effective as in the mouse model, single-dose treatment of guinea pigs 1 day before, or 1 or 2 days after challenge did protect some animals. Interestingly, the protective effects seen in these animal models did not correlate with the in vitro neutralizing activity of the antibodies, suggesting different mechanisms of the neutralization by these antibodies. These results underscore the potential therapeutic utility of monoclonal antibodies for postexposure treatment of Ebola virus infections.
PMID: 17055127 [PubMed - indexed for MEDLINE]

1609. Mol Cell. 2007 Jan 12;25(1):85-97.

Unconventional mechanism of mRNA capping by the RNA-dependent RNA polymerase of vesicular stomatitis virus.

Ogino T(1), Banerjee AK.

Author information: (1)Department of Molecular Genetics, Section of Virology, Lerner Research Institute, Cleveland Clinic, Cleveland, OH 44195, USA.

All known eukaryotic and some viral mRNA capping enzymes (CEs) transfer a GMP moiety of GTP to the 5'-diphosphate end of the acceptor RNA via a covalent enzyme-GMP intermediate to generate the cap structure. In striking contrast, the putative CE of vesicular stomatitis virus (VSV), a prototype of nonsegmented negative-strand (NNS) RNA viruses including rabies, measles, and Ebola, incorporates the GDP moiety of GTP into the cap structure of transcribing mRNAs. Here, we report that the RNA-dependent RNA polymerase L protein of VSV catalyzes the capping reaction by an RNA:GDP polyribonucleotidyltransferase activity, in which a 5'-monophosphorylated viral mRNA-start sequence is transferred to GDP generated from GTP via a covalent enzyme-RNA intermediate. Thus, the L proteins of VSV and, by extension, other NNS RNA viruses represent a new class of viral CEs, which have evolved independently from known eukaryotic CEs.

PMID: 17218273 [PubMed - indexed for MEDLINE]

1610. Proc Natl Acad Sci U S A. 2007 Jan 9;104(2):624-9. Epub 2007 Jan 3.

Crystal structure of the C-terminal domain of Ebola virus VP30 reveals a role in transcription and nucleocapsid association.

Hartlieb B(1), Muziol T, Weissenhorn W, Becker S.

Author information: (1)European Molecular Biology Laboratory (EMBL), 6 Rue Jules Horowitz, 38042 Grenoble, France.

Transcription of the highly pathogenic Ebola virus depends on VP30, a nucleocapsid-associated Ebola virus-specific transcription factor. The transcription activator VP30 was shown to play an essential role in Ebola virus replication, most likely by stabilizing nascent mRNA. Here we present the crystal structure of the C-terminal domain (CTD) of VP30 (VP30(CTD)) at 2.0-A resolution. VP30(CTD) folds independently into a dimeric helical assembly. The VP30(CTD) dimers assemble into hexamers that are present in virions, by an oligomerization domain located in the N terminus of VP30. Mutagenesis of conserved charged amino acids on VP30(CTD) revealed that two regions, namely a basic cluster around Lys-180 and Glu-197, are required for nucleocapsid interaction. However, only mutagenesis of the basic cluster was shown to impair transcription activation, suggesting that both processes are regulated independently. The structure and the mutagenesis results reveal a potential pocket for small-molecule inhibitors that might prevent VP30 activity and thus virus propagation as it has been shown previously by peptides, which interfere with VP30 homooligomerization.

PMCID: PMC2111399 PMID: 17202263 [PubMed - indexed for MEDLINE]

1611. Curr Top Microbiol Immunol. 2007;315:363-87.

Ebolavirus and other filoviruses.

Gonzalez JP(1), Pourrut X, Leroy E.

Author information: (1)Fundamentals and Domains of Disease Emergence Research Unit, RU178, Institute for Research Development, IRD, Paris, France. frjpg@mahidol.ac.th

Since Ebola fever emerged in Central Africa in 1976, a number of studies have been undertaken to investigate its natural history and to characterize its transmission from a hypothetical reservoir host(s) to humans. This research has comprised investigations on a variety of animals and their characterization as intermediate, incidental, amplifying, reservoir, or vector hosts. A viral transmission chain was recently unveiled after a long absence of epidemic Ebola fever. Animal trapping missions were carried out in the Central African rain forest in an area where several epidemics and epizootics had occurred between 2001 and 2005. Among the various animals captured and analyzed, three species of fruit bats (suborder Megachiroptera) were found asymptomatically and naturally infected with Ebola virus: Hypsignathus monstrosus (hammer-headed fruit beats), Epomops franqueti (singing fruit bats), and Myonycteris torquata (little collared fruit bats). From experimental data, serological studies and virus genetic analysis, these findings confirm the importance of these bat species as potential reservoir species of Ebola virus in Central Africa. While feeding bats drop partially eaten fruit and masticated fruit pulp (spats) to the ground, possibly promoting indirect transmission of Ebola virus to certain ground dwelling mammals, if virus is being shed in saliva by chronically and asymptomatically infected bats. Great apes and forest duikers are particularly sensitive to lethal Ebola virus infection. These terrestrial mammals feed on fallen fruits and possibly spats, suggesting a chain of events leading to Ebola virus spillover to these incidental hosts. This chain of events may occur sporadically at different sites and times depending on a combination of the phenology of fruit production by different trees, animal behavior, and various, but as yet still unknown environmental factors, which could include drought. During the reproductive period, infected body fluid can also be shed in the environment and present a potential risk for indirect transmission to other vertebrates.

PMID: 17848072 [PubMed - indexed for MEDLINE]

1612. Genome Biol. 2007;8(8):R174.

The temporal program of peripheral blood gene expression in the response of nonhuman primates to Ebola hemorrhagic fever.

Rubins KH(1), Hensley LE, Wahl-Jensen V, Daddario DiCaprio KM, Young HA, Reed DS, Jahrling PB, Brown PO, Relman DA, Geisbert TW.

Author information: (1)Department of Microbiology and Immunology, 299 Campus Dr, Stanford University School of Medicine, Stanford, California 94305, USA. rubins@wi.mit.edu

BACKGROUND: Infection with Ebola virus (EBOV) causes a fulminant and often fatal hemorrhagic fever. In order to improve our understanding of EBOV pathogenesis and EBOV-host interactions, we examined the molecular features of EBOV infection in vivo. RESULTS: Using high-density cDNA microarrays, we analyzed genome-wide host expression patterns in sequential blood samples from nonhuman primates infected with EBOV. The temporal program of gene expression was strikingly similar between animals. Of particular interest were features of the data that reflect the interferon response, cytokine signaling, and apoptosis. Transcript levels for tumor necrosis factor-alpha converting enzyme (TACE)/alpha-disintegrin and metalloproteinase (ADAM)-17 increased during days 4 to 6 after infection. In addition, the serum concentration of cleaved Ebola glycoprotein (GP2 delta) was elevated in late-stage EBOV infected animals. Of note, we were able to detect changes in gene expression of more than 300 genes before symptoms appeared. CONCLUSION: These results provide the first genome-wide ex vivo analysis of the host response to systemic filovirus infection and disease. These data may elucidate mechanisms of viral pathogenesis and host defense, and may suggest targets for diagnostic and therapeutic development.

PMCID: PMC2375004 PMID: 17725815 [PubMed - indexed for MEDLINE]

1613. J Clin Microbiol. 2007 Jan;45(1):224-6. Epub 2006 Nov 1.

Rapid molecular strategy for filovirus detection and characterization.

Zhai J(1), Palacios G, Towner JS, Jabado O, Kapoor V, Venter M, Grolla A, Briese T, Paweska J, Swanepoel R, Feldmann H, Nichol ST, Lipkin WI.

Author information: (1)Jerome L. and Dawn Greene Infectious Disease Laboratory, Mailman School of Public Health, Columbia University, New York, NY 10032, USA.

Filoviruses have the capacity to cause lethal outbreaks of hemorrhagic fever in primates. Here we present a simple consensus reverse transcription-PCR method for filovirus recognition and characterization and demonstrate its utility with all known filovirus strains. Phylogenetic assignment is achieved by automated web-based sequence analysis of amplification products.

PMCID: PMC1828965 PMID: 17079496 [PubMed - indexed for MEDLINE]

1614. J Virol. 2007 Jan;81(1):182-92. Epub 2006 Oct 25.

The VP35 protein of Ebola virus inhibits the antiviral effect mediated by double-stranded RNA-dependent protein kinase PKR.

Feng Z(1), Cerveny M, Yan Z, He B.

Author information: (1)Department of Microbiology and Immunology (M/C 790), College of Medicine, The University of Illinois at Chicago, 835 South Wolcott Avenue, Chicago, IL 60612, USA.

The VP35 protein of Ebola virus is a viral antagonist of interferon. It acts to block virus or double-stranded RNA-mediated activation of interferon regulatory factor 3, a transcription factor that facilitates the expression of interferon and interferon-stimulated genes. In this report, we show that the VP35 protein is also able to inhibit the antiviral response induced by alpha interferon. This depends on the VP35 function that interferes with the pathway regulated by double-stranded RNA-dependent protein kinase PKR. When expressed in a heterologous system, the VP35 protein enhanced viral polypeptide synthesis and growth in Vero cells pretreated with alpha/beta interferon, displaying an interferon-resistant phenotype. In correlation, phosphorylation of PKR and eIF-2alpha was suppressed in cells expressing the VP35 protein. This activity of the VP35 protein was required for efficient viral replication in PKR+/+ but not PKR-/- mouse embryo fibroblasts. Furthermore, VP35 appears to be a RNA binding protein. Notably, a deletion of amino acids 1 to 200, but not R312A substitution in the RNA binding motif, abolished the ability of the VP35 protein to confer viral resistance to interferon. However, the R312A substitution rendered the VP35 protein unable to inhibit the induction of the beta interferon promoter mediated by virus infection. Together, these results show that the VP35 protein targets multiple pathways of the interferon system.

PMCID: PMC1797262 PMID: 17065211 [PubMed - indexed for MEDLINE]

1615. Med Hypotheses. 2007;68(1):151-7. Epub 2006 Aug 8.

AIDS: caused by development of resistance to drugs in a non-target intracellular parasite.

Parris GE(1).

Author information: (1)9601 Warfield Road, Gaithersburg, MD 20882, United States. antimony_121@hotmail.com

Comment in Med Hypotheses. 2007;68(5):1187-8.

The origin of acquired immune disorder syndrome (AIDS) has been the subject of substantial controversy both in the scientific community and in the popular press. The debate involves the mode of transmission of a simian virus (SIV) to humans. Both major camps in the argument presume that humans are normally free of such viruses and assume that once the simian virus was transmitted, it immediately infected some T-cells and caused the release of toxic agents that killed off bystander (uninfected) T-cells resulting in AIDS. The evolution of the Simian virus (SIV) into a human virus (HIV) is regarded as an artifact. In contrast, a fundamentally different hypothesis has been proposed [Parris GE. Med Hypotheses 2004;62(3):354-7] in which it is presumed that in hyper-endemic areas of malaria (central Africa), all primates (humans and non-human primates) have shared a retrovirus that augments their T-cell response to the malaria parasite. The virus can be called "primate T-cell retrovirus" (PTRV). Over thousands of years the virus has crossed species lines many times (with little effect) and typically adapts to the host quickly. In this model, AIDS is seen to be the result of the development of resistance of the virus (PTRV) to continuous exposure to pro-apoptotic (schizonticidal) aminoquinoline drugs used to prevent malaria. The hypothesis was originally proposed based on biochemical activities of the aminoquinolines (e.g., pamaquine (plasmoquine(TM)), primaquine and chloroquine), but recent publications demonstrated that some of these drugs definitely adversely affect HIV and other viruses and logically would cause them to evolve resistance. Review of the timeline that has been created for the evolution of HIV in humans is also shown to be qualitatively and quantitatively consistent with this hypothesis (and not with either version of the conventional hypothesis). SARS and Ebola also fit this pattern.

PMID: 16893612 [PubMed - indexed for MEDLINE]

1616. Nucleic Acids Res. 2007;35(11):3602-11. Epub 2007 May 7.

Dynamics of filamentous viral RNPs prior to egress.

Santangelo PJ(1), Bao G.

Author information: (1)Wallace H. Coulter Department of Biomedical Engineering, Georgia Institute of Technology and Emory University, 313 Ferst Drive, Atlanta, GA 30332, USA. philip.santangelo@bme.gatech.edu

The final step in the maturation of paramyxoviruses, orthomyxoviruses and viruses of several other families, entails the budding of the viral nucleocapsid through the plasma membrane of the host cell. Many medically important viruses, such as influenza, parainfluenza, respiratory syncytial virus (RSV) and Ebola, can form filamentous particles when budding. Although filamentous virions have been previously studied, details of how viral filaments bud from the plasma membrane remain largely unknown. Using molecular beacon (MB)-fluorescent probes to image the viral genomic RNA (vRNA) of human RSV (hRSV) in live Vero cells, the dynamics of assembled viral filaments was observed to consist of three primary types of motion prior to egress from the plasma membrane: (i) filament projection and rotation, (ii) migration and (iii) non-directed motion. In addition, from information gained by imaging the 3D distribution of cellular

vRNA, observing and characterizing vRNA dynamics, imaging vRNA/Myosin Va colocalization, and studying the effects of cytochalasin D (actin depolymerizing agent) exposure, a model for filamentous virion egress is presented.
PMCID: PMC1920244 PMID: 17485480 [PubMed - indexed for MEDLINE]

1617. PLoS Pathog. 2007 Jan;3(1):e9.

Neutralizing antibody fails to impact the course of Ebola virus infection in monkeys.

Oswald WB(1), Geisbert TW, Davis KJ, Geisbert JB, Sullivan NJ, Jahrling PB, Parren PW, Burton DR.

Author information: (1)Departments of Immunology and Molecular Biology, The Scripps Research Institute, La Jolla, California, United States of America.
Prophylaxis with high doses of neutralizing antibody typically offers protection against challenge with viruses producing acute infections. In this study, we have investigated the ability of the neutralizing human monoclonal antibody, KZ52, to protect against Ebola virus in rhesus macaques. This antibody was previously shown to fully protect guinea pigs from infection. Four rhesus macaques were given 50 mg/kg of neutralizing human monoclonal antibody KZ52 intravenously 1 d before challenge with 1,000 plaque-forming units of Ebola virus, followed by a second dose of 50 mg/kg antibody 4 d after challenge. A control animal was exposed to virus in the absence of antibody treatment. Passive transfer of the neutralizing human monoclonal antibody not only failed to protect macaques against challenge with Ebola virus but also had a minimal effect on the explosive viral replication following infection. We show that the inability of antibody to impact infection was not due to neutralization escape. It appears that Ebola virus has a mechanism of infection propagation in vivo in macaques that is uniquely insensitive even to high concentrations of neutralizing antibody.
PMCID: PMC1779296 PMID: 17238286 [PubMed - indexed for MEDLINE]

1618. PLoS Pathog. 2007 Jan;3(1):e2.

Effective post-exposure treatment of Ebola infection.

Feldmann H(1), Jones SM, Daddario-DiCaprio KM, Geisbert JB, Ströher U, Grolla A, Bray M, Fritz EA, Fernando L, Feldmann F, Hensley LE, Geisbert TW.

Author information: (1)Special Pathogens Program, National Microbiology Laboratory, Public Health Agency of Canada, Winnipeg, Manitoba, Canada. Heinz_Feldmann@phac-aspc.gc.ca
Ebola viruses are highly lethal human pathogens that have received considerable attention in recent years due to an increasing re-emergence in Central Africa and a potential for use as a biological weapon. There is no vaccine or treatment licensed for human use. In the past, however, important advances have been made in developing preventive vaccines that are protective in animal models. In this regard, we showed that a single injection of a live-attenuated recombinant vesicular stomatitis virus vector expressing the Ebola virus glycoprotein completely protected rodents and nonhuman primates from lethal Ebola challenge. In contrast, progress in developing therapeutic interventions against Ebola virus infections has been much slower and there is clearly an urgent need to develop effective post-exposure strategies to respond to future outbreaks and acts of bioterrorism, as well as to treat laboratory exposures. Here we tested the efficacy of the vesicular stomatitis virus-based Ebola vaccine vector in post-exposure treatment in three relevant animal models. In the guinea pig and mouse models it was possible to protect 50% and 100% of the animals, respectively, following treatment as late as 24 h after lethal challenge. More important, four out of eight rhesus macaques were protected if treated 20 to 30 min following an otherwise uniformly lethal infection. Currently, this approach provides the most effective post-exposure treatment strategy for Ebola infections and is particularly suited for use in accidentally exposed individuals and in the control of secondary transmission during naturally occurring outbreaks or deliberate release.
PMCID: PMC1779298 PMID: 17238284 [PubMed - indexed for MEDLINE]

1619. Trans R Soc Trop Med Hyg. 2007 Jan;101(1):64-78. Epub 2006 Sep 28.

Morbidity and mortality of wild animals in relation to outbreaks of Ebola haemorrhagic fever in Gabon, 1994-2003.

Lahm SA(1), Kombila M, Swanepoel R, Barnes RF.

Author information: (1)Institute for Research in Tropical Ecology, Makokou, Gabon. sallyalahm@aol.com
Antibody to Ebola virus was found in 14 (1.2%) of 1147 human sera collected in Gabon in 1981-1997. Six seropositive subjects were bled in the northeast in 1991, more than 3 years prior to recognition of the first known outbreak of Ebola haemorrhagic fever (EHF), whilst eight came from the southwest where the disease has not been recognised. It has been reported elsewhere that 98 carcasses of wild animals were found in systematic studies in northeastern Gabon and adjoining northwestern Republic of the Congo (RoC) during five EHF epidemics in August 2001 to June 2003, with Ebola virus infection being confirmed in 14 carcasses. During the present opportunistic observations, reports were investigated of a further 397 carcasses, mainly gorillas, chimpanzees, mandrills and bush pigs, found by rural residents in 35 incidents in Gabon and RoC during 1994-2003. Sixteen incidents had temporal and/or spatial coincidence with confirmed EHF outbreaks, and the remaining 19 appeared to represent extension of disease from such sites. There appeared to be sustained Ebola virus activity in the northeast in 1994-1999, with sequential spread from 1996 onwards, first westwards, then southerly, and then northeastwards, reaching the Gabon-RoC border in 2001. This implies that there was transmission of infection between wild mammals, but the species involved are highly susceptible and unlikely to be natural hosts of the virus.
PMID: 17010400 [PubMed - indexed for MEDLINE]

1620. Vestn Ross Akad Med Nauk. 2007;(12):40-4.

[Important issues of biological safety].

[Article in Russian]

Onishchenko GG.

The problem of biological security raises alarm due to the real growth of biological threats. Biological security includes a wide scope of problems, the solution of which becomes a part of national security as a necessary condition for the constant development of the country. A number of pathogens, such as human immunodeficiency virus, exotic Ebola and Lassa viruses causing hemorrhagic fever, rotaviruses causing acute intestinal diseases, etc. were first discovered in the last century. Terrorist actions committed in the USA in 2001 using the anthrax pathogen made the problem of biological danger even more important. In Russian Federation, biological threats are counteracted through the united state policy being a part of general state security policy. The biological Security legislation of Russian Federation is chiefly based on the 1992 Federal Law on Security. On the basis of cumulated experience, the President of Russia ratified Basics of Russian Federation's State Policy for Chemical and Biological Security for the Period through 2010 and Beyond on 4 December, 2003. The document determines the main directions and stages of the state development in the area of chemical and biological security. The Federal target program Russian Federation's National Program for Chemical and Biological Security is being developed, and its development is to be completed soon in order to perfect the national system for biological security and fulfill Basics of Russian Federation's State Policy for Chemical and Biological Security for the Period through 2010 and Beyond, ratified by the President. The new global strategy for control over infectious diseases, presented in the materials of Saint Petersburg summit of the Group of Eight, as well as the substantive part of its elements in Sanitary International Standards, are to a large degree an acknowledgement of the Russian Federation's experience and the algorithm for fighting extremely dangerous infections. This Russia's experience has resulted in the following global achievements: smallpox elimination in the USSR (1936); the USSR's suggestions on the program of smallpox elimination in the world and 2 billion doses of the vaccine transferred to the possession of the WHO (since 1958); the global elimination of the disease (1980); effective control over avian influenza at the epizootic stage, recognized internationally at Beijing International Congress, 17-18 January, 2006.

PMID: 18225506 [PubMed - indexed for MEDLINE]

1621. Vopr Virusol. 2007 Jan-Feb;52(1):10-6.

[Molecular mechanisms of Ebola virus reproduction].

[Article in Russian]

Subbotina EL, Chepurnov AA.

The review presents recent data on the molecular mechanisms of the stages of an Ebola virus replication cycle, on the interaction of viral and cellular components at each stage, as well as on the mechanisms responsible for he realization of viral genetic information in the infected cell.

PMID: 17338228 [PubMed - indexed for MEDLINE]

1622. Science. 2006 Dec 8;314(5805):1564.

Ebola outbreak killed 5000 gorillas.

Bermejo M(1), Rodríguez-Teijeiro JD, Illera G, Barroso A, Vilà C, Walsh PD.

Author information: (1)Ecosystèmes Forestiers d'Afrique Centrale (ECOFAC), Box Postale 15115 Libreville, Gabon. magda_bermejo@yahoo.es

Comment in Science. 2006 Dec 8;314(5805):1522-3.

Over the past decade, the Zaire strain of Ebola virus (ZEBOV) has repeatedly emerged in Gabon and Congo. Each human outbreak has been accompanied by reports of gorilla and chimpanzee carcasses in neighboring forests, but both the extent of ape mortality and the causal role of ZEBOV have been hotly debated. Here, we present data suggesting that in 2002 and 2003 ZEBOV killed about 5000 gorillas in our study area. The lag between neighboring gorilla groups in mortality onset was close to the ZEBOV disease cycle length, evidence that group-to-group transmission has amplified gorilla die-offs.

PMID: 17158318 [PubMed - indexed for MEDLINE]

1623. Science. 2006 Dec 8;314(5805):1522-3.

Ecology. Tracking Ebola's deadly march among wild apes.

Vogel G.

Comment on Science. 2006 Dec 8;314(5805):1564.

PMID: 17158293 [PubMed - indexed for MEDLINE]

1624. Biometrics. 2006 Dec;62(4):1170-7.

Statistical inference in a stochastic epidemic SEIR model with control intervention: Ebola as a case study.

Lekone PE(1), Finkenstädt BF.

Author information: (1)Department of Statistics, University of Warwick, Coventry CV4 7AL, UK. lekonepe@mopipi.ub.bw

A stochastic discrete-time susceptible-exposed-infectious-recovered (SEIR) model for infectious diseases is developed with the aim of estimating parameters from daily incidence and mortality time series for an outbreak of Ebola in the Democratic Republic of Congo in 1995. The incidence time series exhibit many low integers as well as zero counts requiring an intrinsically stochastic modeling approach. In order to capture the stochastic nature of the transitions between the compartmental populations in such a model we specify appropriate conditional binomial distributions. In addition, a relatively simple temporally varying transmission rate function is introduced that allows for the effect of control interventions. We develop Markov chain Monte Carlo methods for inference that are used to explore the posterior distribution of the parameters. The algorithm is further extended to integrate numerically over state variables of the model, which are unobserved. This provides a realistic stochastic model that can be used by epidemiologists to study the dynamics of the disease and the effect of control interventions.

PMID: 17156292 [PubMed - indexed for MEDLINE]

1625. Expert Opin Investig Drugs. 2006 Dec;15(12):1523-35.

Progress towards the treatment of Ebola haemorrhagic fever.

Ströher U(1), Feldmann H.

Author information: (1)National Microbiology Laboratory, Public Health Agency of Canada, 1015 Arlington Street, Winnipeg, Manitoba, R3E3R2, Canada. Ute_Stroeher@phac-aspc.gc.ca

Being highly pathogenic for human and nonhuman primates and the subject of former weapon programmes makes Ebola virus one of the most feared pathogens worldwide today. Due to a lack of licensed pre- and postexposure intervention, the current response depends on rapid diagnostics, proper isolation procedures and supportive care of case patients. Consequently, the development of more specific countermeasures is of high priority for the preparedness of many nations. Over the past years, enhanced research efforts directed to better understand virus replication and pathogenesis have identified potential new targets for intervention strategies. The authors discuss the most promising therapeutic approaches for Ebola haemorrhagic fever as judged by their efficacy in animal models. The current development in this field encourages discussions on how to move some of the experimental approaches towards clinical application.

PMID: 17107278 [PubMed - indexed for MEDLINE]

1626. Expert Rev Anti Infect Ther. 2006 Dec;4(6):917-21.

Filoviruses: recent advances and future challenges.

Bray M(1), Pilch R.

Author information: (1)NIAID/NIH, Biodefense Clinical Research Branch, 6700A Rockledge Drive, Room 5128, Bethesda, MD 20892, USA. mbray@niaid.nih.gov

PMID: 17181407 [PubMed - indexed for MEDLINE]

1627. FASEB J. 2006 Dec;20(14):2519-30. Epub 2006 Oct 5.

Implication of a retrovirus-like glycoprotein peptide in the immunopathogenesis of Ebola and Marburg viruses.

Yaddanapudi K(1), Palacios G, Towner JS, Chen I, Sariol CA, Nichol ST, Lipkin WI.

Author information: (1)Jerome L. and Dawn Greene Infectious Disease Laboratory, Mailman School of Public Health, Columbia University, 722 West 168th St., New York, NY 10032, USA.

Ebola and Marburg viruses can cause hemorrhagic fever (HF) outbreaks with high mortality in primates. Whereas Marburg (MARV), Ebola Zaire (ZEBOV), and Ebola Sudan (SEBOV) viruses are pathogenic in humans, apes, and monkeys, Ebola Reston (REBOV) is pathogenic only in monkeys. Early immunosuppression may contribute to pathogenesis by facilitating viral replication. Lymphocyte depletion, intravascular apoptosis, and cytokine dysregulation are prominent in fatal cases. Here we functionally characterize a 17 amino acid domain in filoviral glycoproteins that resembles an immunosuppressive motif in retroviral envelope proteins. Activated human or rhesus peripheral blood mononuclear cells (PBMC) were exposed to inactivated ZEBOV or a panel of 17mer peptides representing all sequenced strains of filoviruses, then analyzed for CD4+ and CD8+ T cell activation, apoptosis, and cytokine expression. Exposure of human and rhesus PBMC to ZEBOV, SEBOV, or MARV peptides or inactivated ZEBOV resulted in decreased expression of activation markers on CD4 and CD8 cells; CD4 and CD8 cell apoptosis as early as 12 h postexposure; inhibition of CD4 and CD8 cell cycle progression; decreased interleukin (IL)-2, IFN-gamma, and IL12-p40 expression; and increased IL-10 expression. In contrast, only rhesus T cells were sensitive to REBOV peptides. These findings are consistent with the observation that REBOV is not pathogenic in humans and have implications for understanding the pathogenesis of filoviral HF.

PMID: 17023517 [PubMed - indexed for MEDLINE]

1628. J Virol. 2006 Dec;80(24):12070-8. Epub 2006 Sep 27.

Mutation of YMYL in the Nipah virus matrix protein abrogates budding and alters subcellular localization.

Ciancanelli MJ(1), Basler CF.

Author information: (1)Department of Microbiology, Box 1124, Mount Sinai School of Medicine, 1 Gustave L. Levy Place, New York, NY 10029, USA.

Matrix (M) proteins reportedly direct the budding of paramyxoviruses from infected cells. In order to begin to characterize the assembly process for the highly lethal, emerging paramyxovirus Nipah virus (NiV), we have examined the budding of NiV M. We demonstrated that expression of the NiV M protein is sufficient to produce budding virus-like particles (VLPs) that are physically and morphologically similar to NiV. We identified in NiV M a sequence, YMYL, with similarity to the YPDL late domain found in the equine infectious anemia virus Gag protein. When the YMYL within NiV M was mutated, VLP release was abolished and M was relocalized to the nucleus, but the mutant M proteins retained oligomerization activity. When YMYL was fused to a late-domain mutant of the Ebola virus VP40 matrix protein, VP40 budding was restored. These results suggest that the YMYL sequence may act as a trafficking signal and a late domain for NiV M.

PMCID: PMC1676283 PMID: 17005661 [PubMed - indexed for MEDLINE]

1629. Klin Mikrobiol Infekc Lek. 2006 Dec;12(6):217-23.

[Ebola and Marburg fever--outbreaks of viral haemorrhagic fever].

[Article in Czech]

Chlíbek R(1), Smetana J, Vacková M.

Author information: (1)Katedra epidemiologie Fakulty vojenského zdravotnictví Univerzity obrany, Hradec Králové. chlibek@pmfhk.cz

With an increasing frequency of traveling and tourism to exotic countries, a new threat-import of rare, very dangerous infections-emerges in humane medicine. Ebola fever and Marburg fever, whose agents come from the same group of Filoviridae family, belong among these diseases. The natural reservoir of these viruses has not yet been precisely determined. The pathogenesis of the diseases is not absolutely clear, there is neither a possibility of vaccination, nor an effective treatment. Fever and haemorrhagic diathesis belong to the basic symptoms of the diseases. Most of the infected persons die, the death rate is 70-88 %. The history of Ebola fever is relatively short-30 years, Marburg fever is known almost 40 years. Hundreds of people have died of these diseases so far. The study involves epidemics recorded in the world and their epidemiological relations. Not a single case has been recorded in the Czech Republic, nevertheless a sick traveler or infected animals are the highest risk of import these diseases. In our conditions, the medical staff belong to a highly endangered group of people because of stringent isolation of patients, strict rules of barrier treatment regime and high infectivity of the diseases. For this reason, the public should be prepared for possible contact with these highly virulent infections.

PMID: 17230375 [PubMed - indexed for MEDLINE]

1630. Clin Vaccine Immunol. 2006 Nov;13(11):1267-77. Epub 2006 Sep 20.

A DNA vaccine for Ebola virus is safe and immunogenic in a phase I clinical trial.

Martin JE(1), Sullivan NJ, Enama ME, Gordon IJ, Roederer M, Koup RA, Bailer RT, Chakrabarti BK, Bailey MA, Gomez PL, Andrews CA, Moodie Z, Gu L, Stein JA, Nabel GJ, Graham BS.

Author information: (1)Vaccine Research Center, National Institute of Allergy and Infectious Diseases, National Institutes, Bethesda, MD 20892-3017, USA.
Ebola viruses represent a class of filoviruses that causes severe hemorrhagic fever with high mortality. Recognized first in 1976 in the Democratic Republic of Congo, outbreaks continue to occur in equatorial Africa. A safe and effective Ebola virus vaccine is needed because of its continued emergence and its potential for use for biodefense. We report the safety and immunogenicity of an Ebola virus vaccine in its first phase I human study. A three-plasmid DNA vaccine encoding the envelope glycoproteins (GP) from the Zaire and Sudan/Gulu species as well as the nucleoprotein was evaluated in a randomized, placebo-controlled, double-blinded, dose escalation study. Healthy adults, ages 18 to 44 years, were randomized to receive three injections of vaccine at 2 mg (n = 5), 4 mg (n = 8), or 8 mg (n = 8) or placebo (n = 6). Immunogenicity was assessed by enzyme-linked immunosorbent assay (ELISA), immunoprecipitation-Western blotting, intracellular cytokine staining (ICS), and enzyme-linked immunospot assay. The vaccine was well-tolerated, with no significant adverse events or coagulation abnormalities. Specific antibody responses to at least one of the three antigens encoded by the vaccine as assessed by ELISA and CD4(+) T-cell GP-specific responses as assessed by ICS were detected in 20/20 vaccinees. CD8(+) T-cell GP-specific responses were detected by ICS assay in 6/20 vaccinees. This Ebola virus DNA vaccine was safe and immunogenic in humans. Further assessment of the DNA platform alone and in combination with replication-defective adenoviral vector vaccines, in concert with challenge and immune data from nonhuman primates, will facilitate evaluation and potential licensure of an Ebola virus vaccine under the Animal Rule.

PMCID: PMC1656552 PMID: 16988008 [PubMed - indexed for MEDLINE]

1631. Emerg Med Clin North Am. 2006 Nov;24(4):1019-33.

Emergency medicine and the public's health: emerging infectious diseases.

Saks MA(1), Karras D.

Author information: (1)Department of Emergency Medicine, Drexel University College of Medicine, Philadelphia, PA 19101, USA. msaks@drexelmed.edu
In recent years, multiple global forces have contributed to the emergence and widespread distribution of previously unknown disease entities. This article discusses Ebola virus, West Nile virus, and Hantavirus as representative emerging infectious diseases. Smallpox is discussed along with concerns about the safety of the smallpox vaccine, given the uncertain risk of bioterrorism and smallpox exposure. ED physicians must become familiar with the presentation, management, and public health impact of all of these entities, as well as understand the potential impact of other emerging infectious diseases.

PMID: 16982350 [PubMed - indexed for MEDLINE]

1632. J Intern Med. 2006 Nov;260(5):399-408.

Zoonotic viral diseases and the frontier of early diagnosis, control and prevention.

Heeney JL(1).

Author information: (1)Department of Virology, BPRC, Rijswijk, and the Department of Medical Microbiology, University of Leiden, Leiden, The Netherlands. heeney@bprc.nl
Public awareness of the human health risks of zoonotic infections has grown in recent years. Currently, concern of H5N1 flu transmission from migratory bird populations has increased with foci of fatal human cases. This comes on the heels of other major zoonotic viral epidemics in the last decade. These include other acute emerging or re-emerging viral diseases such as severe acute respiratory syndrome (SARS), West-Nile virus, Ebola virus, monkeypox, as well as the more inapparent insidious slow viral and prion diseases. Virus infections with zoonotic potential can become serious killers once they are able to establish the necessary adaptations for efficient human-to-human transmission under circumstances sufficient to reach epidemic proportions. The monitoring and early diagnosis of these potential risks are overlapping frontiers of human and veterinary medicine. Here, current viral zoonotics and evolving threats are reviewed.

PMID: 17040245 [PubMed - indexed for MEDLINE]

1633. J Virol Methods. 2006 Nov;137(2):219-28. Epub 2006 Jul 20.

Detection of Ebola virus envelope using monoclonal and polyclonal antibodies in ELISA, surface plasmon resonance and a quartz crystal microbalance immunosensor.

Yu JS(1), Liao HX, Gerdon AE, Huffman B, Scearce RM, McAdams M, Alam SM, Popernack PM, Sullivan NJ, Wright D, Cliffel DE, Nabel GJ, Haynes BF.

Author information: (1)Human Vaccine Institute, Duke University Medical Center, Durham, NC 27710, United States. yu000022@mc.duke.edu
Ebola virus (EBOV) Zaire, Sudan, as well as Ivory Coast are virulent human EBOV species. Both polyclonal and monoclonal antibodies (MAbs) were developed against soluble EBOV envelope glycoprotein (GP) for the study of EBOV envelope diversity and development of diagnostic reagents. Three EBOV Sudan-Gulu GP peptides, from the N-terminus, mid-GP, and C-terminus regions were used to immunize rabbits for the generation of anti-EBOV polyclonal antibodies. Polyclonal antisera raised against the C-terminus peptide could detect both Sudan-Gulu as well as Zaire GPs, while anti-N and mid-region peptide polyclonal sera recognized only EBOV Sudan-Gulu GP. Of the three anti-EBOV GP mouse MAbs produced, MAb 15H10 recognized all human EBOV GP species tested (Zaire, Sudan and Ivory Coast), and as well as reacted with the Reston non-human primate EBOV GPs. In addition, MAb 15H10 bound virion-associated GP of all known EBOV species. MAb 17A3 recognized GPs of both EBOV Sudan-Gulu and Zaire, while MAb 6D11 recognized only EBOV Sudan-Gulu GP. To detect EBOV GP, these antibody

reagents were used in ELISA, surface plasmon resonance and in a quartz crystal microbalance immunosensor. Thus, polyclonal and monoclonal antibodies can be used in combination to identify and differentiate both human and non-human primate EBOV GPs.

PMID: 16857271 [PubMed - indexed for MEDLINE]

1634. Virus Res. 2006 Nov;121(2):205-14. Epub 2006 Jul 12.

Identification of two amino acid residues on Ebola virus glycoprotein 1 critical for cell entry.

Mpanju OM(1), Towner JS, Dover JE, Nichol ST, Wilson CA.

Author information: (1)Gene Transfer and Immunogenicity Branch, Division of Cellular, Tissue and Gene Therapies, Center for Biologics Evaluation and Research, Food and Drug Administration, Bethesda, MD 20892, USA.

Using site-directed mutagenesis and retroviral vector pseudotyping of the wild type or mutated glycoprotein of Zaire ebolavirus (ZEBOV), we analyzed 15 conserved residues in the N-terminus of the filovirus glycoprotein 1 (GP1) in order to identify residues critical for cell entry. Results from infectivity assays and Western blot analyses identified two phenylalanine residues at positions 88 and 159 that appear to be critical for ZEBOV entry in vitro. We extended this observation by introduction of alanines at either position 88 or 159 of Ivory Coast Ebolavirus (CIEBOV) and observed the same phenotype. Further, we showed that introduction of each of the two mutations in a recombinant full-length clone of ZEBOV (Mayinga strain) that also carried the coding sequence for GFP could not be rescued, suggesting the mutants rendered the virus non-infectious. The two phenylalanines that are critical for both ZEBOV and CIEBOV entry are found in two linear domains of GP1 that are highly conserved among filoviruses, and thus could provide a target for rational development of broadly cross-protective vaccines or antiviral therapies.

PMID: 16839637 [PubMed - indexed for MEDLINE]

1635. Vopr Virusol. 2006 Nov-Dec;51(6):4-10.

[The properties of Ebola virus proteins].

[Article in Russian]

Subbotina EL, Kachko AV, Chepurnov AA.

The paper describes the structure and functions of Ebola virus properties. It also presents information on the role of structural (NP, VP40, VP35, GP, VP30, VP24, and L) and secreted (sGP, delta-peptide, GP1, GP(1,2delta), ssGP) proteins in the viral replication cycle and in the pathogenesis of Ebola hemorrhagic fever.

PMID: 17214074 [PubMed - indexed for MEDLINE]

1636. Antimicrob Agents Chemother. 2006 Oct;50(10):3367-74.

Bile salt-stimulated lipase from human milk binds DC-SIGN and inhibits human immunodeficiency virus type 1 transfer to CD4+ T cells.

Naarding MA(1), Dirac AM, Ludwig IS, Speijer D, Lindquist S, Vestman EL, Stax MJ, Geijtenbeek TB, Pollakis G, Hernell O, Paxton WA.

Author information: (1)Department of Human Retrovirology, Academic Medical Center, University of Amsterdam, Meibergdreef 15, 1105 AZ, Amsterdam, the Netherlands.

A wide range of pathogens, including human immunodeficiency virus type 1 (HIV-1), hepatitis C virus, Ebola virus, cytomegalovirus, dengue virus, Mycobacterium, Leishmania, and Helicobacter pylori, can interact with dendritic cell (DC)-specific ICAM3-grabbing nonintegrin (DC-SIGN), expressed on DCs and a subset of B cells. More specifically, the interaction of the gp120 envelope protein of HIV-1 with DC-SIGN can facilitate the transfer of virus to CD4+ T lymphocytes in trans and enhance infection. We have previously demonstrated that a multimeric LeX component in human milk binds to DC-SIGN, preventing HIV-1 from interacting with this receptor. Biochemical analysis reveals that the compound is heat resistant, trypsin sensitive, and larger than 100 kDa, indicating a specific glycoprotein as the inhibitory compound. By testing human milk from three different mothers, we found the levels of DC-SIGN binding and viral inhibition to vary between samples. Using sodium dodecyl sulfate-polyacrylamide gel electrophoresis, Western blotting, and matrix-assisted laser desorption ionization analysis, we identified bile salt-stimulated lipase (BSSL), a Lewis X (LeX)-containing glycoprotein found in human milk, to be the major variant protein between the samples. BSSL isolated from human milk bound to DC-SIGN and inhibited the transfer of HIV-1 to CD4+ T lymphocytes. Two BSSL isoforms isolated from the same human milk sample showed differences in DC-SIGN binding, illustrating that alterations in the BSSL forms explain the differences observed. These results indicate that variations in BSSL lead to alterations in LeX expression by the protein, which subsequently alters the DC-SIGN binding capacity and the inhibitory effect on HIV-1 transfer. Identifying the specific molecular interaction between the different forms may aid in the future design of antimicrobial agents.

PMCID: PMC1610064 PMID: 17005819 [PubMed - indexed for MEDLINE]

1637. Chembiochem. 2006 Oct;7(10):1605-11.

Structure-function analysis of the soluble glycoprotein, sGP, of Ebola virus.

Falzarano D(1), Krokhin O, Wahl-Jensen V, Seebach J, Wolf K, Schnittler HJ, Feldmann H.

Author information: (1)Department of Medical Microbiology, University of Manitoba Winnipeg, Manitoba R3E 0W3, Canada.

In addition to the transmembrane protein, GP(1,2), the Ebola virus glycoprotein gene encodes the soluble glycoproteins sGP and Delta-peptide. Two more soluble proteins, GP(1) and GP(1,2DeltaTM), are generated from GP(1,2) as a result of disulfide-bond instability and proteolytic cleavage, respectively, and are shed from the surface of infected cells. The sGP glycoprotein is secreted as a disulfide-linked homodimer, but there have been conflicting reports on whether it is arranged in a parallel or antiparallel orientation. Off-line HPLC-MALDI-TOF MS (MS/MS) was used to identify the arrangement of all disulfide bonds and simultaneously determine site-specific information regarding N-glycosylation. Our data prove that sGP is a parallel homodimer that contains C53-C53' and C306-C306' disulfide bonds, and although there are six predicted N-linked carbohydrate sites, only five are consistently glycosylated. The disulfide bond arrangement was confirmed by using cysteine to glycine mutations at amino acid positions 53 and 306. The mutants had a reduced ability to rescue the barrier function of TNF-alpha-treated endothelial cells--a function previously reported for sGP. This indicates that these disulfide bonds are critical for the proposed anti-inflammatory function of sGP.

PMID: 16977667 [PubMed - indexed for MEDLINE]

1638. J Am Vet Med Assoc. 2006 Oct 1;229(7):1090-9.

Evaluation of ProMED-mail as an electronic early warning system for emerging animal diseases: 1996 to 2004.

Cowen P(1), Garland T, Hugh-Jones ME, Shimshony A, Handysides S, Kaye D, Madoff LC, Pollack MP, Woodall J.

Author information: (1)ProMED-mail, International Society of Infectious Diseases, 181 Longwood Ave, Boston, MA 02115-2577, USA.

OBJECTIVE: To identify emerging animal and zoonotic diseases and associated geographic distribution, disease agents, animal hosts, and seasonality of reporting in the Program for Monitoring Emerging Diseases (ProMED)-mail electronic early warning system. DESIGN: Retrospective study. SAMPLE POPULATION: 10,490 disease reports. PROCEDURES: Descriptive statistics were collated for all animal disease reports appearing on the ProMED-mail system from January 1, 1996, to December 31, 2004. RESULTS: Approximately 30% of reports concerned events in the United States; reports were next most common in the United Kingdom, Canada, Australia, Russia, and China. Rabies, bovine spongiform encephalopathy, and anthrax were reported consistently over the study period, whereas avian influenza, Ebola virus, and Hantavirus infection were reported frequently in approximately half of the study years. Reports concerning viral agents composed more than half of the postings. Humans affected by zoonotic disease accounted for a third of the subjects. Cattle were affected in 1,080 reports, and wildlife species were affected in 825 reports. For the 10,490 postings studied, there was a retraction rate of 0.01 and a correction rate of 0.02. CONCLUSIONS AND CLINICAL RELEVANCE: ProMED-mail provided global coverage, but gaps in coverage for individual countries were detected. The value of a global electronic reporting system for monitoring emerging diseases over a 9-year period illustrated how new technologies can augment disease surveillance strategies. The number of animal and zoonotic diseases highlights the importance of animals in the study of emerging diseases.

PMID: 17014355 [PubMed - indexed for MEDLINE]

1639. J Virol. 2006 Oct;80(20):10109-16.

Tyro3 family-mediated cell entry of Ebola and Marburg viruses.

Shimojima M(1), Takada A, Ebihara H, Neumann G, Fujioka K, Irimura T, Jones S, Feldmann H, Kawaoka Y.

Author information: (1)Division of Virology, Department of Microbiology and Immunology, Institute of Medical Science, University of Tokyo, 4-6-1 Shirokanedai, Minato-ku, Tokyo 108-8639, Japan.

Filoviruses, represented by the genera Ebolavirus and Marburgvirus, cause a lethal hemorrhagic fever in humans and in nonhuman primates. Although filovirus can replicate in various tissues or cell types in these animals, the molecular mechanisms of its broad tropism remain poorly understood. Here we show the involvement of members of the Tyro3 receptor tyrosine kinase family-Axl, Dtk, and Mer-in cell entry of filoviruses. Ectopic expression of these family members in lymphoid cells, which otherwise are highly resistant to filovirus infection, enhanced infection by pseudotype viruses carrying filovirus glycoproteins on their envelopes. This enhancement was reduced by antibodies to Tyro3 family members, Gas6 ligand, or soluble ectodomains of the members. Live Ebola viruses infected both Axl- and Dtk-expressing cells more efficiently than control cells. Antibody to Axl inhibited infection of pseudotype viruses in a number of Axl-positive cell lines. These results implicate each Tyro3 family member as a cell entry factor in filovirus infection.

PMCID: PMC1617303 PMID: 17005688 [PubMed - indexed for MEDLINE]

1640. J Virol Methods. 2006 Oct;137(1):115-9. Epub 2006 Jul 11.

A luciferase-based budding assay for Ebola virus.

McCarthy SE(1), Licata JM, Harty RN.

Author information: (1)Department of Pathobiology, School of Veterinary Medicine, University of Pennsylvania, 3800 Spruce St., Philadelphia, PA 19104, USA.

The VP40 matrix protein of Ebola virus (EBOV) is capable of budding from mammalian cells as a virus-like particle (VLP) and is the major protein involved in virus egress. A functional budding assay has been developed based upon this characteristic of VP40 to assess the contributions of VP40 sequences as well as host proteins to the budding process. This well-defined assay has been modified for potential use in a high-throughput format in which the detection and quantification of firefly luciferase protein in VLPs represents a direct measure of VP40 budding efficiency. Luciferase was found to be incorporated into budding VP40 VLPs. Furthermore, co-expression of EBOV glycoprotein (GP) enhances release of VLPs containing VP40 and luciferase. In contrast, when luciferase is co-expressed with a budding deficient mutant of VP40, luciferase levels in the VLP fraction decrease significantly. This assay represents a promising high-throughput approach to identify inhibitors of EBOV budding.

PMID: 16837071 [PubMed - indexed for MEDLINE]

1641. Med Trop (Mars). 2006 Oct;66(5):465-8.

[Detection of anti-Lassa antibodies in the Western Forest area of the Ivory Coast].

[Article in French]

Akoua-Koffi C(1), Ter Meulen J, Legros D, Akran V, Aïdara M, Nahounou N, Dogbo P, Ehouman A.

Author information: (1)Laboratoire des arbovirus/entérovirus, Institut Pasteur Côte d'Ivoire. polioci@globeaccess.net

Lassa fever is an African viral hemorrhagic fever (VHF) known to be endemic in a number of West African countries including Nigeria, Sierra Leone, Liberia and Guinea. Despite having common borders with Liberia and Guinea, Côte d'Ivoire has never reported any cases of Lassa fever. In March 2000, as part of a research project on VHF--mainly yellow fever, Lassa fever and Ebola fever--in Guinea and Cote d'Ivoire, an exploratory survey was conducted to assess knowledge about VHF and immunological status against Lassa virus among forest workers in the Duekoue and Guiglo regions. One hundred and sixty-three male forest workers were interviewed using a questionnaire designed to assess risk factors for VHF exposure and personal medical history over the last 12 months.

Detection of IgG antibodies against Lassa virus was performed by immunofluorescence assay with Lassa virus antigens from the Josiah and Las/AV strains. The overall prevalence of IgG antibodies was 26% (42/161). Among the Lassa IgG positive subjects, 38.5% were loggers including 20% that were positive at a serum dilution of 1/40 and 46.7% were national park workers or forest rangers including 69% that were positive at a dilution of 1/40 and more. Forty-one percent of subjects had heard of VHF including 14% who attributed it to animals and 2% who attributed it to plants. Contact with rodents was frequent and more than 50% of subjects had either eaten or skinned rodents. Although the prevalence of anti-Lassa IgG antibodies seemed high in the study population, no conclusion can be about level of exposure to Lassa virus.

PMID: 17201291 [PubMed - indexed for MEDLINE]

1642. PLoS Pathog. 2006 Oct;2(10):e90.

Recent common ancestry of Ebola Zaire virus found in a bat reservoir.

Biek R(1), Walsh PD, Leroy EM, Real LA.

Author information: (1)Center for Disease Ecology, Department of Biology, Emory University, Atlanta, Georgia, USA.

PMCID: PMC1626099 PMID: 17069458 [PubMed - indexed for MEDLINE]

1643. Virology. 2006 Sep 30;353(2):324-32. Epub 2006 Jul 3.

Complex adenovirus-vectored vaccine protects guinea pigs from three strains of Marburg virus challenges.

Wang D(1), Hevey M, Juompan LY, Trubey CM, Raja NU, Deitz SB, Woraratanadharm J, Luo M, Yu H, Swain BM, Moore KM, Dong JY.

Author information: (1)Division of Bio-defense Vaccines, GenPhar Inc., 871 Lowcountry Blvd., Mount Pleasant, SC 29464, USA.

The Marburg virus (MARV), an African filovirus closely related to the Ebola virus, causes a deadly hemorrhagic fever in humans, with up to 90% mortality. Currently, treatment of disease is only supportive, and no vaccines are available to prevent spread of MARV infections. In order to address this need, we have developed and characterized a novel recombinant vaccine that utilizes a single complex adenovirus-vectored vaccine (cAdVax) to overexpress a MARV glycoprotein (GP) fusion protein derived from the Musoke and Ci67 strains of MARV. Vaccination with the cAdVaxM(fus) vaccine led to efficient production of MARV-specific antibodies in both mice and guinea pigs. Significantly, guinea pigs vaccinated with at least 5 x 10(7) pfu of cAdVaxM(fus) vaccine were 100% protected against lethal challenges by the Musoke, Ci67 and Ravn strains of MARV, making it a vaccine with trivalent protective efficacy. Therefore, the cAdVaxM(fus) vaccine serves as a promising vaccine candidate to prevent and contain multi-strain infections by MARV.

PMID: 16820184 [PubMed - indexed for MEDLINE]

1644. Am J Primatol. 2006 Sep;68(9):928-33.

Anthrax in Western and Central African great apes.

Leendertz FH(1), Lankester F, Guislain P, Néel C, Drori O, Dupain J, Speede S, Reed P, Wolfe N, Loul S, Mpoudi-Ngole E, Peeters M, Boesch C, Pauli G, Ellerbrok H, Leroy EM.

Author information: (1)Great Ape Health Monitoring Unit, c/o Max Planck Institute for Evolutionary Anthropology, Leipzig, Germany. LeendertzF@rki.de

During the period of December 2004 to January 2005, Bacillus anthracis killed three wild chimpanzees (Pan troglodytes troglodytes) and one gorilla (Gorilla gorilla gorilla) in a tropical forest in Cameroon. While this is the second anthrax outbreak in wild chimpanzees, this is the first case of anthrax in gorillas ever reported. The number of great apes in Central Africa is dramatically declining and the populations are seriously threatened by diseases, mainly Ebola. Nevertheless, a considerable number of deaths cannot be attributed to Ebola virus and remained unexplained. Our results show that diseases other than Ebola may also threaten wild great apes, and indicate that the role of anthrax in great ape mortality may have been underestimated. These results suggest that risk identification, assessment, and management for the survival of the last great apes should be performed with an open mind, since various pathogens with distinct characteristics in epidemiology and pathogenicity may impact the populations. An animal mortality monitoring network covering the entire African tropical forest, with the dual aims of preventing both great ape extinction and human disease outbreaks, will create necessary baseline data for such risk assessments and management plans.

Copyright 2006 Wiley-Liss, Inc.

PMID: 16900500 [PubMed - indexed for MEDLINE]

1645. J Gen Virol. 2006 Sep;87(Pt 9):2477-85.

Generation of an adenoviral vaccine vector based on simian adenovirus 21.

Roy S(1), Zhi Y, Kobinger GP, Figueredo J, Calcedo R, Miller JR, Feldmann H, Wilson JM.

Author information: (1)Gene Therapy Program, Department of Pathology and Laboratory Medicine, University of Pennsylvania School of Medicine, Philadelphia, PA 19104, USA.

Adenoviral vectors can be used to generate potent humoral and cellular immune responses to transgene products. Use of adenoviral vectors based on non-human isolates may allow for their utilization in populations harbouring neutralizing antibodies to common human serotypes. A vector chimera was constructed using simian adenovirus 22 (a serotype belonging to the species Human adenovirus E) and simian adenovirus 21 (a serotype belonging to the species Human adenovirus B) expressing the Ebola (Zaire) virus glycoprotein (Ad C5/C1-ZGP). This chimeric adenovirus vector was used as a model to test its efficacy as a genetic vaccine and comparisons were made to a vector based on the commonly used human adenovirus C serotype 5 (Adhu5-ZGP). Ebola glycoprotein-specific T- and B-cell responses were measured in B10BR mice vaccinated with either Adhu5-ZGP or Ad C5/C1-ZGP vectors. Both vectors resulted in Ebola glycoprotein-specific gamma interferon-expressing T cells, although the Ad C5/C1-ZGP vector appeared to induce lower frequencies with kinetics slower than those elicited by the Adhu5-ZGP vector. The total immunoglobulin G response to Ebola glycoprotein was similar in sera from mice vaccinated with either vector. Two rhesus macaques vaccinated with the Ad C5/C1-ZGP vector were found to mount T-cell and antibody responses to the Ebola glycoprotein. It was found that a single administration of the chimeric Ad C5/C1-ZGP vector protected mice against a lethal challenge with a mouse-adapted strain of the Ebola (Zaire) virus.

PMID: 16894185 [PubMed - indexed for MEDLINE]

1646. PLoS Pathog. 2006 Sep;2(9):e99.

Assembly and budding of Ebolavirus.

Noda T(1), Ebihara H, Muramoto Y, Fujii K, Takada A, Sagara H, Kim JH, Kida H, Feldmann H, Kawaoka Y.

Author information: (1)Laboratory of Microbiology, Department of Disease Control, Graduate School of Veterinary Medicine, Hokkaido University, Sapporo, Japan.

Ebolavirus is responsible for highly lethal hemorrhagic fever. Like all viruses, it must reproduce its various components and assemble them in cells in order to reproduce infectious virions and perpetuate itself. To generate infectious Ebolavirus, a viral genome-protein complex called the nucleocapsid (NC) must be produced and transported to the cell surface, incorporated into virions, and then released from cells. To further our understanding of the Ebolavirus life cycle, we expressed the various viral proteins in mammalian cells and examined them ultrastructurally and biochemically. Expression of nucleoprotein alone led to the formation of helical tubes, which likely serve as a core for the NC. The matrix protein VP40 was found to be critical for transport of NCs to the cell surface and for the incorporation of NCs into virions, where interaction between nucleoprotein and the matrix protein VP40 is likely essential for these processes. Examination of virus-infected cells revealed that virions containing NCs mainly emerge horizontally from the cell surface, whereas empty virions mainly bud vertically, suggesting that horizontal budding is the major mode of Ebolavirus budding. These data form a foundation for the identification and development of potential antiviral agents to combat the devastating disease caused by this virus.

PMCID: PMC1579243 PMID: 17009868 [PubMed - indexed for MEDLINE]

1647. Virology. 2006 Sep 1;352(2):345-56. Epub 2006 Jun 13.

Modulation of virion incorporation of Ebolavirus glycoprotein: effects on attachment, cellular entry and neutralization.

Marzi A(1), Wegele A, Pöhlmann S.

Author information: (1)Institute for Clinical and Molecular Virology, University Erlangen-Nürnberg, 91054 Erlangen, Germany.

The filoviruses Ebolavirus (EBOV) and Marburgvirus (MARV) cause severe hemorrhagic fever in humans and are potential agents of biological warfare. The envelope glycoprotein (GP) of filoviruses mediates viral entry into cells and is an attractive target for therapeutic intervention and vaccine design. Here, we asked if the efficiency of virion incorporation of EBOV-GP impacts attachment and entry into target cells and modulates susceptibility to neutralizing antibodies. In order to control the level of EBOV-GP expression, we generated cell lines expressing the GPs of the four known EBOV subspecies in an inducible fashion. Regulated expression of GP on the cell surface allowed production of reporter viruses harboring different amounts of GP. A pronounced reduction of virion incorporation of EBOV-GP had relatively little effect on virion infectivity, suggesting that only a few copies of GP might be sufficient for efficient engagement of cellular receptors. In contrast, optimal interactions with cellular attachment factors like the DC-SIGN protein required incorporation of high amounts of GP. Antibody-mediated neutralization of virions bearing high amounts of GP was slightly more efficient than neutralization of virions harboring low amounts of GP, suggesting that the efficiency of GP incorporation into virions might modulate susceptibility to neutralizing antibodies. Finally, regulated expression of GP in permissive 293 cells did not reduce EBOV-GP-driven infection but diminished vesicular stomatitis virus GP (VSV-G) and amphotropic murine leukemia virus (A-MLV) GP mediated entry in a dose-dependent manner. Therefore, intracellular GP does not seem to downmodulate expression of its receptor(s) but might alter expression and/or function of molecules involved in VSV-G and A-MLV-GP-dependent entry. Our results suggest that the efficiency of virion incorporation of GP could impact EBOV attachment to target cells and might modulate control of viral spread by the humoral immune response.

PMID: 16777170 [PubMed - indexed for MEDLINE]

1648. Vopr Virusol. 2006 Sep-Oct;51(5):8-16.

[Hemorrhagic (Marburg, Ebola, Lassa, and Bolivian) fevers: epidemiology, clinical pictures, and treatment].

[Article in Russian]

Borisevich IV, Markin VA, Firsova IV, Evseev AA, Khamitov RA, Maksimov VA.

The evaluation of the biological and epidemiological properties of Ebola, Marburg, Lassa, and Machupo viruses suggests that they are of social importance for health care authorities. The studies have created prerequisites to the development of reliable biosafety means against these pathogens. Particular emphasis is laid on the methods for infection diagnosis and on the studies to design specific protective agents--immunoglobulins and inactivated vaccines.

PMID: 17087059 [PubMed - indexed for MEDLINE]

1649. N Engl J Med. 2006 Aug 31;355(9):866-9.

Marburg hemorrhagic fever--the forgotten cousin strikes.

Feldmann H(1).

Author information: (1)Special Pathogens Program at the National Microbiology Laboratory, Public Health Agency of Canada, Winnipeg, Canada.

Comment on N Engl J Med. 2006 Aug 31;355(9):909-19.

PMID: 16943398 [PubMed - indexed for MEDLINE]

1650. J Biol Chem. 2006 Aug 11;281(32):23083-91. Epub 2006 Jun 7.

Interaction of AMSH with ESCRT-III and deubiquitination of endosomal cargo.

Agromayor M(1), Martin-Serrano J.

Author information: (1)Department of Infectious Diseases, King's College London School of Medicine at Guy's, King's College, and St. Thomas' Hospitals, London SE1 9RT, United Kingdom.
The "class E" vacuolar protein sorting (VPS) pathway mediates sorting of ubiquitinated cargo into the forming vesicles of the multivesicular bodies (MVB), and it is essential for down-regulation of signaling by growth factors and budding of enveloped viruses such as Ebola and HIV-1. Work in yeast has identified DOA4 as a gene that is recruited by the class E machinery to remove ubiquitin from the endosomal cargo before it is incorporated into MVB vesicles, but the identity of the mammalian counterpart is unclear. Here we report the interaction of AMSH (associated molecule with the SH3 domain of STAM), an endosomal deubiquitinating enzyme, with the endodomal sorting complex required for transport (ESCRT-III) subunits CHMP1A, CHMP1B, CHMP2A, and CHMP3. We also show that a catalytically inactive AMSH inhibits retroviral budding in a dominant-negative manner and induces the accumulation of ubiquitinated forms of an endosomal cargo, namely murine leukemia virus Gag. Finally, VPS4 and AMSH compete for binding to the C-terminal regions of CHMP1A and CHMP1B, revealing a coordinated interaction with ESCRT-III. Taken together, these results are consistent with a role of AMSH in the deubiquitination of the endosomal cargo preceding lysosomal degradation.
PMID: 16760479 [PubMed - indexed for MEDLINE]

1651. Endocrinology. 2006 Aug;147(8):3797-808. Epub 2006 May 18.

Functional expression of mouse relaxin and mouse relaxin-3 in the lung from an Ebola virus glycoprotein-pseudotyped lentivirus via tracheal delivery.

Silvertown JD(1), Walia JS, Summerlee AJ, Medin JA.

Author information: (1)Division of Stem Cell and Developmental Biology, Ontario Cancer Institute, University Health Network, Toronto, Ontario, Canada M5G 2M1.
The peptide hormone relaxin is a known modulator of connective tissue and the extracellular matrix by virtue of its ability to regulate matrix metalloproteinases (MMPs). Relaxin knockout mice exhibit age-related pulmonary fibrosis, and delivery of recombinant human H2 relaxin ameliorates fibrotic-like conditions in the mouse lung. We investigated whether lentiviral vectors (LVs) engineering the expression of murine relaxins could induce MMP activity in the mouse lung. Mouse relaxin and mouse relaxin-3 peptides engineered by recombinant LVs were biologically active as shown by stimulation of cAMP from both THP-1 and 293T cells stably expressing relaxin receptor LGR7 and by up-regulation of MMP-2 activity from primary C57BL/6 lung cell cultures. To provide the virions with enhanced tropism for the lung, LVs were pseudotyped with the Zaire strain of the Ebola virus glycoprotein (EboZ GP) and delivered by endotracheal intubation. LVs engineering luciferase pseudotyped with EboZ GP, but not with vesicular stomatitis virus glycoprotein resulted in successful LV transduction and transgene expression in C57BL/6 mouse lung by as early as d 4. Mice treated via tracheal delivery with EboZ GP pseudotyped LVs that engineered expression of mouse relaxins exhibited increased MMP-2 and MMP-9 activity in lung tissue up until the end of our study at d 21. Taken together, this study provides proof-of-principle that relaxin gene expression targeted to the mouse lungs can result in enhanced MMP activity offering potential for alleviating disease conditions characterized by dysregulation of extracellular matrix protein accumulation.
PMID: 16709614 [PubMed - indexed for MEDLINE]

1652. Virology. 2006 Aug 1;351(2):260-70. Epub 2006 May 4.

Ebola virus-like particles produced in insect cells exhibit dendritic cell stimulating activity and induce neutralizing antibodies.

Ye L(1), Lin J, Sun Y, Bennouna S, Lo M, Wu Q, Bu Z, Pulendran B, Compans RW, Yang C.

Author information: (1)Department of Microbiology and Immunology and Emory Vaccine Center, Emory University School of Medicine, Atlanta, GA 30322, USA.
Recombinant baculoviruses (rBV) expressing Ebola virus VP40 (rBV-VP40) or GP (rBV-GP) proteins were generated. Infection of Sf9 insect cells by rBV-VP40 led to assembly and budding of filamentous particles from the cell surface as shown by electron microscopy. Ebola virus-like particles (VLPs) were produced by coinfection of Sf9 cells with rBV-VP40 and rBV-GP, and incorporation of Ebola GP into VLPs was demonstrated by SDS-PAGE and Western blot analysis. Recombinant baculovirus infection of insect cells yielded high levels of VLPs, which were shown to stimulate cytokine secretion from human dendritic cells similar to VLPs produced in mammalian cells. The immunogenicity of Ebola VLPs produced in insect cells was evaluated by immunization of mice. Analysis of antibody responses showed that most of the GP-specific antibodies were of the IgG2a subtype, while no significant level of IgG1 subtype antibodies specific for GP was induced, indicating the induction of a Th1-biased immune response. Furthermore, sera from Ebola VLP immunized mice were able to block infection by Ebola GP pseudotyped HIV virus in a single round infection assay, indicating that a neutralizing antibody against the Ebola GP protein was induced. These results show that production of Ebola VLPs in insect cells using recombinant baculoviruses represents a promising approach for vaccine development against Ebola virus infection.
PMID: 16678231 [PubMed - indexed for MEDLINE]

1653. Curr Biol. 2006 Jul 11;16(13):R489-91.

Gorilla susceptibility to Ebola virus: the cost of sociality.

Caillaud D, Levréro F, Cristescu R, Gatti S, Dewas M, Douadi M, Gautier-Hion A, Raymond M, Ménard N.

PMID: 16824905 [PubMed - indexed for MEDLINE]

1654. Biochim Biophys Acta. 2006 Jul;1762(7):693-703. Epub 2006 Jun 6.

Peptides derived from HIV-1, HIV-2, Ebola virus, SARS coronavirus and coronavirus 229E exhibit high affinity binding to the formyl peptide receptor.

Mills JS(1).

Author information: (1)109 Lewis Hall, Montana State University, Bozeman, MT 59717-3520, USA. umbmj@montana.edu
Peptides derived from the membrane proximal region of fusion proteins of human immunodeficiency viruses 1 and 2, Coronavirus 229 E, severe acute respiratory syndrome coronavirus and Ebola virus were all potent antagonists of the formyl peptide receptor expressed in Chinese hamster ovary cells.

Binding of viral peptides was affected by the naturally occurring polymorphisms at residues 190 and 192, which are located at second extracellular loop-transmembrane helix 5 interface. Substitution of R190 with W190 enhanced the affinity for a severe acute respiratory syndrome coronavirus peptide 6 fold but reduced the affinity for N-formyl-Nle-Leu-Phe by 2.5 fold. A 12 mer peptide derived from coronavirus 229E (ETYIKPWWVWL) was the most potent antagonist of the formyl peptide receptor W190 with a K(i) of 230 nM. Fluorescently labeled ETYIKPWWVWL was effectively internalized by all three variants with EC(50) of approximately 25 nM. An HKU-1 coronavirus peptide, MYVKWPWYVWL, was a potent antagonist but N-formyl-MYVKWPWYVWL was a potent agonist. ETYIKPWWVWL did not stimulate GTPgammaS binding but inhibited the stimulation by formyl-NleLeuPhe. It also blocked beta arrestin translocation and receptor downregulation induced by formyl-Nle-Leu-Phe. This indicates that formyl peptide receptor may be important in viral infections and that variations in its sequence among individuals may affect their likelihood of viral and bacterial infections.

PMCID: PMC2075610 PMID: 16842982 [PubMed - indexed for MEDLINE]

1655. J Virol. 2006 Jul;80(14):7260-4.

Infection of naive target cells with virus-like particles: implications for the function of ebola virus VP24.

Hoenen T(1), Groseth A, Kolesnikova L, Theriault S, Ebihara H, Hartlieb B, Bamberg S, Feldmann H, Ströher U, Becker S.

Author information: (1)Institut für Virologie, Philipps Universität Marburg, Marburg, Germany.

Infectious virus-like particle (iVLP) systems have recently been established for several negative-strand RNA viruses, including the highly pathogenic Zaire ebolavirus (ZEBOV), and allow study of the viral life cycle under biosafety level 2 conditions. However, current systems depend on the expression of viral helper nucleocapsid proteins in target cells, thus making it impossible to determine whether ribonucleoprotein complexes transferred by iVLPs are able to facilitate initial transcription, an indispensable step in natural infection. Here we describe a ZEBOV iVLP system which overcomes this limitation and show that VP24 is essential for the formation of a functional ribonucleoprotein complex.

PMCID: PMC1489071 PMID: 16809331 [PubMed - indexed for MEDLINE]

1656. J Virol. 2006 Jul;80(14):7235-44.

Activation of triggering receptor expressed on myeloid cells-1 on human neutrophils by marburg and ebola viruses.

Mohamadzadeh M(1), Coberley SS, Olinger GG, Kalina WV, Ruthel G, Fuller CL, Swenson DL, Pratt WD, Kuhns DB, Schmaljohn AL.

Author information: (1)U.S. Army Medical Research Institute for Infectious Diseases, 1425 Porter Street, Frederick, MD 21702, USA. Mansour.Mohamadzadeh@amedd.army.mil

Marburg virus (MARV) and Ebola virus (EBOV), members of the viral family Filoviridae, cause fatal hemorrhagic fevers in humans and nonhuman primates. High viral burden is coincident with inadequate adaptive immune responses and robust inflammatory responses, and virus-mediated dysregulation of early host defenses has been proposed. Recently, a novel class of innate receptors called the triggering receptors expressed in myeloid cells (TREM) has been discovered and shown to play an important role in innate inflammatory responses and sepsis. Here, we report that MARV and EBOV activate TREM-1 on human neutrophils, resulting in DAP12 phosphorylation, TREM-1 shedding, mobilization of intracellular calcium, secretion of proinflammatory cytokines, and phenotypic changes. A peptide specific to TREM-1 diminished the release of tumor necrosis factor alpha by filovirus-activated human neutrophils in vitro, and a soluble recombinant TREM-1 competitively inhibited the loss of cell surface TREM-1 that otherwise occurred on neutrophils exposed to filoviruses. These data imply direct activation of TREM-1 by filoviruses and also indicate that neutrophils may play a prominent role in the immune and inflammatory responses to filovirus infections.

PMCID: PMC1489070 PMID: 16809329 [PubMed - indexed for MEDLINE]

1657. J Virol. 2006 Jul;80(13):6497-516.

Marburgvirus genomics and association with a large hemorrhagic fever outbreak in Angola.

Towner JS(1), Khristova ML, Sealy TK, Vincent MJ, Erickson BR, Bawiec DA, Hartman AL, Comer JA, Zaki SR, Ströher U, Gomes da Silva F, del Castillo F, Rollin PE, Ksiazek TG, Nichol ST.

Author information: (1)Special Pathogens Branch, Centers for Disease Control and Prevention, 1600 Clifton Road, Mailstop G14, Atlanta, GA 30333, USA.

In March 2005, the Centers for Disease Control and Prevention (CDC) investigated a large hemorrhagic fever (HF) outbreak in Uige Province in northern Angola, West Africa. In total, 15 initial specimens were sent to CDC, Atlanta, Ga., for testing for viruses associated with viral HFs known to be present in West Africa, including ebolavirus. Marburgvirus was also included despite the fact that the origins of all earlier outbreaks were linked directly to East Africa. Surprisingly, marburgvirus was confirmed (12 of 15 specimens) as the cause of the outbreak. The outbreak likely began in October 2004 and ended in July 2005, and it included 252 cases and 227 (90%) fatalities (report from the Ministry of Health, Republic of Angola, 2005), making it the largest Marburg HF outbreak on record. A real-time quantitative reverse transcription-PCR assay utilized and adapted during the outbreak proved to be highly sensitive and sufficiently robust for field use. Partial marburgvirus RNA sequence analysis revealed up to 21% nucleotide divergence among the previously characterized East African strains, with the most distinct being Ravn from Kenya (1987). The Angolan strain was less different (approximately 7%) from the main group of East African marburgviruses than one might expect given the large geographic separation. To more precisely analyze the virus genetic differences between outbreaks and among viruses within the Angola outbreak itself, a total of 16 complete virus genomes were determined, including those of the virus isolates Ravn (Kenya, 1987) and 05DRC, 07DRC, and 09DRC (Democratic Republic of Congo, 1998) and the reference Angolan virus isolate (Ang1379v). In addition, complete genome sequences were obtained from RNAs extracted from 10 clinical specimens reflecting various stages of the disease and locations within the Angolan outbreak. While the marburgviruses exhibit high overall genetic diversity (up to 22%), only 6.8% nucleotide difference was found between the West African Angolan viruses and the majority of East African viruses, suggesting that the virus reservoir species in these regions are not substantially distinct. Remarkably few nucleotide differences were found among the Angolan clinical specimens (0 to 0.07%), consistent with an outbreak scenario in which a single (or rare) introduction of virus from the reservoir species into the human population was followed by person-to-person transmission with little accumulation of mutations. This is in contrast to the 1998 to 2000 marburgvirus outbreak, where evidence of several virus genetic lineages (with up to 21% divergence) and multiple virus introductions into the human population was found.

PMCID: PMC1488971 PMID: 16775337 [PubMed - indexed for MEDLINE]

1658. J Virol. 2006 Jul;80(13):6430-40.

Reverse genetic generation of recombinant Zaire Ebola viruses containing disrupted IRF-3 inhibitory domains results in attenuated virus growth in vitro and higher levels of IRF-3 activation without inhibiting viral transcription or replication.

Hartman AL(1), Dover JE, Towner JS, Nichol ST.

Author information: (1)Special Pathogens Branch, Division of Viral and Rickettsial Diseases, National Center for Infectious Diseases, Centers for Disease Control and Prevention, 1600 Clifton Road, MS G-14, Atlanta, GA 30329, USA.

The VP35 protein of Zaire Ebola virus is an essential component of the viral RNA polymerase complex and also functions to antagonize the cellular type I interferon (IFN) response by blocking activation of the transcription factor IRF-3. We previously mapped the IRF-3 inhibitory domain within the C terminus of VP35. In the present study, we show that mutations that disrupt the IRF-3 inhibitory function of VP35 do not disrupt viral transcription/replication, suggesting that the two functions of VP35 are separable. Second, using reverse genetics, we successfully recovered recombinant Ebola viruses containing mutations within the IRF-3 inhibitory domain. Importantly, we show that the recombinant viruses were attenuated for growth in cell culture and that they activated IRF-3 and IRF-3-inducible gene expression at levels higher than that for Ebola virus containing wild-type VP35. In the context of Ebola virus pathogenesis, VP35 may function to limit early IFN-beta production and other antiviral signals generated from cells at the primary site of infection, thereby slowing down the host's ability to curb virus replication and induce adaptive immunity.

PMCID: PMC1488969 PMID: 16775331 [PubMed - indexed for MEDLINE]

1659. J Virol. 2006 Jul;80(13):6305-17.

The signal peptide of the ebolavirus glycoprotein influences interaction with the cellular lectins DC-SIGN and DC-SIGNR.

Marzi A(1), Akhavan A, Simmons G, Gramberg T, Hofmann H, Bates P, Lingappa VR, Pöhlmann S.

Author information: (1)Institute for Clinical and Molecular Virology and Nikolaus-Fiebiger-Center, University Erlangen-Nürnberg, Glückstrasse 6, 91054 Erlangen, Germany.

The C-type lectins DC-SIGN and DC-SIGNR (collectively referred to as DC-SIGN/R) bind to the ebolavirus glycoprotein (EBOV-GP) and augment viral infectivity. DC-SIGN/R strongly enhance infection driven by the GP of EBOV subspecies. Zaire (ZEBOV) but have a much less pronounced effect on infection mediated by the GP of EBOV subspecies. Sudan (SEBOV). For this study, we analyzed the determinants of the differential DC-SIGN/R interactions with ZEBOV- and SEBOV-GP. The efficiency of DC-SIGN engagement by ZEBOV-GP was dependent on the rate of GP incorporation into lentiviral particles, while appreciable virion incorporation of SEBOV-GP did not allow robust DC-SIGN/R usage. Forced incorporation of high-mannose carbohydrates into SEBOV-GP augmented the engagement of DC-SIGN/R to the levels observed with ZEBOV-GP, indicating that appropriate glycosylation of SEBOV-GP is sufficient for efficient DC-SIGN/R usage. However, neither signals for N-linked glycosylation unique to SEBOV- or ZEBOV-GP nor the highly variable and heavily glycosylated mucin-like domain modulated the interaction with DC-SIGN/R. In contrast, analysis of chimeric GPs identified the signal peptide as a determinant of DC-SIGN/R engagement. Thus, ZEBOV- but not SEBOV-GP was shown to harbor high-mannose carbohydrates, and GP modification with these glycans was controlled by the signal peptide. These results suggest that the signal peptide governs EBOV-GP interactions with DC-SIGN/R by modulating the incorporation of high-mannose carbohydrates into EBOV-GP. In summary, we identified the level of GP incorporation into virions and signal peptide-controlled glycosylation of GP as determinants of attachment factor engagement.

PMCID: PMC1488929 PMID: 16775318 [PubMed - indexed for MEDLINE]

1660. PLoS Pathog. 2006 Jul;2(7):e73.

Molecular determinants of Ebola virus virulence in mice.

Ebihara H(1), Takada A, Kobasa D, Jones S, Neumann G, Theriault S, Bray M, Feldmann H, Kawaoka Y.

Author information: (1)Institute of Medical Science, University of Tokyo, Tokyo, Japan.

Zaire ebolavirus (ZEBOV) causes severe hemorrhagic fever in humans and nonhuman primates, with fatality rates in humans of up to 90%. The molecular basis for the extreme virulence of ZEBOV remains elusive. While adult mice resist ZEBOV infection, the Mayinga strain of the virus has been adapted to cause lethal infection in these animals. To understand the pathogenesis underlying the extreme virulence of Ebola virus (EBOV), here we identified the mutations responsible for the acquisition of the high virulence of the adapted Mayinga strain in mice, by using reverse genetics. We found that mutations in viral protein 24 and in the nucleoprotein were primarily responsible for the acquisition of high virulence. Moreover, the role of these proteins in virulence correlated with their ability to evade type I interferon-stimulated antiviral responses. These findings suggest a critical role for overcoming the interferon-induced antiviral state in the pathogenicity of EBOV and offer new insights into the pathogenesis of EBOV infection.

PMCID: PMC1513261 PMID: 16848640 [PubMed - indexed for MEDLINE]

1661. Vopr Virusol. 2006 Jul-Aug;51(4):32-7.

[Hematological and immunological parameters during Ebola virus passages in guinea-pigs].

[Article in Russian]

Dadaeva AA, Sizikova LP, Subbotina EL, Chepurnov AA.

The trend in hematological and immunological parameters during Ebola virus passages in guinea-pigs indicated that pathophysiological changes occurred just during the second passage and further became stronger. The increase of some parameters and their correlation with the occurrence of fatal outcomes allowed the authors to reveal the most significant changes as increased juvenile platelets, whole blood virus appearance, higher echinocytes, a rise in the pro mil of blast cells and megakaryocytes in the bone marrow, and decreased neutrophilic phagocytic activity. Viral acquisition of the properties of lethality to guinea-pigs depends on the fine mechanisms responsible for viral interaction with host cells, which may lead to viral genetic changes during passages.

PMID: 16929596 [PubMed - indexed for MEDLINE]

1662. J Infect Dis. 2006 Jun 15;193(12):1650-7. Epub 2006 May 10.

Postexposure protection of guinea pigs against a lethal ebola virus challenge is conferred by RNA interference.

Geisbert TW(1), Hensley LE, Kagan E, Yu EZ, Geisbert JB, Daddario-DiCaprio K, Fritz EA, Jahrling PB, McClintock K, Phelps JR, Lee AC, Judge A, Jeffs LB, MacLachlan I.

Author information: (1)United States Army Medical Research Institute of Infectious Diseases, Fort Detrick, Maryland 21702-5011, USA. tom.geisbert@amedd.army.mil

BACKGROUND: Ebola virus (EBOV) infection causes a frequently fatal hemorrhagic fever (HF) that is refractory to treatment with currently available antiviral therapeutics. RNA interference represents a powerful, naturally occurring biological strategy for the inhibition of gene expression and has demonstrated utility in the inhibition of viral replication. Here, we describe the development of a potential therapy for EBOV infection that is based on small interfering RNAs (siRNAs). METHODS: Four siRNAs targeting the polymerase (L) gene of the Zaire species of EBOV (ZEBOV) were either complexed with polyethylenimine (PEI) or formulated in stable nucleic acid-lipid particles (SNALPs). Guinea pigs were treated with these siRNAs either before or after lethal ZEBOV challenge. RESULTS: Treatment of guinea pigs with a pool of the L gene-specific siRNAs delivered by PEI polyplexes reduced plasma viremia levels and partially protected the animals from death when administered shortly before the ZEBOV challenge. Evaluation of the same pool of siRNAs delivered using SNALPs proved that this system was more efficacious, as it completely protected guinea pigs against viremia and death when administered shortly after the ZEBOV challenge. Additional experiments showed that 1 of the 4 siRNAs alone could completely protect guinea pigs from a lethal ZEBOV challenge. CONCLUSIONS: Further development of this technology has the potential to yield effective treatments for EBOV HF as well as for diseases caused by other agents that are considered to be biological threats.

PMID: 16703508 [PubMed - indexed for MEDLINE]

1663. J Biol Chem. 2006 Jun 9;281(23):15951-8. Epub 2006 Apr 4.

Conserved receptor-binding domains of Lake Victoria marburgvirus and Zaire ebolavirus bind a common receptor.

Kuhn JH(1), Radoshitzky SR, Guth AC, Warfield KL, Li W, Vincent MJ, Towner JS, Nichol ST, Bavari S, Choe H, Aman MJ, Farzan M.

Author information: (1)Department of Microbiology and Molecular Genetics, Harvard Medical School, New England Primate Research Center, Southborough, Massachusetts 01772, USA.

The GP(1,2) envelope glycoproteins (GP) of filoviruses (marburg- and ebolaviruses) mediate cell-surface attachment, membrane fusion, and entry into permissive cells. Here we show that a 151-amino acid fragment of the Lake Victoria marburgvirus GP1 subunit bound filovirus-permissive cell lines more efficiently than full-length GP1. An homologous 148-amino acid fragment of the Zaire ebolavirus GP1 subunit similarly bound the same cell lines more efficiently than a series of longer GP1 truncation variants. Neither the marburgvirus GP1 fragment nor that of ebolavirus bound a nonpermissive lymphocyte cell line. Both fragments specifically inhibited replication of infectious Zaire ebolavirus, as well as entry of retroviruses pseudotyped with either Lake Victoria marburgvirus or Zaire ebolavirus GP(1,2). These studies identify the receptor-binding domains of both viruses, indicate that these viruses utilize a common receptor, and suggest that a single small molecule or vaccine can be developed to inhibit infection of all filoviruses.

PMID: 16595665 [PubMed - indexed for MEDLINE]

1664. Clin Infect Dis. 2006 Jun 1;42(11):1521-6. Epub 2006 Apr 26.

Detection of Ebola virus in oral fluid specimens during outbreaks of Ebola virus hemorrhagic fever in the Republic of Congo.

Formenty P(1), Leroy EM, Epelboin A, Libama F, Lenzi M, Sudeck H, Yaba P, Allarangar Y, Boumandouki P, Nkounkou VB, Drosten C, Grolla A, Feldmann H, Roth C.

Author information: (1)World Health Organization, Department of Communicable Diseases Surveillance and Response, Geneva, Switzerland. formentyp@who.int

BACKGROUND: Patients who have refused to provide blood samples has meant that there have been significant delays in confirming outbreaks of Ebola virus hemorrhagic fever (EVHF). During the 2 EVHF outbreaks in the Republic of Congo in 2003, we assessed the use of oral fluid specimens versus serum samples for laboratory confirmation of cases of EVHF. METHODS: Serum and oral fluid specimens were obtained from 24 patients with suspected Ebola and 10 healthy control subjects. Specimens were analyzed for immunoglobulin G antibodies by enzyme-linked immunosorbent assay (ELISA) and for Ebola virus by antigen detection ELISA and reverse-transcriptase polymerase chain reaction (RT-PCR). Oral fluid specimens were collected with a commercially available collection device. RESULTS: We failed to detect antibodies against Ebola in the oral fluid specimens obtained from patients whose serum samples were seropositive. All patients with positive serum RT-PCR results also had positive results for their oral fluid specimens. CONCLUSIONS: This study demonstrates the usefulness of oral fluid samples for the investigation of Ebola outbreaks, but further development in antibodies and antigen detection in oral fluid specimens is needed before these samples are used for filovirus surveillance activities in Africa.

PMID: 16652308 [PubMed - indexed for MEDLINE]

1665. J Virol. 2006 Jun;80(11):5168-78.

Ebola virus VP35 protein binds double-stranded RNA and inhibits alpha/beta interferon production induced by RIG-I signaling.

Cárdenas WB(1), Loo YM, Gale M Jr, Hartman AL, Kimberlin CR, Martínez-Sobrido L, Saphire EO, Basler CF.

Author information: (1)Department of Microbiology, Mount Sinai School of Medicine, 1 Gustave L. Levy Place, New York, NY 10029, USA.

The Ebola virus (EBOV) VP35 protein blocks the virus-induced phosphorylation and activation of interferon regulatory factor 3 (IRF-3), a transcription factor critical for the induction of alpha/beta interferon (IFN-alpha/beta) expression. However, the mechanism(s) by which this blockage occurs remains incompletely defined. We now provide evidence that VP35 possesses double-stranded RNA (dsRNA)-binding activity. Specifically, VP35 bound to poly(rI) . poly(rC)-coated Sepharose beads but not control beads. In contrast, two VP35 point mutants, R312A and K309A, were found to be greatly impaired in their dsRNA-binding activity. Competition assays showed that VP35 interacted specifically with poly(rI) . poly(rC), poly(rA) . poly(rU), or in vitro-transcribed dsRNAs derived from EBOV sequences, and not with single-stranded RNAs (ssRNAs) or double-stranded DNA. We then screened wild-type and mutant VP35s for their ability to target different components of the signaling pathways that activate IRF-3. These experiments indicate that VP35 blocks activation of IRF-3 induced by overexpression of RIG-I, a cellular helicase recently implicated in the activation of IRF-3 by either virus or dsRNA. Interestingly, the VP35 mutants impaired for dsRNA binding have a decreased but measurable IFN antagonist activity in these assays. Additionally, wild-type and dsRNA-binding-mutant VP35s were found to have equivalent abilities to inhibit activation of the IFN-beta promoter induced by overexpression of IPS-I, a recently identified signaling molecule downstream of RIG-I, or by overexpression of the IRF-3 kinases IKKepsilon and TBK-I. These data support the hypothesis that dsRNA binding may contribute to VP35 IFN antagonist function. However, additional mechanisms of inhibition, at a point proximal to the IRF-3 kinases, most likely also exist.
PMCID: PMC1472134 PMID: 16698997 [PubMed - indexed for MEDLINE]

1666. J Virol. 2006 Jun;80(11):5156-67.

Ebola virus VP24 binds karyopherin alpha1 and blocks STAT1 nuclear accumulation.

Reid SP(1), Leung LW, Hartman AL, Martinez O, Shaw ML, Carbonnelle C, Volchkov VE, Nichol ST, Basler CF.

Author information: (1)Department of Microbiology, Box 1124, Mount Sinai School of Medicine, 1 Gustave L. Levy Place, New York, NY 10029, USA.

Ebola virus (EBOV) infection blocks cellular production of alpha/beta interferon (IFN-alpha/beta) and the ability of cells to respond to IFN-alpha/beta or IFN-gamma. The EBOV VP35 protein has previously been identified as an EBOV-encoded inhibitor of IFN-alpha/beta production. However, the mechanism by which EBOV infection inhibits responses to IFNs has not previously been defined. Here we demonstrate that the EBOV VP24 protein functions as an inhibitor of IFN-alpha/beta and IFN-gamma signaling. Expression of VP24 results in an inhibition of IFN-induced gene expression and an inability of IFNs to induce an antiviral state. The VP24-mediated inhibition of cellular responses to IFNs correlates with the impaired nuclear accumulation of tyrosine-phosphorylated STAT1 (PY-STAT1), a key step in both IFN-alpha/beta and IFN-gamma signaling. Consistent with this proposed function for VP24, infection of cells with EBOV also confers a block to the IFN-induced nuclear accumulation of PY-STAT1. Further, VP24 is found to specifically interact with karyopherin alpha1, the nuclear localization signal receptor for PY-STAT1, but not with karyopherin alpha2, alpha3, or alpha4. Overexpression of VP24 results in a loss of karyopherin alpha1-PY-STAT1 interaction, indicating that the VP24-karyopherin alpha1 interaction contributes to the block to IFN signaling. These data suggest that VP24 is likely to be an important virulence determinant that allows EBOV to evade the antiviral effects of IFNs.
PMCID: PMC1472181 PMID: 16698996 [PubMed - indexed for MEDLINE]

1667. J Virol. 2006 Jun;80(11):5135-44.

Ebola virus VP35-VP40 interaction is sufficient for packaging 3E-5E minigenome RNA into virus-like particles.

Johnson RF(1), McCarthy SE, Godlewski PJ, Harty RN.

Author information: (1)Department of Pathobiology, School of Veterinary Medicine, University of Pennsylvania, 3800 Spruce St., Philadelphia, PA 19104, USA.

The packaging of viral genomic RNA into nucleocapsids and subsequently into virions is not completely understood. Phosphoprotein (P) and nucleoprotein (NP) interactions link NP-RNA complexes with P-L (polymerase) complexes to form viral nucleocapsids. The nucleocapsid then interacts with the viral matrix protein, leading to specific packaging of the nucleocapsid into the virion. A mammalian two-hybrid assay and confocal microscopy were used to demonstrate that Ebola virus VP35 and VP40 interact and colocalize in transfected cells. VP35 was packaged into budding virus-like particles (VLPs) as observed by protease protection assays. Moreover, VP40 and VP35 were sufficient for packaging an Ebola virus minigenome RNA into VLPs. Results from immunoprecipitation-reverse transcriptase PCR experiments suggest that VP35 confers specificity of the nucleocapsid for viral genomic RNA by direct VP35-RNA interactions.
PMCID: PMC1472164 PMID: 16698994 [PubMed - indexed for MEDLINE]

1668. PLoS Med. 2006 Jun;3(6):e177. Epub 2006 May 16.

Immune protection of nonhuman primates against Ebola virus with single low-dose adenovirus vectors encoding modified GPs.

Sullivan NJ(1), Geisbert TW, Geisbert JB, Shedlock DJ, Xu L, Lamoreaux L, Custers JH, Popernack PM, Yang ZY, Pau MG, Roederer M, Koup RA, Goudsmit J, Jahrling PB, Nabel GJ.

Author information: (1)Vaccine Research Center, National Institute of Allergy and Infectious Diseases, National Institutes of Health, Bethesda, Maryland, USA.

BACKGROUND: Ebola virus causes a hemorrhagic fever syndrome that is associated with high mortality in humans. In the absence of effective therapies for Ebola virus infection, the development of a vaccine becomes an important strategy to contain outbreaks. Immunization with DNA and/or replication-defective adenoviral vectors (rAd) encoding the Ebola glycoprotein (GP) and nucleoprotein (NP) has been previously shown to confer specific protective immunity in nonhuman primates. GP can exert cytopathic effects on transfected cells in vitro, and multiple GP forms have been identified in nature, raising the question of which would be optimal for a human vaccine. METHODS AND FINDINGS: To address this question, we have explored the efficacy of mutant GPs from multiple Ebola virus strains with reduced in vitro cytopathicity and analyzed their protective effects in the primate challenge model, with or without NP. Deletion of the GP transmembrane domain eliminated in vitro cytopathicity but reduced its protective efficacy by at least one order of magnitude. In contrast, a point mutation was identified that abolished this cytopathicity but retained immunogenicity and conferred immune protection in the absence of NP. The minimal effective rAd dose was established at 10(10) particles, two logs lower than that used previously. CONCLUSIONS: Expression of specific GPs alone vectored by rAd are sufficient to confer protection against lethal challenge in a relevant nonhuman primate model. Elimination of NP from the vaccine and dose reductions to 10(10) rAd particles do not diminish protection and simplify the vaccine, providing the basis for selection of a human vaccine candidate.

PMCID: PMC1459482 PMID: 16683867 [PubMed - indexed for MEDLINE]

1669. Toxicol Sci. 2006 Jun;91(2):610-9. Epub 2006 Mar 28.

Biodistribution of DNA plasmid vaccines against HIV-1, Ebola, Severe Acute Respiratory Syndrome, or West Nile virus is similar, without integration, despite differing plasmid backbones or gene inserts.

Sheets RL(1), Stein J, Manetz TS, Duffy C, Nason M, Andrews C, Kong WP, Nabel GJ, Gomez PL.

Author information: (1)U.S. Public Health Service, Vaccine Production Program, NIH/NIAID/Vaccine Research Center, Bethesda, Maryland 20892-7628, USA. rsheets@niaid.nih.gov

The Vaccine Research Center has developed a number of vaccine candidates for different diseases/infectious agents (HIV-1, Severe Acute Respiratory Syndrome virus, West Nile virus, and Ebola virus, plus a plasmid cytokine adjuvant-IL-2/Ig) based on a DNA plasmid vaccine platform. To support the clinical development of each of these vaccine candidates, preclinical studies have been performed in mice or rabbits to determine where in the body these plasmid vaccines would biodistribute and how rapidly they would clear. In the course of these studies, it has been observed that regardless of the gene insert (expressing the vaccine immunogen or cytokine adjuvant) and regardless of the promoter used to drive expression of the gene insert in the plasmid backbone, the plasmid vaccines do not biodistribute widely and remain essentially in the site of injection, in the muscle and overlying subcutis. Even though approximately 10(14) molecules are inoculated in the studies in rabbits, by day 8 or 9 (approximately 1 week postinoculation), already all but on the order of 10(4)-10(6) molecules per microgram of DNA extracted from tissue have been cleared at the injection site. Over the course of 2 months, the plasmid clears from the site of injection with only a small percentage of animals (generally 10-20%) retaining a small number of copies (generally around 100 copies) in the muscle at the injection site. This pattern of biodistribution (confined to the injection site) and clearance (within 2 months) is consistent regardless of differences in the promoter in the plasmid backbone or differences in the gene insert being expressed by the plasmid vaccine. In addition, integration has not been observed with plasmid vaccine candidates inoculated i.m. by Biojector 2000 or by needle and syringe. These data build on the repeated-dose toxicology studies performed (see companion article, Sheets et al., 2006) to demonstrate the safety and suitability for investigational human use of DNA plasmid vaccine candidates for a variety of infectious disease prevention indications.

PMCID: PMC2377020 PMID: 16569729 [PubMed - indexed for MEDLINE]

1670. Toxicol Sci. 2006 Jun;91(2):620-30. Epub 2006 Mar 28.

Toxicological safety evaluation of DNA plasmid vaccines against HIV-1, Ebola, Severe Acute Respiratory Syndrome, or West Nile virus is similar despite differing plasmid backbones or gene-inserts.

Sheets RL(1), Stein J, Manetz TS, Andrews C, Bailer R, Rathmann J, Gomez PL.

Author information: (1)U.S. Public Health Service, Vaccine Production Program, NIH/NIAID/Vaccine Research Center, Bethesda, Maryland 20892-7628, USA. rsheets@niaid.nih.gov

The Vaccine Research Center has developed a number of vaccine candidates for different diseases/infectious agents (HIV-1, Severe Acute Respiratory Syndrome virus, West Nile virus, and Ebola virus, plus a plasmid cytokine adjuvant-IL-2/Ig) based on a DNA plasmid vaccine platform. To support the clinical development of each of these vaccine candidates, preclinical studies were performed to screen for potential toxicities (intrinsic and immunotoxicities). All treatment-related toxicities identified in these repeated-dose toxicology studies have been confined primarily to the sites of injection and seem to be the result of both the delivery method (as they are seen in both control and treated animals) and the intended immune response to the vaccine (as they occur with greater frequency and severity in treated animals). Reactogenicity at the site of injection is generally seen to be reversible as the frequency and severity diminished between doses and between the immediate and recovery termination time points. This observation also correlated with the biodistribution data reported in the companion article (Sheets et al., 2006), in which DNA plasmid vaccine was shown to remain at the site of injection, rather than biodistributing widely, and to clear over time. The results of these safety studies have been submitted to the Food and Drug Administration to support the safety of initiating clinical studies with these and related DNA plasmid vaccines. Thus far, standard repeated-dose toxicology studies have not identified any target organs for toxicity (other than the injection site) for our DNA plasmid vaccines at doses up to 8 mg per immunization, regardless of disease indication (i.e., expressed gene-insert) and despite differences (strengths) in the promoters used to drive this expression. As clinical data accumulate with these products, it will be possible to retrospectively compare the safety profiles of the products in the clinic to the results of the repeated-dose toxicology studies, in order to determine the utility of such toxicology studies for signaling potential immunotoxicities or intrinsic toxicities from DNA vaccines. These data build on the biodistribution studies performed (see companion article, Sheets et al., 2006) to demonstrate the safety and suitability for investigational human use of DNA plasmid vaccine candidates for a variety of infectious disease prevention indications.

PMCID: PMC2366098 PMID: 16569728 [PubMed - indexed for MEDLINE]

1671. Uirusu. 2006 Jun;56(1):117-24.

[Properties of the Ebola virus glycoprotein].

[Article in Japanese]

Takada A(1).

Author information: (1)Department of Global Epidemiology, Hokkaido University Research Center for Zoonosis Control, Kita-18, Nishi-9, Kita-ku, Sapporo 060-0818, Japan. atakada@czc.hokudai.ac.jp

In central and west Africa, Ebola virus, a member of the filovirus group, has produced sporadic outbreaks of lethal disease. This virus causes hemorrhagic fever in humans and nonhuman primates, resulting in mortality rates of up to 90%. Although there are no satisfactory biologic explanations for this extreme virulence, it has been suggested that functions of the envelope glycoprotein are likely to play important roles in the pathogenicity of Ebola virus.

PMID: 17038820 [PubMed - indexed for MEDLINE]

1672. Virol J. 2006 May 23;3:31.

Effect of Ebola virus proteins GP, NP and VP35 on VP40 VLP morphology.

Johnson RF(1), Bell P, Harty RN.

Author information: (1)Department of Pathobiology, School of Veterinary Medicine, University of Pennsylvania, 3800 Spruce St., Philadelphia, PA 19104, USA. rfj@vet.upenn.edu

Recently we described a role for Ebola virus proteins, NP, GP, and VP35 in enhancement of VP40 VLP budding. To explore the possibility that VLP structure was altered by co-expression of EBOV proteins leading to the observed enhancement of VP40 VLP budding, we performed density gradient analysis as well as electron microscopy studies. Our data suggest that VP40 is the major determinant of VLP morphology, as co-expression of NP, GP and VP35 did not significantly change VLP density, length, and diameter. Ultra-structural changes were noted in the core of the VLPs when NP was co-expressed with VP40. Overall, these findings indicate that major changes in morphology of VP40 VLPs were likely not responsible for enhanced budding of VP40 VLPs in the presence of GP, NP and/or VP35.

PMCID: PMC1502131 PMID: 16719918 [PubMed - indexed for MEDLINE]

1673. Int Immunol. 2006 May;18(5):741-53. Epub 2006 Mar 28.

Functional comparison of mouse CIRE/mouse DC-SIGN and human DC-SIGN.

Caminschi I(1), Corbett AJ, Zahra C, Lahoud M, Lucas KM, Sofi M, Vremec D, Gramberg T, Pöhlmann S, Curtis J, Handman E, van Dommelen SL, Fleming P, Degli-Esposti MA, Shortman K, Wright MD.

Author information: (1)Walter and Eliza Hall Institute of Medical Research Melbourne, Victoria 3050, Australia. caminschi@wehi.edu.au

CIRE/mDC-SIGN is a C-type lectin we originally identified as a molecule differentially expressed by mouse dendritic cell (DC) populations. Immunostaining with a CIRE/mDC-SIGN-specific mAb revealed that CIRE/mDC-SIGN is indeed on the surface of some CD4+, CD4- 8- DCs and plasmacytoid pre-DCs, but not on CD8+ DCs. It has been proposed that CIRE/mDC-SIGN is the functional orthologue of human DC-SIGN (hDC-SIGN), a molecule that both enhances T cell responses and facilitates antigen uptake. We assessed if CIRE/mDC-SIGN and hDC-SIGN exhibit functional similarities. CIRE/mDC-SIGN is down-regulated upon activation, but unlike hDC-SIGN, incubation with IL-4 and IL-13 did not enhance CIRE/mDC-SIGN expression, indicating differences in gene regulation. Like hDC-SIGN, CIRE/mDC-SIGN bound mannosylated residues. However, we could detect no role for CIRE/mDC-SIGN in T cell-DC interactions and the protein did not bind to pathogens known to interact with hDC-SIGN, including Leishmania mexicana, cytomegalovirus, HIV and lentiviral particles bearing the Ebolavirus glycoprotein. The binding of CIRE/mDC-SIGN to hDC-SIGN ligands was not rescued when CIRE/mDC-SIGN was engineered to express the stalk region of hDC-SIGN. We conclude that there are significant differences in the fine specificity of the C-type lectin domains of hDC-SIGN and CIRE/mDC-SIGN and that these two molecules may not be functional orthologues.

PMID: 16569675 [PubMed - indexed for MEDLINE]

1674. J Gen Virol. 2006 May;87(Pt 5):1247-57.

Ebola virus glycoprotein GP is not cytotoxic when expressed constitutively at a moderate level.

Alazard-Dany N(1), Volchkova V, Reynard O, Carbonnelle C, Dolnik O, Ottmann M, Khromykh A, Volchkov VE.

Author information: (1)Filovirus Laboratory, Claude Bernard University Lyon 1, INSERM U758, IFR 128 BioSciences Lyon-Gerland, France.

Transient expression of Ebola virus (EBOV) glycoprotein GP causes downregulation of surface proteins, cell rounding and detachment, a phenomenon believed to play a central role in the pathogenicity of the virus. In this study, evidence that moderate expression of GP does not result in such morphological changes was provided. It was shown that GP continuously produced in 293T cells from the Kunjin virus replicon was correctly processed and transported to the plasma membrane without affecting the surface expression of beta1 and alpha5 integrins and major histocompatibility complex I molecules. The level of GP expression in Kunjin replicon GP-expressing cells was similar to that observed in cells infected with EBOV early in infection and lower than that produced in cells transfected with plasmid DNA, phCMV-GP, expressing GP from a strong promoter. Importantly, transient transfection of Kunjin replicon GP-expressing cells with GP-coding plasmid DNA resulted in overexpression of GP, which lead to the downregulation of surface molecules and massive rounding and detachment of transfected cells. Here, it was also demonstrated that cell rounding and downregulation of the surface markers are the late events in EBOV infection, whereas synthesis and massive release of virus particles occur at early steps and do not cause significant cytotoxic effects. These findings indicate that the synthesis of EBOV GP in virus-infected cells is controlled well by several mechanisms that do not allow GP overexpression and hence the early appearance of its cytotoxic properties.

PMID: 16603527 [PubMed - indexed for MEDLINE]

1675. Trends Mol Med. 2006 May;12(5):206-15. Epub 2006 Apr 17.

Ebola virus: unravelling pathogenesis to combat a deadly disease.

Hoenen T(1), Groseth A, Falzarano D, Feldmann H.

Author information: (1)Special Pathogens Program, National Microbiology Laboratory, Public Health Agency of Canada, 1015 Arlington St., Winnipeg, MB R3E 3R2, Canada.

Ebola virus (EBOV) causes severe haemorrhagic fever leading to up to 90% lethality. Increasingly frequent outbreaks and the placement of EBOV in the category A list of potential biothreat agents have boosted interest in this virus. Furthermore, development of new technologies (e.g. reverse genetics systems) and extensive studies on Ebola haemorrhagic fever (EHF) in animal models have substantially expanded the knowledge on the pathogenic mechanisms that underlie this disease. Two major factors in EBOV pathogenesis are the impairment of the immune response and vascular dysfunction. Here, we attempt to summarize the current knowledge on EBOV pathogenesis focusing on these two factors and on recent progress in the development of vaccines and potential therapeutics.

PMID: 16616875 [PubMed - indexed for MEDLINE]

1676. Lancet. 2006 Apr 29;367(9520):1373-4.

Good news for Marburg virus workers.

Becker S(1).

Author information: (1)Robert Koch Institute, Berlin 13353, Germany. beckerst@rki.de

Comment on Lancet. 2006 Apr 29;367(9520):1399-404.

PMID: 16650630 [PubMed - indexed for MEDLINE]

1677. Virology. 2006 Apr 10;347(2):354-63. Epub 2006 Jan 18.

Impact of polymorphisms in the DC-SIGNR neck domain on the interaction with pathogens.

Gramberg T(1), Zhu T, Chaipan C, Marzi A, Liu H, Wegele A, Andrus T, Hofmann H, Pöhlmann S.

Author information: (1)Institute for Clinical and Molecular Virology, University Erlangen-Nürnberg, 91054 Erlangen, Germany.

The lectins DC-SIGN and DC-SIGNR augment infection by human immunodeficiency virus (HIV), Ebolavirus (EBOV) and other pathogens. The neck domain of these proteins drives multimerization, which is believed to be required for efficient recognition of multivalent ligands. The neck domain of DC-SIGN consists of seven sequence repeats with rare variations. In contrast, the DC-SIGNR neck domain is polymorphic and, in addition to the wild type (wt) allele with seven repeat units, allelic forms with five and six sequence repeats are frequently found. A potential association of the DC-SIGNR genotype and risk of HIV-1 infection is currently under debate. Therefore, we investigated if DC-SIGNR alleles with five and six repeat units exhibit defects in pathogen capture. Here, we show that wt DC-SIGNR and patient derived alleles with five and six repeats bind viral glycoproteins, augment viral infection and tetramerize with comparable efficiency. Moreover, coexpression of wt DC-SIGNR and alleles with five repeats did not decrease the interaction with pathogens compared to expression of each allele alone, suggesting that potential formation of hetero-oligomers does not appreciably reduce pathogen binding, at least under conditions of high expression. Thus, our results do not provide evidence for diminished pathogen capture by DC-SIGNR alleles with five and six repeat units. Albeit, we cannot exclude that subtle, but in vivo relevant differences remained undetected, our analysis suggests that indirect mechanisms could account for the association of polymorphisms in the DC-SIGNR neck region with reduced risk of HIV-1 infection.

PMID: 16413044 [PubMed - indexed for MEDLINE]

1678. Vaccine. 2006 Apr 5;24(15):2975-86. Epub 2005 Dec 9.

De novo syntheses of Marburg virus antigens from adenovirus vectors induce potent humoral and cellular immune responses.

Wang D(1), Schmaljohn AL, Raja NU, Trubey CM, Juompan LY, Luo M, Deitz SB, Yu H, Woraratanadharm J, Holman DH, Moore KM, Swain BM, Pratt WD, Dong JY.

Author information: (1)Division of Biodefense Vaccines, GenPhar Inc., 871 Lowcountry Blvd., Mount Pleasant, SC 29464, USA.

Marburg virus (MARV) is an African filovirus that causes a deadly hemorrhagic fever in humans, with up to 90% mortality. Currently, there are no MARV vaccines or therapies approved for human use. We hypothesized that developing a vaccine that induces a de novo synthesis of MARV antigens in vivo will lead to strong induction of both a humoral and cell-mediated immune response against MARV. Here, we develop and characterize three novel gene-based vaccine candidates which express the viral glycoprotein (GP) from either the Ci67, Ravn or Musoke strain of MARV. Immunization of mice with complex adenovirus (Ad)-based vaccine candidates (cAdVax vaccines), led to efficient production of both antibodies and cytotoxic T lymphocytes (CTL) specific to Musoke strain GP and Ci67 strain GP, respectively. Antibody responses were also shown to be cross-reactive across the MARV strains, but not cross-reactive to Ebola virus, a related filovirus. Additionally, three 1 x 10(8)pfu doses of vaccine vector were demonstrated to be safe in mice, as this did not lead to any detectable toxicity in liver or spleen. These promising results indicate that a cAdVax-based vaccine could be effective for induction of both humoral and cell-mediated immune responses to multiple strains of the Marburg virus.

PMID: 16530297 [PubMed - indexed for MEDLINE]

1679. Clin Vaccine Immunol. 2006 Apr;13(4):444-51.

Laboratory diagnostic systems for Ebola and Marburg hemorrhagic fevers developed with recombinant proteins.

Saijo M(1), Niikura M, Ikegami T, Kurane I, Kurata T, Morikawa S.

Author information: (1)Department of Virology 1, National Institute of Infectious Diseases, 4-7-1 Gakuen, Musashimurayama, Tokyo 208-0011, Japan. msaijo@nih.go.jp

PMCID: PMC1459631 PMID: 16603611 [PubMed - indexed for MEDLINE]

1680. Curr Opin Mol Ther. 2006 Apr;8(2):93-103.

Antisense treatments for biothreat agents.

Warfield KL(1), Panchal RG, Aman MJ, Bavari S.

Author information: (1)U.S. Army Medical Research Institute of Infectious Diseases, Fort Detrick, Frederick, MD 21702, USA.

Antisense oligomers (ASOs) represent a promising technology to treat viral and bacterial infections, and have already been shown to be successful against a variety of pathogens in cell culture studies and nonhuman primate models of infection. For these reasons, antisense technologies are being pursued as treatments against biothreat agents such as Ebola virus, dengue virus and Bacillus anthracis. Several generations of modified oligonucleotides have been developed to maximize nuclease resistance, target affinity, potency, cell entry, and other pharmacokinetic properties. First-generation ASOs contain phosphorothioate modifications to increase stability through nuclease resistance. Further chemical modifications in second-generation ASOs include 2'-O-methyl and 2'-O-methoxy-ethyl oligos, which increase nuclease resistance and oligo:RNA binding affinities. Third-generation ASOs contain a variety of chemical modifications that enhance stability, affinity and bioavailability. A fourth class of oligonucleotide-based compounds consists of small interfering RNAs, which have recently become widely used for gene knockdown in vitro and in vivo. This review focuses on the third-generation phosphorodiamidate morpholino oligomers, which are nonionic and contain a morpholine ring instead of a ribose, as well as phosphorodiamidate linkages in place of phosphorothioates. Multiple antisense oligomer-based therapeutics are being developed for use against biothreat agents, and antisense drugs will likely become a critical member of our arsenal in the defense against highly pathogenic, emerging or genetically engineered pathogens.

PMID: 16610760 [PubMed - indexed for MEDLINE]

1681. J Virol. 2006 Apr;80(8):4174-8.

Role of endosomal cathepsins in entry mediated by the Ebola virus glycoprotein.

Schornberg K(1), Matsuyama S, Kabsch K, Delos S, Bouton A, White J.

Author information: (1)Department of Microbiology, University of Virginia, 1300 Jefferson Park Ave., Charlottesville, Virginia 22908-0734, USA.

Using chemical inhibitors and small interfering RNA (siRNA), we have confirmed roles for cathepsin B (CatB) and cathepsin L (CatL) in Ebola virus glycoprotein (GP)-mediated infection. Treatment of Ebola virus GP pseudovirions with CatB and CatL converts GP1 from a 130-kDa to a 19-kDa species. Virus with 19-kDa GP1 displays significantly enhanced infection and is largely resistant to the effects of the CatB inhibitor and siRNA, but it still requires a low-pH-dependent endosomal/lysosomal function. These and other results support a model in which CatB and CatL prime GP by generating a 19-kDa intermediate that can be acted upon by an as yet unidentified endosomal/lysosomal enzyme to trigger fusion.

PMCID: PMC1440424 PMID: 16571833 [PubMed - indexed for MEDLINE]

1682. J Virol. 2006 Apr;80(8):3743-51.

Functional mapping of the nucleoprotein of Ebola virus.

Watanabe S(1), Noda T, Kawaoka Y.

Author information: (1)Department of Pathobiological Sciences, School of Veterinary Medicine, University of Wisconsin--Madison, 2015 Linden Dr., Madison, Wisconsin 53706, USA.

At 739 amino acids, the nucleoprotein (NP) of Ebola virus is the largest nucleoprotein of the nonsegmented negative-stranded RNA viruses, and like the NPs of other viruses, it plays a central role in virus replication. Huang et al. (Y. Huang, L. Xu, Y. Sun, and G. J. Nabel, Mol. Cell 10:307-316, 2002) previously demonstrated that NP, together with the minor matrix protein VP24 and polymerase cofactor VP35, is necessary and sufficient for the formation of nucleocapsid-like structures that are morphologically indistinguishable from those seen in Ebola virus-infected cells. They further showed that NP is O glycosylated and sialylated and that these modifications are important for interaction between NP and VP35. However, little is known about the structure-function relationship of Ebola virus NP. Here, we examined the glycosylation of Ebola virus NP and further investigated its properties by generating deletion mutants to define the region(s) involved in NP-NP interaction (self-assembly), in the formation of nucleocapsid-like structures, and in the replication of the viral genome. We were unable to identify the types of glycosylation and sialylation, although we did confirm that Ebola virus NP was glycosylated. We also determined that the region from amino acids 1 to 450 is important for NP-NP interaction (self-assembly). We further demonstrated that these amino-terminal 450 residues and the following 150 residues are required for the formation of nucleocapsid-like structures and for viral genome replication. These data advance our understanding of the functional region(s) of Ebola virus NP, which in turn should improve our knowledge of the Ebola virus life cycle and its extreme pathogenicity.

PMCID: PMC1440433 PMID: 16571791 [PubMed - indexed for MEDLINE]

1683. Med Sci (Paris). 2006 Apr;22(4):411-5.

[Sphingolipids, vehicle for pathogenic agents and cause of genetic diseases].

[Article in French]

Fasano C(1), Hiol A, Miolan JP, Niel JP.

Author information: (1)Département de Pharmacologie, Faculté de Médecine, Université de Montréal, Québec, Canada.

Sphingolipids are present in all eukaryotic cells and share a sphingoid base : sphingosine. They were first discovered in 1884 and for a long time they were thought to participate to membrane structure only. Recently it has been established that they are mainly located in particular areas of the membrane called rafts which are signalling platforms. It has also been demonstrated that sphingolipids are receptors and second messengers. They play a crucial role in cellular functioning and are necessary to maintenance and developing of living organisms. However due to their receptor properties, they are also gateway for penetration of pathogenic agents such as virus (Ebola, HIV) or toxins (botulinium, tetanus). These agents first bind to glycosphingolipids or proteins mainly located in rafts. The complex so formed is required for the crossing of the membrane by the pathogenic agent. Sphingolipids metabolism is regulated by numerous enzymes. A failure in the activity of one of them induces an accumulation of sphingolipids known as sphingolipidoses. These are genetic diseases having severe consequences for the survival of the organism. The precise mechanisms of the sphingolipidoses are still mainly unknown which explains why few therapeutic strategies are available. These particular properties of lipids rafts and sphingolipids explain why a growing number of studies in the medical and scientific fields are devoted to them.

PMID: 16597411 [PubMed - indexed for MEDLINE]

1684. Med Sci (Paris). 2006 Apr;22(4):405-10.

[Ebola and Marburg viruses: the humans strike back].

[Article in French]

Alazard-Dany N(1), Ottmann Terrangle M, Volchkov V.

Author information: (1)Laboratoire des Filovirus, Inserm U758, ENS Lyon, IFR 128 BioSciences Lyon-Gerland, Université Claude Bernard Lyon I, France.

Ebola and Marburg viruses are the causative agents of rapidly progressive hemorrhagic fevers with high mortality rates. Pre- or post-exposure treatments against the diseases are currently not available for human use. In the field, establishment of strict quarantine measures preventing further virus transmission are still the only way to fight the infections. However, our knowledge of Ebola and Marburg viruses has markedly increased as a result of two recent discoveries discussed in this review. Chandran et al. have elucidated the mechanism by which Ebola GP is converted to a fusion-active form. Infectivity of Ebola virus was shown to be dependent on the cleavage of GP by cellular endosomal proteases, cathepsin B and L, thus opening new therapeutic approaches options. As for Jones SM et al., they have successfully vaccinated monkeys with recombinant vesicular stomatitis virus expressing Ebola or Marburg virus surface glycoprotein GP, a promising vaccine approach.

PMID: 16597410 [PubMed - indexed for MEDLINE]

1685. Med Trop (Mars). 2006 Apr;66(2):119-24.

[Chiroptera and zoonosis: an emerging problem on all five continents].

[Article in French]

Hance P(1), Garnotel E, Morillon M.

Author information: (1)Service de biologie, HIA Laveran, Marseille, France. biologie.alaveran@mageos.com

Zoonosis is the cause of the vast majority of emerging diseases. Bats that occupy the second place in the mammal class play an important role. Whether they belong to the microchiroptera suborder or to the megachiroptera suborder, bats on all five continents have been implicated in transmission of numerous pathogens including not only viruses such as Lyssavirus (e.g. rabies), Hepanivirus (e.g. Hendra and Nipah virus) and recently coronavirus (e.g. SARS-like coronavirus and Ebola virus) but also fungus such as histoplasmosis. By modifying environmental conditions and encroaching on their biotope, human intervention has probably contributed to the introduction of chiropteras into an epidemiologic chain in which they previously had no place, thus promoting the emergence of new pathogens.

PMID: 16775933 [PubMed - indexed for MEDLINE]

1686. Virology. 2006 Mar 15;346(2):394-401. Epub 2005 Dec 13.

Chimpanzee adenovirus vaccine protects against Zaire Ebola virus.

Kobinger GP(1), Feldmann H, Zhi Y, Schumer G, Gao G, Feldmann F, Jones S, Wilson JM.

Author information: (1)Special Pathogens Program, National Microbiology Laboratory, Health Canada, Canadian Science Centre for Human and Animal Health, University of Manitoba, Winnipeg, Canada.

This study evaluated the use of a chimpanzee-based adenovirus vaccine in mouse and Guinea pigs models of Zaire Ebola virus (ZEBOV) infection. Vaccine vector expressing the envelope glycoprotein of ZEBOV was created from the molecular clone of chimpanzee adenovirus pan7 (AdC7). AdC7 vaccine stimulated robust T and B cell responses to ZEBOV in naïve mice inducing complete protection to an otherwise lethal challenge of ZEBOV. Complete protection to Zaire Ebola virus was also observed in Guinea pigs vaccinated with a relatively low dose of AdC7 (5 x 10(9)/kg). Pre-existing immunity to AdHu5 was generated in mice following pre-exposure to AdHu5 or administration of pooled human immune globulin. Pre-existing immunity to human adenoviruses severely compromised the efficacy of the human AdHu5 vaccine but not the chimpanzee AdC7 vaccine. These results validate further development of Chimpanzee-based vaccine and highlight the impact of pre-existing immunity to the vaccine carrier.

PMID: 16356525 [PubMed - indexed for MEDLINE]

1687. Antimicrob Agents Chemother. 2006 Mar;50(3):984-93.

VP35 knockdown inhibits Ebola virus amplification and protects against lethal infection in mice.

Enterlein S(1), Warfield KL, Swenson DL, Stein DA, Smith JL, Gamble CS, Kroeker AD, Iversen PL, Bavari S, Mühlberger E.

Author information: (1)Department of Virology, Philipps-University Marburg, Hans-Meerwein-Str. 3, 35043 Marburg, Germany.

Phosphorodiamidate morpholino oligomers (PMO) are a class of uncharged single-stranded DNA analogs modified such that each subunit includes a phosphorodiamidate linkage and morpholine ring. PMO antisense agents have been reported to effectively interfere with the replication of several positive-strand RNA viruses in cell culture. The filoviruses, Marburg virus and Ebola virus (EBOV), are negative-strand RNA viruses that cause up to 90% lethality in human outbreaks. There is currently no commercially available vaccine or efficacious therapeutic for any filovirus. In this study, PMO conjugated to arginine-rich cell-penetrating peptide (P-PMO) and nonconjugated PMO were assayed for the ability to inhibit EBOV infection in cell culture and in a mouse model of lethal EBOV infection. A 22-mer P-PMO designed to base pair with the translation start site region of EBOV VP35 positive-sense RNA generated sequence-specific and time- and dose-dependent inhibition of EBOV amplification in cell culture. The same oligomer provided complete protection to mice when administered before or after an otherwise lethal infection of EBOV. A corresponding nonconjugated PMO, as well as nonconjugated truncated versions of 16 and

19 base residues, provided length-dependent protection to mice when administered prophylactically. Together, these data suggest that antisense PMO and P-PMO have the potential to control EBOV infection and are promising therapeutic candidates.
PMCID: PMC1426423 PMID: 16495261 [PubMed - indexed for MEDLINE]
1688. Bull Acad Natl Med. 2006 Mar;190(3):597-608; discussion 609, 625-7.

[Emerging viral diseases].
[Article in French]

Bricaire F(1), Bossi P.
Author information: (1)Service des Maladies infectieuses et tropicales - Groupe Hospitalier de la Pitié-Salpêtrière, 47 bld de l'Hôpital, 75015 Paris.
Emerging and re-emerging infectious diseases have again entered the public arena in recent years. This is due to factors such as evolving lifestyles, ecological and socio-political upheavals, and recent diagnostic advances. Numerous pathogens, including viruses like West Nile, Chikungunya and Japanese encephalitis on the one hand, and hemorrhagic fever viruses like Ebola and Maburg, are particular concerns. Recently, the Corona virus responsible for SARS, which caused an epidemic sufficiently worrisome to challenge crisis management concepts, was successfully isolated. It is in this context that so-called "bird flu'", may be on the verge of causing a human pandemic. Pox and Monkeypox are virtually emerging viruses that have potential for use in bioterrorism. The management and treatment of these emerging infectious diseases calls for new approaches, organizations and infrastructures.
PMID: 17140098 [PubMed - indexed for MEDLINE]
1689. J Virol. 2006 Mar;80(6):3009-20.

Global suppression of the host antiviral response by Ebola- and Marburgviruses: increased antagonism of the type I interferon response is associated with enhanced virulence.

Kash JC(1), Mühlberger E, Carter V, Grosch M, Perwitasari O, Proll SC, Thomas MJ, Weber F, Klenk HD, Katze MG.
Author information: (1)Department of Microbiology, School of Medicine, University of Washington, Box 358070, Seattle, Washington 98195-8070, USA. jkash@u.washington.edu
We studied the effect of filovirus infection on host cell gene expression by characterizing the regulation of gene expression responses in human liver cells infected with Zaire Ebolavirus (ZEBOV), Reston Ebolavirus (REBOV), and Marburgvirus (MARV), using transcriptional profiling and bioinformatics. Expression microarray analysis demonstrated that filovirus infection resulted in the up-regulation of immune-related genes and the down-regulation of many coagulation and acute-phase proteins. These studies further revealed that a common feature of filovirus virulence is suppression of key cellular antiviral responses, including TLR-, interferon (IFN) regulatory factor 3-, and PKR-related pathways. We further showed that ZEBOV and MARV were more potent antagonists of the IFN response and inhibited the expression of most of the IFN-stimulated genes (ISGs) observed in mock-infected IFN-alpha-2b treated cells, compared to REBOV infection, which activated more than 20% of these ISGs. Finally, we examined IFN-related gene expression in filovirus-infected cells treated with IFN-alpha-2b. These experiments revealed that a majority of genes induced in mock-infected cells treated with type I IFN were antagonized in treated ZEBOV- and MARV-infected cells, while in contrast, REBOV infection resulted in a significant increase in ISG expression. Analysis of STAT1 and -2 phosphorylation following IFN treatment showed a significant reduction of STAT phosphorylation for MARV but not for ZEBOV and REBOV, indicating that different mechanisms might be involved in antagonizing IFN signaling pathways by the different filovirus species. Taken together, these studies showed a correlation between antagonism of type I IFN responses and filovirus virulence.
PMCID: PMC1395418 PMID: 16501110 [PubMed - indexed for MEDLINE]
1690. J Virol. 2006 Mar;80(6):2815-22.

Detection of cell-cell fusion mediated by Ebola virus glycoproteins.

Bär S(1), Takada A, Kawaoka Y, Alizon M.
Author information: (1)Department of Cell Biology, Institut Cochin, INSERM U567, CNRS UMR 8104, Université René Descartes, Paris, France. s.baer@dkfz-heidelberg.de
Ebola viruses (EboV) are enveloped RNA viruses infecting cells by a pH-dependent process mediated by viral glycoproteins (GP) involving endocytosis of virions and their routing into acidic endosomes. As with well-characterized pH-dependent viral entry proteins, in particular influenza virus hemagglutinin, it is thought that EboV GP require activation by low pH in order to mediate fusion of the viral envelope with the membrane of endosomes. However, it has not yet been possible to confirm the direct role of EboV GP in membrane fusion and the requirement for low-pH activation. It was in particular not possible to induce formation of syncytia by exposing cells expressing EboV GP to acidic medium. Here, we have used an assay based on the induction of a beta-galactosidase (lacZ) reporter gene in target cells to detect cytoplasmic exchanges, indicating membrane fusion, with cells expressing EboV GP (Zaire species). Acidic activation of GP-expressing cells was required for efficient fusion with target cells. The direct role of EboV GP in this process is indicated by its inhibition by anti-GP antibodies and by the lack of activity of mutant GP normally expressed at the cell surface but defective for virus entry. Fusion was not observed when target cells underwent acidic treatment, for example, when they were placed in coculture with GP-expressing cells before the activation step. This unexpected feature, possibly related to the nature of the EboV receptor, could explain the impossibility of inducing formation of syncytia among GP-expressing cells.
PMCID: PMC1395460 PMID: 16501090 [PubMed - indexed for MEDLINE]
1691. J Virol. 2006 Mar;80(6):2738-46.

Development of a cAdVax-based bivalent ebola virus vaccine that induces immune responses against both the Sudan and Zaire species of Ebola virus.

Wang D(1), Raja NU, Trubey CM, Juompan LY, Luo M, Woraratanadharm J, Deitz SB, Yu H, Swain BM, Moore KM, Pratt WD, Hart MK, Dong JY.

Author information: (1)Division of Biodefense Vaccines, GenPhar, Inc., 871 Lowcountry Blvd., Mount Pleasant, South Carolina 29464, USA.
Ebola virus (EBOV) causes a severe hemorrhagic fever for which there are currently no vaccines or effective treatments. While lethal human outbreaks have so far been restricted to sub-Saharan Africa, the potential exploitation of EBOV as a biological weapon cannot be ignored. Two species of EBOV, Sudan ebolavirus (SEBOV) and Zaire ebolavirus (ZEBOV), have been responsible for all of the deadly human outbreaks resulting from this virus. Therefore, it is important to develop a vaccine that can prevent infection by both lethal species. Here, we describe the bivalent cAdVaxE(GPs/z) vaccine, which includes the SEBOV glycoprotein (GP) and ZEBOV GP genes together in a single complex adenovirus-based vaccine (cAdVax) vector. Vaccination of mice with the bivalent cAdVaxE(GPs/z) vaccine led to efficient induction of EBOV-specific antibody and cell-mediated immune responses to both species of EBOV. In addition, the cAdVax technology demonstrated induction of a 100% protective immune response in mice, as all vaccinated C57BL/6 and BALB/c mice survived challenge with a lethal dose of ZEBOV (30,000 times the 50% lethal dose). This study demonstrates the potential efficacy of a bivalent EBOV vaccine based on a cAdVax vaccine vector design.
PMCID: PMC1395467 PMID: 16501083 [PubMed - indexed for MEDLINE]

1692. J Virol. 2006 Mar;80(5):2267-79.

A single intranasal inoculation with a paramyxovirus-vectored vaccine protects guinea pigs against a lethal-dose Ebola virus challenge.

Bukreyev A(1), Yang L, Zaki SR, Shieh WJ, Rollin PE, Murphy BR, Collins PL, Sanchez A.

Author information: (1)National Institute of Allergy and Infectious Diseases, National Institutes of Health, Bethesda, MD 20892, USA. abukreyev@niaid.nih.gov
To determine whether intranasal inoculation with a paramyxovirus-vectored vaccine can induce protective immunity against Ebola virus (EV), recombinant human parainfluenza virus type 3 (HPIV3) was modified to express either the EV structural glycoprotein (GP) by itself (HPIV3/EboGP) or together with the EV nucleoprotein (NP) (HPIV3/EboGP-NP). Expression of EV GP by these recombinant viruses resulted in its efficient incorporation into virus particles and increased cytopathic effect in Vero cells. HPIV3/EboGP was 100-fold more efficiently neutralized by antibodies to EV than by antibodies to HPIV3. Guinea pigs infected with a single intranasal inoculation of 10(5.3) PFU of HPIV3/EboGP or HPIV3/EboGP-NP showed no apparent signs of disease yet developed a strong humoral response specific to the EV proteins. When these animals were challenged with an intraperitoneal injection of 10(3) PFU of EV, there were no outward signs of disease, no viremia or detectable EV antigen in the blood, and no evidence of infection in the spleen, liver, and lungs. In contrast, all of the control animals died or developed severe EV disease following challenge. The highly effective immunity achieved with a single vaccine dose suggests that intranasal immunization with live vectored vaccines based on recombinant respiratory viruses may be an advantageous approach to inducing protective responses against severe systemic infections, such as those caused by hemorrhagic fever agents.
PMCID: PMC1395378 PMID: 16474134 [PubMed - indexed for MEDLINE]

1693. Med Health R I. 2006 Mar;89(3):89.

A bat out of hell.

Aronson SM.
PMID: 16596929 [PubMed - indexed for MEDLINE]

1694. Sci Am. 2006 Mar;294(3):24, 248.

Going to bat.

Choi CQ.
PMID: 16502604 [PubMed - indexed for MEDLINE]

1695. Virology. 2006 Feb 20;345(2):482-91. Epub 2005 Nov 17.

Evidence that multiple defects in murine DC-SIGN inhibit a functional interaction with pathogens.

Gramberg T(1), Caminschi I, Wegele A, Hofmann H, Pöhlmann S.

Author information: (1)Institute for Clinical and Molecular Virology, University Erlangen-Nürnberg, 91054 Erlangen, Germany.
Certain viruses, bacteria, fungi and parasites target dendritic cells through the interaction with the cellular attachment factor DC-SIGN, making this C-type lectin an attractive target for therapeutic intervention. Studies on DC-SIGN function would be greatly aided by the establishment of a mouse model, however, it is unclear if the murine (m) homologue of human (h) DC-SIGN also binds to pathogens. Here, we investigated the interaction of mDC-SIGN, also termed CIRE, with the Ebolavirus glycoprotein (EBOV-GP), a ligand of hDC-SIGN. We found that mDC-SIGN neither binds EBOV-GP nor enhances infection by reporterviruses pseudotyped with EBOV-GP. Analysis of chimeras between mDC-SIGN and hDC-SIGN provided evidence that determinants in the carbohydrate recognition domain and in the neck domain of mDC-SIGN inhibit a functional interaction with EBOV-GP. Moreover, mDC-SIGN was found be monomeric, suggesting that lack of multimerization, which is believed to be required for efficient pathogen recognition by hDC-SIGN, might be one factor that prevents binding of mDC-SIGN to EBOV-GP. Our results suggest that mDC-SIGN on murine dendritic cells is not an adequate model for pathogen interactions with hDC-SIGN.
PMID: 16297949 [PubMed - indexed for MEDLINE]

1696. Expert Rev Anti Infect Ther. 2006 Feb;4(1):67-76.

Development of treatment strategies to combat Ebola and Marburg viruses.

Paragas J(1), Geisbert TW.

Author information: (1)Virology Division, US Army Medical Research Institute of Infectious Diseases, Fort Detrick, MD 21702-5011, USA. jason.paragas@amedd.army.mil
Ebola and Marburg viruses are emerging/re-emerging pathogens that pose a significant threat to human health. These naturally occurring viral infections frequently cause a lethal hemorrhagic fever in humans and nonhuman primates. The disastrous consequences of infection with these viruses have been

pursued as potential biological weapons. To date, there are no therapeutic options available for the prophylaxis or treatment of infected individuals. The recognition that Ebola and Marburg viruses may be exploited as biological weapons has resulted in major efforts to develop modalities to counter infection. In this review, select technologies and approaches will be highlighted as part of the critical path for the development of therapeutics to ameliorate the invariably devastating outcomes of human filoviral infections.

PMID: 16441210 [PubMed - indexed for MEDLINE]

1697. Expert Rev Anti Infect Ther. 2006 Feb;4(1):57-66.

Development of human monoclonal antibodies against diseases caused by emerging and biodefense-related viruses.

Zhu Z(1), Dimitrov AS, Chakraborti S, Dimitrova D, Xiao X, Broder CC, Dimitrov DS.

Author information: (1)Protein Interactions Group, CCRNP, BRP, SAIC-Frederick, Inc., NCI-Frederick, NIH Bldg 469, Rm 139, PO Box B, MD 21702-1201, USA. zhongyuzhu@ncifcrf.gov

Polyclonal antibodies have a century-old history of being effective against some viruses; recently, monoclonal antibodies (mAbs) have also shown success. The humanized mAb Synagis (palivizumab), which is still the only mAb against a viral disease approved by the US FDA, has been widely used as a prophylactic measure against respiratory syncytial virus infections in neonates and immunocompromised individuals. The first fully human mAbs against two other paramyxoviruses, Hendra and Nipah virus, which can cause high (up to 75%) mortality, were recently developed; one of them, m101, showed exceptional potency against infectious virus. In an amazing pace of research, several potent human mAbs targeting the severe acute respiratory syndrome coronavirus S glycoprotein that can affect infections in animal models have been developed months after the virus was identified in 2003. A potent humanized mAb with therapeutic potential was recently developed against the West Nile virus. The progress in developing neutralizing human mAbs against Ebola, Crimean-Congo hemorrhagic fever, vaccinia and other emerging and biodefense-related viruses is slow. A major problem in the development of effective therapeutic agents against viruses, including therapeutic antibodies, is the viruses' heterogeneity and mutability. A related problem is the low binding affinity of crossreactive antibodies able to neutralize a variety of primary isolates. Combinations of mAbs or mAbs with other drugs, and/or the identification of potent new mAbs and their derivatives that target highly conserved viral structures, which are critical for virus entry into cells, are some of the possible solutions to these problems, and will continue to be a major focus of antiviral research.

PMID: 16441209 [PubMed - indexed for MEDLINE]

1698. J Virol. 2006 Feb;80(4):1734-41.

Time- and temperature-dependent activation of hepatitis C virus for low-pH-triggered entry.

Tscherne DM(1), Jones CT, Evans MJ, Lindenbach BD, McKeating JA, Rice CM.

Author information: (1)Laboratory of Virology and Infectious Diseases, Center for the Study of Hepatitis C, The Rockefeller University, 1230 York Avenue, New York, NY 10021, USA.

Hepatitis C virus (HCV) is an important human pathogen associated with chronic liver disease. Recently, based on a genotype 2a isolate, tissue culture systems supporting complete replication and infectious virus production have been developed. In this study, we used cell culture-produced infectious HCV to analyze the viral entry pathway into Huh-7.5 cells. Bafilomycin A1 and concanamycin A, inhibitors of vacuolar ATPases, prevented HCV entry when they were present prior to infection and had minimal effect on downstream replication events. HCV entry therefore appears to be pH dependent, requiring an acidified intracellular compartment. For many other enveloped viruses, acidic pH triggers an irreversible conformational change, which promotes virion-endosomal membrane fusion. Such viruses are often inactivated by low pH. In the case of HCV, exposure of virions to acidic pH followed by return to neutral pH did not affect their infectivity. This parallels the observation made for the related pestivirus bovine viral diarrhea virus. Low pH could activate the entry of cell surface-bound HCV but only after prolonged incubation at 37 degrees C. This suggests that there are rate-limiting, postbinding events that are needed to render HCV competent for low-pH-triggered entry. Such events may involve interaction with a cellular coreceptor or other factors but do not require cathepsins B and L, late endosomal proteases that activate Ebola virus and reovirus for entry.

PMCID: PMC1367161 PMID: 16439530 [PubMed - indexed for MEDLINE]

1699. Med Sci (Paris). 2006 Feb;22(2):206-11.

[Scientific progress and new biological weapons].

[Article in French]

Berche P(1).

Author information: (1)Service de microbiologie, Hôpital Necker- Enfants-malades, 149, rue de Sèvres, 75015 Paris, France. berche@necker.fr

The biological weapons are different from conventional weapons, because living germs hold an extraordinary and predictable potential for multiplication, propagation and genetic variation during their dissemination in a susceptible population. Only natural pathogens (1rst generation weapons) have been used in the past (smallpox virus, plague, anthrax, toxins...). However, new threats are emerging, due to the rapid progress of scientific knowledge and its exponential worldwide diffusion. It is possible to synthesize microorganisms from in silico sequences widely diffused on Internet (poliovirus, influenza...), thus resulting in the accessibility of very dangerous virus confined today in high-security laboratories (virus Ebola...). It is possible also to "improve" pathogens by genetic manipulations, becoming more resistant or virulent (2nd generation weapons). Finally, one can now create de novo new pathogens by molecular breeding (DNA shuffling), potentially highly dangerous for naive populations (3rd generation weapons). Making biological weapons does not require too much technological resources and appears accessible to terrorists, due to low cost and easy use. Although the destructive consequences are difficult to predict, the psychological and social damages should be considerable, because of the highly emotional burden in the population associated to the transgression by man of a taboo of life.

PMID: 16457765 [PubMed - indexed for MEDLINE]

1700. Trends Parasitol. 2006 Feb;22(2):51-4. Epub 2006 Jan 10.

New medicines from nature's armamentarium.

Crump A(1).

Author information: (1)crumpa@easynet.co.uk

Nature frequently unleashes a barrage of new and frightening diseases against humans--such as HIV, severe acquired respiratory syndrome, Ebola virus and avian flu recently--in addition to the seemingly ever-present scourges such as malaria and tuberculosis. Fortunately, nature also provides the wherewithal to help conquer the diseases that it sets loose. All that is needed is the human ingenuity to discover, develop and apply the solutions in an optimal fashion. Participants at the 9th Max Tishler Memorial Symposium (Tokyo, July 2005) were told about several new advances in the search for new anti-infective drugs derived from natural sources and were able to learn how one of the most effective drugs ever, ivermectin, made its way through what was, at the time, uncharted territory and how precedents were set at nearly every stage to form a model for all subsequent public-private partnerships.

PMID: 16406332 [PubMed - indexed for MEDLINE]

1701. Online J Issues Nurs. 2006 Jan 31;11(1):2.

Emerging infectious diseases at the beginning of the 21st century.

Lashley FR(1).

Author information: (1)College of Nursing at Rutgers, New Jersey, USA. flashley@rutgers.edu

The emergence and re-emergence of infectious diseases involves many interrelated factors. Global interconnectedness continues to increase with international travel and trade; economic, political, and cultural interactions; and human-to-human and animal-to-human interactions. These interactions include the accidental and deliberate sharing of microbial agents and antimicrobial resistance and allow the emergence of new and unrecognized microbial disease agents. As the 21st century begins, already new agents have been identified, and new outbreaks have occurred. Solutions to limiting the spread of emerging infectious diseases will require cooperative efforts among many disciplines and entities worldwide. This article defines emerging infectious diseases, summarizes historical background, and discusses factors that contribute to emergence. Seven agents that have made a significant appearance, particularly in the 21st century, are reviewed, including: Ebola and Marburg hemorrhagic fevers, human monkeypox, bovine spongiform encephalopathy, severe acute respiratory syndrome (SARS), West Nile virus, and avian influenza. The article provides for each agent a brief historical background, case descriptions, and health care implications.

PMID: 16629503 [PubMed - indexed for MEDLINE]

1702. Virology. 2006 Jan 5;344(1):64-70.

Filovirus assembly and budding.

Hartlieb B(1), Weissenhorn W.

Author information: (1)Institut für Virologie, Robert-Koch-Str. 17, 35037 Marburg, Germany.

Filoviruses belong to the order of negative-stranded non-segmented RNA viruses and are classified into two genera, Ebola and Marburg viruses. They have a characteristic filamentous shape, which is largely determined by the matrix protein VP40. Although VP40 is the main driving force for assembly and budding from the host cell, the production of infectious virus involves an intricate interplay between all viral structural proteins in addition to cellular factors, e.g., those that normally function in multi-vesicular body biogenesis. As a consequence, assembly and budding steps are defined to specific cellular compartments, and the recent progress in understanding how the different components are assembled into stable enveloped virus particles is reviewed.

PMID: 16364737 [PubMed - indexed for MEDLINE]

1703. Acta Biochim Pol. 2006;53(4):617-26. Epub 2006 Nov 27.

Structural studies of algal lectins with anti-HIV activity.

Ziółkowska NE(1), Wlodawer A.

Author information: (1)Protein Structure Section, Macromolecular Crystallography Laboratory, National Cancer Institute, Frederick, MD, USA.

A number of antiviral lectins, small proteins that bind carbohydrates found on viral envelopes, are currently in pre-clinical trials as potential drugs for prevention of transmission of human immunodeficiency virus (HIV) and other enveloped viruses, such as the Ebola virus and the coronavirus responsible for severe acute respiratory syndrome (SARS). Lectins of algal origin whose antiviral properties make them candidate agents for prevention of viral transmission through topical applications include cyanovirin-N, Microcystis viridis lectin, scytovirin, and griffithsin. Although all these proteins exhibit significant antiviral activity, their structures are unrelated and their mode of binding of carbohydrates differs significantly. This review summarizes the current state of knowledge of the structures of algal lectins, their mode of binding of carbohydrates, and their potential medical applications.

PMID: 17128290 [PubMed - indexed for MEDLINE]

1704. Adv Exp Med Biol. 2006;582:35-44.

Viral haemorrhagic fevers caused by Lassa, Ebola and Marburg viruses.

Curtis N(1).

Author information: (1)Department of Paediatrics, University of Melbourne, Parkville, Australia.

PMID: 16802617 [PubMed - indexed for MEDLINE]

1705. An R Acad Nac Med (Madr). 2006;123(3):631-45.

[The primordial reservoir in the infectious contagion cicle. The avian influenza model].

[Article in Spanish]

Suárez Fernández G.

An update of the role of the primordial reservoir in the biological cycle of the process of infection and contagion is made, using diseases of very frequent incidence at the present moment in the Mediterranean Area and the Iberian Peninsula. These diseases are, amongst others Severe and Acute Respiratory Syndrome (SARS), Rabies, Lyme disease, African Horse Sickness, Blue Tongue, African Swine Fever, Ebola Hemorrhagic Fever, Hantavirosis, and Avian Influenza. The zoonoses classification proposed by the WHO Control Center in Athens in 1994 for the Mediterranean Area, based on the type of reservoir, the importance of the process and the type of transmission, and not focusing on the etiological agent, is very positively valued. Finally, the problem of Avian Influenza and the real risk posed by aquatic migratory birds in the diffusion and contagion of the present Avian Influence epidemics is reviewed.

PMID: 17451102 [PubMed - indexed for MEDLINE]

1706. Curr Med Chem. 2006;13(29):3529-52.

Antiviral properties of deazaadenine nucleoside derivatives.

Vittori S(1), Dal Ben D, Lambertucci C, Marucci G, Volpini R, Cristalli G.

Author information: (1)Dipartimento di Scienze Chimiche, via S. Agostino 1, University of Camerino, I-62032, Camerino, Italy. sauro.vittori@unicam.it

Viral infections have menaced human beings since time immemorial, and even today new viral strains that cause lethal diseases are being discovered with alarming frequency. One major example is HIV, the etiological agent of AIDS, which spread up in the last two decades. Very recently, other virus based diseases such as avian flu have spread fear around the world, and hemorrhagic fevers from central Africa serious threaten human health because of their very deadly effects. New antiviral agents are still greatly needed to counter these menaces. Many scientists are involved in this field of research, and many of the recently discovered effective antiviral compounds are nucleoside analogues. Among those derivatives, deazapurine nucleoside analogues have demonstrated potent inhibitory effect of viral replication. This review reports on recently generated data from preparing and testing deazapurine nucleoside derivatives as inhibitors in virus replication systems. Although most of the reported data have been produced in antiHIV, antiHCMV, and antiHSV biological testing, very recently other new important fields of application have been discovered, all in topical subjects of strong interest. In fact, deazapurine nucleosides have been found to be active as chemotherapeutics for some veterinary systemic viral infections, for which no antiviral drugs are licensed yet. Furthermore, they demonstrated efficacy in the inhibition of Hepatitis C virus replication. Finally, these compounds showed high potency as virucides against Ebola Virus, curing Ebola infected mice with a single dose administration.

PMID: 17168721 [PubMed - indexed for MEDLINE]

1707. J Immunol. 2006 Jan 1;176(1):426-40.

Internalizing antibodies to the C-type lectins, L-SIGN and DC-SIGN, inhibit viral glycoprotein binding and deliver antigen to human dendritic cells for the induction of T cell responses.

Dakappagari N(1), Maruyama T, Renshaw M, Tacken P, Figdor C, Torensma R, Wild MA, Wu D, Bowdish K, Kretz-Rommel A.

Author information: (1)Alexion Antibody Technologies, San Diego, CA 92121, USA.

The C-type lectin L-SIGN is expressed on liver and lymph node endothelial cells, where it serves as a receptor for a variety of carbohydrate ligands, including ICAM-3, Ebola, and HIV. To consider targeting liver/lymph node-specific ICAM-3-grabbing nonintegrin (L-SIGN) for therapeutic purposes in autoimmunity and infectious disease, we isolated and characterized Fabs that bind strongly to L-SIGN, but to a lesser degree or not at all to dendritic cell-specific ICAM-grabbing nonintegrin (DC-SIGN). Six Fabs with distinct relative affinities and epitope specificities were characterized. The Fabs and those selected for conversion to IgG were tested for their ability to block ligand (HIV gp120, Ebola gp, and ICAM-3) binding. Receptor internalization upon Fab binding was evaluated on primary human liver sinusoidal endothelial cells by flow cytometry and confirmed by confocal microscopy. Although all six Fabs internalized, three Fabs that showed the most complete blocking of HIVgp120 and ICAM-3 binding to L-SIGN also internalized most efficiently. Differences among the Fab panel in the ability to efficiently block Ebola gp compared with HIVgp120 suggested distinct binding sites. As a first step to consider the potential of these Abs for Ab-mediated Ag delivery, we evaluated specific peptide delivery to human dendritic cells. A durable human T cell response was induced when a tetanus toxide epitope embedded into a L-SIGN/DC-SIGN-cross-reactive Ab was targeted to dendritic cells. We believe that the isolated Abs may be useful for selective delivery of Ags to DC-SIGN- or L-SIGN-bearing APCs for the modulation of immune responses and for blocking viral infections.

PMID: 16365436 [PubMed - indexed for MEDLINE]

1708. J Virol. 2006 Jan;80(2):1038-43.

Rescue of recombinant Marburg virus from cDNA is dependent on nucleocapsid protein VP30.

Enterlein S(1), Volchkov V, Weik M, Kolesnikova L, Volchkova V, Klenk HD, Mühlberger E.

Author information: (1)Department of Virology, Philipps University Marburg, Robert-Koch-Str. 17, 35037 Marburg, Germany.

Here we report recovery of infectious Marburg virus (MARV) from a full-length cDNA clone. Compared to the wild-type virus, recombinant MARV showed no difference in terms of morphology of virus particles, intracellular distribution in infected cells, and growth kinetics. The nucleocapsid protein VP30 of MARV and Ebola virus (EBOV) contains a Zn-binding motif which is important for the function of VP30 as a transcriptional activator in EBOV, whereas its role for MARV is unclear. It has been reported previously that MARV VP30 is able to support transcription in an EBOV-specific minigenome system. When the Zn-binding motif was destroyed, MARV VP30 was shown to be inactive in the EBOV system. While it was not possible to rescue recombinant MARV when the VP30 plasmid was omitted from transfection, MARV VP30 with a destroyed Zn-binding motif and EBOV VP30 were able to mediate virus recovery. In contrast, rescue of recombinant EBOV was not supported by EBOV VP30 containing a mutated Zn-binding domain.

PMCID: PMC1346851 PMID: 16379005 [PubMed - indexed for MEDLINE]

1709. J Virol. 2006 Jan;80(1):460-73.

Nonstructural protein 3 of bluetongue virus assists virus release by recruiting ESCRT-I protein Tsg101.

Wirblich C(1), Bhattacharya B, Roy P.

Author information: (1)Department of Infectious and Tropical Diseases, London School of Hygiene and Tropical Medicine, London, United Kingdom.

The release of Bluetongue virus (BTV) and other members of the Orbivirus genus from infected host cells occurs predominantly by cell lysis, and in some cases, by budding from the plasma membrane. Two nonstructural proteins, NS3 and NS3A, have been implicated in this process. Here we show that both proteins bind to human Tsg101 and its ortholog from Drosophila melanogaster with similar strengths in vitro. This interaction is mediated by a conserved PSAP motif in NS3 and appears to play a role in virus release. The depletion of Tsg101 with small interfering RNA inhibits the release of BTV and African horse sickness virus, a related orbivirus, from HeLa cells up to fivefold and threefold, respectively. Like most other viral proteins which recruit Tsg101, NS3 also harbors a PPXY late-domain motif that allows NS3 to bind NEDD4-like ubiquitin ligases in vitro. However, the late-domain motifs in NS3 do not function as effectively in facilitating the release of mini Gag virus-like particles from 293T cells as the late domains from human immunodeficiency virus type 1, human T-cell leukemia virus, and Ebola virus. A mutagenesis study showed that the arginine residue in the PPRY motif is responsible for the low activity of the NS3 late-domain motifs. Our data suggest that the BTV late-domain motifs either recruit an antagonist that interferes with budding or fail to recruit an agonist which is different from NEDD4.

PMCID: PMC1317520 PMID: 16352570 [PubMed - indexed for MEDLINE]

1710. Med Sci (Paris). 2006 Jan;22(1):78-9.

[Bats, reserves of the Ebola virus: the mystery is dissipated].

[Article in French]

Leroy E(1), Pourrut X, Gonzalez JP.

Author information: (1)Institut de Recherche pour le Développement (IRD), UR178, Centre International de Recherches Médicales de Franceville, BP769, Gabon. Eric.Leroy@ird.fr

PMID: 16386226 [PubMed - indexed for MEDLINE]

1711. PLoS Pathog. 2006 Jan;2(1):e1. Epub 2006 Jan 13.

Gene-specific countermeasures against Ebola virus based on antisense phosphorodiamidate morpholino oligomers.

Warfield KL(1), Swenson DL, Olinger GG, Nichols DK, Pratt WD, Blouch R, Stein DA, Aman MJ, Iversen PL, Bavari S.

Author information: (1)US Army Medical Research Institute of Infectious Diseases, Fort Detrick, Frederick, Maryland, USA.

The filoviruses Marburg virus and Ebola virus (EBOV) quickly outpace host immune responses and cause hemorrhagic fever, resulting in case fatality rates as high as 90% in humans and nearly 100% in nonhuman primates. The development of an effective therapeutic for EBOV is a daunting public health challenge and is hampered by a paucity of knowledge regarding filovirus pathogenesis. This report describes a successful strategy for interfering with EBOV infection using antisense phosphorodiamidate morpholino oligomers (PMOs). A combination of EBOV-specific PMOs targeting sequences of viral mRNAs for the viral proteins (VPs) VP24, VP35, and RNA polymerase L protected rodents in both pre- and post-exposure therapeutic regimens. In a prophylactic proof-of-principal trial, the PMOs also protected 75% of rhesus macaques from lethal EBOV infection. The work described here may contribute to development of designer, "druggable" countermeasures for filoviruses and other microbial pathogens.

PMCID: PMC1326218 PMID: 16415982 [PubMed - indexed for MEDLINE]

1712. Trop Doct. 2006 Jan;36(1):1-4.

A clinical guide to viral haemorrhagic fevers: Ebola, Marburg and Lassa.

Jeffs B(1).

Author information: (1)Medicens Sans Frontieres, Spain. BENJAMIN.JEFFS@lshtm.ac.uk

The viral haemorrhagic fevers are a group of diseases that share many clinical features. Ebola, Marburg and Lassa are diseases that cause a relatively small number of deaths globally, but pose special risks to medical staff due to the ease of transmission, and can have a profound impact to the communities they affect. This article gives a brief overview of diseases caused by the Ebola, Marburg and Lassa viruses. It gives some practical advice to the clinician on the diagnosis and management of these diseases.

PMID: 16483416 [PubMed - indexed for MEDLINE]

1713. Vector Borne Zoonotic Dis. 2006 Winter;6(4):315-24.

Public health awareness of emerging zoonotic viruses of bats: a European perspective.

van der Poel WH(1), Lina PH, Kramps JA.

Author information: (1)Animal Sciences Group, Wageningen University Research, Lelystad, The Netherlands. wim.vanderpoel@wur.nl

Bats classified in the order Chiroptera are the most abundant and widely distributed non-human mammalian species in the world. Several bat species are reservoir hosts of zoonotic viruses and therefore can be a public health hazard. Lyssaviruses of different genotypes have emerged from bats in America (Genotype 1 rabies virus; RABV), Europe (European bat lyssavirus; EBLV), and Australia (Australian bat lyssavirus; ABLV), whereas Nipah virus is the most important recent zoonosis of bat origin in Asia. Furthermore, some insectivorous bat species may be important reservoirs of SARS coronavirus, whereas Ebola virus has been detected in some megachiropteran fruit bats. Thus far, European bat lyssavirus (EBLV) is the only zoonotic virus that has been detected in bats in Europe. New zoonotic viruses may emerge from bat reservoirs and known ones may spread to a wider geographical range. To assess future threats posed by zoonotic viruses of bats, there is a need for accurate knowledge of the factors underlying disease emergence, for an effective surveillance programme, and for a rapid response system. In Europe, primary efforts should be focussed on the implementation of effective passive and active surveillance systems for

EBLVs in the Serotine bat, Eptesicus serotinus, and Myotis species (i.e., M. daubentonii and M. dasycneme). Apart from that, detection methods for zoonotic viruses that may emerge from bats should be implemented. Analyses of data from surveillance studies can shed more light on the dynamics of bat viruses, (i.e., population persistence of viruses in bats). Subsequently, studies will have to be performed to assess the public health hazards of such viruses (i.e., infectivity and risk of infection to people). With the knowledge generated from this kind of research, a rapid response system can be set up to enhance public health awareness of emerging zoonotic viruses of bats.

PMID: 17187565 [PubMed - indexed for MEDLINE]

1714. Viral Immunol. 2006 Winter;19(4):602-12.

Filoviruses and the balance of innate, adaptive, and inflammatory responses.

Mohamadzadeh M(1), Chen L, Olinger GG, Pratt WD, Schmaljohn AL.

Author information: (1)US Army Medical Research Institute for Infectious Diseases, Frederick, MD 21702, USA. mansour.mohamadzadeh@det.amedd.army.mil

The Filoviruses Marburg virus and Ebola virus are among the deadliest of human pathogens, causing fulminant hemorrhagic fevers typified by overmatched specific immune responses and profuse inflammatory responses. Keys to both vaccination and treatment may reside, first, in the understanding of immune dysfunctions that parallel Filoviral disease and, second, in devising ways to redirect and restore normal immune function as well as to mitigate inflammation. Here, we describe how Filoviral infections may subvert innate immune responses through perturbances of dendritic cells and neutrophils, with particular emphasis on the downstream effects on adaptive immunity and inflammation. We suggest that pivotal events may be subject to therapeutic intervention as Filoviruses encounter immune processes.

PMID: 17201655 [PubMed - indexed for MEDLINE]

1715. Br Med Bull. 2005 Dec 22;73-74:123-37. Print 2005.

Lessons from nosocomial viral haemorrhagic fever outbreaks.

Fisher-Hoch SP(1).

Author information: (1)Department of Epidemiology, University of Texas Houston Health Science Center, School of Public Health, Brownsville Campus, Brownsville, TX, USA susan.p.fisher-hoch@utb.edu

The outbreak of Marburg haemorrhagic fever in Angola in 2004-2005 shows once again the devastating and rapid spread of viral haemorrhagic fevers in medical settings where hygiene practices are poorly applied or ignored. The legacy of years of war and poverty in Angola has resulted in very poor medical education and services. The initial high rate of infection among infants in Angola may have been related to poor hospital practices, possibly administration of vaccines. Though the outbreak in Angola was in a part of Africa not previously known to have filovirus infection, prior ecological modelling had predicted this location and many others. Prevention of future outbreaks will not be easy. The urgent need is dissemination of knowledge and the training, discipline and resources for good clinical practice. Educating the public to demand higher standards could be a powerful tool. Good practices are difficult to establish and maintain on the scale needed.

PMID: 16373655 [PubMed - indexed for MEDLINE]

1716. Virol J. 2005 Dec 20;2:92.

Packaging of actin into Ebola virus VLPs.

Han Z(1), Harty RN.

Author information: (1)Department of Pathobiology, School of Veterinary Medicine, University of Pennsylvania, Philadelphia, PA 19104, USA. ziyinghan@yahoo.com

The actin cytoskeleton has been implicated in playing an important role assembly and budding of several RNA virus families including retroviruses and paramyxoviruses. In this report, we sought to determine whether actin is incorporated into Ebola VLPs, and thus may play a role in assembly and/or budding of Ebola virus. Our results indicated that actin and Ebola virus VP40 strongly co-localized in transfected cells as determined by confocal microscopy. In addition, actin was packaged into budding VP40 VLPs as determined by a functional budding assay and protease protection assay. Co-expression of a membrane-anchored form of Ebola virus GP enhanced the release of both VP40 and actin in VLPs. Lastly, disruption of the actin cytoskeleton with latrunculin-A suggests that actin may play a functional role in budding of VP40/GP VLPs. These data suggest that VP40 may interact with cellular actin, and that actin may play a role in assembly and/or budding of Ebola VLPs.

PMCID: PMC1334228 PMID: 16367999 [PubMed - indexed for MEDLINE]

1717. Curr Drug Targets Infect Disord. 2005 Dec;5(4):307-400.

Developments in antiviral drug design, discovery and development in 2004.

Meanwell NA(1), Belema M, Carini DJ, D'Andrea SV, Kadow JF, Krystal M, Naidu BN, Regueiro-Ren A, Scola PM, Sit SY, Walker MA, Wang T, Yeung KS.

Author information: (1)Department of Chemistry, The Bristol-Myers Squibb Pharmaceutical Research Institute, Wallingford, CT 06492, USA. Nicholas.Meanwell@bms.com

This article summarizes key aspects of progress made during 2004 toward the design, discovery and development of antiviral agents for clinical use. Important developments in the identification, characterization and clinical utility of inhibitors of human immunodeficiency virus; the hepatitis viruses, hepatitis B, hepatitis C; the herpes family of viruses, herpes simplex viruses 1 and 2, varicella zoster virus, Epstein-Barr virus and human cytomegalovirus; the respiratory viruses, influenza, respiratory syncytial virus, human metapneumovirus, picornaviruses, measles and the severe acute respiratory syndrome coronavirus; human papilloma virus; rotavirus; Ebola virus and West Nile virus, are reviewed.

PMID: 16535860 [PubMed - indexed for MEDLINE]

1718. Curr Mol Med. 2005 Dec;5(8):761-72.

Ebola and Marburg viruses: pathogenesis and development of countermeasures.

Hensley LE(1), Jones SM, Feldmann H, Jahrling PB, Geisbert TW.

Author information: (1)Virology Division, U.S. Army Medical Research Institute of Infectious Diseases, 1425 Porter Street, Fort Detrick, MD 21702-5011, USA.

Ebola and Marburg viruses, family Filoviridae, are among the best known examples of emerging and re-emerging pathogens. Although outbreaks have been sporadic and geographically restricted to areas of Central Africa, the hemorrhagic fevers caused by these viruses are remarkably severe and are associated with high case fatality rates often exceeding 80 percent. In addition to humans, these viruses have decimated populations of wild apes in Central Africa. Currently, there are no vaccines or effective therapies available for human use. Progress in understanding the geneses of the pathophysiological changes that make filoviral infections of humans so destructive has been slow, primarily because these viruses require special containment for safe research. However, an increasing understanding of the molecular mechanisms of filoviral pathogenesis, facilitated by the development of new tools to elucidate critical regulatory elements in the viral life cycle, is providing new targets that can be exploited for therapeutic interventions. In addition, substantial progress has been made in developing recombinant vaccines against these viruses.

PMID: 16375711 [PubMed - indexed for MEDLINE]

1719. Nature. 2005 Dec 1;438(7068):575-6.

Fruit bats as reservoirs of Ebola virus.

Leroy EM(1), Kumulungui B, Pourrut X, Rouquet P, Hassanin A, Yaba P, Délicat A, Paweska JT, Gonzalez JP, Swanepoel R.

Author information: (1)Centre International de Recherches Médicales de Franceville, BP 769 Franceville, Gabon. eric.leroy@ird.fr

The first recorded human outbreak of Ebola virus was in 1976, but the wild reservoir of this virus is still unknown. Here we test for Ebola in more than a thousand small vertebrates that were collected during Ebola outbreaks in humans and great apes between 2001 and 2003 in Gabon and the Republic of the Congo. We find evidence of asymptomatic infection by Ebola virus in three species of fruit bat, indicating that these animals may be acting as a reservoir for this deadly virus.

PMID: 16319873 [PubMed - indexed for MEDLINE]

1720. Nihon Rinsho. 2005 Dec;63(12):2161-6.

[Clinical aspects of viral hemorrhagic fever].

[Article in Japanese]

Saijo M(1).

Author information: (1)Department of Virology I, National Institute of Infectious Diseases.

Viral hemorrhagic fever (VHF) is defined as virus infections that usually cause pyrexia and hemorrhagic symptoms with multiple organ failure. VHF includes following viral infections: Ebola hemorrhagic fever (EHF), Marburg hemorrhagic fever (MHF), Crimean-Congo hemorrhagic fever (CCHF) and Lassa fever. In particular, the causative agents of EHF, MHF, CCHF, and Lassa fever are Ebola, Marburg, CCHF, Lassa viruses, respectively, and regarded as biosafety level-4 pathogens because of their high virulence to humans. Recently, relatively large outbreaks of EHF and MHF have occurred in Africa, and areas of EHF- and MHF-outbreaks seem to be expanding. Although outbreaks of VHF have not been reported in Japan, there is a possibility that the deadly hemorrhagic fever viruses would be introduced to Japan in future. Therefore, preparedness for possible future outbreaks of VHF is necessary in areas without VHF outbreaks.

PMID: 16363689 [PubMed - indexed for MEDLINE]

1721. Nihon Rinsho. 2005 Dec;63(12):2154-60.

[Countermeasure against viral hemorrhagic fever at the border in Japan].

[Article in Japanese]

Iwasaki E(1).

Author information: (1)Sendai Quarantine Station.

Human have struggled against many infectious diseases such as cholera, plague, dysentery and yellow fever for a long time. And we have spent a lot of energy to control these infectious diseases and developed various tool for them. One of these efforts was Quarantine system that was established in 14th century in Europe. But during recent days, we are suffering from newly emerged diseases. These new infectious diseases are zoonosis and most of them are serious and highly infectious. Viral hemorrhagic fever such as Ebola hemorrhagic fever, Marburg hemorrhagic fever and Lassa fever are typical these emerging serious diseases, and these outbreak always have occurred in Africa and neighboring countries. Fortunately we have never experienced any case, but as these diseases are so serious, we are so nervous diseases entering in Japan. Against these serious diseases, in Japan, Quarantine Station are doing screening examination at airport and port by questionnaire and measuring body temperature, because these viral hemorrhagic fever patients show high fever. If people were suspected viral hemorrhagic fever at Quarantine Station at the border, they will be leaded to hospital for further examination and treatment as soon as possible.

PMID: 16363688 [PubMed - indexed for MEDLINE]

1722. Immunogenetics. 2005 Nov;57(10):730-8. Epub 2005 Nov 8.

Analysis of the expressed heavy chain variable-region genes of Macaca fascicularis and isolation of monoclonal antibodies specific for the Ebola virus' soluble glycoprotein.

Druar C(1), Saini SS, Cossitt MA, Yu F, Qiu X, Geisbert TW, Jones S, Jahrling PB, Stewart DI, Wiersma EJ.

Author information: (1)Cangene Corporation, 3404 American Drive, Mississauga, Ontario L4V 1T4, Canada.

The cynomolgus macaque, Macaca fascicularis, is frequently used in immunological and other biomedical research as a model for man; understanding it's antibody repertoire is, therefore, of fundamental interest. The expressed variable-region gene repertoire of a single M. fascicularis, which was immune to the Ebola virus, was studied. Using 5' rapid amplification of cDNA ends with immunoglobulin (Ig)G-specific primers, we obtained 30 clones encoding full-length variable, diversity, and joining domains. Similar to the human V(H) repertoire, the M. fascicularis repertoire utilized numerous immunoglobulin heavy variable (IGHV) gene fragments, with the V(H)3 (41%), V(H)4 (39%), and V(H)1 (14%) subgroups used more frequently than the V(H)5 (3.9%) or V(H)7 (1.7%) subgroups. Diverse immunoglobulin heavy joining (IGHJ) fragments also appeared to be utilized, including a putative homolog of JH5beta gene segment identified in the related species Macaca mulatta, Rhesus macaque, but not in humans. Although the diverse V region genes in the IgG antibody repertoire of M. fascicularis had likely undergone somatic hypermutations (SHMs), they nevertheless showed high nucleotide identity with the corresponding human germline genes, 80-89% for IGHV and 72-92% for IGHJ. M. fascicularis and human V(H) genes were also similar in other aspects: length of complementarity-determining regions and framework regions, and distribution of consensus sites for SHMs. Finally, we demonstrated that monoclonal antibodies (mAbs) specific for an Ebola protein could be obtained from M. fascicularis tissue samples by phage display technology. In summary, the study provides new insight into the M. fascicularis V region gene repertoire and further supports the idea that macaque-derived mAbs may be of therapeutic value to humans.

PMID: 16215733 [PubMed - indexed for MEDLINE]

1723. J Clin Invest. 2005 Nov;115(11):3256-64. Epub 2005 Oct 20.

Lewis X component in human milk binds DC-SIGN and inhibits HIV-1 transfer to CD4+ T lymphocytes.

Naarding MA(1), Ludwig IS, Groot F, Berkhout B, Geijtenbeek TB, Pollakis G, Paxton WA.

Author information: (1)Department of Human Retrovirology, Academic Medical Center, University of Amsterdam, Amsterdam, The Netherlands.

DC-specific ICAM3-grabbing non-integrin (DC-SIGN), which is expressed on DCs, can interact with a variety of pathogens such as HIV-1, hepatitis C, Ebola, cytomegalovirus, Dengue virus, Mycobacterium, Leishmania, and Candida albicans. We demonstrate that human milk can inhibit the DC-SIGN-mediated transfer of HIV-1 to CD4+ T lymphocytes as well as viral transfer by both immature and mature DCs. The inhibitory factor directly interacted with DC-SIGN and prevented the HIV-1 gp120 envelope protein from binding to the receptor. The human milk proteins lactoferrin, alpha-lactalbumin, lysozyme, beta-casein, and secretory leukocyte protease inhibitor did not bind DC-SIGN or demonstrate inhibition of viral transfer. The inhibitory effect could be fully alleviated with an Ab recognizing the Lewis X (LeX) sugar epitope, commonly found in human milk. LeX in polymeric form or conjugated to protein could mimic the inhibitory activity, whereas free LeX sugar epitopes could not. We reveal that a LeX motif present in human milk can bind to DC-SIGN and thereby prevent the capture and subsequent transfer of HIV-1 to CD4+ T lymphocytes. The presence of such a DC-SIGN-binding molecule in human milk may both influence antigenic presentation and interfere with pathogen transfer in breastfed infants.

PMCID: PMC1257537 PMID: 16239964 [PubMed - indexed for MEDLINE]

1724. J Virol. 2005 Nov;79(22):14244-52.

Predicted inactivation of viruses of relevance to biodefense by solar radiation.

Lytle CD(1), Sagripanti JL.

Author information: (1)Edgewood Chemical Biological Center, U.S. Army, Aberdeen Proving Ground, Maryland 21010-5424, USA.

UV radiation from the sun is the primary germicide in the environment. The goal of this study was to estimate inactivation of viruses by solar exposure. We reviewed published reports on 254-nm UV inactivation and tabulated the sensitivities of a wide variety of viruses, including those with double-stranded DNA, single-stranded DNA, double-stranded RNA, or single-stranded RNA genomes. We calculated D(37) values (fluence producing on average one lethal hit per virion and reducing viable virus to 37%) from all available data. We defined size-normalized sensitivity (SnS) by multiplying UV(254) sensitivities (D(37) values) by the genome size, and SnS values were relatively constant for viruses with similar genetic composition. In addition, SnS values were similar for complete virions and their defective particles, even when the corresponding D(37) values were significantly different. We used SnS to estimate the UV(254) sensitivities of viruses for which the genome composition and size were known but no UV inactivation data were available, including smallpox virus, Ebola, Marburg, Crimean-Congo, Junin, and other hemorrhagic viruses, and Venezuelan equine encephalitis and other encephalitis viruses. We compiled available data on virus inactivation as a function of wavelength and calculated a composite action spectrum that allowed extrapolation from the 254-nm data to solar UV. We combined our estimates of virus sensitivity with solar measurements at different geographical locations to predict virus inactivation. Our predictions agreed with the available experimental data. This work should be a useful step to understanding and eventually predicting the survival of viruses after their release in the environment.

PMCID: PMC1280232 PMID: 16254359 [PubMed - indexed for MEDLINE]

1725. J Virol. 2005 Nov;79(22):14189-96.

Protective cytotoxic T-cell responses induced by venezuelan equine encephalitis virus replicons expressing Ebola virus proteins.

Olinger GG(1), Bailey MA, Dye JM, Bakken R, Kuehne A, Kondig J, Wilson J, Hogan RJ, Hart MK.

Author information: (1)United States Army Medical Research Institute of Infectious Diseases, Division of Virology, 1425 Porter Street, Frederick, MD 21702-5011, USA.

Infection with Ebola virus causes a severe disease accompanied by high mortality rates, and there are no licensed vaccines or therapies available for human use. Filovirus vaccine research efforts still need to determine the roles of humoral and cell-mediated immune responses in protection from Ebola virus infection. Previous studies indicated that exposure to Ebola virus proteins expressed from packaged Venezuelan equine encephalitis virus replicons elicited protective immunity in mice and that antibody-mediated protection could only be demonstrated after vaccination against the glycoprotein. In this study, the murine CD8(+) T-cell responses to six Ebola virus proteins were examined. CD8(+) T cells specific for Ebola virus glycoprotein, nucleoprotein, and viral proteins (VP24, VP30, VP35, and VP40) were identified by intracellular cytokine assays using splenocytes from vaccinated mice. The cells were expanded by restimulation with peptides and demonstrated cytolytic activity. Adoptive transfer of the CD8(+) cytotoxic T cells protected filovirus naïve mice from challenge with Ebola virus. These data support a role for CD8(+) cytotoxic T cells as part of a protective mechanism induced by vaccination against six Ebola virus proteins and provide additional evidence that cytotoxic T-cell responses can contribute to protection from filovirus infections.

PMCID: PMC1280180 PMID: 16254354 [PubMed - indexed for MEDLINE]

1726. PLoS Biol. 2005 Nov;3(11):e371. Epub 2005 Oct 25.

Wave-like spread of Ebola Zaire.

Walsh PD(1), Biek R, Real LA.

Author information: (1)Max-Planck-Institute for Evolutionary Primatology, Leipzig, Germany. walsh@eva.mpg.de

In the past decade the Zaire strain of Ebola virus (ZEBOV) has emerged repeatedly into human populations in central Africa and caused massive die-offs of gorillas and chimpanzees. We tested the view that emergence events are independent and caused by ZEBOV variants that have been long resident at each locality. Phylogenetic analyses place the earliest known outbreak at Yambuku, Democratic Republic of Congo, very near to the root of the ZEBOV tree, suggesting that viruses causing all other known outbreaks evolved from a Yambuku-like virus after 1976. The tendency for earlier outbreaks to be directly ancestral to later outbreaks suggests that outbreaks are epidemiologically linked and may have occurred at the front of an advancing wave. While the ladder-like phylogenetic structure could also bear the signature of positive selection, our statistical power is too weak to reach a conclusion in this regard. Distances among outbreaks indicate a spread rate of about 50 km per year that remains consistent across spatial scales. Viral evolution is clocklike, and sequences show a high level of small-scale spatial structure. Genetic similarity decays with distance at roughly the same rate at all spatial scales. Our analyses suggest that ZEBOV has recently spread across the region rather than being long persistent at each outbreak locality. Controlling the impact of Ebola on wild apes and human populations may be more feasible than previously recognized.

PMCID: PMC1262627 PMID: 16231972 [PubMed - indexed for MEDLINE]

1727. Wkly Epidemiol Rec. 2005 Oct 28;80(43):370-5.

Outbreak of Ebola haemorrhagic fever in Yambio, south Sudan, April - June 2004.

[Article in English, French]

[No authors listed]

PMID: 16285261 [PubMed - indexed for MEDLINE]

1728. Virology. 2005 Oct 25;341(2):179-89. Epub 2005 Aug 10.

Homo-oligomerization facilitates the interferon-antagonist activity of the ebolavirus VP35 protein.

Reid SP(1), Cárdenas WB, Basler CF.

Author information: (1)Department of Microbiology, Box 1124, Mount Sinai School of Medicine, 1 Gustave L. Levy Place, New York, NY 10029, USA.

We have identified a putative coiled-coil motif within the amino-terminal half of the ebolavirus VP35 protein. Cross-linking studies demonstrated the ability of VP35 to form trimers, consistent with the presence of a functional coiled-coil motif. VP35 mutants lacking the coiled-coil motif or possessing a mutation designed to disrupt coiled-coil function were defective in oligomerization, as deduced by co-immunoprecipitation studies. VP35 inhibits signaling that activates interferon regulatory factor 3 (IRF-3) and inhibits (IFN)-alpha/beta production. Experiments comparing the ability of VP35 mutants to block IFN responses demonstrated that the VP35 amino-terminus, which retains the putative coiled-coil motif, was unable to inhibit IFN responses, whereas the VP35 carboxy-terminus weakly inhibited the activation of IFN responses. IFN-antagonist function was restored when a heterologous trimerization motif was fused to the carboxy-terminal half of VP35, suggesting that an oligomerization function at the amino-terminus facilitates an "IFN-antagonist" function exerted by the carboxy-terminal half of VP35.

PMCID: PMC3955989 PMID: 16095644 [PubMed - indexed for MEDLINE]

1729. Crit Care Clin. 2005 Oct;21(4):765-83, vii.

Hemorrhagic fever viruses.

Pigott DC(1).

Author information: (1)Department of Emergency Medicine, The University of Alabama at Birmingham, 619 South 19th Street, Birmingham, AL 35249-7013, USA. dpigott@uabmc.edu

This article reviews the epidemiology, pathophysiology, and clinical management of patients with suspected or confirmed viral hemorrhagic fever infection. The focus is on clinical management based on case series from naturally occuring outbreaks of viral hemorrhagic fever infection as well as imported cases of viral hemorrhagic fever encountered in industrialized nations. The potential risk of bioterrorism involving these agents is discussed as well as emergency department and critical care management of isolated cases or larger outbreaks. Important aspects of management, including recognition of infected patients, isolation and decontamination procedures, as well as available vaccines and therapies are emphasized.

PMID: 16168314 [PubMed - indexed for MEDLINE]

1730. J Transcult Nurs. 2005 Oct;16(4):289-97.

Providing care and facing death: nursing during Ebola outbreaks in central Africa.

Hewlett BL(1), Hewlett BS.

Author information: (1)Oregon State University, USA.

Few studies have focused on describing the experiences of health care workers during rapid killing epidemics. In this article, the views and experiences of nurses during three outbreaks of Ebola hemorrhagic fever (EHF) in Central Africa are examined. These three outbreaks occurred in Kikwit, Democratic Republic of Congo (DRC, 1995); Gulu, Uganda (2000-2001); and Republic of Congo (ROC, 2003). Open-ended and semistructured interviews with individuals and small groups were conducted during the outbreaks in Uganda and ROC; data from DRC are extracted from published sources. Three key themes emerged from the interviews: (a) lack of protective gear, basic equipment, and other resources necessary to provide care, especially during the early phases of the outbreaks; (b) stigmatization by family, coworkers, and community; and (c) exceptional commitment to the nursing profession in a context where the lives of the health care workers were in jeopardy.
PMID: 16160191 [PubMed - indexed for MEDLINE]

1731. J Vet Med Educ. 2005 Fall;32(3):342-4.
Developing scientist leaders for tumultuous times.
Woteki CE(1).

Author information: (1)College of Agriculture, Iowa State University, 138 Curtiss Hall, Ames, IA 50011-1050, USA.

Leadership is a quality that can be learned. It is a behavior that one practices, and, after lots of practice, it becomes a habit. This is a lesson I learned from my father, who was a career pilot in the US Air Force and instilled this into me and my siblings from a very early age. It is also something I have learned in observing others. I have frequently asked why some people from certain disciplinary backgrounds seem to have an advantage in the leadership area. Think of the backgrounds of our Presidents, for example; so many of them have been attorneys. Members of Congress, as well, also frequently come from that disciplinary background. Key decision makers in government frequently come from economics backgrounds. I have also asked why this is the case. Frequently, the answer seems to be that these disciplines define themselves as being those that create leaders, not that they limit their members' aspirations. Why are so few veterinarians in leadership positions? It seems quite a paradox that they are not. The assets of an education in veterinary medicine are many. The education provides a very broad background in systems biology, medicine, and public health. There are many career paths for veterinarians. Most choose private practice, but, beyond that, career paths exist in industry, particularly the biomedical industry; in trade associations; in government and industry research; and in public health and regulatory positions. There are also many opportunities in academia, certainly in colleges of veterinary medicine but, beyond that, also in human medicine and in the biology disciplines. International opportunities also exist in governmental and non-governmental organizations, such as the Food and Agriculture Organization at the United Nations and the World Health Organization, and in advocacy and lobbying. Veterinarians are also making news these days. The emerging zoonotic diseases that have seized headlines in papers around the world give prominence to veterinarians and the skills they bring to bear in fighting current outbreaks and preventing future outbreaks of these diseases, such as SARS, Ebola, West Nile virus, and even HIV/AIDS.
PMID: 16261495 [PubMed - indexed for MEDLINE]

1732. Virus Res. 2005 Oct;113(1):16-25.
Complete genome sequence of an Ebola virus (Sudan species) responsible for a 2000 outbreak of human disease in Uganda.
Sanchez A(1), Rollin PE.

Author information: (1)Special Pathogens Branch, Division of Viral and Rickettsial Diseases, National Center for Infectious Diseases, Centers for Disease Control and Prevention, 1600 Clifton Road N.E., Building 15, Atlanta, GA 30333, USA. ASanchez1@cdc.gov

The entire genomic RNA of the Gulu (Uganda 2000) strain of Ebola virus was sequenced and compared to the genomes of other filoviruses. This data represents the first comprehensive genetic analysis for a representative isolate of the Sudan species of Ebola virus. The genome organization of the Sudan species is nearly identical to that of the Zaire species, but the presence of a gene overlap (between GP and VP30 genes) and a longer trailer sequence distinguish it from that of the Reston species. As has been observed with other filoviruses, stemloop structures were predicted to form at the 5' end of Ebola Sudan mRNA molecules, and the genomic RNA termini showed a high degree of sequence complimentarity. Comparisons of the amino acid sequences of encoded gene products shows that there is a comparable level of identity or similarity between Ebola virus species, with Sudan and Zaire actually showing a slightly closer relationship to the Reston species than to one another. These comparisons also indicated that the VP24 is the most conserved Ebola virus protein (followed closely by the VP40 and L proteins), while the GP is the least conserved gene product. The most divergent regions were seen in the C-terminus of GP1 (mucin-like region) and within the C-terminal third of the nucleoprotein sequence.
PMID: 16139097 [PubMed - indexed for MEDLINE]

1733. J Am Chem Soc. 2005 Sep 28;127(38):13126-7.
Inhibiting HIV fusion with a beta-peptide foldamer.
Stephens DM(1), Kim S, Welch BD, Hodsdon ME, Kay MS, Schepartz A.

Author information: (1)Department of Chemistry, , Yale University, New Haven, Connecticut 06520-8107, USA.

Linear peptides derived from the HIV gp41 C-terminus (C-peptides), such as the 36-residue Fuzeon, are potent HIV fusion inhibitors. These molecules bind to the N-peptide region of gp41 and inhibit an intramolecular protein-protein interaction that powers fusion of the viral and host cell membranes. The N-peptide region contains a surface pocket that is occupied in the post-fusion state by three alpha-helical residues found near the gp41 C-terminus: Trp628, Trp631, and Ile635- the WWI epitope. Here, we describe a set of beta3-decapeptides (betaWWI-1-4) in which the WWI epitope is presented on one face of a short 14-helix stabilized by macrodipole neutralization and side chain-side chain salt bridges. betaWWI-1-4 bind in vitro to IZN17, a validated gp41 model, and inhibit syncytia formation in cell culture. Molecules lacking a complete WWI functional epitope neither bind IZN17 nor inhibit syncytia formation. These results provide evidence that short beta-peptide 14-helices can inhibit an intramolecular protein-protein interaction in vivo. Molecules related to betaWWI-1-4 could represent starting points for the development of highly potent inhibitors or antigens effective against HIV or other viruses, including SARS, Ebola, HRSV, and influenza, that employ common fusion mechanisms.

PMCID: PMC2873035 PMID: 16173723 [PubMed - indexed for MEDLINE]

1734. Bull Soc Pathol Exot. 2005 Sep;98(3):244-54.

[Training the trainers seminar and analysis of the Ebola virus hemorrhagic fever outbreaks in central Africa from 2001 to 2004. (Brazzaville, Républic of Congo, April 6-8, 2004].

[Article in French]

Formenty P(1), Epelboin A, Allarangar Y, Libama F, Boumandouki P, Koné L, Molamou A, Gami N, Mombouli JV, Martinez MG, Ngampo S.

Author information: (1)OMS Genève, CDS/CSR/ARO, Suisse.

PMID: 16267969 [PubMed - indexed for MEDLINE]

1735. Bull Soc Pathol Exot. 2005 Sep;98(3):239-43.

Climate-based health monitoring systems for eco-climatic conditions associated with infectious diseases.

Pinzon E(1), Wilson JM, Tucker CJ.

Author information: (1)Science Systems and Applications, Inc. (SSAI), USA. Jorge.E.Pinzon.l@gsfc.nasa.gov

Despite a century of confidence and optimism in modern medicine and technology inspired by their often successful prevention and control efforts, infectious diseases remain an omnipresent, conspicuous major challenge to public health. Effective detection and control of infectious diseases require predictive and proactive efficient methods that provide early warning of an epidemic activity. Of particular relevance to these efforts is linking information at the landscape and coarser scales to data at the scale of the epidemic activity. In recent years, landscape epidemiology has used satellite remote sensing and geographic information systems as the technology capable of providing, from local to global scales, spatial and temporal climatic patterns that may influence the intensity of a vector-borne disease and predicts risk conditions associated with an epidemic. This article provides a condensed, and selective look at classical material and recent research about remote sensing and GIS (geographic information system) applications in public health.

PMID: 16267968 [PubMed - indexed for MEDLINE]

1736. Bull Soc Pathol Exot. 2005 Sep;98(3):237-8.

Ebola and great apes in Central Africa: current status and future needs.

Karesh W(1), Reed P.

Author information: (1)Field Veterinary Program Wildlife Conservation Society, 2300 Southern Blvd, Bronx, NY 10460, USA. wkaresh@wcs.org

PMID: 16267967 [PubMed - indexed for MEDLINE]

1737. Bull Soc Pathol Exot. 2005 Sep;98(3):230-6.

Medical anthropology and Ebola in Congo: cultural models and humanistic care.

Hewlett BS(1), Epelboin A, Hewlett BL, Formenty P.

Author information: (1)Department of Anthropology, Washington State University, 14204 NE Salmon Creek, Vancouver, WA 98686, USA. hewlett@vancouver.wsu.edu

Seldom have medical anthropologists been involved in efforts to control high mortality diseases such as Ebola hemorrhagic fever (EHF) This paper describes the results of two distinct but complementary interventions during the first phases of an outbreak in the Republic of Congo in 2003. The first approach emphasized understanding local peoples cultural models and political-economic explanations for the disease while the second approach focused on providing more humanitarian care of patients by identifying and incorporating local beliefs and practices into patient care and response efforts.

PMID: 16267966 [PubMed - indexed for MEDLINE]

1738. Bull Soc Pathol Exot. 2005 Sep;98(3):224-9.

[Multiple Ebola virus haemorrhagic fever outbreaks in Gabon, from October 2001 to April 2002].

[Article in French]

Nkoghe D(1), Formenty P, Leroy EM, Nnegue S, Edou SY, Ba JI, Allarangar Y, Cabore J, Bachy C, Andraghetti R, de Benoist AC, Galanis E, Rose A, Bausch D, Reynolds M, Rollin P, Choueibou C, Shongo R, Gergonne B, Koné LM, Yada A, Roth C, Mve MT.

Author information: (1)Ministère de la santé publique, Libreville, Gabon.

Outbreaks of Ebola virus haemorrhagic fever have been reported from 1994 to 1996 in the province of Ogooué Ivindo, a forest zone situated in the Northeast of Gabon. Each time, the great primates had been identified as the initial source of human infection. End of November 2001 a new alert came from this province, rapidly confirmed as a EVHV outbreak. The response was given by the Ministry of Health with the help of an international team under the aegis of WHO. An active monitoring system was implemented in the three districts hit by the epidemic (Zadié, Ivindo and Mpassa) to organize the detection of cases and their follow-up. A case definition has been set up, the suspected cases were isolated at hospital, at home or in lazarets and serological tests were performed. These tests consisted of the detection of antigen or specific IgG and the RT-PCR. A classification of cases was made according to the results of biological tests, clinical and epidemiological data. The contact subjects were kept watch over for 21 days. 65 cases were recorded among which 53 deaths. The first human case, a hunter died on the 28th of October 2001. The epidemic spreads over through family transmission and nosocomial contamination. Four distinct primary foci have been identified together with an isolated case situated in the South East of Gabon, 580 km away from the epicenter. Deaths happened within a delay of 6 days. The last death has been recorded on the 22nd of March 2002 and the end of the outbreak was declared on the 6th of May 2002. The epidemic spreads over the Gabon just next. Unexplained deaths of animals had been mentionned in the nearby forests as soon as August 2001: great primates and cephalophus. Samples taken from their carcasses confirmed a concomitant animal epidemic.

PMID: 16267965 [PubMed - indexed for MEDLINE]

1739. Bull Soc Pathol Exot. 2005 Sep;98(3):218-23.

[Clinical management of patients and deceased during the Ebola outbreak from October to December 2003 in Republic of Congo].

[Article in French]

Boumandouki P(1), Formenty P, Epelboin A, Campbell P, Atsangandoko C, Allarangar Y, Leroy EM, Kone ML, Molamou A, Dinga-Longa O, Salemo A, Kounkou RY, Mombouli V, Ibara JR, Gaturuku P, Nkunku S, Lucht A, Feldmann H.

Author information: (1)(Ministère de la santé et de la population, Brazzaville, Congo.

Outbreaks of Ebola virus hemorrhagic fever (EVHF) have been reported since 2001 in the Cuvette Ouest department, a forested area located in the Western North of Congo. At the end of October 2003 a new alarm came from this department which was quickly confirmed as being an epidemic of EVHF. The outbreak response was organized by the ministry of health with the assistance of an international team under the aegis of WHO. The case management of suspect cases was done in an isolation ward set up at the hospital; when patients refused to go to the ward for care they were isolated in their house according to a protocol "transmission risks reduction at home". Safe burials were performed by specialized teams which respected the major aspects of the funeral to allow the process of mourning of the families. An active surveillance system was set up in order to organize the detection of new cases and the follow-up of their contacts. A case definition was adopted. From October 11 to December 2, 2003, 35 cases including 29 deaths were reported, 16 cases were laboratory confirmed. The first four cases had been exposed to monkey meat (Cercopithecus nictitans). The epidemic spread was due to family transmission. The population interpretation of the disease, in particular questions around wizards and evil-minded persons, is a factor which must be taken into account by the medical teams during communication meetings for behavioral change of the populations. The case management of patient in isolation wards to prevent the transmission of the virus in the community remains the most effective means to dam up Ebola virus hemorrhagic fever outbreaks. The good perception by the community of the safe funerary procedures is an important aspect in the establishment of confidence relations with the local population.

PMID: 16267964 [PubMed - indexed for MEDLINE]

1740. Bull Soc Pathol Exot. 2005 Sep;98(3):210-7.

Ebola virus circulation in Africa: a balance between clinical expression and epidemiological silence.

Gonzalez JP(1), Herbreteau V, Morvan J, Leroy EM.

Author information: (1)Institut de recherche pour le développement (IRD), Unité de recherche 178.

Nearly thirty years after the first epidemics, Ebola virus (EBOV) remains hardly described, its transmission unclear and its reservoir elusive. Soon after the Ebola fever outbreak and virus discovery in 1976 and in order to investigate the distribution of EBOV in Central Africa, several countries including a range of ecological zones were investigated in the early 1980s, using extensive survey: Central African Republic (CAR), Cameroon, Chad, Congo, Gabon and Equatorial Guinea. Since 1992, ELISA antibody test along with a RT-PCR have been used to detect specific virus antibodies and characterize viral RNA. The widely separated geographic locations of outbreaks have suggested that the reservoir and the transmission cycle of EBOV are probably closely associated with the rain forest ecosystem, what is supported by the distribution of antibodies. The fact that outbreaks seldom occur suggests the presence of a rare or ecologically isolated animal reservoir having few contacts with humans and non-human primates. However various serological investigations showed a high prevalence in humans without any pathology reported. This suggests a circulation of both pathogenic and non-pathogenic strains as well as more frequent contacts with man than expected, and could partially explain fifteen years of Ebola fever silence between the emergence and re-emergence of Ebola virus in the Congolese basin. Nowadays, largely enlightened by the study of recent epizootic and epidemic manifestations of EBOV in Gabon and neighboring countries, EBOV natural history starts to be understood as for the fundamentals of epizootic in non-human primates and chains of transmission.

PMID: 16267963 [PubMed - indexed for MEDLINE]

1741. Bull Soc Pathol Exot. 2005 Sep;98(3):205-9.

Laboratory diagnosis of Ebola and Marburg hemorrhagic fever.

Grolla A(1), Lucht A, Dick D, Strong JE, Feldmann H.

Author information: (1)National Microbiology Laboratory, Public Health Agency of Canada, Winnipeg, Manitoba, Canada.

The control of Filovirus outbreaks can be greatly enhanced by timely laboratory confirmation of infection or the identification of alternative disease processes. The status of current laboratory diagnostics for Ebola and Marburg virus infections is discussed in terms of the assays available and their interpretation. In addition, the role of field-based laboratory support and its limitations and capabilities in an outbreak response setting, especially in regards to real-time PCR and immunofiltration assays, is presented.

PMID: 16267962 [PubMed - indexed for MEDLINE]

1742. J Gen Virol. 2005 Sep;86(Pt 9):2535-42.

Mannose-binding lectin binds to Ebola and Marburg envelope glycoproteins, resulting in blocking of virus interaction with DC-SIGN and complement-mediated virus neutralization.

Ji X(1), Olinger GG, Aris S, Chen Y, Gewurz H, Spear GT.

Author information: (1)Rush St Luke's Medical Center, Department of Immunology and Microbiology, 1653 W. Congress Parkway, Chicago, IL 60612, USA.

Mannose-binding lectin (MBL), a serum lectin that mediates innate immune functions including activation of the lectin complement pathway, binds to carbohydrates expressed on some viral glycoproteins. In this study, the ability of MBL to bind to virus particles pseudotyped with Ebola and Marburg envelope glycoproteins was evaluated. Virus particles bearing either Ebola (Zaire strain) or Marburg (Musoke strain) envelope glycoproteins bound at significantly higher levels to immobilized MBL compared with virus particles pseudotyped with vesicular stomatitis virus glycoprotein or with no virus glycoprotein. As observed in previous studies, Ebola-pseudotyped virus bound to cells expressing the lectin DC-SIGN (dendritic cell-specific intercellular adhesion molecule 3-grabbing non-integrin). However, pre-incubation of virus with MBL blocked DC-SIGN-mediated binding to cells, suggesting that the two lectins bind at the same or overlapping sites on the Ebola glycoprotein. Neutralization experiments showed that virus pseudotyped with Ebola or Marburg (Musoke) glycoprotein was neutralized by complement, while the Marburg (Ravn strain) glycoprotein-pseudotyped virus was less sensitive to neutralization. Neutralization was partially mediated through the lectin complement pathway, since a complement source deficient in MBL was significantly less effective at neutralizing viruses pseudotyped with filovirus glycoproteins and addition of purified MBL to the MBL-deficient complement increased neutralization. These experiments demonstrated that MBL binds to filovirus envelope glycoproteins resulting in important biological effects and suggest that MBL can interact with filoviruses during infection in humans.

PMID: 16099912 [PubMed - indexed for MEDLINE]

1743. J Virol. 2005 Sep;79(18):11742-51.

Rab9 GTPase is required for replication of human immunodeficiency virus type 1, filoviruses, and measles virus.

Murray JL(1), Mavrakis M, McDonald NJ, Yilla M, Sheng J, Bellini WJ, Zhao L, Le Doux JM, Shaw MW, Luo CC, Lippincott-Schwartz J, Sanchez A, Rubin DH, Hodge TW.

Author information: (1)National Center for HIV, STD, and TB Prevention, Centers for Disease Control and Prevention, Atlanta, Georgia 30333, USA.

Rab proteins and their effectors facilitate vesicular transport by tethering donor vesicles to their respective target membranes. By using gene trap insertional mutagenesis, we identified Rab9, which mediates late-endosome-to-trans-Golgi-network trafficking, among several candidate host genes whose disruption allowed the survival of Marburg virus-infected cells, suggesting that Rab9 is utilized in Marburg replication. Although Rab9 has not been implicated in human immunodeficiency virus (HIV) replication, previous reports suggested that the late endosome is an initiation site for HIV assembly and that TIP47-dependent trafficking out of the late endosome to the trans-Golgi network facilitates the sorting of HIV Env into virions budding at the plasma membrane. We examined the role of Rab9 in the life cycles of HIV and several unrelated viruses, using small interfering RNA (siRNA) to silence Rab9 expression before viral infection. Silencing Rab9 expression dramatically inhibited HIV replication, as did silencing the host genes encoding TIP47, p40, and PIKfyve, which also facilitate late-endosome-to-trans-Golgi vesicular transport. In addition, silencing studies revealed that HIV replication was dependent on the expression of Rab11A, which mediates trans-Golgi-to-plasma-membrane transport, and that increased HIV Gag was sequestered in a CD63+ endocytic compartment in a cell line stably expressing Rab9 siRNA. Replication of the enveloped Ebola, Marburg, and measles viruses was inhibited with Rab9 siRNA, although the non-enveloped reovirus was insensitive to Rab9 silencing. These results suggest that Rab9 is an important cellular target for inhibiting diverse viruses and help to define a late-endosome-to-plasma-membrane vesicular transport pathway important in viral assembly.

PMCID: PMC1212642 PMID: 16140752 [PubMed - indexed for MEDLINE]

1744. Med Trop (Mars). 2005 Sep;65(4):349-54.

[Isolated case of haemorrhagic fever observed in Gabon during the 2002 outbreak of Ebola but distant from epidemic zones].

[Article in French]

Nkoghe D(1), Nnegue S, Mve MT, Formenty P, Thompson G, Iba Ba J, Okome Nkoumou M, Leroy E.

Author information: (1)Ministère de la Santé Publique, Libreville, Gabon dnkoghe@hotmail.com

During the last outbreak of Ebola virus haemorrhagic fever that occurred concurrently in Gabon and Congo, several primary foci were identified in the Ogooue Ivindo province (Northeast Gabon), where previous outbreaks had occurred. A 48-year-old woman living in Franceville located 580 Km from the epicentre presented fever with haemorrhagic signs. She was evacuated to Libreville where Ebola infection was suspected. Diagnosis was confirmed at the Centre International de Recherches Médicales of Franceville on the basis of detection of specific antibodies. Symptoms had already subsided by the time diagnosis was documented. An epidemiological investigation was undertaken to identify the source of contamination and detect secondary cases. No human or nonhuman primate source of contamination could be formally identified. Direct contact with the virus reservoir could not be ruled out. No secondary cases were detected. The favourable outcome, absence of secondary, and failure to identify a source of contamination suggest that epidemiologically undefined cases may go unnoticed during and outside of outbreaks.

PMID: 16548488 [PubMed - indexed for MEDLINE]

1745. Nature. 2005 Sep 1;437(7055):20-2.

What the chimp means to me.

Pilcher H, Check E.

PMID: 16136103 [PubMed - indexed for MEDLINE]

1746. Vopr Virusol. 2005 Sep-Oct;50(5):25-9.

[Human recombinant antibodies to Ebola virus: preparation and characteristics].

[Article in Russian]

Tikunova NV, Batanova TA, Chepurnov AA.

Human recombinant antibodies against a purified Ebola virus (EV) lysate were selected from a combinatorial library of scFv-antibodies using the phage display technique. Nine unique antibodies were identified after sequencing the Vh- and Vl-genes encoding the selected antibodies. Solid-phase enzyme immunoassay (EIA) indicated that these antibodies were able to bind both inactivated and native EV. Immunoblotting showed that 6 antibodies identified nucleoprotein (NP), one antibody did VP24 and another antibody did VP40. One of the selected antibodies reacted with two EP proteins: VP24 and VP40. Solid-phase EIA demonstrated cross-reactivity with Marburg virus (MAR) and defined VP24 MAR as a target protein for the antibody.

PMID: 16250595 [PubMed - indexed for MEDLINE]

1747. Curr Opin Investig Drugs. 2005 Aug;6(8):823-30.

Therapy and prophylaxis of Ebola virus infections.

Feldmann H(1), Jones SM, Schnittler HJ, Geisbert T.

Author information: (1)Special Pathogens Program, National Microbiology Laboratory, Public Health Agency of Canada, Winnipeg, Canada. Heinz_Feldmann@phac-aspc.gc.ca

The first cases of Ebola hemorrhagic fever were reported from Sudan and Zaire (now Democratic Republic of the Congo) in 1976, but the virus has only received significant attention since 1995. Until recently, the development of therapeutics or vaccines was not considered a priority. The knowledge gained during the past decade on the biology and pathogenesis of Ebola virus has led to the development of therapeutic strategies that are currently being investigated. Considering the aggressive nature of Ebola infections, in particular the rapid and overwhelming viral burdens, early diagnosis will play a significant role in determining the success of any intervention strategy. Advanced understanding of the immune response has produced several vaccine candidates of which a few can be considered for further evaluation. This review will summarize and discuss the current therapeutic and prophylactic strategies for Ebola hemorrhagic fever.

PMID: 16121689 [PubMed - indexed for MEDLINE]

1748. Int J Biochem Cell Biol. 2005 Aug;37(8):1560-6. Epub 2005 Mar 7.

Ebola virus: the role of macrophages and dendritic cells in the pathogenesis of Ebola hemorrhagic fever.

Bray M(1), Geisbert TW.

Author information: (1)Biodefense Clinical Research Branch, Office of Clinical Research, National Institute of Allergy and Infectious Diseases, National Institutes of Health, Bethesda, MD 20892, USA. mbray@niaid.nih.gov

Ebola hemorrhagic fever is a severe viral infection characterized by fever, shock and coagulation defects. Recent studies in macaques show that major features of illness are caused by effects of viral replication on macrophages and dendritic cells. Infected macrophages produce proinflammatory cytokines, chemokines and tissue factor, attracting additional target cells and inducing vasodilatation, increased vascular permeability and disseminated intravascular coagulation. However, they cannot restrict viral replication, possibly because of suppression of interferon responses. Infected dendritic cells also secrete proinflammatory mediators, but cannot initiate antigen-specific responses. In consequence, virus disseminates to these and other cell types throughout the body, causing multifocal necrosis and a syndrome resembling septic shock. Massive "bystander" apoptosis of natural killer and T cells further impairs immunity. These findings suggest that modifying host responses would be an effective therapeutic strategy, and treatment of infected macaques with a tissue-factor inhibitor reduced both inflammation and viral replication and improved survival.

PMID: 15896665 [PubMed - indexed for MEDLINE]

1749. J Virol. 2005 Aug;79(16):10660-71.

The Ebola virus genomic replication promoter is bipartite and follows the rule of six.

Weik M(1), Enterlein S, Schlenz K, Mühlberger E.

Author information: (1)Department of Virology, Philipps University Marburg, Robert-Koch-Str.17, 35037 Marburg, Germany.

In this work we investigated the cis-acting signals involved in replication of Ebola virus (EBOV) genomic RNA. A set of mingenomes with mutant 3' ends were generated and used in a reconstituted replication and transcription system. Our results suggest that the EBOV genomic replication promoter is bipartite, consisting of a first element located within the leader region of the genome and a second, downstream element separated by a spacer region. While proper spacing of the two promoter elements is a prerequisite for replication, the nucleotide sequence of the spacer is not important. Replication activity was only observed when six or a multiple of six nucleotides were deleted or inserted, while all other changes in length abolished replication completely. These data indicate that the EBOV replication promoter obeys the rule of six, although the genome length is not divisible by six. The second promoter element is located in the 3' nontranslated region of the first gene and consists of eight UN5 hexamer repeats, where N is any nucleotide. However, three consecutive hexamers, which could be located anywhere within the promoter element, were sufficient to support replication as long as the hexameric phase was preserved. By using chemical modification assays, we could demonstrate that nucleotides 5 to 44 of the EBOV leader are involved in the formation of a stable secondary structure. Formation of the RNA stem-loop occurred independently of the presence of the trailer, indicating that a panhandle structure is not formed between the 3' and 5' ends.

PMCID: PMC1182658 PMID: 16051858 [PubMed - indexed for MEDLINE]

1750. J Virol. 2005 Aug;79(16):10442-50.

Effects of Ebola virus glycoproteins on endothelial cell activation and barrier function.

Wahl-Jensen VM(1), Afanasieva TA, Seebach J, Ströher U, Feldmann H, Schnittler HJ.

Author information: (1)Special Pathogens Program, National Microbiology Laboratory, Public Health Agency of Canada, Winnipeg, Manitoba.

Ebola virus causes severe hemorrhagic fever with high mortality rates in humans and nonhuman primates. Vascular instability and dysregulation are disease-decisive symptoms during severe infection. While the transmembrane glycoprotein GP(1,2) has been shown to cause endothelial cell destruction, the role of the soluble glycoproteins in pathogenesis is largely unknown; however, they are hypothesized to be of biological relevance in terms of target cell activation and/or increase of endothelial permeability. Here we show that virus-like particles (VLPs) consisting of the Ebola virus matrix protein VP40 and GP(1,2) were able to activate endothelial cells and induce a decrease in barrier function as determined by impedance spectroscopy and hydraulic conductivity measurements. In contrast, the soluble glycoproteins sGP and delta-peptide did not activate endothelial cells or change the endothelial barrier function. The VLP-induced decrease in barrier function was further enhanced by the cytokine tumor necrosis factor alpha (TNF-alpha), which is known to induce a long-lasting decrease in endothelial cell barrier function and is hypothesized to play a key role in Ebola virus pathogenesis. Surprisingly, sGP, but not delta-peptide, induced a recovery of endothelial barrier function following treatment with TNF-alpha. Our results demonstrate that Ebola virus GP(1,2) in its particle-associated form mediates endothelial cell activation and a decrease in endothelial cell barrier function. Furthermore, sGP, the major soluble glycoprotein of Ebola virus, seems to possess an anti-inflammatory role by protecting the endothelial cell barrier function.

PMCID: PMC1182673 PMID: 16051836 [PubMed - indexed for MEDLINE]

1751. J Virol. 2005 Aug;79(16):10300-7.

Ebola virus VP40 late domains are not essential for viral replication in cell culture.

Neumann G(1), Ebihara H, Takada A, Noda T, Kobasa D, Jasenosky LD, Watanabe S, Kim JH, Feldmann H, Kawaoka Y.

Author information: (1)Department of Pathobiological Sciences, School of Veterinary Medicine, University of Wisconsin-Madison, 2015 Linden Dr., Madison, WI 53706, USA.

Ebola virus particle formation and budding are mediated by the VP40 protein, which possesses overlapping PTAP and PPXY late domain motifs (7-PTAPPXY-13). These late domain motifs have also been found in the Gag proteins of retroviruses and the matrix proteins of rhabdo- and arenaviruses. While in vitro studies suggest a critical role for late domain motifs in the budding of these viruses, including Ebola virus, it remains unclear as to whether the VP40 late domains play a role in Ebola virus replication. Alteration of both late domain motifs drastically reduced VP40 particle formation in vitro. However, using reverse genetics, we were able to generate recombinant Ebola virus containing mutations in either or both of the late domains. Viruses containing mutations in one or both of their late domain motifs were attenuated by one log unit. Transmission and scanning electron microscopy did not reveal appreciable differences between the mutant and wild-type viruses released from infected cells. These findings indicate that the Ebola VP40 late domain motifs enhance virus replication but are not absolutely required for virus replication in cell culture.

PMCID: PMC1182630 PMID: 16051823 [PubMed - indexed for MEDLINE]

1752. Protein Sci. 2005 Aug;14(8):1975-92.

The intrinsically disordered C-terminal domain of the measles virus nucleoprotein interacts with the C-terminal domain of the phosphoprotein via two distinct sites and remains predominantly unfolded.

Bourhis JM(1), Receveur-Bréchot V, Oglesbee M, Zhang X, Buccellato M, Darbon H, Canard B, Finet S, Longhi S.

Author information: (1)Architecture et Fonction des Macromolécules Biologiques (AFMB), UMR 6098 CNRS at Universités Aix-Marseille I et II, ESIL, Campus de Luminy, 13288 Marseille Cedex 09, France.

Measles virus is a negative-sense, single-stranded RNA virus within the Mononegavirales order,which includes several human pathogens, including rabies, Ebola, Nipah, and Hendra viruses. The measles virus nucleoprotein consists of a structured N-terminal domain, and of an intrinsically disordered C-terminal domain, N(TAIL) (aa 401-525), which undergoes induced folding in the presence of the C-terminal domain (XD, aa 459-507) of the viral phosphoprotein. With in N(TAIL), an alpha-helical molecular recognition element (alpha-MoRE, aa 488-499) involved in binding to P and in induced folding was identified and then observed in the crystal structure of XD. Using small-angle X-ray scattering, we have derived a low-resolution structural model of the complex between XD and N(TAIL), which shows that most of N(TAIL) remains disordered in the complex despite P-induced folding within the alpha-MoRE. The model consists of an extended shape accommodating the multiple conformations adopted by the disordered N-terminal region of N(TAIL), and of a bulky globular region, corresponding to XD and to the C terminus of N(TAIL) (aa 486-525). Using surface plasmon resonance, circular dichroism, fluorescence spectroscopy, and heteronuclear magnetic resonance, we show that N(TAIL) has an additional site (aa 517-525) involved in binding to XD but not in the unstructured-to-structured transition. This work provides evidence that intrinsically disordered domains can establish complex interactions with their partners, and can contact them through multiple sites that do not all necessarily gain regular secondary structure.

PMCID: PMC2279309 PMID: 16046624 [PubMed - indexed for MEDLINE]

1753. Thromb Haemost. 2005 Aug;94(2):254-61.

The contribution of the endothelium to the development of coagulation disorders that characterize Ebola hemorrhagic fever in primates.

Hensley LE(1), Geisbert TW.

Author information: (1)Virology Division, U.S. Army Medical Research Institute of Infectious Diseases, Fort Detrick, MD, USA.

Recently, there have been substantial developments in the understanding of Ebola hemorrhagic fever pathogenesis, but there are still major gaps. These infections occur in underdeveloped areas of the world, and much of our knowledge of naturally occurring disease is derived from sporadic outbreaks that occurred decades in the past. Recently conducted laboratory animal studies have provided insight into Ebola pathogenesis and may help guide clinical investigations of disease using contemporary methodologies that were not available previously. A better understanding of the relevant host and viral factors that influence clinical and virologic outcome will be critical to our ability to combat this aggressive pathogen. This article reviews the most relevant information relating to the postulated pathogenesis of this disease, focusing on the role of the endothelium in contributing to the coagulation disorders that characterize Ebola hemorrhagic fever in primates. Some of the remaining and key unanswered questions relating to the role of the vascular system in the pathogenesis of this disease, that need to be addressed in further research, are highlighted.

PMID: 16113813 [PubMed - indexed for MEDLINE]

1754. J Immunol. 2005 Jul 15;175(2):1184-91.

Induction of humoral and CD8+ T cell responses are required for protection against lethal Ebola virus infection.

Warfield KL(1), Olinger G, Deal EM, Swenson DL, Bailey M, Negley DL, Hart MK, Bavari S.

Author information: (1)U.S. Army Medical Research Institute of Infectious Diseases, 1425 Porter Street, Frederick, MD 21702, USA.

Ebola virus (EBOV)-like particles (eVLP), composed of the EBOV glycoprotein and matrix viral protein (VP)40 with a lipid membrane, are a highly efficacious method of immunization against EBOV infection. The exact requirements for immunity against EBOV infection are poorly defined at this time. The goal of this work was to determine the requirements for EBOV immunity following eVLP vaccination. Vaccination of BALB/c or C57BL/6 mice with eVLPs in conjunction with QS-21 adjuvant resulted in mixed IgG subclass responses, a Th1-like memory cytokine response, and protection from lethal EBOV challenge. Further, this vaccination schedule led to the generation of both CD4(+) and CD8(+) IFN-gamma(+) T cells recognizing specific peptides within glycoprotein and VP40. The transfer of both serum and splenocytes, but not serum or splenocytes alone, from eVLP-vaccinated mice conferred protection against lethal EBOV infection in these studies. B cells were required for eVLP-mediated immunity to EBOV because B cell-deficient mice vaccinated with eVLPs were not protected from lethal EBOV challenge. We also found that CD8(+), but not CD4(+), T cells are absolutely required for eVLP-mediated protection against EBOV infection. Further, eVLP-induced protective mechanisms were perforin-independent, but IFN-gamma-dependent. Taken together, both EBOV-specific humoral and cytotoxic CD8(+) T cell responses are critical to mediate protection against filoviruses following eVLP vaccination.

PMID: 16002721 [PubMed - indexed for MEDLINE]

1755. JAMA. 2005 Jul 13;294(2):163-4.

Vaccines against Ebola and Marburg viruses show promise in primate studies.

Hampton T.

PMID: 16014579 [PubMed - indexed for MEDLINE]

1756. J Gen Virol. 2005 Jul;86(Pt 7):1869-77.

Paramyxovirus mRNA editing, the "rule of six" and error catastrophe: a hypothesis.

Kolakofsky D(1), Roux L, Garcin D, Ruigrok RW.

Author information: (1)Department of Microbiology and Molecular Medicine, Université de Genève, Geneva, Switzerland. daniel.kolakofsky@medecine.unige.ch

The order Mononegavirales includes three virus families that replicate in the cytoplasm: the Paramyxoviridae, composed of two subfamilies, the Paramyxovirinae and Pneumovirinae, the Rhabdoviridae and the Filoviridae. These viruses, also called non-segmented negative-strand RNA viruses (NNV), contain five to ten tandemly linked genes, which are separated by conserved junctional sequences that act as mRNA start and poly(A)/stop sites. For the NNV, downstream mRNA synthesis depends on termination of the upstream mRNA, and all NNV RNA-dependent RNA polymerases reiteratively copy ("stutter" on) a short run of template uridylates during transcription to polyadenylate and terminate their mRNAs. The RNA-dependent RNA polymerase of a subset of the NNV, all members of the Paramyxovirinae, also stutter in a very controlled fashion to edit their phosphoprotein gene mRNA, and Ebola virus, a filovirus, carries out a related process on its glycoprotein mRNA. Remarkably, all viruses that edit their phosphoprotein mRNA are also governed by the "rule of six", i.e. their genomes must be of polyhexameric length (6n+0) to replicate efficiently. Why these two seemingly unrelated processes are so tightly linked in the Paramyxovirinae has been an enigma. This paper will review what is presently known about these two processes that are unique to viruses of this subfamily, and will discuss whether this enigmatic linkage could be due to the phenomenon of RNA virus error catastrophe.

PMID: 15958664 [PubMed - indexed for MEDLINE]

1757. J Immunol. 2005 Jul 1;175(1):413-20.

Novel innate immune functions for galectin-1: galectin-1 inhibits cell fusion by Nipah virus envelope glycoproteins and augments dendritic cell secretion of proinflammatory cytokines.

Levroney EL(1), Aguilar HC, Fulcher JA, Kohatsu L, Pace KE, Pang M, Gurney KB, Baum LG, Lee B.

Author information: (1)Department of Microbiology, Immunology, and Molecular Genetics, David Geffen School of Medicine at University of California, Los Angeles, CA 90095, USA.

Galectin-1 (gal-1), an endogenous lectin secreted by a variety of cell types, has pleiotropic immunomodulatory functions, including regulation of lymphocyte survival and cytokine secretion in autoimmune, transplant disease, and parasitic infection models. However, the role of gal-1 in viral infections is unknown. Nipah virus (NiV) is an emerging pathogen that causes severe, often fatal, febrile encephalitis. The primary targets of NiV are endothelial cells. NiV infection of endothelial cells results in cell-cell fusion and syncytia formation triggered by the fusion (F) and attachment (G) envelope glycoproteins of NiV that bear glycan structures recognized by gal-1. In the present study, we report that NiV envelope-mediated cell-cell fusion is blocked by gal-1. This inhibition is specific to the Paramyxoviridae family because gal-1 did not inhibit fusion triggered by envelope glycoproteins of other viruses, including two retroviruses and a pox virus, but inhibited fusion triggered by envelope glycoproteins of the related Hendra virus and another paramyxovirus. The physiologic dimeric form of gal-1 is required for fusion inhibition because a monomeric gal-1 mutant had no inhibitory effect on cell fusion. gal-1 binds to specific N-glycans on NiV glycoproteins and aberrantly oligomerizes NiV-F and NiV-G, indicating a mechanism for fusion inhibition. gal-1 also increases dendritic cell production of proinflammatory cytokines such as IL-6, known to be protective in the setting of other viral diseases such as Ebola infections. Thus, gal-1 may have direct antiviral effects and may also augment the innate immune response against this emerging pathogen.

PMID: 15972675 [PubMed - indexed for MEDLINE]

1758. J Struct Biol. 2005 Jul;151(1):30-40.

An all-atom model of the pore-like structure of hexameric VP40 from Ebola: structural insights into the monomer-hexamer transition.

Nguyen TL(1), Schoehn G, Weissenhorn W, Hermone AR, Burnett JC, Panchal RG, McGrath C, Zaharevitz DW, Aman MJ, Gussio R, Bavari S.

Author information: (1)Target Structure-Based Drug Discovery Group, Developmental Therapeutics Program, SAIC, National Cancer Institute, Frederick, MD 21702, USA.

The matrix protein VP40 is an indispensable component of viral assembly and budding by the Ebola virus. VP40 is a monomer in solution, but can fold into hexameric and octameric states, two oligomeric conformations that play central roles in the Ebola viral life cycle. While the X-ray structures of monomeric and octameric VP40 have been determined, the structure of hexameric VP40 has only been solved by three-dimensional electron microscopy (EM) to a resolution of approximately 30 A. In this paper, we present the refinement of the EM reconstruction of truncated hexameric VP40 to approximately 20 A and the construction of an all-atom model (residues 44-212) using the EM model at approximately 20 A and the X-ray structure of monomeric VP40 as templates. The hexamer model suggests that the monomer-hexamer transition involves a conformational change in the N-terminal domain that is not evident during octamerization and therefore, may provide the basis for elucidating the biological function of VP40.

PMID: 15908231 [PubMed - indexed for MEDLINE]

1759. J Virol Methods. 2005 Jul;127(1):1-9. Epub 2005 Apr 25.

Analysis of Ebola virus and VLP release using an immunocapture assay.

Kallstrom G(1), Warfield KL, Swenson DL, Mort S, Panchal RG, Ruthel G, Bavari S, Aman MJ.

Author information: (1)Division of Virology, U.S. Army Medical Research Institute of Infectious Diseases, Fort Detrick, MD 21702, USA.

Ebola virus (EBOV), an emerging pathogen, is the causative agent of a rapidly progressive hemorrhagic fever with high mortality rates. There are currently no approved vaccines or treatments available for Ebola hemorrhagic fever. Standard plaque assays are currently the only reliable techniques for enumerating the virus. Effective drug-discovery screening as well as target identification and validation require simple and more rapid detection methods. This report describes the development of a rapid ELISA that measures virus release with high sensitivity. This assay detects both Ebola virus and EBOV-like particles (VLPs) directly from cell-culture supernatants with the VP40 matrix protein serving as antigen. Using this assay, the contribution of the EBOV nucleocapsid (NC) proteins in VLP release was determined. These findings indicate that a combination of NC proteins together with the envelope components is optimal for VLP formation and release, a finding that is important for vaccination with Ebola VLPs. Furthermore, this assay can be used in surrogate models in non-biocontainment environment, facilitating both basic research on the mechanism of EBOV assembly and budding as well as drug-discovery research.

PMID: 15893559 [PubMed - indexed for MEDLINE]

1760. Nat Med. 2005 Jul;11(7):720-1.

A single shot against Ebola and Marburg virus.

Baize S.

Comment on Nat Med. 2005 Jul;11(7):786-90.

PMID: 16015361 [PubMed - indexed for MEDLINE]

1761. Nat Med. 2005 Jul;11(7):786-90. Epub 2005 Jun 5.

Live attenuated recombinant vaccine protects nonhuman primates against Ebola and Marburg viruses.

Jones SM(1), Feldmann H, Ströher U, Geisbert JB, Fernando L, Grolla A, Klenk HD, Sullivan NJ, Volchkov VE, Fritz EA, Daddario KM, Hensley LE, Jahrling PB, Geisbert TW.

Author information: (1)Special Pathogens Program, National Microbiology Laboratory, Public Health Agency of Canada, 1015 Arlington Street, Winnipeg, Manitoba R3E 3R2, Canada.

Comment in Nat Med. 2005 Jul;11(7):720-1.

Vaccines and therapies are urgently needed to address public health needs stemming from emerging pathogens and biological threat agents such as the filoviruses Ebola virus (EBOV) and Marburg virus (MARV). Here, we developed replication-competent vaccines against EBOV and MARV based on attenuated recombinant vesicular stomatitis virus vectors expressing either the EBOV glycoprotein or MARV glycoprotein. A single intramuscular injection of the EBOV or MARV vaccine elicited completely protective immune responses in nonhuman primates against lethal EBOV or MARV challenges. Notably, vaccine vector shedding was not detectable in the monkeys and none of the animals developed fever or other symptoms of illness associated with vaccination. The EBOV vaccine induced humoral and apparent cellular immune responses in all vaccinated monkeys, whereas the MARV vaccine induced a stronger humoral than cellular immune response. No evidence of EBOV or MARV replication was detected in any of the protected animals after challenge. Our data suggest that these vaccine candidates are safe and highly efficacious in a relevant animal model.

PMID: 15937495 [PubMed - indexed for MEDLINE]

1762. N Engl J Med. 2005 Jun 23;352(25):2645-6.

How Ebola virus infects cells.

Kawaoka Y(1).

Author information: (1)International Research Center for Infectious Diseases and the Division of Virology, the Department of Microbiology and Immunology, Institute of Medical Science, University of Tokyo, Tokyo.

PMID: 15972874 [PubMed - indexed for MEDLINE]

1763. N Engl J Med. 2005 Jun 23;352(25):2571-3.

Marburg and Ebola--arming ourselves against the deadly filoviruses.

Peters CJ(1).

Author information: (1)Center for Biodefense and Emerging Infectious Diseases, University of Texas Medical Branch, Galveston, USA.

PMID: 15972860 [PubMed - indexed for MEDLINE]
1764. Adv Drug Deliv Rev. 2005 Jun 17;57(9):1247-65. Epub 2005 Apr 18.

Particulate delivery systems for biodefense subunit vaccines.

Bramwell VW(1), Eyles JE, Oya Alpar H.

Author information: (1)School of Pharmacy, University of London, 29-39 Brunswick Square, London, WCIN IAX, UK.

Expanding identification of potentially protective subunit antigens and correlates of protection has provided a basis for the introduction of safer vaccines. Despite encouraging results in animal models, the significant potential of particulate delivery systems in vaccine design has not yet translated into effective vaccines available for use in humans. This review article will focus on the current status of the development of particulate vaccines, mainly liposomes and bio-degradable polymers, against potential agents for biowarfare: plague, anthrax, botulinum, and smallpox; and filoviruses: Marburg and Ebola.

PMID: 15935873 [PubMed - indexed for MEDLINE]
1765. Science. 2005 Jun 10;308(5728):1643-5. Epub 2005 Apr 14.

Endosomal proteolysis of the Ebola virus glycoprotein is necessary for infection.

Chandran K(1), Sullivan NJ, Felbor U, Whelan SP, Cunningham JM.

Author information: (1)Department of Medicine, Brigham and Women's Hospital and Harvard Medical School, Boston, MA 02115, USA.

Ebola virus (EboV) causes rapidly fatal hemorrhagic fever in humans and there is currently no effective treatment. We found that the infection of African green monkey kidney (Vero) cells by vesicular stomatitis viruses bearing the EboV glycoprotein (GP) requires the activity of endosomal cysteine proteases. Using selective protease inhibitors and protease-deficient cell lines, we identified an essential role for cathepsin B (CatB) and an accessory role for cathepsin L (CatL) in EboV GP-dependent entry. Biochemical studies demonstrate that CatB and CatL mediate entry by carrying out proteolysis of the EboV GP subunit GP1 and support a multistep mechanism that explains the relative contributions of these enzymes to infection. CatB and CatB/CatL inhibitors diminish the multiplication of infectious EboV-Zaire in cultured cells and may merit investigation as anti-EboV drugs.

PMID: 15831716 [PubMed - indexed for MEDLINE]
1766. Virology. 2005 Jun 5;336(2):291-8.

Functional characterization of Ebola virus L-domains using VSV recombinants.

Irie T(1), Licata JM, Harty RN.

Author information: (1)Department of Pathobiology, School of Veterinary Medicine, University of Pennsylvania, 3800 Spruce Street, Philadelphia, PA 19104-6049, USA.

VSV recombinants containing the overlapping L-domain sequences from Ebola virus VP40 (PTAPPEY) were recovered by reverse-genetics. Replication kinetics of M40-WT, M40-P24L, and M40-Y30A were indistinguishable from VSV-WT in BHK-21 cells, whereas the double mutant (M40-P2728A) was defective in budding. Insertion of the Ebola L-domain region into VSV M protein was sufficient to alter the dependence on host proteins for efficient budding. Indeed, M40 recombinants containing a functional PTAP motif specifically incorporated endogenous tsg101 into budding virions and were dependent on tsg101 expression for efficient budding. Thus, VSV represents an excellent negative-sense RNA virus model for elucidating the functional aspects and diverse host interactions associated with the L-domains of Ebola virus.

PMCID: PMC2929245 PMID: 15892969 [PubMed - indexed for MEDLINE]
1767. Expert Rev Vaccines. 2005 Jun;4(3):429-40.

Filovirus-like particles as vaccines and discovery tools.

Warfield KL(1), Swenson DL, Demmin G, Bavari S.

Author information: (1)United States Army Medical Research Institute of Infectious Diseases, Fort Detrick, MD 21702-5011, USA.
kelly.warfield@det.amedd.army.mil

Ebola and Marburg viruses are members of the family Filoviridae, which cause severe hemorrhagic fevers in humans. Filovirus outbreaks have been sporadic, with mortality rates currently ranging from 30 to 90%. Unfortunately, there is no efficacious human therapy or vaccine available to treat disease caused by either Ebola or Marburg virus infection. Expression of the filovirus matrix protein, VP40, is sufficient to drive spontaneous production and release of virus-like particles (VLPs) that resemble the distinctively filamentous infectious virions. The addition of other filovirus proteins, including virion proteins (VP)24, 30 and 35 and glycoprotein, increases the efficiency of VLP production and results in particles containing multiple filovirus antigens. Vaccination with Ebola or Marburg VLPs containing glycoprotein and VP40 completely protects rodents from lethal challenge with the homologous virus. These candidate vaccines are currently being tested for immunogenicity and efficacy in nonhuman primates. Furthermore, the Ebola and Marburg VLPs are being used as a surrogate model to further understand the filovirus life cycle, with the goal of developing rationally designed vaccines and therapeutics. Thus, in addition to their use as a vaccine, VLPs are currently being used as tools to learn lessons about filovirus pathogenesis, immunology, replication and assembly requirements.

PMID: 16026254 [PubMed - indexed for MEDLINE]
1768. Microbes Infect. 2005 Jun;7(7-8):1005-14.

The natural history of Ebola virus in Africa.

Pourrut X(1), Kumulungui B, Wittmann T, Moussavou G, Délicat A, Yaba P, Nkoghe D, Gonzalez JP, Leroy EM.

Author information: (1)Centre International de Recherches Médicales de Franceville, Gabon.

Several countries spanning the equatorial forest regions of Africa have had outbreaks of Ebola hemorrhagic fever over the last three decades. This article is an overview of the many published investigations of how Ebola virus circulates in its natural environment, focusing on the viral reservoir, susceptible animal species, environmental conditions favoring inter-species transmission, and how the infection is transmitted to humans. Major breakthroughs have been made in recent years but many outstanding questions must be dealt with if we are to prevent human outbreaks by interfering with the viral life cycle.

PMID: 16002313 [PubMed - indexed for MEDLINE]

1769. Vaccine. 2005 Apr 27;23(23):3033-42.

Virus-like particles exhibit potential as a pan-filovirus vaccine for both Ebola and Marburg viral infections.

Swenson DL(1), Warfield KL, Negley DL, Schmaljohn A, Aman MJ, Bavari S.

Author information: (1)United States Army Medical Research Institute of Infectious Diseases, 1425 Porter Street, Frederick, MD 21702-5011, USA. dana.swenson@det.amedd.army.mil

A safe and effective pan-filovirus vaccine is highly desirable since the filoviruses Ebola virus (EBOV) and Marburg virus (MARV) cause highly lethal disease typified by unimpeded viral replication and severe hemorrhagic fever. Previously, we showed that expression of the homologous glycoprotein (GP) and matrix protein VP40 from a single filovirus, either EBOV or MARV, resulted in formation of wild-type virus-like particles (VLPs) in mammalian cells. When used as a vaccine, the wild-type VLPs protected from homologous filovirus challenge. The aim of this work was to generate a multi-agent vaccine that would simultaneously protect against multiple and diverse members of the Filoviridae family. Our initial approach was to construct hybrid VLPs containing heterologous viral proteins, of EBOV and MARV, and test the efficacy of the hybrid VLPs in a guinea pig model. Our data indicate that vaccination with GP was required and sufficient to protect against a homologous filovirus challenge, as heterologous wild-type VLPs or hybrid VLPs that did not contain the homologous GP failed to protect. Alternately, we vaccinated guinea pigs with a mixture of wild-type Ebola and Marburg VLPs. Vaccination with a single dose of the multivalent VLP vaccine elicited strong immune responses to both viruses and protected animals against EBOV and MARV challenge. This work provides a critical foundation towards the development of a pan-filovirus vaccine that is safe and effective for use in primates and humans.

PMID: 15811650 [PubMed - indexed for MEDLINE]

1770. J Immunol. 2005 Apr 1;174(7):4198-202.

CD8-mediated protection against Ebola virus infection is perforin dependent.

Gupta M(1), Greer P, Mahanty S, Shieh WJ, Zaki SR, Ahmed R, Rollin PE.

Author information: (1)Special Pathogens Branch, Division of Viral and Rickettsial Diseases, National Center for Infectious Diseases, Centers for Disease Control and Prevention, Atlanta, GA 30333, USA. mgupta@cdc.gov

CD8 T cells have been shown to play an important role in the clearance and protection against fatal Ebola virus infection. In this study, we examined the mechanisms by which CD8 T cells mediate this protection. Our data demonstrate that all normal mice infected s.c. with a mouse-adapted Ebola virus survived the infection, as did 100% of mice deficient in Fas and 90% of those deficient in IFN-gamma. In contrast, perforin-deficient mice uniformly died after s.c. challenge. Perforin-deficient mice failed to clear viral infection even though they developed normal levels of neutralizing anti-Ebola Abs and 5- to 10-fold higher levels of IFN-gamma than control mice. Using MHC class I tetramers, we have also shown that perforin-deficient mice have 2- to 4-fold higher numbers of Ebola-specific CD8s than control mice. These findings suggest that the clearance of Ebola virus is perforin-dependent and provide an additional example showing that this basic immunologic mechanism is not limited to the clearance of noncytopathic viruses.

PMID: 15778381 [PubMed - indexed for MEDLINE]

1771. J Virol. 2005 Apr;79(8):4793-805.

Comprehensive analysis of ebola virus GP1 in viral entry.

Manicassamy B(1), Wang J, Jiang H, Rong L.

Author information: (1)Department of Microbiology and Immunology, College of Medicine, University of Illinois at Chicago, E829 MSB, 835 S. Wolcott Ave., Chicago, IL 60612, USA.

Ebola virus infection is initiated by interactions between the viral glycoprotein GP1 and its cognate receptor(s), but little is known about the structure and function of GP1 in viral entry, partly due to the concern about safety when working with the live Ebola virus and the difficulty of manipulating the RNA genome of Ebola virus. In this study, we have used a human immunodeficiency virus-based pseudotyped virus as a surrogate system to dissect the role of Ebola virus GP1 in viral entry. Analysis of more than 100 deletion and amino acid substitution mutants of GP1 with respect to protein expression, processing, viral incorporation, and viral entry has allowed us to map the region of GP1 responsible for viral entry to the N-terminal 150 residues. Furthermore, six amino acids in this region have been identified as critical residues for early events in Ebola virus entry, and among these, three are clustered and are implicated as part of a potential receptor-binding pocket. In addition, substitutions of some 30 residues in GP1 are shown to adversely affect GP1 expression, processing, and viral incorporation, suggesting that these residues are involved in the proper folding and/or overall conformation of GP. Sequence comparison of the GP1 proteins suggests that the majority of the critical residues for GP folding and viral entry identified in Ebola virus GP1 are conserved in Marburg virus. These results provide information for elucidating the structural and functional roles of the filoviral glycoproteins and for developing potential therapeutics to block viral entry.

PMCID: PMC1069533 PMID: 15795265 [PubMed - indexed for MEDLINE]

1772. J Virol. 2005 Apr;79(8):4709-19.

Association of ebola virus matrix protein VP40 with microtubules.

Ruthel G(1), Demmin GL, Kallstrom G, Javid MP, Badie SS, Will AB, Nelle T, Schokman R, Nguyen TL, Carra JH, Bavari S, Aman MJ.

Author information: (1)USAMRIID, 1425 Porter St., Frederick, MD 21702, USA.

Viruses exploit a variety of cellular components to complete their life cycles, and it has become increasingly clear that use of host cell microtubules is a vital part of the infection process for many viruses. A variety of viral proteins have been identified that interact with microtubules, either directly or via a microtubule-associated motor protein. Here, we report that Ebola virus associates with microtubules via the matrix protein VP40. When transfected into mammalian cells, a fraction of VP40 colocalized with microtubule bundles and VP40 coimmunoprecipitated with tubulin. The degree of colocalization and microtubule bundling in cells was markedly intensified by truncation of the C terminus to a length of 317 amino acids. Further truncation to 308 or fewer amino acids abolished the association with microtubules. Both the full-length and the 317-amino-acid truncation mutant stabilized microtubules against depolymerization with nocodazole. Direct physical interaction between purified VP40 and tubulin proteins was demonstrated in vitro. A region of moderate homology to the tubulin binding motif of the microtubule-associated protein MAP2 was identified in VP40. Deleting this region resulted in loss of microtubule stabilization against drug-induced depolymerization. The presence of VP40-associated microtubules in cells continuously treated with nocodazole suggested that VP40 promotes tubulin polymerization. Using an in vitro polymerization assay, we demonstrated that VP40 directly enhances tubulin polymerization without any cellular mediators. These results suggest that microtubules may play an important role in the Ebola virus life cycle and potentially provide a novel target for therapeutic intervention against this highly pathogenic virus.
PMCID: PMC1069569 PMID: 15795257 [PubMed - indexed for MEDLINE]

1773. J Virol. 2005 Apr;79(7):4425-33.

RNA polymerase I-driven minigenome system for Ebola viruses.

Groseth A(1), Feldmann H, Theriault S, Mehmetoglu G, Flick R.

Author information: (1)National Laboratory for Zoonotic Diseases and Special Pathogens, National Microbiology Laboratory, Public Health Agency of Canada, Winnipeg, MB R3E 3R2, Canada.

In general, Ebola viruses are well known for their ability to cause severe hemorrhagic fever in both human and nonhuman primates. However, despite substantial sequence homology to other members of the family Filoviridae, Reston ebolavirus displays reduced pathogenicity for nonhuman primates and has never been demonstrated to cause clinical disease in humans, despite its ability to cause infection. In order to develop a tool to explore potential roles for transcription and replication in the reduced pathogenicity of Reston ebolavirus, we developed an RNA polymerase I (Pol I)-driven minigenome system. Here we demonstrate successful Reston ebolavirus minigenome rescue, including encapsidation, transcription, and replication, as well as the packaging of minigenome transcripts into progeny particles. The Pol I-driven Reston ebolavirus minigenome system provides a higher signal intensity with less background (higher signal-to-noise ratio) than a comparable T7-driven Reston ebolavirus minigenome system which was developed simultaneously. Successful Reston ebolavirus minigenome rescue was also achieved by the use of helper plasmids derived from the closely related Zaire ebolavirus or the more distantly related Lake Victoria marburgvirus. The use of heterologous helper plasmids in the Reston ebolavirus minigenome system yielded levels of reporter expression which far exceeded the level produced by the homologous helper plasmids. This comparison between minigenomes and helper plasmids from different filovirus species and genera indicates that inherent differences in the transcription and/or replication capacities of the ribonucleoprotein complexes of pathogenic and apathogenic filoviruses may exist, as these observations were confirmed in a Lake Victoria marburgvirus minigenome system.
PMCID: PMC1061559 PMID: 15767442 [PubMed - indexed for MEDLINE]

1774. MMWR Morb Mortal Wkly Rep. 2005 Apr 1;54(12):308-9.

Outbreak of Marburg virus hemorrhagic fever--Angola, October 1, 2004-March 29, 2005

Centers for Disease Control and Prevention (CDC).

On March 23, 2005, the World Health Organization (WHO) confirmed Marburg virus (family Filoviridae, which includes Ebola virus) as the causative agent of an outbreak of viral hemorrhagic fever (VHF) in Uige Province in northern Angola. Testing conducted by CDC's Special Pathogens Branch detected the presence of virus in nine of 12 clinical specimens from patients who died during the outbreak.
PMID: 15800477 [PubMed - indexed for MEDLINE]

1775. J Infect Dis. 2005 Mar 15;191(6):964-8. Epub 2005 Feb 8.

Low seroprevalence of IgG antibodies to Ebola virus in an epidemic zone: Ogooué-Ivindo region, Northeastern Gabon, 1997.

Heffernan RT(1), Pambo B, Hatchett RJ, Leman PA, Swanepoel R, Ryder RW.

Author information: (1)Department of Epidemiology and Public Health, Division of Epidemiology of Microbial Diseases, Yale University School of Medicine, New Haven, Connecticut, USA.

A population-based serosurvey was performed to determine the seroprevalence of antibodies to Ebola virus (EBO) in a region that has experienced multiple epidemics of EBO hemorrhagic fever. Of 2533 residents in 8 villages, serum samples from 979 (38.6%) were tested by enzyme-linked immunosorbent assay for immunoglobulin (Ig) G and IgM antibodies to Ebola-Zaire (EBO-Z) virus. Fourteen samples (1.4%) were found positive for IgG antibodies, and 4 of these (.4%) were samples from survivors of an epidemic of EBO hemorrhagic fever. Seroprevalence based on the remaining 10 IgG-seropositive individuals with no history of exposure to EBO was 1.0% (exact binomial 95% confidence interval, 0.5%-1.9%). No serum samples were found positive for IgM antibodies to EBO-Z virus. The low seroprevalence suggests that, outside of recognized outbreaks, human exposure to EBO in this epidemic zone is rare.
PMID: 15717273 [PubMed - indexed for MEDLINE]

1776. Emerg Infect Dis. 2005 Mar;11(3):385-90.

Ebola virus antibody prevalence in dogs and human risk.

Allela L(1), Boury O, Pouillot R, Délicat A, Yaba P, Kumulungui B, Rouquet P, Gonzalez JP, Leroy EM.

Author information: (1)Centre International de Recherches Médicales de Franceville, Franceville, Gabon.

During the 2001-2002 outbreak in Gabon, we observed that several dogs were highly exposed to Ebola virus by eating infected dead animals. To examine whether these animals became infected with Ebola virus, we sampled 439 dogs and screened them by Ebola virus-specific immunoglobulin (Ig) G assay, antigen detection, and viral polymerase chain reaction amplification. Seven (8.9%) of 79 samples from the 2 main towns, 15 (15.2%) of 99 samples from Mekambo, and 40 (25.2%) of 159 samples from villages in the Ebola virus-epidemic area had detectable Ebola virus-IgG, compared to only 2 (2%) of 102 samples from France. Among dogs from villages with both infected animal carcasses and human cases, seroprevalence was 31.8%. A significant positive direct association existed between seroprevalence and the distances to the Ebola virus-epidemic area. This study suggests that dogs can be infected by Ebola virus and that the putative infection is asymptomatic.

PMCID: PMC3298261 PMID: 15757552 [PubMed - indexed for MEDLINE]

1777. J Public Health (Oxf). 2005 Mar;27(1):120-4.

Communicable disease and health protection quarterly review: July to September 2004 from the Health Protection Agency, Communicable Disease Surveillance Centre.

Health Protection Agency, Communicable Disease Surveillance Centre.

PMID: 15749727 [PubMed - indexed for MEDLINE]

1778. J Vet Med Sci. 2005 Mar;67(3):325-8.

Nucleocapsid-like structures of Ebola virus reconstructed using electron tomography.

Noda T(1), Aoyama K, Sagara H, Kida H, Kawaoka Y.

Author information: (1)Laboratory of Microbiology, Department of Disease Control, Graduate School of Veterinary Medicine, Hokkaido University, Sapporo 060-0818, Japan.

Electron tomography (ET) is a new technique for high resolution, three-dimensional (3D) reconstruction of pleiomorphic macromolecular complexes, such as virus components. By employing this technique, we resolved the 3D structure of Ebola virus nucleocapsid-like (NC-like) structures in the cytoplasm of cells expressing NP, VP24, and VP35: the minimum components required to form these NC-like structures. Reconstruction of these tubular NC-like structures of Ebola virus showed them to be composed of left-handed helices spaced at short intervals, which is structurally consistent with other non-segmented negative-strand RNA viruses.

PMID: 15805739 [PubMed - indexed for MEDLINE]

1779. Trans R Soc Trop Med Hyg. 2005 Mar;99(3):226-33.

The disease profile of poverty: morbidity and mortality in northern Uganda in the context of war, population displacement and HIV/AIDS.

Accorsi S(1), Fabiani M, Nattabi B, Corrado B, Iriso R, Ayella EO, Pido B, Onek PA, Ogwang M, Declich S.

Author information: (1)Istituto Superiore di Sanità, National Centre for Epidemiology, Surveillance and Health Promotion, Viale Regina Elena 299, 00161 Rome, Italy.

The population of Gulu District (northern Uganda) has been severely incapacitated by war, epidemics and social disruption. This study is aimed at describing disease patterns and trends in this area through a retrospective analysis of discharge records for 155205 in-patients of Lacor Hospital in the period 1992-2002. The burden of infectious diseases in childhood is overwhelming, with malaria accounting for the steepest increase in admissions. Admissions for war-related injuries and malnutrition fluctuated with the intensity of the war and the severity of famine. Emerging and re-emerging infections, such as HIV/AIDS, tuberculosis and Ebola, accounted for a heavy disease burden; however, there has been a trend for admissions related to HIV/AIDS and tuberculosis to decrease since the implementation of community-based services. Vulnerable groups (infants, children and women) accounted for 79.8% of admissions. Long-term war, population displacement, the collapse of social structures and the breakdown of the health system place people at a much greater risk of persistent, emerging and re-emerging infectious diseases, malnutrition and war-related injuries, shaping the 'disease profile of poverty'. Most of the disease burden results from infectious diseases of childhood, whose occurrence could be dramatically reduced by low-cost and effective preventive and curative interventions.

PMID: 15653126 [PubMed - indexed for MEDLINE]

1780. Virology. 2005 Feb 5;332(1):406-17.

A reconstituted replication and transcription system for Ebola virus Reston and comparison with Ebola virus Zaire.

Boehmann Y(1), Enterlein S, Randolf A, Mühlberger E.

Author information: (1)Department of Virology, Philipps University Marburg, Robert-Koch-Str. 17, 35037 Marburg, Germany. boehmann@cervi-lyon.inserm.fr

The only known filovirus, which presumably is not pathogenic for humans, is Ebola virus (EBOV) Reston. When EBOV Reston and the highly pathogenic EBOV Zaire were grown in cell culture, comparison of the replication kinetics showed a clear growth impairment of EBOV Reston, indicating that the replication cycle of EBOV Reston might be delayed. In addition, the cytopathic effect caused by the virus was much milder with EBOV Reston than with EBOV Zaire. To compare replication and transcription of EBOV Reston and Zaire, a reconstituted minigenomic replication and transcription system based on reverse genetics has been established for EBOV Reston. This system was used to exchange the EBOV Zaire and EBOV Reston nucleocapsid (NC) proteins NP, VP35, VP30, and L, which catalyze replication and transcription. Furthermore, chimeric minigenomes were constructed containing the cis-acting replication signals of EBOV Zaire combined with those of EBOV Reston. Surprisingly, the cis-acting signals as well as almost all NC proteins could be exchanged between EBOV Reston and Zaire, suggesting a high degree of functional homology of the replication/transcription complexes of EBOV Zaire and EBOV Reston. Only the combination of EBOV Zaire VP35 and EBOV Reston L did not result in replication and transcription activity. Although these two proteins did not constitute an active polymerase complex, it was shown by immunofluorescence analysis that they were still able to interact.

PMID: 15661171 [PubMed - indexed for MEDLINE]
1781. Virology. 2005 Feb 5;332(1):20-7.

Generation of eGFP expressing recombinant Zaire ebolavirus for analysis of early pathogenesis events and high-throughput antiviral drug screening.

Towner JS(1), Paragas J, Dover JE, Gupta M, Goldsmith CS, Huggins JW, Nichol ST.

Author information: (1)Special Pathogens Branch, Division of Viral and Rickettsial Diseases, NCID, Centers for Disease Control and Prevention, Atlanta, GA 30333, USA.

Zaire ebolavirus causes large outbreaks of severe and usually fatal hemorrhagic disease in humans for which there is no effective treatment or cure. To facilitate examination of early critical events in viral pathogenesis and to identify antiviral compounds, a recombinant Zaire ebolavirus was engineered to express a foreign protein, eGFP, to provide a rapid and sensitive means to monitor virus replication in infected cells. This genetically engineered virus represents the first insertion of a foreign gene into ebolavirus. We show that Ebola-eGFP virus (EboZ-eGFP) infects known early targets of human infections and serves as an ideal model to screen antiviral compounds in less time than any previously published assay.

PMID: 15661137 [PubMed - indexed for MEDLINE]
1782. Emerg Infect Dis. 2005 Feb;11(2):283-90.

Wild animal mortality monitoring and human Ebola outbreaks, Gabon and Republic of Congo, 2001-2003.

Rouquet P(1), Froment JM, Bermejo M, Kilbourn A, Karesh W, Reed P, Kumulungui B, Yaba P, Délicat A, Rollin PE, Leroy EM.

Author information: (1)Centre International de Recherches Médicales de Franceville, (CIRMF) BP 769, Franceville, Gabon. p.rouquent@cirmf.org

All human Ebola virus outbreaks during 2001-2003 in the forest zone between Gabon and Republic of Congo resulted from handling infected wild animal carcasses. After the first outbreak, we created an Animal Mortality Monitoring Network in collaboration with the Gabonese and Congolese Ministries of Forestry and Environment and wildlife organizations (Wildlife Conservation Society and Programme de Conservation et Utilisation Rationnelle des Ecosystemes Forestiers en Afrique Centrale) to predict and possibly prevent human Ebola outbreaks. Since August 2001, 98 wild animal carcasses have been recovered by the network, including 65 great apes. Analysis of 21 carcasses found that 10 gorillas, 3 chimpanzees, and 1 duiker tested positive for Ebola virus. Wild animal outbreaks began before each of the 5 human Ebola outbreaks. Twice we alerted the health authorities to an imminent risk for human outbreaks, weeks before they occurred.

PMCID: PMC3320460 PMID: 15752448 [PubMed - indexed for MEDLINE]
1783. J Virol. 2005 Feb;79(4):2413-9.

Role of Ebola virus secreted glycoproteins and virus-like particles in activation of human macrophages.

Wahl-Jensen V(1), Kurz SK, Hazelton PR, Schnittler HJ, Ströher U, Burton DR, Feldmann H.

Author information: (1)Special Pathogens Program, National Microbiology Laboratory, University of Manitoba, Winnipeg, Manitoba, Canada.

Ebola virus, a member of the family Filoviridae, causes one of the most severe forms of viral hemorrhagic fever. In the terminal stages of disease, symptoms progress to hypotension, coagulation disorders, and hemorrhages, and there is prominent involvement of the mononuclear phagocytic and reticuloendothelial systems. Cells of the mononuclear phagocytic system are primary target cells and producers of inflammatory mediators. Ebola virus efficiently produces four soluble glycoproteins during infection: sGP, delta peptide (Delta-peptide), GP(1), and GP(1,2Delta). While the presence of these glycoproteins has been confirmed in blood (sGP) and in vitro systems, it is hypothesized that they are of biological relevance in pathogenesis, particularly target cell activation. To gain insight into their function, we expressed the four soluble glycoproteins in mammalian cells and purified and characterized them. The role of the transmembrane glycoprotein in the context of virus-like particles was also investigated. Primary human macrophages were treated with glycoproteins and virus-like particles and subsequently tested for activation by detection of several critical proinflammatory cytokines (tumor necrosis factor alpha, interleukin-6 [IL-6], and IL-1 beta) and the chemokine IL-8. The presentation of the glycoprotein was determined to be critical since virus-like particles, but not soluble glycoproteins, induced high levels of activation. We propose that the presentation of GP(1,2) in the rigid form such as that observed on the surface of particles is critical for initiating a sufficient signal for the activation of primary target cells. The secreted glycoproteins do not appear to play any role in exogenous activation of these cells during Ebola virus infection.

PMCID: PMC546544 PMID: 15681442 [PubMed - indexed for MEDLINE]
1784. J Virol. 2005 Feb;79(3):1898-905.

VP40 octamers are essential for Ebola virus replication.

Hoenen T(1), Volchkov V, Kolesnikova L, Mittler E, Timmins J, Ottmann M, Reynard O, Becker S, Weissenhorn W.

Author information: (1)Institut für Virologie, Robert-Koch-Str. 17, 35037 Marburg, Germany.

Matrix protein VP40 of Ebola virus is essential for virus assembly and budding. Monomeric VP40 can oligomerize in vitro into RNA binding octamers, and the crystal structure of octameric VP40 has revealed that residues Phe125 and Arg134 are the most important residues for the coordination of a short single-stranded RNA. Here we show that full-length wild-type VP40 octamers bind RNA upon HEK 293 cell expression. While the Phe125-to-Ala mutation resulted in reduced RNA binding, the Arg134-to-Ala mutation completely abolished RNA binding and thus octamer formation. The absence of octamer formation, however, does not affect virus-like particle (VLP) formation, as the VLPs generated from the expression of wild-type VP40 and mutated VP40 in HEK 293 cells showed similar morphology and abundance and no significant difference in size. These results strongly indicate that octameric VP40 is dispensable for VLP formation. The cellular localization of mutant VP40 was different from that of wild-type VP40. While wild-type VP40 was present in small patches predominantly at the plasma membrane, the octamer-negative mutants were found in larger aggregates at the periphery of the cell and in the perinuclear region. We next introduced the Arg134-to-Ala and/or the Phe125-to-Ala mutation into the Ebola virus genome. Recombinant wild-type virus and virus expressing the VP40 Phe125-to-Ala mutation were both rescued. In contrast, no recombinant virus expressing the VP40 Arg134-to-Ala mutation could be recovered. These results suggest that RNA binding of VP40 and therefore octamer formation are essential for the Ebola virus life cycle.

PMCID: PMC544139 PMID: 15650213 [PubMed - indexed for MEDLINE]

1785. Acta Microbiol Immunol Hung. 2005;52(3-4):273-89.

Interferon: ten stories in one. A short review of some of the highlights in the history of an almost quinquagenarian.

De Clercq E(1).

Author information: (1)Rega Institute for Medical Research, KU Leuven, Belgium.

This short review article on some pertinent observations in the unfolding story of interferon is dedicated to Professor Ilona Béládi on the occasion of her 80th birthday. This by no means covers the whole story on interferon. It just highlights some of the more striking findings made with interferon (or its inducers) over a time span of almost 50 years since its original discovery (in 1957) by Isaacs and Lindenmann. These observations concern (i) the induction of interferon by synthetic polyanions such as polyacrylic acid and polymethacrylic acid; (ii) the prolonged antiviral activity shown by polyacrylic acid in vivo; (iii) the interferon-inducing ability of double-stranded RNAs such as poly(I) x poly(C) and (iv) mismatched derivatives thereof (i.e. ampligen); (v) the cloning and expression of interferon-beta, and (vi) its usefulness in the treatment of multiple sclerosis; (vii) the potential of (pegylated) interferon-alpha in the treatment of hepatitis C and (viii) the therapy/prophylaxis of SARS; (ix) the efficacy of interferon (inducers) in the experimental treatment of flavivirus encephalitis and enterovirus myocarditis; and, finally, (x) the role of interferon in the activity shown by S-adenosylhomocysteine inhibitors such as 3-deazaneplanocin A against experimental Ebola virus infections in mice.

PMID: 16400870 [PubMed - indexed for MEDLINE]

1786. Arch Virol Suppl. 2005;(19):157-77.

The role of reverse genetics systems in determining filovirus pathogenicity.

Theriault S(1), Groseth A, Artsob H, Feldmann H.

Author information: (1)National Laboratory for Zoonotic Diseases and Special Pathogens, National Microbiology Laboratory, Public Health Agency of Canada, Winnipeg, Manitoba, Canada.

The family Filoviridae is comprised of two genera: Marburgvirus and Ebolavirus. To date minigenome systems have been developed for two Ebola viruses (Reston ebolavirus and Zaire ebolavirus [ZEBOV]) as well as for Lake Victoria marburgvirus, the sole member of the Marburgvirus genus. The use of these minigenome systems has helped characterize functions for many viral proteins in both genera and have provided valuable insight towards the development of an infectious clone system in the case of ZEBOV. The recent development of two such infectious clone systems for ZEBOV now allow effective strategies for experimental mutagenesis to study the biology and pathogenesis of one of the most lethal human pathogens.

PMID: 16355872 [PubMed - indexed for MEDLINE]

1787. Curr Top Med Chem. 2005;5(13):1191-203.

Recent advances in antiviral nucleoside and nucleotide therapeutics.

Simons C(1), Wu Q, Htar TT.

Author information: (1)Medicinal Chemistry Division, Welsh School of Pharmacy, Cardiff University, King Edward VII Avenue, Cardiff CF10 3XF, UK. SimonsC@Cardiff.ac.uk

Recent developments in nucleoside/nucleotide therapeutics and antiviral drug targets are described covering progress in the development of nucleoside/nucleotide mimetics for the treatment of influenza virus, human immunodeficiency virus type 1, hepatitis B and C virus, herpes virus infections; including herpes simplex virus, cytomegalovirus and varicella zoster virus infections, and the highly pathogenic poxviruses (variola, vaccinia and monkey pox) and filoviruses (Ebola and Marburg).

PMID: 16305526 [PubMed - indexed for MEDLINE]

1788. Healthc Q. 2005;8(4):20, 22.

Taking down Goliaths: new vaccines may spell the end for Ebola, Marburg and Lassa virus infections.

Singh B(1).

Author information: (1)CIHR, Institute of Infection and Immunity.

PMID: 16323509 [PubMed - indexed for MEDLINE]

1789. Hum Gene Ther. 2005 Jan;16(1):49-56.

Transduction of the choroid plexus and ependyma in neonatal mouse brain by vesicular stomatitis virus glycoprotein-pseudotyped lentivirus and adeno-associated virus type 5 vectors.

Watson DJ(1), Passini MA, Wolfe JH.

Author information: (1)Department of Pathobiology and Walter Flato Goodman Center for Comparative Medical Genetics, School of Veterinary Medicine, University of Pennsylvania, Philadelphia, PA 19104, USA.

Evaluation of gene transfer into the developing mouse brain has shown that when adeno-associated virus serotype 1 (AAV1) or AAV2 vectors are injected into the cerebral lateral ventricles at birth, widespread parenchymal transduction occurs. Lentiviral vectors have not been tested by this route. In this study, we found that injection of lentiviral vectors pseudotyped with vesicular stomatitis virus glycoprotein (VSV-G) resulted in targeted transduction of the ependymal cells lining the ventricular system and the choroid plexus along the entire rostrocaudal axis of the brain, whereas a Mokola pseudotype transduced only a few cells after injection into the neonatal ventricle. In contrast, when lentiviral vectors pseudotyped with either VSV-G or Mokola glycoprotein are injected into the adult mouse brain, they transduce similar patterns of cells. An Ebola-Zaire-pseudotyped vector did not transduce any neonatal CNS cells, as was also the case for adult parenchymal injections. Long-term gene expression (12 months) occurred with a constitutively active mammalian promoter and a self-inactivating long terminal repeat (LTR), whereas the cytomegalovirus promoter in a vector with an intact LTR was expressed only in short-term experiments. We found that an AAV5 vector also targeted the ependymal and choroid plexus cells throughout the ventricular system. This vector exhibited limited penetration from the ventricle to other structures, which was significantly different from the previously reported patterns of transduction after intraventricular injection of AAV1 and AAV2 vectors.

PMID: 15703488 [PubMed - indexed for MEDLINE]

1790. ILAR J. 2005;46(1):15-22.

Demand for nonhuman primate resources in the age of biodefense.

Patterson JL(1), Carrion R Jr.

Author information: (1)Department of Virology and Immunology, Southwest Foundation for Biomedical Research, San Antonio, Texas, USA.

The demand for nonhuman primates will undoubtedly increase to meet biomedical needs in this current age of biodefense. The availability of funding has increased the research on select agents and has created a requirement to validate results in relevant primate models. This review provides a description of current and potential biological threats that are likely to require nonhuman primates for the development of vaccines and therapeutics. Primates have been an invaluable resource in the dissection of viral disease pathogenesis as well as in testing vaccine efficacy. DNA vaccine approaches have been studied successfully for Ebola, Lassa, and anthrax in nonhuman primate models. Nonhuman primate research with monkeypox has provided insight into the role of cytokines in limiting disease severity. Biodefense research that has focused on select agents of bacterial origin has also benefited from nonhuman primate studies. Rhesus macaques have traditionally been the model of choice for anthrax research and have yielded successful findings in vaccine development. In plague research, African green monkeys have contributed to vaccine development. However, the disadvantages of current vaccines will undoubtedly require the generation of new vaccines, thus increasing the need for nonhuman primate research. Unfortunately, the current biosafety level (BSL)-3 and BSL-4 facilities equipped to perform this research are limited, which may ultimately impede progress in this era of biodefense.

PMID: 15644560 [PubMed - indexed for MEDLINE]

1791. Immunobiology. 2005;210(5):321-33.

Human dendritic cells and macrophages exhibit different intracellular processing pathways for soluble and liposome-encapsulated antigens.

Peachman KK(1), Rao M, Alving CR, Palmer DR, Sun W, Rothwell SW.

Author information: (1)Department of Vaccine Production and Delivery, Division of Retrovirology, Walter Reed Army Institute of Research, US Military HIV Research Program, 13 Taft Court Suite 200, Rockville, MD 20850, USA. Kristina.Peachman@na.amedd.army.mil

The intracellular fates of soluble and liposomal antigens in human macrophages and dendritic cells are not well defined. Previous studies using murine macrophages have demonstrated that liposomal antigens can enter the MHC class I pathway. The Golgi complex is a major organelle in this pathway. Phagocytosis of the antigens is followed by translocation of antigen-derived peptides to the trans-Golgi where they can complex with MHC class I molecules. In contrast, soluble antigens are normally processed through the MHC class II pathway. Therefore, in the present study, ovalbumin and a synthetic Ebola peptide were used either in a soluble form or encapsulated in liposomes to investigate the intracellular trafficking and localization of these antigens to the Golgi complex in human macrophages and dendritic cells. While liposome-encapsulated antigens were transported to the trans-Golgi region in 59-78% of macrophages, soluble antigens remained diffuse throughout the cytoplasm with only 3-11% of the macrophages exhibiting trans-Golgi localization. The majority of dendritic cells localized both soluble (Ebola, 75%; ovalbumin, 84%) and liposomal antigens (58% and 65%), and irradiated Ebola virus to the trans-Golgi. These studies demonstrate that the intracellular fate of soluble and liposomal antigens can differ depending upon the antigen-presenting cell.

PMID: 16164039 [PubMed - indexed for MEDLINE]

1792. J Gene Med. 2005 Jan;7(1):50-8.

Transduction of satellite cells after prenatal intramuscular administration of lentiviral vectors.

MacKenzie TC(1), Kobinger GP, Louboutin JP, Radu A, Javazon EH, Sena-Esteves M, Wilson JM, Flake AW.

Author information: (1)The Children's Institute for Surgical Science, Children's Hospital of Philadelphia, Philadelphia, 3615 Civic Center Blvd., Philadelphia, PA 19104-4318, USA.

BACKGROUND: We have previously reported long-term expression of lacZ in myocytes after in utero intramuscular injection of Mokola and Ebola pseudotyped lentiviral vectors. In further experiments, we have noted that these vectors also transduce small cells at the periphery of the muscle fibers that have the morphology of satellite cells, or muscle stem cells. In this study we performed experiments to further define the morphology and function of these cells. METHODS: Balb/c mice at 14-15 days gestation were injected intramuscularly with Ebola or Mokola pseudotyped lentiviral vectors carrying CMV-lacZ. Animals were harvested at various time points, muscles were stained with X-gal, and processed for electron microscopy (EM) and immunofluorescence. To determine whether transduced satellite cells were functionally capable of regenerating injured muscles, animals were injected with notexin in the same area 8 weeks after the in utero injection of viral vector. RESULTS: Transmission EM of transduced cells confirmed the ultrastructural appearance of satellite cells. Double immunofluorescence for beta-galactosidase and satellite cell markers demonstrated co-localization of these markers in transduced cells. In the notexin-injured animals, small blue cells were seen at the areas of regeneration that co-localized beta-galactosidase with markers of regenerating satellite cells. Central nucleated blue fibers were seen at late time points, indicating regenerated muscle fibers arising from a transduced satellite cell. CONCLUSIONS: This study demonstrates transduction of muscle satellite cells following prenatal viral vector mediated gene transfer. These findings may have important implications for gene therapy strategies directed toward muscular dystrophy.

PMID: 15515139 [PubMed - indexed for MEDLINE]

1793. J Virol. 2005 Jan;79(2):918-26.

Studies of ebola virus glycoprotein-mediated entry and fusion by using pseudotyped human immunodeficiency virus type 1 virions: involvement of cytoskeletal proteins and enhancement by tumor necrosis factor alpha.

Yonezawa A(1), Cavrois M, Greene WC.

Author information: (1)Gladstone Institute of Virology and Immunology, 1650 Owens St., San Francisco, CA 94158, USA.

The Ebola filoviruses are aggressive pathogens that cause severe and often lethal hemorrhagic fever syndromes in humans and nonhuman primates. To date, no effective therapies have been identified. To analyze the entry and fusion properties of Ebola virus, we adapted a human immunodeficiency virus type 1 (HIV-1) virion-based fusion assay by substituting Ebola virus glycoprotein (GP) for the HIV-1 envelope. Fusion was detected by cleavage of the fluorogenic substrate CCF2 by beta-lactamase-Vpr incorporated into virions and released as a result of virion fusion. Entry and fusion induced by the Ebola virus GP occurred with much slower kinetics than with vesicular stomatitis virus G protein (VSV-G) and were blocked by depletion of membrane cholesterol and by inhibition of vesicular acidification with bafilomycin A1. These properties confirmed earlier studies and validated the assay for exploring other properties of Ebola virus GP-mediated entry and fusion. Entry and fusion of Ebola virus GP pseudotypes, but not VSV-G or HIV-1 Env pseudotypes, were impaired in the presence of the microtubule-disrupting agent nocodazole but were enhanced in the presence of the microtubule-stabilizing agent paclitaxel (Taxol). Agents that impaired microfilament function, including cytochalasin B, cytochalasin D, latrunculin A, and jasplakinolide, also inhibited Ebola virus GP-mediated entry and fusion. Together, these findings suggest that both microtubules and microfilaments may play a role in the effective trafficking of vesicles containing Ebola virions from the cell surface to the appropriate acidified vesicular compartment where fusion occurs. In terms of Ebola virus GP-mediated entry and fusion to various target cells, primary macrophages proved highly sensitive, while monocytes from the same donors displayed greatly reduced levels of entry and fusion. We further observed that tumor necrosis factor alpha, which is released by Ebola virus-infected monocytes/macrophages, enhanced Ebola virus GP-mediated entry and fusion to human umbilical vein endothelial cells. Thus, Ebola virus infection of one target cell may induce biological changes that facilitate infection of secondary target cells that play a key role in filovirus pathogenesis. Finally, these studies indicate that pseudotyping in the HIV-1 virion-based fusion assay may be a valuable approach to the study of entry and fusion properties mediated through the envelopes of other viral pathogens.

PMCID: PMC538559 PMID: 15613320 [PubMed - indexed for MEDLINE]

1794. J Virol. 2005 Jan;79(1):547-53.

Ebola virus glycoprotein toxicity is mediated by a dynamin-dependent protein-trafficking pathway.

Sullivan NJ(1), Peterson M, Yang ZY, Kong WP, Duckers H, Nabel E, Nabel GJ.

Author information: (1)Vaccine Research Center, National Institute for Allergy and Infectious Disease, National Institutes of Health, Bethesda, Maryland 20814, USA.

Ebola virus infection causes a highly lethal hemorrhagic fever syndrome associated with profound immunosuppression through its ability to induce widespread inflammation and cellular damage. Though GP, the viral envelope glycoprotein, mediates many of these effects, the molecular events that underlie Ebola virus cytopathicity are poorly understood. Here, we define a cellular mechanism responsible for Ebola virus GP cytotoxicity. GP selectively decreased the expression of cell surface molecules that are essential for cell adhesion and immune function. GP dramatically reduced levels of alphaVbeta3 without affecting the levels of alpha2beta1 or cadherin, leading to cell detachment and death. This effect was inhibited in vitro and in vivo by brefeldin A and was dependent on dynamin, the GTPase. GP also decreased cell surface expression of major histocompatibility complex class I molecules, which alters recognition by immune cells, and this effect was also dependent on the mucin domain previously implicated in GP cytotoxicity. By altering the trafficking of select cellular proteins, Ebola virus GP inflicts cell damage and may facilitate immune escape by the virus.

PMCID: PMC538691 PMID: 15596847 [PubMed - indexed for MEDLINE]

1795. Lancet Neurol. 2005 Jan;4(1):12-3.

Infections of the nervous system.

Gendelman HE(1), Persidsky Y.

Author information: (1)Center for Neurovirology and Neurodegenerative Disorders and Department of Pharmacology, University of Nebraska Medical Center, Omaha NE, USA. hegendel@unmc.edu

PMID: 15620853 [PubMed - indexed for MEDLINE]

1796. Mini Rev Med Chem. 2005 Jan;5(1):21-31.

The highly specific carbohydrate-binding protein cyanovirin-N: structure, anti-HIV/Ebola activity and possibilities for therapy.

Barrientos LG(1), Gronenborn AM.

Author information: (1)Laboratory of Chemical Physics, NIDDK, National Institutes of Health, Bethesda, MD 20892, USA. lbarrientosl@cdc.gov

Cyanovirin-N (CV-N), a cyanobacterial lectin, is a potent viral entry inhibitor currently under development as a microbicide against a broad spectrum of enveloped viruses. CV-N was originally identified as a highly active anti-HIV agent and later, as a virucidal agent against other unrelated enveloped viruses such as Ebola, and possibly other viruses. CV-N's antiviral activity appears to involve unique recognition of N-linked high-mannose oligosaccharides, Man-8 and Man-9, on the viral surface glycoproteins. Due to its distinct mode of action and opportunities for harnessing the associated interaction for therapeutic intervention, a substantial body of research on CV-N has accumulated since its discovery in 1997. In this review we focus in particular on structural studies on CV-N and their relationship to biological activity.

PMID: 15638789 [PubMed - indexed for MEDLINE]

1797. Nucleosides Nucleotides Nucleic Acids. 2005;24(10-12):1395-415.

John Montgomery's legacy: carbocyclic adenosine analogues as SAH hydrolase inhibitors with broad-spectrum antiviral activity.

De Clercq E(1).

Author information: (1)Rega Institute for Medical Research, Department of Microbiology and Immunology, K.U. Letven, Minderbroedersstraat 10, B-3000 Leuven, Belgium. erik.declercq@rega.kuleuven.be

Ever since the S-adenosylhomocysteine (AdoHcy, SAH) hydrolase was recognized as a pharmacological target for antiviral agents (J. A. Montgomery et al., J. Med. Chem. 25:626-629, 1982), an increasing number of adenosine, acyclic adenosine, and carbocyclic adenosine analogues have been described as potent SAH hydrolase inhibitors endowed with broad-spectrum antiviral activity. The antiviral activity spectrum of the SAH hydrolase inhibitors include pox-, rhabdo-, filo-, arena-, paramyxo-, reo-, and retroviruses. Among the most potent SAH hydrolase inhibitors and antiviral agents rank carbocyclic 3-deazaadenosine (C-c3 Ado), neplanocin A, 3-deazaneplanocin A, the 5'-nor derivatives of carbocyclic adenosine (C-Ado, aristeromycin), and the 2-halo (i.e., 2-fluoro) and 6'-R-alkyl (i.e., 6'-R-methyl) derivatives of neplanocin A. These compounds are particularly active against poxviruses (i.e., vaccinia virus), and rhabdoviruses (i.e., vesicular stomatitis virus). The in vivo efficacy of C-c3 Ado and 3-deazaneplanocin A has been established in mouse models for vaccinia virus, vesicular stomatitis virus, and Ebola virus. SAH hydrolase inhibitors such as C-c3Ado and 3-deazaneplanocin A should in thefirst place be considered for therapeutic (or prophylactic) use against poxvirus infections, including smallpox, and hemorrhagic fever virus infections such as Ebola.

PMID: 16438025 [PubMed - indexed for MEDLINE]

1798. Stud Health Technol Inform. 2005;116:217-22.

Using blood glucose data as an indicator for epidemic disease outbreaks.

Arsand E(1), Walseth OA, Andersson N, Fernando R, Granberg O, Bellika JG, Hartvigsen G.

Author information: (1)Norwegian Centre for Telemedicine, University hospital of North Norway, Tromsø, Norway.

In the future, transfer of vital sensor data from patients to the public health care system is likely to become commonplace. Systems for automatic transfer of sensor data are now at the prototype stage. As electronic health record (EHR) systems adapt such functionality, widespread use may become an actuality in the foreseeable future.To prevent spreading of diseases, an early detection of infection is important. At the time an outbreak is diagnosed, many people may already be infected due to the incubation period. This study suggests an approach for detecting an epidemic outbreak at an early stage by monitoring blood glucose data collected from people with diabetes. Continuous analysis of blood glucose data may have the potential to prevent large outbreaks of infectious diseases, such as different strains of Influenza, Cholera, Plague, Ebola, Anthrax and SARS.When a person gets infected, the blood glucose value increases. If the blood glucose data from a large number of patients with diabetes are collected in a central database, it may be possible to detect an epidemic disease outbreak at an early stage. Advanced data analysis on the data may detect predominant numbers of incidences, indicating a possible outbreak. This gives the health authorities the possibilities to take actions to limit the outbreak and its consequences for all the inhabitants in an affected area.At the Norwegian Centre for Telemedicine, a mobile system for automatic transfer of blood glucose values has been constructed. By using wireless communication standards such as Bluetooth and GSM, the system transfers blood glucose data to an electronic health record system. Combined with a system accessing and querying data from EHR systems for patient surveillance we are extending our work into an Epidemic Disease Detection using blood Glucose (EDDG) system.

PMID: 16160262 [PubMed - in process]

1799. Euro Surveill. 2004 Dec 15;9(12):E11-2.

Bichat guidelines for the clinical management of haemorrhagic fever viruses and bioterrorism-related haemorrhagic fever viruses.

Bossi P(1), Tegnell A, Baka A, Van Loock F, Hendriks J, Werner A, Maidhof H, Gouvras G; Task Force on Biological and Chemical Agent Threats, Public Health Directorate, European Commission, Luxembourg.

Author information: (1)Task Force on Biological and Chemical Agent Threats, Public Health Directorate, European Commission, Luxembourg. philippe.bossi@psl.ap-hop-paris.fr

Haemorrhagic fever viruses (HFVs) are a diverse group of viruses that cause a clinical disease associated with fever and bleeding disorder. HFVs that are associated with a potential biological threat are Ebola and Marburg viruses (Filoviridae), Lassa fever and New World arenaviruses (Machupo, Junin, Guanarito and Sabia viruses) (Arenaviridae), Rift Valley fever (Bunyaviridae) and yellow fever, Omsk haemorrhagic fever, and Kyanasur Forest disease (Flaviviridae). In terms of biological warfare concerning dengue, Crimean-Congo haemorrhagic fever and Hantaviruses, there is not sufficient knowledge to include them as a major biological threat. Dengue virus is the only one of these that cannot be transmitted via aerosol. Crimean-Congo haemorrhagic fever and the agents of haemorrhagic fever with renal syndrome appear difficult to weaponise. Ribavirin is recommended for the treatment and the prophylaxis of the arenaviruses and the bunyaviruses, but is not effective for the other families. All patients must be isolated and receive intensive supportive therapy.

PMID: 15677844 [PubMed - indexed for MEDLINE]

1800. J Virol Methods. 2004 Dec 15;122(2):131-9.

Optimized large-scale production of high titer lentivirus vector pseudotypes.

Sena-Esteves M(1), Tebbets JC, Steffens S, Crombleholme T, Flake AW.

Author information: (1)Department of Surgery, The Children's Hospital of Philadelphia, Abramson Research Center, 3615 Civic Center Blvd., Philadelphia, PA 19104, USA. msesteves@partners.org

The goal of the present study was to develop an efficient transient transfection method for large-scale production of high titer lentivirus vector stocks of eight different pseudotypes. The envelope genes used for this purpose were those from VSV-G, Mokola, Rabies, MLV-Ampho, MLV-10A1, LCMV-WE, and LCMV-Arm53b. All envelopes were cloned into phCMV, which yielded lentivirus vector titers one, two, or three orders of magnitude higher than the original plasmids for the Rabies, MLV-10A1, and MLV-Ampho envelopes, respectively. When these newly constructed envelope expression plasmids were used for packaging, treatment with sodium butyrate resulted in almost five-fold increase in titers for some of the pseudotypes, had no effect for others (VSV-G and Rabies), and negatively impacted titers for the LCMV-derived pseudotypes. Production of vectors in serum-free media yielded titers only slightly lower than those obtained in the presence of serum. The efficiency of concentrating vector supernatants by ultracentrifugation or ultrafiltration was compared, with higher recovery efficiencies for the latter method, but the highest titers for most pseudotypes were obtained by ultracentrifugation. The best conditions for each individual pseudotype yielded lentivirus vector stocks with titers above $1 \times 10(9)$ tu/mL for most pseudotypes, and higher than $1 \times 10(10)$ tu/mL for VSV-G.
PMID: 15542136 [PubMed - indexed for MEDLINE]

1801. Wkly Epidemiol Rec. 2004 Dec 3;79(49):435-9.

Ebola haemorrhagic fever--fact sheet revised in May 2004.

[Article in English, French]

[No authors listed]

PMID: 15638356 [PubMed - indexed for MEDLINE]

1802. Emerg Infect Dis. 2004 Dec;10(12):2094-9.

Exposure to nonhuman primates in rural Cameroon.

Wolfe ND(1), Prosser TA, Carr JK, Tamoufe U, Mpoudi-Ngole E, Torimiro JN, LeBreton M, McCutchan FE, Birx DL, Burke DS.

Author information: (1)Johns Hopkins Bloomberg School of Public Health, Baltimore, Maryland 21205, USA. nwolfe@jhsph.edu

Exposure to nonhuman primates has led to the emergence of important diseases, including Ebola hemorrhagic fever, AIDS, and adult T-cell leukemia. To determine the extent of exposure to nonhuman primates, persons were examined in 17 remote villages in Cameroon that represented three habitats (savanna, gallery forest, and lowland forest). Questionnaire data were collected to assess whether persons kept wild animal pets; hunted and butchered wild game; had experienced bites, scratches, or injuries from live animals; or had been injured during hunting or butchering. While all villages had substantial exposure to nonhuman primates, higher rates of exposure were seen in lowland forest sites. The study demonstrates that exposure is not limited to small groups of hunters. A high percentage of rural villagers report exposure to nonhuman primate blood and body fluids and risk acquiring infectious diseases.
PMCID: PMC3323379 PMID: 15663844 [PubMed - indexed for MEDLINE]

1803. Emerg Infect Dis. 2004 Dec;10(12):2073-81.

Potential mammalian filovirus reservoirs.

Peterson AT(1), Carroll DS, Mills JN, Johnson KM.

Author information: (1)University of Kansas, Lawrence, Kansas 66045, USA. town@ku.edu

Ebola and Marburg viruses are maintained in unknown reservoir species; spillover into human populations results in occasional human cases or epidemics. We attempted to narrow the list of possibilities regarding the identity of those reservoir species. We made a series of explicit assumptions about the reservoir: it is a mammal; it supports persistent, largely asymptomatic filovirus infections; its range subsumes that of its associated filovirus; it has coevolved with the virus; it is of small body size; and it is not a species that is commensal with humans. Under these assumptions, we developed priority lists of mammal clades that coincide distributionally with filovirus outbreak distributions and compared these lists with those mammal taxa that have been tested for filovirus infection in previous epidemiologic studies. Studying the remainder of these taxa may be a fruitful avenue for pursuing the identity of natural reservoirs of filoviruses.
PMCID: PMC3323391 PMID: 15663841 [PubMed - indexed for MEDLINE]

1804. J Clin Microbiol. 2004 Dec;42(12):5472-6.

Sequencing needs for viral diagnostics.

Gardner SN(1), Lam MW, Mulakken NJ, Torres CL, Smith JR, Slezak TR.

Author information: (1)Computations, Lawrence Livermore National Laboratory, P.O. Box 808, L-174, Livermore, CA 94551, USA. gardner26@llnl.gov

We built a system to guide decisions regarding the amount of genomic sequencing required to develop diagnostic DNA signatures, which are short sequences that are sufficient to uniquely identify a viral species. We used our existing DNA diagnostic signature prediction pipeline, which selects regions of a target species genome that are conserved among strains of the target (for reliability, to prevent false negatives) and unique relative to other species (for specificity, to avoid false positives). We performed simulations, based on existing sequence data, to assess the number of genome sequences of a target species and of close phylogenetic relatives (near neighbors) that are required to predict diagnostic signature regions that are conserved among strains of the target species and unique relative to other bacterial and viral species. For DNA viruses such as variola (smallpox), three target genomes provide sufficient guidance for selecting species-wide signatures. Three near-neighbor genomes are critical for species specificity. In contrast, most RNA viruses require four target genomes and no near-neighbor genomes, since lack of conservation among strains is more limiting than uniqueness. Severe acute respiratory syndrome and Ebola Zaire are exceptional, as additional target genomes currently do not improve predictions, but near-neighbor sequences are urgently needed. Our results also indicate that double-stranded DNA viruses are more conserved among strains than are RNA viruses, since in most cases there was at least one conserved signature candidate for the DNA viruses and zero conserved signature candidates for the RNA viruses.
PMCID: PMC535215 PMID: 15583268 [PubMed - indexed for MEDLINE]

1805. J Infect Dis. 2004 Dec 1;190(11):1895-9. Epub 2004 Nov 3.

A serological survey of Ebola virus infection in central African nonhuman primates.

Leroy EM(1), Telfer P, Kumulungui B, Yaba P, Rouquet P, Roques P, Gonzalez JP, Ksiazek TG, Rollin PE, Nerrienet E.

Author information: (1)Centre International de Recherches Medicales de Franceville, Institut de Recherche pour le Developpement, UR034, Franceville, Gabon. eric.leroy@ird.fr.

Comment in J Infect Dis. 2004 Dec 1;190(11):1893-4.

We used an ELISA to determine the prevalence of IgG antibodies specific for the Zaire subtype of Ebola virus in 790 nonhuman primates, belonging to 20 species, studied between 1985 and 2000 in Cameroon, Gabon, and the Republic of Congo. The seroprevalence rate of Ebola antibody in wild-born chimpanzees was 12.9%, indicating that (1) Ebola virus circulates in the forests of a large region of central Africa, including countries such as Cameroon, where no human cases of Ebola infections have been reported; (2) Ebola virus was present in the area before recent outbreaks in humans; (3) chimpanzees are continuously in contact with the virus; and (4) nonlethal Ebola infection can occur in chimpanzees. These results, together with the unexpected detection of Ebola-specific IgG in other species (5 drills, 1 baboon, 1 mandrill, and 1 Cercopithecus), may help to narrow the search for the reservoir of Ebola virus. They also suggest that future Ebola outbreaks may occur anywhere in the central African forest region.

PMID: 15529251 [PubMed - indexed for MEDLINE]

1806. J Infect Dis. 2004 Dec 1;190(11):1893-4. Epub 2004 Nov 3.

Ebola virus ecology.

McCormick JB.

Comment on J Infect Dis. 2004 Dec 1;190(11):1895-9.

PMID: 15529250 [PubMed - indexed for MEDLINE]

1807. Nat Med. 2004 Dec;10(12 Suppl):S110-21.

Exotic emerging viral diseases: progress and challenges.

Geisbert TW(1), Jahrling PB.

Author information: (1)Virology Division, US Army Medical Research Institute of Infectious Diseases, 1425 Porter Street, Fort Detrick, Maryland 21702-5011, USA. tom.geisbert@amedd.army.mil

The agents causing viral hemorrhagic fever (VHF) are a taxonomically diverse group of viruses that may share commonalities in the process whereby they produce systemic and frequently fatal disease. Significant progress has been made in understanding the biology of the Ebola virus, one of the best known examples. This knowledge has guided our thinking about other VHF agents, including Marburg, Lassa, the South American arenaviruses, yellow fever, Crimean-Congo and Rift Valley fever viruses. Comparisons among VHFs show that a common pathogenic feature is their ability to disable the host immune response by attacking and manipulating the cells that initiate the antiviral response. Of equal importance, these comparisons highlight critical gaps in our knowledge of these pathogens.

PMID: 15577929 [PubMed - indexed for MEDLINE]

1808. PLoS Med. 2004 Dec;1(3):e59.

Containing the threat--don't forget Ebola.

Cohen J(1).

Author information: (1)Brighton and Sussex Medical School, Brighton, United Kingdom. j.cohen@bsms.ac.uk

PMCID: PMC539049 PMID: 15630468 [PubMed - indexed for MEDLINE]

1809. Soc Sci Med. 2004 Dec;59(12):2561-71.

Representations of SARS in the British newspapers.

Washer P(1).

Author information: (1)Academic Centre for Medical Education, University College London, Archway Campus, Highgate Hill, London N19 3LW, UK. peter.washer@ucl.ac.uk

In the Spring of 2003, there was a huge interest in the global news media following the emergence of a new infectious disease: severe acute respiratory syndrome (SARS). This study examines how this novel disease threat was depicted in the UK newspapers, using social representations theory and in particular existing work on social representations of HIV/AIDS and Ebola to analyse the meanings of the epidemic. It investigates the way that SARS was presented as a dangerous threat to the UK public, whilst almost immediately the threat was said to be 'contained' using the mechanism of 'othering': SARS was said to be unlikely to personally affect the UK reader because the Chinese were so different to 'us'; so 'other'. In this sense, the SARS scare, despite the remarkable speed with which it was played out in the modern global news media, resonates with the meanings attributed to other epidemics of infectious diseases throughout history. Yet this study also highlights a number of differences in the social representations of SARS compared with earlier epidemics. In particular, this study examines the phenomena of 'emerging and re-emerging infectious diseases' over the past 30 or so years and suggests that these have impacted on the faith once widely held that Western biomedicine could 'conquer' infectious disease.

PMID: 15474209 [PubMed - indexed for MEDLINE]

1810. Virus Res. 2004 Dec;106(2):181-8.

Filovirus budding.

Jasenosky LD(1), Kawaoka Y.

Author information: (1)Department of Pathobiological Sciences, School of Veterinary Medicine, University of Wisconsin-Madison, 2015 Linden Drive West, Madison, WI 53706, USA.

Family Filoviridae, which includes Ebola virus (EBOV) and Marburg virus (MARV), is a growing threat to human and non-human primate populations in central Africa. Although many facets of the filovirus life cycle remain to be deciphered, a great deal has been learned in recent years. In particular, a clearer understanding of the roles played by viral, as well as cellular, proteins in the assembly and budding processes has been achieved. This review will discuss the current state of filovirus budding research, with especial emphasis placed on the viral matrix protein VP40 and its relationship with the cellular vesicular sorting pathway. Possible budding functions of the viral glycoprotein (GP), as well as the membrane-associated viral protein 24 (VP24), will also be described, and a model for filovirus budding will be proposed.

PMID: 15567496 [PubMed - indexed for MEDLINE]

1811. Nihon Naika Gakkai Zasshi. 2004 Nov 10;93(11):2303-8.

[Viral hemorrhagic fevers--Ebola hemorrhagic fever, Marburg virus disease, and Lassa fever].

[Article in Japanese]

Taniguchi K.

PMID: 15624463 [PubMed - indexed for MEDLINE]

1812. Proc Natl Acad Sci U S A. 2004 Nov 2;101(44):15748-53. Epub 2004 Oct 20.

CD209L (L-SIGN) is a receptor for severe acute respiratory syndrome coronavirus.

Jeffers SA(1), Tusell SM, Gillim-Ross L, Hemmila EM, Achenbach JE, Babcock GJ, Thomas WD Jr, Thackray LB, Young MD, Mason RJ, Ambrosino DM, Wentworth DE, Demartini JC, Holmes KV.

Author information: (1)Department of Microbiology and Molecular Biology Program, University Colorado Health Sciences Center, 4200 East 9th Avenue, Denver, CO 80262, USA.

Angiotensin-converting enzyme 2 (ACE2) is a receptor for SARS-CoV, the novel coronavirus that causes severe acute respiratory syndrome [Li, W. Moore, M. J., Vasilieva, N., Sui, J., Wong, S. K., Berne, M. A., Somasundaran, M., Sullivan, J. L., Luzuriaga, K., Greenough, T. C., et al. (2003) Nature 426, 450-454]. We have identified a different human cellular glycoprotein that can serve as an alternative receptor for SARS-CoV. A human lung cDNA library in vesicular stomatitis virus G pseudotyped retrovirus was transduced into Chinese hamster ovary cells, and the cells were sorted for binding of soluble SARS-CoV spike (S) glycoproteins, S(590) and S(1180). Clones of transduced cells that bound SARS-CoV S glycoprotein were inoculated with SARS-CoV, and increases in subgenomic viral RNA from 1-16 h or more were detected by multiplex RT-PCR in four cloned cell lines. Sequencing of the human lung cDNA inserts showed that each of the cloned cell lines contained cDNA that encoded human CD209L, a C-type lectin (also called L-SIGN). When the cDNA encoding CD209L from clone 2.27 was cloned and transfected into Chinese hamster ovary cells, the cells expressed human CD209L glycoprotein and became susceptible to infection with SARS-CoV. Immunohistochemistry showed that CD209L is expressed in human lung in type II alveolar cells and endothelial cells, both potential targets for SARS-CoV. Several other enveloped viruses including Ebola and Sindbis also use CD209L as a portal of entry, and HIV and hepatitis C virus can bind to CD209L on cell membranes but do not use it to mediate virus entry. Our data suggest that the large S glycoprotein of SARS-CoV may use both ACE2 and CD209L in virus infection and pathogenesis.

PMCID: PMC524836 PMID: 15496474 [PubMed - indexed for MEDLINE]

1813. Am J Trop Med Hyg. 2004 Nov;71(5):664-74.

Trigger events: enviroclimatic coupling of Ebola hemorrhagic fever outbreaks.

Pinzon JE(1), Wilson JM, Tucker CJ, Arthur R, Jahrling PB, Formenty P.

Author information: (1)Biospheric Sciences Branch, Laboratory for Terrestrial Physics, National Aeronautics and Space Administration-Goddard Space Flight Center, Greenbelt, MD 20771, USA. pinzon@negev.gsfc.nasa.gov

We use spatially continuous satellite data as a correlate of precipitation within tropical Africa and show that the majority of documented Ebola hemorrhagic fever outbreaks were closely associated with sharply drier conditions at the end of the rainy season. We propose that these trigger events may enhance transmission of Ebola virus from its cryptic reservoir to humans. These findings suggest specific directions to help understand the sylvatic cycle of the virus and may provide early warning tools to detect possible future outbreaks of this enigmatic disease.

PMID: 15569802 [PubMed - indexed for MEDLINE]

1814. Emerg Med Clin North Am. 2004 Nov;22(4):1051-65, ix-x.

Deadly viral syndrome mimics.

Lowenstein R(1).

Author information: (1)Department of Emergency Medicine, Boston Medical Center, Dowling 1 South, 1 Boston Medical Center Place, Boston, MA 02118, USA. Robert.lowenstein@bmc.org

Upper respiratory tract infections (ie, "the common cold") have several hundred causes, the most common of which include rhino-virus, coronavirus, and respiratory syncytial virus. The clinical presentation varies with symptoms. Every emergency department, no matter what the demographics, cares for patients with this constellation of symptoms. Emergency physicians examine, diagnose, and treat these disorders frequently. With increasing burdens being placed on emergency physicians, it is possible to assume a diagnosis of upper respiratory tract infection without generating a complete differential diagnosis. The challenge is to identify and recognize the distinctions between an innocuous upper respiratory tract infection and a life-threatening disease "mimic" or entities. This article discusses some of these life-threatening mimics.

PMID: 15474781 [PubMed - indexed for MEDLINE]

1815. J Virol. 2004 Nov;78(22):12277-87.

Multivesicular bodies as a platform for formation of the Marburg virus envelope.

Kolesnikova L(1), Berghöfer B, Bamberg S, Becker S.

Author information: (1)Institut für Virologie der Philipps-Universität Marburg, Robert-Koch-Strasse 17, D-35037 Marburg, Germany.

The Marburg virus (MARV) envelope consists of a lipid membrane and two major proteins, the matrix protein VP40 and the glycoprotein GP. Both proteins use different intracellular transport pathways: GP utilizes the exocytotic pathway, while VP40 is transported through the retrograde late endosomal pathway. It is currently unknown where the proteins combine to form the viral envelope. In the present study, we identified the intracellular site where the two major envelope proteins of MARV come together as peripheral multivesicular bodies (MVBs). Upon coexpression with VP40, GP is redistributed from the trans-Golgi network into the VP40-containing MVBs. Ultrastructural analysis of MVBs suggested that they provide the platform for the formation of membrane structures that bud as virus-like particles from the cell surface. The virus-like particles contain both VP40 and GP. Single expression of GP also resulted in the release of particles, which are round or pleomorphic. Single expression of VP40 led to the release of filamentous structures that closely resemble viral particles and contain traces of endosomal marker proteins. This finding indicated a central role of VP40 in the formation of the filamentous structure of MARV particles, which is similar to the role of the related Ebola virusVP40. In MARV-infected cells, VP40 and GP are colocalized in peripheral MVBs as well. Moreover, intracellular budding of progeny virions into MVBs was frequently detected. Taken together, these results demonstrate an intracellular intersection between GP and VP40 pathways and suggest a crucial role of the late endosomal compartment for the formation of the viral envelope.

PMCID: PMC525088 PMID: 15507615 [PubMed - indexed for MEDLINE]

1816. J Virol. 2004 Nov;78(21):12090-5.

DC-SIGN and DC-SIGNR interact with the glycoprotein of Marburg virus and the S protein of severe acute respiratory syndrome coronavirus.

Marzi A(1), Gramberg T, Simmons G, Möller P, Rennekamp AJ, Krumbiegel M, Geier M, Eisemann J, Turza N, Saunier B, Steinkasserer A, Becker S, Bates P, Hofmann H, Pöhlmann S.

Author information: (1)Institute for Clinical and Molecular Virology, University Erlangen-Nürnberg, Nikolaus-Fiebiger-Center, Glückstrasse 6, D-91054 Erlangen, Germany.

The lectins DC-SIGN and DC-SIGNR can augment viral infection; however, the range of pathogens interacting with these attachment factors is incompletely defined. Here we show that DC-SIGN and DC-SIGNR enhance infection mediated by the glycoprotein (GP) of Marburg virus (MARV) and the S protein of severe acute respiratory syndrome coronavirus and might promote viral dissemination. SIGNR1, a murine DC-SIGN homologue, also enhanced infection driven by MARV and Ebola virus GP and could be targeted to assess the role of attachment factors in filovirus infection in vivo.

PMCID: PMC523257 PMID: 15479853 [PubMed - indexed for MEDLINE]

1817. Lancet Infect Dis. 2004 Nov;4(11):704-8.

Seasonality of infectious diseases and severe acute respiratory syndrome-what we don't know can hurt us.

Dowell SF(1), Ho MS.

Author information: (1)International Emerging Infections Program, Thai Ministry of Public Health and the US Centers for Disease Control and Prevention, Nonthaburi, Thailand. scottd@tuc.or.th

The novel severe acute respiratory syndrome (SARS) coronavirus caused severe disease and heavy economic losses before apparently coming under complete control. Our understanding of the forces driving seasonal disappearance and recurrence of infectious diseases remains fragmentary, thus limiting any predictions about whether, or when, SARS will recur. It is true that most established respiratory pathogens of human beings recur in wintertime, but a new appreciation for the high burden of disease in tropical areas reinforces questions about explanations resting solely on cold air or low humidity. Seasonal variation in host physiology may also contribute. Newly emergent zoonotic diseases such as ebola or pandemic strains of influenza have recurred in unpredictable patterns. Most established coronaviruses exhibit winter seasonality, with a unique ability to establish persistent infections in a minority of infected animals. Because SARS coronavirus RNA can be detected in the stool of some individuals for at least 9 weeks, recurrence of SARS from persistently shedding human or animal reservoirs is biologically plausible.

PMID: 15522683 [PubMed - indexed for MEDLINE]

1818. Med Microbiol Immunol. 2004 Nov;193(4):181-7. Epub 2003 Oct 31.

Production of monoclonal antibodies and development of an antigen capture ELISA directed against the envelope glycoprotein GP of Ebola virus.

Lucht A(1), Grunow R, Otterbein C, Möller P, Feldmann H, Becker S.

Author information: (1)Bundeswehr Institute of Microbiology, Neuherbergstrasse 11, 80937 Munich, Germany. andreaslu@gmx.de

Ebola virus (EBOV) causes severe outbreaks of Ebola hemorrhagic fever in endemic regions of Africa and is considered to be of impact for other parts of the world as an imported viral disease. To develop a new diagnostic test, monoclonal antibodies to EBOV were produced from mice immunized with inactivated EBOV species Zaire. Antibodies directed against the viral glycoprotein GP were characterized by ELISA, Western blot and immunofluorescence analyses. An antigen capture ELISA was established, which is specific for EBOV-Zaire and shows a sensitivity of approximately 10(3) plaque-forming units/ml. Since the ELISA is able to detect even SDS-inactivated EBOV in spiked human sera, it could complement the existing diagnostic tools in the field and in routine laboratories where high containment facilities are not available.

PMID: 14593476 [PubMed - indexed for MEDLINE]

1819. Virus Res. 2004 Nov;106(1):43-50.

Rescue of Ebola virus from cDNA using heterologous support proteins.

Theriault S(1), Groseth A, Neumann G, Kawaoka Y, Feldmann H.

Author information: (1)Special Pathogens Program, National Laboratory for Zoonotic Diseases and Special Pathogens, National Microbiology Laboratory, Health Canada, Canada.

Using the infectious clone for Zaire ebolavirus, the functional specificity of viral proteins of the ribonucleoprotein complex in transcription/replication was investigated by substituting them with heterologous proteins derived from closely (Reston ebolavirus) and distantly related filoviruses (Marburgvirus). The data clearly demonstrated that transcription/replication are neither strictly species-specific nor genus-specific. Protein interactions between the nucleoprotein NP and the virion protein VP35 and the polymerase L and VP35 seemed to be the most critical steps. In contrast to previous data, viral proteins were able to target heterologous filovirus RNA. Together these results indicated that protein-protein interactions are more critical than protein-RNA interactions.

PMID: 15522446 [PubMed - indexed for MEDLINE]

1820. Virology. 2004 Oct 25;328(2):177-84.

A C-terminal basic amino acid motif of Zaire ebolavirus VP35 is essential for type I interferon antagonism and displays high identity with the RNA-binding domain of another interferon antagonist, the NS1 protein of influenza A virus.

Hartman AL(1), Towner JS, Nichol ST.

Author information: (1)Special Pathogens Branch, Division of Viral and Rickettsial Diseases, National Center for Infectious Diseases, Centers for Disease Control and Prevention, 1600 Clifton Road MS G-14 Atlanta, GA 30329, USA. biq7@cdc.gov

The ebolavirus VP35 protein antagonizes the cellular type I interferon response by blocking phosphorylation of IRF-3, a transcription factor that turns on the expression of a large number of antiviral genes. To identify the domain of VP35 responsible for interferon antagonism, we generated mutations within the VP35 gene and found that a C-terminal basic amino acid motif is required for inhibition of ISG56 reporter gene expression as well as IFN-beta production. Remarkably, this basic amino acid motif displayed high sequence identity with part of the N-terminal RNA-binding domain of another interferon-antagonist, the NS1 protein of influenza A virus.

PMID: 15464838 [PubMed - indexed for MEDLINE]

1821. Biochem Biophys Res Commun. 2004 Oct 15;323(2):696-702.

Disulfide bond assignment of the Ebola virus secreted glycoprotein SGP.

Barrientos LG(1), Martin AM, Rollin PE, Sanchez A.

Author information: (1)Special Pathogens Branch, Division of Viral and Rickettsial Diseases, Scientific Resources Program, National Center for Infectious Diseases, Centers for Disease Control and Prevention, Atlanta, GA, USA.

The non-structural glycoprotein (SGP) of Ebola virus (EboV) is secreted in large amounts from infected cells as a disulfide-linked homodimer. In this communication, highly purified SGP, derived from Vero E6 cultures infected with the Zaire species of EboV, was used to determine the correct localization of inter- and intrachain disulfide bonds. Matrix-assisted laser desorption/ionization-time-of-flight mass spectrometry analysis of proteolytic cleavage fragments indicates that all cysteines (six per monomeric unit) form unique disulfide bonds. Monomers of the SGP homodimer are joined in a parallel manner by two intersubunit disulfide bonds formed between paired N-terminal and C-terminal cysteines (C53-C53' and C306-C306'). The remaining cysteines are involved in intrachain disulfide bonding (paired as C108-C135 and C121-C147), which resembles the disulfide bond topology of fibronectin type II domains. The findings presented here provide the foundation for future studies aimed at defining the structural and functional properties of SGP.

Copyright 2004 Elsevier Inc.

PMID: 15369806 [PubMed - indexed for MEDLINE]

1822. Clin Microbiol Infect. 2004 Oct;10(10):945-8.

Sequence and structure relatedness of matrix protein of human respiratory syncytial virus with matrix proteins of other negative-sense RNA viruses.

Latiff K(1), Meanger J, Mills J, Ghildyal R.

Author information: (1)Children's Virology Research Unit, Macfarlane Burnet Institute of Medical Research and Public Health, Monash University, Melbourne, Australia.

Matrix proteins of viruses within the order Mononegavirales have similar functions and play important roles in virus assembly. Protein sequence alignment, phylogenetic tree derivation, hydropathy profiles and secondary structure prediction were performed on selected matrix protein sequences, using human respiratory syncytial virus matrix protein as the reference. No general conservation of primary, secondary or tertiary structure was found, except for a broad similarity in the hydropathy pattern correlating with the fact that all the proteins studied are membrane-associated. Interestingly, the matrix proteins of Ebola virus and human respiratory syncytial virus shared secondary structure homology.

PMID: 15373896 [PubMed - indexed for MEDLINE]

1823. J Virol. 2004 Oct;78(19):10370-7.

Analysis of human peripheral blood samples from fatal and nonfatal cases of Ebola (Sudan) hemorrhagic fever: cellular responses, virus load, and nitric oxide levels.

Sanchez A(1), Lukwiya M, Bausch D, Mahanty S, Sanchez AJ, Wagoner KD, Rollin PE.

Author information: (1)Special Pathogens Branch, Division of Viral and Rickettsial Diseases, National Center for Infectious Diseases, Centers for Disease Control and Prevention, Atlanta, GA 30333, USA. ASanchez1@cdc.gov

Peripheral blood samples obtained from patients during an outbreak of Ebola virus (Sudan species) disease in Uganda in 2000 were used to phenotype peripheral blood mononuclear cells (PBMC), quantitate gene expression, measure antigenemia, and determine nitric oxide levels. It was determined that as the severity of disease increased in infected patients, there was a corresponding increase in antigenemia and leukopenia. Blood smears revealed thrombocytopenia, a left shift in neutrophils (in some cases degenerating), and atypical lymphocytes. Infected patients who died had reduced numbers of T cells, CD8(+) T cells, and activated (HLA-DR(+)) CD8(+) T cells, while the opposite was noted for patients who survived the disease. Expression levels of cytokines, Fas antigen, and Fas ligand (TaqMan quantitation) in PBMC from infected patients were not significantly different from those in uninfected patients (treated in the same isolation wards), nor was there a significant increase in expression compared to healthy volunteers (United States). This unresponsive state of PBMC from infected patients despite high levels of circulating antigen and virus replication suggests that some form of immunosuppression had developed. Ebola virus RNA levels (virus load) in PBMC specimens were found to be much higher in infected patients who died than patients who survived the disease. Similarly, blood levels of nitric oxide were much higher in fatal cases (increasing with disease severity), and extremely elevated levels (>/=150 microM) would have negatively affected vascular tone and contributed to virus-induced shock.

PMCID: PMC516433 PMID: 15367603 [PubMed - indexed for MEDLINE]

1824. Sci Am. 2004 Oct;291(4):20, 24.

An uncertain defense. How do you test that a human Ebola vaccine works? You don't.

Gibbs WW.

PMID: 15487661 [PubMed - indexed for MEDLINE]

1825. Structure. 2004 Oct;12(10):1799-807.

Flipping the switch from monomeric to dimeric CV-N has little effect on antiviral activity.

Barrientos LG(1), Lasala F, Delgado R, Sanchez A, Gronenborn AM.

Author information: (1)Laboratory of Chemical Physics, National Institute of Diabetes and Digestive and Kidney Diseases, National Institutes of Health, Bethesda, MD 20892, USA. lbarrientos1@cdc.gov

Cyanovirin-N can exist in solution in monomeric and domain-swapped dimeric forms, with HIV-antiviral activity being reported for both. Here we present results for CV-N variants that form stable solution dimers: the obligate dimer [DeltaQ50]CV-N and the preferential dimer [S52P]CV-N. These variants exhibit comparable DeltaG values (10.6 +/- 0.5 and 9.4 +/- 0.5 kcal.mol(-1), respectively), similar to that of stabilized, monomeric [P51G]CV-N (9.8 +/- 0.5 kcal.mol(-1)), but significantly higher than wild-type CV-N (4.1 +/- 0.2 kcal.mol(-1)). During folding/unfolding, no stably folded monomer was observed under any condition for the obligate dimer [DeltaQ50]CV-N, whereas two monomeric, metastable species were detected for [S52P]CV-N at low concentrations. This is in contrast to our previous results for [P51G]CV-N and wild-type CV-N, for which the dimeric forms were found to be the metastable species. The dimeric mutants exhibit comparable antiviral activity against HIV and Ebola, similar to that of wild-type CV-N and the stabilized [P51G]CV-N variant.

Copyright 2004 Elsevier Ltd.

PMID: 15458629 [PubMed - indexed for MEDLINE]

1826. Trends Microbiol. 2004 Oct;12(10):433-7.

Ebola virus ecology: a continuing mystery.

Feldmann H(1), Wahl-Jensen V, Jones SM, Ströher U.

Author information: (1)Special Pathogens Program, National Microbiology Laboratory, Health Canada, Winnipeg, Manitoba R3E 3R2, Canada. Heinz_Feldmann@hc-sc.gc.ca

PMID: 15381189 [PubMed - indexed for MEDLINE]

1827. Expert Rev Mol Med. 2004 Sep 21;6(20):1-24.

Ebola virus: new insights into disease aetiopathology and possible therapeutic interventions.

Geisbert TW(1), Hensley LE.

Author information: (1)Department of Viral Pathology and Ultrastructure, Virology Division, United States Army Medical Research Institute of Infectious Diseases, Fort Detrick, MD 21702-5011, USA. tom.geisbert@amedd.army.mil

Ebola virus (EBOV) gained public notoriety in the last decade largely as a consequence of the highly publicized isolation of a new EBOV species in a suburb of Washington, DC, in 1989, together with the dramatic clinical presentation of EBOV infection and high case-fatality rate in Africa (near 90% in some outbreaks), and the unusual and striking morphology of the virus. Furthermore, there are no vaccines or effective therapies currently available. Progress in understanding the origins of the pathophysiological changes that make EBOV infections of humans so devastating has been slow, primarily because these viruses require special containment for safe research. However, an increasing understanding of the mechanisms of EBOV pathogenesis, facilitated by the development of new tools to elucidate critical regulatory elements in the viral life cycle, is providing new targets that can be exploited for therapeutic interventions. Notably, identifying factors triggering the haemorrhagic complications that characterise EBOV infections led to the development of a strategy to modulate coagulopathy; this therapeutic modality successfully mitigated the effects of EBOV haemorrhagic fever in nonhuman primates. This review summarises our current understanding of EBOV pathogenesis and discusses various approaches to therapeutic intervention based on our current understanding of how EBOV produces a lethal infection.

PMID: 15383160 [PubMed - indexed for MEDLINE]

1828. J Biol Chem. 2004 Sep 17;279(38):40204-8. Epub 2004 Jul 19.

High resolution crystal structure of human Rab9 GTPase: a novel antiviral drug target.

Chen L(1), DiGiammarino E, Zhou XE, Wang Y, Toh D, Hodge TW, Meehan EJ.

Author information: (1)Laboratory for Structural Biology, Department of Chemistry, Graduate Programs of Biotechnology, Chemistry and Materials Science, University of Alabama in Huntsville, Huntsville, Alabama 35899, USA.

Rab GTPases and their effectors facilitate vesicular transport by tethering donor vesicles to their respective target membranes. Rab9 mediates late endosome to trans-Golgi transport and has recently been found to be a key cellular component for human immunodeficiency virus-1, Ebola, Marburg, and measles virus replication, suggesting that it may be a novel target in the development of broad spectrum antiviral drugs. As part of our structure-based drug design program, we have determined the crystal structure of a C-terminally truncated human Rab9 (residues 1-177) to 1.25-A resolution. The overall structure shows a characteristic nucleotide binding fold consisting of a six-stranded beta-sheet surrounded by five alpha-helices with a tightly bound GDP molecule in the active site. Structure-based sequence alignment of Rab9 with other Rab proteins reveals that its active site consists of residues highly conserved in the Rab GTPase family, implying a common catalytic mechanism. However, Rab9 contains seven regions that are significantly different in conformation from other Rab proteins. Some of those regions coincide with putative effector-binding sites and switch I and switch II regions identified by structure/sequence alignments. The Rab9 structure at near atomic resolution provides an excellent model for structure-based antiviral drug design.

PMID: 15263003 [PubMed - indexed for MEDLINE]

1829. Vaccine. 2004 Sep 3;22(25-26):3495-502.

Marburg virus-like particles protect guinea pigs from lethal Marburg virus infection.

Warfield KL(1), Swenson DL, Negley DL, Schmaljohn AL, Aman MJ, Bavari S.

Author information: (1)United States Army Medical Research Institute of Infectious Diseases, 1425 Porter Street, Frederick, MD 21702-5011, USA. kelly.warfield@det.amedd.army.mil

Ongoing outbreaks of filoviruses in Africa and concerns about their use in bioterrorism attacks have led to intense efforts to find safe and effective vaccines to prevent the high mortality associated with these viruses. We previously reported the generation of virus-like particles (VLPs) for the filoviruses, Marburg (MARV) and Ebola (EBOV) virus, and that vaccinating mice with Ebola VLPs (eVLPs) results in complete survival from a lethal EBOV challenge. The objective of this study was to determine the efficacy of Marburg VLPs (mVLPs) as a potential vaccine against lethal MARV infection in a guinea pig model. Guinea pigs vaccinated with mVLPs or inactivated MARV developed MARV-specific antibody titers, as tested by ELISA or plaque-reduction and neutralization assays and were completely protected from a MARV challenge over 2000 LD50. While eVLP vaccination induced high EBOV-specific antibody responses, it did not cross-protect against MARV challenge in guinea pigs. Vaccination with mVLP or eVLP induced proliferative responses in vitro only upon re-exposure to the homologous antigen and this recall proliferative response was dependent on the presence of CD4+ T cells. Taken together with our previous work, these findings suggest that VLPs are a promising vaccine candidate for the deadly filovirus infections.

PMID: 15308377 [PubMed - indexed for MEDLINE]

1830. MMW Fortschr Med. 2004 Sep 2;146(35-36):4-6.

[Threat or creation of panic? Disease agents as terror weapons].

[Article in German]

Holzgreve H.

PMID: 15540528 [PubMed - indexed for MEDLINE]

1831. Antiviral Res. 2004 Sep;63(3):209-15.

Application of real-time PCR for testing antiviral compounds against Lassa virus, SARS coronavirus and Ebola virus in vitro.

Günther S(1), Asper M, Röser C, Luna LK, Drosten C, Becker-Ziaja B, Borowski P, Chen HM, Hosmane RS.

Author information: (1)Department of Virology, Bernhard-Nocht-Institute of Tropical Medicine, Bernhard-Nocht-Strasse 74, D-20359 Hamburg, Germany.

This report describes the application of real-time PCR for testing antivirals against highly pathogenic viruses such as Lassa virus, SARS coronavirus and Ebola virus. The test combines classical cell culture with a quantitative real-time PCR read-out. The assay for Lassa virus was validated with ribavirin, which showed an IC(50) of 9 micrograms/ml. Small-scale screening identified a class of imidazole nucleoside/nucleotide analogues with antiviral activity against Lassa virus. The analogues contained either dinitrile or diester groups at the imidazole 4,5-positions, and many of which possessed an acyclic sugar or sugar phosphonate moiety at the imidazole 1-position. The IC(50) values of the most active compounds ranged from 5 to 21 micrograms/ml. The compounds also inhibited replication of SARS coronavirus and Ebola virus in analogous assays, although to a lesser extent than Lassa virus.

PMID: 15451189 [PubMed - indexed for MEDLINE]

1832. Chin Med J (Engl). 2004 Sep;117(9):1395-400.

DC-SIGN: binding receptors for hepatitis C virus.

Wang QC(1), Feng ZH, Nie QH, Zhou YX.

Author information: (1)PLA Center for Diagnosis and Treatment for Infectious Diseases, Tangdu Hospital, Fourth Military Medical University, Xi'an 710038, China. Quanchuwang998@hotmail.com

OBJECTIVE: To review the recent developments in and research into binding receptors of hepatitis C virus (HCV) and especially the role of dendritic cell-specific adhesion receptor (DC-SIGN) in HCV. DATA SOURCES: Both Chinese- and English-language literature was searched using MEDLINE (2000 - 2003) and the databank of Chinese-language literature (2000 - 2003). STUDY SELECTION: Relevant articles on DC-SIGN and HCV binding receptors in recent domestic and foreign literature were selected. DATA EXTRACTION: Data were mainly extracted from 40 articles which are listed in the references section of this review. RESULTS: DC-SIGN, a dendritic cell-specific adhesion receptor and a type II transmembrane mannose-binding C-type lectin, is very important in the function of dendritic cells (DC), both in mediating naïve T cell interactions through ICAM-3 and as a rolling receptor that mediates the DC-specific ICAM-2-dependent migration processes. It can be used by HCV and other viral and bacterial pathogens including human immunodeficiency virus (HIV), Ebola virus, CMV and Mycobacterium tuberculosis to facilitate infection. Both DC-SIGN and DC-SIGNR can act either in cis, by concentrating virus on target cells, or in trans, by transmission of bound virus to a target cell expressing appropriate entry receptors. Recent report showed that DC-SIGN not only plays a role in entry into DC, HCV E2 interaction with DC-SIGN might also be detrimental to the interaction of DC with T cells during antigen presentation. CONCLUSIONS: DC-SIGNs are high-affinity binding receptors for HCV. The clinical strategies that target DC-SIGN may be successful in restricting HCV dissemination and pathogenesis as well as directing the migration of DCs to manipulate appropriate immune responses in autoimmunity and tumorigenic situations.

PMID: 15377434 [PubMed - indexed for MEDLINE]

1833. Clin Lab Med. 2004 Sep;24(3):825-38, viii.

Emerging infections in animals--potential new zoonoses?

Torres-Vélez F(1), Brown C.

Author information: (1)Department of Pathology, College of Veterinary Medicine, University of Georgia, Athens, GA 30602-7388, USA.

It is well recognized that most emerging diseases of humans are zoonotic, and that the forces working to create emerging diseases in humans are also operating in animal populations. However, what is often overlooked is that emerging human diseases are usually preceded by the emergence of the same pathogen in an animal population. In fact, the developing disease in animals acts as a link allowing the disease to take hold and wreck havoc in public health. Numerous examples--Rift Valley fever, monkeypox, Nipah, and Ebola--serve to underscore this linkage and to highlight the increasing interconnectedness of animal and human health.

PMID: 15325066 [PubMed - indexed for MEDLINE]

1834. J Antimicrob Chemother. 2004 Sep;54(3):579-81. Epub 2004 Aug 12.

Glycodendritic structures: promising new antiviral drugs.

Rojo J(1), Delgado R.

Author information: (1)Grupo de Carbohidratos, Instituto de Investigaciones Químicas, CSIC, Isla de la Cartuja, Americo Vespucio s/n, Sevilla, Spain. javier.rojo@iiq.csic.es

DC-SIGN, a C-type lectin expressed by dendritic cells, is able to recognize high mannosylated glycoproteins at the surface of a broad range of pathogens including viruses, bacteria, fungi and parasites. For at least some of these agents this interaction appears to be an important part of the infection process. Therefore, this lectin might be considered in the design of new antiviral drugs. In this manner, multivalent carbohydrate systems based on dendrimers and dendritic polymers are promising candidates as antiviral drugs. Boltorn hyperbranched dendritic polymers functionalized with mannose have been used to inhibit DC-SIGN-mediated infection in an Ebola-pseudotyped viral model. Their physiological solubility, lack of toxicity and especially their low price suggest the application of these glycodendritic polymers for possible formulation as microbicides.

PMID: 15308605 [PubMed - indexed for MEDLINE]

1835. Trends Immunol. 2004 Sep;25(9):461-4.

Emerging roles of tissue factor in viral hemorrhagic fever.

Ruf W(1).

Author information: (1)Department of Immunology, The Scripps Research Institute, 10550 North Torrey Pines Road, La Jolla, CA 92037, USA. ruf@scripps.edu

Activation of coagulation by tissue factor (TF) is frequently observed in sepsis syndrome and is documented in certain viral hemorrhagic fevers. Coagulation protease complexes signal by activating the G-protein coupled, protease-activated receptors that regulate inflammation. Blockade of TF attenuates lethality in experimental models of Ebola virus infection but - similar to findings in bacterial sepsis - reduction of inflammation, rather than attenuation of coagulation, predicts survival of treated animals. Thus, targeting TF appears to aid the antiviral immune response in hemorrhagic fevers, and further studies are encouraged to define how TF-dependent signaling regulates immunity.

PMID: 15324737 [PubMed - indexed for MEDLINE]

1836. Virology. 2004 Sep 1;326(2):280-7.

Ebola and Marburg virus-like particles activate human myeloid dendritic cells.

Bosio CM(1), Moore BD, Warfield KL, Ruthel G, Mohamadzadeh M, Aman MJ, Bavari S.

Author information: (1)Clinical Research Management, Frederick, MD 21702, USA.

The filoviruses, Ebola (EBOV) and Marburg (MARV), are potential global health threats, which cause deadly hemorrhagic fevers. Although both EBOV and MARV logarithmically replicate in dendritic cells (DCs), these viruses do not elicit DC cytokine secretion and fail to activate and mature infected DCs. Here, we employed virus-like particles (VLPs) of EBOV and MARV to investigate whether these genome-free particles maintain similar immune evasive properties as authentic filoviruses. Confocal microscopy indicated that human myeloid-derived DCs readily took up VLPs. However, unlike EBOV and MARV, VLPs induced maturation of DCs including upregulation of costimulatory molecules (CD40, CD80, CD86), major histocompatibility complex (MHC) class I and II surface antigens, and the late DC maturation marker CD83. The chemokine receptors CCR5 and CCR7 were also modulated on VLP-stimulated DCs, indicating that DC could migrate following VLP exposure. Furthermore, VLPs also elicited DC secretion of the pro-inflammatory cytokines TNF-alpha, IL-8, IL-6, and MIP-1alpha. Most significantly, in stark contrast to DC treated with intact EBOV or MARV, DC stimulated with EBOV or MARV VLPs showed enhanced ability to support human

T-cell proliferation in an allogenic mixed lymphocyte response (MLR). Thus, our findings suggest that unlike EBOV and MARV, VLPs are effective stimulators of DCs and have potential in enhancing innate and adaptive immune responses.

PMID: 15302213 [PubMed - indexed for MEDLINE]

1837. Bull Soc Pathol Exot. 2004 Aug;97(3):207-12.

[Bacterial and viral epidemics of zoonotic origin; the role of hunting and cutting up wild animals].

[Article in French]

Chastel C(1), Charmot G.

Author information: (1)Laboratoire de virologie, Faculté de médecine, 22 Av. Camille Desmoulins, F-29 285 Brest, France. chastelc@aol.com

Since the Prehistoric times hunting has been a vital activity for man. However, this may account for the contamination of the hunter, his family and relatives. Infections may occur by direct contact with blood or tissues of infected animal during handling and cutting up preys and when preparing or eating meat, or also when bitten by injured animal. Apes and antelopes hunting in sub-Saharan Africa proves to be particularly important since it has been well established that the recent or previous emergence of some viral zoonosis (Ebola, Aids, T lymphotropic viruses and Monkeypox) resulted from hunting and poaching. Moreover predation among different species of non human primates such as that practised by chimpanzees against monkeys, has led to the construction of recombinant simian Lentiviruses, such as SIV cpz able to infect man and then spread over the entire mankind as it was the case with HIV-I. SARS is another possible example of the zoonotic risks represented by the sale, handling and cutting up Chinese wild animals such as Himalayan civets for culinary purposes.

PMID: 15462204 [PubMed - indexed for MEDLINE]

1838. Bull Soc Pathol Exot. 2004 Aug;97(3):199-205.

[Epidemics of Ebola haemorrhagic fever in Gabon (1994-2002). Epidemiologic aspects and considerations on control measures].

[Article in French]

Milleliri JM(1), Tévi-Benissan C, Baize S, Leroy E, Georges-Courbot MC.

Author information: (1)IMTSSA - Le Pharo -Allée du Médecin Colonel Jamot - BP 46, 13998 Marseille Armées, France. j-m.milleliri@wanadoo.fr

Based on the description of the four Ebola haemorrhagic fever epidemics (EHF) occurred in Gabon between 1994 and 2002, the authors are considering the cultural and psycho-sociological aspects accounting for the difficulty to implement control measures. On the whole, the result of these raging epidemics came up to 207 cases and 150 dead (lethality: 72%). Analysing precisely the aspects of the third epidemic and pointing up the possible factors explaining its spreading far beyond its epicentre, the authors bring about the limits of measures not always understood by local populations. The discussion will deal with the possibilities of a better surveillance, a quick management of intervention means including a regional permanent pre-alert and taking into account the issue raised by the possible Ebola virus endemic.

PMID: 15462203 [PubMed - indexed for MEDLINE]

1839. Lancet Infect Dis. 2004 Aug;4(8):487-98.

Pathogenesis of filoviral haemorrhagic fevers.

Mahanty S(1), Bray M.

Author information: (1)Malaria Vaccine Development Unit, at the National Institute of Allergy and Infectious Diseases, National Institutes of Health, Rockville, MD 20852, USA.

The filoviruses, marburgvirus and ebolavirus, cause epidemics of haemorrhagic fever with high case-fatality rates. The severe illness results from a complex of pathogenetic mechanisms that enable the virus to suppress innate and adaptive immune responses, infect and kill a broad variety of cell types, and elicit strong inflammatory responses and disseminated intravascular coagulation, producing a syndrome resembling septic shock. Most experimental data have been obtained on Zaire ebolavirus, which causes uniformly lethal disease in experimentally infected non-human primates but produces a broader range of outcomes in naturally infected human beings. 10-30% of patients can survive the illness by mobilising adaptive immune responses, and there is limited evidence that mild or symptomless infections also occur. The other filoviruses that have caused human disease, Sudan ebolavirus, Ivory Coast ebolavirus, and marburgvirus, produce a similar illness but with somewhat lower case-fatality rates. Variations in outcome during an epidemic might be due partly to genetically determined differences in innate immune responses to the viruses. Recent studies in non-human primates have shown that blocking of certain host responses, such as the coagulation cascade, can result in reduced viral replication and improved host survival.

PMID: 15288821 [PubMed - indexed for MEDLINE]

1840. Rev Sci Tech. 2004 Aug;23(2):497-511.

The role of wildlife in emerging and re-emerging zoonoses.

Bengis RG(1), Leighton FA, Fischer JR, Artois M, Mörner T, Tate CM.

Author information: (1)Veterinary Investigation Centre, PO Box 12, Skukuza, Kruger National Park, 1350, South Africa.

There are huge numbers of wild animals distributed throughout the world and the diversity of wildlife species is immense. Each landscape and habitat has a kaleidoscope of niches supporting an enormous variety of vertebrate and invertebrate species, and each species or taxon supports an even more impressive array of macro- and micro-parasites. Infectious pathogens that originate in wild animals have become increasingly important throughout the world in recent decades, as they have had substantial impacts on human health, agricultural production, wildlife-based economies and wildlife conservation. The emergence of these pathogens as significant health issues is associated with a range of causal factors, most of them linked to the sharp and exponential rise of global human activity. Among these causal factors are the burgeoning human population, the increased frequency and speed of local and international travel, the increase in human-assisted movement of animals and animal products, changing agricultural practices that favour the transfer of pathogens between wild and domestic animals, and a range of environmental changes that alter the distribution of wild hosts and vectors and thus facilitate the transmission of infectious agents. Two different patterns of transmission of pathogens from wild animals to humans are evident among these emerging zoonotic diseases. In one pattern, actual transmission of the pathogen to humans is a rare event but, once it has occurred, human-to-human transmission maintains the infection for some period of time or permanently. Some examples of pathogens with this pattern of transmission are human immunodeficiency virus/acquired immune deficiency syndrome, influenza A, Ebola virus and severe acute respiratory syndrome. In the second pattern, direct or vector-mediated animal-to-human transmission is the usual source of human infection. Wild animal populations are the principal reservoirs of the pathogen and human-to-human disease transmission is rare. Examples of pathogens with this pattern of transmission include rabies and other lyssaviruses, Nipah virus, West Nile virus, Hantavirus, and the agents of Lyme borreliosis, plague, tularemia, leptospirosis and ehrlichiosis. These zoonotic diseases from wild animal sources all have trends that are rising sharply upwards. In this paper, the authors discuss the causal factors associated with the emergence or re-emergence of these zoonoses, and highlight a selection to provide a composite view of their range, variety and origins. However, most of these diseases are covered in more detail in dedicated papers elsewhere in this Review.

PMID: 15702716 [PubMed - indexed for MEDLINE]

1841. J Exp Med. 2004 Jul 19;200(2):169-79. Epub 2004 Jul 12.

Role of natural killer cells in innate protection against lethal ebola virus infection.

Warfield KL(1), Perkins JG, Swenson DL, Deal EM, Bosio CM, Aman MJ, Yokoyama WM, Young HA, Bavari S.

Author information: (1)United States Army Medical Research Institute of Infectious Diseases, 1425 Porter St., Frederick, MD 21702, USA.

Ebola virus is a highly lethal human pathogen and is rapidly driving many wild primate populations toward extinction. Several lines of evidence suggest that innate, nonspecific host factors are potentially critical for survival after Ebola virus infection. Here, we show that nonreplicating Ebola virus-like particles (VLPs), containing the glycoprotein (GP) and matrix protein virus protein (VP)40, administered 1-3 d before Ebola virus infection rapidly induced protective immunity. VLP injection enhanced the numbers of natural killer (NK) cells in lymphoid tissues. In contrast to live Ebola virus, VLP treatment of NK cells enhanced cytokine secretion and cytolytic activity against NK-sensitive targets. Unlike wild-type mice, treatment of NK-deficient or -depleted mice with VLPs had no protective effect against Ebola virus infection and NK cells treated with VLPs protected against Ebola virus infection when adoptively transferred to naive mice. The mechanism of NK cell-mediated protection clearly depended on perforin, but not interferon-gamma secretion. Particles containing only VP40 were sufficient to induce NK cell responses and provide protection from infection in the absence of the viral GP. These findings revealed a decisive role for NK cells during lethal Ebola virus infection. This work should open new doors for better understanding of Ebola virus pathogenesis and direct the development of immunotherapeutics, which target the innate immune system, for treatment of Ebola virus infection.

PMCID: PMC2212007 PMID: 15249592 [PubMed - indexed for MEDLINE]

1842. J Theor Biol. 2004 Jul 7;229(1):119-26.

The basic reproductive number of Ebola and the effects of public health measures: the cases of Congo and Uganda.

Chowell G(1), Hengartner NW, Castillo-Chavez C, Fenimore PW, Hyman JM.

Author information: (1)Center for Nonlinear Studies (MS B258), Los Alamos National Laboratory, Los Alamos, NM 87545, USA. gc82@cornell.edu

Despite improved control measures, Ebola remains a serious public health risk in African regions where recurrent outbreaks have been observed since the initial epidemic in 1976. Using epidemic modeling and data from two well-documented Ebola outbreaks (Congo 1995 and Uganda 2000), we estimate the number of secondary cases generated by an index case in the absence of control interventions R0. Our estimate of R0 is 1.83 (SD 0.06) for Congo (1995) and 1.34 (SD 0.03) for Uganda (2000). We model the course of the outbreaks via an SEIR (susceptible-exposed-infectious-removed) epidemic model that includes a smooth transition in the transmission rate after control interventions are put in place. We perform an uncertainty analysis of the basic reproductive number R0 to quantify its sensitivity to other disease-related parameters. We also analyse the sensitivity of the final epidemic size to the time interventions begin and provide a distribution for the final epidemic size. The control measures implemented during these two outbreaks (including education and contact tracing followed by quarantine) reduce the final epidemic size by a factor of 2 relative the final size with a 2-week delay in their implementation.

Copyright 2004 Elsevier Ltd.

PMID: 15178190 [PubMed - indexed for MEDLINE]

1843. FEBS Lett. 2004 Jul 2;569(1-3):261-6.

Roles of a conserved proline in the internal fusion peptide of Ebola glycoprotein.

Gómara MJ(1), Mora P, Mingarro I, Nieva JL.

Author information: (1)Unidad de Biofísica (CSIC-UPV/EHU) y Departamento de Bioquímica, Universidad del País Vasco, Aptdo. 644, 48080 Bilbao, Spain.

The structural determinants underlying the functionality of viral internal fusion peptides (IFPs) are not well understood. We have compared EBOwt (GAAIGLAWIPYFGPAAE), representing the IFP of the Ebola fusion protein GP, and EBOwt (GAAIGLAWIPYFGRAAE) derived from a non-functional mutant with conserved Pro537 substituted by Arg. P537R substitution did not abrogate peptide-membrane association, but interfered with the ability to induce bilayer destabilization. Structural determinations suggest that Pro537 is required to preserve a membrane-perturbing local conformation in apolar environments.

PMID: 15225645 [PubMed - indexed for MEDLINE]

1844. Dermatol Clin. 2004 Jul;22(3):291-302, vi.

Other viral bioweapons: Ebola and Marburg hemorrhagic fever.

Salvaggio MR(1), Baddley JW.

Author information: (1)Division of Infectious Diseases, Department of Medicine, University of Alabama at Birmingham, 1900 University Boulevard, 229 Tinsley Harrison Tower, Birmingham, AL 35294, USA.

The term viral hemorrhagic fever refers to a clinical syndrome characterized by acute onset of fever accompanied by nonspecific findings of malaise, prostration, diarrhea,and headache. Patients frequently show signs of increased vascular permeability, and many develop bleeding diatheses. The hemorrhagic fever viruses represent potential agents for biologic warfare because of capability of aerosol transmission, high morbidity,and mortality associated with infection, and ability to replicate in cell culture in high concentrations. Herein we discuss the Filoviridae, the agents of Ebola and Marburg hemorrhagic fevers.
PMID: 15207310 [PubMed - indexed for MEDLINE]

1845. J Virol. 2004 Jul;78(14):7344-51.

Contribution of ebola virus glycoprotein, nucleoprotein, and VP24 to budding of VP40 virus-like particles.

Licata JM(1), Johnson RF, Han Z, Harty RN.

Author information: (1)Department of Pathobiology, School of Veterinary Medicine, University of Pennsylvania, 3800 Spruce St, Philadelphia, PA 19104-6049, USA.

The VP40 matrix protein of Ebola virus buds from cells in the form of virus-like particles (VLPs) and plays a central role in virus assembly and budding. In this study, we utilized a functional budding assay and cotransfection experiments to examine the contributions of the glycoprotein (GP), nucleoprotein (NP), and VP24 of Ebola virus in facilitating release of VP40 VLPs. We demonstrate that VP24 alone does not affect VP40 VLP release, whereas NP and GP enhance release of VP40 VLPs, individually and to a greater degree in concert. We demonstrate further the following: (i). VP40 L domains are not required for GP-mediated enhancement of budding; (ii). the membrane-bound form of GP is necessary for enhancement of VP40 VLP release; (iii). NP appears to physically interact with VP40 as judged by detection of NP in VP40-containing VLPs; and (iv). the C-terminal 50 amino acids of NP may be important for interacting with and enhancing release of VP40 VLPs. These findings provide a more complete understanding of the role of VP40 and additional Ebola virus proteins during budding.
PMCID: PMC434112 PMID: 15220407 [PubMed - indexed for MEDLINE]

1846. Lancet Infect Dis. 2004 Jul;4(7):388.

Sudan Ebola outbreak of known strain.

Bosch X.

PMID: 15252932 [PubMed - indexed for MEDLINE]

1847. BMJ. 2004 Jun 19;328(7454):1456.

Crisis in western Sudan is delaying help for south of country.

Moszynski P.

PMCID: PMC428543 PMID: 15205280 [PubMed - indexed for MEDLINE]

1848. Clin Infect Dis. 2004 Jun 15;38(12):1731-5. Epub 2004 May 24.

Crimean-Congo hemorrhagic fever: prevention and control limitations in a resource-poor country.

Smego RA Jr(1), Sarwari AR, Siddiqui AR.

Author information: (1)Department of Medicine, University of North Dakota School of Medicine and Health Sciences, Fargo, ND, 58102, USA. rsmego@medicine.nodak.edu

In autumn 2000, an outbreak of Crimean-Congo hemorrhagic fever (CCHF) occurred in Pakistan and involved nosocomial cases due to human-to-human transmission at a tertiary care hospital in Karachi. During a hospital-based investigation, 6 serologically confirmed cases (i.e., patients seropositive for CCHF antigen or anti-CCHF immunoglobulin M antibodies by means of a capture enzyme-linked immunosorbent assay [ELISA]) and 3 clinically confirmed cases (i.e., patients with negative ELISA for CCHF but with relevant epidemiologic exposures and compatible clinical disease) of CCHF were identified. The outbreak originated in rural Balochistan, a region of known CCHF endemicity where miniepidemics regularly occur, and subsequently spread to the urban centers of Quetta and Karachi. This outbreak demonstrated the capacities and weaknesses associated with a developing country's response to hemorrhagic fever epidemics. We describe aspects of disease prevention, control challenges, and political obstacles posed by illness associated with what we refer to as the "Asian Ebola virus."
PMID: 15227619 [PubMed - indexed for MEDLINE]

1849. Biophys J. 2004 Jun;86(6):3744-9.

Molecular dynamics simulation of lipid reorientation at bilayer edges.

Kasson PM(1), Pande VS.

Author information: (1)Department of Chemistry, Stanford University, Stanford, California, USA.

Understanding cellular membrane processes is critical for the study of events such as viral entry, neurotransmitter exocytosis, and immune activation. Supported lipid bilayers are commonly used to model these membrane processes experimentally. Despite the relative simplicity of such a system, many important structural and dynamic parameters are not experimentally observable with current techniques. Computational approaches allow the development of a high-resolution model of bilayer processes. We have performed molecular dynamics simulations of dimyristoylphosphatidylcholine (DMPC) bilayers to model the creation of bilayer gaps-a common process in bilayer patterning-and to analyze their structure and dynamics. We propose a model for gap formation in which the bilayer edges form metastable micelle-like structures on a nanosecond timescale. Molecules near edges structurally resemble lipids in ungapped bilayers but undergo small-scale motions more rapidly. These data suggest that lipids may undergo rapid local rearrangements during membrane fusion, facilitating the formation of fusion intermediates thought key to the infection cycle of viruses such as influenza, Ebola, and HIV.
PMCID: PMC1304275 PMID: 15189870 [PubMed - indexed for MEDLINE]

1850. J Virol. 2004 Jun;78(11):5554-63.

Context-dependent effects of L domains and ubiquitination on viral budding.

Martin-Serrano J(1), Perez-Caballero D, Bieniasz PD.

Author information: (1)Aaron Diamond AIDS Research Center, 455 First Ave., New York, NY 10021, USA.

Many enveloped viruses encode late assembly domains, or L domains, that facilitate virion egress. PTAP-type L domains act by recruiting the ESCRT-I (endosomal sorting complex required for transport I) component Tsg101, and YPXL/LXXLF-type L domains recruit AIP-I/ALIX, both of which are class E vacuolar protein sorting (VPS) factors, normally required for the generation of vesicles within endosomes. The binding cofactors for PPXY-type L domains have not been unambiguously resolved but may include Nedd4-like ubiquitin ligases. Largely because they act as autonomous binding sites for host factors, L domains are generally transferable and active in a context-independent manner. Ebola virus matrix protein (EbVP40) contains two overlapping L-domain motifs within the sequence ILPTAPPEYMEA. Here, we show that both motifs are required for efficient EbVP40 budding. However, upon transplantation into two different retroviral contexts, the relative contributions of the PTAP and PPEY motifs differ markedly. In a murine leukemia virus carrying the EbVP40 sequence, both motifs contributed to overall L domain activity, and budding proceeded in a partly Tsg101-independent manner. Conversely, when transplanted into the context of human immunodeficiency virus type 1 (HIV-1), EbVP40 L-domain activity was entirely due to a PTAP-Tsg101 interaction. In fact, a number of PPXY-type L domains were inactive in the context of HIV-1. Surprisingly, PTAP and YPXL-type L domains that simulated HIV-1 budding reduced the amount of ubiquitin conjugated to Gag, while inactive PPXY-type L domains increased Gag ubiquitination. These observations suggest that active L domains recruit deubiquitinating enzymes as a consequence of class E VPS factor recruitment. Moreover, context-dependent L-domain function may reflect distinct requirements for host functions during the morphogenesis of different viral particles or the underlying presence of additional, as yet undiscovered L domains.

PMCID: PMC415830 PMID: 15140952 [PubMed - indexed for MEDLINE]

1851. EMBO J. 2004 May 19;23(10):2175-84. Epub 2004 Apr 22.

Ectodomain shedding of the glycoprotein GP of Ebola virus.

Dolnik O(1), Volchkova V, Garten W, Carbonnelle C, Becker S, Kahnt J, Ströher U, Klenk HD, Volchkov V.

Author information: (1)Institut für Virologie, Philipps-Universität Marburg, Marburg, Germany.

In this study, release of abundant amounts of the Ebola virus (EBOV) surface glycoprotein GP in a soluble form from virus-infected cells was investigated. We demonstrate that the mechanism responsible for the release of GP is ectodomain shedding mediated by cellular sheddases. Proteolytic cleavage taking place at amino-acid position D637 removes the transmembrane anchor and liberates complexes consisting of GP1 and truncated GP2 (GP(2delta)) subunits from the cell surface. We show that tumor necrosis factor alpha-converting enzyme (TACE), a member of the ADAM family of zinc-dependent metalloproteases, is involved in EBOV GP shedding. This finding shows for the first time that virus-encoded surface glycoproteins are substrates for ADAMs. Furthermore, we provide evidence that shed GP is present in significant amounts in the blood of virus-infected animals and that it may play an important role in the pathogenesis of infection by efficiently blocking the activity of virus-neutralizing antibodies.

PMCID: PMC424403 PMID: 15103332 [PubMed - indexed for MEDLINE]

1852. J Clin Virol. 2004 May;30(1):94-9.

Rapid detection protocol for filoviruses.

Weidmann M(1), Mühlberger E, Hufert FT.

Author information: (1)Department of Virology, Institute of Medical Microbiology and Hygiene, University of Freiburg, Hermann-Herder-Street 11, 79104 Freiburg, Germany. Weidmann@ukl.uni-freiburg.de

BACKGROUND: The incidence of filovirus disease outbreaks has been increasing in recent years. Although there have been advances in the developments of diagnostics, field tests are rare. Apart from family members of infected patients, health care workers are at high risk of being infected during the initial phase of an outbreak. RT-PCR has been shown to be helpful in containing outbreaks. OBJECTIVES: To develop Taqman-RT-PCR for the detection of Ebola-Zaire virus (EBOV-Z), Ebola-Sudan virus (EBOV-S) and Marburg virus (MBGV). STUDY DESIGN: Quantitative Taqman-RT-PCRs for the detection of these viruses were developed and established on a portable Smartcycler TD. RESULTS AND CONCLUSIONS: All three assays were highly sensitive and specific. The mobility of the assay system may help to contain future outbreaks.

PMID: 15072761 [PubMed - indexed for MEDLINE]

1853. J Infect. 2004 May;48(4):347-53.

Organisation of health care during an outbreak of Marburg haemorrhagic fever in the Democratic Republic of Congo, 1999.

Colebunders R(1), Sleurs H, Pirard P, Borchert M, Libande M, Mustin JP, Tshomba A, Kinuani L, Olinda LA, Tshioko F, Muyembe-Tamfum JJ.

Author information: (1)Médecins sans Frontières, Dupréstraat 94, B-1090 Brussel, Belgium. bcoleb@itg.be

Organising health care was one of the tasks of the International Scientific and Technical Committee during the 1998-1999 outbreak in Durba/Watsa, in the north-eastern province (Province Orientale), Democratic Republic of Congo. With the logistical support of Médecins sans Frontières (MSF), two isolation units were created: one at the Durba Reference Health Centre and the other at the Okimo Hospital in Watsa. Between May 6th, the day the isolation unit was installed and May 19th, 15 patients were admitted to the Durba Health Centre. In only four of them were the diagnosis of Marburg haemorrhagic fever (MHF) confirmed by laboratory examination. Protective equipment was distributed to health care workers and family members caring for patients. Information about MHF, modes of transmission and the use of barrier nursing techniques was provided to health care workers and sterilisation procedures were reviewed. In contrast to Ebola outbreaks, there was little panic among health care workers and the general public in Durba and all health services remained operational.

PMID: 15066337 [PubMed - indexed for MEDLINE]

1854. J Virol. 2004 May;78(10):5458-65.

Properties of replication-competent vesicular stomatitis virus vectors expressing glycoproteins of filoviruses and arenaviruses.

Garbutt M(1), Liebscher R, Wahl-Jensen V, Jones S, Möller P, Wagner R, Volchkov V, Klenk HD, Feldmann H, Ströher U.

Author information: (1)Special Pathogens Program, National Microbiology Laboratory, Health Canada, Winnipeg, Manitoba, Canada R3E 3R2.

Replication-competent recombinant vesicular stomatitis viruses (rVSVs) expressing the type I transmembrane glycoproteins and selected soluble glycoproteins of several viral hemorrhagic fever agents (Marburg virus, Ebola virus, and Lassa virus) were generated and characterized. All recombinant viruses exhibited rhabdovirus morphology and replicated cytolytically in tissue culture. Unlike the rVSVs with an additional transcription unit expressing the soluble glycoproteins, the viruses carrying the foreign transmembrane glycoproteins in replacement of the VSV glycoprotein were slightly attenuated in growth. Biosynthesis and processing of the foreign glycoproteins were authentic, and the cell tropism was defined by the transmembrane glycoprotein. None of the rVSVs displayed pathogenic potential in animals. The rVSV expressing the Zaire Ebola virus transmembrane glycoprotein mediated protection in mice against a lethal Zaire Ebola virus challenge. Our data suggest that the recombinant VSV can be used to study the role of the viral glycoproteins in virus replication, immune response, and pathogenesis.

PMCID: PMC400370 PMID: 15113924 [PubMed - indexed for MEDLINE]

1855. FEMS Microbiol Lett. 2004 Apr 15;233(2):179-86.

Structural studies on the Ebola virus matrix protein VP40 indicate that matrix proteins of enveloped RNA viruses are analogues but not homologues.

Timmins J(1), Ruigrok RW, Weissenhorn W.

Author information: (1)European Molecular Biology Laboratory, Grenoble, France.

Matrix proteins are the driving force of assembly of enveloped viruses. Their main function is to interact with and polymerize at cellular membranes and link other viral components to the matrix-membrane complex resulting in individual particle shapes and ensuring the integrity of the viral particle. Although matrix proteins of different virus families show functional analogy, they share no sequence or structural homology. Their diversity is also evident in that they use a variety of late domain motifs to commit the cellular vacuolar protein sorting machinery to virus budding. Here, we discuss the structural and functional aspects of teh filovirus matrix protein VP40 and compare them to other known matrix protein structures from vesicular stomatitis virus adn retroviral matrix protein.

PMID: 15108720 [PubMed - indexed for MEDLINE]

1856. J Infect Dis. 2004 Apr 15;189(8):1440-3. Epub 2004 Apr 1.

In vitro evaluation of cyanovirin-N antiviral activity, by use of lentiviral vectors pseudotyped with filovirus envelope glycoproteins.

Barrientos LG(1), Lasala F, Otero JR, Sanchez A, Delgado R.

Author information: (1)Special Pathogens Branch, Division of Viral and Rickettsial Diseases, National Center for Infectious Diseases, Centers for Disease Control and Prevention, Atlanta, Georgia 30333, USA. lbarrientosl@cdc.gov

Cyanovirin-N (CV-N) has been shown to inhibit Ebola Zaire virus (EboZV) infection, both in vitro and in vivo, through its ability to bind to oligomannoses-8/9 on the EboZV surface glycoprotein (GP). Here, we report the in vitro potency of CV-N to inhibit EboZV GP- and Marburg virus GP-pseudotyped viruses (EC50 approximately 40-60 nmol/L and approximately 6-25 nmol/L, respectively) from mediating gene transduction into HeLa cells. In addition, we provide evidence that CV-N can effectively inhibit DC-SIGN-mediated EboZV infection. Our data emphasize both the utility of GP-pseudotyped vectors in the assessment of compounds that affect cell entry by filovirus and the use of CV-N as a reagent for the probing of carbohydrate-dependent interactions at viral entry.

PMID: 15073681 [PubMed - indexed for MEDLINE]

1857. Virology. 2004 Apr 10;321(2):181-8.

Ebola virus glycoprotein-mediated anoikis of primary human cardiac microvascular endothelial cells.

Ray RB(1), Basu A, Steele R, Beyene A, McHowat J, Meyer K, Ghosh AK, Ray R.

Author information: (1)Department of Pathology, Saint Louis University, St. Louis, MO 63110, USA. rayrb@slu.edu

Ebola virus glycoprotein (EGP) has been implicated for the induction of cytotoxicity and injury in vascular cells. On the other hand, EGP has also been suggested to induce massive cell rounding and detachment from the plastic surface by downregulating cell adhesion molecules without causing cytotoxicity. In this study, we have examined the cytotoxic role of EGP in primary endothelial cells by transduction with a replication-deficient recombinant adenovirus expressing EGP (Ad-EGP). Primary human cardiac microvascular endothelial cells (HCMECs) transduced with Ad-EGP displayed loss of cell adhesion from the plastic surface followed by cell death. Transfer of conditioned medium from EGP-transduced HCMEC into naive cells did not induce loss of adhesion or cell death, suggesting that EGP needs to be expressed intracellularly to exert its cytotoxic effect. Subsequent studies suggested that HCMEC death occurred through apoptosis. Results from this study shed light on the EGP-induced anoikis in primary human cardiac endothelial cells, which may have significant pathological consequences.

PMID: 15051379 [PubMed - indexed for MEDLINE]

1858. J Clin Microbiol. 2004 Apr;42(4):1753-5.

First international quality assurance study on the rapid detection of viral agents of bioterrorism.

Niedrig M(1), Schmitz H, Becker S, Günther S, ter Meulen J, Meyer H, Ellerbrok H, Nitsche A, Gelderblom HR, Drosten C.

Author information: (1)Robert Koch-Institute, Berlin, Germany.

We have conducted an international quality assurance study of filovirus, Lassa virus, and orthopox virus PCR with 24 participants. Of the participating laboratories, 45.8 and 66.7% detected virus in all plasma samples, which contained > or = 5,000 and > or = 100,000 copies per ml, respectively. Sensitivity levels were not significantly different between viruses. False-negative results were attributable to a lack of sensitivity.
PMCID: PMC387573 PMID: 15071040 [PubMed - indexed for MEDLINE]

1859. J Virol. 2004 Apr;78(8):4330-41.

Rapid diagnosis of Ebola hemorrhagic fever by reverse transcription-PCR in an outbreak setting and assessment of patient viral load as a predictor of outcome.

Towner JS(1), Rollin PE, Bausch DG, Sanchez A, Crary SM, Vincent M, Lee WF, Spiropoulou CF, Ksiazek TG, Lukwiya M, Kaducu F, Downing R, Nichol ST.

Author information: (1)Special Pathogens Branch, Division of Viral and Rickettsial Diseases, National Center for Infectious Diseases, Centers for Disease Control and Prevention, Atlanta, Georgia 30333, USA.

The largest outbreak on record of Ebola hemorrhagic fever (EHF) occurred in Uganda from August 2000 to January 2001. The outbreak was centered in the Gulu district of northern Uganda, with secondary transmission to other districts. After the initial diagnosis of Sudan ebolavirus by the National Institute for Virology in Johannesburg, South Africa, a temporary diagnostic laboratory was established within the Gulu district at St. Mary's Lacor Hospital. The laboratory used antigen capture and reverse transcription-PCR (RT-PCR) to diagnose Sudan ebolavirus infection in suspect patients. The RT-PCR and antigen-capture diagnostic assays proved very effective for detecting ebolavirus in patient serum, plasma, and whole blood. In samples collected very early in the course of infection, the RT-PCR assay could detect ebolavirus 24 to 48 h prior to detection by antigen capture. More than 1,000 blood samples were collected, with multiple samples obtained from many patients throughout the course of infection. Real-time quantitative RT-PCR was used to determine the viral load in multiple samples from patients with fatal and nonfatal cases, and these data were correlated with the disease outcome. RNA copy levels in patients who died averaged 2 log(10) higher than those in patients who survived. Using clinical material from multiple EHF patients, we sequenced the variable region of the glycoprotein. This Sudan ebolavirus strain was not derived from either the earlier Boniface (1976) or Maleo (1979) strain, but it shares a common ancestor with both. Furthermore, both sequence and epidemiologic data are consistent with the outbreak having originated from a single introduction into the human population.
PMCID: PMC374287 PMID: 15047846 [PubMed - indexed for MEDLINE]

1860. World J Gastroenterol. 2004 Apr 1;10(7):925-9.

DC-SIGN: binding receptor for HCV?

Feng ZH(1), Wang QC, Nie QH, Jia ZS, Zhou YX.

Author information: (1)The Center of Diagnosis and Treatment for Infectious Diseases of PLA, Tangdu Hospital, Fourth Military Medical University, Xi'an 710038, Shaanxi Province, China. fengzh@fmmu.edu.cn

DC-SIGN, a dendritic Cell-specific adhesion receptor and a type II transmembrane mannose-binding C-type lectin, is very important in the function of DC, both in mediating naive T cell interactions through ICAM-3 and as a rolling receptor that mediates the DC-specific ICAM-2-dependent migration processes. It can be used by viral and bacterial pathogens including Human Immunodeficiency Virus (HIV), HCV, Ebola Virus, CMV and Mycobacterium tuberculosis to facilitate infection. Both DC-SIGN and DC-SIGNR can act either in cis, by concentrating virus on target cells, or in trans, by transmission of bound virus to a target cell expressing appropriate entry receptors. Recent work showed that DC-SIGN are high-affinity binding receptors for HCV. Besides playing a role in entry into DC, HCV E2 interaction with DC-SIGN might also be detrimental for the interaction of DC with T cells during antigen presentation. The clinical strategies that target DC-SIGN may be successful in restricting HCV dissemination and pathogenesis as well as directing the migration of DCs to manipulate appropriate immune responses in autoimmunity and tumorigenic situations.
PMID: 15052667 [PubMed - indexed for MEDLINE]

1861. Expert Opin Biol Ther. 2004 Mar;4(3):329-36.

Ebola virus glycoproteins: guidance devices for targeting gene therapy vectors.

Sanders DA(1).

Author information: (1)Markey Center for Structural Biology, Department of Biological Sciences, Lilly Hall, Purdue University, 915 W. State Street, West Lafayette, IN 47907-2054, USA. retrovir@purdue.edu

Replacing the native viral envelope protein on the surface of a retrovirus or lentivirus with the glycoprotein of a foreign enveloped virus, a process called pseudotyping, can expand the set of potential target cells for a viral vector or can restrict entry to specific cells. The Ebola virus glycoprotein, because of its evolutionary origins and the route of viral entry promoted by it, possesses distinct advantages in forming the outer shell of such pseudotyped retroviruses for gene therapy applications. Studies of the transduction of human airway epithelia by lentivirus pseudotyped with a modified Ebola virus glycoprotein from which the region of O- glycosylation has been removed have demonstrated that such recombinant viruses possess particular promise for the treatment of cystic fibrosis. This result highlights the synergism between basic studies of virus entry and gene therapy advances.
PMID: 15006727 [PubMed - indexed for MEDLINE]

1862. J Clin Invest. 2004 Mar;113(5):649.

Viral star wars.

Goodman L.
PMCID: PMC351332 PMID: 14991058 [PubMed - indexed for MEDLINE]

1863. J Virol. 2004 Mar;78(6):2943-7.

Human macrophage C-type lectin specific for galactose and N-acetylgalactosamine promotes filovirus entry.

Takada A(1), Fujioka K, Tsuiji M, Morikawa A, Higashi N, Ebihara H, Kobasa D, Feldmann H, Irimura T, Kawaoka Y.

Author information: (1)Division of Virology, Department of Microbiology and Immunology, Institute of Medical Science, University of Tokyo, Tokyo 108-8639, Japan.

Filoviruses cause lethal hemorrhagic disease in humans and nonhuman primates. An initial target of filovirus infection is the mononuclear phagocytic cell. Calcium-dependent (C-type) lectins such as dendritic cell- or liver/lymph node-specific ICAM-3 grabbing nonintegrin (DC-SIGN or L-SIGN, respectively), as well as the hepatic asialoglycoprotein receptor, bind to Ebola or Marburg virus glycoprotein (GP) and enhance the infectivity of these viruses in vitro. Here, we demonstrate that a recently identified human macrophage galactose- and N-acetylgalactosamine-specific C-type lectin (hMGL), whose ligand specificity differs from DC-SIGN and L-SIGN, also enhances the infectivity of filoviruses. This enhancement was substantially weaker for the Reston and Marburg viruses than for the highly pathogenic Zaire virus. We also show that the heavily glycosylated, mucin-like domain on the filovirus GP is required for efficient interaction with this lectin. Furthermore, hMGL, like DC-SIGN and L-SIGN, is present on cells known to be major targets of filoviruses (i.e., macrophages and dendritic cells), suggesting a role for these C-type lectins in viral replication in vivo. We propose that filoviruses use different C-type lectins to gain cellular entry, depending on the cell type, and promote efficient viral replication.

PMCID: PMC353724 PMID: 14990712 [PubMed - indexed for MEDLINE]

1864. J Virol. 2004 Mar;78(6):2657-65.

Budding of PPxY-containing rhabdoviruses is not dependent on host proteins TGS101 and VPS4A.

Irie T(1), Licata JM, McGettigan JP, Schnell MJ, Harty RN.

Author information: (1)Department of Pathobiology, School of Veterinary Medicine, University of Pennsylvania, Philadelphia, Pennsylvania 19104, USA.

Erratum in J Virol. 2004 May;78(10):5532.

Viral matrix proteins of several enveloped RNA viruses play important roles in virus assembly and budding and are by themselves able to bud from the cell surface in the form of lipid-enveloped, virus-like particles (VLPs). Three motifs (PT/SAP, PPxY, and YxxL) have been identified as late budding domains (L-domains) responsible for efficient budding. L-domains can functionally interact with cellular proteins involved in vacuolar sorting (VPS4A and TSG101) and endocytic pathways (Nedd4), suggesting involvement of these pathways in virus budding. Ebola virus VP40 has overlapping PTAP and PPEY motifs, which can functionally interact with TSG101 and Nedd4, respectively. As for vesicular stomatitis virus (VSV), a PPPY motif within M protein can interact with Nedd4. In addition, M protein has a PSAP sequence downstream of the PPPY motif, but the function of PSAP in budding is not clear. In this study, we compared L-domain functions between Ebola virus and VSV by constructing a chimeric M protein (M40), in which the PPPY motif of VSV M is replaced by the L domains of VP40. The budding efficiency of M40 was 10-fold higher than that of wild-type (wt) M protein. Overexpression of a dominant negative mutant of VPS4A or depletion of cellular TSG101 reduced the budding of only M40-containing VLPs but not that of wt M VLPs or live VSV. These findings suggest that the PSAP motif of M protein is not critical for budding and that there are fundamental differences between PTAP-containing viruses (Ebola virus and human immunodeficiency virus type 1) and PPPY-containing viruses (VSV and rabies virus) regarding their dependence on specific host factors for efficient budding.

PMCID: PMC353768 PMID: 14990685 [PubMed - indexed for MEDLINE]

1865. Vopr Virusol. 2004 Mar-Apr;49(2):21-5.

[Dynamics of complement hemolytic activity in experimental Ebola infection].

[Article in Russian]

Zabavichene NM, Chepurnov AA.

The dynamic hemolytic activity of complements (HAC) was investigated in blood of guinea pigs in lethal and non-lethal Ebola infection. The increasing HAC dynamic activity in the animal blood was found to correlate with the infection lethal course. HAC as observed in animals with lethal infection was sweepingly increasing after they, were infected with Ebola virus, and yet after 15 hours from the infection time the complement activity parameters topped 2-fold the basic values in 100% of guinea pigs. They began to be dropping by the end of day 1, their decrease reached, when the incubation time was over (days 3-4 after infection) the basic value, after which they continued to go down to the zero value in 2-3 days before the lethal outcome. The described phenomenon, like the phenomenon of accelerated death, was even more pronounced, when the animals were infected after a single immunization by activated Ebola virus. In case, guinea pigs were infected by a non-lethal Ebola virus strain, the compliment synthesis was observed to be activated only at the end of the incubation period; the process was accompanied with a gradual raise and with a plateau-type or wave-type increase of the complement during the treatment time--it was equally accompanied with normalizing activity parameters during recovery. The detected specificity could be important in prognosticating a disease outcome. A reliable correlation was demonstrated between the complement hemolytic activity and the level of circulating immune complexes in blood of experimental animals, which can be traced both in lethal and non-lethal infection.

PMID: 15106379 [PubMed - indexed for MEDLINE]

1866. Vopr Virusol. 2004 Mar-Apr;49(2):11-7.

[Strain differences related to Ebola virus reproduction in peritoneal macrophages and in aorta explants of guinea pigs].

[Article in Russian]

Dadaeva AA, Sizikova LP, Chepurnov AA.

Reproduction of the Ebola strains (ES) virus causing lethality in guinea pigs as well as in peritoneal macrophages and aorta explants of animals was investigated in vitro and in vivo; besides, production of interferon-gamma (IFN-gamma) and of tumor necrosis factor-alpha (TNF-alpha) by macrophages and endotheliocytes of guinea pigs was also studied. The interplay "macrophage--ES" by the example of 2 models of susceptibility to ES demonstrates that the ES

lethality is not unambiguously related only with a level of virus reproduction in macrophages. The interplay "endotheliocyte--ES" is indicative of that the ES lethality is inversely dependent on a level of production of the IFN-gamma and of TNF-alpha by endotheliocytes. In general, the Eboly fever lethality is not conditioned only by the ability or inability of ES to reproduce in macrophages and endotheliocytes; it also depends on a variety of pathogenetic factors, one of which could be the cytotoxic action of immune complexes shaping in the process of infection progression.
PMID: 15106377 [PubMed - indexed for MEDLINE]

1867. Fortune. 2004 Feb 23;149(4):34.

By the numbers. The bird flu that's sweeping across Asia.

Stires D.

PMID: 14983665 [PubMed - indexed for MEDLINE]

1868. JAMA. 2004 Feb 4;291(5):549-50.

Ebola vaccines tested in humans, monkeys.

Vastag B.

PMID: 14762022 [PubMed - indexed for MEDLINE]

1869. Curr Opin Mol Ther. 2004 Feb;6(1):6-7.

Web alert. Molecular, viral and cell-based vaccines for disease prevention and therapy.

Stephens AC(1).

Author information: (1)Academic Department of Paediatrics, Imperial College London, St Mary's Campus, 2nd Floor, Medical School, Norfolk Place, Paddington, London W2 1 PG, UK. a.stephens@imperial.ac.uk

PMID: 15011774 [PubMed - indexed for MEDLINE]

1870. Hum Gene Ther. 2004 Feb;15(2):211-9.

Transduction of human islets with pseudotyped lentiviral vectors.

Kobinger GP(1), Deng S, Louboutin JP, Vatamaniuk M, Matschinsky F, Markmann JF, Raper SE, Wilson JM.

Author information: (1)Gene Therapy Program, Division of Medical Genetics, Department of Medicine, University of Pennsylvania Health System, Philadelphia, PA 19104, USA.

Type I diabetes is caused by an autoimmune-mediated elimination of insulin-secreting pancreatic islets. Genetic modification of islets offers a powerful molecular tool for improving our understanding of islet biology. Moreover, efficient genetic engineering of islets could allow for evaluation of new strategies aimed at preventing islet destruction. The present study evaluated the ability of a human immunodeficiency virus (HIV)-based lentiviral vector pseudotyped with various viral envelopes to target human islets ex vivo, with the goal of improving efficiency while minimizing toxicity. Transfer of the enhanced green fluorescent protein reporter gene in human islets was first evaluated with an HIV-based vector pseudotyped with the vesicular stomatitis virus (VSV), murine leukemia virus, Ebola, rabies, Mokola, or lymphocytic choriomeningitis virus (LCMV) envelope glycoprotein to optimize transduction efficiency. Results indicated that LCMV-pseudotyped vector transduced insulin-secreting beta cells with the highest efficiency. Moreover, toxicity associated with transduction of islets was found to be lower with LCMV-pseudotyped vector than with VSV-G-pseudotyped vector, the second most efficient vector for islet transduction. Overall, our study describes an improved methodology for achieving safe and efficient gene transfer into cells of human islets.
PMID: 14975193 [PubMed - indexed for MEDLINE]

1871. J Virol. 2004 Feb;78(4):2131-6.

Distribution of hydrophobic residues is crucial for the fusogenic properties of the Ebola virus GP2 fusion peptide.

Adam B(1), Lins L, Stroobant V, Thomas A, Brasseur R.

Author information: (1)Centre de Biophysique Moléculaire Numérique, FSAGX, 5030 Gembloux, Leuven, Belgium.

The lipid-destabilizing properties of the N-terminal domain of the GP2 of Ebola virus were investigated. Our results suggest that the domain of Ebola virus needed for fusion is shorter than that previously reported. The fusogenic properties of this domain are related to its oblique orientation at the lipid/water interface owing to an asymmetric distribution of the hydrophobic residues when helical.
PMCID: PMC369453 PMID: 14747578 [PubMed - indexed for MEDLINE]

1872. Lancet Infect Dis. 2004 Feb;4(2):69.

Infectious disease surveillance update.

Das P.

PMID: 14964186 [PubMed - indexed for MEDLINE]

1873. Trends Biochem Sci. 2004 Feb;29(2):80-7.

The kindest cuts of all: crystal structures of Kex2 and furin reveal secrets of precursor processing.

Rockwell NC(1), Thorner JW.

Author information: (1)Department of Molecular and Cell Biology, Division of Biochemistry and Molecular Biology, University of California at Berkeley, Room 16, Barker Hall, Berkeley, CA 94720-3202, USA.

Pro-hormone or pro-protein convertases are a conserved family of eukaryotic serine proteases found in the secretory pathway. These endoproteases mature precursors for peptides and proteins that perform a wide range of physiologically important and clinically relevant functions. The first member of this family to be identified was Kex2 in the yeast Saccharomyces cerevisiae. One mammalian member of this family - furin - is responsible for processing substrates that include insulin pro-receptor, human immunodeficiency virus gp160 glycoprotein, Ebola virus glycoprotein, and anthrax protective antigen. Recent determination of the crystal structures for the catalytic core domains of both Kex2 and furin - the first for any members of this family - provide remarkable insights and a new level of understanding of substrate specificity and catalysis by the pro-protein convertases.

PMID: 15102434 [PubMed - indexed for MEDLINE]

1874. Science. 2004 Jan 16;303(5656):387-90.

Multiple Ebola virus transmission events and rapid decline of central African wildlife.

Leroy EM(1), Rouquet P, Formenty P, Souquière S, Kilbourne A, Froment JM, Bermejo M, Smit S, Karesh W, Swanepoel R, Zaki SR, Rollin PE.

Author information: (1)Institut de Recherche pour le Développement, UR034, Centre International de Recherches Médicales de Franceville, BP 769 Franceville, Gabon. Eric.Leroy@ird.fr

Erratum in Science. 2004 Jan 20;303(5658):628.

Comment in Science. 2004 Jan 16;303(5656):298-9.

Several human and animal Ebola outbreaks have occurred over the past 4 years in Gabon and the Republic of Congo. The human outbreaks consisted of multiple simultaneous epidemics caused by different viral strains, and each epidemic resulted from the handling of a distinct gorilla, chimpanzee, or duiker carcass. These animal populations declined markedly during human Ebola outbreaks, apparently as a result of Ebola infection. Recovered carcasses were infected by a variety of Ebola strains, suggesting that Ebola outbreaks in great apes result from multiple virus introductions from the natural host. Surveillance of animal mortality may help to predict and prevent human Ebola outbreaks.

PMID: 14726594 [PubMed - indexed for MEDLINE]

1875. Science. 2004 Jan 16;303(5656):298-9.

Epidemiology. Ebola outbreaks may have had independent sources.

Vogel G.

Comment on Science. 2004 Jan 16;303(5656):387-90.

PMID: 14726565 [PubMed - indexed for MEDLINE]

1876. Lancet. 2004 Jan 10;363(9403):136.

Space agency donates satellites to help study Ebola.

Bosch X.

PMID: 14733196 [PubMed - indexed for MEDLINE]

1877. Virology. 2004 Jan 5;318(1):224-30.

Identification of murine T-cell epitopes in Ebola virus nucleoprotein.

Simmons G(1), Lee A, Rennekamp AJ, Fan X, Bates P, Shen H.

Author information: (1)Department of Microbiology, School of Medicine, University of Pennsylvania, Philadelphia, PA 19104-6076, USA.

CD8 T cells play an important role in controlling Ebola infection and in mediating vaccine-induced protective immunity, yet little is known about antigenic targets in Ebola that are recognized by CD8 T cells. Overlapping peptides were used to identify major histocompatibility complex class I-restricted epitopes in mice immunized with vectors encoding Ebola nucleoprotein (NP). CD8 T-cell responses were mapped to a H-2(d)-restricted epitope (NP279-288) and two H-2(b)-restricted epitopes (NP44-52 and NP288-296). The identification of these epitopes will facilitate studies of immune correlates of protection and the evaluation of vaccine strategies in murine models of Ebola infection.

PMID: 14972550 [PubMed - indexed for MEDLINE]

1878. Biosecur Bioterror. 2004;2(3):186-91.

Marburg and Ebola viruses as aerosol threats.

Leffel EK(1), Reed DS.

Author information: (1)Center for Aerobiological Sciences, U.S. Army Medical Research Institute of Infectious Diseases, Fort Detrick, Frederick, Maryland 21702-5011, USA.

Ebola and Marburg viruses are the sole members of the genus Filovirus in the family Filoviridae. There has been considerable media attention and fear generated by outbreaks of filoviruses because they can cause a severe viral hemorrhagic fever (VHF) syndrome that has a rapid onset and high mortality. Although they are not naturally transmitted by aerosol, they are highly infectious as respirable particles under laboratory conditions. For these and other reasons, filoviruses are classified as category A biological weapons. However, there is very little data from animal studies with aerosolized filoviruses. Animal models of filovirus exposure are not well characterized, and there are discrepancies between these models and what has been observed in human outbreaks. Building on published results from aerosol studies, as well as a review of the history, epidemiology, and disease course of naturally occurring outbreaks, we offer an aerobiologist's perspective on the threat posed by aerosolized filoviruses.

PMID: 15588056 [PubMed - indexed for MEDLINE]

1879. Emerg Infect Dis. 2004 Jan;10(1):40-7.

Ecologic and geographic distribution of filovirus disease.

Peterson AT(1), Bauer JT, Mills JN.

Author information: (1)Department of Ecology and Evolutionary Biology, University of Kansas, Lawrence, Kansas, USA. town@ku.edu

We used ecologic niche modeling of outbreaks and sporadic cases of filovirus-associated hemorrhagic fever (HF) to provide a large-scale perspective on the geographic and ecologic distributions of Ebola and Marburg viruses. We predicted that filovirus would occur across the Afrotropics: Ebola HF in the humid rain forests of central and western Africa, and Marburg HF in the drier and more open areas of central and eastern Africa. Most of the predicted geographic extent of Ebola HF appear to have been observed; Marburg HF has the potential to occur farther south and east. Ecologic conditions appropriate for Ebola HF are also present in Southeast Asia and the Philippines, where Ebola Reston is hypothesized to be distributed. This first large-scale ecologic analysis provides a framework for a more informed search for taxa that could constitute the natural reservoir for this virus family.

PMCID: PMC3322747 PMID: 15078595 [PubMed - indexed for MEDLINE]

1880. IDrugs. 2004 Jan;7(1):42-4.

British society for immunology-annual conference 2003.

Worker C(1).

Author information: (1)CharlotteWorker@aol.com

PMID: 14968818 [PubMed - indexed for MEDLINE]

1881. Immunol Res. 2004;29(1-3):1-18.

Use of recombinant cytokines for optimized induction of antiviral immunity against SIV in the nonhuman primate model of human AIDS.

Ansari AA(1), Mayne AE, Onlamoon N, Pattanapanyasat K, Mori K, Villinger F.

Author information: (1)Department of Pathology and Laboratory Medicine, Emory University School of Medicine, 1639 Pierce Drive, Atlanta, GA 30322, USA. pathaaa@emory.edu

Outbreaks of infectious diseases such as HIV and the much televised and attention-getting outbreaks of diseases such as Ebola, Hantaviruses, and the most recent outbreak of SARS have induced a significant new interest in the formulations and more importantly the science of vaccinology, which has previously to a large extent been conducted empirically. Our laboratory has focused on the use of recombinant nonhuman primate cytokines as adjunctive therapies for inducing antigen-specific immune responses in monkeys because most recombinant human cytokines appear to be immunogenic. This article provides a summary of our work with such cytokines, which includes attempts to define optimum dosing schedules that lead to optimal primary and lasting memory antigen-specific immune responses.

PMID: 15181266 [PubMed - indexed for MEDLINE]

1882. Int J Infect Dis. 2004 Jan;8(1):27-37.

Containing a haemorrhagic fever epidemic: the Ebola experience in Uganda (October 2000-January 2001).

Lamunu M(1), Lutwama JJ, Kamugisha J, Opio A, Nambooze J, Ndayimirije N, Okware S.

Author information: (1)Uganda Ministry of Health, Kampala, Uganda. mlamunu@yahoo.co.uk

INTRODUCTION: The Ebola virus, belonging to the family of filoviruses, was first recognized in 1976 when it caused concurrent outbreaks in Yambuku in the Democratic Republic of Congo (DRC), and in the town of Nzara in Sudan. Both countries share borders with Uganda. A total of 425 cases and 224 deaths attributed to Ebola haemorrhagic fever (EHF) were recorded in Uganda in 2000/01. Although there was delayed detection at the community level, prompt and efficient outbreak investigation led to the confirmation of the causative agent on 14 October 2000 by the National Institute of Virology in South Africa, and the subsequent institution of control interventions. CONTROL INTERVENTIONS: Public health interventions to contain the epidemic aimed at minimizing transmission in the health care setting and in the community, reducing the case fatality rate due to the epidemic, strengthening co-ordination for the response and building capacity for on-going surveillance and control. Co-ordination of the control interventions was organized through the Interministerial Committee, National Ebola Task Force, District Ebola Task Forces, and the Technical Committees at national and district levels. The World Health Organization (WHO) under the Global Outbreak Alert and Response Network co-ordinated the international response. The post-outbreak control interventions addressed weaknesses prior to outbreak detection and aimed at improving preparations for future outbreak detection and response. Challenges to control efforts included inadequate and poor quality protective materials, deaths of health workers, numerous rumors and the rejection of convalescent cases by members of the community. CONCLUSIONS: This was recognized as the largest reported outbreak of EHF in the world. Control interventions were very successful in containing the epidemic. The community structures used to contain the epidemic have continued to perform well after containment of the outbreak, and have proved useful in the identification of other outbreaks. This was also the first outbreak response co-ordinated by the WHO under the Global Outbreak Alert and Response Network, a voluntary organization recently created to co-ordinate technical and financial resources to developing countries during outbreaks.

PMID: 14690778 [PubMed - indexed for MEDLINE]

1883. J Virol. 2004 Jan;78(2):999-1005.

Production of novel ebola virus-like particles from cDNAs: an alternative to ebola virus generation by reverse genetics.

Watanabe S(1), Watanabe T, Noda T, Takada A, Feldmann H, Jasenosky LD, Kawaoka Y.

Author information: (1)Department of Pathobiological Sciences, School of Veterinary Medicine, University of Wisconsin-Madison, Madison, Wisconsin 53706, USA.

We established a plasmid-based system for generating infectious Ebola virus-like particles (VLPs), which contain an Ebola virus-like minigenome consisting of a negative-sense copy of the green fluorescent protein gene. This system produced nearly 10(3) infectious particles per ml of supernatant, equivalent to the titer of Ebola virus generated by a reverse genetics system. Interestingly, infectious Ebola VLPs were generated, even without expression of VP24. Transmission and scanning electron microscopic analyses showed that the morphology of the Ebola VLPs was indistinguishable from that of authentic Ebola virus. Thus, this system allows us to study Ebola virus entry, replication, and assembly without biosafety level 4 containment. Furthermore, it may be useful in vaccine production against this highly pathogenic agent.

PMCID: PMC368804 PMID: 14694131 [PubMed - indexed for MEDLINE]
1884. J Virol. 2004 Jan;78(2):958-67.

Persistent infection with ebola virus under conditions of partial immunity.

Gupta M(1), Mahanty S, Greer P, Towner JS, Shieh WJ, Zaki SR, Ahmed R, Rollin PE.

Author information: (1)Special Pathogens Branch, Division of Viral and Rickettsial Diseases, National Center for Infectious Diseases, Centers for Disease Control and Prevention, Atlanta, Georgia 30333, USA. mgupta@cdc.gov

Ebola hemorrhagic fever in humans is associated with high mortality; however, some infected hosts clear the virus and recover. The mechanisms by which this occurs and the correlates of protective immunity are not well defined. Using a mouse model, we determined the role of the immune system in clearance of and protection against Ebola virus. All CD8 T-cell-deficient mice succumbed to subcutaneous infection and had high viral antigen titers in tissues, whereas mice deficient in B cells or CD4 T cells cleared infection and survived, suggesting that CD8 T cells, independent of CD4 T cells and antibodies, are critical to protection against subcutaneous Ebola virus infection. B-cell-deficient mice that survived the primary subcutaneous infection (vaccinated mice) transiently depleted or not depleted of CD4 T cells also survived lethal intraperitoneal rechallenge for >/==" BORDER="0">25 days. However, all vaccinated B-cell-deficient mice depleted of CD8 T cells had high viral antigen titers in tissues following intraperitoneal rechallenge and died within 6 days, suggesting that memory CD8 T cells by themselves can protect mice from early death. Surprisingly, vaccinated B-cell-deficient mice, after initially clearing the infection, were found to have viral antigens in tissues later (day 120 to 150 post-intraperitoneal infection). Furthermore, following intraperitoneal rechallenge, vaccinated B-cell-deficient mice that were transiently depleted of CD4 T cells had high levels of viral antigen in tissues earlier (days 50 to 70) than vaccinated undepleted mice. This demonstrates that under certain immunodeficiency conditions, Ebola virus can persist and that loss of primed CD4 T cells accelerates the course of persistent infections. These data show that CD8 T cells play an important role in protection against acute disease, while both CD4 T cells and antibodies are required for long-term protection, and they provide evidence of persistent infection by Ebola virus suggesting that under certain conditions of immunodeficiency a host can harbor virus for prolonged periods, potentially acting as a reservoir.

PMCID: PMC368745 PMID: 14694127 [PubMed - indexed for MEDLINE]
1885. Lancet Infect Dis. 2004 Jan;4(1):7.

Infectious disease surveillance update.

Das P.

PMID: 14725281 [PubMed - indexed for MEDLINE]
1886. Med Trop (Mars). 2004;64(4):331-3.

[Ebola virus hemorrhagic fever: another deadly strike in Sudan].

[Article in French]

Thill M(1), Tolou H.

Author information: (1)Service de Virologie, Institut de médecine tropicale du service de santé des armées, BP 46, 13998 Marseille Armées, France. imtssa.vro@wanadoo.fr

PMID: 15615380 [PubMed - indexed for MEDLINE]
1887. Med Trop (Mars). 2004;64(2):199-204.

[Practical guidelines for the management of Ebola infected patients in the field].

[Article in French]

Nkoghé D(1), Formenty P, Nnégué S, Mvé MT, Hypolite I, Léonard P, Leroy E; Comité International de Coordination Technique et Scientifique.

Author information: (1)Ministère de la Santé Publique, Libreville, Gabon. dnkoghe@hotmail.com

Ebola hemorrhagic fever appears after an incubation of 3 days to 3 weeks. The first symptoms are fever accompanied by general and hemorrhagic signs leading to death in 50 to 90% of cases. During epidemics definition of cases permits prompt diagnosis. Due to the high risk of person-to-person and nosocomial transmission associated with Ebola hemorrhagic fever, management is based on isolation of patients and institution of protected care. Hands and soiled material are often decontaminated using sodium hypochlorite. Patient waste is decontaminated and incinerated. Treatment is essentially supportive. There is currently no vaccine available. Persons having been in close contact with patient should be kept under medical surveillance for 21 days. Recovering patients should use condoms for three months. Bodies of deceased patients should be handled by trained teams and buried quickly.

PMID: 15460155 [PubMed - indexed for MEDLINE]
1888. Med Trop (Mars). 2004;64(2):127-31.

[New form of hemorraghic fever in Zaire].

[Article in French]

Raffier G(1).

Author information: (1)SSA. gilbert.raffier@wanadoo.fr

The purpose of this report is to describe the events that occurred immediately before and during the first weeks of the Ebola virus epicemic in the Democratic Republic of the Congo (formerly Zaire) in September and October 1976. By October 4 Dr Raffier and Dr Ruppol were already on hand at the epicenter of the epicemic in the Equator region about 1000 km from Kinshasa. They had been mandated by the State Health Commissioner to conduct a firsthand assessment of the reportedly disastrous local conditions and to implement emergency measures necessary to reassure the population. It was immediately understood to take all steps to prevent mass migration and to collect specimens necessary for rapid identification of the cause of an exceptionally serious crisis situation.

Traveling by plane and helicopter the two physicians went to the cities of Bumba and Lissala as well as to many surrounding villages including Yambouku where the first case was reported. Upon returning to Kinshash on October 9, specimens were sent to the CDC in Atlanta where the offending virus was identified. Authorities in Paris and Bruxelles were alerted of the emergency in order to secure the assistance of various specialists incuding virologists, epidemiologists, biologists and entomologists. Most of the new staff arrived on October 23 and were joined by colleagues from the United States, Belgium, and Canada as well as one specialist from South Africa on October 30. These experts were then able to form an International Medical Comission for an in depth assessment of this new epidemic outbreak.

PMID: 15460138 [PubMed - indexed for MEDLINE]

1889. Nucleosides Nucleotides Nucleic Acids. 2004;23(1-2):67-76.

L-deaza-5'-noraisteromycin.

Yin X(1), Schneller SW.

Author information: (1)Department of Chemistry, Auburn University, Auburn, Alabama 36849, USA.

(+/-)-1-Deazaaristeromycin (4) has been reported to be an inactivator of S-adenosylhomocysteine (AdoHcy) hydrolase and, as a consequence, to affect S-adenosylmethionine (AdoMet) mediated macromolecular biomethylations. To extend this to our program focused on 5'-noraristeromycin derivatives as inhibitors of the same hydrolase enzyme as potential antiviral agents, both enantiomers of 1-deaza-5'-noraristeromycin (5 and 20) have been prepared. Compounds 5 and 20 were evaluated against the following viruses: vaccinia, cowpox, monkeypox, Ebola, herpes simplex type 1 and 2, human cytomegalovirus, Epstein Barr, varicella zoster, hepatitis B, hepatitis C, HIV-1 and HIV-2, adenovirus type 1, measles, Pichinde, parainfluenza type 3, influenza A (H1N1 and H3N2), influenza B, Venezuelan equine encephalitis, rhinovirus type 2, respiratory syncytial, yellow fever, and West Nile. No activity was found nor was there any cytotoxicity to the viral host cells.

PMID: 15043137 [PubMed - indexed for MEDLINE]

1890. Protein Eng Des Sel. 2004 Jan;17(1):107-12.

Prediction of proprotein convertase cleavage sites.

Duckert P(1), Brunak S, Blom N.

Author information: (1)Center for Biological Sequence Analysis, BioCentrum-DTU, Technical University of Denmark, Building 208, DK-2800 Lyngby, Denmark. Many secretory proteins and peptides are synthesized as inactive precursors that in addition to signal peptide cleavage undergo post-translational processing to become biologically active polypeptides. Precursors are usually cleaved at sites composed of single or paired basic amino acid residues by members of the subtilisin/kexin-like proprotein convertase (PC) family. In mammals, seven members have been identified, with furin being the one first discovered and best characterized. Recently, the involvement of furin in diseases ranging from Alzheimer's disease and cancer to anthrax and Ebola fever has created additional focus on proprotein processing. We have developed a method for prediction of cleavage sites for PCs based on artificial neural networks. Two different types of neural networks have been constructed: a furin-specific network based on experimental results derived from the literature, and a general PC-specific network trained on data from the Swiss-Prot protein database. The method predicts cleavage sites in independent sequences with a sensitivity of 95% for the furin neural network and 62% for the general PC network. The ProP method is made publicly available at http://www.cbs.dtu.dk/services/ProP.

PMID: 14985543 [PubMed - indexed for MEDLINE]

1891. Verh K Acad Geneeskd Belg. 2004;66(5-6):384-405; discussion 406.

Epidemiology: past, present and future.

Kesteloot H(1).

Author information: (1)Department of Epidemiology, School of Public Health, KULeuven, Kapucijnenvoer 35-B 3000 Leuven.

Epidemiology in the past was concerned essentially by the study of infectious diseases which were the cause of huge mortalities especially since urbanisation was initiated. Epidemics of pest, typhus, cholera, influenza a.o. were common. The epidemics were halted by better hygiene, vaccination and antibiotics. Since the second world war epidemiology was dominated by an "epidemic" of new chronic diseases, especially heart disease and cancer. This was due to an increase in life span and to an increase in smoking habits and in the intake of saturated fat and a too small intake of fruit and vegetables combined with a too high intake of salt (NaCl). Gradually epidemiology evolved as the study of the causes, the distribution, the risk factors and the prevention of chronic diseases, but also including accidents, suicide, depression a.o., diseases with a mass occurrence at the population level. The importance of nutrition as a determinant of health gradually became recognized, but remains undervalued by the medical profession. Mortality at the population level follows some simple mathematical laws and can be represented accurately (r2>0.99) between the ages of 35 and 84 year by either Gompertz equations (ln mortality versus age) or by a polynomial equation (ln mortality versus, age2). This is valid for all populations and both sexes and remains valid at times of great and rapid changes in mortality. This shows that measures for prevention should be directed towards the total population. The future of epidemiology should be directed towards the slowing of the ageing process at the population level by a healthy life style consisting of: not smoking, avoiding obesity, a fair amount of physical activity and a healthy nutrition i.e little salt, little saturated fat, an adequate amount of omega-3 fatty acids and a large amount of fruit and vegetables, with an occasional glass of red wine. This contains the secret of a long and healthy life. Conceptually it will be important to determine whether a maximum human life span, genetically determined, exists. A maximal rectangularization of the mortality curve should then be the ultimate goal. At the same time the possible re-emergence of old and new infectious diseases (SARS, Ebola, BSE, AIDS) should be kept in mind.

PMID: 15641567 [PubMed - indexed for MEDLINE]

1892. Vestn Ross Akad Med Nauk. 2004;(8):7-11.

[Functional activity of peritoneal macrophages in experimental Ebola fever].

[Article in Russian]

Dadaeva AA, Sizikova LP, Chepurnov AA.

The phagocytic activity of peritoneal macrophages (a representative of mononuclear phagocytes) as well as the TNF-alpha were studied in animals with different susceptibility to Ebola virus (EV). The results denote the following: 1. Phagocytosis activation by peritoneal macrophages after EV is introduced into the body correlates directly with a susceptibility degree of an animal to EV. 2. The EV content in peritoneal lavage is inversely dependent on a phagocytic activity of peritoneal macrophages. The TNF-alpha activity increases, in blood serum of body susceptible to EV, 500-fold versus the unsusceptible body. Therefore, production of endogenous TNF-alpha can be interpreted as the development of body's immune protection but not as a reason for the development of vascular shock. Presumably, the nonspecific immunity factors condition the EV susceptibility.

PMID: 15455683 [PubMed - indexed for MEDLINE]

1893. Viral Immunol. 2004;17(3):390-400.

Depletion of peripheral blood T lymphocytes and NK cells during the course of ebola hemorrhagic Fever in cynomolgus macaques.

Reed DS(1), Hensley LE, Geisbert JB, Jahrling PB, Geisbert TW.

Author information: (1)Center for Aerobiological Sciences, U.S. Army Medical Research Institute of Infectious Diseases, Fort Detrick, Frederick, Maryland, USA. doug.reed@det.amedd.army.mil

During the course of an experimentally induced Ebola virus (EBOVA) infection of cynomolgus macaques, peripheral blood mononuclear cells were isolated and characterized by multi-color flow cytometry. Both CD4+ and CD8+ lymphocyte counts decreased 60-70% during the first 4 days after infection. Among CD8+ lymphocytes, this decline was greatest among the CD8(lo) population, which was composed mostly of CD3- CD16+ NK cells. In contrast, the number of CD20+ B lymphocytes in the blood did not significantly change during the course of the infection. Phenotypic analysis of T lymphocyte subsets by flow cytometry failed to show evidence of a robust immune response to the infection. Apoptosis could be detected as early as day 2 postinfection among the CD8+ and CD16+ subsets of lymphocytes. Increased expression of CD95 (Fas) suggests that apoptosis may be induced via signaling through the Fas/Fas-L cascade. In contrast, the number of HLA-DR+ cells increased tenfold in the blood during the course of infection. These data suggest that EBOV may block dendritic cell maturation after infection, thereby inhibiting activation of lymphocytes and eliminating those subsets that are most likely to be capable of mounting an effective response to the virus.

PMID: 15357905 [PubMed - indexed for MEDLINE]

1894. Vnitr Lek. 2004 Jan;50(1):76.

[An effective vaccine against Ebola hemorrhagic fever].

[Article in Czech]

Pospísil L.

PMID: 15049337 [PubMed - indexed for MEDLINE]

1895. Proc Natl Acad Sci U S A. 2003 Dec 23;100(26):15936-41. Epub 2003 Dec 12.

In vivo oligomerization and raft localization of Ebola virus protein VP40 during vesicular budding.

Panchal RG(1), Ruthel G, Kenny TA, Kallstrom GH, Lane D, Badie SS, Li L, Bavari S, Aman MJ.

Author information: (1)Developmental Therapeutics Program, Target Structure Based Drug Discovery Group, Science Applications International Corporation, National Cancer Institute, Frederick, MD 21702-1201, USA.

The matrix protein VP40 plays a critical role in Ebola virus assembly and budding, a process that utilizes specialized membrane domains known as lipid rafts. Previous studies with purified protein suggest a role for oligomerization of VP40 in this process. Here, we demonstrate VP40 oligomers in lipid rafts of mammalian cells, virus-like particles, and in the authentic Ebola virus. By mutagenesis, we identify several critical C-terminal sequences that regulate oligomerization at the plasma membrane, association with detergent-resistant membranes, and vesicular release of VP40, directly linking these phenomena. Furthermore, we demonstrate the active recruitment of TSG101 into lipid rafts by VP40. We also report the successful application of the biarsenic fluorophore, FlAsH, combined with a tetracysteine tag for imaging of Ebola VP40 in live cells.

PMCID: PMC307671 PMID: 14673115 [PubMed - indexed for MEDLINE]

1896. Proc Natl Acad Sci U S A. 2003 Dec 23;100(26):15889-94. Epub 2003 Dec 12.

Ebola virus-like particles protect from lethal Ebola virus infection.

Warfield KL(1), Bosio CM, Welcher BC, Deal EM, Mohamadzadeh M, Schmaljohn A, Aman MJ, Bavari S.

Author information: (1)US Army Medical Research Institute of Infectious Diseases, Frederick, MD 21702, USA.

The filovirus Ebola causes hemorrhagic fever with 70-80% human mortality. High case-fatality rates, as well as known aerosol infectivity, make Ebola virus a potential global health threat and possible biological warfare agent. Development of an effective vaccine for use in natural outbreaks, response to biological attack, and protection of laboratory workers is a higher national priority than ever before. Coexpression of the Ebola virus glycoprotein (GP) and matrix protein (VP40) in mammalian cells results in spontaneous production and release of virus-like particles (VLPs) that resemble the distinctively filamentous infectious virions. VLPs have been tested and found efficacious as vaccines for several viruses, including papillomavirus, HIV, parvovirus, and rotavirus. Herein, we report that Ebola VLPs (eVLPs) were immunogenic in vitro as eVLPs matured and activated mouse bone marrow-derived dendritic cells, assessed by increases in cell-surface markers CD40, CD80, CD86, and MHC class I and II and secretion of IL-6, IL-10, macrophage inflammatory protein (MIP)-1alpha, and tumor necrosis factor alpha by the dendritic cells. Further, vaccinating mice with eVLPs activated CD4+ and CD8+ T cells, as well as CD19+ B cells. After vaccination with eVLPs, mice developed high titers of Ebola virus-specific antibodies, including neutralizing antibodies. Importantly, mice vaccinated with eVLPs

were 100% protected from an otherwise lethal Ebola virus inoculation. Together, our data suggest that eVLPs represent a promising vaccine candidate for protection against Ebola virus infections and a much needed tool to examine the genesis and nature of immune responses to Ebola virus.
PMCID: PMC307663 PMID: 14673108 [PubMed - indexed for MEDLINE]

1897. Lancet. 2003 Dec 13;362(9400):1953-8.

Treatment of Ebola virus infection with a recombinant inhibitor of factor VIIa/tissue factor: a study in rhesus monkeys.

Geisbert TW(1), Hensley LE, Jahrling PB, Larsen T, Geisbert JB, Paragas J, Young HA, Fredeking TM, Rote WE, Vlasuk GP.

Author information: (1)Virology Division, US Army Medical Research Institute of Infectious Diseases, Fort Detrick, MD 21702, USA. tom.geisbert@amedd.army.mil
BACKGROUND: Infection with the Ebola virus induces overexpression of the procoagulant tissue factor in primate monocytes and macrophages, suggesting that inhibition of the tissue-factor pathway could ameliorate the effects of Ebola haemorrhagic fever. Here, we tested the notion that blockade of fVIIa/tissue factor is beneficial after infection with Ebola virus. METHODS: We used a rhesus macaque model of Ebola haemorrhagic fever, which produces near 100% mortality. We administered recombinant nematode anticoagulant protein c2 (rNAPc2), a potent inhibitor of tissue factor-initiated blood coagulation, to the macaques either 10 min (n=6) or 24 h (n=3) after a high-dose lethal injection of Ebola virus. Three animals served as untreated Ebola virus-positive controls. Historical controls were also used in some analyses. FINDINGS: Both treatment regimens prolonged survival time, with a 33% survival rate in each treatment group. Survivors are still alive and healthy after 9 months. All but one of the 17 controls died. The mean survival for the six rNAPc2-treated macaques that died was 11.7 days compared with 8.3 days for untreated controls (p=0.0184). rNAPc2 attenuated the coagulation response as evidenced by modulation of various important coagulation factors, including plasma D dimers, which were reduced in nearly all treated animals; less prominent fibrin deposits and intravascular thromboemboli were observed in tissues of some animals that succumbed to Ebola virus. Furthermore, rNAPc2 attenuated the proinflammatory response with lower plasma concentrations of interleukin 6 and monocyte chemoattractant protein-1 (MCP-1) noted in the treated than in the untreated macaques. INTERPRETATION: Post-exposure protection with rNAPc2 against Ebola virus in primates provides a new foundation for therapeutic regimens that target the disease process rather than viral replication.
PMID: 14683653 [PubMed - indexed for MEDLINE]

1898. MedGenMed. 2003 Dec 3;5(4):24.

Conference report - I. Investigating new vaccines: Ebola and HIV: highlights from the Viral Vaccine Meeting; October 25-28, 2003; Barcelona, Spain.

Armandola E(1).

Author information: (1)European Patent Office, Munich, Germany.
PMID: 14745371 [PubMed - indexed for MEDLINE]

1899. Am J Pathol. 2003 Dec;163(6):2371-82.

Pathogenesis of Ebola hemorrhagic fever in primate models: evidence that hemorrhage is not a direct effect of virus-induced cytolysis of endothelial cells.

Geisbert TW(1), Young HA, Jahrling PB, Davis KJ, Larsen T, Kagan E, Hensley LE.

Author information: (1)United States Army Medical Institute of Infectious Diseases, Fort Detrick, MD 21702-5011, USA. tom.geisbert@amedd.army.mil
Ebola virus (EBOV) infection causes a severe and often fatal hemorrhagic disease in humans and nonhuman primates. Whether infection of endothelial cells is central to the pathogenesis of EBOV hemorrhagic fever (HF) remains unknown. To clarify the role of endothelial cells in EBOV HF, we examined tissues of 21 EBOV-infected cynomolgus monkeys throughout time, and also evaluated EBOV infection of primary human umbilical vein endothelial cells and primary human lung-derived microvascular endothelial cells in vitro. Results showed that endothelial cells were not early cellular targets of EBOV in vivo, as viral replication was not consistently observed until day 5 after infection, a full day after the onset of disseminated intravascular coagulation. Moreover, the endothelium remained relatively intact even at terminal stages of disease. Although human umbilical vein endothelial cells and human lung-derived microvascular endothelial cells were highly permissive to EBOV replication, significant cytopathic effects were not observed. Analysis of host cell gene response at 24 to 144 hours after infection showed some evidence of endothelial cell activation, but changes were unremarkable considering the extent of viral replication. Together, these data suggest that coagulation abnormalities associated with EBOV HF are not the direct result of EBOV-induced cytolysis of endothelial cells, and are likely triggered by immune-mediated mechanisms.
PMCID: PMC1892396 PMID: 14633609 [PubMed - indexed for MEDLINE]

1900. Am J Pathol. 2003 Dec;163(6):2347-70.

Pathogenesis of Ebola hemorrhagic fever in cynomolgus macaques: evidence that dendritic cells are early and sustained targets of infection.

Geisbert TW(1), Hensley LE, Larsen T, Young HA, Reed DS, Geisbert JB, Scott DP, Kagan E, Jahrling PB, Davis KJ.

Author information: (1)United States Army Medical Institute of Infectious Diseases, Fort Detrick, MD 21702-5011, USA. tom.geisbert@amedd.army.mil
Ebola virus (EBOV) infection causes a severe and fatal hemorrhagic disease that in many ways appears to be similar in humans and nonhuman primates; however, little is known about the development of EBOV hemorrhagic fever. In the present study, 21 cynomolgus monkeys were experimentally infected with EBOV and examined sequentially over a 6-day period to investigate the pathological events of EBOV infection that lead to death. Importantly, dendritic cells in lymphoid tissues were identified as early and sustained targets of EBOV, implicating their important role in the immunosuppression characteristic of EBOV infections. Bystander lymphocyte apoptosis, previously described in end-stage tissues, occurred early in the disease-course in intravascular and extravascular locations. Of note, apoptosis and loss of NK cells was a prominent finding, suggesting the importance of innate immunity in determining the fate of the host. Analysis of peripheral blood mononuclear cell gene expression showed temporal increases in tumor necrosis factor-related apoptosis-inducing ligand and Fas transcripts, revealing a possible mechanism for the observed bystander apoptosis, while up-regulation of NAIP and cIAP2 mRNA suggest that

EBOV has evolved additional mechanisms to resist host defenses by inducing protective transcripts in cells that it infects. The sequence of pathogenetic events identified in this study should provide new targets for rational prophylactic and chemotherapeutic interventions.
PMCID: PMC1892369 PMID: 14633608 [PubMed - indexed for MEDLINE]
1901. Antimicrob Agents Chemother. 2003 Dec;47(12):3970-2.

Mannosyl glycodendritic structure inhibits DC-SIGN-mediated Ebola virus infection in cis and in trans.

Lasala F(1), Arce E, Otero JR, Rojo J, Delgado R.

Author information: (1)Laboratorio de Microbiología Molecular, Servicio de Microbiología, Hospital Universitario 12 de Octubre, Madrid, Spain.

We have designed a glycodendritic structure, BH30sucMan, that blocks the interaction between dendritic cell-specific intercellular adhesion molecule 3-grabbing nonintegrin (DC-SIGN) and Ebola virus (EBOV) envelope. BH30sucMan inhibits DC-SIGN-mediated EBOV infection at nanomolar concentrations. BH30sucMan may counteract important steps of the infective process of EBOV and, potentially, of microorganisms shown to exploit DC-SIGN for cell entry and infection.
PMCID: PMC296220 PMID: 14638512 [PubMed - indexed for MEDLINE]
1902. Curr Opin Allergy Clin Immunol. 2003 Dec;3(6):467-73.

Chemokine regulation of inflammation during acute viral infection.

Glass WG(1), Rosenberg HF, Murphy PM.

Author information: (1)Laboratory of Host Defenses, National Institute of Allergy and Infectious Diseases, National Institutes of Health, Bethesda, Maryland 20892, USA.

PURPOSE OF REVIEW: Chemokines are important inflammatory mediators, and regulate disease due to viral infection. This article will discuss scientific papers published primarily since June 2002 that have introduced new concepts in how chemokines regulate the inflammatory response to specific viruses. RECENT FINDINGS: Acute respiratory viruses commonly induce inflammatory chemokines such as CCL3 (also known as macrophage inflammatory protein-1alpha) and CCL5 (RANTES), which can amplify inflammatory responses leading to immunopathology. Where single agent therapy fails, combination antiviral and anti-CCL3 treatment is synergistic and able to prevent mortality in mice infected with the highly lethal pneumonia virus of mice. Human herpesvirus-6 also induces production of CCL3 and CCL5, which are able to block HIV-1 replication in coinfected human lymphoid tissue. On this basis, Margolis has proposed a new and general approach to the treatment and prevention of infection by viral pathogens. SUMMARY: Inflammatory chemokines play both beneficial and harmful roles in infectious diseases caused by viruses. Blocking them or using them as immunomodulators, depending on the virus, may be rational approaches to treatment or prevention of disease. With regard to blockade, combination antiviral/antichemokine therapy is a new strategy worth considering as a general therapeutic approach to viral infections, including severe acute respiratory syndrome (SARS). With regard to immunomodulation, use of weak or attenuated viruses to skew the local cytokine network to a configuration able to inhibit a pathogen is a new and interesting concept, but is fraught with important safety issues. Identifying master chemokines to target or exploit in human viral infection is a major opportunity and challenge for clinical immunologists.
PMID: 14612671 [PubMed - indexed for MEDLINE]
1903. Curr Opin Biotechnol. 2003 Dec;14(6):641-6.

Emerging viral infections in a rapidly changing world.

Kuiken T(1), Fouchier R, Rimmelzwaan G, Osterhaus A.

Author information: (1)Department of Virology, Erasmus Medical Center, PO Box 1738, 3000 DR, Rotterdam, The Netherlands. t.kuiken@erasmusmc.nl
Emerging viral infections in both humans and animals have been reported with increased frequency in recent years. Recent advances have been made in our knowledge of some of these, including severe acute respiratory syndrome-associated coronavirus, influenza A virus, human metapneumovirus, West Nile virus and Ebola virus. Research efforts to mitigate their effects have concentrated on improved surveillance and diagnostic capabilities, as well as on the development of vaccines and antiviral agents. More attention needs to be given to the identification of the underlying causes for the emergence of infectious diseases, which are often related to anthropogenic social and environmental changes. Addressing these factors might help to decrease the rate of emergence of infectious diseases and allow the transition to a more sustainable society.
PMID: 14662395 [PubMed - indexed for MEDLINE]
1904. Emerg Infect Dis. 2003 Dec;9(12):1531-7.

Risk factors for Marburg hemorrhagic fever, Democratic Republic of the Congo.

Bausch DG(1), Borchert M, Grein T, Roth C, Swanepoel R, Libande ML, Talarmin A, Bertherat E, Muyembe-Tamfum JJ, Tugume B, Colebunders R, Kondé KM, Pirad P, Olinda LL, Rodier GR, Campbell P, Tomori O, Ksiazek TG, Rollin PE.

Author information: (1)Centers for Disease Control and Prevention, Atlanta, Georgia, USA. dbausch@Tulane.edu
We conducted two antibody surveys to assess risk factors for Marburg hemorrhagic fever in an area of confirmed Marburg virus transmission in the Democratic Republic of the Congo. Questionnaires were administered and serum samples tested for Marburg-specific antibodies by enzyme-linked immunosorbent assay. Fifteen (2%) of 912 participants in a general village cross-sectional antibody survey were positive for Marburg immunoglobulin G antibody. Thirteen (87%) of these 15 were men who worked in the local gold mines. Working as a miner (odds ratio [OR] 13.9, 95% confidence interval [CI] 3.1 to 62.1) and receiving injections (OR 7.4, 95% CI 1.6 to 33.2) were associated with a positive antibody result. All 103 participants in a targeted antibody survey of healthcare workers were antibody negative. Primary transmission of Marburg virus to humans likely occurred via exposure to a still unidentified reservoir in the local mines. Secondary transmission appears to be less common with Marburg virus than with Ebola virus, the other known filovirus.
PMCID: PMC3034318 PMID: 14720391 [PubMed - indexed for MEDLINE]

1905. Expert Rev Vaccines. 2003 Dec;2(6):777-89.

Towards a vaccine against Ebola virus.

Geisbert TW(1), Jahrling PB.

Author information: (1)Virology Division, United States Army Medical Research Institute of Infectious Diseases, Fort Detrick, MD 21702-5011, USA.
tom.geisbert@amedd.army.mil

Ebola virus infection causes hemorrhagic fever with high mortality rates in humans and nonhuman primates. Currently, there are no vaccines or therapies approved for human use. Outbreaks of Ebola virus have been infrequent, largely confined to remote locations in Africa and quarantine of sick patients has been effective in controlling epidemics. In the past, this small global market has generated little commercial interest for developing an Ebola virus vaccine. However, heightened awareness of bioterrorism advanced by the events surrounding September 11, 2001, concomitant with knowledge that the former Soviet Union was evaluating Ebola virus as a weapon, has dramatically changed perspectives regarding the need for a vaccine against Ebola virus. This review takes a brief historic look at attempts to develop an efficacious vaccine, provides an overview of current vaccine candidates and highlights strategies that have the greatest potential for commercial development.

PMID: 14711361 [PubMed - indexed for MEDLINE]

1906. J Infect Dis. 2003 Dec 1;188(11):1630-8. Epub 2003 Nov 14.

Ebola and Marburg viruses replicate in monocyte-derived dendritic cells without inducing the production of cytokines and full maturation.

Bosio CM(1), Aman MJ, Grogan C, Hogan R, Ruthel G, Negley D, Mohamadzadeh M, Bavari S, Schmaljohn A.

Author information: (1)United States Army Medical Research Institute of Infectious Diseases, Frederick, Maryland 21702-5011, USA.

Comment in J Infect Dis. 2003 Dec 1;188(11):1613-7.

Ebola virus (EBOV) and Marburg virus (MARV) cause rapidly progressive hemorrhagic fever with high mortality and may possess specialized mechanisms to evade immune destruction. We postulated that immune evasion could be due to the ability of EBOV and MARV to interfere with dendritic cells (DCs), which link innate and adaptive immune responses. We demonstrate that EBOV and MARV infected and replicated in primary human DCs without inducing cytokine secretion. Infected DC cultures supported exponential viral growth without releasing interferon (IFN)-alpha and were impaired in IFN-alpha production if treated with double-stranded RNA. Moreover, EBOV and MARV impaired the ability of DCs to support T cell proliferation, and infected, immature DCs underwent an anomalous maturation. These findings may explain the profound virulence of EBOV and MARV--DCs are disabled, and an effective early host response is delayed by the necessary reliance on less-efficient secondary mechanisms.

PMID: 14639532 [PubMed - indexed for MEDLINE]

1907. J Infect Dis. 2003 Dec 1;188(11):1618-29. Epub 2003 Nov 14.

Mechanisms underlying coagulation abnormalities in ebola hemorrhagic fever: overexpression of tissue factor in primate monocytes/macrophages is a key event.

Geisbert TW(1), Young HA, Jahrling PB, Davis KJ, Kagan E, Hensley LE.

Author information: (1)Virology Division, United States Army Medical Research Institute of Infectious Diseases, Fort Detrick, Maryland, USA 21702-5011.
tom.geisbert@amedd.army.mil.

Comment in J Infect Dis. 2003 Dec 1;188(11):1613-7.

Disseminated intravascular coagulation is a prominent manifestation of Ebola virus (EBOV) infection. Here, we report that tissue factor (TF) plays an important role in triggering the hemorrhagic complications that characterize EBOV infections. Analysis of samples obtained from 25 macaques showed increased levels of TF associated with lymphoid macrophages, whereas analysis of peripheral blood-cell RNA showed increased levels of TF transcripts by day 3. Plasma from macaques contained increased numbers of TF-expressing membrane microparticles. Dysregulation of the fibrinolytic system developed during the course of infection, including a rapid decrease in plasma levels of protein C. Infection of primary human monocytes/macrophages (PHMs) was used to further evaluate the role of TF in EBOV infections. Analysis of PHM RNA at 1-48 h showed increased TF transcripts, whereas levels of TF protein were dramatically increased by day 2. Thus, chemotherapeutic strategies aimed at controlling overexpression of TF may ameliorate the effects of EBOV hemorrhagic fever.

PMID: 14639531 [PubMed - indexed for MEDLINE]

1908. J Infect Dis. 2003 Dec 1;188(11):1613-7. Epub 2003 Nov 14.

Ebola hemorrhagic fever and septic shock.

Bray M, Mahanty S.

Comment on J Infect Dis. 2003 Dec 1;188(11):1618-29. J Infect Dis. 2003 Dec 1;188(11):1630-8.

PMID: 14639530 [PubMed - indexed for MEDLINE]

1909. J Okla State Med Assoc. 2003 Dec;96(12):575-8.

Terrorism symposium update and conclusion.

Bronze MS(1), Huycke MM, Greenfield RA.

Author information: (1)Infectious Diseases Section, Department of Medicine, College of Medicine, University of Oklahoma Health Sciences Center, USA.

PMID: 14965028 [PubMed - indexed for MEDLINE]

1910. J Virol. 2003 Dec;77(24):13433-8.

Folate receptor alpha and caveolae are not required for Ebola virus glycoprotein-mediated viral infection.

Simmons G(1), Rennekamp AJ, Chai N, Vandenberghe LH, Riley JL, Bates P.

416

Author information: (1)Department of Microbiology. Abramson Family Cancer Research Institute, University of Pennsylvania, School of Medicine, Philadelphia, Pennsylvania 19104-6076, USA.

Folate receptor alpha (FRalpha) has been described as a factor involved in mediating Ebola virus entry into cells (6). Furthermore, it was suggested that interaction with FRalpha results in internalization and subsequent viral ingress into the cytoplasm via caveolae (9). Descriptions of cellular receptors for Ebola virus and its entry mechanisms are of fundamental importance, particularly with the advent of vectors bearing Ebola virus glycoprotein (GP) being utilized for gene transfer into cell types such as airway epithelial cells. Thus, the ability of FRalpha to mediate efficient entry of viral pseudotypes carrying GP was investigated. We identified cell lines and primary cell types such as macrophages that were readily infected by GP pseudotypes despite lacking detectable surface FRalpha, indicating that this receptor is not essential for Ebola virus infection. Furthermore, we find that T-cell lines stably expressing FRalpha are not infectible, suggesting that FRalpha is also not sufficient to mediate entry. T-cell lines lack caveolae, the predominant route of FRalpha-mediated folate metabolism. However, the coexpression of FRalpha with caveolin-1, the major structural protein of caveolae, was not able to rescue infectivity in a T-cell line. In addition, other cell types lacking caveolae are fully infectible by GP pseudotypes. Finally, a panel of ligands to and soluble analogues of FRalpha were unable to inhibit infection on a range of cell lines, questioning the role of FRalpha as an important factor for Ebola virus entry.
PMCID: PMC296046 PMID: 14645601 [PubMed - indexed for MEDLINE]
1911. Med Sci (Paris). 2003 Dec;19(12):1183-4.

[Ebola hemorrhagic fever: a unique efficacious vaccine dose in primates].

[Article in French]
Baize S, Deubel V.
PMID: 14691739 [PubMed - indexed for MEDLINE]
1912. Science. 2003 Nov 14;302(5648):1141-2.

Virology. New vaccine and treatment excite Ebola researchers.

Enserink M.
PMID: 14615510 [PubMed - indexed for MEDLINE]
1913. J Biol Chem. 2003 Nov 7;278(45):44567-73. Epub 2003 Aug 27.

Crystal structure of the measles virus phosphoprotein domain responsible for the induced folding of the C-terminal domain of the nucleoprotein.

Johansson K(1), Bourhis JM, Campanacci V, Cambillau C, Canard B, Longhi S.

Author information: (1)Architecture et Fonction des Macromolécules Biologiques, UMR 6098 CNRS et Université Aix-Marseille, 13288 Marseille 09, France.
Measles virus is a negative-sense, single-stranded RNA virus belonging to the Mononegavirales order which comprises several human pathogens such as Ebola, Nipah, and Hendra viruses. The phosphoprotein of measles virus is a modular protein consisting of an intrinsically disordered N-terminal domain (Karlin, D., Longhi, S., Receveur, V., and Canard, B. (2002) Virology 296, 251-262) and of a C-terminal moiety (PCT) composed of alternating disordered and globular regions. We report the crystal structure of the extreme C-terminal domain (XD) of measles virus phosphoprotein (aa 459-507) at 1.8 A resolution. We have previously reported that the C-terminal domain of measles virus nucleoprotein, NTAIL, is intrinsically unstructured and undergoes induced folding in the presence of PCT (Longhi, S., Receveur-Brechot, V., Karlin, D., Johansson, K., Darbon, H., Bhella, D., Yeo, R., Finet, S., and Canard, B. (2003) J. Biol. Chem. 278, 18638-18648). Using far-UV circular dichroism, we show that within PCT, XD is the region responsible for the induced folding of NTAIL. The crystal structure of XD consists of three helices, arranged in an anti-parallel triple-helix bundle. The surface of XD formed between helices alpha2 and alpha3 displays a long hydrophobic cleft that might provide a complementary hydrophobic surface to embed and promote folding of the predicted alpha-helix of NTAIL. We present a tentative model of the interaction between XD and NTAIL. These results, beyond presenting the first measles virus protein structure, shed light both on the function of the phosphoprotein at the molecular level and on the process of induced folding.
PMID: 12944395 [PubMed - indexed for MEDLINE]
1914. Emerg Infect Dis. 2003 Nov;9(11):1430-7.

Ebola hemorrhagic fever transmission and risk factors of contacts, Uganda.

Francesconi P(1), Yoti Z, Declich S, Onek PA, Fabiani M, Olango J, Andraghetti R, Rollin PE, Opira C, Greco D, Salmaso S.
Author information: (1)Istituto Superiore di Sanità, Rome, Italy.
From August 2000 through January 2001, a large epidemic of Ebola hemorrhagic fever occurred in Uganda, with 425 cases and 224 deaths. Starting from three laboratory-confirmed cases, we traced the chains of transmission for three generations, until we reached the primary case-patients (i.e., persons with an unidentified source of infection). We then prospectively identified the other contacts in whom the disease had developed. To identify the risk factors associated with transmission, we interviewed both healthy and ill contacts (or their proxies)who had been reported by the case-patients (or their proxies) and who met the criteria set for contact tracing during surveillance. The patterns of exposure of 24 case-patients and 65 healthy contacts were defined, and crude and adjusted prevalence proportion ratios (PPR) were estimated for different types of exposure. Contact with the patient's body fluids (PPR = 4.61%, 95% confidence interval 1.73 to 12.29) was the strongest risk factor, although transmission through fomites also seems possible.
PMCID: PMC3035551 PMID: 14718087 [PubMed - indexed for MEDLINE]
1915. Mol Ther. 2003 Nov;8(5):777-89.

Lentiviral vectors pseudotyped with minimal filovirus envelopes increased gene transfer in murine lung.

Medina MF(1), Kobinger GP, Rux J, Gasmi M, Looney DJ, Bates P, Wilson JM.
Author information: (1)Division of Medical Genetics, Philadelphia, Pennsylvania 19104, USA.

A human immunodeficiency virus (HIV)-based vector pseudotyped with the Ebola Zaire (EboZ) viral envelope glycoprotein (GP) was recently shown to transduce murine airway epithelia cells in vivo. In this study, the vector was further redesigned to improve gene transfer and also to increase safety. We used mutant EboZ envelopes for pseudotyping, which resulted in higher titers and increased transduction of airway cells in vivo compared to vectors pseudotyped with wild-type EboZ GP. As these envelopes lack regions associated with toxicity of the wild-type EboZ GP, they should also be safer to use for pseudotyping of lentiviral vectors. In addition, lentiviral vectors were created based on feline immunodeficiency virus and shown to have similar efficiency of transduction compared to HIV-based vectors. The creation of lentiviral vectors with highly engineered EboZ envelopes improved the performance of the system and should also increase its safety since only minimal regions of the EboZ envelope, which lack the toxic domain, are used.

PMID: 14599811 [PubMed - indexed for MEDLINE]

1916. Nucleosides Nucleotides Nucleic Acids. 2003 Nov;22(11):1995-2001.

5'-nor carbocyclic ribavirin.

Tuncbilek M(1), Schneller SW.

Author information: (1)Department of Chemistry, Auburn University, Auburn, Alabama 36849, USA.

An efficient synthesis of 5'-nor carbocyclic ribavirin (4) is described in 13 steps from conveniently available (+)-(1R,4S)-4-hydroxy-2-cyclopenten-1-yl acetate (6). Compound 4 was evaluated against the following viruses: herpes simplex type 1 and 2, vaccinia, cowpox, smallpox, Ebola, hepatitis B, hepatitis C, adenovirus type 1, influenza A (H1N1 and H3N2), influenza B, parainfluenza type 3, Pichinde, Punta Toro A, respiratory syncytial, rhinovirus type 2, Venezuelan equine encephalitis, yellow fever, and West Nile. No activity was found nor was there any cytotoxicity to the viral host cells.

PMID: 14680022 [PubMed - indexed for MEDLINE]

1917. Rev Med Virol. 2003 Nov-Dec;13(6):387-98.

Antibody-dependent enhancement of viral infection: molecular mechanisms and in vivo implications.

Takada A(1), Kawaoka Y.

Author information: (1)Division of Virology, Department of Microbiology and Immunology, Institute of Medical Science, University of Tokyo, Tokyo 108-8639, Japan. atakada@ims.u-tokyo.ac.jp

Besides the common receptor/coreceptor-dependent mechanism of cellular attachment, some viruses rely on antiviral antibodies for their efficient entry into target cells. This mechanism, known as antibody-dependent enhancement (ADE) of viral infection, depends on the cross-linking of complexes of virus-antibody or virus-activated complement components through interaction with cellular molecules such as Fc receptors or complement receptors, leading to enhanced infection of susceptible cells. Recent studies have suggested that additional mechanisms underlie ADE: involvement of complement component C1q and its receptor (Ebola virus), antibody-mediated modulation of the interaction between viral protein and its coreceptor (human immunodeficiency virus) and suppression of cellular antiviral genes by the replication of viruses entering cells via ADE (Ross River virus). Since ADE is exploited by a variety of viruses and has been associated with disease exacerbation, it may have broad relevance to the pathogenesis of viral infection and antiviral strategies.

Copyright 2003 John Wiley & Sons, Ltd.

PMID: 14625886 [PubMed - indexed for MEDLINE]

1918. Proc Natl Acad Sci U S A. 2003 Oct 28;100(22):12978-83. Epub 2003 Oct 16.

The small RING finger protein Z drives arenavirus budding: implications for antiviral strategies.

Perez M(1), Craven RC, de la Torre JC.

Author information: (1)Department of Neuropharmacology, The Scripps Research Institute, 10550 North Torrey Pines Road, La Jolla, CA 92037, USA.

By using a reverse genetics system that is based on the prototypic arenavirus lymphocytic choriomeningitis virus (LCMV), we have identified the arenavirus small RING finger Z protein as the main driving force of virus budding. Both LCMV and Lassa fever virus (LFV) Z proteins exhibited self-budding activity, and both substituted efficiently for the late domain that is present in the Gag protein of Rous sarcoma virus. LCMV and LFV Z proteins contain proline-rich motifs that are characteristic of late domains. Mutations in the PPPY motif of LCMV Z severely impaired the formation of virus-like particles. LFV Z contains two different proline-rich motifs, PPPY and PTAP, which are separated by eight amino acids. Mutational analysis revealed that both motifs are required for efficient LFV Z-mediated budding. Both LCMV and LFV Z proteins recruited to the plasma membrane Tsg101, which is a component of the class E vacuolar protein sorting machinery that has been implicated in budding of HIV and Ebola virus. Targeting of Tsg101 by RNA interference caused a strong reduction in Z-mediated budding. These results indicate that Z is the arenavirus functional counterpart of the matrix proteins found in other negative strand enveloped RNA viruses. Moreover, members of the vacuolar protein sorting pathway appear to play an important role in arena-virus budding. These findings open possibilities for antiviral strategies to combat LFV and other hemorrhagic fever arenaviruses.

PMCID: PMC240730 PMID: 14563923 [PubMed - indexed for MEDLINE]

1919. J Biol Chem. 2003 Oct 24;278(43):41830-6. Epub 2003 Aug 11.

Oligomerization of Ebola virus VP30 is essential for viral transcription and can be inhibited by a synthetic peptide.

Hartlieb B(1), Modrof J, Mühlberger E, Klenk HD, Becker S.

Author information: (1)Institut für Virologie der Philipps-Universität Marburg, Robert-Koch-Strasse 17, 35037 Marburg, Germany.

Transcription of Ebola virus (EBOV)-specific mRNA is driven by the nucleocapsid proteins NP, VP35, and L. This process is further dependent on VP30, an essential EBOV-specific transcription factor. The present study addresses the self-assembly of VP30 and the functional significance of this process for viral transcription and propagation. Essential for oligomerization of VP30 is a region spanning amino acids 94-112. Within this region a cluster of four leucine residues is of critical importance. Mutation of only one of these leucine residues resulted in oligomerization-deficient VP30 molecules that were no longer able

to support EBOV-specific transcription. The essential role of homo-oligomerization for the function of VP30 was further corroborated by the finding that mixed VP30 oligomers consisting of VP30 and transcriptionally inactive VP30 mutants were impaired in their ability to support EBOV transcription. The dominant negative effect of these VP30 mutants was dependent on their ability to bind to VP30. The oligomerization of VP30 could be dose dependently inhibited by a 25-mer peptide (E30pep-wt) derived from the presumed oligomerization domain (IC50,1 mum). A control peptide (E30pep-3LA), in which three leucines were changed to alanine, had no inhibitory effect. Thus, E30pep-wt seemed to bind efficiently to VP30 and consequently blocked the oligomerization of the protein. When E30pep-wt was transfected into EBOV-infected cells, the peptide inhibited viral replication suggesting that inhibition of VP30 oligomerization represents a target for EBOV antiviral drugs.
PMID: 12912982 [PubMed - indexed for MEDLINE]

1920. Bioorg Med Chem. 2003 Oct 15;11(21):4599-613.
A system of protein target sequences for anti-RNA-viral chemotherapy by a vitamin B6-derived zinc-chelating trioxa-adamantane-triol.
Kesel AJ(1).
Author information: (1)Chammünsterstr. 47, D-81827 München, Germany. andreas.kesel@t-online.de
#NAME? #NAME? #NAME? #NAME? PMID: 14527557 [PubMed - indexed for MEDLINE] #NAME?

1921. Emerg Infect Dis. 2003 Oct;9(10):1242-8.
Cultural contexts of Ebola in northern Uganda.
Hewlett BS(1), Amola RP.
Author information: (1)Department of Anthropology, Washington State University, 14204 NE Salmon Creek Avenue, Vancouver, WA 98686, USA. hewlett@vancouver.wsu.edu
PMCID: PMC3033100 PMID: 14609458 [PubMed - indexed for MEDLINE]

1922. Structure. 2003 Oct;11(10):1219-26.
Crystal structure of the borna disease virus nucleoprotein.
Rudolph MG(1), Kraus I, Dickmanns A, Eickmann M, Garten W, Ficner R.
Author information: (1)Department of Molecular Structural Biology, Institute for Microbiology and Genetics, GZMB, Georg-August University, 37077 Göttingen, Germany.
Comment in Structure. 2003 Oct;11(10):1194-6.
Borna disease virus (BDV) causes an infection of the central nervous system in a wide range of vertebrates, which can fatally progress to an immune-mediated disease, called Borna disease. BDV is a member of the Mononegavirales, which also includes the highly infectious measles and Ebola viruses. The viral nucleoproteins are central to transcription, replication, and packaging of the RNA genome. We present the X-ray structure of the BDV nucleoprotein determined at 1.76 A resolution. The structure reveals a novel fold, organized into two distinct domains, and an assembly into a planar homotetramer. Surface potential calculations strongly support an RNA binding model with the RNA wrapping around the outside of the tetramer, although a positively charged central channel in the tetramer could fit single-stranded RNA in an alternative binding mode. This first structure of an RNA virus nucleoprotein provides a paradigmatic model for RNA packaging and replication of single-stranded RNA viruses.
PMID: 14527390 [PubMed - indexed for MEDLINE]

1923. Vaccine. 2003 Sep 8;21(25-26):4071-80.
Comparison of individual and combination DNA vaccines for B. anthracis, Ebola virus, Marburg virus and Venezuelan equine encephalitis virus.
Riemenschneider J(1), Garrison A, Geisbert J, Jahrling P, Hevey M, Negley D, Schmaljohn A, Lee J, Hart MK, Vanderzanden L, Custer D, Bray M, Ruff A, Ivins B, Bassett A, Rossi C, Schmaljohn C.
Author information: (1)Virology Division, United States Army Medical Research Institute of Infectious Diseases, Fort Detrick, Frederick, MD 21702-5011, USA.
Multiagent DNA vaccines for highly pathogenic organisms offer an attractive approach for preventing naturally occurring or deliberately introduced diseases. Few animal studies have compared the feasibility of combining unrelated gene vaccines. Here, we demonstrate that DNA vaccines to four dissimilar pathogens that are known biowarfare agents, Bacillus anthracis, Ebola (EBOV), Marburg (MARV), and Venezuelan equine encephalitis virus (VEEV), can elicit protective immunity in relevant animal models. In addition, a combination of all four vaccines is shown to be equally as effective as the individual vaccines for eliciting immune responses in a single animal species. These results demonstrate for the first time the potential of combined DNA vaccines for these agents and point to a possible method of rapid development of multiagent vaccines for disparate pathogens such as those that might be encountered in a biological attack.
PMID: 12922144 [PubMed - indexed for MEDLINE]

1924. Int Nurs Rev. 2003 Sep;50(3):156-66.
Surviving Ebola: understanding experience through artistic expression.
Locsin RC(1), Barnard A, Matua AG, Bongomin B.
Author information: (1)Christine E. Lynn College of Nursing, Florida Atlantic University, 777 Glades Road, Boca Raton, FL 33431-0091, USA. locsin@fau.edu
BACKGROUND: A dearth of knowledge and information exist about the understanding of the experience of surviving a life-threatening illness such as Ebola Hemorrhagic Fever (Ebola). OBJECTIVES: To understand the ways in which survivors of Ebola understood the experience of surviving a life-threatening illness. METHODS: Eleven participants were asked to illustrate their understanding of the experience of surviving Ebola. (Only six of the drawings are published in this paper.) Using drawings and interviews as data, a phenomenographic approach was used to guide the research process and to analyse data. RESULTS: Analysis revealed four ways of understanding the experience. These are described as categories of descriptions or conceptions, namely, escape in peaceful awareness,

hope for a world outside of fear, persistence in defying death, and constant fear of dying. Importantly, the structure and referential aspects of the experiences are portrayed in the form of an outcome space, which is the understanding of the experience of living as survivors of Ebola, described as both "living in fear of the predatory spectre", while simultaneously "living in constant hopefulness". This experience is illustrated as paradoxically living in fear while concurrently hoping for life. DISCUSSION: Understanding the experience of survivors of a life-threatening illness is significant to nursing and its practice. Critical to this significance is its influence on the practice of compassionate and competent nursing.

PMID: 12930284 [PubMed - indexed for MEDLINE]

1925. J Virol. 2003 Sep;77(18):9987-92.

Nedd4 regulates egress of Ebola virus-like particles from host cells.

Yasuda J(1), Nakao M, Kawaoka Y, Shida H.

Author information: (1)Division of Molecular Virology, Institute for Genetic Medicine, Hokkaido University, N15 W7, Kita-ku, Sapporo 060-0815, Japan. j-yasuda@imm.hokudai.ac.jp

Ebola virus budding is mediated by two proline-rich motifs, PPxY and PTAP, within the viral matrix protein VP40. We have previously shown that a Nedd4-like protein BUL1, but not Nedd4, positively regulates budding of type D retrovirus Mason-Pfizer monkey virus (J. Yasuda, E. Hunter, M. Nakao, and H. Shida, EMBO Rep. 3:636-640, 2002). Here, we report that the cellular E3 ubiquitin ligase Nedd4 regulates budding of VP40-induced virus-like particles (VLPs) through interaction with the PPxY motif. Mutation of the active site cysteine (C894A), resulting in abrogation of ubiquitin ligase activity, impaired the function of Nedd4 on budding. In addition, the WW domains of Nedd4 are essential for binding to the viral PPxY motif, and a small fragment of Nedd4 containing only WW domains significantly inhibited Ebola VLP budding in a dominant-negative manner. Our findings suggest that the viruses containing PPxY as an L-domain motif specifically use E3 in the process of virus budding. We also examined the effects of overexpression of Tsg101 and its mutant. As expected, Tsg101 enhanced VP40-induced VLP release, and TsgDeltaC, which lacks its C-terminal half, inhibited VLP release. These results indicate that Nedd4, together with Tsg101, plays an important role in Ebola virus budding.

PMCID: PMC224586 PMID: 12941909 [PubMed - indexed for MEDLINE]

1926. J Virol. 2003 Sep;77(18):9733-7.

Ebola virus pathogenesis: implications for vaccines and therapies.

Sullivan N(1), Yang ZY, Nabel GJ.

Author information: (1)Vaccine Research Center, National Institute of Allergy and Infectious Diseases, National Institutes of Health, Building 40, Room 4502, MSC 3005, 40 Convent Drive, Bethesda, MD 20892-3005, USA.

PMCID: PMC224575 PMID: 12941881 [PubMed - indexed for MEDLINE]

1927. J Virol. 2003 Sep;77(17):9542-52.

Specific association of glycoprotein B with lipid rafts during herpes simplex virus entry.

Bender FC(1), Whitbeck JC, Ponce de Leon M, Lou H, Eisenberg RJ, Cohen GH.

Author information: (1)Department of Microbiology, School of Dental Medicine, University of Pennsylvania, Philadelphia, Pennsylvania 19104, USA. fbender@biochem.dental.upen.edu

Herpes simplex virus (HSV) entry requires the interaction of glycoprotein D (gD) with a cellular receptor such as herpesvirus entry mediator (HVEM or HveA) or nectin-1 (HveC). However, the fusion mechanism is still not understood. Since cholesterol-enriched cell membrane lipid rafts are involved in the entry of other enveloped viruses such as human immunodeficiency virus and Ebola virus, we tested whether HSV entry proceeds similarly. Vero cells and cells expressing either HVEM or nectin-1 were treated with cholesterol-sequestering drugs such as methyl-beta-cyclodextrin or nystatin and then exposed to virus. In all cases, virus entry was inhibited in a dose-dependent manner, and the inhibitory effect was fully reversible by replenishment of cholesterol. To examine the association of HVEM and nectin-1 with lipid rafts, we analyzed whether they partitioned into nonionic detergent-insoluble glycolipid-enriched membranes (DIG). There was no constitutive association of either receptor with DIG. Binding of soluble gD or virus to cells did not result in association of nectin-1 with the raft-containing fractions. However, during infection, a fraction of gB but not gC, gD, or gH associated with DIG. Similarly, when cells were incubated with truncated soluble glycoproteins, soluble gB but not gC was found associated with DIG. Together, these data favor a model in which HSV uses gB to rapidly mobilize lipid rafts that may serve as a platform for entry and cell signaling. It also suggests that gB may interact with a cellular molecule associated with lipid rafts.

PMCID: PMC187402 PMID: 12915568 [PubMed - indexed for MEDLINE]

1928. Semin Respir Infect. 2003 Sep;18(3):206-15.

Ebola hemorrhagic fever in the era of bioterrorism.

Polesky A(1), Bhatia G.

Author information: (1)Santa Clara County Tuberculosis Clinic, Santa Clara Valley Health and Hospital System, San Jose, CA, USA. Andrea.Polesky@hhs.co.santa-clara.ca.us

Viral hemorrhagic fevers are among a small group of infectious diseases considered potential candidates for use as agents of bioterrorism. Ebola hemorrhagic fever, the focus of this article, has the highest mortality rate of the viral hemorrhagic fevers and has no effective treatment. It is transmitted easily to family members and health care professionals not following universal precautions. The history of this infection, its clinical presentation, and epidemiology are discussed. Attention is paid to the immunopathogenesis of the disease with a focus on pulmonary involvement. Recommendations for infection control and Ebola virus' potential as a bioterrorism agent are addressed.

PMID: 14505282 [PubMed - indexed for MEDLINE]
1929. Wkly Epidemiol Rec. 2003 Aug 15;78(33):285-9.

Outbreak(s) of Ebola haemorrhagic fever in the Republic of the Congo, January-April 2003.

[Article in English, French]

[No authors listed]

PMID: 14509121 [PubMed - indexed for MEDLINE]
1930. Nature. 2003 Aug 7;424(6949):681-4.

Accelerated vaccination for Ebola virus haemorrhagic fever in non-human primates.

Sullivan NJ(1), Geisbert TW, Geisbert JB, Xu L, Yang ZY, Roederer M, Koup RA, Jahrling PB, Nabel GJ.

Author information: (1)Vaccine Research Center, National Institute of Allergy and Infectious Diseases, National Institutes of Health, Bldg. 40, Room 4502, MSC 3005, 40 Convent Drive, Bethesda, Maryland 20892-3005, USA.

Comment in Nature. 2003 Aug 7;424(6949):602.

Containment of highly lethal Ebola virus outbreaks poses a serious public health challenge. Although an experimental vaccine has successfully protected non-human primates against disease, more than six months was required to complete the immunizations, making it impractical to limit an acute epidemic. Here, we report the development of accelerated vaccination against Ebola virus in non-human primates. The antibody response to immunization with an adenoviral (ADV) vector encoding the Ebola glycoprotein (GP) was induced more rapidly than with DNA priming and ADV boosting, but it was of lower magnitude. To determine whether this earlier immune response could nonetheless protect against disease, cynomolgus macaques were challenged with Ebola virus after vaccination with ADV-GP and nucleoprotein (NP) vectors. Protection was highly effective and correlated with the generation of Ebola-specific CD8(+) T-cell and antibody responses. Even when animals were immunized once with ADV-GP/NP and challenged 28 days later, they remained resistant to challenge with either low or high doses of virus. This accelerated vaccine provides an intervention that may help to limit the epidemic spread of Ebola, and is applicable to other viruses.

PMID: 12904795 [PubMed - indexed for MEDLINE]
1931. Nature. 2003 Aug 7;424(6949):602.

Fast vaccine offers hope in battle with Ebola.

Clarke T, Knight J.

Comment on Nature. 2003 Aug 7;424(6949):681-4.

PMID: 12904747 [PubMed - indexed for MEDLINE]
1932. Acta Trop. 2003 Aug;87(3):321-9.

Elaboration of laboratory strains of Ebola virus and study of pathophysiological reactions of animals inoculated with these strains.

Chepurnov AA(1), Zubavichene NM, Dadaeva AA.

Author information: (1)State Research Center of Virology and Biotechnology, Vector, Koltsovo, Novosibirsk 630559, Russia. chepurnov@vector.nsc.ru

Selective passages in animals and cell cultures were used to produce a set of Ebola virus (EBO) laboratory strains with changed virulence for some animal genera. Comparative study of the genomes of wild-type EBO and selected variants formed the basis for studying the molecular causes of EBO virulence. Investigation of pathophysiological reactions of the animals inoculated with these strains allowed some key factors in Ebola fever pathogenesis to be determined.

PMID: 12875925 [PubMed - indexed for MEDLINE]
1933. Acta Trop. 2003 Aug;87(3):315-20.

Inactivation of Ebola virus with a surfactant nanoemulsion.

Chepurnov AA(1), Bakulina LF, Dadaeva AA, Ustinova EN, Chepurnova TS, Baker JR Jr.

Author information: (1)State Research Center of Virology and Biotechnology Vector, Koltsovo, Novosibirsk region 630559, Russia. chepurnov@vector.nsc.ru

Hemorrhagic fever caused by Ebola virus (EBO) is a highly contagious infection. This necessitates that the contaminated instruments, clothes, and hospital premises must be completely disinfected. Nanoemulsions are a new form of disinfectant composed of detergents and vegetable oil suspended in water. The antiviral activity of nanoemulsion ATB has been investigated against EBO. The nanoemulsion was tested against two preparations of EBO (strain Zaire) obtained from Vero cell culture fluid (EBO-zc) and from blood of infected monkeys (EBO-zb). The nanoemulsion ATB was virucidal against both preparations of EBO, inactivating the purified virus within 20 min even when diluted 1:100 with the growth medium. Inactivation of the virus in tissue preparations was also complete, but required 1:10 dilutions with media or higher. After treatment with ATB (10 and 1% concentrations), no EBO was apparent even after two passages in Vero cell culture. These data indicate that the nanoemulsion is an effective disinfectant for EBO. Because of the excellent biocompatibility of nanoemulsions, studies are planned to determine whether the nanoemulsion-killed virus is suitable for developing a vaccine against EBO.

PMID: 12875924 [PubMed - indexed for MEDLINE]
1934. Can Commun Dis Rep. 2003 Aug 1;29(15):129-33.

Outbreak(s) of Ebola hemorrhagic fever, Congo and Gabon, October 2001 to July 2002

[Article in English, French]

[No authors listed]

PMID: 12916393 [PubMed - indexed for MEDLINE]
1935. Nat Rev Immunol. 2003 Aug;3(8):677-85.

Ebola virus: from discovery to vaccine.

Feldmann H(1), Jones S, Klenk HD, Schnittler HJ.

Author information: (1)Department of Medical Microbiology, University of Manitoba, Winnipeg, Canada. heinz_feldmann@hc-sc.gc.ca

Ebola virus, being highly pathogenic for humans and non-human primates and the subject of former weapons programmes, is now one of the most feared pathogens worldwide. In addition, the lack of pre- and post-exposure interventions makes the development of rapid diagnostics, new antiviral agents and protective vaccines a priority for many nations. Further insight into the ecology, immunology and pathogenesis of Ebola virus will promote the delivery of these urgently required tools.

PMID: 12974482 [PubMed - indexed for MEDLINE]

1936. Virology. 2003 Aug 1;312(2):415-24.

Protection from lethal infection is determined by innate immune responses in a mouse model of Ebola virus infection.

Mahanty S(1), Gupta M, Paragas J, Bray M, Ahmed R, Rollin PE.

Author information: (1)Special Pathogens Branch, Division of Viral and Rickettsial Diseases, National Centers for Infectious Diseases, Centers for Disease Control & Prevention, Atlanta, GA 30333, USA. smahanty@niaid.nih.gov

A mouse-adapted strain of Ebola Zaire virus produces a fatal infection when BALB/cj mice are infected intraperitoneally (ip) but subcutaneous (sc) infection with the same virus fails to produce illness and confers long-term protection from lethal ip rechallenge. To identify immune correlates of protection in this model, we compared viral replication and cytokine/chemokine responses to Ebola virus in mice infected ip (10 PFU/mouse), or sc (100 PFU/mouse) and sc "immune" mice rechallenged ip (10(6) PFU/mouse) at several time points postinfection (pi). Ebola viral antigens were detected in the serum, liver, spleen, and kidneys of ip-infected mice by day 2 pi, increasing up to day 6. Sc-infected mice and immune mice rechallenged ip had no detectable viral antigens until day 6 pi, when low levels of viral antigens were detected in the livers of sc-infected mice only. TNF-alpha and MCP-1 were detected earlier and at significantly higher levels in the serum and tissues of ip-infected mice than in sc-infected or immune mice challenged ip. In contrast, high levels of IFN-alpha and IFN-gamma were found in tissues within 2 days after challenge in sc-infected and immune mice but not in ip-infected mice. Mice became resistant to ip challenge within 48 h of sc infection, coinciding with the rise in tissue IFN-alpha levels. In this model of Ebola virus infection, the nonlethal sc route of infection is associated with an attenuated inflammatory response and early production of antiviral cytokines, particularly IFN-alpha, as compared with lethal ip infection.

PMID: 12919746 [PubMed - indexed for MEDLINE]

1937. Virology. 2003 Aug 1;312(2):359-68.

Oligomerization and polymerization of the filovirus matrix protein VP40.

Timmins J(1), Schoehn G, Kohlhaas C, Klenk HD, Ruigrok RW, Weissenhorn W.

Author information: (1)European Molecular Biology Laboratory, 6 rue Jules Horowitz, 38042 Grenoble, France.

The matrix protein VP40 from Ebola virus plays an important role in the assembly process of virus particles by interacting with cellular factors, cellular membranes, and the ribonuclearprotein particle complex. Here we show that the N-terminal domain of VP40 folds into a mixture of two different oligomeric states in vitro, namely hexameric and octameric ringlike structures, as detected by gel filtration chromatography, chemical cross-linking, and electron microscopy. Octamer formation depends largely on the interaction with nucleic acids, which in turn confers in vitro SDS resistance. Refolding experiments with a nucleic acid free N-terminal domain preparation reveal a mostly dimeric form of VP40, which is transformed into an SDS resistant octamer upon incubation with E. coli nucleic acids. In addition, we demonstrate that the N-terminal domain of Marburg virus VP40 also folds into ringlike structures, similar to Ebola virus VP40. Interestingly, Marburg virus VP40 rings reveal a high tendency to polymerize into rods composed of stacked rings. These results may suggest distinct roles for different oligomeric forms of VP40 in the filovirus life cycle.

PMID: 12919741 [PubMed - indexed for MEDLINE]

1938. Lancet. 2003 Jul 19;362(9379):222.

African countries to cooperate on epidemic control. Experts hope that sharing expertise and resources will help control disease outbreaks in the region.

Wendo C.

PMID: 12889467 [PubMed - indexed for MEDLINE]

1939. JAMA. 2003 Jul 16;290(3):317-9.

An Ebola epidemic simmers in Africa: in remote region, outbreak shows staying power.

Thacker PD.

PMID: 12865357 [PubMed - indexed for MEDLINE]

1940. Drug Discov Today. 2003 Jul 15;8(14):609-10.

Ebola glycoprotein: the key to successful gene therapy?

Sutherland S.

PMID: 12867139 [PubMed - indexed for MEDLINE]

1941. APMIS. 2003 Jul-Aug;111(7-8):698-714.

Pathogens target DC-SIGN to influence their fate DC-SIGN functions as a pathogen receptor with broad specificity.

Geijtenbeek TB(1), van Kooyk Y.

Author information: (1)Department of Molecular Cell Biology, Vrije Universiteit Medical Center Amsterdam, Amsterdam, The Netherlands.

Dendritic cells (DC) are vital in the defense against pathogens. To sense pathogens DC express pathogen recognition receptors such as toll-like receptors (TLR) and C-type lectins that recognize different fragments of pathogens, and subsequently activate or present pathogen fragments to T cells. It is now becoming evident that some pathogens subvert DC functions to escape immune surveillance. HIV-I targets the DC-specific C-type lectin DC-SIGN to hijack DC for viral dissemination. HIV-I binding to DC-SIGN protects HIV-I from antigen processing and facilitates its transport to lymphoid tissues, where DC-SIGN promotes HIV-I infection of T cells. Recent studies demonstrate that DC-SIGN is a more universal pathogen receptor that also recognizes Ebola, cytomegalovirus and mycobacteria. Mycobacterium tuberculosis targets DC-SIGN by a mechanism that is distinct from that of HIV-I, leading to inhibition of the immunostimulatory function of DC and pathogen survival. Thus, a better understanding of DC-SIGN-pathogen interactions and their effects on DC function is necessary to combat infections.

PMID: 12974773 [PubMed - indexed for MEDLINE]

1942. Clin Diagn Lab Immunol. 2003 Jul;10(4):552-7.

Antigen capture enzyme-linked immunosorbent assay for specific detection of Reston Ebola virus nucleoprotein.

Ikegami T(1), Niikura M, Saijo M, Miranda ME, Calaor AB, Hernandez M, Acosta LP, Manalo DL, Kurane I, Yoshikawa Y, Morikawa S.

Author information: (1)Special Pathogens Laboratory, Department of Virology I, National Institute of Infectious Diseases, Musashimurayama, Tokyo 208-0011, Japan.

Antigen capture enzyme-linked immunosorbent assay (ELISA) is one of the most useful methods to detect Ebola virus rapidly. We previously developed an antigen capture ELISA using a monoclonal antibody (MAb), 3-3D, which reacted not only to the nucleoprotein (NP) of Zaire Ebola virus (EBO-Z) but also to the NPs of Sudan (EBO-S) and Reston Ebola (EBO-R) viruses. In this study, we developed antigen capture ELISAs using two novel MAbs, Res2-6C8 and Res2-1D8, specific to the NP of EBO-R. Res2-6C8 and Res2-1D8 recognized epitopes consisting of 4 and 8 amino acid residues, respectively, near the C-terminal region of the EBO-R NP. The antigen capture ELISAs using these two MAbs detected the EBO-R NP in the tissues from EBO-R-infected cynomolgus macaques. The antigen capture ELISAs using Res2-6C8 and Res2-1D8 are useful for the rapid detection of the NP in EBO-R-infected cynomolgus macaques.

PMCID: PMC164255 PMID: 12853385 [PubMed - indexed for MEDLINE]

1943. J Virol. 2003 Jul;77(14):7945-56.

The Ebola virus VP35 protein inhibits activation of interferon regulatory factor 3

Basler CF(1), Mikulasova A, Martinez-Sobrido L, Paragas J, Mühlberger E, Bray M, Klenk HD, Palese P, García-Sastre A.

Author information: (1)Department of Microbiology, Mount Sinai School of Medicine, I Gustave L. Levy Place, New York, NY 10029, USA. chris.basler@mssm.edu

The Ebola virus VP35 protein was previously found to act as an interferon (IFN) antagonist which could complement growth of influenza delNSI virus, a mutant influenza virus lacking the influenza virus IFN antagonist protein, NSI. The Ebola virus VP35 could also prevent the virus- or double-stranded RNA-mediated transcriptional activation of both the beta IFN (IFN-beta) promoter and the IFN-stimulated ISG54 promoter (C. Basler et al., Proc. Natl. Acad. Sci. USA 97:12289-12294, 2000). We now show that VP35 inhibits virus infection-induced transcriptional activation of IFN regulatory factor 3 (IRF-3)-responsive mammalian promoters and that VP35 does not block signaling from the IFN-alpha/beta receptor. The ability of VP35 to inhibit this virus-induced transcription correlates with its ability to block activation of IRF-3, a cellular transcription factor of central importance in initiating the host cell IFN response. We demonstrate that VP35 blocks the Sendai virus-induced activation of two promoters which can be directly activated by IRF-3, namely, the ISG54 promoter and the ISG56 promoter. Further, expression of VP35 prevents the IRF-3-dependent activation of the IFN-alpha4 promoter in response to viral infection. The inhibition of IRF-3 appears to occur through an inhibition of IRF-3 phosphorylation. VP35 blocks virus-induced IRF-3 phosphorylation and subsequent IRF-3 dimerization and nuclear translocation. Consistent with these observations, Ebola virus infection of Vero cells activated neither transcription from the ISG54 promoter nor nuclear accumulation of IRF-3. These data suggest that in Ebola virus-infected cells, VP35 inhibits the induction of antiviral genes, including the IFN-beta gene, by blocking IRF-3 activation.

PMCID: PMC161945 PMID: 12829834 [PubMed - indexed for MEDLINE]

1944. J Virol. 2003 Jul;77(13):7539-44.

Antibody-dependent enhancement of Ebola virus infection.

Takada A(1), Feldmann H, Ksiazek TG, Kawaoka Y.

Author information: (1)Division of Virology, Department of Microbiology and Immunology, Institute of Medical Science, University of Tokyo, Tokyo 108-8639, Japan. atakada@ims.u-tokyo.ac.jp

Most strains of Ebola virus cause a rapidly fatal hemorrhagic disease in humans, yet there are still no biologic explanations that adequately account for the extreme virulence of these emerging pathogens. Here we show that Ebola Zaire virus infection in humans induces antibodies that enhance viral infectivity. Plasma or serum from convalescing patients enhanced the infection of primate kidney cells by the Zaire virus, and this enhancement was mediated by antibodies to the viral glycoprotein and by complement component C1q. Our results suggest a novel mechanism of antibody-dependent enhancement of Ebola virus infection, one that would account for the dire outcome of Ebola outbreaks in human populations.

PMCID: PMC164833 PMID: 12805454 [PubMed - indexed for MEDLINE]

1945. J Virol Methods. 2003 Jul;111(1):21-8.

Development, characterization and use of monoclonal VP40-antibodies for the detection of Ebola virus.

Lucht A(1), Grunow R, Möller P, Feldmann H, Becker S.

Author information: (1)Bundeswehr Institute of Microbiology, Neuherbergstrasse II, D-80937 München, Germany. andreaslu@gmx.de

Ebola virus (EBOV) causes uncommon but dramatic outbreaks in remote regions of Africa, where diagnostic facilities are limited. In order to develop diagnostic tests, which can be handled and distributed easily, monoclonal antibodies (mAbs) to EBOV, species Zaire, were produced from mice immunized with inactivated viral particles. Nine stable hybridoma cell lines were obtained producing specific mAbs directed against the viral structural protein VP40. These mAbs were characterized by enzyme-linked immunosorbent, immunoblot and immunofluorescence assays. Subsequently, an antigen capture enzyme-linked immunosorbent assay was established, which detects VP40 of all known species of EBOV. This assay could detect viral material in spiked human serum that has been sodium dodecylsulfate-inactivated. The established enzyme-linked immunosorbent assay therefore has the ability to become a very useful tool for obtaining an accurate diagnosis in the field, limiting the risk of laboratory infections.
PMID: 12821193 [PubMed - indexed for MEDLINE]
1946. Nat Rev Immunol. 2003 Jul;3(7):557-68.

Pathogens: raft hijackers.

Mañes S(1), del Real G, Martínez-A C.

Author information: (1)Department of Immunology and Oncology, Centro Nacional de Biotecnología/Spanish Council for Scientific Research, Campus de la Universidad Autónoma de Madrid, Cantoblanco, Madrid E-28049, Spain.

Throughout evolution, organisms have developed immune-surveillance networks to protect themselves from potential pathogens. At the cellular level, the signalling events that regulate these defensive responses take place in membrane rafts--dynamic microdomains that are enriched in cholesterol and glycosphingolipids--that facilitate many protein-protein and lipid-protein interactions at the cell surface. Pathogens have evolved many strategies to ensure their own survival and to evade the host immune system, in some cases by hijacking rafts. However, understanding the means by which pathogens exploit rafts might lead to new therapeutic strategies to prevent or alleviate certain infectious diseases, such as those caused by HIV-I or Ebola virus.
PMID: 12876558 [PubMed - indexed for MEDLINE]
1947. Nat Struct Biol. 2003 Jul;10(7):520-6.

The crystal structure of the proprotein processing proteinase furin explains its stringent specificity.

Henrich S(1), Cameron A, Bourenkov GP, Kiefersauer R, Huber R, Lindberg I, Bode W, Than ME.

Author information: (1)Max-Planck-Institut für Biochemie, Abt. Strukturforschung, Am Klopferspitz 18A, 82152 Martinsried, Germany.

Erratum in Nat Struct Biol. 2003 Aug;10(8):669.

In eukaryotes, many essential secreted proteins and peptide hormones are excised from larger precursors by members of a class of calcium-dependent endoproteinases, the prohormone-proprotein convertases (PCs). Furin, the best-characterized member of the mammalian PC family, has essential functions in embryogenesis and homeostasis but is also implicated in various pathologies such as tumor metastasis, neurodegeneration and various bacterial and viral diseases caused by such pathogens as anthrax and pathogenic Ebola virus strains. Furin cleaves protein precursors with narrow specificity following basic Arg-Xaa-Lys/Arg-Arg-like motifs. The 2.6 A crystal structure of the decanoyl-Arg-Val-Lys-Arg-chloromethylketone (dec-RVKR-cmk)-inhibited mouse furin ectodomain, the first PC structure, reveals an eight-stranded jelly-roll P domain associated with the catalytic domain. Contoured surface loops shape the active site by cleft, thus explaining furin's stringent requirement for arginine at P1 and P4, and lysine at P2 sites by highly charge-complementary pockets. The structure also explains furin's preference for basic residues at P3, P5 and P6 sites. This structure will aid in the rational design of antiviral and antibacterial drugs.
PMID: 12794637 [PubMed - indexed for MEDLINE]
1948. Wkly Epidemiol Rec. 2003 Jun 27;78(26):223-8.

Outbreak(s) of Ebola haemorrhagic fever, Congo and Gabon, October 2001-July 2002.

[Article in English, French]

[No authors listed]

PMID: 15571171 [PubMed - indexed for MEDLINE]
1949. Science. 2003 Jun 13;300(5626):1645.

Conservation biology. Can great apes be saved from Ebola?

Vogel G.

PMID: 12805515 [PubMed - indexed for MEDLINE]
1950. Epidemiol Bull. 2003 Jun;24(2):4-5.

Case definitions. Ebola-Marburg viral diseases.

[No authors listed]

PMID: 15112622 [PubMed - indexed for MEDLINE]
1951. Epidemiol Infect. 2003 Jun;130(3):533-9.

Immunoglobulin G enzyme-linked immunosorbent assay using truncated nucleoproteins of Reston Ebola virus.

Ikegami T(1), Saijo M, Niikura M, Miranda ME, Calaor AB, Hernandez M, Manalo DL, Kurane I, Yoshikawa Y, Morikawa S.

Author information: (1)Special Pathogens Laboratory, Department of Virology I, National Institute of Infectious Diseases, 4-7-I Gakuen, Musashimurayama, Tokyo 208-0011, Japan.

We developed an immunoglobulin G (IgG) enzyme-linked immunosorbent assay (ELISA), using partial recombinant nucleoproteins (rNP) of Reston Ebola virus (EBO-R) and Zaire Ebola virus (EBO-Z). We examined the reaction of 10 sera from cynomolgus macaques naturally infected with EBO-R to each of the partial rNP in the IgG ELISA. All the sera reacted to the C-terminal halves of the rNP of both EBO-R and EBO-Z. Most of the sera reacted to the RdeltaC (amino acid (aa) 360-739), and Rdelta6 (aa 451-551) and/or Rdelta8 (aa 631-739) at a higher dilution than to the corresponding truncated rNPs of EBO-Z. The results indicate that this IgG ELISA is useful for detecting EBO-R specific antibody, and may have a potential to discriminate EBO-R infection from other subtypes.

PMCID: PMC2869991 PMID: 12825739 [PubMed - indexed for MEDLINE]

1952. Microbes Infect. 2003 Jun;5(7):639-49.

Molecular mechanisms of filovirus cellular trafficking.

Aman MJ(1), Bosio CM, Panchal RG, Burnett JC, Schmaljohn A, Bavari S.

Author information: (1)Clinical Research Management Inc., 1425 Porter Street, Frederick, MD 21702, USA. amanm@ncifcrf.gov

Erratum in Microbes Infect. 2003 Nov;5(13):1287.

The filoviruses, Ebola and Marburg, are two of the most pathogenic viruses, causing lethal hemorrhagic fever in humans. Recent discoveries suggest that filoviruses, along with other phylogenetically or functionally related viruses, utilize a complex mechanism of replication exploiting multiple cellular components including lipid rafts, endocytic compartments, and vacuolar protein sorting machinery. In this review, we summarize these recent findings and discuss the implications for vaccine and therapeutics development.

PMID: 12787740 [PubMed - indexed for MEDLINE]

1953. Thromb Haemost. 2003 Jun;89(6):967-72.

Viral hemorrhagic fever--a vascular disease?

Schnittler HJ(1), Feldmann H.

Author information: (1)Institute of Physiology, Medical Faculty Carl Gustav Carus, Technical University Dresden, Fiedlerstrasse 42, 01307 Dresden, Germany. hans.schnittler@mailbox.tu-dresden.de

The syndrome of "viral hemorrhagic fever" in man caused by certain viruses, such as Ebola, Lassa, Dengue, and Crimean-Congo hemorrhagic fever viruses, is often associated with a shock syndrome of undetermined pathogenesis. However, the vascular system, particularly the vascular endothelium, seems to be directly and indirectly targeted by all these viruses. Here we briefly summarize the current knowledge on Marburg and Ebola virus infections, the prototype viral hemorrhagic fever agents, and formulate a working hypothesis for the pathogenesis of viral hemorrhagic fever. Infections with filoviruses show lethality up to 89% and in severe cases lead to a shock syndrome associated with hypotension, coagulation disorders and an imbalance of fluid distribution between the intravascular and extravascular tissue space. The primary target cells for filoviruses are mononuclear phagocytotic cells which are activated upon infection and release certain cytokines and chemokines. These mediators indirectly target the endothelium and are thought to play a key role in the pathogenesis of filoviral hemorrhagic fever. In addition, direct infection and subsequent destruction of endothelial cells might contribute to the pathogenesis. Filoviruses, particularly Ebola virus, encode nonstructural glycoproteins which are released from infected host cells. Their function as potential determinants in pathogenicity remains to be investigated.

PMID: 12783108 [PubMed - indexed for MEDLINE]

1954. MedGenMed. 2003 May 29;5(2):20.

Biodefense research: new tricks to fight old enemies.

Mariani SM(1); American Association of Immunologists.

Author information: (1)Medscape General Medicine.

PMID: 14603119 [PubMed - indexed for MEDLINE]

1955. Harefuah. 2003 May;142(5):324-5, 400.

[Why viral (SARS, Ebola and AIDS) epidemics now?].

[Article in Hebrew]

Shoenfeld Y(1), Shemer J.

Author information: (1)Sackler Faculty of Medicine, Tel Aviv University, Israel.

In the last three decades we have seen several viral (and bacterial; i.e. TB) epidemics which took place at an era where we would have expected the eradication of many infectious diseases. There are many hypotheses to explain this paradox; 1) Is it the hygiene theory, namely extensive use of wide spread and too potent antibiotics which eliminate protective infecting agent? And hence the beneficial effect of probiotics? Is it the widespread use of vaccine? Is it a mistake or a terror acts of leakage of viral mutant from research or other laboratories? Be it as it may, the globalization and the employment of long distance flights make the spread easy to extreme points in the globe (Shanghai-Toronto). The new epidemiology? Immunology fields will have to deal with these novel aspects to combat and to prevent more events.

PMID: 12803050 [PubMed - indexed for MEDLINE]

1956. Int J Parasitol. 2003 May;33(5-6):583-95.

Vaccine research efforts for filoviruses.

Hart MK(1).

Author information: (1)Virology Division, United States Army Medical Research Institute of Infectious Diseases, 1425 Porter Street, Fort Detrick, Frederick, MD 21702-5011, USA. marykate.hart@amedd.army.mil

Ebola and Marburg viruses belong to the family Filoviridae, and cause acute, frequently fatal, haemorrhagic fever in humans and non-human primates. No vaccines are available for human use. This review describes the status of research efforts to develop vaccines for these viruses and to identify the immune mechanisms of protection. The vaccine approaches discussed include DNA-based vaccines, and subunit vaccines vectored by adenovirus, alphavirus replicons, and vaccinia virus.

PMID: 12782057 [PubMed - indexed for MEDLINE]

1957. J Virol. 2003 May;77(10):5902-10.

Lentivirus vectors pseudotyped with filoviral envelope glycoproteins transduce airway epithelia from the apical surface independently of folate receptor alpha.

Sinn PL(1), Hickey MA, Staber PD, Dylla DE, Jeffers SA, Davidson BL, Sanders DA, McCray PB Jr.

Author information: (1)Program in Gene Therapy, Department of Pediatrics, University of Iowa College of Medicine, Iowa City, Iowa 52242, USA.

The practical application of gene therapy as a treatment for cystic fibrosis is limited by poor gene transfer efficiency with vectors applied to the apical surface of airway epithelia. Recently, folate receptor alpha (FR alpha), a glycosylphosphatidylinositol-linked surface protein, was reported to be a cellular receptor for the filoviruses. We found that polarized human airway epithelia expressed abundant FR alpha on their apical surface. In an attempt to target these apical receptors, we pseudotyped feline immunodeficiency virus (FIV)-based vectors by using envelope glycoproteins (GPs) from the filoviruses Marburg virus and Ebola virus. Importantly, primary cultures of well-differentiated human airway epithelia were transduced when filovirus GP-pseudotyped FIV was applied to the apical surface. Furthermore, by deleting a heavily O-glycosylated extracellular domain of the Ebola GP, we improved the titer of concentrated vector severalfold. To investigate the folate receptor dependence of gene transfer with the filovirus pseudotypes, we compared gene transfer efficiency in immortalized airway epithelium cell lines and primary cultures. By utilizing phosphatidylinositol-specific phospholipase C (PI-PLC) treatment and FR alpha-blocking antibodies, we demonstrated FR alpha-dependent and -independent entry by filovirus glycoprotein-pseudotyped FIV-based vectors in airway epithelia. Of particular interest, entry independent of FR alpha was observed in primary cultures of human airway epithelia. Understanding viral vector binding and entry pathways is fundamental for developing cystic fibrosis gene therapy applications.

PMCID: PMC154009 PMID: 12719583 [PubMed - indexed for MEDLINE]

1958. Lancet Infect Dis. 2003 May;3(5):267.

Infectious disease surveillance update.

Das P.

PMID: 12726968 [PubMed - indexed for MEDLINE]

1959. Mil Med. 2003 May;168(5):368-72.

U.S. military officer participation in the Centers for Disease Control and Prevention's Epidemic Intelligence Service (1951-2001).

Noah DL(1), Ostroff SM, Cropper TL, Thacker SB.

Author information: (1)Office of the Air Force Surgeon General HQ USAF/SG 110 Luke Avenue, Room 400, Bolling Air Force Base, Washington, DC 20332-7050, USA.

The Epidemic Intelligence Service (EIS) was created in 1951 to provide epidemiologists to investigate natural and intentional disease epidemics. From an initial class of 23 U.S. citizens, the program has evolved into a globally recognized, hands-on learning experience, accepting approximately 65 to 75 new officers each year. The first U.S. military epidemic intelligence service officer (EISO) was accepted into the program in 1994. Since that time, 12 such officers have completed, or have begun, EIS training. They have comprised 2.1% of all EISOs from 1994 to 2001 and 0.47% of all EISOs. This total has included nine Air Force veterinarians, one Army veterinarian, one Army physician, and one Navy physician. Each military EISO had the opportunity to lead investigations of significant public health events (e.g., Ebola, monkeypox, malaria, Nipah virus, West Nile fever, and anthrax outbreaks). All graduates from the military returned to active duty assignments in operational medical units, research institutes, or the intelligence community.

PMID: 12775171 [PubMed - indexed for MEDLINE]

1960. Science. 2003 Apr 11;300(5617):232.

Conservation biology. Ebola, hunting push ape populations to the brink.

Kaiser J.

PMID: 12690159 [PubMed - indexed for MEDLINE]

1961. Nature. 2003 Apr 10;422(6932):551.

Ape populations decimated by hunting and Ebola virus.

Whitfield J.

Comment on Nature. 2003 Apr 10;422(6932):611-4.

PMID: 12686965 [PubMed - indexed for MEDLINE]

1962. Nature. 2003 Apr 10;422(6932):611-4. Epub 2003 Apr 6.

Catastrophic ape decline in western equatorial Africa.

Walsh PD(1), Abernethy KA, Bermejo M, Beyers R, De Wachter P, Akou ME, Huijbregts B, Mambounga DI, Toham AK, Kilbourn AM, Lahm SA, Latour S, Maisels F, Mbina C, Mihindou Y, Obiang SN, Effa EN, Starkey MP, Telfer P, Thibault M, Tutin CE, White LJ, Wilkie DS.

Author information: (1)Department of Ecology and Evolutionary Biology, Guyot Hall, Princeton, New Jersey 08540, USA. pwalsh@princeton.edu

Comment in Nature. 2003 Apr 10;422(6932):551.

Because rapidly expanding human populations have devastated gorilla (Gorilla gorilla) and common chimpanzee (Pan troglodytes) habitats in East and West Africa, the relatively intact forests of western equatorial Africa have been viewed as the last stronghold of African apes. Gabon and the Republic of Congo alone are thought to hold roughly 80% of the world's gorillas and most of the common chimpanzees. Here we present survey results conservatively indicating that ape populations in Gabon declined by more than half between 1983 and 2000. The primary cause of the decline in ape numbers during this period was commercial hunting, facilitated by the rapid expansion of mechanized logging. Furthermore, Ebola haemorrhagic fever is currently spreading through ape populations in Gabon and Congo and now rivals hunting as a threat to apes. Gorillas and common chimpanzees should be elevated immediately to 'critically endangered' status. Without aggressive investments in law enforcement, protected area management and Ebola prevention, the next decade will see our closest relatives pushed to the brink of extinction.

PMID: 12679788 [PubMed - indexed for MEDLINE]

1963. BMC Microbiol. 2003 Apr 4;3:6.

Ebola virus infection inversely correlates with the overall expression levels of promyelocytic leukaemia (PML) protein in cultured cells.

Björndal AS(1), Szekely L, Elgh F.

Author information: (1)Centre for Microbiological Preparedness, Swedish Institute for Infectious Disease Control (SMI), Nobels väg 18, 17182 Solna, Sweden. Asa.Bjorndal@mtc.ki.se

BACKGROUND: Ebola virus causes severe, often fatal hemorrhagic fever in humans. The mechanism of escape from cellular anti-viral mechanisms is not yet fully understood. The promyelocytic leukaemia (PML) associated nuclear body is part of the interferon inducible cellular defense system. Several RNA viruses have been found to interfere with the anti-viral function of the PML body. The possible interaction between Ebola virus and the PML bodies has not yet been explored. RESULTS: We found that two cell lines, Vero E6 and MCF7, support virus production at high and low levels respectively. The expression of viral proteins was visualized and quantified using high resolution immunofluorescence microscopy. Ebola encoded NP and VP35 accumulated in cytoplasmic inclusion bodies whereas VP40 was mainly membrane associated but it was also present diffusely in the cytoplasm as well as in the euchromatic areas of the nucleus. The anti-VP40 antibody also allowed the detection of extracellular virions. Interferon-alpha treatment decreased the production of all three viral proteins and delayed the development of cytopathic effects in both cell lines. Virus infection and interferon-alpha treatment induced high levels of PML protein expression in MCF7 but much less in Vero E6 cells. No disruption of PML bodies, a common phenomenon induced by a variety of different viruses, was observed. CONCLUSION: We have established a simple fixation and immunofluorescence staining procedure that allows specific co-detection and precise sub-cellular localization of the PML nuclear bodies and the Ebola virus encoded proteins NP, VP35 and VP40 in formaldehyde treated cells. Interferon-alpha treatment delays virus production in vitro. Intact PML bodies may play an anti-viral role in Ebola infected cells.

PMCID: PMC154099 PMID: 12697055 [PubMed - indexed for MEDLINE]

1964. Biol Res Nurs. 2003 Apr;4(4):276-81.

Ebola virus: immune mechanisms of protection and vaccine development.

Nyamathi AM(1), Fahey JL, Sands H, Casillas AM.

Author information: (1)School of Nursing, University of California, Los Angeles, Room 2-250, Factor Building, Box 951720, Los Angeles, CA 90095-1702, USA. anyamath@sonnet.ucla.edu

Vaccination is one of our most powerful antiviral strategies. Despite the emergence of deadly viruses such as Ebola virus, vaccination efforts have focused mainly on childhood communicable diseases. Although Ebola virus was once believed to be limited to isolated outbreaks in distant lands, forces of globalization potentiate outbreaks anywhere in the world through incidental transmission. Moreover, since this virus has already been transformed into weapon-grade material, the potential exists for it to be used as a biological weapon with catastrophic consequences for any population vulnerable to attack. Ebola hemorrhagic fever (EHF) is a syndrome that can rapidly lead to death within days of symptom onset. The disease directly affects the immune system and vascular bed, with correspondingly high mortality rates. Patients with severe disease produce dangerously high levels of inflammatory cytokines, which destroy normal tissue and microcirculation, leading to profound capillary leakage, renal failure, and disseminated intravascular coagulation. Vaccine development has been fraught with obstacles, primarily of a biosafety nature. Case reports of acutely ill patients with EHF showing improvement with the transfusion of convalescent plasma are at odds with animal studies demonstrating further viral replication with the same treatment. Using mRNA extracted from bone marrow of Ebola survivors, human monoclonal antibodies against Ebola virus surface protein have been experimentally produced and now raise the hope for the development of a safe vaccine.

PMID: 12698920 [PubMed - indexed for MEDLINE]

1965. Biol Res Nurs. 2003 Apr;4(4):268-75.

A current review of Ebola virus: pathogenesis, clinical presentation, and diagnostic assessment.

Casillas AM(1), Nyamathi AM, Sosa A, Wilder CL, Sands H.

Author information: (1)University of California, Los Angeles, School of Medicine, Room 52-175, Center for Health Sciences, Los Angeles, CA 90095, USA. acasillas@mednet.ucla.edu

Ebola hemorrhagic fever (EHF) is an acute viral syndrome that presents with fever and an ensuing bleeding diathesis that is marked by high mortality in human and nonhuman primates. Fatality rates are between 50% and 100%. Due to its lethal nature, this filovirus is classified as a biological class 4 pathogen. The natural reservoir of the virus is unknown. As a result, little is understood about how Ebola virus is transmitted or how it replicates in its host. Although the primary source of infection is unknown, the epidemiologic mode of transmission is well defined. A variety of tests have proven to be specific and useful for Ebola virus identification. There is no FDA-approved antiviral treatment for EHF. Incubation ranges from 2 to 21 days. Patients who are able to mount an immune response to the virus will begin to recover in 7 to 10 days and start a period of prolonged convalescence. Supportive management of infected patients is the primary method of treatment, with particular attention to maintenance of hydration, circulatory volume, blood pressure, and the provision of supplemental

oxygen. Since there is no specific treatment outside of supportive management and palliative care, containment of this potentially lethal virus is paramount. In almost all outbreaks of EHF, the fatality rate among health care workers with documented infections was higher than that of non-health care workers.
PMID: 12698919 [PubMed - indexed for MEDLINE]

1966. J Med Virol. 2003 Apr;69(4):503-9.

Polystyrene derivatives substituted with arginine interact with Babanki (Togaviridae) and Kedougou (Flaviviridae) viruses.

Imbert-Laurenceau E(1), Crepinior J, Crance JM, Jouan A, Migonney V.

Author information: (1)Laboratoire des Systèmes Macromoléculaires et Immunovirologie Humaine, Ecole Normale Supérieure, Lyon, France. emmanuelle.laurenceau@ens-lyon.fr

Outbreaks of new or old diseases appear primarily in tropical zones such as Africa, south and central America, or Asia. Among these diseases, those induced by Arboviruses (the best known of which are being yellow fever, dengue, Ebola, and Sindbis) are under intensive observation by the World Health Organization. Rapid isolation and identification of the viral species is the first step in the diagnosis, study, and control of epidemics. One major problem with the isolation of viruses is capturing sufficient numbers of viral particles to test. The work presented in this report addresses this question. We have tested the interaction between Babanki (Togaviridae), Kedougou (Flaviviridae) viruses, and a range of insoluble polystyrene derivatives substituted with arginine groups. Insoluble functionalized copolymers were found to develop specific interactions with viruses through chemical groups present on their surfaces. The adsorption of viruses varied according to the percentage of arginine substituted onto the polymer, with a maximum value for both viruses of about 20% of grafting rate. It was also found that the Kedougou virus displayed the highest affinity for this polymer.

PMID: 12601758 [PubMed - indexed for MEDLINE]

1967. J Virol. 2003 Apr;77(8):4794-804.

Role of ESCRT-I in retroviral budding.

Martin-Serrano J(1), Zang T, Bieniasz PD.

Author information: (1)Aaron Diamond AIDS Research Center and The Rockefeller University, New York, New York 10016, USA.

Retroviral late-budding (L) domains are required for the efficient release of nascent virions. The three known types of L domain, designated according to essential tetrapeptide motifs (PTAP, PPXY, or YPDL), each bind distinct cellular cofactors. We and others have demonstrated that recruitment of an ESCRT-I subunit, Tsg101, a component of the class E vacuolar protein sorting (VPS) machinery, is required for the budding of viruses, such as human immunodeficiency virus type I (HIV-I) and Ebola virus, that encode a PTAP-type L domain, but subsequent events remain undefined. In this study, we demonstrate that VPS28, a second component of ESCRT-I, binds to a sequence close to the Tsg101 C terminus and is therefore recruited to the plasma membrane by HIV-I Gag. In addition, we show that Tsg101 exhibits a multimerization activity. Using a complementation assay in which Tsg101 is artificially recruited to sites of HIV-I assembly, we demonstrate that the integrity of the VPS28 binding site within Tsg101 is required for particle budding. In addition, mutation of a putative leucine zipper or residues important for Tsg101 multimerization also impairs the ability of Tsg101 to support HIV-I budding. A minimal multimerizing Tsg101 domain is a dominant negative inhibitor of PTAP-mediated HIV-I budding but does not inhibit YPDL-type or PPXY-type L-domain function. Nevertheless, YDPL-type L-domain activity is inhibited by expression of a catalytically inactive mutant of the class E VPS ATPase VPS4. These results indicate that all three classes of retroviral L domains require a functioning class E VPS pathway in order to effect budding. However, the PTAP-type L domain appears to be unique in its requirement for an intact, or nearly intact, ESCRT-I complex.
PMCID: PMC152150 PMID: 12663786 [PubMed - indexed for MEDLINE]

1968. Microbes Infect. 2003 Apr;5(5):379-85.

Serological reactivity of baculovirus-expressed Ebola virus VP35 and nucleoproteins.

Groen J(1), van den Hoogen BG, Burghoorn-Maas CP, Fooks AR, Burton J, Clegg CJ, Zeller H, Osterhaus AD.

Author information: (1)Institute of Virology, Erasmus MC, Dr. Molenwaterplein 40, 3015GD, Rotterdam, The Netherlands.

Ebola virus (EBOV) is a member of the family Filoviridae and is classified as a biosafety level 4 virus. This classification makes the preparation of antigen and performance of diagnostic assays time-consuming and complicated. The objective of this study was to evaluate the value of EBOV immunoassays based on recombinant nucleoprotein (r-NP) and recombinant VP35 (r-VP35) using large serum panels of African origin and from primates. Furthermore, we investigated whether the results obtained with EBOV r-VP35 enzyme-linked immunosorbent assay (ELISA) could improve on the findings obtained with the EBOV r-NP ELISA. The full-length EBOV NP and VP35 of the EBOV subtype Zaire were expressed as histidine-tagged recombinant proteins in the baculovirus expression system. The antigenic reactivity and specificity of these recombinant proteins were determined by Western blotting and ELISA using EBOV specific monoclonal antibodies. The results obtained with the r-NP and r-VP35 ELISAs were compared with the results obtained in an indirect immunofluorescence assay based on native EBOV subtype Zaire. EBOV specific monoclonal antibodies reacted specifically with the respective proteins in both Western blot and ELISA. Five hundred and twenty six samples from humans and primates were tested with r-NP and r-VP35 ELISAs. Monkey serum samples positive for EBOV subtype Reston and Zaire were both positive in the EBOV r-NP ELISA, whereas only the EBOV Zaire infected monkeys were positive in the r-VP35 ELISA. The sensitivity and specificity values of the EBOV recombinants' ELISAs compared to those of the immunofluorescence assay were 92% and 99% for r-NP and 44% and 100% for r-VP35. r-NP ELISA proved to be a sensitive and specific assay for EBOV diagnosis and for epidemiological studies for both EBOV subtypes Reston and Zaire. The use of r-VP35 in an ELISA format has no additional value for EBOV serodiagnosis.
PMID: 12737993 [PubMed - indexed for MEDLINE]

1969. Sante Publique. 2003 Apr;15 Spec No:151-5.

Changing world, changing doctors, changing education!

van Ree JW(1).

Author information: (1)Maastricht University, Dep. General Practice, Vocational Training P. de Bijeplein I, Paviljoen.-POB 616, 6200 MD Maastricht, The Netherlands.

Future developments in the community will underline the need to provide a community-oriented health care system in which public health doctors collaborate with general practitioners, as the hospital-based health care system that currently exists in many countries will not be able to solve the problems of health care in the future. Increasing populations, increasing mobility all over the world, spread of new diseases (aids/hiv and ebola virus for example) will have great impact on our societies and the expectations of the societies and patients of their doctors. Most societies in which our young doctors will serve, expect their adults to live on healthily into their 80th. That means that the society of the future will be a double aging society (more older people who are older than before) with all concomitant burdens of degenerative chronic diseases. How should we handle the problems in 2025 when our capacities stay restricted to what we once learned in 2002? For this purpose the medical faculties have to change their curricula. The medical faculties will have to educate different kind of doctors, different from the doctors they have educated for many decades. These doctors must collaborate with other health care workers in primary health care teams. Collaboration in these teams requires mutual trust, win-win situations and agreement on the principles of health promotion programs. Only by collaboration between public health care and individual, personal health care it will be possible to achieve unity for health for all people. In the future both public health doctors and general practitioners need each other's complementary support and since they share the same area of interest, they need to work together.

PMID: 12784489 [PubMed - indexed for MEDLINE]

1970. Structure. 2003 Apr;11(4):423-33.

The matrix protein VP40 from Ebola virus octamerizes into pore-like structures with specific RNA binding properties.

Gomis-Rüth FX(1), Dessen A, Timmins J, Bracher A, Kolesnikowa L, Becker S, Klenk HD, Weissenhorn W.

Author information: (1)European Molecular Biology Laboratory (EMBL), 6 rue Jules Horowitz, 38042, Grenoble, France.

The Ebola virus membrane-associated matrix protein VP40 is thought to be crucial for assembly and budding of virus particles. Here we present the crystal structure of a disk-shaped octameric form of VP40 formed by four antiparallel homodimers of the N-terminal domain. The octamer binds an RNA triribonucleotide containing the sequence 5'-U-G-A-3' through its inner pore surface, and its oligomerization and RNA binding properties are facilitated by two conformational changes when compared to monomeric VP40. The selective RNA interaction stabilizes the ring structure and confers in vitro SDS resistance to octameric VP40. SDS-resistant octameric VP40 is also found in Ebola virus-infected cells, which suggests that VP40 has an additional function in the life cycle of the virus besides promoting virus assembly and budding off the plasma membrane.

PMID: 12679020 [PubMed - indexed for MEDLINE]

1971. Trends Mol Med. 2003 Apr;9(4):153-9.

A fatal attraction: Mycobacterium tuberculosis and HIV-1 target DC-SIGN to escape immune surveillance.

van Kooyk Y(1), Appelmelk B, Geijtenbeek TB.

Author information: (1)Department of Molecular Cell Biology, Vrije Universiteit Medical Center Amsterdam, v.d. Boechorststraat 7, 1081 BT Amsterdam, The Netherlands.

Dendritic cells (DCs) are vital in the defense against pathogens. However, it is becoming increasingly clear that some pathogens subvert DC functions to escape immune surveillance. For example, HIV-1 targets the DC-specific C-type lectin DC-SIGN (DC-specific intercellular-adhesion-molecule-3-grabbing nonintegrin) to hijack DCs for viral dissemination. Binding to DC-SIGN protects HIV-1 from antigen processing and facilitates its transport to lymphoid tissues, where DC-SIGN promotes HIV-1 infection of T cells. Recent studies demonstrate that DC-SIGN is a universal pathogen receptor that also recognizes Ebola, cytomegalovirus and mycobacteria. Mycobacterium tuberculosis targets DC-SIGN by a mechanism that is distinct from that of HIV-1, leading to inhibition of the immunostimulatory function of DC and, hence, promotion of pathogen survival. A better understanding of DC-SIGN-pathogen interactions and their effects on DC function should help to combat infections.

PMID: 12727141 [PubMed - indexed for MEDLINE]

1972. Virus Res. 2003 Apr;92(2):213-7.

Vaccine for AIDS and Ebola virus infection.

Nabel GJ(1).

Author information: (1)Vaccine Research Center, National Institutes of Allergy and Infectious Diseases, National Institutes of Health, 40 Convent Drive, Bethesda, MD 20892-3005, USA. gnabel@nih.gov

Ebola virus and HIV present challenges for vaccine development because natural immunity to these viruses is difficult to find, and there are no immune correlates of protection in humans. Modern molecular genetic, virologic and immune analyses have been used to rationally identify promising approaches based on animal model and human clinical studies. Improved vaccine candidates have been defined for HIV, and a promising Ebola vaccine have conferred protection in non-human primates. Further evaluation in humans will allow an assessment of their potential efficacy and point the way to the development of more successful vaccines.

PMID: 12686432 [PubMed - indexed for MEDLINE]

1973. Virus Res. 2003 Apr;92(2):187-93.

Comparison of the protective efficacy of DNA and baculovirus-derived protein vaccines for EBOLA virus in guinea pigs.

Mellquist-Riemenschneider JL(1), Garrison AR, Geisbert JB, Saikh KU, Heidebrink KD, Jahrling PB, Ulrich RG, Schmaljohn CS.

Author information: (1)Department of Molecular Virology, Virology Division, Division U.S. Army Medical Research Institute of Infectious Diseases, 1301 Ditto Ave., Ft. Detrick, Frederick 21702, MD, USA.

The filoviruses Ebola virus (EBOV) and Marburg virus (MARV) cause severe hemorrhagic fever in humans for which no vaccines are available. Previously, a priming dose of a DNA vaccine expressing the glycoprotein (GP) gene of MARV followed by boosting with recombinant baculovirus-derived GP protein was found to confer protective immunity to guinea pigs (Hevey et al., 2001. Vaccine 20, 568-593). To determine whether a similar prime-boost vaccine approach would be effective for EBOV, we generated and characterized recombinant baculoviruses expressing full-length EBOV GP (GP(1,2)) or a terminally-deleted GP (GPa-) and examined their immunogenicity in guinea pigs. As expected, cells infected with the GPa- recombinant secreted more GP(1) than those infected with the GP(1,2) recombinant. In lectin binding studies, the insect cell culture-derived GPs were found to differ from mammalian cell derived virion GP, in that they had no complex/hybrid N-linked glycans or glycans containing sialic acid. Despite these differences, the baculovirus-derived GPs were able to bind monoclonal antibodies to five distinct epitopes on EBOV GP, indicating that the antigenic structures of the proteins remain intact. As a measure of the ability of the baculovirus-derived proteins to elicit cell-mediated immune responses, we evaluated the T-cell stimulatory capacity of the GPa- protein in cultured human dendritic cells. Increases in cytotoxicity as compared to controls suggest that the baculovirus proteins have the capacity to evoke cell-mediated immune responses. Guinea pigs vaccinated with the baculovirus-derived GPs alone, or in a DNA prime-baculovirus protein boost regimen developed antibody responses as measured by ELISA and plaque reduction neutralization assays; however, incomplete protection was achieved when the proteins were given alone or in combination with DNA vaccines. These data indicate that a vaccine approach that was effective for MARV is not effective for EBOV in guinea pigs.
PMID: 12686428 [PubMed - indexed for MEDLINE]
1974. Lancet. 2003 Mar 22;361(9362):1020.

Death toll continues to climb in Congo Ebola outbreak.

Frankish H.
PMID: 12660066 [PubMed - indexed for MEDLINE]
1975. J Immunol. 2003 Mar 15;170(6):2797-801.

Cutting edge: impairment of dendritic cells and adaptive immunity by Ebola and Lassa viruses.

Mahanty S(1), Hutchinson K, Agarwal S, McRae M, Rollin PE, Pulendran B.

Author information: (1)Special Pathogens Branch, Division of Viral and Rickettsial Diseases, National Center for Infectious Diseases, Centers for Disease Control and Prevention, Atlanta, GA 30333, USA. smahanty@cdc.gov

Acute infection of humans with Ebola and Lassa viruses, two principal etiologic agents of hemorrhagic fevers, often results in a paradoxical pattern of immune responses: early infection, characterized by an outpouring of inflammatory mediators such as TNF-alpha, IL-1 beta, and IL-6, vs late stage infections, which are associated with poor immune responses. The mechanisms underlying these diverse outcomes are poorly understood. In particular, the role played by cells of the innate immune system, such as dendritic cells (DC), is not known. In this study, we show that Ebola and Lassa viruses infect human monocyte-derived DC and impair their function. Monocyte-derived DC exposed to either virus fail to secrete proinflammatory cytokines, do not up-regulate costimulatory molecules, and are poor stimulators of T cells. These data represent the first evidence for a mechanism by which Ebola and Lassa viruses target DC to impair adaptive immunity.
PMID: 12626527 [PubMed - indexed for MEDLINE]
1976. Antiviral Res. 2003 Mar;58(1):47-56.

Cyanovirin-N binds to the viral surface glycoprotein, GP1,2 and inhibits infectivity of Ebola virus.

Barrientos LG(1), O'Keefe BR, Bray M, Sanchez A, Gronenborn AM, Boyd MR.

Author information: (1)Laboratory of Chemical Physics, National Institute of Diabetes and Digestive and Kidney Diseases, National Institutes of Health, Bethesda, MD, USA.

Ebola virus (Ebo) causes severe hemorrhagic fever and high mortality in humans. There are currently no effective therapies. Here, we have explored potential anti-Ebo activity of the human immunodeficiency virus (HIV)-inactivating protein cyanovirin-N (CV-N). CV-N is known to potently inhibit the infectivity of a broad spectrum of HIV strains at the level of viral entry. This involves CV-N binding to N-linked high-mannose oligossacharides on the viral glycoprotein gp120. The Ebola envelope contains somewhat similar oligosaccharide constituents, suggesting possible susceptibility to inhibition by CV-N. Our initial results revealed that CV-N had both in vitro and in vivo antiviral activity against the Zaire strain of the Ebola virus (Ebo-Z). Addition of CV-N to the cell culture medium at the time of Ebo-Z infection inhibited the development of viral cytopathic effects (CPEs). CV-N also delayed the death of Ebo-Z-infected mice, both when given as a series of daily subcutaneous injections and when the virus was incubated ex vivo together with CV-N before inoculation into the mice. Furthermore, similar to earlier results with HIV gp120, CV-N bound with considerable affinity to the Ebola surface envelope glycoprotein, GP(1,2). Competition experiments with free oligosaccharides were consistent with the view that carbohydrate-mediated CV-N/GP(1,2) interactions involve oligosaccharides residing on the Ebola viral envelope. Overall, these studies broaden the range of viruses known to be inhibited by CV-N, and further implicate carbohydrate moieties on viral surface proteins as common viral molecular targets for this novel protein.
PMID: 12719006 [PubMed - indexed for MEDLINE]
1977. J Virol. 2003 Mar;77(5):3334-8.

Ebola virus transcription activator VP30 is a zinc-binding protein.

Modrof J(1), Becker S, Mühlberger E.

Author information: (1)Institut für Virologie der Philipps-Universität Marburg, 35037 Marburg, Germany.
Ebola virus VP30 is an essential activator of viral transcription. In viral particles, VP30 is closely associated with the nucleocapsid complex. A conspicuous structural feature of VP30 is an unconventional zinc-binding Cys(3)-His motif comprising amino acids 68 to 95. By using a colorimetric zinc-binding assay we found that the VP30-specific Cys(3)-His motif stoichiometrically binds zinc ions in a one-to-one relationship. Substitution of the conserved cysteines and the histidine within the motif led to a complete loss of the capacity for zinc binding. Functional analyses revealed that none of the tested mutations of the proposed zinc-coordinating residues influenced binding of VP30 to nucleocapsid-like particles but, concerning its role in activating viral transcription, all resulted in a protein that was inactive.
PMCID: PMC149768 PMID: 12584359 [PubMed - indexed for MEDLINE]
1978. Nihon Rinsho. 2003 Mar;61 Suppl 3:544-9.

[Ebola virus and Marburg virus].
[Article in Japanese]
Morikawa S(1).
Author information: (1)Department of Virology I, National Institute of Infectious Diseases.
PMID: 12718026 [PubMed - indexed for MEDLINE]
1979. Virology. 2003 Feb 15;306(2):210-8.

Analysis of the role of predicted RNA secondary structures in Ebola virus replication.
Crary SM(1), Towner JS, Honig JE, Shoemaker TR, Nichol ST.
Author information: (1)Special Pathogens Branch, Division of Viral and Rickettsial Diseases, Centers for Disease Control and Prevention, Atlanta, GA 30333, USA.
Thermodynamic modeling of Ebola viral RNA predicts the formation of RNA stem-loop structures at the 3' and 5' termini and panhandle structures between the termini of the genomic (or antigenomic) RNAs. Sequence analysis showed a high degree of identity among Ebola Zaire, Sudan, Reston, and Cote d'Ivoire subtype viruses in their 3' and 5' termini (18 nucleotides in length) and within a second region (internal by approximately 20 nucleotides). While base pairing of the two conserved regions could lead to the formation of the base of the putative stem-loop or panhandle structures, the intervening sequence variation altered the predictions for the rest of the structures. Using an in vivo minigenome replication system, we engineered mutations designed to disrupt potential base pairing in the viral RNA termini. Analysis of these variants by screening for enhanced green fluorescent protein reporter expression and by quantitation of minigenomic RNA levels demonstrated that the upper portions of the putative panhandle and 3' genomic structures can be destabilized without affecting virus replication.
PMID: 12642094 [PubMed - indexed for MEDLINE]
1980. J Mol Biol. 2003 Feb 14;326(2):493-502.

Ebola virus matrix protein VP40 interaction with human cellular factors Tsg101 and Nedd4.
Timmins J(1), Schoehn G, Ricard-Blum S, Scianimanico S, Vernet T, Ruigrok RW, Weissenhorn W.
Author information: (1)European Molecular Biology Laboratory, 6 rue Jules Horowitz, 38042 Grenoble, France.
The Ebola virus matrix protein VP40 is a major viral structural protein and plays a central role in virus assembly and budding at the plasma membrane of infected cells. For efficient budding, a full amino terminus of VP40 is required, which includes a PPXY and a PT/SAP motif, both of which have been proposed to interact with cellular proteins. Here, we report that Ebola VP40 can interact with cellular factors human Nedd4 and Tsg101 in vitro. We show that WW domain 3 of human Nedd4 is necessary and sufficient for binding to the PPXY motif of VP40, which requires an oligomeric conformation of VP40. Single particle electron microscopy reconstructions indicate that WW3 of Nedd4 is in close contact with the N-terminal domain of hexameric VP40. In contrast, the ubiquitin enzyme variant domain of Tsg101 was sufficient for binding to the PT/SAP motif of VP40, regardless of the oligomeric state of the matrix protein. These results suggest that hNedd4 and Tsg101 may play complimentary roles at a late stage of the assembly process, by recruiting cellular factors of two independent pathways to the site of budding at the plasma membrane.
PMID: 12559917 [PubMed - indexed for MEDLINE]
1981. Curr Opin Investig Drugs. 2003 Feb;4(2):172-8.

Therapeutic options for diseases due to potential viral agents of bioterrorism.
Bronze MS(1), Greenfield RA.
Author information: (1)Department of Medicine, University of Oklahoma Health Sciences Center, Williams Pavilion, Room WP2080, 920 Stanton Young Blvd, Oklahoma City, OK 73190, USA. Michael-Bronze@OUHSC.edu
The etiologic agents of smallpox and viral hemorrhagic fever have emerged as potential agents of bioterrorism due to their virulence, potential for human to human dissemination and limited strategies for treatment and prevention. Cidofovir has shown significant promise in animal models, and limited case reports in humans are encouraging. Ribavirin is the treatment of choice for certain hemorrhagic fever viral infections, but has no current application to Ebola and Marburg infections. Current vaccine strategies for smallpox are effective, but carry significant risk for complications. Licensed vaccines for hemorrhagic fever viruses are limited to yellow fever, but animal studies are promising. Genomic analysis of the viral pathogen and the animal model response to infection may provide valuable information enabling the development of novel treatment and prevention strategies. Current knowledge of these strategies is reviewed.
PMID: 12669378 [PubMed - indexed for MEDLINE]
1982. J Virol. 2003 Feb;77(3):1812-9.

431

Overlapping motifs (PTAP and PPEY) within the Ebola virus VP40 protein function independently as late budding domains: involvement of host proteins TSG101 and VPS-4.

Licata JM(1), Simpson-Holley M, Wright NT, Han Z, Paragas J, Harty RN.

Author information: (1)Department of Pathobiology, School of Veterinary Medicine, University of Pennsylvania, Philadelphia, Pennsylvania 19104-6049, USA.

The VP40 protein of Ebola virus can bud from mammalian cells in the form of lipid-bound, virus-like particles (VLPs), and late budding domains (L-domains) are conserved motifs (PTAP, PPxY, or YxxL; where "x" is any amino acid) that facilitate the budding of VP40-containing VLPs. VP40 is unique in that potential overlapping L-domains with the sequences PTAP and PPEY are present at amino acids 7 to 13 of VP40 (PTAPPEY). L-domains are thought to function by interacting with specific cellular proteins, such as the ubiquitin ligase Nedd4, and a component of the vacuolar protein sorting (vps) pathway, tsg101. Mutational analysis of the PTAPPEY sequence of VP40 was performed to understand further the contribution of each individual motif in promoting VP40 budding. In addition, the contribution of tsg101 and a second member of the vps pathway, vps4, in facilitating budding was addressed. Our results indicate that (i) both the PTAP and PPEY motifs contribute to efficient budding of VP40-containing VLPs; (ii) PTAP and PPEY can function as L-domains when separated and moved from the N terminus (amino acid position 7) to the C terminus (amino acid position 316) of full-length VP40; (iii) A VP40-PTAP/tsg101 interaction recruits tsg101 into budding VLPs; (iv) a VP40-PTAP/tsg101 interaction recruits VP40 into lipid raft microdomains; and (v) a dominant-negative mutant of vps4 (E228Q), but not wild-type vps4, significantly inhibited the budding of Ebola virus (Zaire). These results provide important insights into the complex interplay between viral and host proteins during the late stages of Ebola virus budding.

PMCID: PMC140960 PMID: 12525615 [PubMed - indexed for MEDLINE]

1983. J Virol. 2003 Feb;77(3):1793-800.

Biochemical and functional characterization of the Ebola virus VP24 protein: implications for a role in virus assembly and budding.

Han Z(1), Boshra H, Sunyer JO, Zwiers SH, Paragas J, Harty RN.

Author information: (1)Laboratory 412. Laboratory 413, Department of Pathobiology, School of Veterinary Medicine, University of Pennsylvania, Philadelphia, Pennsylvania 19104-6049, USA.

The VP24 protein of Ebola virus is believed to be a secondary matrix protein and minor component of virions. In contrast, the VP40 protein of Ebola virus is the primary matrix protein and the most abundant virion component. The structure and function of VP40 have been well characterized; however, virtually nothing is known regarding the structure and function of VP24. Wild-type and mutant forms of VP24 were expressed in mammalian cells to gain a better understanding of the biochemical and functional nature of this viral protein. Results from these experiments demonstrated that (i) VP24 localizes to the plasma membrane and perinuclear region in both transfected and Ebola virus-infected cells, (ii) VP24 associates strongly with lipid membranes, (iii) VP24 does not contain N-linked sugars when expressed alone in mammalian cells, (iv) VP24 can oligomerize when expressed alone in mammalian cells, (v) progressive deletions at the N terminus of VP24 resulted in a decrease in oligomer formation and a concomitant increase in the formation of high-molecular-weight aggregates, and (vi) VP24 was present in trypsin-resistant virus like particles released into the media covering VP24-transfected cells. These data indicate that VP24 possesses structural features commonly associated with viral matrix proteins and that VP24 may have a role in virus assembly and budding.

PMCID: PMC140957 PMID: 12525613 [PubMed - indexed for MEDLINE]

1984. Pol Merkur Lekarski. 2003 Feb;14(80):146-9.

[Viral hemorrhagic fevers as a biological weapon].

[Article in Polish]

Grygorczuk S(1), Hermanowska-Szpakowicz T.

Author information: (1)Klinika Chorób Zakaznych i Neuroinfekcji Akademii Medycznej w Białymstoku.

Viral haemorrhagic fevers are zoonoses caused by a group of phylogenetically diverse RNA-viruses, capable of causing serious haemorrhagic complications in humans. The West-African Ebola and Marburg viruses pose the most significant threat because of their easy spreading through direct contact with the ill person and high death rate reaching 90%. They are considered among the most dangerous agents possibly used in bioterrorist attack and have been studied as a part of the Soviet biological weapons programme. The first symptoms of the Ebola haemorrhagic fever appear 4 to 16 days after the infection and are rather unspecific (fever, flu-like and gastrointestinal symptoms, cough, sore throat, conjunctivitis). Within a few days the disease leads to weight loss, haemorrhagic complications and circulatory insufficiency. The infection may be transmitted through direct contact with the patient, his/her body fluids and cadavers; droplet transmission is much less likely. There is no specific prophylaxis nor treatment; still, isolation of patients and use of personal protection means by persons providing care to patients seem efficient in stopping the infection. The knowledge of the biology and epidemiology of Filoviridae is still limited, which makes the results of bioterrorist attack using these pathogens hard to predict.

PMID: 12728677 [PubMed - indexed for MEDLINE]

1985. FEBS Lett. 2003 Jan 30;535(1-3):23-8.

Calcium-dependent conformational changes of membrane-bound Ebola fusion peptide drive vesicle fusion.

Suárez T(1), Gómara MJ, Goñi FM, Mingarro I, Muga A, Pérez-Payá E, Nieva JL.

Author information: (1)Unidad de Biofísica (CSIC-UPV/EHU) y Departamento de Bioquímica, Universidad del País Vasco, Aptdo. 644, 48080, Bilbao, Spain.

The fusogenic subdomain of the Ebola virus envelope glycoprotein is an internal sequence located ca. 20 residues downstream the N-terminus of the glycoprotein transmembrane subunit. Partitioning of the Ebola fusion peptide into membranes containing phosphatidylinositol in the absence of Ca2+ stabilizes an alpha-helical conformation, and gives rise to vesicle efflux but not vesicle fusion. In the presence of millimolar Ca2+ the membrane-bound peptide adopts an extended beta-structure, and induces inter-vesicle mixing of lipids. The peptide conformational polymorphism may be related to the flexibility of the virus-cell intermembrane fusogenic complex.

PMID: 12560072 [PubMed - indexed for MEDLINE]

1986. Virology. 2003 Jan 5;305(1):115-23.

DC-SIGN and DC-SIGNR bind ebola glycoproteins and enhance infection of macrophages and endothelial cells.

Simmons G(1), Reeves JD, Grogan CC, Vandenberghe LH, Baribaud F, Whitbeck JC, Burke E, Buchmeier MJ, Soilleux EJ, Riley JL, Doms RW, Bates P, Pöhlmann S.

Author information: (1)Department of Molecular Histopathology, University of Cambridge, Cambridge, CB2 1QP, United Kingdom.

Ebola virus exhibits a broad cellular tropism in vitro. In humans and animal models, virus is found in most tissues and organs during the latter stages of infection. In contrast, a more restricted cell and tissue tropism is exhibited early in infection where macrophages, liver, lymph node, and spleen are major initial targets. This indicates that cellular factors other than the broadly expressed virus receptor(s) modulate Ebola virus tropism. Here we demonstrate that the C-type lectins DC-SIGN and DC-SIGNR avidly bind Ebola glycoproteins and greatly enhance transduction of primary cells by Ebola virus pseudotypes and infection by replication-competent Ebola virus. DC-SIGN and DC-SIGNR are expressed in several early targets for Ebola virus infection, including dendritic cells, alveolar macrophages, and sinusoidal endothelial cells in the liver and lymph node. While DC-SIGN and DC-SIGNR do not directly mediate Ebola virus entry, their pattern of expression in vivo and their ability to efficiently capture virus and to enhance infection indicate that these attachment factors can play an important role in Ebola transmission, tissue tropism, and pathogenesis.

PMID: 12504546 [PubMed - indexed for MEDLINE]

1987. FEBS Lett. 2003 Jan 2;533(1-3):47-53.

Pre-transmembrane sequence of Ebola glycoprotein. Interfacial hydrophobicity distribution and interaction with membranes.

Sáez-Cirión A(1), Gómara MJ, Agirre A, Nieva JL.

Author information: (1)Unidad de Biofísica (CSIC-UPV/EHU) and Departamento de Bioquímica, Universidad del País Vasco, Aptdo. 644, 48080, Bilbao, Spain.

The membrane-interacting domain that precedes the transmembrane anchor of Ebola glycoprotein has been characterized. This aromatic-rich region is predicted to bind the membrane interface adopting an alpha-helical structure. Peptides representing either the Ebola glycoprotein pre-transmembrane sequence, or a 'scrambled' control with a different hydrophobic-at-interface moment, have been studied. Insertion into lipid monolayers, changes in intrinsic fluorescence and in infrared spectra demonstrated that only the wild-type peptide bound the interface under equilibrium conditions and adopted an alpha-helical conformation. The presence of the raft-associated lipid sphingomyelin did not affect membrane insertion, but it stimulated highly the membrane-destabilizing capacity of the pre-transmembrane sequence. A parallel study of the effects of the viral sequence and of melittin suggests that Ebola glycoprotein pre-transmembrane sequence might target membranes inherently prone to destabilization by lytic peptides.

PMID: 12505157 [PubMed - indexed for MEDLINE]

1988. Annu Rev Microbiol. 2003;57:343-67.

Measles virus 1998-2002: progress and controversy.

Rall GF(1).

Author information: (1)Division of Basic Science, Fox Chase Cancer Center, 7701 Burholme Avenue, Philadelphia, Pennsylvania 19111, USA. gf_rall@fccc.edu

Despite the extensive media exposure that viruses such as West Nile, Norwalk, and Ebola have received lately, and the emerging threat that old pathogens may reappear as new agents of terrorism, measles virus (MV) persists as one of the leading causes of death by infectious agents worldwide, approaching the annual mortality rate of human immunodeficiency virus (HIV)-1. For most MV victims, fatality is indirect: Virus-induced transient immunosuppression predisposes the individual to opportunistic infections that, left untreated, can result in mortality. In rare cases, MV may also cause progressive neurodegenerative disease. During the past five years (1998-2002), development of animal models and the application of reverse genetics and immunological assays have collectively contributed to major progress in our understanding of MV biology and pathogenesis. Nevertheless, questions and controversies remain that are the basis for future research. In this review, major advances and current debates are discussed, including MV receptor usage, the cellular basis of immunosuppression, the suspected role of MV in "nonviral" diseases such as multiple sclerosis and Paget's disease, and the controversy surrounding MV vaccine safety.

PMID: 14527283 [PubMed - indexed for MEDLINE]

1989. Antiviral Res. 2003 Jan;57(1-2):53-60.

Defense against filoviruses used as biological weapons.

Bray M(1).

Author information: (1)Medical Officer, Biodefense Clinical Research Branch, OCR/OD/NIAID/NIH, 6700A Rockledge Drive, Room 5132, Bethesda, MD 20892, USA. mbray@niaid.nih.gov

The filoviruses, Marburg and Ebola, are classified as Category A biowarfare agents by the Centers for Disease Control. Most known human infections with these viruses have been fatal, and no vaccines or effective therapies are currently available. Filoviruses are highly infectious by the airborne route in the laboratory, but investigations of African outbreaks have shown that person-to-person spread requires direct contact with virus-containing material. In consequence, filovirus epidemics can be halted by isolating patients and instituting standard infection control and barrier nursing procedures. The filovirus disease syndrome resembles that caused by other hemorrhagic fever viruses, necessitating studies in a biocontainment laboratory to confirm the diagnosis. Some progress has been made in developing vaccines and antiviral drugs, but efforts are hindered by the limited number of maximum containment laboratories.

Terrorists might have great difficulty acquiring a filovirus for use as a weapon, but my attempt to do so because of the agents' ability to inspire fear. Accurate information is the best tool to prevent panic in the event of an attack.

PMID: 12615303 [PubMed - indexed for MEDLINE]

1990. Biosecur Bioterror. 2003;1(4):233-7.

Interview with David L. Heymann, MD, representative for polio eradication and former Executive Director, Communicable Diseases, World Health Organization. Interview by Madeline Drexler.

Heymann DL.

PMID: 15040202 [PubMed - indexed for MEDLINE]

1991. Clin Diagn Lab Immunol. 2003 Jan;10(1):83-7.

Analysis of linear B-cell epitopes of the nucleoprotein of ebola virus that distinguish ebola virus subtypes.

Niikura M(1), Ikegami T, Saijo M, Kurata T, Kurane I, Morikawa S.

Author information: (1)Department of Virology, National Institute of Infectious Diseases, Tokyo 208-0011, Japan.

Ebola virus consists of four genetically distinguishable subtypes. We developed monoclonal antibodies (MAbs) to the nucleoprotein (NP) of Ebola virus Zaire subtype and analyzed their cross-reactivities to the Reston and Sudan subtypes. We further determined the epitopes recognized by these MAbs. Three MAbs reacted with the three major subtypes and recognized a fragment containing 110 amino acids (aa) at the C-terminal extremity. They did not show specific reactivities to any 10-aa short peptides in Pepscan analyses, suggesting that these MAbs recognize conformational epitope(s) located within this region. Six MAbs recognized a fragment corresponding to aa 361 to 461 of the NP. Five of these six MAbs showed specific reactivities in Pepscan analyses, and the epitopes were identified in two regions, aa 424 to 430 and aa 451 to 455. Three MAbs that recognized the former epitope region cross-reacted with all three subtypes, and one that recognized the same epitope region was Zaire specific. One MAb, which recognized the latter epitope region, was reactive with Zaire and Sudan subtypes but not with the Reston subtype. These results suggest that Ebola virus NP has at least two linear epitope regions and that the recognition of the epitope by MAbs can vary even within the same epitope region. These MAbs showing different subtype specificities might be useful reagents for developing an immunological system to identify Ebola virus subtypes.

PMCID: PMC145268 PMID: 12522044 [PubMed - indexed for MEDLINE]

1992. Drug Discov Today. 2003 Jan 1;8(1):22-30.

Examining unmet needs in infectious disease.

Snell NJ(1).

Author information: (1)National Heart and Lung Institute, Imperial College School of Medicine, Dovehouse Street, SW3 6LY, London, UK. noel.snell@astrazeneca.com

In the past 30 years, more than 30 new aetiological agents of infectious disease have been identified. Some of these are responsible for entirely novel and life-threatening disorders, such as AIDS, Ebola fever, hantavirus pulmonary syndrome and Nipah virus encephalitis. During the same period, some longstanding infectious diseases (such as tuberculosis) have became resurgent, as a result of a combination of complacency, increased travel and social dislocation, and also increasing drug resistance. This review looks at some of the key unmet needs in this therapeutic area and discusses strategies to address them.

PMID: 12546988 [PubMed - indexed for MEDLINE]

1993. Intervirology. 2003;46(2):71-8.

Viral zoonoses - a threat under control?

Ludwig B(1), Kraus FB, Allwinn R, Doerr HW, Preiser W.

Author information: (1)Institute for Medical Virology, Johann Wolfgang Goethe University, Frankfurt am Main, Germany. B.Ludwing@em.uni-frankfurt.de

Despite intensive research and considerable effort to eradicate infectious diseases, modern medicine has failed to control many infectious diseases which have been thought to be easy to overcome with advances in medical science and technology. In fact, infectious diseases remain a dominant feature in public health considerations for the 21st century. Some infectious agents already known to be pathogenic have gained increasing importance in recent decades due to changes in disease patterns. Furthermore, many new, previously unknown infectious agents with a high pathogenic potential have been identified. Nearly all of these emergent disease episodes have involved zoonotic or species-jumping infectious agents. The complex interaction of factors like environmental and ecological changes, social factors, decline of health care, human demographics and behaviour influences the emergence of re-emergence of such diseases. Viruses, especially RNA viruses with their ability to adapt quickly to changing environmental conditions, are among the most prominent examples of emerging pathogens. In this review, we present the important examples of zoonotic viruses and discuss the factors playing a key role in the emergence and resurgence of these diseases.

Copyright 2003 S. Karger AG, Basel

PMID: 12684545 [PubMed - indexed for MEDLINE]

1994. J Virol. 2003 Jan;77(2):1501-11.

Newcastle disease virus (NDV)-based assay demonstrates interferon-antagonist activity for the NDV V protein and the Nipah virus V, W, and C proteins.

Park MS(1), Shaw ML, Muñoz-Jordan J, Cros JF, Nakaya T, Bouvier N, Palese P, García-Sastre A, Basler CF.

Author information: (1)Department of Microbiology, Mount Sinai School of Medicine, New York, New York 10029, USA.

We have generated a recombinant Newcastle disease virus (NDV) that expresses the green fluorescence protein (GFP) in infected chicken embryo fibroblasts (CEFs). This virus is interferon (IFN) sensitive, and pretreatment of cells with chicken alpha/beta IFN (IFN-alpha/beta) completely blocks viral GFP expression. Prior transfection of plasmid DNA induces an IFN response in CEFs and blocks NDV-GFP replication. However, transfection of known inhibitors of the IFN-alpha/beta system, including the influenza A virus NS1 protein and the Ebola virus VP35 protein, restores NDV-GFP replication. We therefore conclude that the NDV-GFP virus could be used to screen proteins expressed from plasmids for the ability to counteract the host cell IFN response. Using this system, we show that expression of the NDV V protein or the Nipah virus V, W, or C proteins rescues NDV-GFP replication in the face of the transfection-induced IFN response. The V and W proteins of Nipah virus, a highly lethal pathogen in humans, also block activation of an IFN-inducible promoter in primate cells. Interestingly, the amino-terminal region of the Nipah virus V protein, which is identical to the amino terminus of Nipah virus W, is sufficient to exert the IFN-antagonist activity. In contrast, the anti-IFN activity of the NDV V protein appears to be located in the carboxy-terminal region of the protein, a region implicated in the IFN-antagonist activity exhibited by the V proteins of mumps virus and human parainfluenza virus type 2.
PMCID: PMC140815 PMID: 12502864 [PubMed - indexed for MEDLINE]

1995. J Virol. 2003 Jan;77(2):1337-46.

Differential N-linked glycosylation of human immunodeficiency virus and Ebola virus envelope glycoproteins modulates interactions with DC-SIGN and DC-SIGNR.

Lin G(1), Simmons G, Pöhlmann S, Baribaud F, Ni H, Leslie GJ, Haggarty BS, Bates P, Weissman D, Hoxie JA, Doms RW.

Author information: (1)Hematology-Oncology Division, Department of Medicine, University of Pennsylvania, Philadelphia 19104, USA.

The C-type lectins DC-SIGN and DC-SIGNR [collectively referred to as DC-SIGN(R)] bind and transmit human immunodeficiency virus (HIV) and simian immunodeficiency virus to T cells via the viral envelope glycoprotein (Env). Other viruses containing heavily glycosylated glycoproteins (GPs) fail to interact with DC-SIGN(R), suggesting some degree of specificity in this interaction. We show here that DC-SIGN(R) selectively interact with HIV Env and Ebola virus GPs containing more high-mannose than complex carbohydrate structures. Modulation of N-glycans on Env or GP through production of viruses in different primary cells or in the presence of the mannosidase I inhibitor deoxymannojirimycin dramatically affected DC-SIGN(R) infectivity enhancement. Further, murine leukemia virus, which typically does not interact efficiently with DC-SIGN(R), could do so when produced in the presence of deoxymannojirimycin. We predict that other viruses containing GPs with a large proportion of high-mannose N-glycans will efficiently interact with DC-SIGN(R), whereas those with solely complex N-glycans will not. Thus, the virus-producing cell type is an important factor in dictating both N-glycan status and virus interactions with DC-SIGN(R), which may impact virus tropism and transmissibility in vivo.
PMCID: PMC140807 PMID: 12502850 [PubMed - indexed for MEDLINE]

1996. J Virol. 2003 Jan;77(2):1069-74.

Identification of protective epitopes on ebola virus glycoprotein at the single amino acid level by using recombinant vesicular stomatitis viruses.

Takada A(1), Feldmann H, Stroeher U, Bray M, Watanabe S, Ito H, McGregor M, Kawaoka Y.

Author information: (1)Division of Virology, Department of Microbiology and Immunology, Institute of Medical Science, University of Tokyo, Japan.

Ebola virus causes lethal hemorrhagic fever in humans, but currently there are no effective vaccines or antiviral compounds for this infectious disease. Passive transfer of monoclonal antibodies (MAbs) protects mice from lethal Ebola virus infection (J. A. Wilson, M. Hevey, R. Bakken, S. Guest, M. Bray, A. L. Schmaljohn, and M. K. Hart, Science 287:1664-1666, 2000). However, the epitopes responsible for neutralization have been only partially characterized because some of the MAbs do not recognize the short synthetic peptides used for epitope mapping. To identify the amino acids recognized by neutralizing and protective antibodies, we generated a recombinant vesicular stomatitis virus (VSV) containing the Ebola virus glycoprotein-encoding gene instead of the VSV G protein-encoding gene and used it to select escape variants by growing it in the presence of a MAb (133/3.16 or 226/8.1) that neutralizes the infectivity of the virus. All three variants selected by MAb 133/3.16 contained a single amino acid substitution at amino acid position 549 in the GP2 subunit. By contrast, MAb 226/8.1 selected three different variants containing substitutions at positions 134, 194, and 199 in the GP1 subunit, suggesting that this antibody recognized a conformational epitope. Passive transfer of each of these MAbs completely protected mice from a lethal Ebola virus infection. These data indicate that neutralizing antibody cocktails for passive prophylaxis and therapy of Ebola hemorrhagic fever can reduce the possibility of the emergence of antigenic variants in infected individuals.
PMCID: PMC140786 PMID: 12502822 [PubMed - indexed for MEDLINE]

1997. J Virol. 2003 Jan;77(1):799-803.

Overcoming immunity to a viral vaccine by DNA priming before vector boosting.

Yang ZY(1), Wyatt LS, Kong WP, Moodie Z, Moss B, Nabel GJ.

Author information: (1)Vaccine Research Center, National Institute of Allergy and Infectious Diseases, National Institutes of Health, Bethesda, Maryland 20892-3005, USA.

Replication-defective adenovirus (ADV) and poxvirus vectors have shown potential as vaccines for pathogens such as Ebola or human immunodeficiency virus in nonhuman primates, but prior immunity to the viral vector in humans may limit their clinical efficacy. To overcome this limitation, the effect of prior viral exposure on immune responses to Ebola virus glycoprotein (GP), shown previously to protect against lethal hemorrhagic fever in animals, was studied. Prior exposure to ADV substantially reduced the cellular and humoral immune responses to GP expressed by ADV, while exposure to vaccinia inhibited vaccine-induced cellular but not humoral responses to GP expressed by vaccinia. This inhibition was largely overcome by priming with a DNA expression vector before boosting with the viral vector. Though heterologous viral vectors for priming and boosting can also overcome this effect, the paucity of such clinical viral vectors may limit their use. In summary, it is possible to counteract prior viral immunity by priming with a nonviral, DNA vaccine.

PMCID: PMC140625 PMID: 12477888 [PubMed - indexed for MEDLINE]

1998. Ky Nurse. 2003 Jan-Mar;51(1):12.

Infectious disease (Ebola virus).

Murphy L(1), Newcomb R.

Author information: (1)College Health Science, Department of Baccalaureate and Graduate Nursing Program, Eastern Kentucky University, Richmond, KY 40475, USA.

PMID: 12655811 [PubMed - indexed for MEDLINE]

1999. Med Trop (Mars). 2003;63(3):291-5.

[Outbreak of Ebola hemorrhagic fever in the Republic of the Congo, 2003: a new strategy?].

[Article in French]

Formenty P(1), Libama F, Epelboin A, Allarangar Y, Leroy E, Moudzeo H, Tarangonia P, Molamou A, Lenzi M, Ait-Ikhlef K, Hewlett B, Roth C, Grein T.

Author information: (1)Département des Maladies transmissibles, Surveillance et Action, Organisation Mondiale de la Santé, Genève, Suisse. formentyp@who.int

This article describes the last Ebola haemorrhagic fever (EHF) outbreak that occurred in the Cuvette Ouest Region of the Republic of Congo from January to April 2003. Epidemiological study demonstrated that the first patient, in whom diagnosis was made retrospectively, became ill on December 25, 2002. Subsequently until May 7, 2003, a total of 143 cases were recorded in the Mbomo and Kéllé health districts including 129 fatalities. Thirteen cases were laboratory confirmed and 130 were epidemiologically linked. Fifty-three percent of patients were male. Age ranged form 5 days to 80 years. Transmission involved direct contact with an infected person especially within families. Epidemiological data traced introduction of Ebola virus into the population to three primary cases mainly involving hunters. In all three cases development of the disease followed contact with non-human primates (gorillas) and other mammals (antelope) that had either been killed or found dead. Three health care workers were infected during the epidemic but nosocomial transmission played a minor role in the epidemic. On June 5, the Minister of Health and Population of the Congo Republic officially declared that the outbreak of EHF was over in the Cuvette Ouest Region. The last case was recorded on April 22 in the small village of Ndjoukou.

PMID: 14579469 [PubMed - indexed for MEDLINE]

2000. Mol Gen Mikrobiol Virusol. 2003;(2):38-40, backcover.

[Analysis of antigenic determinant profiles of the Ebola virus VP35 protein N-terminal region using its short recombinant fragments].

[Article in Russian]

Rudzevich TN, Ternovoĭ VA, Kazachinskaia EI, Razumov IA, Chepurnov AA, Loktev VB, Netesov SV.

cDNA of fragments of gene VP35 of the Ebola virus (EV) were expressed in vector pQE30 for the purpose of isolation of recombinant fragments of protein VP35. Five short affinity-purified fragments of the EV VP35 protein were analyzed, by using the methods of IEA and immunoblotting, with polyclonal antiviral sera (PAS) against EV and with hybrid monoclonal antibodies (Mabs) 1C6 and 6F7 specific to EV VP35 protein. All fragments of protein VP35 with an intact N-terminal region and removed C-terminal region were found to interact effectively with PAS and with Mabs 1C6 and 6F7. Rec86N, the smallest of the above fragments, comprised the initial 86 amino acid residues of the VP35 N-terminal region. A removal of 36 amino acid residues from the N-terminal region of Rec310N, the largest recombinant fragment, resulted in a loss of interaction with Mabs 1C6 and 6F7, while the interaction with polyclonal antibodies remained intact. The obtained results show that the initial 86 amino acid residues of the N-terminal region of EV VP35 are of the key importance in forming the antigenic structure of VP35 and that they contain multiple B-cell epitopes. Finally, the initial 36 amino acids of VP35 predetermine the shaping-up of two antigenic determinants for Mabs 1C6 and 6F7.

PMID: 12800775 [PubMed - indexed for MEDLINE]

2001. Vopr Virusol. 2003 Jan-Feb;48(1):43-4.

[Titration of Ebola and Marburg viruses by plaque formation under semi liquid agar].

[Article in Russian]

Ustinova EN, Shestopalov AM, Bakulina LF, Chepurnov AA.

The method of titration of Ebola and Marburg viruses using plaque formation under semifluid agar cover is considered. Advantages of this method over conventional method of titration of these viruses with the use of hard agar cover are discussed.

PMID: 12608062 [PubMed - indexed for MEDLINE]

2002. Vopr Virusol. 2003 Jan-Feb;48(1):21-4.

[In vitro synthesis of immunoglobulins caused by an inactivated Ebola virus].

[Article in Russian]

Tuzova MN, Gaĭdul' KV, Chepurnov AA.

An in vitro model Ebola infection was used to study the humoral response of human mononuclear cells to stimulation by purified inactivated Ebola virus antigen. Inactivated Ebola virus was cocultivated with human mononuclear cells in the presence or absence of B-cell mitogen LPS E. coli: B5. An increase in the rate of synthesis of immunoglobulins (both IgG and, to a less extent, other classes) was observed. The Ebola virus proteins were suggested to exert no suppression effect on B-cells. The IgM/IgG synthesis was evaluated by EIA in supernatants after 7 days of cultivation. It was concluded that Ebola fever is accompanied by active humoral immune response, which provides a promising basis for further search of the methods of treatment of this disease.

PMID: 12608056 [PubMed - indexed for MEDLINE]

2003. Am J Nurs. 2002 Dec;102(12):49-52.

Ebola.

Easter A(1).

Author information: (1)College of Nursing, University of Arkansas for Medical Sciences,

PMID: 12473930 [PubMed - indexed for MEDLINE]

2004. Emerg Infect Dis. 2002 Dec;8(12):1521-3.

Ebola-Poe: a modern-day parallel of the red death?

Vora SK, Ramanan SV.

PMCID: PMC2738525 PMID: 12508799 [PubMed - indexed for MEDLINE]

2005. J Virol. 2002 Dec;76(24):12463-72.

Covalent modifications of the ebola virus glycoprotein.

Jeffers SA(1), Sanders DA, Sanchez A.

Author information: (1)Department of Biological Sciences, Purdue University, 1392 Lilly Hall, West Lafayette, IN 47907, USA.

The role of covalent modifications of the Ebola virus glycoprotein (GP) and the significance of the sequence identity between filovirus and avian retrovirus GPs were investigated through biochemical and functional analyses of mutant GPs. The expression and processing of mutant GPs with altered N-linked glycosylation, substitutions for conserved cysteine residues, or a deletion in the region of O-linked glycosylation were analyzed, and virus entry capacities were assayed through the use of pseudotyped retroviruses. Cys-53 was the only GP(1) (approximately 130 kDa) cysteine residue whose replacement resulted in the efficient secretion of GP(1), and it is therefore proposed that it participates in the formation of the only disulfide bond linking GP(1) to GP(2) (approximately 24 kDa). We propose a complete cystine bridge map for the filovirus GPs based upon our analysis of mutant Ebola virus GPs. The effect of replacement of the conserved cysteines in the membrane-spanning region of GP(2) was found to depend on the nature of the substitution. Mutations in conserved N-linked glycosylation sites proved generally, with a few exceptions, innocuous. Deletion of the O-linked glycosylation region increased GP processing, incorporation into retrovirus particles, and viral transduction. Our data support a common evolutionary origin for the GPs of Ebola virus and avian retroviruses and have implications for gene transfer mediated by Ebola virus GP-pseudotyped retroviruses.

PMCID: PMC136726 PMID: 12438572 [PubMed - indexed for MEDLINE]

2006. Trop Med Int Health. 2002 Dec;7(12):1068-75.

An outbreak of Ebola in Uganda.

Okware SI(1), Omaswa FG, Zaramba S, Opio A, Lutwama JJ, Kamugisha J, Rwaguma EB, Kagwa P, Lamunu M.

Author information: (1)Uganda Ministry of Health, Kampala, Uganda.

An outbreak of Ebola disease was reported from Gulu district, Uganda, on 8 October 2000. The outbreak was characterized by fever and haemorrhagic manifestations, and affected health workers and the general population of Rwot-Obillo, a village 14 km north of Gulu town. Later, the outbreak spread to other parts of the country including Mbarara and Masindi districts. Response measures included surveillance, community mobilization, case and logistics management. Three coordination committees were formed: National Task Force (NTF), a District Task Force (DTF) and an Interministerial Task Force (IMTF). The NTF and DTF were responsible for coordination and follow-up of implementation of activities at the national and district levels, respectively, while the IMTF provided political direction and handled sensitive issues related to stigma, trade, tourism and international relations. The international response was coordinated by the World Health Organization (WHO) under the umbrella organization of the Global Outbreak and Alert Response Network. A WHO/CDC case definition for Ebola was adapted and used to capture four categories of cases, namely, the 'alert', 'suspected', 'probable' and 'confirmed cases'. Guidelines for identification and management of cases were developed and disseminated to all persons responsible for surveillance, case management, contact tracing and Information Education Communication (IEC). For the duration of the epidemic that lasted up to 16 January 2001, a total of 425 cases with 224 deaths were reported countrywide. The case fatality rate was 53%. The attack rate (AR) was highest in women. The average AR for Gulu district was 12.6 cases/10 000 inhabitants when the contacts of all cases were considered and was 4.5 cases/10 000 if limited only to contacts of laboratory confirmed cases. The secondary AR was 2.5% when nearly 5000 contacts were followed up for 21 days. Uganda was finally declared Ebola free on 27 February 2001, 42 days after the last case was reported. The Government's role in coordination of both local and international support was vital. The NTF and the corresponding district committees harmonized implementation of a mutually agreed programme. Community mobilization using community-based resource persons and political organs, such as Members of Parliament was effective in getting information to the public. This was critical in controlling the epidemic. Past experience in epidemic management has shown that in the absence of regular provision of information to the public, there are bound to be deleterious rumours. Consequently rumour was managed by frank and open discussion of the epidemic, providing daily updates, fact sheets and press releases. Information was regularly disseminated to communities through mass media and press conferences. Thus all levels of the community spontaneously demonstrated solidarity and response to public health interventions. Even in areas of relative insecurity, rebel abductions diminished considerably.

PMID: 12460399 [PubMed - indexed for MEDLINE]

2007. Ned Tijdschr Geneeskd. 2002 Nov 16;146(46):2183-8.

[How to treat a patient with indications for an infectious viral hemorrhagic fever].

[Article in Dutch]

Visser LG(1), Schippers EF, Swaan CM, van den Broek PJ.

Author information: (1)Leids Universitair Medisch Centrum, afd. Infectieziekten, Postbus 9600, 2300 RC Leiden.

Comment in Ned Tijdschr Geneeskd. 2003 Feb 1;147(5):221-2.

Comment on Ned Tijdschr Geneeskd. 2002 Nov 16;146(46):2201-4.

Lassa, Ebola, Marburg and Crimean-Congo haemorrhagic fever viruses are the most important causes of viral haemorrhagic fever which is transmitted from person to person through contact with blood or excreta. A non-specific fever may be the initial symptom of viral haemorrhagic fever. By means of carefully noting where the patient has travelled, possible exposure to ill persons, vectors or an animal reservoir, and the incubation period (< or = 21 days versus longer), it is possible to estimate the risk of infection with one of these viruses. Using this approach it is possible to diagnose high-risk patients in good time and to take appropriate measures.
PMID: 12467160 [PubMed - indexed for MEDLINE]

2008. Virology. 2002 Nov 10;303(1):9-14.

Evidence against Ebola virus sGP binding to human neutrophils by a specific receptor.

Sui J(1), Marasco WA.

Author information: (1)Department of Cancer Immunology & AIDS, Dana-Farber Cancer Institute, Harvard Medical School, 44 Binney Street, Boston, Massachusetts, 02115, USA.

The issue of whether Ebola secretory glycoprotein (sGP) binds to human neutrophils via the IgG Fc receptor IIIb (FcgammaRIIIb, CD16b) or other receptors has been controversial. To clarify this, FACS analysis, an sGP absorption assay, and direct binding of (125)I-sGP to neutrophils were performed. Results from FACS analysis demonstrated that limited washing conditions leads to the nonspecific formation of immune complexes on the neutrophil surface and this, but not a specific interaction between sGP and CD16b, is responsible for the previous observations. An sGP absorption assay also demonstrated that sGP is not specifically bound but is nonspecifically proteolysed by proteases released from neutrophils. Finally, there was no difference in (125)I-sGP binding to neutrophils compared to other control cell types. Taken together, these results demonstrate that neutrophils do not express a specific receptor for Ebola virus sGP. It is unlikely that sGP plays a role in the Ebola virus pathogenesis through interfering with the innate immunity by targeting neutrophils.
PMID: 12482654 [PubMed - indexed for MEDLINE]

2009. J Clin Microbiol. 2002 Nov;40(11):4394-5.

False-negative results of PCR assay with plasma of patients with severe viral hemorrhagic fever.

Drosten C, Panning M, Guenther S, Schmitz H.

PMCID: PMC139694 PMID: 12409441 [PubMed - indexed for MEDLINE]

2010. J Gen Virol. 2002 Nov;83(Pt 11):2635-62.

A decade after the generation of a negative-sense RNA virus from cloned cDNA - what have we learned?

Neumann G(1), Whitt MA, Kawaoka Y.

Author information: (1)Department of Pathobiological Sciences, School of Veterinary Medicine, University of Wisconsin, 2015 Linden Drive West, Madison 53706, USA.

Since the first generation of a negative-sense RNA virus entirely from cloned cDNA in 1994, similar reverse genetics systems have been established for members of most genera of the Rhabdo- and Paramyxoviridae families, as well as for Ebola virus (Filoviridae). The generation of segmented negative-sense RNA viruses was technically more challenging and has lagged behind the recovery of nonsegmented viruses, primarily because of the difficulty of providing more than one genomic RNA segment. A member of the Bunyaviridae family (whose genome is composed of three RNA segments) was first generated from cloned cDNA in 1996, followed in 1999 by the production of influenza virus, which contains eight RNA segments. Thus, reverse genetics, or the de novo synthesis of negative-sense RNA viruses from cloned cDNA, has become a reliable laboratory method that can be used to study this large group of medically and economically important viruses. It provides a powerful tool for dissecting the virus life cycle, virus assembly, the role of viral proteins in pathogenicity and the interplay of viral proteins with components of the host cell immune response. Finally, reverse genetics has opened the way to develop live attenuated virus vaccines and vaccine vectors.
PMID: 12388800 [PubMed - indexed for MEDLINE]

2011. Nat Struct Biol. 2002 Nov;9(11):812-7.

Structure of the Tsg101 UEV domain in complex with the PTAP motif of the HIV-1 p6 protein.

Pornillos O(1), Alam SL, Davis DR, Sundquist WI.

Author information: (1)Department of Biochemistry, University of Utah, Salt Lake City, Utah 84132, USA.

The structural proteins of HIV and Ebola display PTAP peptide motifs (termed 'late domains') that recruit the human protein Tsg101 to facilitate virus budding. Here we present the solution structure of the UEV (ubiquitin E2 variant) binding domain of Tsg101 in complex with a PTAP peptide that spans the late domain of HIV-1 p6(Gag). The UEV domain of Tsg101 resembles E2 ubiquitin-conjugating enzymes, and the PTAP peptide binds in a bifurcated groove above the vestigial enzyme active site. Each PTAP residue makes important contacts, and the Ala 9-Pro 10 dipeptide binds in a deep pocket of the UEV domain that resembles the X-Pro binding pockets of SH3 and WW domains. The structure reveals the molecular basis of HIV PTAP late domain function and represents an attractive starting point for the design of novel inhibitors of virus budding.
PMID: 12379843 [PubMed - indexed for MEDLINE]

2012. Exp Anim. 2002 Oct;51(5):447-55.

Histopathology of natural Ebola virus subtype Reston infection in cynomolgus macaques during the Philippine outbreak in 1996.

Ikegami T(1), Miranda ME, Calaor AB, Manalo DL, Miranda NJ, Niikura M, Saijo M, Une Y, Nomura Y, Kurane I, Ksiazek TG, Yoshikawa Y, Morikawa S.

Author information: (1)Special Pathogens Laboratory, Department of Virology I, National Institute of Infectious Diseases, 4-7-1 Gakuen, Musashimurayama, Tokyo 208-0011, Japan.

We investigated the livers, spleens, kidneys and lungs collected from 24 cynomolgus macaques (Macaca fascicularis) naturally infected with Ebola virus subtype Reston (EBO-R) during the Philippine outbreak in 1996, in order to reveal the histopathologic findings. These macaques showed necrotic hepatocytes with inclusions, slight to massive fibrin deposition in splenic cords, depletion of lymphoid cells in the white pulp of the spleen, and fibrin thrombi in some organs. Immunohistochemical analysis using anti-leukocyte antigen L1 antibody revealed an increase in blood-derived macrophages/monocytes in the livers, kidneys and lungs of EBO-R infected macaques. EBO-R NP antigens were detected in the macrophages/monocytes, endothelial cells and fibroblasts in the liver, spleen, kidney and lung. These results indicate that EBO-R infection is characterized by systemic coagulopathy and an increase in blood-derived macrophages/monocytes in accordance with the EBO-R propagation in macrophages/monocytes.

PMID: 12451705 [PubMed - indexed for MEDLINE]

2013. Med Microbiol Immunol. 2002 Oct;191(2):63-74. Epub 2002 Sep 3.

Emerging and re-emerging infectious diseases.

Feldmann H, Czub M, Jones S, Dick D, Garbutt M, Grolla A, Artsob H.

In human history, numerous infectious diseases have emerged and re-emerged. Aside from many others, the so-called 'exotic' agents in particular are a threat to our public health systems due to limited experience in case management and lack of appropriate resources. Many of these agents are zoonotic in origin and transmitted from animals to man either directly or via vectors. The reservoirs are often infected subclinically or asymptomatically and the distribution of the diseases basically reflects the range and the population dynamics of their reservoir hosts. As examples, emergence/re-emergence is discussed here for diseases caused by filoviruses, hantaviruses, paramyxoviruses, flaviviruses and Yersinia pestis. In addition, bioterrorism is addressed as one factor which has now to be considered in infectious disease emergence/re-emergence. Preparedness for known and unknown infectious diseases will be a top priority for our public health systems in the beginning of the millennium.

PMID: 12410344 [PubMed - indexed for MEDLINE]

2014. Nat Rev Mol Cell Biol. 2002 Oct;3(10):753-66.

Furin at the cutting edge: from protein traffic to embryogenesis and disease.

Thomas G(1).

Author information: (1)Vollum Institute, 3181 SW Sam Jackson Park Road, Portland, Oregon 97239, USA. thomasg@ohsu.edu

Furin catalyses a simple biochemical reaction--the proteolytic maturation of proprotein substrates in the secretory pathway. But the simplicity of this reaction belies furin's broad and important roles in homeostasis, as well as in diseases ranging from Alzheimer's disease and cancer to anthrax and Ebola fever. This review summarizes various features of furin--its structural and enzymatic properties, intracellular localization, trafficking, substrates, and roles in vivo.

PMCID: PMC1964754 PMID: 12360192 [PubMed - indexed for MEDLINE]

2015. J Biol Chem. 2002 Sep 27;277(39):36766-9. Epub 2002 Jul 16.

Dendritic cell (DC)-specific intercellular adhesion molecule 3 (ICAM-3)-grabbing nonintegrin (DC-SIGN, CD209), a C-type surface lectin in human DCs, is a receptor for Leishmania amastigotes.

Colmenares M(1), Puig-Kröger A, Pello OM, Corbí AL, Rivas L.

Author information: (1)Centro de Investigaciones Biológicas, Consejo Superior de Investigaciones Científicas, Velázquez 144, 28006 Madrid, Spain.

Dendritic cells (DCs) play a critical role in the initiation of the immunological response against Leishmania parasites. However, the receptors involved in amastigote-dendritic cell interaction are unknown, especially in absence of opsonizing antibodies. We have studied the interaction of Leishmania pifanoi axenic amastigotes with the C-type lectin DC-specific intercellular adhesion molecule (ICAM)-3-grabbing nonintegrin (DC-SIGN, CD209), a receptor for ICAM-2, ICAM-3, human immunodeficiency virus gp120, and Ebola virus. L. pifanoi amastigotes interact with immature human dendritic cells and CD209-transfected K562 cells in a time- and dose-dependent manner. Leishmania amastigote binding to human dendritic cells and DC-SIGN-transfected cells is inhibited by a function-blocking DC-SIGN-specific monoclonal antibody. More importantly, this monoclonal antibody dramatically reduces internalization of Leishmania amastigotes by immature human DCs. These results constitute the first description of a nonviral pathogen ligand for DC-SIGN and provide evidence for a relevant role of DC-SIGN in Leishmania amastigote uptake by dendritic cells. Our finding has important implications for Leishmania host-cell interaction and the immunoregulation of cutaneous leishmaniasis.

PMID: 12122001 [PubMed - indexed for MEDLINE]

2016. Biochim Biophys Acta. 2002 Sep 13;1577(2):337-53.

Transcriptional control of the RNA-dependent RNA polymerase of vesicular stomatitis virus.

Barr JN(1), Whelan SP, Wertz GW.

Author information: (1)Department of Microbiology, BBRB 17, Room 366, University of Alabama School of Medicine, 845 19th Street S., Birmingham, AL 35294, USA.

The nonsegmented negative strand (NNS) RNA viruses include some of the mosr problematic human, animal and plant pathogens extant: for example, rabies virus, Ebola virus, respiratory syncytial virus, the parainfluenza viruses, measles and infectious hemapoietic necrosis virus. The key feature of transcriptional control in the NNS RNA viruses is polymerase entry at a single 3' proximal site followed by obligatory sequential transcription of the linear array of genes. The levels of gene expression are primarily regulated by their position on the genome. The promoter proximal gene is transcribed in greatest abundance and each successive downstream gene is synthesized in progressively lower amounts due to attenuation of transcription at each successive gene junction. In addition,

NNS RNA virus gene expression is regulated by cis-acting sequences that reside at the beginning and end of each gene and the intergenic junctions. Using vesicular stomatitis virus (VSV), the prototypic NNS, many of these control elements have been identified.The signals for transcription initiation and 5' end modification and for 3' end polyadenylation and termination have been elucidated. The sequences that determine the ability of the polymerase to slip on the template to generate polyadenylate have been identified and polyadenylation has been shown to be template dependent and integral to the termination process. Transcriptional termination is a key element in control of gene expression of the negative strand RNA viruses and a means by which expression of individual genes may be silenced or regulated within the framework of a single transcriptional promoter. In addition, the fundamental question of the site of entry of the polymerase during transcription has been reexamined and our understanding of the process altered and updated. The ability to engineer changes into infectious viruses has confirmed the action of these elements and as a consequence, it has been shown that transcriptional control is key to controlling the outcome of a viral infection. Finally, the principles of transcriptional regulation have been utilized to develop a new paradigm for systematic attenuation of virulence to develop live attenuated viral vaccines.
PMID: 12213662 [PubMed - indexed for MEDLINE]

2017. J Biol Chem. 2002 Sep 6;277(36):33099-104. Epub 2002 Jun 6.

Phosphorylation of VP30 impairs ebola virus transcription.

Modrof J(1), Mühlberger E, Klenk HD, Becker S.

Author information: (1)Institut für Virologie der Philipps-Universität Marburg, Robert-Koch-Strasse 17, Marburg 35037, Germany.

Transcription of the highly pathogenic Ebola virus (EBOV) is dependent on VP30, a constituent of the viral nucleocapsid complex. Here we present evidence that phosphorylation of VP30, which takes place at six N-terminal serine residues and one threonine residue, is of functional significance. Replacement of the phosphoserines by alanines resulted in an only slightly phosphorylated VP30 (VP30(6A)) that is still able to activate EBOV-specific transcription in a plasmid-based minigenome system. VP30(6A), however, did not bind to inclusions that are induced by the major nucleocapsid protein NP. Three intracellular phosphatases (PP1, PP2A, and PP2C) have been determined to dephosphorylate VP30. The presence of okadaic acid (OA), an inhibitor of PP1 and PP2A, had the same negative effect on transcription activation by VP30 as the substitution of the six phosphoserines for aspartate residues. OA, however, did not impair transcription when VP30 was replaced by VP30(6A). In EBOV-infected cells, OA blocked virus growth dose-dependently. The block was mediated by the extensive phosphorylation of VP30, which is evidenced by the result that expression of VP30(6A), in trans, led to the progression of EBOV infection in the presence of OA. In conclusion, phosphorylation of VP30 was shown to regulate negatively transcription activation and positively binding to the NP inclusions.
PMID: 12052831 [PubMed - indexed for MEDLINE]

2018. Acta Clin Belg. 2002 Sep-Oct;57(5):233-40.

Imported viral haemorrhagic fever with a potential for person-to-person transmission: review and recommendations for initial management of a suspected case in Belgium.

Colebunders R(1), Van Esbroeck M, Moreau M, Borchert M.

Author information: (1)Departement Klinische Wetenschappen, Instituut voor Tropische Geneeskunde Nationalestraat 155, B-2000 Antwerpen. bcoleb@itg.be
Viral haemorrhagic fevers are caused by a wide range of viruses. There are 4 types of viruses well known to spread from person to person and able to cause nosocomial outbreaks with a high case fatality rate: an arenavirus (Lassa fever and more exceptionally the Junin and Machupo virus), a bunyavirus (Crimean-Congo haemorrhagic fever) and the Filoviridae (Ebola and Marburg viruses). So far there have been only a limited number of imported cases of viral haemorrhagic fever in industrialized countries. In recent years an increasing number of outbreaks of filovirus infections have occurred in Africa and in 2000 5 cases of Lassa fever were brought from Sierra Leone to Europe. Therefore European physicians should consider the possibility of a viral haemorrhagic fever in an acutely ill patient just returning from Africa or South-America with fever for which there is no obvious cause. Such patients should be questioned for risk factors for viral haemorrhagic fever. Using universal precautions for handling blood and body fluids and barrier nursing techniques there is little risk that if a patient with viral haemorrhagic fever arrives in Belgium there will be secondary cases.
PMID: 12534129 [PubMed - indexed for MEDLINE]

2019. J Virol. 2002 Sep;76(18):9176-85.

Induction of immune responses in mice and monkeys to Ebola virus after immunization with liposome-encapsulated irradiated Ebola virus: protection in mice requires CD4(+) T cells.

Rao M(1), Bray M, Alving CR, Jahrling P, Matyas GR.

Author information: (1)Department of Membrane Biochemistry, Walter Reed Army Institute of Research, Silver Spring, Maryland 20910-7500, USA. Mangala.Rao@Na.Amedd.Army.Mil
Ebola Zaire virus (EBO-Z) causes severe hemorrhagic fever in humans, with a high mortality rate. It is thought that a vaccine against EBO-Z may have to induce both humoral and cell-mediated immune responses to successfully confer protection. Because it is known that liposome-encapsulated antigens induce both antibody and cellular responses, we evaluated the protective efficacy of liposome-encapsulated irradiated EBO-Z [L(EV)], which contains all of the native EBO-Z proteins. In a series of experiments, mice immunized intravenously with L(EV) were completely protected (94/94 mice) against illness and death when they were challenged with a uniformly lethal mouse-adapted variant of EBO-Z. In contrast, only 55% of mice immunized intravenously with nonencapsulated irradiated virus (EV) survived challenge, and all became ill. Treatment with anti-CD4 antibodies before or during immunization with L(EV) eliminated protection, while treatment with anti-CD8 antibodies had no effect, thus indicating a requirement for CD4(+) T lymphocytes for successful immunization. On the other hand, treatment with either anti-CD4 or anti-CD8 antibodies after immunization did not abolish the protection. After immunization with L(EV), antigen-specific gamma interferon (IFN gamma)-secreting CD4(+) T lymphocytes were induced as analyzed by enzyme-linked immunospot assay. Anti-CD4 monoclonal antibody

treatment abolished IFN gamma production (80 to 90% inhibition compared to that for untreated mice). Mice immunized with L(EV), but not EV, developed cytotoxic T lymphocytes specific to two peptides (amino acids [aa] 161 to 169 and aa 231 to 239) present in the amino-terminal end of the EBO-Z surface glycoprotein. Because of the highly successful results in the mouse model, L(EV) was also tested in three cynomolgus monkeys. Although immunization of the monkeys with L(EV)-induced virus-neutralizing antibodies against EBO-Z caused a slight delay in the onset of illness, it did not prevent death.

PMCID: PMC136452 PMID: 12186901 [PubMed - indexed for MEDLINE]

2020. J Virol. 2002 Sep;76(18):9135-42.

Quantitative expression and virus transmission analysis of DC-SIGN on monocyte-derived dendritic cells.

Baribaud F(1), Pöhlmann S, Leslie G, Mortari F, Doms RW.

Author information: (1)Department of Microbiology, University of Pennsylvania, Philadelphia, Pennsylvania 19104, USA.

The C-type lectins DC-SIGN and DC-SIGNR efficiently bind human immunodeficiency virus (HIV) and simian immunodeficiency virus (SIV) strains and can transmit bound virus to adjacent CD4-positive cells. DC-SIGN also binds efficiently to the Ebola virus glycoprotein, enhancing Ebola virus infection. DC-SIGN is thought to be responsible for the ability of dendritic cells (DCs) to capture HIV and transmit it to T cells, thus promoting HIV dissemination in vitro and perhaps in vivo as well. To investigate DC-SIGN function and expression levels on DCs, we characterized a panel of monoclonal antibodies (MAbs) directed against the carbohydrate recognition domain of DC-SIGN. Using quantitative fluorescence-activated cell sorter technology, we found that DC-SIGN is highly expressed on immature monocyte-derived DCs, with at least 100,000 copies and often in excess of 250,000 copies per DC. There was modest variation (three- to fourfold) in DC-SIGN expression levels between individuals and between DCs isolated from the same individual at different times. Several MAbs efficiently blocked virus binding to cell lines expressing human or rhesus DC-SIGN, preventing HIV and SIV transmission. Interactions with Ebola virus pseudotypes were also blocked efficiently. Despite their ability to block virus-DC-SIGN interactions on cell lines, these antibodies only inhibited transmission of virus from DCs by approximately 50% or less. These results indicate that factors other than DC-SIGN may play important roles in the ability of DCs to capture and transmit HIV.

PMCID: PMC136426 PMID: 12186897 [PubMed - indexed for MEDLINE]

2021. J Virol. 2002 Sep;76(17):8532-9.

Ebola virus VP30-mediated transcription is regulated by RNA secondary structure formation.

Weik M(1), Modrof J, Klenk HD, Becker S, Mühlberger E.

Author information: (1)Institut für Virologie der Philipps-Universität Marburg, 35037 Marburg, Germany.

The nucleocapsid protein VP30 of Ebola virus (EBOV), a member of the Filovirus family, is known to act as a transcription activator. By using a reconstituted minigenome system, the role of VP30 during transcription was investigated. We could show that VP30-mediated transcription activation is dependent on formation of a stem-loop structure at the first gene start site. Destruction of this secondary structure led to VP30-independent transcription. Analysis of the transcription products of bicistronic minigenomes with and without the ability to form the secondary structure at the first transcription start signal revealed that transcription initiation at the first gene start site is a prerequisite for transcription of the second gene, independent of the presence of VP30. When the transcription start signal of the second gene was exchanged with the transcription start signal of the first gene, transcription of the second gene also was regulated by VP30, indicating that the stem-loop structure of the first transcription start site acts autonomously and independently of its localization on the RNA genome. Our results suggest that VP30 regulates a very early step of EBOV transcription, most likely by inhibiting pausing of the transcription complex at the RNA structure of the first transcription start site.

PMCID: PMC136988 PMID: 12163572 [PubMed - indexed for MEDLINE]

2022. Mol Ther. 2002 Sep;6(3):349-58.

Efficient transduction of liver and muscle after in utero injection of lentiviral vectors with different pseudotypes.

MacKenzie TC(1), Kobinger GP, Kootstra NA, Radu A, Sena-Esteves M, Bouchard S, Wilson JM, Verma IM, Flake AW.

Author information: (1)Children's Institute for Surgical Science, Children's Hospital of Philadelphia, Philadelphia, Pennsylvania 19104, USA.

In this study we investigate the efficacy of lentiviral vectors of different pseudotypes for gene transfer to tissues of the preimmune fetus. BALB/c fetuses at 14-15 days' gestation received lentiviral vectors carrying the transgene lacZ under the control of the human cytomegalovirus (CMV) promoter by intramuscular (i.m.) or intrahepatic (i.h.) injection. We pseudotyped the lentiviral vectors with vesicular stomatitis virus (VSV-G), with Mokola virus, or with Ebola virus envelope glycoproteins. We harvested the pups at time points between 5 days and 9 months following injection and performed a detailed histologic assessment. The efficiency and distribution of transduction after in utero administration was highly dependent upon the route of administration and the pseudotype of vector used. Biodistribution studies showed widespread distribution of vector sequences in multiple tissues, albeit at very low levels, and transduced cells were found in significant numbers only in liver, heart, and muscle. Overall, VSV-G was the most efficient in transducing hepatocytes, whereas Mokola and Ebola were more efficient in transducing myocytes. Transduction of cardiomyocytes was observed after both i.m. and i.h. injection of all three vectors. Our findings of long-term transduction of skeletal myocytes and cardiomyocytes after in utero administration suggest a novel strategy for the treatment of congenital muscular dystrophies.

PMID: 12231171 [PubMed - indexed for MEDLINE]

2023. Revolution. 2002 Sep-Oct;3(5):15-7.

The ultimate sacrifice.

Manz G.

One hundred seventy-three people died in the outbreak, including a doctor and 12 nurses. Belluz said more people were saved from infection or death because of the extraordinary job of containing the disease and educating people about what they should and shouldn't do.

PMID: 12402626 [PubMed - indexed for MEDLINE]

2024. Virology. 2002 Sep 1;300(2):236-43.

Detection of antibodies against the four subtypes of ebola virus in sera from any species using a novel antibody-phage indicator assay.

Meissner F(1), Maruyama T, Frentsch M, Hessell AJ, Rodriguez LL, Geisbert TW, Jahrling PB, Burton DR, Parren PW.

Author information: (1)Department of Immunology and Molecular Biology, the Scripps Research Institute, La Jolla, California 92037, USA.

The natural host for Ebola virus, presumed to be an animal, has not yet been identified despite an extensive search following several major outbreaks in Africa. A straightforward approach used to determine animal contact with Ebola virus is by assessing the presence of specific antibodies in serum. This approach however has been made very difficult by the absence of specific reagents required for the detection of antibodies from the majority of wild animal species. In this study, we isolated a human monoclonal antibody Fab fragment, KZ51, that reacts with an immunodominant epitope on Ebola virus nucleoprotein (NP) that is conserved on all four Ebola virus subtypes. The antibody KZ51 represents a major specificity as sera from all convalescent patients tested (10/10) and sera from guinea pigs infected with each of the four Ebola virus subtypes competed strongly with KZ51 for binding to radiation-inactivated Ebola virus. These features allowed us to develop a novel assay for the detection of seroconversion irrespective of Ebola virus subtype or animal species. In this assay, the binding of KZ51 Fab-phage particles is used as an indicator assay and the presence of specific antibodies against Ebola virus in sera is indicated by binding competition. A prominent feature of the assay is that the Fab-phage particles may be prestained with a dye so that detection of binding can be directly determined by visual inspection. The assay is designed to be both simple and economical to enable its use in the field.

PMID: 12350354 [PubMed - indexed for MEDLINE]

2025. Vopr Virusol. 2002 Sep-Oct;47(5):29-31.

[Effect of Ebola virus antigen on proliferative response of human lymphocytes in vitro: imbalance in production of tumor necrosis factor alpha and interleukin-1].

[Article in Russian]

Tuzova MN, Sukhenko TG, Chepurnov AA.

An in vitro model infection caused by Ebola virus (EV) showed a high production of tumor necrosis factor-alpha by human peripheral lymphocytes concurrently with a simultaneous reduction in the synthesis of interleukin-1 in response EV antigen stimulation. This may be an important factor in that VE suppresses the body's immunological resistance, which in turn causes unterferon deficiency and suppresses the formation of T helper cells.

PMID: 12522966 [PubMed - indexed for MEDLINE]

2026. Zh Mikrobiol Epidemiol Immunobiol. 2002 Sep-Oct;(5):116-22.

[Filovirus haemorrhagic fevers: Ebola fever].

[Article in Russian]

Titenko AM(1).

Author information: (1)Research Institute for Plague Control of Siberia and the Far East, Irkutsk, Russia.

Epidemiological issues, clinical course and laboratory diagnostics of Ebola haemorrhagic fever are reviewed. The structural features of virions and genetic variants of the virus are described along with ecology of Ebola virus. The data on Ebola fever global morbidity are also presented.

PMID: 12525016 [PubMed - indexed for MEDLINE]

2027. Zh Mikrobiol Epidemiol Immunobiol. 2002 Sep-Oct;(5):25-9.

[Sanitary control of the territory: data bases on the spread of some quarantine infections].

[Article in Russian]

Prometnoĭ VI(1), Golubev BP, Moskovitina EA.

Author information: (1)Research Institute for Plague Control, Rostov-on-Don, Russia.

The data bases (DB) on the spread of plague, yellow fever and contagious virus hemorrhagic fevers (CVHF) in foreign countries have been created. These DB contain information on the main international air and sea ports and their relationships with natural focal territories. The data base "Sanitary control. Yellow fever" contains information on different species serving as vectors for yellow fever virus. Information on the circulation of the causative agents of Ebola fever, Lassa fever and Marburg disease in African countries has been introduced into DB, the differentiation of countries by the degree of the potential danger of the CVHF spread has been made.

PMID: 12524996 [PubMed - indexed for MEDLINE]

2028. Nature. 2002 Aug 22;418(6900):808.

Anthrax case provokes doubt among experts.

Knight J, Check E.

PMID: 12192379 [PubMed - indexed for MEDLINE]

2029. Blood. 2002 Aug 1;100(3):823-32.

Lentiviral vectors pseudotyped with a modified RD114 envelope glycoprotein show increased stability in sera and augmented transduction of primary lymphocytes and CD34+ cells derived from human and nonhuman primates.

Sandrin V(1), Boson B, Salmon P, Gay W, Nègre D, Le Grand R, Trono D, Cosset FL.

Author information: (1)Vectorologie Rétrovirale & Thérapie Génique, U412 INSERM, IFR 74, Ecole Normale Supérieure de Lyon, Lyon, France.

Generating lentiviral vectors pseudotyped with different viral glycoproteins (GPs) may modulate the physicochemical properties of the vectors, their interaction with the host immune system, and their host range. We have investigated the capacity of a panel of GPs of both retroviral (amphotropic murine leukemia virus [MLV-A]; gibbon ape leukemia virus [GALV]; RD114, feline endogenous virus) and nonretroviral (fowl plague virus [FPV]; Ebola virus [EboV]; vesicular stomatitis virus [VSV]; lymphocytic choriomeningitis virus [LCMV]) origins to pseudotype lentiviral vectors derived from simian immunodeficiency virus (SIVmac251). SIV vectors were efficiently pseudotyped with the FPV hemagglutinin, VSV-G, LCMV, and MLV-A GPs. In contrast, the GALV and RD114 GPs conferred much lower infectivity to the vectors. Capitalizing on the conservation of some structural features in the transmembrane domains and cytoplasmic tails of the incorporation-competent MLV-A GP and in RD114 and GALV GPs, we generated chimeric GPs encoding the extracellular and transmembrane domains of GALV or RD114 GPs fused to the cytoplasmic tail (designated TR) of MLV-A GP. Importantly, SIV-derived vectors pseudotyped with these GALV/TR and RD114/TR GP chimeras had significantly higher titers than vectors coated with the parental GPs. Additionally, RD114/TR-pseudotyped vectors were efficiently concentrated and were resistant to inactivation induced by the complement of both human and macaque sera, indicating that modified RD114 GP-pseudotyped lentiviral vectors may be of particular interest for in vivo gene transfer applications. Furthermore, as compared to vectors pseudotyped with other retroviral GPs or with VSV-G, RD114/TR-pseudotyped vectors showed augmented transduction of human and macaque primary blood lymphocytes and CD34+ cells.

PMID: 12130492 [PubMed - indexed for MEDLINE]

2030. Clin Microbiol Infect. 2002 Aug;8(8):489-503.

Anthrax, tularemia, plague, ebola or smallpox as agents of bioterrorism: recognition in the emergency room.

Cunha BA(1).

Author information: (1)Infectious Disease Division, Winthrop-University Hospital, Mineola and State University of New York School of Medicine, Stony Brook, New York 11501, USA.

Bioterrorism has become a potential diagnostic consideration in infectious diseases. This article reviews the clinical presentation and differential diagnosis of potential bioterrorist agents when first presenting to the hospital in the emergency room setting. The characteristic clinical features of inhalation anthrax, tularemic pneumonia, plague pneumonia, including laboratory and radiographic finding, are discussed. Ebola vieus and smallpox are also discussed as potential bioterrorist-transmitted infections from the clinical and epidemiologic standpoint. In addition to the clinical features of the infectious diseases mentioned, the article discusses the infectious disease control and epidemiologic implications of these agents when employed as bioterrorist agents. The review concludes with suggestions for postexposure prophylaxis and therapy.

PMID: 12197871 [PubMed - indexed for MEDLINE]

2031. Expert Opin Ther Targets. 2002 Aug;6(4):423-31.

The role of DC-SIGN and DC-SIGNR in HIV and Ebola virus infection: can potential therapeutics block virus transmission and dissemination?

Baribaud F(1), Doms RW, Pöhlmann S.

Author information: (1)Department of Microbiology, University of Pennsylvania, 225 Johnson Pavilion, 3610 Hamilton Walk, Philadelphia, PA 19104, USA.

Sexual transmission of HIV requires that the virus crosses mucosal barriers and disseminates into lymphoid tissue, the major site of viral replication. To achieve this, HIV might engage DC-SIGN, a calcium dependent lectin that is expressed on mucosal dendritic cells (DCs), which binds avidly to HIV. DC-SIGN and other attachment factors are likely to account for the well-known ability of DCs to enhance infection of T cells by HIV. Attachment of HIV to DC-SIGN might thus enhance viral spread in mucosal tissues and, by taking advantage of the inherent capacity of DCs to migrate into lymphoid tissue, might promote viral dissemination within the host. DC-SIGN and a related molecule, termed DC-SIGNR, also enhance infection by Ebola virus. The expression of these lectins on early targets of Ebola virus infection, like liver endothelial cells and alveolar macrophages, suggests an important role for DC-SIGN and DC-SIGNR in the establishment of Ebola infection. This article reviews the interaction of DC-SIGN and DC-SIGNR with HIV and Ebola, discusses the mechanism of DC-SIGN-mediated viral transmission and examines how this process could be inhibited by potential therapeutics.

PMID: 12223058 [PubMed - indexed for MEDLINE]

2032. Mol Cell. 2002 Aug;10(2):307-16.

The assembly of Ebola virus nucleocapsid requires virion-associated proteins 35 and 24 and posttranslational modification of nucleoprotein.

Huang Y(1), Xu L, Sun Y, Nabel GJ.

Author information: (1)Vaccine Research Center, National Institutes of Allergy and Infectious Diseases, National Institutes of Health, Bethesda, MD 20892, USA.

Ebola virus encodes seven viral structural and regulatory proteins that support its high rates of replication, but little is known about nucleocapsid assembly of this virus in infected cells. We report here that three viral proteins are necessary and sufficient for formation of Ebola virus particles and that intracellular posttranslational modification regulates this process. Expression of the nucleoprotein (NP) and virion-associated proteins VP35 and VP24 led to spontaneous assembly of nucleocapsids in transfected 293T cells by transmission electron microscopy. A specific biochemical interaction of these three proteins was demonstrated, and, interestingly, O-glycosylation and sialation of NP were demonstrated and necessary for their association. This distinct mechanism of regulation for filovirus assembly suggests new approaches for viral therapies and vaccines for Ebola and related viruses.

PMID: 12191476 [PubMed - indexed for MEDLINE]

2033. Virus Res. 2002 Aug;87(2):155-63.

Molecular characterization of an isolate from the 1989/90 epizootic of Ebola virus Reston among macaques imported into the United States.

Groseth A(1), Ströher U, Theriault S, Feldmann H.

Author information: (1)Special Pathogens Program, Canadian Science Centre for Human and Animal Health, 1015 Arlington Street, Winnipeg, Manitoba, Canada R3E 3R2.

We have determined the entire genomic sequence of the Pennsylvania strain, which was isolated along with the Virginia strain during the emergence of Ebola virus Reston in 1989/90 in the United States. Thus, either the Pennsylvania or Virginia strain, neither of which had been previously molecularly characterized, can be considered as the prototype for Ebola virus Reston. Comparative analysis showed a high degree of homology to the concomitantly analyzed and recently published Philippine strain of EBOV Reston from 1996 (Ikegami et al., Arch. Virol., 146 (2001) 2021). In comparison to EBOV Zaire, strain Mayinga, conservation could be found within the open reading frames, the 3' leader and 5' trailer region and the transcriptional signals, whereas the non-coding and intergenic regions did not show any homology. This clearly supports that EBOV Reston is a distinct species within the genus Ebola-like virus but which seems to be similar to other members with respect to transcription and replication strategies. The sequence determination provides the basis for the development of a reverse genetics system for Ebola virus Reston, which is needed to study differences in pathogenicity among filoviruses.
PMID: 12191779 [PubMed - indexed for MEDLINE]

2034. Antiviral Res. 2002 Jul;55(1):151-9.

3-deazaneplanocin A induces massively increased interferon-alpha production in Ebola virus-infected mice.

Bray M(1), Raymond JL, Geisbert T, Baker RO.

Author information: (1)Virology Division, Department of Viral Therapeutics, United States Army Medical Research Institute of Infectious Diseases, Fort Detrick, Frederick, MD 21702-5011, USA. mike.bray@det.amedd.army.mil

3-deazaneplanocin A, an analog of adenosine, is a potent inhibitor of Ebola virus replication. A single dose early in infection prevents illness and death in Ebola virus-infected mice. The ability of this and similar compounds to block both RNA and DNA viruses has been attributed to the inhibition of a cellular enzyme, S-adenosylhomocysteine hydrolase (SAH), indirectly resulting in reduced methylation of the 5' cap of viral messenger RNA. However, we found that the protective effect of the drug resulted from massively increased production of interferon-alpha in Ebola-infected, but not uninfected mice. Peak interferon levels increased with the extent of disease at the time of treatment, indicating that production was boosted only in virus-infected cells. Ebola virus has been shown to suppress innate antiviral mechanisms of the type I interferon response. 3-deazaneplanocin A appears to reverse such suppression, restricting viral dissemination. Further development should focus on identifying adenosine analogues that produce a similar effect in Ebola virus-infected primates.
PMID: 12076759 [PubMed - indexed for MEDLINE]

2035. J Clin Microbiol. 2002 Jul;40(7):2323-30.

Rapid detection and quantification of RNA of Ebola and Marburg viruses, Lassa virus, Crimean-Congo hemorrhagic fever virus, Rift Valley fever virus, dengue virus, and yellow fever virus by real-time reverse transcription-PCR.

Drosten C(1), Göttig S, Schilling S, Asper M, Panning M, Schmitz H, Günther S.

Author information: (1)Bernhard-Nocht-Institute of Tropical Medicine, Hamburg, Germany. drosten@bni.uni-hamburg.de

Viral hemorrhagic fevers (VHFs) are acute infections with high case fatality rates. Important VHF agents are Ebola and Marburg viruses (MBGV/EBOV), Lassa virus (LASV), Crimean-Congo hemorrhagic fever virus (CCHFV), Rift Valley fever virus (RVFV), dengue virus (DENV), and yellow fever virus (YFV). VHFs are clinically difficult to diagnose and to distinguish; a rapid and reliable laboratory diagnosis is required in suspected cases. We have established six one-step, real-time reverse transcription-PCR assays for these pathogens based on the Superscript reverse transcriptase-Platinum Taq polymerase enzyme mixture. Novel primers and/or 5'-nuclease detection probes were designed for RVFV, DENV, YFV, and CCHFV by using the latest DNA database entries. PCR products were detected in real time on a LightCycler instrument by using 5'-nuclease technology (RVFV, DENV, and YFV) or SybrGreen dye intercalation (MBGV/EBOV, LASV, and CCHFV). The inhibitory effect of SybrGreen on reverse transcription was overcome by initial immobilization of the dye in the reaction capillaries. Universal cycling conditions for SybrGreen and 5'-nuclease probe detection were established. Thus, up to three assays could be performed in parallel, facilitating rapid testing for several pathogens. All assays were thoroughly optimized and validated in terms of analytical sensitivity by using in vitro-transcribed RNA. The >or=95% detection limits as determined by probit regression analysis ranged from 1,545 to 2,835 viral genome equivalents/ml of serum (8.6 to 16 RNA copies per assay). The suitability of the assays was exemplified by detection and quantification of viral RNA in serum samples of VHF patients.
PMCID: PMC120575 PMID: 12089242 [PubMed - indexed for MEDLINE]

2036. J Virol. 2002 Jul;76(13):6841-4.

C-type lectins DC-SIGN and L-SIGN mediate cellular entry by Ebola virus in cis and in trans.

Alvarez CP(1), Lasala F, Carrillo J, Muñiz O, Corbí AL, Delgado R.

Author information: (1)Laboratory of Molecular Microbiology, Dept. of Microbiology, Hospital 12 de Octubre, 28041 Madrid, Spain.

Ebola virus is a highly lethal pathogen responsible for several outbreaks of hemorrhagic fever. Here we show that the primate lentiviral binding C-type lectins DC-SIGN and L-SIGN act as cofactors for cellular entry by Ebola virus. Furthermore, DC-SIGN on the surface of dendritic cells is able to function as a trans receptor, binding Ebola virus-pseudotyped lentiviral particles and transmitting infection to susceptible cells. Our data underscore a role for DC-SIGN and L-SIGN in the infective process and pathogenicity of Ebola virus infection.
PMCID: PMC136246 PMID: 12050398 [PubMed - indexed for MEDLINE]

2037. Nat Med. 2002 Jul;8(7):645-6.

Ebola vaccine gets corporate backer.

Dove A.
PMID: 12091886 [PubMed - indexed for MEDLINE]

2038. Trop Doct. 2002 Jul;32(3):181-2.

Defend the human rights of the Ebola victims!

Jeppsson A.
PMID: 12139173 [PubMed - indexed for MEDLINE]

2039. J Virol. 2002 Jun;76(12):6408-12.

Pre- and postexposure prophylaxis of Ebola virus infection in an animal model by passive transfer of a neutralizing human antibody.

Parren PW(1), Geisbert TW, Maruyama T, Jahrling PB, Burton DR.

Author information: (1)Department of Immunology, The Scripps Research Institute, La Jolla, California 92037, USA.

A neutralizing human monoclonal antibody, KZ52, protects guinea pigs from lethal Ebola Zaire virus challenge. Administration before or up to 1 h after challenge resulted in dose-dependent protection by the antibody. Interestingly, some antibody-treated animals survived despite developing high-level viremia, suggesting that the mechanism of protection by KZ52 may extend beyond reduction of viremia by virus neutralization. KZ52 is a promising candidate for immunoprophylaxis of Ebola virus infection.

PMCID: PMC136210 PMID: 12021376 [PubMed - indexed for MEDLINE]

2040. J Virol. 2002 Jun;76(11):5472-9.

Late assembly domain function can exhibit context dependence and involves ubiquitin residues implicated in endocytosis.

Strack B(1), Calistri A, Göttlinger HG.

Author information: (1)Department of Cancer Immunology and AIDS, Dana-Farber Cancer Institute, Harvard Medical School, Boston, Massachusetts 02115, USA.
Retroviral Gag polyproteins contain regions that promote the separation of virus particles from the plasma membrane and from each other. These Gag regions are often referred to as late assembly (L) domains. The L domain of human immunodeficiency virus type 1 (HIV-1) is in the C-terminal p6(gag) domain and harbors an essential P(T/S)APP motif, whereas the L domains of oncoretroviruses are in the N-terminal half of the Gag precursor and have a PPXY core motif. We recently observed that L domains induce the ubiquitination of a minimal HIV-1 Gag construct and that point mutations which abolish L domain activity prevent Gag ubiquitination. In that study, a peptide from the Ebola virus L domain with overlapping P(T/S)APP and PPXY motifs showed exceptional activity in promoting Gag ubiquitination and the release of virus-like particles. We now show that a substitution which disrupts the PPXY motif but leaves the P(T/S)APP motif intact abolishes L domain activity in the minimal Gag context, but not in the context of a near full-length HIV-1 Gag precursor. Our results reveal that the P(T/S)APP motif does not function autonomously and indicate that the HIV-1 nucleocapsid-p1 region, which is proximal to p6(gag), can cooperate with the conserved L domain core motif. We have also examined the effects of ubiquitin mutants on virus-like particle production, and the results indicate that residues required for the endocytosis function of ubiquitin are also involved in virus budding.

PMCID: PMC137019 PMID: 11991975 [PubMed - indexed for MEDLINE]

2041. Med Educ. 2002 Jun;36(6):555-60.

Serious, frightening and interesting conditions: differences in values and attitudes between first-year and final-year medical students.

Brorsson A(1), Hellquist G, Björkelund C, Råstam L.

Author information: (1)Department of Community Medicine, Lund University, Malmö, Sweden.
CONTEXT AND OBJECTIVE: During medical education and training, the values and attitudes of medical students are shaped both by knowledge and by role models. In this study, the aim was to compare the views of first- and final-year students concerning patients with different medical conditions. PARTICIPANTS AND METHOD: In the spring of 1998 all first- and final-year medical students at Göteborg and Lund Universities, Sweden, were invited to answer a questionnaire. A total of 20 medical conditions were to be rated on visual analogue scales, according to three aspects: their perceived seriousness, the student's own fear of them and interest in working with these conditions in the future. RESULTS: The overall response rate was 75%. Concerning seriousness, there was a high degree of concordance between the first- and final-year students. Concerning their own fear, the concordance was less pronounced. When the conditions were rated from the aspect of interest, for the final-year students, gastric or duodenal ulcer replaced infection with Ebola virus for the first-year students, among the five highest-ranked conditions. The correlations between seriousness and fear were lower among the final-year students, but this reached statistical significance only in a few cases. DISCUSSION: A reasonable interpretation of the results is that the values and attitudes of the students were influenced by increased knowledge, as well as by role models encountered during the clinical parts of the training. Conditions less likely to be contracted become less feared, and conditions with effective treatment become more interesting; and the converse was true for each of these changes.

PMID: 12047671 [PubMed - indexed for MEDLINE]

2042. Emerg Infect Dis. 2002 May;8(5):503-7.

Evaluation in nonhuman primates of vaccines against Ebola virus.

Geisbert TW(1), Pushko P, Anderson K, Smith J, Davis KJ, Jahrling PB.

Author information: (1)U.S. Army Medical Research Institute of Infectious Diseases, 1425 Porter Street, Fort Detrick, MD 21702-5011, USA.
tom.geisbert@amedd.army.mil
Ebola virus (EBOV) causes acute hemorrhagic fever that is fatal in up to 90% of cases in both humans and nonhuman primates. No vaccines or treatments are available for human use. We evaluated the effects in nonhuman primates of vaccine strategies that had protected mice or guinea pigs from lethal EBOV infection. The following immunogens were used: RNA replicon particles derived from an attenuated strain of Venezuelan equine encephalitis virus (VEEV) expressing EBOV glycoprotein and nucleoprotein; recombinant Vaccinia virus expressing EBOV glycoprotein; liposomes containing lipid A and inactivated EBOV; and a concentrated, inactivated whole-virion preparation. None of these strategies successfully protected nonhuman primates from robust challenge with EBOV. The disease observed in primates differed from that in rodents, suggesting that rodent models of EBOV may not predict the efficacy of candidate vaccines in primates and that protection of primates may require different mechanisms.

PMCID: PMC3369765 PMID: 11996686 [PubMed - indexed for MEDLINE]

2043. J Virol. 2002 May;76(10):5266-70.

Association of the caveola vesicular system with cellular entry by filoviruses.

Empig CJ(1), Goldsmith MA.

Author information: (1)Gladstone Institute of Virology and Immunology, San Francisco, California 94141-9100, USA.

The filoviruses Ebola Zaire virus and Marburg virus are believed to infect target cells through endocytic vesicles, but the details of this pathway are unknown. We used a pseudotyping strategy to investigate the cell biology of filovirus entry. We observed that specific inhibitors of the caveola system, including cholesterol-sequestering drugs and phorbol esters, inhibited the entry of filovirus pseudotypes into human cells. We also measured slower cell entry kinetics for both filovirus pseudotypes than for pseudotypes of vesicular stomatitis virus (VSV), which has been recognized to exploit the clathrin-mediated entry pathway. Finally, visualization by immunofluorescence and confocal microscopy revealed that the filovirus pseudotypes colocalized with the caveola protein marker caveolin-1 but that VSV pseudotypes did not. Collectively, these results provide evidence suggesting that filoviruses use caveolae to gain entry into cells.

PMCID: PMC136134 PMID: 11967340 [PubMed - indexed for MEDLINE]

2044. J Virol. 2002 May;76(10):4855-65.

Ebola virus VP40 drives the formation of virus-like filamentous particles along with GP.

Noda T(1), Sagara H, Suzuki E, Takada A, Kida H, Kawaoka Y.

Author information: (1)Laboratory of Microbiology, Department of Disease Control, Graduate School of Veterinary Medicine, Hokkaido University, Sapporo 060-0818, Japan.

Using biochemical assays, it has been demonstrated that expression of Ebola virus VP40 alone in mammalian cells induced production of particles with a density similar to that of virions. To determine the morphological properties of these particles, cells expressing VP40 and the particles released from the cells were examined by electron microscopy. VP40 induced budding from the plasma membrane of filamentous particles, which differed in length but had uniform diameters of approximately 65 nm. When the Ebola virus glycoprotein (GP) responsible for receptor binding and membrane fusion was expressed in cells, we found pleomorphic particles budding from the plasma membrane. By contrast, when GP was coexpressed with VP40, GP was found on the filamentous particles induced by VP40. These results demonstrated the central role of VP40 in formation of the filamentous structure of Ebola virions and may suggest an interaction between VP40 and GP in morphogenesis.

PMCID: PMC136157 PMID: 11967302 [PubMed - indexed for MEDLINE]

2045. Mol Ther. 2002 May;5(5 Pt 1):528-37.

Targeted transduction patterns in the mouse brain by lentivirus vectors pseudotyped with VSV, Ebola, Mokola, LCMV, or MuLV envelope proteins.

Watson DJ(1), Kobinger GP, Passini MA, Wilson JM, Wolfe JH.

Author information: (1)Department of Pathobiology and Center for Comparative Medical Genetics, School of Veterinary Medicine, University of Pennsylvania, Philadelphia, Pennsylvania 19104, USA.

Lentiviral vectors have proven to be promising tools for transduction of central nervous system (CNS) cells in vivo and in vitro. In this study, CNS transduction patterns of lentiviral vectors pseudotyped with envelope glycoproteins from Ebola virus, murine leukemia virus (MuLV), lymphocytic choriomeningitis virus (LCMV), or the rabies-related Mokola virus were compared to a vector pseudotyped with the vesicular stomatitis virus glycoprotein (VSV-G). Mokola-, LCMV-, and VSV-G-pseudotyped vectors transduced similar populations, including striatum, thalamus, and white matter. Mokola-pseudotyped vectors were the most efficient of the three. MuLV-pseudotyped lentivirus efficiently transduced striatum and hippocampal dentate gyrus. In contrast, no transduction resulted from injection of Ebola-pseudotyped virus in the CNS. The same pattern was observed in vitro with primary cultured oligodendrocytes. LCMV, MuLV, and Ebola pseudotypes were the most stable. These results demonstrate that targeted transduction in the CNS can be achieved using specific envelope glycoproteins to pseudotype lentiviral vectors, and support the use of Mokola-pseudotyped and MuLV-pseudotyped lentiviral vectors as efficient and stable alternatives to VSV-G-pseudotyped vectors for experiments in the mouse CNS.

PMID: 11991743 [PubMed - indexed for MEDLINE]

2046. Servir. 2002 May-Jun;50(3):132-5.

[Ebola fever, an out of control epidemic?].

[Article in Portuguese]

Zeller H.

PMID: 12229031 [PubMed - indexed for MEDLINE]

2047. Trends Biochem Sci. 2002 May;27(5):222-4.

Viral RNA-polymerases -- a predicted 2'-O-ribose methyltransferase domain shared by all Mononegavirales.

Ferron F(1), Longhi S, Henrissat B, Canard B.

Author information: (1)Architecture et Fonction des Macromolécules Biologiques, UMR 6098, CNRS, and Universitées Aix-Marseille I and II, ESIL, 163, Avenue de Luminy, Case 925, F-13288 Marseille Cedex 9, France.

The Mononegavirales virus group comprises several major human pathogens, including measles, rabies and Ebola viruses. This article reports a computational analysis of the C-terminal region of RNA-dependent RNA-polymerases from Mononegavirales. Using a combination of sequence similarity and threading analysis, a 2'-O-ribose methyltransferase domain was identified that is involved in the capping of viral mRNAs.

PMID: 12076527 [PubMed - indexed for MEDLINE]
2048. Science. 2002 Apr 12;296(5566):279.

Virology. Rafting with Ebola.

Freed EO(1).

Author information: (1)Laboratory of Molecular Microbiology, National Institute of Allergy and Infectious Diseases, National Institutes of Health, Bethesda, MD 20892-0460, USA. efreed@nih.gov

PMID: 11951027 [PubMed - indexed for MEDLINE]
2049. Clin Exp Immunol. 2002 Apr;128(1):163-8.

Inflammatory responses in Ebola virus-infected patients.

Baize S(1), Leroy EM, Georges AJ, Georges-Courbot MC, Capron M, Bedjabaga I, Lansoud-Soukate J, Mavoungou E.

Author information: (1)Centre International de Recherches Médicales de Franceville (CIRMF), Franceville, Gabon, France. baize@cervi-lyon.inserm.fr

Ebola virus subtype Zaire (Ebo-Z) induces acute haemorrhagic fever and a 60-80% mortality rate in humans. Inflammatory responses were monitored in victims and survivors of Ebo-Z haemorrhagic fever during two recent outbreaks in Gabon. Survivors were characterized by a transient release in plasma of interleukin-1beta (IL-1beta), IL-6, tumour necrosis factor-alpha (TNFalpha), macrophage inflammatory protein-1alpha (MIP-1alpha) and MIP-1beta early in the disease, followed by circulation of IL-1 receptor antagonist (IL-1RA) and soluble receptors for TNFalpha (sTNF-R) and IL-6 (sIL-6R) towards the end of the symptomatic phase and after recovery. Fatal infection was associated with moderate levels of TNFalpha and IL-6, and high levels of IL-10, IL-1RA and sTNF-R, in the days before death, while IL-1beta was not detected and MIP-1alpha and MIP-1beta concentrations were similar to those of endemic controls. Simultaneous massive activation of monocytes/macrophages, the main target of Ebo-Z, was suggested in fatal infection by elevated neopterin levels. Thus, presence of IL-1beta and of elevated concentrations of IL-6 in plasma during the symptomatic phase can be used as markers of non-fatal infection, while release of IL-10 and of high levels of neopterin and IL-1RA in plasma as soon as a few days after the disease onset is indicative of a fatal outcome. In conclusion, recovery from Ebo-Z infection is associated with early and well-regulated inflammatory responses, which may be crucial in controlling viral replication and inducing specific immunity. In contrast, defective inflammatory responses and massive monocyte/macrophage activation were associated with fatal outcome.

PMCID: PMC1906357 PMID: 11982604 [PubMed - indexed for MEDLINE]
2050. Exp Anim. 2002 Apr;51(2):173-9.

Chronological and spatial analysis of the 1996 Ebola Reston virus outbreak in a monkey breeding facility in the Philippines.

Miranda ME(1), Yoshikawa Y, Manalo DL, Calaor AB, Miranda NL, Cho F, Ikegami T, Ksiazek TG.

Author information: (1)Veterinary Research Department, Research Institute for Tropical Medicine, Alabang, Muntinlupa City, Philippines 1770.

To describe the transmission pattern of natural infection with Ebola Reston (EBO-R) virus in a breeding colony, the chronological and spatial analysis of mortality during the 1996 EBO-R virus outbreak was done in this study. The EBO-R virus infection among monkeys in the facility was widespread. Over a period of 3 months, 14 out of 21 occupied units were contaminated with antigen positive animals. A large number of wild-caught monkeys were involved in this outbreak suggesting that wild-caught monkeys have a high susceptibility to EBO-R virus infection. In this outbreak, morbidity patterns for individual animal units were very different regardless of the type and size of cages, individual or gang cages. The results suggest that not only the cage size but also poor animal husbandry practices may be risk factors for the spread of EBO-R infection.

PMID: 12012728 [PubMed - indexed for MEDLINE]
2051. Int J Trauma Nurs. 2002 Apr-Jun;8(2):51-3.

Transporting patients with lethal contagious infections.

Marklund LA(1).

Author information: (1)Operational Medicine Division, United States Army Medical Research Institute of Infectious Diseases, USA. leroy.marklund@det.amedd.army.mil

PMID: 12000908 [PubMed - indexed for MEDLINE]
2052. Int J Trauma Nurs. 2002 Apr-Jun;8(2):36-41.

Ebola fever: the African emergency.

Bruce J(1), Brysiewicz P.

Author information: (1)Department of Nursing Education, University of the Witwatersrand, Johannesburg, South Africa.

The Ebola virus produces one of Africa's most lethal viral hemorrhagic fever (VHF) infections. Statistically, Ebola fever is at the bottom of Africa's list of infectious diseases, but the speed with which it induces agonizing death puts Ebola fever at the top of Africa's emergencies. Many aspects of the virus are unknown and have eluded medical scientists for 3 decades. Hence enormous difficulties may be encountered in treating, preventing, and controlling Ebola fever. In this article, the origin of the disease is traced, followed by a description of the Ebola fever triad, with some insights into the perspectives that may complicate treatment and control of the disease. The clinical manifestations are described in relation to the progression of the disease. Patients with the Ebola virus are admitted to the hospital as an emergency with the activation of a disaster-type plan of action.

PMID: 12000905 [PubMed - indexed for MEDLINE]
2053. J Virol. 2002 Apr;76(8):3952-64.

Requirements for budding of paramyxovirus simian virus 5 virus-like particles.

Schmitt AP(1), Leser GP, Waning DL, Lamb RA.

Author information: (1)Howard Hughes Medical Institute, Northwestern University, Evanston, Illinois 60208-3500, USA.

Enveloped viruses are released from infected cells after coalescence of viral components at cellular membranes and budding of membranes to release particles. For some negative-strand RNA viruses (e.g., vesicular stomatitis virus and Ebola virus), the viral matrix (M) protein contains all of the information needed for budding, since virus-like particles (VLPs) are efficiently released from cells when the M protein is expressed from cDNA. To investigate the requirements for budding of the paramyxovirus simian virus 5 (SV5), its M protein was expressed in mammalian cells, and it was found that SV5 M protein alone could not induce vesicle budding and was not secreted from cells. Coexpression of M protein with the viral hemagglutinin-neuraminidase (HN) or fusion (F) glycoproteins also failed to result in significant VLP release. It was found that M protein in the form of VLPs was only secreted from cells, with an efficiency comparable to authentic virus budding, when M protein was coexpressed with one of the two glycoproteins, HN or F, together with the nucleocapsid (NP) protein. The VLPs appeared similar morphologically to authentic virions by electron microscopy. CsCl density gradient centrifugation indicated that almost all of the NP protein in the cells had assembled into nucleocapsid-like structures. Deletion of the F and HN cytoplasmic tails indicated an important role of these cytoplasmic tails in VLP budding. Furthermore, truncation of the HN cytoplasmic tail was found to be inhibitory toward budding, since it prevented coexpressed wild-type (wt) F protein from directing VLP budding. Conversely, truncation of the F protein cytoplasmic tail was not inhibitory and did not affect the ability of coexpressed wt HN protein to direct the budding of particles. Taken together, these data suggest that multiple viral components, including assembled nucleocapsids, have important roles in the paramyxovirus budding process.

PMCID: PMC136107 PMID: 11907235 [PubMed - indexed for MEDLINE]

2054. Lancet Infect Dis. 2002 Apr;2(4):203.

Infectious disease surveillance update.

Das P.

PMID: 11937416 [PubMed - indexed for MEDLINE]

2055. Nat Med. 2002 Apr;8(4):313.

Ebola: small, but real progress.

Birmingham K, Cooney S.

PMID: 11927920 [PubMed - indexed for MEDLINE]

2056. Nurs Sci Q. 2002 Apr;15(2):123-30.

Ebola at Mbarara, Uganda: aesthetic expressions of the lived worlds of people waiting to know.

Locsin RC(1).

Author information: (1)Florida Atlantic University, Boca Raton, USA.

The Ebola epidemic of 2000 was a disastrous experience for the people of Uganda. Prior outbreaks in neighboring African sub-Saharan countries heightened the realization of death from this devastating disease. Waiting to know is a phenomenon described as an excruciating inactivity uniquely experienced by individuals who were exposed to persons with Ebola but who had not yet exhibited signs and symptoms of the disease. In the recent Ebola epidemic in Uganda, contact persons described their experience of waiting to know as "helplessness in anticipation and fear of dying or premature death; agonizing and languishing over losing relatives, friends, and loved ones; trusting no one; and helplessness and hopelessness with the persisting time." In this column, these experiences will be discussed, and visual artworks will further illustrate the lived experience of waiting to know. Human and artistic expressions facilitate understanding of lived experience, and understanding is known to inspire meaningful, compassionate, and competent nursing practice.

PMID: 11949481 [PubMed - indexed for MEDLINE]

2057. JAMA. 2002 Mar 20;287(11):1381-2.

Surprise finding spurs Ebola researchers' hopes.

Vastag B.

PMID: 11903010 [PubMed - indexed for MEDLINE]

2058. J Exp Med. 2002 Mar 4;195(5):593-602.

Lipid raft microdomains: a gateway for compartmentalized trafficking of Ebola and Marburg viruses.

Bavari S(1), Bosio CM, Wiegand E, Ruthel G, Will AB, Geisbert TW, Hevey M, Schmaljohn C, Schmaljohn A, Aman MJ.

Author information: (1)Dept. of Cell Biology and Biochemistry, U.S. Army Medical Research Institute of Infectious Diseases, Frederick, MD 21702-5011, USA. bavaris@ncifcrf.gov

Spatiotemporal aspects of filovirus entry and release are poorly understood. Lipid rafts act as functional platforms for multiple cellular signaling and trafficking processes. Here, we report the compartmentalization of Ebola and Marburg viral proteins within lipid rafts during viral assembly and budding. Filoviruses released from infected cells incorporated raft-associated molecules, suggesting that viral exit occurs at the rafts. Ectopic expression of Ebola matrix protein and glycoprotein supported raft-dependent release of filamentous, virus-like particles (VLPs), strikingly similar to live virus as revealed by electron microscopy. Our findings also revealed that the entry of filoviruses requires functional rafts, identifying rafts as the site of virus attack. The identification of rafts as the gateway for the entry and exit of filoviruses and raft-dependent generation of VLPs have important implications for development of therapeutics and vaccination strategies against infections with Ebola and Marburg viruses.

PMCID: PMC2193767 PMID: 11877482 [PubMed - indexed for MEDLINE]

2059. Adler Mus Bull. 2002 Mar;28(1):16-20.

An ICN remembers: a glimpse of the history of infection control in South Africa.

Pearse J.

PMID: 20329340 [PubMed - indexed for MEDLINE]

2060. Euro Surveill. 2002 Mar;7(3):42-4.

Management of viral haemorrhagic fevers in Switzerland.

Hugonnet S(1), Sax H, Pittet D.

Author information: (1)Infection Control Programme and Medical Intensive Care Unit, Department of Internal Medicine, University of Geneva Hospitals, Geneva, Switzerland.

Over the past years, there have been very few imported cases of VHF in Switzerland: one confirmed and four suspected cases of Ebola fever in Basel in 1994, two suspected cases of Ebola and Lassa fevers in Lausanne in 2000, and in the same year, six suspected cases of Lassa fever in Geneva. Given the considerable diversity in the management of patients with suspected or confirmed VHF, national guidelines are needed, as well as the establishment of a national reference centre.

PMID: 12631944 [PubMed - indexed for MEDLINE]

2061. Euro Surveill. 2002 Mar;7(3):33-6.

Ebola in Africa--discoveries in the past decade.

Arthur RR(1).

Author information: (1)Global Alert and Response, Department of Communicable Disease Surveillance and Response World Health Organization, Geneva, Switzerland.

Within the past decade, Ebola haemorrhagic fever (EHF) has been recognised for the first time in four countries. Our understanding of the epidemiology, clinical aspects, laboratory diagnosis and control measures for EHF has improved considerably as a result of the outbreaks in these countries and the re-emergence that has occurred in another. The coordinated international responses to several of the large EHF outbreaks serve as models for controlling epidemics of other communicable diseases. This report is a chronological overview of the EHF outbreaks in Africa during the past decade, including the recent epidemics in Gabon and the Republic of the Congo, and highlights new discoveries and some of the remaining challenges.

PMID: 12631942 [PubMed - indexed for MEDLINE]

2062. Euro Surveill. 2002 Mar;7(3):31-2.

Viral haemorrhagic fevers in Europe--effective control requires a co-ordinated response.

Crowcroft NS(1), Morgan D, Brown D.

Author information: (1)Health Laboratory Service, CDSC, London, United Kingdom.

Viral haemorrhagic fevers (VHF) have attracted the attention of the medical world and general public for many reasons, some based in reality and more on misinformation. They are amongst the highest profile infections in the public mind, because they are thought to be highly infectious and to kill most of their victims in a dramatic way (1,2). To add to the intrigue, mysteries remain about the source of some of the viruses involved. They emerge and re-emerge in many countries, most recently Ebola in Uganda in 2000 (3) and Gabon in 2001/02 (4), and Congo Crimean Haemorrhagic Fever (CCHF) in Kosovo (5) and Pakistan in 2001 (6). Large outbreaks have affected populations in endemic areas, living mainly in inaccessible areas or refugee camps where living conditions are very difficult. Poorly resourced medical facilities have played a role in amplifying transmission and infection control measures have been difficult or virtually impossible to establish. These viruses are likely to remain a threat until the reservoir is identified and as long as endemic areas are afflicted with ecological change, poverty and social instability. Recent events since September 11 2001 remind us of their potential to be used as weapons, and that fear can present a risk to public health.

PMID: 12631941 [PubMed - indexed for MEDLINE]

2063. Immunol Lett. 2002 Mar 1;80(3):169-79.

Proinflammatory response during Ebola virus infection of primate models: possible involvement of the tumor necrosis factor receptor superfamily.

Hensley LE(1), Young HA, Jahrling PB, Geisbert TW.

Author information: (1)Pathology Division, US Army Medical Research Institute of Infectious Diseases (USAMRIID), Attn: MCMR-UIP-D, 1425 Porter Street, Fort Detrick, MD 21702-5011, USA. lisa.hensley@amedd.army.mil

Ebola virus (EBOV) infections are characterized by dysregulation of normal host immune responses. Insight into the mechanism came from recent studies in nonhuman primates, which showed that EBOV infects cells of the mononuclear phagocyte system (MPS), resulting in apoptosis of bystander lymphocytes. In this study, we evaluated serum levels of cytokines/chemokines in EBOV-infected nonhuman primates, as possible correlates of this bystander apoptosis. Increased levels of interferon (IFN)-alpha, IFN-beta, interleukin (IL)-6, IL-18, MIP-1alpha, and MIP-1beta were observed in all EBOV-infected monkeys, indicating the occurrence of a strong proinflammatory response. To investigate the mechanism(s) involved in lymphoid apoptosis, soluble Fas (sFas) and nitrate accumulation were measured. sFas was detected in 4/9 animals, while, elevations of nitrate accumulation occurred in 3/3 animals. To further evaluate the potential role of these factors in the observed bystander apoptosis and intact animals, in vitro cultures were prepared of adherent human monocytes/macrophages (PHM), and monocytes differentiated into immature dendritic cells (DC). These cultures were infected with EBOV and analyzed for cytokine/chemokine induction and expression of apoptosis-related genes. In addition, the in vitro EBOV infection of peripheral blood mononuclear cells (PBMC) resulted in strong cytokine/chemokine induction, a marked increase in lactate dehydrogenase (LDH) activity, and an increase in the number of apoptotic lymphocytes examined by electron microscopy. Increased levels of sFAS were detected in PHM cultures, although, 90% of EBOV-infected PHM were positive for tumor necrosis factor (TNF)-related apoptosis-inducing ligand (TRAIL) by immunohistochemistry, RNA analysis, and flow cytometry. Inactivated EBOV also

effected increased TRAIL expression in PHM, suggesting that the TNF receptor superfamily may be involved in apoptosis of the host lymphoid cells, and that induction may occur independent of viral replication. In further studies with infected PHM, expression of MHC II was remarkably suppressed after 6 days, an additional correlate of immunological dysregulation. In conclusion, our findings suggest that infection of mononuclear phagocytes is critical, triggering a cascade of events involving cytokines/chemokines and oxygen free radicals. It is the consequence of these events rather than direct viral infection that results in much of the observed pathology. Identification of cytokine/chemokine, nitric oxide, and reactive oxygen species involvement in the observed filoviral pathogenesis may lend insight into the rational design of therapeutic countermeasures of filoviral pathogenesis.
PMID: 11803049 [PubMed - indexed for MEDLINE]
2064. J Virol. 2002 Mar;76(5):2518-28.

Ebola virus glycoproteins induce global surface protein down-modulation and loss of cell adherence.

Simmons G(1), Wool-Lewis RJ, Baribaud F, Netter RC, Bates P.

Author information: (1)Department of Microbiology, School of Medicine, University of Pennsylvania, 303A Johnson Pavilion, 3610 Hamilton Walk, Philadelphia, PA 19104-6076, USA.

The Ebola virus envelope glycoprotein (GP) derived from the pathogenic Zaire subtype mediates cell rounding and detachment from the extracellular matrix in 293T cells. In this study we provide evidence that GPs from the other pathogenic subtypes, Sudan and Côte d'Ivoire, as well as from Reston, a strain thought to be nonpathogenic in humans, also induced cell rounding, albeit at lower levels than Zaire GP. Sequential removal of regions of potential O-linked glycosylation at the C terminus of GP1 led to a step-wise reduction in cell detachment without obviously affecting GP function, suggesting that such modifications are involved in inducing the detachment phenotype. While causing cell rounding and detachment in 293T cells, Ebola virus GP did not cause an increase in cell death. Indeed, following transient expression of GP, cells were able to readhere and continue to divide. Also, the rounding effect was not limited to 293T cells. Replication-deficient adenovirus vectors expressing Ebola virus GP induced the loss of cell adhesion in a range of cell lines and primary cell types, including those with proposed relevance to Ebola virus infection in vivo, such as endothelial cells and macrophages. In both transfected 293T and adenovirus-infected Vero cells, a reduction in cell surface expression of adhesion molecules such as integrin beta1 concurrent with the loss of cell adhesion was observed. A number of other cell surface molecules, however, including major histocompatibility complex class I and the epidermal growth factor receptor, were also down-modulated, suggesting a global mechanism for surface molecule down-regulation.
PMCID: PMC153797 PMID: 11836430 [PubMed - indexed for MEDLINE]
2065. Lancet Infect Dis. 2002 Mar;2(3):133.

Infectious disease surveillance update.

Das P.
PMID: 11944179 [PubMed - indexed for MEDLINE]
2066. Soc Sci Med. 2002 Mar;54(6):955-69.

Representations of far-flung illnesses: the case of Ebola in Britain.

Joffe H(1), Haarhoff G.

Author information: (1)Department of Psychology, University College London, UK. h.joffe@ucl.ac.uk

In western cultures lay people are faced with a plethora of far-flung illnesses, relayed to them by the mass media. A number of social scientists have called for scrutiny of the link between people's patterns of thinking concerning such events, and the messages to which they are exposed. Using the outbreaks of Ebola in Africa in the mid-1990s as a vehicle, the study examines how British broadsheets and their readers, and British tabloids and their readers, make sense of this far-flung illness. Existing work on early representations of HIV/AIDS in the west is utilised to inform the research questions. In particular, this study investigates whether Ebola is constructed as a threat, how media and lay representations of Ebola interact, and whether there are different pockets of shared thinking, or a more uniform representation, in relation to Ebola in Britain. An analysis of the themes in 48 broadsheet and tabloid articles, and 50 interviews with their readers, reveals a common picture in which Ebola is represented as African. associated with African practices, and seen as posing little threat to Britain. However, group differences exist, and are characterised by a more essentialised vision of Ebola in the tabloids and their readers, in contrast to a focus on structural features linked to Ebola's escalation in the broadsheets and their readers. In terms of the media-mind relationship, beyond the similarities found between media type and their respective readers' ideas, certain key differences exist: While the newspapers make Ebola 'real' by referring to its potential to globalise. as well as to how it can be contained, lay thinkers feel detached from it, and draw an analogy between Ebola and science fiction. This is discussed as a method of symbolic coping on the part of the readers, as well as in terms of the power exerted by media imagery on lay representations of Ebola.
PMID: 11996028 [PubMed - indexed for MEDLINE]
2067. Vopr Virusol. 2002 Mar-Apr;47(2):45-8.

[Sensitizing and virus-neutralizing characteristics of goat immunoglobulins to Ebola virus].

[Article in Russian]

Zubavichene NM, Dedkova LM, Sergeev NN, Ofitserov VI.

Sensitizing and virus-neutralizing properties of IgG isolated from the sera of goats immunized with Ebola virus and a relevant gammaglobulin prepared by ethanol fractionation were compared. The ratio of the virus-neutralizing activities of subclasses IgG2, IgG1a, and IgG1b was 100:10:1. Anaphylactogenic activity of IgG2 in the immediate type hypersensitivity test in guinea pigs was 2-fold lower than that of IgG1a and IgG1b. Goat gammaglobulin to Ebola virus, consisting from IgG2 antibodies by more than 50%, possessed virus-neutralizing and sensitizing characteristics compatible to IgG2.
PMID: 12046470 [PubMed - indexed for MEDLINE]

2068. Lancet. 2002 Feb 23;359(9307):712.

Re-emergence of ebola haemorrhagic fever in Gabon.

Leroy EM, Souquière S, Rouquet P, Drevet D.

PMID: 11879899 [PubMed - indexed for MEDLINE]

2069. AIDS Alert. 2002 Feb;17(2):24-5, 14.

HIV/Ebola comparison could spur new treatments.

Bieniasz P.

A researcher has discovered a link between HIV and Ebola virus: Both viruses use the same method to spread through the human body.

PMID: 11862746 [PubMed - indexed for MEDLINE]

2070. Cancer Biother Radiopharm. 2002 Feb;17(1):19-28.

Mitogen therapy for biological warfare/terrorist attacks and viral hemorrhagic fever control.

Wimer BM.

Ken Alibek was for 17 years a leader in Biopreparat, the Soviet Union's top secret agency involved in developing and stockpiling the most lethal bacteria, viruses, and toxins in the history of mankind before he defected with his family to the United States in 1992. Very contrite when he discovered he had been misled to believe that his efforts had been essential to the survival of his homeland, Alibek has become active sounding an alarm about, among other things, thousands of unemployed Russian scientists who have been seeking survival by selling their destructive expertise to rouge states and bioterrorists. Working full time in devising protective measures that might help control the damaging effects of terrorist attacks, Alibek has placed strong emphasis on stimulating nonspecific immunities of victims mainly with interleukins and other cytokines. A more productive alternative would be giving mitogens such as PHA and PWM to reinforce vaccine and antibiotic actions, at the same time stimulating protective immune, myelopoietic, and lymphopoietic responses. A key objective would be to find an effective management for the dreaded viral hemorrhagic fevers. Using Ebola infection as an experimental model, Yang et al. have shown that PHA can block both the viral secretions that inhibit neutrophil immune responses and the viral transmembrane glycoprotein that facilitates damage of the human endothelial cells responsible for the lethal hemorrhagic manifestations. Normal serum glycoproteins have in the past been clearly shown to inhibit the functions of PHA, thereby increasing dosage requirements. Extrapolation of this interaction with serum glycoproteins suggests that PHA given intravenously in adequate dosage should readily be able to block the deleterious Ebola virus glycoprotein effects. Data in an extensive classification of the hemorrhagic fever viruses recently presented by Barry make it possible to predict that mitogen therapy should be effective for virtually all of the disorders included. Therapeutic trials should best start with intravenous administration of PHA since this is the mitogen about which most is known and the only one given to humans, although the nonagglutinating advantages of fraction i.v. of PHA should be evaluated as a replacement. Functioning in a different mode, PWM has the advantage of much greater potency, and can be given either intravenously or orally, since these appear to be equally effective routes of administration. The best means of properly integrating the use of these mitogens needs to be determined.

PMID: 11915170 [PubMed - indexed for MEDLINE]

2071. Lancet Infect Dis. 2002 Feb;2(2):69.

Infectious disease surveillance update.

Das P.

PMID: 11901651 [PubMed - indexed for MEDLINE]

2072. Lancet Infect Dis. 2002 Feb;2(2):69.

Jungle conceals Ebola origins.

Kerr C.

PMID: 11901650 [PubMed - indexed for MEDLINE]

2073. Virology. 2002 Feb 1;293(1):15-9.

Evidence against an important role for infectivity-enhancing antibodies in Ebola virus infections.

Geisbert TW(1), Hensley LE, Geisbert JB, Jahrling PB.

Author information: (1)Pathology Division, U.S. Army Medical Research Institute of Infectious Diseases, Fort Detrick, Maryland 21702-5011, USA. tom.geisbert@amedd.army.mil

The neutralizing and enhancing activities of Ebola virus (EBOV)-specific antibodies were tested among four murine antibodies specific to the surface glycoprotein (GP), a recombinant human monoclonal antibody specific to GP, a polyclonal equine IgG, and serum obtained from a convalescent monkey. All but one of these antibodies neutralized EBOV infectivity of primary human monocytes/macrophages or Vero cells. None of the antibodies enhanced EBOV infectivity in these cells. Taken together with in vivo observations that early deaths were not observed in animals immunized with various viral vectors expressing EBOV GP, it is unlikely that any EBOV-enhancing antibodies profoundly affected EBOV pathogenesis.

PMID: 11853394 [PubMed - indexed for MEDLINE]

2074. Anaesthesist. 2002 Jan;51(1):50-2.

["Biological" but deadly. Potential biological weapons].

[Article in German]

Schroeder I(1).

Author information: (1)ingo.schroeder@springer.de

PMID: 11968178 [PubMed - indexed for MEDLINE]

2075. Clin Diagn Lab Immunol. 2002 Jan;9(1):19-27.

Viral replication and host gene expression in alveolar macrophages infected with Ebola virus (Zaire strain).

Gibb TR(1), Norwood DA Jr, Woollen N, Henchal EA.

Author information: (1)Diagnostic Systems Division, United States Army Medical Research Institute of Infectious Diseases, Fort Detrick, MD 21702-5011, USA. tammy.gibb@sbccom.apgea.army.mil

In order to characterize the cellular response to and identify potential diagnostic markers for the early detection of Ebola virus, an in vitro culture system involving nonhuman primate alveolar macrophages was developed. Ebola virus replication in the alveolar macrophages was characterized by plaque assay, immunohistochemical analysis, and in situ hybridization. Fluorogenic 5'-nuclease assays specific for nonhuman primate proinflammatory cytokines and chemokines were designed and used to evaluate mRNA transcription in macrophages infected with Ebola virus. Transient increases in cytokine and chemokine mRNA levels were observed immediately following exposure to Ebola virus. At 2 h postexposure, levels of cytokine and chemokine mRNAs were markedly reduced. Although Ebola virus infection of alveolar macrophages failed to induce a sustained increase in proinflammatory cytokine and chemokine mRNA transcription (potentially reducing the use of these markers as diagnostic tools), the fluorogenic 5'-nuclease assays developed may have prognostic value for individuals infected with Ebola virus. Recently published data have indicated that persons who remain asymptomatic after exposure to Ebola virus are capable of mounting an early proinflammatory cytokine response and that those who become clinically ill are not. If implemented immediately after exposure, these assays could be used to predict which individuals will be more likely to remain asymptomatic as opposed to those who will be more likely to develop clinical signs and eventually succumb to the virus.

PMCID: PMC119875 PMID: 11777824 [PubMed - indexed for MEDLINE]

2076. J Adv Nurs. 2002 Jan;37(2):173-81.

The lived experience of waiting-to-know: Ebola at Mbarara, Uganda--hoping for life, anticipating death.

Locsin RC(1), Matua AG.

Author information: (1)Department of Nursing, Faculty of Medicine, Mbarara University of Science and Technology, Mbarara, Uganda. locsin@fau.edu

PURPOSE PF THE STUDY: The purpose of the study was to describe the phenomenon of 'waiting to know'. It is a phenomenon uniquely experienced by persons who had been exposed to patients with Ebola Hemorrhagic Fever (Ebola) but who have not yet exhibited signs and symptoms of the disease.RESEARCH METHOD/ANALYSIS: The phenomenological human science approach was used using the four life worlds as guides for reflection. These are spatiality, corporeality, temporality, and relationality. PARTICIPANTS: Seven health care personnel were selected through professional networking. They were preferred because of their exposure to patients with Ebola during the epidemic at Mbarara, Uganda. RESULTS/FINDINGS: Written descriptions of the experience of 'waiting to know' whether exposure to patients with Ebola causes these participants to be infected, were obtained and analysed. Through immersion with the written descriptions, the following themes emerged: helplessness in anticipation and fear of dying or premature death; agonizing and languishing over losing relatives, friends, and loved ones; trusting no one, and; helplessness and hopelessness with the persistence of time.

PMID: 11851785 [PubMed - indexed for MEDLINE]

2077. J Gen Virol. 2002 Jan;83(Pt 1):67-73.

Sequence analysis of the GP, NP, VP40 and VP24 genes of Ebola virus isolated from deceased, surviving and asymptomatically infected individuals during the 1996 outbreak in Gabon: comparative studies and phylogenetic characterization.

Leroy EM(1), Baize S, Mavoungou E, Apetrei C.

Author information: (1)Centre International de Recherches Médicales de Franceville, BP 769 Franceville, Gabon. leroy@cirmf.sci.ga

The aims of this study were to determine if the clinical outcome of Ebola virus (EBOV) infection is associated with virus genetic structure and to document the genetic changes in the Gabon strains of EBOV by sequencing the GP, NP, VP40 and VP24 genes from deceased and surviving symptomatic and asymptomatic individuals. GP and NP sequences were identical in the three groups of patients and only one silent substitution occurred in the VP40 and VP24 genes in asymptomatic individuals. A strain from an asymptomatic individual had a reverse substitution to the Gabon-94 sequence, indicating that minor virus variants may cocirculate during an outbreak. These results suggest that the different clinical outcomes of EBOV infection do not result from virus mutations. Phylogenetic analysis confirmed that Gabon-96 belonged to the Zaire subtype of EBOV and revealed that synonymous substitution rates were higher than nonsynonymous substitution rates in the GP, VP40 and VP24 genes. In contrast, nonsynonymous substitutions predominated over synonymous substitutions in the NP gene of the two Gabon strains, pointing to divergent evolution of these strains and to selective pressures on this gene.

PMID: 11752702 [PubMed - indexed for MEDLINE]

2078. J Virol. 2002 Jan;76(1):406-10.

Reverse genetics demonstrates that proteolytic processing of the Ebola virus glycoprotein is not essential for replication in cell culture.

Neumann G(1), Feldmann H, Watanabe S, Lukashevich I, Kawaoka Y.

Author information: (1)Department of Pathobiological Sciences, School of Veterinary Medicine, University of Wisconsin-Madison, Madison, Wisconsin 53706, USA.

Ebola virus, a prime example of an emerging pathogen, causes fatal hemorrhagic fever in humans and in nonhuman primates. Identification of major determinants of Ebola virus pathogenicity has been hampered by the lack of effective strategies for experimental mutagenesis. Here we exploit a reverse genetics system that allows the generation of Ebola virus from cloned cDNA to engineer a mutant Ebola virus with an altered furin recognition motif in the glycoprotein (GP). When expressed in cells, the GP of the wild type, but not of the mutant, virus was cleaved into GP1 and GP2. Although posttranslational furin-mediated cleavage of GP was thought to be an essential step in Ebola virus infection, generation of a viable mutant Ebola virus lacking a furin recognition motif in the GP cleavage site demonstrates that GP cleavage is not essential for replication of Ebola virus in cell culture.

PMCID: PMC135697 PMID: 11739705 [PubMed - indexed for MEDLINE]

2079. Lancet Infect Dis. 2002 Jan;2(1):7.

Infectious disease surveillance update.

Shapiro DS.

PMID: 11892498 [PubMed - indexed for MEDLINE]

2080. Med Trop (Mars). 2002;62(3):295-300.

[Ebola: a virus endemic to central Africa?].

[Article in French]

Georges-Courbot MC(1), Leroy E, Zeller H.

Author information: (1)Centre National de Référence des Fièvres Hémorragiques Virales, Unité de Biologie des Infections virales émergentes, CRMPL, Laboratoire P4 Jean Mérieux, 21 Avenue Tony Garnier, 69365 Lyon. mgeorges@cervi-lyon.inserm.fr

From October 2001 to March 2002, an outbreak of Ebola haemorrhagic fever occurred in the North-Eastern Gabon (63 cases) and neighbouring Congo (57 cases). It was the fourth epidemic in North Eastern Gabon since 1994. Meanwhile this outbreak differed from the previous epidemics: at least five different emerging sources of the virus in the human population were observed from the local fauna resulting in fears of an endemic Ebola virus in the area. The control of the outbreak was uneasy because of the unfriendly attitude of the local population related to the restrictive measures for the isolation of suspected patients and the epidemiological surveillance. Such rejection process emphasizes the need of a continuous increasing public awareness.

PMID: 12244929 [PubMed - indexed for MEDLINE]

2081. Microbiol Immunol. 2002;46(9):633-8.

Development of an immunofluorescence method for the detection of antibodies to Ebola virus subtype Reston by the use of recombinant nucleoprotein-expressing HeLa cells.

Ikegami T(1), Saijo M, Niikura M, Miranda ME, Calaor AB, Hernandez M, Manalo DL, Kurane I, Yoshikawa Y, Morikawa S.

Author information: (1)Department of Virology I, National Institute of Infectious Diseases, Musashimurayama, Tokyo, Japan.

An indirect immunofluorescent assay (IFA) to detect Ebola virus subtype Reston (EBO-R) antibodies was developed by the use of a HeLa cell line stably expressing EBO-R nucleoprotein (NP). This IFA has a high specificity for the detection of EBO-R IgG antibodies in both hyperimmune rabbit sera and monkey sera collected during an EBO-R outbreak in the Philippines in 1996. Furthermore, this IFA showed a higher sensitivity for the detection of EBO-R antibodies than did the IFA using HeLa cells expressing the NP of Ebola virus subtype Zaire. These results suggest that this new IFA is useful for seroepidemiological studies of EBO-R infection among monkeys.

PMID: 12437031 [PubMed - indexed for MEDLINE]

2082. Nat Biotechnol. 2002 Jan;20(1):21-5.

Bioterrorism--biotechnology to the rescue?

Niiler E(1).

Author information: (1)eniiler@home.com

PMID: 11753354 [PubMed - indexed for MEDLINE]

2083. Trop Doct. 2002 Jan;32(1):10-5.

The outbreak and control of Ebola viral haemorrhagic fever in a Ugandan medical school.

Bitekyerezo M(1), Kyobutungi C, Kizza R, Mugeni J, Munyarugero E, Tirwomwe F, Twongyeirwe E, Muhindo G, Nakibuuka V, Nakate M, John L, Ruiz A, Frame K, Priotto G, Pepper L, Kabakyenga J, Baingana S, Ledo D.

Author information: (1)Mbarara University Teaching Hospital, Uganda.

Uganda has just experienced the largest outbreak of Ebola haemorrhagic fever (EHF) ever recorded. Mbarara University Teaching Hospital (MUTH) is responsible for training approximately one-third of Uganda's doctors. Mbarara is located in SouthWest Uganda, 614 km from Gulu, the main epicentre of the outbreak. On 23 October a patient was admitted to the medical ward of MUTH with an acute fever. He soon exhibited haemorrhagic symptoms and died. He was later confirmed to have suffered Ebola. Three more patients subsequently contracted the disease. All died. There were no further cases in Mbarara. No members of staff or medical student was infected. We give details of the clinical features of those patients who contracted the disease, the setting up of an Ebola isolation unit, the case surveillance and the search for the source of the outbreak. The implications for similar institutions in East Africa are discussed.

PMID: 11991014 [PubMed - indexed for MEDLINE]

2084. Wiad Lek. 2002;55 Suppl 1(Pt 2):686-93.

[The restructuring of national sanitary inspectorate with regard to environmental hazards and health needs of the population].

[Article in Polish]

Grabowski ML(1).

Author information: (1)Głównego Inspektoratu Sanitarnego w Warszawie. grabowski@gis.mz.gov.pl

The article presents the history of Polish sanitary and epidemiological services from 1918 until contemporary times. Emphasizing many achievements of National Sanitary Inspectorate, which are responsible for the low sick-rate of infectious diseases in Poland, the article also points to the increasing number and growing severity of environmental hazards in recent years. The article discusses problems caused by the "old" infectious diseases, which, though until recently regarded as passed, are posing threats to the society nowadays (e.g. TB, pestis, cholera). Equally, the article highlights problems caused by the "new" highly infectious diseases (e.g. Ebola fever, AIDS). Moreover, the article focuses on the particularly relevant subject of tackling biological weapons, the use of which can be traced past the recent events after September 11 and back to the Middle Ages. Finally, the article stresses the role of sanitary and epidemiological services in fighting recent animal epidemics, such as foot-and-mouth disease and mad cow disease. Discussing particular cases of the environmental hazards mentioned above, recorded in Poland, the article emphasizes the importance of the proper staff selection for National Sanitary Inspectorate. In the past decade in Poland, Sanitary Inspectors were selected mostly with regard to their political orientation, rather than their professional background. The author of the article hopes that human life and health will be treated with more respect in Poland in the neart future and the positions of Sanitary Inspectors will be given to professionals with proper epidemiological preparation. Radical changes in the policy of staff selection, modernization of training programs, as well as creation of a more practical structure of National Sanitary Inspectorate are the necessary conditions for transforming sanitary and epidemiological services in Poland into reliable and prestigious institutions, capable of dealing with the environmental hazards of the twenty-first century.

PMID: 17474584 [PubMed - indexed for MEDLINE]

2085. Zh Mikrobiol Epidemiol Immunobiol. 2002 Jan-Feb;(1):91-8.

[Viral haemorrhagic fevers--evolution of the epidemic potential].

[Article in Russian]

Markin VA(1), Markov VI.

Author information: (1)Center of Special Laboratory, Diagnostics and Treatment of Particularly Dangerous and Exotic Infectious Diseases, Sergiev Posad, Moscow Region, Russia.

In this review modern data on dangerous and particularly dangerous viral haemorrhagic fevers caused by a group of viruses belonging to the families of phylo-, arena-, flavi-, bunya- and togaviruses are presented. Morbidity rates and epidemics caused by Marburg virus, Ebola fever virus, Lassa fever virus, Argentinian and Bolivian haemorrhagic fever viruses, dengue haemorrhagic fever virus, Crimean haemorrhagic fever virus, Hantaviruses are analyzed. Mechanisms of the evolution of the epidemic manifestation of these infections are considered. The importance of the development of tools and methods of diagnosis, rapid prevention and treatment of exotic haemorrhagic fevers is emphasized.

PMID: 11949268 [PubMed - indexed for MEDLINE]

2086. Tidsskr Nor Laegeforen. 2001 Dec 10;121(30):3538-43.

[Microorganisms strike back--infectious diseases during the last 50 years].

[Article in Norwegian]

Solberg CO(1).

Author information: (1)Medisinsk avdeling Haukeland Sykehus 5021 Bergen. claus.solberg@haukeland.no

In the first half of the 20th century, improved living conditions, preventive measures, vaccines and antibiotics led to a marked reduction in morbidity and mortality from infectious diseases. It was predicted that the conquest of all infectious diseases was imminent. However, 50 years later, in 1999, they were still the major cause of disease worldwide, and caused nearly one third of all deaths (a total of 55.9 million). The eradication of smallpox in the 1970s and the approaching eradication of poliomyelitis represent major achievements. The prevalence of measles, pertussis and tetanus neonatorum is also markedly reduced, but still 1.5 million children in developing countries die each year because of lack of vaccines. Malaria and tuberculosis are re-emerging. Tuberculosis and HIV/AIDS are the diseases with known aetiology that cause most deaths, altogether 5 million each year. Respiratory and gastrointestinal infections cause 6.5 million deaths annually. Infections in the immunocompromised host have become a trade mark of today's advanced medicine. Almost every year, new diseases related to new micro-organisms are described; over the last 30 years, approximately 40 new diseases/micro-organisms have been diagnosed. Among the best known are HIV/AIDS, peptic ulcer caused by Helicobacter pylori, Legionnaires' disease, borreliosis (Lyme disease), hepatitis C, gastroenteritis caused by rotavirus, and Ebola haemorrhagic fever. Antimicrobial resistance development of micro-organisms has become one of the major health problems worldwide; a number of preventive measures are being introduced.

PMID: 11808014 [PubMed - indexed for MEDLINE]

2087. Afr Health Sci. 2001 Dec;1(2):60-5.

Ebola haemorrhagic fever among hospitalised children and adolescents in northern Uganda: epidemiologic and clinical observations.

Mupere E(1), Kaducu OF, Yoti Z.

Author information: (1)Gulu Regional Referral Hospital Northern Uganda, P. O. Box 160, Gulu, Uganda. mupez@yahoo.com

BACKGROUND: A unique feature of previous Ebola outbreaks has been the relative sparing of children. For the first time, an out break of an unusual illness-Ebola haemorrhagic fever occurred in Northern Uganda Gulu district. OBJECTIVES: To describe the epidemiologic and clinical aspects of hospitalised children and adolescents on the isolation wards. METHODS: A retrospective descriptive survey of hospital records for hospitalised children and adolescents under 18 years on the isolation wards in Gulu, Northern Uganda was conducted. All patient test notes were consecutively reviewed and non was excluded because being deficient. RESULTS: Analysis revealed that 90 out of the 218 national laboratory confirmed Ebola cases were children and adolescents with a case fatality of 40%. The mean age was 8.2 years +/- SD 5.6 with a range of 16.99 years. The youngest child on the isolation wards was 3 days old. The under fives contributed the highest admission (35%) among children and adolescents; and case fatality because of prolonged close contact with the seropositive relatives among the laboratory confirmed cases. All (100%) Ebola positive children and adolescents were febrile while only 16% had hemorrhagic manifestations. CONCLUSION: Similar to previous Ebola outbreaks, a relative sparing of children in this outbreak was observed. The under fives were at an increased risk of

contact with the sick and dying. RECOMMENDATIONS: Strategies to shield children from exposure to dying and sick Ebola relatives are recommended in the event of future Ebola outbreaks. Health education to children and adolescents to avoid contact with sick and their body fluids should be emphasized.
PMCID: PMC2141551 PMID: 12789118 [PubMed - indexed for MEDLINE]

2088. Bull Exp Biol Med. 2001 Dec;132(6):1182-6.

Study of the pathogenesis of Ebola fever in laboratory animals with different sensitivity to this virus.

Chepurnov AA(1), Dadaeva AA, Kolesnikov SI.

Author information: (1)Laboratory of Especially Dangerous Viral Infection, Vektor State Research Center for Virology and Biotechnology, Ministry of Health, Kol'tsovo, Novosibirsk Region. chepurnov@vector.nsc.ru

Pathophysiological parameters were compared in animals with different sensitivity to Ebola virus infected with this virus. Analysis of the results showed the differences in immune reactions underlying the difference between Ebola-sensitive and Ebola-resistant animals. No neutrophil activation in response to Ebola virus injection was noted in Ebola-sensitive animal. Phagocytic activity of neutrophils in these animals inversely correlated with animal sensitivity to Ebola virus. Animal susceptibility to Ebola virus directly correlated with the decrease in the number of circulating T and B cells. We conclude that the immune system plays the key role in animal susceptibility and resistance to Ebola virus.
PMID: 12152882 [PubMed - indexed for MEDLINE]

2089. J Virol. 2001 Dec;75(23):11709-19.

Identification, phylogeny, and evolution of retroviral elements based on their envelope genes.

Bénit L(1), Dessen P, Heidmann T.

Author information: (1)Unité des Rétrovirus Endogènes et Eléments Rétroïdes des Eucaryotes Supérieurs, CNRS UMR 1573, Institut Gustave Roussy, 94805 Villejuif Cedex, France.

Phylogenetic analyses of retroviral elements, including endogenous retroviruses, have relied essentially on the retroviral pol gene expressing the highly conserved reverse transcriptase. This enzyme is essential for the life cycle of all retroid elements, but other genes are also endowed with conserved essential functions. Among them, the transmembrane (TM) subunit of the envelope gene is involved in virus entry through membrane fusion. It has also been reported to contain a domain, named the immunosuppressive domain, that has immunosuppressive properties most probably essential for virus spread within the host. This domain is conserved among a large series of retroviral elements, and we have therefore attempted to generate phylogenetic links between retroviral elements identified from databases following tentative alignments of the immunosuppressive domain and adjacent sequences. This allowed us to unravel a conserved organization among TM domains, also found in the Ebola and Marburg filoviruses, and to identify a large number of human endogenous retroviruses (HERVs) from sequence databases. The latter elements are part of previously identified families of HERVs, and some of them define new families. A general phylogenetic analysis based on the TM proteins of retroelements, and including those with no clearly identified immunosuppressive domain, could then be derived and compared with pol-based phylogenetic trees, providing a comprehensive survey of retroelements and definitive evidence for recombination events in the generation of both the endogenous and the present-day infectious retroviruses.
PMCID: PMC114757 PMID: 11689652 [PubMed - indexed for MEDLINE]

2090. J Virol. 2001 Dec;75(23):11677-85.

Individual and bivalent vaccines based on alphavirus replicons protect guinea pigs against infection with Lassa and Ebola viruses.

Pushko P(1), Geisbert J, Parker M, Jahrling P, Smith J.

Author information: (1)Virology Division, United States Army Medical Research Institute for Infectious Diseases, Fort Detrick, Frederick, Maryland 21702, USA. peter.pushko@amedd.army.mil

Lassa and Ebola viruses cause acute, often fatal, hemorrhagic fever diseases, for which no effective vaccines are currently available. Although lethal human disease outbreaks have been confined so far to sub-Saharan Africa, they also pose significant epidemiological concern worldwide as demonstrated by several instances of accidental importation of the viruses into North America and Europe. In the present study, we developed experimental individual vaccines for Lassa virus and bivalent vaccines for Lassa and Ebola viruses that are based on an RNA replicon vector derived from an attenuated strain of Venezuelan equine encephalitis virus. The Lassa and Ebola virus genes were expressed from recombinant replicon RNAs that also encoded the replicase function and were capable of efficient intracellular self-amplification. For vaccinations, the recombinant replicons were incorporated into virus-like replicon particles. Guinea pigs vaccinated with particles expressing Lassa virus nucleoprotein or glycoprotein genes were protected from lethal challenge with Lassa virus. Vaccination with particles expressing Ebola virus glycoprotein gene also protected the animals from lethal challenge with Ebola virus. In order to evaluate a single vaccine protecting against both Lassa and Ebola viruses, we developed dual-expression particles that expressed glycoprotein genes of both Ebola and Lassa viruses. Vaccination of guinea pigs with either dual-expression particles or with a mixture of particles expressing Ebola and Lassa virus glycoprotein genes protected the animals against challenges with Ebola and Lassa viruses. The results showed that immune responses can be induced against multiple vaccine antigens coexpressed from an alphavirus replicon and suggested the possibility of engineering multivalent vaccines based upon alphavirus vectors for arenaviruses, filoviruses, and possibly other emerging pathogens.
PMCID: PMC114754 PMID: 11689649 [PubMed - indexed for MEDLINE]

2091. Mol Diagn. 2001 Dec;6(4):323-33.

Biological agents: weapons of warfare and bioterrorism.

Broussard LA(1).

Author information: (1)Department of Clinical Laboratory Sciences, Louisiana State University Health Sciences Center, New Orleans, LA 70112, USA. lbrous@lsuhsc.edu

The use of microorganisms as agents of biological warfare is considered inevitable for several reasons, including ease of production and dispersion, delayed onset, ability to cause high rates of morbidity and mortality, and difficulty in diagnosis. Biological agents that have been identified as posing the greatest threat are variola major (smallpox), Bacillus anthracis (anthrax), Yersinia pestis (plague), Clostridium botulinum toxin (botulism), Francisella tularensis (tularaemia), filoviruses (Ebola hemorrrhagic fever and Marburg hemorrhagic fever), and arenaviruses Lassa (Lassa fever) and Junin (Argentine hemorrhagic fever). The pathogenesis, clinical manifestations, diagnosis, and treatment of these agents are discussed. Rapid identification and diagnosis using molecular diagnostic techniques such as PCR is an essential element in the establishment of coordinated laboratory response systems and is the focus of current research and development. Molecular techniques for detection and identification of these organisms are reviewed.

PMID: 11774197 [PubMed - indexed for MEDLINE]

2092. Nat Med. 2001 Dec;7(12):1313-9.

HIV-1 and Ebola virus encode small peptide motifs that recruit Tsg101 to sites of particle assembly to facilitate egress.

Martin-Serrano J(1), Zang T, Bieniasz PD.

Author information: (1)Aaron Diamond AIDS Research Center and The Rockefeller University, New York, New York, USA.

Comment in Nat Med. 2001 Dec;7(12):1278-80.

Retroviral Gag proteins encode sequences, termed late domains, which facilitate the final stages of particle budding from the plasma membrane. We report here that interactions between Tsg101, a factor involved in endosomal protein sorting, and short peptide motifs in the HIV-1 Gag late domain and Ebola virus matrix (EbVp40) proteins are essential for efficient egress of HIV-1 virions and Ebola virus-like particles. EbVp40 recruits Tsg101 to sites of particle assembly and a short, EbVp40-derived Tsg101-binding peptide sequence can functionally substitute for the HIV-1 Gag late domain. Notably, recruitment of Tsg101 to assembling virions restores budding competence to a late-domain-defective HIV-1 in the complete absence of viral late domain. These studies define an essential virus-host interaction that is conserved in two unrelated viruses. Because the Tsg101 is recruited by small, conserved viral sequence motifs, agents that mimic these structures are potential inhibitors of the replication of these lethal human pathogens.

PMID: 11726971 [PubMed - indexed for MEDLINE]

2093. Nat Med. 2001 Dec;7(12):1278-80.

HIV-1 and Ebola virus: the getaway driver nabbed.

Luban J.

Comment on Nat Med. 2001 Dec;7(12):1313-9.

PMID: 11726960 [PubMed - indexed for MEDLINE]

2094. Nursing. 2001 Dec;31(12):30.

Ebola: preparing for the worst.

McConnell EA.

PMID: 11921713 [PubMed - indexed for MEDLINE]

2095. Virus Res. 2001 Nov 28;80(1-2):117-23.

Symposium on Marburg and Ebola viruses.

Klenk HD(1), Feldmann H.

Author information: (1)Institut für Virologie, Philipps-Universität, Robert-Koch-Str. 17, D-35037, Marburg, Germany.

PMID: 11597757 [PubMed - indexed for MEDLINE]

2096. Clin Infect Dis. 2001 Nov 15;33(10):1707-12. Epub 2001 Oct 10.

Viral hemorrhagic fever hazards for travelers in Africa.

Isaäcson M(1).

Author information: (1)Department of Clinical Microbiology and Infectious Diseases, South African Institute for Medical Research, Johannesburg, South Africa. misaacson@worldonline.co.za

This short review covers 6 viral hemorrhagic fevers (VHFs) that are known to occur in Africa: yellow fever, Rift Valley fever, Crimean-Congo hemorrhagic fever, Lassa fever, Marburg virus disease, and Ebola hemorrhagic fever. All of these have at one time or another affected travelers, often the adventurous kind who are "roughing it" in rural areas, who should therefore be made aware by their physicians or travel health clinics about their potential risk of exposure to any VHF along their travel route and how to minimize the risk. A significant proportion of VHF cases involving travelers have affected expatriate health care workers who were nosocomially exposed in African hospitals or clinics. The VHFs are associated with a high case-fatality rate but are readily prevented by well-known basic precautions.

PMID: 11595975 [PubMed - indexed for MEDLINE]

2097. Cell Mol Life Sci. 2001 Nov;58(12-13):1826-41.

Ebola virus: the search for vaccines and treatments.

Wilson JA(1), Bosio CM, Hart MK.

Author information: (1)Virology Division, United States Army Medical Research Institute of Infectious Diseases, Fort Detrick, Frederick, Maryland 21702-5011, USA.

Ebola viruses belong to the family Filoviridae, which are among the most virulent infectious agents known. These viruses cause acute, and frequently fatal, hemorrhagic fever in humans and nonhuman primates. Currently, no vaccines or treatments are available for human use. This review describes Ebola viruses, with a particular focus on the status of research efforts to develop vaccines and therapeutics and to identify the immune mechanisms of protection.
PMID: 11766882 [PubMed - indexed for MEDLINE]

2098. J Clin Microbiol. 2001 Nov;39(11):4125-30.

Development and evaluation of a fluorogenic 5' nuclease assay to detect and differentiate between Ebola virus subtypes Zaire and Sudan.

Gibb TR(1), Norwood DA Jr, Woollen N, Henchal EA.

Author information: (1)Diagnostic Systems Division, United States Army Medical Research Institute of Infectious Diseases, Fort Detrick, Maryland 21702-5011, USA. Tammy.Gibb@SBCCOM.APGEA.ARMY.MIL

The ability to rapidly recognize Ebola virus infections is critical to quickly limit further spread of the disease. A rapid, sensitive, and specific laboratory diagnostic test is needed to confirm outbreaks of Ebola virus infection and to distinguish it from other diseases that can cause similar clinical symptoms. A one-tube reverse transcription-PCR assay for the identification of Ebola virus subtype Zaire (Ebola Zaire) and Ebola virus subtype Sudan (Ebola Sudan) was developed and evaluated by using the ABI PRISM 7700 sequence detection system. This assay uses one common primer set and two differentially labeled fluorescent probes to simultaneously detect and differentiate these two subtypes of Ebola virus. The sensitivity of the primer set was comparable to that of previously designed primer sets, as determined by limit-of-detection experiments. This assay is unique in its ability to simultaneously detect and differentiate Ebola Zaire and Ebola Sudan. In addition, this assay is compatible with emerging rapid nucleic acid analysis platforms and therefore may prove to be a very useful diagnostic tool for the control and management of future outbreaks.
PMCID: PMC88497 PMID: 11682540 [PubMed - indexed for MEDLINE]

2099. J Comp Pathol. 2001 Nov;125(4):243-53.

Haematological, biochemical and coagulation changes in mice, guinea-pigs and monkeys infected with a mouse-adapted variant of Ebola Zaire virus.

Bray M(1), Hatfill S, Hensley L, Huggins JW.

Author information: (1)Virology Division, United States Army Medical Research Institute of Infectious Diseases (USAMRIID), Fort Detrick, Frederick, Maryland 21702-5011, USA.

Ebola Zaire virus from the 1976 outbreak (EBO-Z) was recently adapted to the stage of lethal virulence in BALB/c mice through serial passage. In the present study, various parameters were examined in groups of mice and guinea-pigs and in three rhesus monkeys after infection with mouse-adapted EBO-Z. The virus caused fatal disease not only in mice but also in guinea-pigs, in which the course of illness resembled that produced by guinea-pig-adapted EBO-Z. Mice, guinea-pigs and monkeys showed similar haematological and biochemical disturbances, but coagulopathy was less striking in mice than in the other two species. The virus caused severe illness in all three monkeys, one of which died. In the lethally infected monkey the degree of viraemia and the haematological, serum biochemical and coagulation changes were greater than in the other two animals, an observation that may prove to be of value in predicting fatal outcome. All three monkeys developed disseminated intravascular coagulation. The two survivors were completely resistant to challenge one year later with non-adapted EBO-Z. In general, the clinical and pathological changes produced in the three species resembled those previously described in guinea-pigs and non-human primates infected with non-mouse-adapted EBO-Z. It was noteworthy, however, that mouse-adaptation appeared to have resulted in a degree of attenuation for monkeys.
Copyright Harcourt Publishers Ltd.
PMID: 11798241 [PubMed - indexed for MEDLINE]

2100. J Comp Pathol. 2001 Nov;125(4):233-42.

Pathogenesis of experimental Ebola Zaire virus infection in BALB/c mice.

Gibb TR(1), Bray M, Geisbert TW, Steele KE, Kell WM, Davis KJ, Jaax NK.

Author information: (1)Diagnostic Systems, United States Army Medical Research Institute of Infectious Diseases (USAMRIID), Fort Detrick, Frederick, Maryland 21702-5011, USA.

Guinea-pigs and non-human primates have traditionally been used as animal models for studying Ebola Zaire virus (EBO-Z) infections. The virus was also recently adapted to the stage of lethal virulence in BALB/c mice. This murine model is now in use for testing antiviral medications and vaccines. However, the pathological features of EBO-Z infection in mice have not yet been fully described. To identify sites of viral replication and characterize sequential morphological changes in BALB/c mice, adult female mice were infected with mouse-adapted EBO-Z and killed in groups each day for 5 days post-infection. Tissues were examined by light microscopy, immunohistochemistry, electron microscopy and in-situ hybridization. As in guinea-pigs and non-human primates, cells of the mononuclear phagocytic system were the earliest targets of infection. Viral replication was observed by day 2 in macrophages in lymph nodes and spleen. By the time of onset of illness and weight loss (day 3), the infection had spread to hepatocytes and adrenal cortical cells, and to macrophages and fibroblast-like cells in many organs. Severe lymphocytolysis was observed in the spleen, lymph nodes and thymus. There was minimal infection of endothelial cells. All of these changes resembled those observed in EBO-Z-infected guinea-pigs and non-human primates. In contrast to the other animal models, however, there was little fibrin deposition in the late stage of disease. The availability of immunodeficient, gene-knockout and transgenic mice will make the mouse model particularly useful for studying the early steps of Ebola pathogenesis.
Copyright Harcourt Publishers Ltd.
PMID: 11798240 [PubMed - indexed for MEDLINE]

2101. J Med Virol. 2001 Nov;65(3):561-6.

Multiplex analysis of cytokines in the blood of cynomolgus macaques naturally infected with Ebola virus (Reston serotype).

Hutchinson KL(1), Villinger F, Miranda ME, Ksiazek TG, Peters CJ, Rollin PE.

Author information: (1)Special Pathogens Branch, Division of Viral and Rickettsial Diseases, Centers for Disease Control and Prevention, 1600 Clifton Road NE, Mail stop G14, Atlanta, GA 30333, USA. khutchinson@cdc.gov

Ebola virus (EBO) causes the most severe form of viral hemorrhagic fever in humans and nonhuman primates with up to 90% of infections culminating in death. The requirement of maximum containment laboratories for Ebola virus research has limited opportunities to study the pathogenesis of EBO infections. While tissue damage does occur, often it would appear not to be sufficient to explain death, indicating that soluble mediators play an important role in disease progression. In previous studies, fatal human infections with the Zaire subtype of Ebola (EBO-Z) were associated with an increase in the levels of inflammatory cytokines. In this investigation, a new multiplex assay was developed and used to measure circulating levels of cytokines and chemokines in cynomolgus macaques infected with the Reston subtype of EBO (EBO-R). Increased levels of IL-6, TNF-alpha, IFN-gamma, IL-2, IL-4, IL-8, IL-10, and GM-CSF were detected in infected animals, and the increase in circulating cytokines correlated with an increase in circulating viral antigen. Blood samples from animals showing high levels of cytokines were also tested for the chemokines: MCP-1, IL-1beta, MIP-1alpha, MIP-1beta, IP-10, and RANTES. High levels of MCP-1 and MIP-1beta, and RANTES were found in infected primates and, while levels were more variable, IL-1beta was detected only in infected animals.

PMID: 11596094 [PubMed - indexed for MEDLINE]

2102. J Virol. 2001 Nov;75(22):11025-33.

Infection and activation of monocytes by Marburg and Ebola viruses.

Ströher U(1), West E, Bugany H, Klenk HD, Schnittler HJ, Feldmann H.

Author information: (1)Institut für Virologie, Philipps-Universität, D-35037 Marburg, Germany.

In this study we investigated the effects of Marburg virus and Ebola virus (species Zaire and Reston) infections on freshly isolated suspended monocytes in comparison to adherent macrophages under culture conditions. Our data showed that monocytes are permissive for both filoviruses. As is the case in macrophages, infection resulted in the activation of monocytes which was largely independent of virus replication. The activation was triggered similarly by Marburg and Ebola viruses, species Zaire and Reston, as indicated by the release of the proinflammatory cytokines interleukin-1beta (IL-1beta), tumor necrosis factor alpha, and IL-6 as well as the chemokines IL-8 and gro-alpha. Our data suggest that infected monocytes may play an important role in the spread of filoviruses and in the pathogenesis of filoviral hemorrhagic disease.

PMCID: PMC114683 PMID: 11602743 [PubMed - indexed for MEDLINE]

2103. Vopr Virusol. 2001 Nov-Dec;46(6):43-5.

[Dynamics of expression of Marburg and Ebola virus antigens in infected Vero cells].

[Article in Russian]

Titenko AM, Andaev EI, Borisova TI.

Time course of Marburg and Ebola virus antigens expression in Vero cells was studied by indirect immunofluorescence test. The maximum accumulation of virus specific antigens in Vero cells infected with a high dose was observed after 48-54 h of incubation. It is essential for laboratory diagnosis that virus specific antigens can present as incorporations of different shape and size, starting from small hardly discernible granules (immediately after the virus adsorption) to large lumps, cords, accumulations, and diffuse fluorescence.

PMID: 11785389 [PubMed - indexed for MEDLINE]

2104. Lancet. 2001 Oct 20;358(9290):1350.

Caring for the survivors of Uganda's Ebola epidemic one year on.

Wendo C.

PMID: 11684230 [PubMed - indexed for MEDLINE]

2105. Arch Virol. 2001 Oct;146(10):2021-7.

Genome structure of Ebola virus subtype Reston: differences among Ebola subtypes. Brief report.

Ikegami T(1), Calaor AB, Miranda ME, Niikura M, Saijo M, Kurane I, Yoshikawa Y, Morikawa S.

Author information: (1)Department of Virology I, National Institute of Infectious Diseases, Tokyo, Japan.

We determined the complete genome sequence of Ebola virus subtype Reston (EBO-R) in the Philippines in 1996. The deduced transcriptional signals were highly conserved among Ebola viruses except for the stop signal of L genes. The intergenic regions were composed of 4 to 7 nucleotides, and of 2 characteristic overlaps and a long intergenic region. The glycoprotein (GP) had several amino acid differences from EBO-R isolated in 1989 and 1992. The variety of GP sequences strongly suggests the independent introduction of EBO-R from unknown natural reservoirs in 1996.

PMID: 11722021 [PubMed - indexed for MEDLINE]

2106. Curr Opin Infect Dis. 2001 Oct;14(5):513-8.

Recent advances in vaccines against viral haemorrhagic fevers.

Baize S(1), Marianneau P, Georges-Courbot MC, Deubel V.

Author information: (1)Unit of Biology of Emerging Viral Infections, Mérieux-Pasteur Research Centre, Lyon, France.

Development of vaccines against viral haemorrhagic fevers is a public health priority. Recent advances in our knowledge of pathogenesis and of the immune responses elicited by these viruses emphasize the crucial role of the immune system in the control of infection, but also its probable involvement in pathogenesis. Several vaccine candidates against viral haemorrhagic fevers have been evaluated in animals during the past year. Together, these data suggest that a vaccine approach against viral haemorrhagic fevers is feasible, should induce well-balanced immune responses with cellular and humoral components, and should avoid the potential deleterious effects that are associated with such immune responses.

PMID: 11964870 [PubMed - indexed for MEDLINE]

2107. Indian J Pathol Microbiol. 2001 Oct;44(4):391-2.

Bioterrorism.

Shahi SK, Ranga S, Gupta P.

PMID: 12035346 [PubMed - indexed for MEDLINE]

2108. J Nippon Med Sch. 2001 Oct;68(5):370-5.

Ebola hemorrhagic fever (EHF): mechanism of transmission and pathogenicity.

Mwanatambwe M(1), Yamada N, Arai S, Shimizu-Suganuma M, Shichinohe K, Asano G.

Author information: (1)Department of Pathology, Nippon Medical School, Tokyo, Japan.

Hemorrhagic fevers represent a wide spectrum of viral infectious diseases, out-breaking mostly as epidemics, some of them being highly lethal. They range from those caused by bunyaviridae, associated with renal or pulmonary syndromes and those recently emerging and caused by the filoviridae family of thread-like viruses. Among the latter, Ebola hemorrhagic fever (EHF) bears the highest mortality and morbidity rates. One form of the disease has been documented only in monkeys. The human form, has occurred mainly in areas surrounding rain forests in central Africa. Patients present with signs of hemorrhagic diathesis, fever, diarrhea and neurological disorders, leading sometimes to confusion with local endemic diseases. Fatal victims of the disease die of dehydration. Poor hygienic conditions facilitate the spread of the virus. Biologically, the virus seems to target both the host blood coagulative and immune defense systems. Intensive epidemiologic search have failed to establish the definitive natural host of the virus. Twice, with a 19-year interval, major outbreaks have taken place in the Democratic Republic of the Congo. The second major outbreak in the northwestern city of Kikwit in April 1995 will serve here to elucidate the mechanism of the viral infection.

PMID: 11598619 [PubMed - indexed for MEDLINE]

2109. Nihon Koshu Eisei Zasshi. 2001 Oct;48(10):853-9.

[Epidemics and related cultural factors for Ebola hemorrhagic fever in Gabon].

[Article in Japanese]

Kunii O(1), Kita E, Shibuya K.

Author information: (1)Department of International Community Health, Graduate School of Medicine, The University of Tokyo.

OBJECTIVE: The Republic of Gabon experienced epidemics of Ebola hemorrhagic fever (EHF) three times between 1994 and 1997. This study aimed at exploring cultural factors related to the outbreaks. METHODS: We collected information about EHF epidemics from the Gabon Ministry of Health, district hospitals and other facilities and conducted in-depth interviews with 20 villagers and 2 traditional healers in the village where the third epidemic occurred. RESULTS: All three epidemics were supposed to have direct or indirect relationship with great apes, the victims having cooked or eaten chimpanzees meat. Although the reuse of syringes and needles in hospitals which had worsened past EHF outbreaks in Sudan and Zaire did not contribute to the outbreak in Gabon, traditional practices as family members remaining close to the patient to nurse him/her, and hugging and touching the dead at funerals were suspected to be crucial sources of infection. Interviews with traditional healers revealed that traditional treatment methods as cutting a patient' skin with an unsterilized knife and applying blood to the skin were risky and might have been contributory factors in the deaths of one traditionals healer and his assistant in the third EHF outbreak. In one village where EHF had reached epidemic proportions, in-depth interviews were conducted with 2 traditional healers and 20 persons of mean age 33 (20-46) years with a sampling method of selecting every tenth household from the entrance. Even though they lived in a village suffering an EHF outbreak, only two thirds of them knew the name of the disease and about half of them could not explain what kind of disease it was. One quarter felt it was fatal and another quarter felt fearful. Three persons thought it had been due to evil spirits; others responded the mosquitoes or patient's sweat/saliva were the cause. CONCLUSIONS: This study showed that cultural factors might be very crucial to EHF outbreaks in developing countries. Quick intervention with health education is needed to disseminate appropriate knowledge and persuade people that traditional practices could carry a high risk of infection.

PMID: 11725529 [PubMed - indexed for MEDLINE]

2110. Trends Microbiol. 2001 Oct;9(10):506-11.

The pathogenesis of Ebola hemorrhagic fever.

Takada A(1), Kawaoka Y.

Author information: (1)Division of Virology, Department of Microbiology and Immunology, Institute of Medical Science, University of Tokyo, Tokyo 108-8639, Japan.

Ebola virus causes lethal hemorrhagic disease in humans, yet there are still no satisfactory biological explanations to account for its extreme virulence. This review focuses on recent findings relevant to understanding the pathogenesis of Ebola virus infection and developing vaccines and effective therapy. The available data suggest that the envelope glycoprotein and the interaction of some viral proteins with the immune system are likely to play important roles in the extraordinary pathogenicity of this virus. There are also indications that genetically engineered vaccines, including plasmid DNA and viral vectors expressing Ebola virus proteins, and passive transfer of neutralizing antibodies could be feasible options for the control of Ebola virus-associated disease.

PMID: 11597453 [PubMed - indexed for MEDLINE]

2111. J Clin Microbiol. 2001 Sep;39(9):3267-71.

Detection of Ebola viral antigen by enzyme-linked immunosorbent assay using a novel monoclonal antibody to nucleoprotein.

Niikura M(1), Ikegami T, Saijo M, Kurane I, Miranda ME, Morikawa S.

Author information: (1)Department of Virology I, National Institute of Infectious Diseases, Tokyo, Japan.

With the increase in international traffic, the risk of introducing rare but severe infectious diseases like Ebola hemorrhagic fever is increasing all over the world. However, the system for the diagnosis of Ebola virus infection is available in a limited number of countries. In the present study, we developed an Ebola virus antigen-detection enzyme-linked immunosorbent assay (ELISA) system using a novel monoclonal antibody (MAb) to the nucleoprotein (NP). This antibody recognized an epitope defined by a 26-amino-acid stretch near the C terminus of NP. In a sandwich ELISA system with the MAb, as little as 30 ng of purified recombinant NP (rNP) was detected. Although this MAb was prepared by immunization with rNP of subtype Zaire, it also reacted to the corresponding region of NP derived from the Reston and Sudan subtypes. These results suggest that our ELISA system should work with three of four Ebola subtypes. Furthermore, our ELISA system detected the NP in subtype Reston-infected monkey specimens, while the background level in noninfected specimens was very low, suggesting the usefulness of the ELISA for laboratory diagnosis with clinical specimens.

PMCID: PMC88329 PMID: 11526161 [PubMed - indexed for MEDLINE]

2112. Vopr Virusol. 2001 Sep-Oct;46(5):25-31.

[Antigenic structure of Ebola virus VP35 protein].

[Article in Russian]

Kazachinskaia EI, Ternovoĭ VA, Rudzevich TN, Netesov SV, Chepurnov AA, Razumov IA.

Antigenic structure of Ebola virus (EV) (strain Mayinga) nucleocapsid protein VP35 was analyzed using monoclonal antibodies to EV VP35 and polyclonal antibodies to EV. EV protein VP35 was shown to have antigenic sites inducing the production of antibodies in animals. For better characterization of protein VP35 antigenic structure. EV gene encoding the full-length VP35 was cloned in vector pQE31 as a recombinant fusion protein (rec.VP35). The antigenic and immunogenic properties of rec.VP35 and EV VP35 were compared by ELISA and Western blot analysis with polyclonal and monoclonal antibodies. Antibodies of positive sera and VP35 MAbs cross reacted with the analyzed antigens. The topography of epitopes on EV VP35 and rec.VP35 was studied using MAbs and polyclonal antibodies to rec.VP35 in a competitive antibody binding assay. Two epitopes of one site were identified on these proteins. These epitopes are present on infectious virion protein VP35 and are stable during physicochemical exposures.

PMID: 11715705 [PubMed - indexed for MEDLINE]

2113. Curr Opin Infect Dis. 2001 Aug;14(4):467-80.

Emerging viral infections.

Lee LM(1), Henderson DK.

Author information: (1)Office of the Deputy Director for Clinical Care, Warren Grant Magnuson Clinical Center, National Institutes of Health, Bethesda, Maryland 20892, USA.

The past decade has witnessed the emergence of several significant viral pathogens and the further evolution of additional viral pathogens. Transmitted by a variety of differing routes, these organisms have presented substantial intellectual challenges to medicine of the 20th and 21st centuries. As perhaps the benchmark pathogen of the past decade, HIV has provided medicine and society with a most formidable opponent, and one that has yet to be fully conquered. Nonetheless, a variety of additional viral pathogens have also perplexed medicine over the past 10-15 years.

PMID: 11964867 [PubMed - indexed for MEDLINE]

2114. Virology. 2001 Aug 1;286(2):384-90.

Vaccine potential of Ebola virus VP24, VP30, VP35, and VP40 proteins.

Wilson JA(1), Bray M, Bakken R, Hart MK.

Author information: (1)Virology Division, United States Army Medical Research Institute of Infectious Diseases, 1425 Porter Street, Fort Detrick, Frederick, Maryland 21702-5011, USA.

Previous vaccine efforts with Ebola virus Zaire (EBOV-Z) emphasized the potential protective efficacies of immune responses to the surface glycoprotein and the nucleoprotein. To determine whether the VP24, VP30, VP35, and VP40 proteins are also capable of eliciting protective immune responses, these genes were expressed from alphavirus replicons and used to vaccinate BALB/c and C57BL/6 mice. Although all of the VP proteins were capable of inducing protective immune responses, no single VP protein protected both strains of mice tested. VP24, VP30, and VP40 induced protective immune responses in BALB/c mice, whereas C57BL/6 mice survived challenge only after vaccination with VP35. Passive transfer of immune sera to the VP proteins did not protect unvaccinated mice from lethal disease. The demonstration that the VP proteins are capable of eliciting protective immune responses to EBOV-Z indicates that they may be important components of a vaccine designed to protect humans from Ebola hemorrhagic fever.

PMID: 11485406 [PubMed - indexed for MEDLINE]

2115. Cell. 2001 Jul 13;106(1):117-26.

Folate receptor-alpha is a cofactor for cellular entry by Marburg and Ebola viruses.

Chan SY(1), Empig CJ, Welte FJ, Speck RF, Schmaljohn A, Kreisberg JF, Goldsmith MA.

Author information: (1)Gladstone Institute of Virology and Immunology, San Francisco, CA 94141, USA.

Human infections by Marburg (MBG) and Ebola (EBO) viruses result in lethal hemorrhagic fever. To identify cellular entry factors employed by MBG virus, noninfectible cells transduced with an expression library were challenged with a selectable pseudotype virus packaged by MBG glycoproteins (GP). A cDNA encoding the folate receptor-alpha (FR-alpha) was recovered from cells exhibiting reconstitution of viral entry. A FR-alpha cDNA was recovered in a similar strategy employing EBO pseudotypes. FR-alpha expression in Jurkat cells facilitated MBG or EBO entry, and FR-blocking reagents inhibited infection by MBG or EBO. Finally, FR-alpha bound cells expressing MBG or EBO GP and mediated syncytia formation triggered by MBG GP. Thus, FR-alpha is a significant cofactor for cellular entry for MBG and EBO viruses.

PMID: 11461707 [PubMed - indexed for MEDLINE]

2116. Science. 2001 Jul 13;293(5528):191.

Virology. New finding heats up the hot zone.

Cohen J.

PMID: 11452091 [PubMed - indexed for MEDLINE]

2117. Ann Pharm Fr. 2001 Jul;59(4):246-77.

[The worldwide challenges of "new" or reemerging communicable diseases at the dawn of the 21st century].

[Article in French]

Werner GH(1).

Author information: (1)Membre Associé Libre de l'Académie nationale de Pharmacie.

In the first part of this review, AIDS, prion diseases, Hantavirus and arbovirus infections, Ebola hemorrhagic fever, legionellosis, hepatitis C, enterotoxigenic Escherichia coli infections, Lyme disease, tuberculosis have provided alarming examples of emerging or reemerging infectious diseases. In this second part, the stress is placed on the reemergence of diphtheria and of serious streptococcal infections, on bartonelloses, Chlamydia infections, fungal infections, while malaria and cholera are still prevalent in several areas. The increasing resistance of too many pathogens to antimicrobial agents is a major source of concern, directly related to the challenge of nosocomial infections. An infectious cause has been demonstrated (or strongly suspected) for various diseases and the scope of infectiology keeps widening, while the threat of bioterrorism cannot be neglected. The causes of the emergence or reemergence of infectious diseases are multiple and diverse, often in direct relation with human activities (population migrations, changes in husbandry or farming practices, worldwide exchanges of goods and foods, inadequate uses of antibiotics) but also with climatic variations in several areas. The challenge represented by this unexpected comeback of infections to the forefront of human and animal pathology can only be met with a significant improvement of hygienic practices, cessation of certain dangerous behaviors and also, of course, with the development of novel antimicrobial molecules (acting on original targets) as well as of a whole series of new specific vaccines.

PMID: 11468579 [PubMed - indexed for MEDLINE]

2118. Antivir Chem Chemother. 2001 Jul;12(4):251-8.

Intracellular phosphorylation of carbocyclic 3-deazaadenosine, an anti-Ebola virus agent.

Smee DF(1), Bray M, Huggins JW.

Author information: (1)Virology Division, US Army Medical Research Institute of Infectious Diseases, Frederick, MD, USA. dsmee@cc.usu.edu

Carbocyclic 3-deazaadenosine (C-c3Ado) is a potent inhibitor of Ebola virus in mice by infrequent dosing, even though its half life in plasma is only 23-28 min. This prompted studies to determine whether C-c3Ado undergoes intracellular metabolism to derivatives that may promote in vivo activity. In cells, radiolabelled compound readily underwent metabolism to monophosphate, diphosphate and triphosphate (C-c3ATP) forms, with C-c3ATP being the major metabolite detected. A non-polar metabolite was also detected both inside and outside treated cells. The retention time of C-c3ATP was similar but not identical to ATP on a strong anion exchange high performance liquid chromatography (HPLC) column or on a DEAE-Sephadex open column. C-c3ATP and ATP were susceptible to degradation to their respective nucleosides by bovine alkaline phosphatase. Intracellular formation of C-c3ATP reached a plateau by about 4 h after treatment of monkey (Vero 76) and mouse (Balb/3T3 clone A31) cells with 10 or 100 microM extracellular compound. Phosphorylation was linearly dose responsive at 1, 3 and 10 microM. However, the extent of phosphorylation decreased with increasingly higher concentrations (30, 100 and 300 microM). When compound was removed from the medium, the nucleoside cleared the cells within 1 min, whereas C-c3ATP had a half life of decay of 2-3 h in five cell lines. Phosphorylation of C-c3Ado to C-c3ATP was not inhibited by cotreatment of cells (at a 20:1 ratio) with adenosine, guanosine, inosine, xanthosine, cytidine or uridine. There was no evidence of incorporation of C-c3Ado (10 microM) into macromolecules of cells over 72 h, whereas adenosine was readily incorporated. C-c3ATP may represent a form of C-c3Ado that might contribute to extending its intracellular half life or otherwise exhibit antiviral activity and/or toxicity.

PMID: 11771734 [PubMed - indexed for MEDLINE]

2119. J Am Acad Nurse Pract. 2001 Jul;13(7):291-2.

Ebola and Marburg hemorrhagic fevers.

Roberts A(1), Kemp C.

Author information: (1)Louise Herrington School of Nursing, Baylor University, USA. amy_roberts@baylor.edu

PMID: 11930600 [PubMed - indexed for MEDLINE]

2120. J Biol Regul Homeost Agents. 2001 Jul-Sep;15(3):314-21.

The model of response to viral haemorrhagic fevers of the National Institute for Infectious Diseases "Lazzaro Spallanzani".

Armignacco O(1), Lauria FN, Puro V, Macrì G, Petrecchia A, Ippolito G.

Author information: (1)National Institute for Infectious Diseases Lazzaro Spallanzani-IRCCS, Rome, Italy.

Viral haemorrhagic fevers (VHF) are severe and life-threatening diseases caused by a range of viruses. However, only four agents of VHF are known to be readily capable of person-to-person spread: Lassa virus, Crimean/Congo haemorrhagic fever virus, Ebola and Marburg viruses. Diseases caused by these viruses are endemic only in few areas in the world, most notably Africa and some rural parts of the Middle East and Eastern Europe. Nonetheless, the

increasing volume of international travel presents a greater likelihood for the importation of these infections or of suspected cases in non endemic countries. Four conditions can lead to the importation and to the subsequent recognition of VHF within Europe: 1) patients arriving as a result of a planned medical evacuation; 2) persons who became sick on route to their destination; 3) persons discovered ill when entering a country, for example during routine clinical examination at the airport; 4) persons becoming sick after their arrival. Public health implications and the risk of secondary spread of pathogens in the above reported circumstances are very different. Similarly, preparedness and response should vary. This paper summarizes the present knowledge on the four VHF capable of person-to-person spread, describes the high isolation area constructed at the Italian National Institute for Infectious Diseases Lazzaro Spallanzani in Rome to respond to the occurrence of VHF. A brief overview of procedures and equipment adopted is provided.
PMID: 11693443 [PubMed - indexed for MEDLINE]
2121. J Health Commun. 2001 Jul-Sep;6(3):281-94.
An "Urban legend" of global proportion: an analysis of nonfiction accounts of the Ebola virus.
Weldon RA(1).

Author information: (1)Department of Communication, 10 Strickler Hall, University of Louisville, Louisville, KY 40292, USA. Rebecca.Weldon@Louisville.edu
Using Brunvald's (1981) six criteria of successful urban legends, this study explores nonfiction accounts of the Ebola virus. Focusing particularly on Richard Preston's book The Hot Zone (1994), this study addresses the social construction of the predatorial virus, demonstrating how events are constructed as social problems via media representations, and reality is transformed into legend. The implications of these depictions of the predatorial virus are discussed, along with exploring the effects of mass media reports on health care beliefs and practices. Likewise, implications regarding these stories, cultural beliefs and values are discussed.
PMID: 11550594 [PubMed - indexed for MEDLINE]
2122. Am J Med. 2001 Jun 1;110(8):674-5.
Ebola-Athens preemergence?
Olson PE, Benenson AS, Genovese EN, Earhart KC.
Comment on Am J Med. 2000 Oct 1;109(5):391-7.
PMID: 11388345 [PubMed - indexed for MEDLINE]
2123. Clin Exp Immunol. 2001 Jun;124(3):453-60.
Early immune responses accompanying human asymptomatic Ebola infections.
Leroy EM(1), Baize S, Debre P, Lansoud-Soukate J, Mavoungou E.
Author information: (1)Centre International de Recherches Médicales de Franceville, BP 769, Franceville, Gabon. leroy@cirmf.sci.ga
In a recent study we identified certain asymptomatic individuals infected by Ebola virus (EBOV) who mounted specific IgG and early and strong inflammatory responses. Here, we further characterized the primary immune response to EBOV during the course of asymptomatic infection in humans. Inflammatory responses occurred in temporal association with anti-inflammatory phase composed by soluble antagonist IL-1RA, circulating TNF receptors, IL-10 and cortisol. At the end of the inflammatory process, mRNA expression of T-cell cytokines (IL-2 and IL-4) and activation markers (CD28, CD40L and CTLA4) was up-regulated, strongly suggesting T-cell activation. This T-cell activation was followed by EBOV-specific IgG responses (mainly IgG3 ang IgG1), and by marked and sustained up-regulation of IFN gamma, FasL and perforin mRNA expression, suggesting activation of cytotoxic cells. The terminal down-regulation of these latter markers coincided with the release of the apoptotic marker 41/7 NMP in blood and with the disappearance of viral RNA from PBMC, suggesting that infected cells are eliminated by cytotoxic mechanisms. Finally, RT-PCR analysis of TCR-V beta repertoire usage showed that TCR-V beta 12 mRNA was never expressed during the infection. Taken together, these findings improve our understanding about immune response during human asymptomatic Ebola infection, and throw new light on protection against Ebola virus.
PMCID: PMC1906073 PMID: 11472407 [PubMed - indexed for MEDLINE]
2124. J Gen Virol. 2001 Jun;82(Pt 6):1365-73.
The role of the Type I interferon response in the resistance of mice to filovirus infection.
Bray M(1).
Author information: (1)Department of Viral Therapeutics, Virology Division, United States Army Medical Research Institute of Infectious Diseases, 1425 Porter Street, Fort Detrick, Frederick, MD 21702-5011, USA. mike.bray@det.amedd.army.mil
Adult immunocompetent mice inoculated with Ebola (EBO) or Marburg (MBG) virus do not become ill. A suckling-mouse-passaged variant of EBO Zaire '76 ('mouse-adapted EBO-Z') causes rapidly lethal infection in adult mice after intraperitoneal (i.p.) inoculation, but does not cause apparent disease when inoculated subcutaneously (s.c.). A series of experiments showed that both forms of resistance to infection are mediated by the Type I interferon response. Mice lacking the cell-surface IFN-alpha/beta receptor died within a week after inoculation of EBO-Z '76, EBO Sudan, MBG Musoke or MBG Ravn, or after s.c. challenge with mouse-adapted EBO-Z. EBO Reston and EBO Ivory Coast did not cause illness, but immunized the mice against subsequent challenge with mouse-adapted EBO-Z. Normal adult mice treated with antibodies against murine IFN-alpha/beta could also be lethally infected with i.p.-inoculated EBO-Z '76 or EBO Sudan and with s.c.-inoculated mouse-adapted EBO-Z. Severe combined immunodeficient (SCID) mice became ill 3-4 weeks after inoculation with EBO-Z '76, EBO Sudan or MBG Ravn, but not the other viruses. Treatment with anti-IFN-alpha/beta antibodies markedly accelerated the course of EBO-Z '76 infection. Antibody treatment blocked the effect of a potent antiviral drug, 3-deazaneplanocin A, indicating that successful filovirus therapy may require the active participation of the Type I IFN response. Mice lacking an IFN-alpha/beta response resemble primates in their susceptibility to rapidly progressive,

overwhelming filovirus infection. The outcome of filovirus transfer between animal species appears to be determined by interactions between the virus and the innate immune response.
PMID: 11369881 [PubMed - indexed for MEDLINE]

2125. J Virol. 2001 Jun;75(11):5205-14.

Ebola virus VP40-induced particle formation and association with the lipid bilayer.

Jasenosky LD(1), Neumann G, Lukashevich I, Kawaoka Y.

Author information: (1)Department of Pathobiological Sciences, School of Veterinary Medicine, University of Wisconsin-Madison, Madison, Wisconsin 53706, USA. Viral protein 40 (VP40) of Ebola virus appears equivalent to matrix proteins of other viruses, yet little is known about its role in the viral life cycle. To elucidate the functions of VP40, we investigated its ability to induce the formation of membrane-bound particles when it was expressed apart from other viral proteins. We found that VP40 is indeed able to induce particle formation when it is expressed in mammalian cells, and this process appeared to rely on a conserved N-terminal PPXY motif, as mutation or loss of this motif resulted in markedly reduced particle formation. These findings demonstrate that VP40 alone possesses the information necessary to induce particle formation, and this process most likely requires cellular WW domain-containing proteins that interact with the PPXY motif of VP40. The ability of VP40 to bind cellular membranes was also studied. Flotation gradient analysis indicated that VP40 binds to membranes in a hydrophobic manner, as NaCl at 1 M did not release the protein from the lipid bilayer. Triton X-114 phase-partitioning analysis suggested that VP40 possesses only minor features of an integral membrane protein. We confirmed previous findings that truncation of the 50 C-terminal amino acids of VP40 results in decreased association with cellular membranes and demonstrated that this deletion disrupts hydrophobic interactions of VP40 with the lipid bilayer, as well as abolishing particle formation. Truncation of the 150 C-terminal amino acids or 100 N-terminal amino acids of VP40 enhanced the protein's hydrophobic association with cellular membranes. These data suggest that VP40 binds the lipid bilayer in an efficient yet structurally complex fashion.
PMCID: PMC114926 PMID: 11333902 [PubMed - indexed for MEDLINE]

2126. Virology. 2001 May 25;284(1):20-5.

Monocyte-derived human macrophages and peripheral blood mononuclear cells infected with ebola virus secrete MIP-1alpha and TNF-alpha and inhibit poly-IC-induced IFN-alpha in vitro.

Gupta M(1), Mahanty S, Ahmed R, Rollin PE.

Author information: (1)Emory Vaccine Center, Emory University School of Medicine, Atlanta, Georgia 30322, USA.
Ebola virus infection of humans is associated with high levels of circulating inflammatory chemokines and cytokines. We demonstrate that direct infection of human PBMC results in the induction of MCP-1, MIP-1alpha, RANTES, and TNF-alpha as early as 24 h p.i. in response to live virus. Monocyte-derived macrophages infected with live Ebola-virus secreted MIP-1alpha and TNF-alpha specifically while RANTES and MCP-1 were secreted by with both live or inactivated virus stimulation and do not require viral replication. Type I interferons (IFN-alpha and -beta), IL-1beta and IL-10, were not induced by Ebola virus. Furthermore, live virus infection of both PBMCs and monocytes-derived macrophages inhibited IFN-alpha induced by double-stranded RNA in vitro. These data provide the first direct evidence of a role for macrophages in the pathogenesis to Ebola virus and suggest that Ebola virus can inhibit cellular antiviral mechanisms mediated by type I interferons.
Copyright 2001 Academic Press.
PMID: 11352664 [PubMed - indexed for MEDLINE]

2127. Ann Pharm Fr. 2001 May;59(3):147-75.

[The worldwide challenges of "new" or reemerging communicable diseases at the dawn of the 21st century].

[Article in French]

Werner GH(1).

Author information: (1)Membre Associé Libre de l'Académie nationale de Pharmacie.
In spite of the very significant advances made during the 20 th century in the prevention and the treatment of communicable diseases, infections are still today, even in developed countries, a major cause of morbidity and mortality. New infectious diseases have emerged (AIDS, legionellosis, exterotoxigenic E. coli, Ebola fever), others have significantly reemerged (tuberculosis, diphtheria, Bartonella infections) or have seen their geographic distribution widen considerably (dengue, Hantavirus, West Nile Virus, Lyme disease). New and widespread hepatotropic viruses (mainly hepatitis C) have been identified, while the bacterial cause (Helicobacter pylori) of gastric ulcer was demonstrated. The second part of this review will deal with other examples of emerging or reemerging infections and with the problem of the increasing resistance of pathogens to antimicrobial agents. It will analyse the multiple causes of these various phenomena and describe the diverse strategies which should become available for the prevention and/or treatment of these numerous infectious diseases.
PMID: 11427818 [PubMed - indexed for MEDLINE]

2128. Arch Pathol Lab Med. 2001 May;125(5):625-30.

Ebola virus glycoprotein demonstrates differential cellular localization in infected cell types of nonhuman primates and guinea pigs.

Steele K(1), Crise B, Kuehne A, Kell W.

Author information: (1)Department of Pathology, Uniformed Services University of the Health Sciences, 4301 Jones Bridge Road, Bethesda, MD 20814, USA. ksteele@usuhs.mil
BACKGROUND: In vitro studies have previously shown that Ebola virus glycoprotein (GP) is rapidly processed and largely released from infected cells, whereas other viral proteins, such as VP40, accumulate within cells. OBJECTIVE: To determine infected cell types in which Ebola virus GP and VP40, individually, localize

in vivo. METHODS: Immunohistochemistry and in situ hybridization using GP- and VP40-specific antibodies and genetic probes were used to analyze archived tissues of experimentally infected nonhuman primates and guinea pigs and Vero E6 and 293 cells infected in vitro. RESULTS: The GP antigen was consistently present in hepatocytes, adrenal cortical cells, fibroblasts, fibroblastic reticular cells, ovarian thecal cells, and several types of epithelial cells, but was not detected in macrophages and blood monocytes of animals, nor in Vero cells and 293 cells. All GP-positive and GP-negative cell types analyzed contained VP40 antigen and both GP and VP40 RNAs. CONCLUSIONS: Ebola virus GP appears to selectively accumulate in many cell types infected in vivo, but not in macrophages and monocytes. This finding suggests that many cell types may have a GP-processing pathway that differs from the pathway described by previous in vitro studies. Differential cellular localization of GP could be relevant to the pathogenesis of Ebola hemorrhagic fever.
PMID: 11300932 [PubMed - indexed for MEDLINE]

2129. Dokl Biochem Biophys. 2001 May-Jun;378:195-7.

Recombinant monoclonal human antibodies against Ebola virus.

Tikunova NV(1), Kolokol'tsov AA, Chepurnov AA.

Author information: (1)State Research Center of Virology and Biotechnology Vektor, Kol'tsovo, Novosibirsk Oblast, 360559 Russia.

PMID: 11712178 [PubMed - indexed for MEDLINE]

2130. J Virol. 2001 May;75(10):4649-54.

Passive transfer of antibodies protects immunocompetent and imunodeficient mice against lethal Ebola virus infection without complete inhibition of viral replication.

Gupta M(1), Mahanty S, Bray M, Ahmed R, Rollin PE.

Author information: (1)Special Pathogens Branch, Division of Viral and Rickettsial Diseases, National Center for Infectious Diseases, Centers for Disease Control and Prevention, Atlanta, Georgia 30333, USA.

Ebola hemorrhagic fever is a severe, usually fatal illness caused by Ebola virus, a member of the filovirus family. The use of nonhomologous immune serum in animal studies and blood from survivors in two anecdotal reports of Ebola hemorrhagic fever in humans has shown promise, but the efficacy of these treatments has not been demonstrated definitively. We have evaluated the protective efficacy of polyclonal immune serum in a mouse model of Ebola virus infection. Our results demonstrate that mice infected subcutaneously with live Ebola virus survive infection and generate high levels of anti-Ebola virus immunoglobulin G (IgG). Passive transfer of immune serum from these mice before challenge protected upto 100% of naive mice against lethal Ebola virus infection. Protection correlated with the level of anti-Ebola virus IgG titers, and passive treatment with high-titer antiserum was associated with a delay in the peak of viral replication. Transfer of immune serum to SCID mice resulted in 100% survival after lethal challenge with Ebola virus, indicating that antibodies alone can protect from lethal disease. Thus antibodies suppress or delay viral growth, provide protection against lethal Ebola virus infection, and may not require participation of other immune components for protection.
PMCID: PMC114218 PMID: 11312335 [PubMed - indexed for MEDLINE]

2131. Nurs Stand. 2001 Apr 25-May 1;15(32):40-2.

Ebola haemorrhagic fever.

Walker L(1).

Author information: (1)Patient Care Services, Aga Khan Hospital, Dar es Salaam, Tanzania, East Africa. lisawafrica@hotmail.com

This article focuses on the management of a patient who was admitted to The Aga Khan Hospital in Dar es Salaam, Tanzania, with suspected Ebola haemorrhagic fever (Ebola HF). It defines the disease, symptoms and how it is spread, diagnosed, treated and prevented. Recommendations are made for management of Ebola HF in a hospital setting.
PMID: 12216182 [PubMed - indexed for MEDLINE]

2132. Virology. 2001 Apr 25;283(1):1-6.

Vesicular release of ebola virus matrix protein VP40.

Timmins J(1), Scianimanico S, Schoehn G, Weissenhorn W.

Author information: (1)EMBL, 6 rue Jules Horowitz, 38042 Grenoble, France.

We have analysed the expression and cellular localisation of the matrix protein VP40 from Ebola virus. Full-length VP40 and an N-terminal truncated construct missing the first 31 residues [VP40(31-326)] both locate to the plasma membrane of 293T cells when expressed transiently, while a C-terminal truncation of residues 213 to 326 [VP40(31-212)] shows only expression in the cytoplasm, when analysed by indirect immunofluorescence and plasma membrane preparations. In addition, we find that full-length VP40 [VP40(1-326)] and VP40(31-326) are both released into the cell culture supernatant and float up in sucrose gradients. The efficiency of their release, however, is dependent on the presence of the N-terminal 31 residues. VP40 that is released into the supernatant is resistant to trypsin digestion, a finding that is consistent with the formation of viruslike particles detected by electron microscopy. Together, these results provide strong evidence that Ebola virus VP40 is sufficient for virus assembly and budding from the plasma membrane.
Copyright 2001 Academic Press.
PMID: 11312656 [PubMed - indexed for MEDLINE]

2133. Lakartidningen. 2001 Apr 11;98(15):1812.

[Ebola: second or third when it comes to the most lethal viral infections].

[Article in Swedish]

Jeppsson A.

PMID: 11374012 [PubMed - indexed for MEDLINE]

2134. Lakartidningen. 2001 Apr 11;98(15):1810.

[Alarmingly protracted ebola epidemics in Uganda].

[Article in Swedish]

Jeppsson A.

PMID: 11374011 [PubMed - indexed for MEDLINE]

2135. CMAJ. 2001 Apr 3;164(7):1031-2.

Canada's Ebola scare over but questions just beginning.

Kilpatrick K.

PMCID: PMC80935 PMID: 11314433 [PubMed - indexed for MEDLINE]

2136. Epidemiol Mikrobiol Imunol. 2001 Apr;50(2):54-66.

[Ebola fever: an emerging disease].

[Article in Czech]

Jezek Z.

One of the most fatal diseases encountered by mankind so far is Ebola fever. Ebola fever is caused by a highly pathogenic virus from the Filoviridae family which is found in nature in four different sub-types which differ among others also by their pathogenicity for man. The hitherto detected EBO sub-types are stable do not change in the course of an epidemic nor in the course of the patient's illness, nor during passage of the virus from one subject to another. The author presents a historical review of epidemics, nosocomial and laboratory infections, spread and epizoonosis caused by the Ebola virus. The author presents a detailed clinical picture describing the frequency and evolution of different clinical symptoms and signs based on the observation of 103 patients infected with the Ebola virus in Kikwit, Zaire (nowadays Democratic Republic of Congo) in 1995. In the laboratory diagnosis individual tests are mentioned assessing the presence of the virus, viral antigens and antibodies, incl. the most recent immunohistochemical test. The author mentions the problem of patient care and his therapy, incl. available antiviral drugs and passive immunotherapy. He also discusses the possibility and probability of spread of the Ebola virus into our environment. He mentions principles for transport of subjects with suspected disease, demands for their strict isolation and maximum protection of the attending staff incl. barrier nursing technique. The author discusses also principles of epidemiological work, detection and isolation of sources, identification and follow up of contacts and epidemiological supervision of affected areas. Past epidemics made it possible to assemble many scientific findings and practical experience. These make it possible to cope nowadays with any attack of the Ebola virus not only in areas of its epizootic occurrence.

PMID: 11329728 [PubMed - indexed for MEDLINE]

2137. J Pharmacol Exp Ther. 2001 Apr;297(1):1-10.

2001 ASPET Otto Krayer Award Lecture. Molecular targets for antiviral agents.

De Clercq E(1).

Author information: (1)Rega Institute for Medical Research, Katholieke Universiteit Leuven, Minderbroedersstraat 10, B-3000 Leuven, Belgium. erik.declercq@rega.kuleuven.ac.be

Erratum in J Pharmacol Exp Ther 2001 Jun;297(3):1227.

There are a number of virus-specific processes within the virus replicative cycle or virus-infected cell that have proven to be attractive targets for chemotherapeutic intervention, i.e., virus adsorption and entry into the cells, reverse (RNA --> DNA) transcription, viral DNA polymerization, and cellular enzymatic reactions that are associated with viral DNA and RNA synthesis and viral mRNA maturation (i.e., methylation). A variety of chemotherapeutic agents, both nucleoside (and nucleotide) and non-nucleoside entities, have been identified that specifically interact with these viral targets, that selectively inhibit virus replication, and that are either used or considered for clinical use in the treatment of virus infections in humans. Their indications encompass virtually all major human viral pathogens, including human immunodeficiency virus (HIV), hepatitis B virus (HBV), herpes simplex virus (HSV), varicella-zoster virus (VZV), cytomegalovirus (CMV), human papilloma virus (HPV), orthomyxoviruses (influenza A and B), paramyxoviruses [e.g., respiratory syncytial virus (RSV)] and hemorrhagic fever viruses (such as Ebola virus).

PMID: 11259521 [PubMed - indexed for MEDLINE]

2138. J Virol. 2001 Apr;75(8):4014-8.

Human immunodeficiency virus type 1 particles pseudotyped with envelope proteins that fuse at low pH no longer require Nef for optimal infectivity.

Chazal N(1), Singer G, Aiken C, Hammarskjöld ML, Rekosh D.

Author information: (1)Myles H. Thaler Center for AIDS and Human Retrovirus Research, University of Virginia, Charlottesville, Virginia 22908, USA.

We have investigated the effects of Nef on infectivity in the context of various viral envelope proteins. These experiments were performed with a minimal vector system where Nef is the only accessory protein present. Our results support the hypothesis that the route of entry influences the ability of Nef to enhance human immunodeficiency virus (HIV) infectivity. We show that HIV particles pseudotyped with Ebola virus glycoprotein or vesicular stomatitis virus glycoprotein (VSV-G), which fuse at low pH, do not require Nef for optimal infectivity. In contrast, Nef significantly enhances the infectivity of virus particles that contain envelope proteins that fuse at neutral pH (CCR5-dependent HIV Env, CXCR4-dependent HIV Env, or amphotropic murine leukemia virus Env). In addition, our results demonstrate that virus particles containing mixed CXCR4-dependent HIV and VSV-G envelope proteins show a conditional requirement for Nef for optimal infectivity, depending on which protein is allowed to facilitate entry.

PMCID: PMC114896 PMID: 11264394 [PubMed - indexed for MEDLINE]

2139. Can Commun Dis Rep. 2001 Mar 15;27(6):49-53.

Outbreak of Ebola hemorrhagic fever, Uganda, August 2000-January 2001.

[Article in English, French]

[No authors listed]

PMID: 11428235 [PubMed - indexed for MEDLINE]

2140. Science. 2001 Mar 9;291(5510):1965-9. Epub 2001 Feb 1.

Recovery of infectious Ebola virus from complementary DNA: RNA editing of the GP gene and viral cytotoxicity.

Volchkov VE(1), Volchkova VA, Muhlberger E, Kolesnikova LV, Weik M, Dolnik O, Klenk HD.

Author information: (1)Institut für Virologie, Philipps-Universität, Robert-Koch-Strasse 17, 35037 Marburg, Germany. viktor.volchkov@ens-lyon.fr

To study the mechanisms underlying the high pathogenicity of Ebola virus, we have established a system that allows the recovery of infectious virus from cloned cDNA and thus permits genetic manipulation. We created a mutant in which the editing site of the gene encoding envelope glycoprotein (GP) was eliminated. This mutant no longer expressed the nonstructural glycoprotein sGP. Synthesis of GP increased, but most of it accumulated in the endoplasmic reticulum as immature precursor. The mutant was significantly more cytotoxic than wild-type virus, indicating that cytotoxicity caused by GP is down-regulated by the virus through transcriptional RNA editing and expression of sGP.

PMID: 11239157 [PubMed - indexed for MEDLINE]

2141. CMAJ. 2001 Mar 6;164(5):685.

Ebola erupts again.

Weir E.

PMCID: PMC80845 PMID: 11258226 [PubMed - indexed for MEDLINE]

2142. J Virol. 2001 Mar;75(6):2660-4.

Protection from Ebola virus mediated by cytotoxic T lymphocytes specific for the viral nucleoprotein.

Wilson JA(1), Hart MK.

Author information: (1)Virology Division, U.S. Army Medical Research Institute of Infectious Diseases, Fort Detrick, Frederick, Maryland 21702-5011, USA.

Cytotoxic T lymphocytes (CTLs) are proposed to be critical for protection from intracellular pathogens such as Ebola virus. However, there have been no demonstrations that protection against Ebola virus is mediated by Ebola virus-specific CTLs. Here, we report that C57BL/6 mice vaccinated with Venezuelan equine encephalitis virus replicons encoding the Ebola virus nucleoprotein (NP) survived lethal challenge with Ebola virus. Vaccination induced both antibodies to the NP and a major histocompatibility complex class I-restricted CTL response to an 11-amino-acid sequence in the amino-terminal portion of the Ebola virus NP. Passive transfer of polyclonal NP-specific antiserum did not protect recipient mice. In contrast, adoptive transfer of CTLs specific for the Ebola virus NP protected unvaccinated mice from lethal Ebola virus challenge. The protective CTLs were CD8(+), restricted to the D(b) class I molecule, and recognized an epitope within amino acids 43 to 53 (VYQVNNLEEIC) in the Ebola virus NP. The demonstration that CTLs can prevent lethal Ebola virus infection affects vaccine development in that protective cellular immune responses may be required for optimal protection from Ebola virus.

PMCID: PMC115890 PMID: 11222689 [PubMed - indexed for MEDLINE]

2143. J Virol. 2001 Mar;75(5):2324-30.

Infectivity-enhancing antibodies to Ebola virus glycoprotein.

Takada A(1), Watanabe S, Okazaki K, Kida H, Kawaoka Y.

Author information: (1)Laboratory of Microbiology, Department of Disease Control, Graduate School of Veterinary Medicine, Hokkaido University, Sapporo 060-0818, Japan.

Ebola virus causes severe hemorrhagic fever in primates, resulting in mortality rates of up to 100%, yet there are no satisfactory biologic explanations for this extreme virulence. Here we show that antisera produced by DNA immunization with a plasmid encoding the surface glycoprotein (GP) of the Zaire strain of Ebola virus enhances the infectivity of vesicular stomatitis virus pseudotyped with the GP. Substantially weaker enhancement was observed with antiserum to the GP of the Reston strain, which is much less pathogenic in humans than the Ebola Zaire and Sudan viruses. The enhancing activity was abolished by heat but was increased in the presence of complement system inhibitors, suggesting that heat-labile factors other than the complement system are required for this effect. We also generated an anti-Zaire GP monoclonal antibody that enhanced viral infectivity and another that neutralized it, indicating the presence of distinct epitopes for these properties. Our findings suggest that antibody-dependent enhancement of infectivity may account for the extreme virulence of the virus. They also raise issues about the development of Ebola virus vaccines and the use of passive prophylaxis or therapy with Ebola virus GP antibodies.

PMCID: PMC114815 PMID: 11160735 [PubMed - indexed for MEDLINE]

2144. Mayo Clin Health Lett. 2001 Mar;19(3):7.

Exotic diseases. Are they spreading to a town near you?

[No authors listed]

PMID: 11242844 [PubMed - indexed for MEDLINE]

2145. Nat Biotechnol. 2001 Mar;19(3):225-30.

Filovirus-pseudotyped lentiviral vector can efficiently and stably transduce airway epithelia in vivo.

Kobinger GP(1), Weiner DJ, Yu QC, Wilson JM.

Author information: (1)Institute for Human Gene Therapy and Department of Molecular and Cellular Engineering, University of Pennsylvania Health System, Philadelphia, PA 19104, USA.

Traditional gene therapy vectors have demonstrated limited utility for treatment of chronic lung diseases such as cystic fibrosis (CF). Herein we describe a vector based on a Filovirus envelope protein-pseudotyped HIV vector, which we chose after systematically evaluating multiple strategies. The vector efficiently transduces intact airway epithelium from the apical surface, as demonstrated in both in vitro and in vivo model systems. This shows the potential of pseudotyping in expanding the utility of lentiviral vectors. Pseudotyped lentiviral vectors may hold promise for the treatment of CF.
PMID: 11231554 [PubMed - indexed for MEDLINE]

2146. Vet Pathol. 2001 Mar;38(2):203-15.

Cutaneous DNA vaccination against Ebola virus by particle bombardment: histopathology and alteration of CD3-positive dendritic epidermal cells.

Steele KE(1), Stabler K, VanderZanden L.

Author information: (1)Division of Pathology, US Army Medical Research Institute of Infectious Diseases, Fort Detrick, MD, USA. ksteele@usuhs.mil

We analyzed the localization of gold particles, expression of immunogenic protein, and histopathologic changes after vaccinating guinea pigs and mice with a DNA vaccine to the Ebola virus glycoprotein administered by cutaneous particle bombardment. Gold particles were deposited in all layers of the epidermis and in the dermis. Those in the epidermis were lost as the damaged layers sloughed, while those in the dermis were phagocytized by macrophages. Glycoprotein was demonstrated by immunohistochemistry primarily in keratinocytes in the epidermis and hair follicle epithelium and less frequently in dermal macrophages, fibroblasts, sebocytes, and cells that appeared to be Langerhans cells. The number of cells that expressed glycoprotein increased between 4 and 8 hours postvaccination, then decreased to near zero by 48 hours. The vaccine sites were histologically divisible into three zones. The central portion, zone 1, contained the most gold particles in the dermis and epidermis and had extensive tissue damage, including full-thickness epidermal necrosis. Zone 2 contained fewer gold particles in the epidermis and dermis and had less extensive necrosis. The majority of cells in which glycoprotein was expressed were in zone 2. Zone 3 contained gold particles only in the epidermis and had necrosis of only a few scattered cells. Regeneration of the epidermis in damaged areas was evident at 24 hours postvaccination and was essentially complete by day 5 in the mice and day 10 in the guinea pigs. Inflammatory changes were characterized by hemorrhage, edema, and infiltrates of neutrophils initially and by infiltrates of lymphocytes and macrophages at later times. In zone 1, inflammation affected both the epidermis and dermis. Peripherally, inflammation was relatively limited to the epidermis. CD3-positive dendritic epidermal cells were demonstrated in the epidermis and superficial hair follicles of unvaccinated immunocompetent mice and beige mice but not of SCID mice. These cells disappeared from all but the most peripheral portions of the vaccine sites of vaccinated mice within 24 hours. They reappeared slowly, failing to reach numbers comparable with unvaccinated mice by 35 days postvaccination. The epidermis of control guinea pigs also had CD3-positive cells, but they did not have dendrites. These findings should contribute to a better understanding of the mechanisms operating in response to DNA vaccination by particle bombardment.
PMID: 11280377 [PubMed - indexed for MEDLINE]

2147. Virology. 2001 Mar 1;281(1):102-8.

In vitro dissection of the membrane and RNP binding activities of influenza virus M1 protein.

Baudin F(1), Petit I, Weissenhorn W, Ruigrok RW.

Author information: (1)EMBL Grenoble Outstation, B.P. 156, 38042 Grenoble Cedex 9, France.

Spontaneous proteolysis of influenza virus M1 protein during crystallisation has defined an N-terminal domain of amino acids 1--164. Full-length M1, the N-terminal domain, and the C-terminal part of M1 (residues 165--252) were produced in Escherichia coli. In vitro tests showed that only full-length M1 and its N-terminal domain bind to negatively charged liposomes and that only full-length M1 and its C-terminal part bind to RNP. However, only full-length M1 had transcription inhibition activity. Several independent experimental approaches indicate that in vitro transcription inhibition occurs through polymerisation/aggregation of M1 onto RNP, or of M1 onto M1 already bound to RNP, rather than by binding to a specific active site on the nucleoprotein or the polymerase. The structure/function of influenza virus M1 will be compared with that of the Ebola virus matrix protein, VP40.

Copyright 2001 Academic Press.

PMID: 11222100 [PubMed - indexed for MEDLINE]

2148. JAMA. 2001 Feb 28;285(8):1010-2.

From the Centers for Disease Control and Prevention. Outbreak of Ebola hemorrhagic fever--Uganda, August 2000-January 2001.

[No authors listed]

PMID: 11263418 [PubMed - indexed for MEDLINE]

2149. MMWR Morb Mortal Wkly Rep. 2001 Feb 9;50(5):73-7.

Outbreak of Ebola hemorrhagic fever Uganda, August 2000-January 2001.

Centers for Disease Control and Prevention (CDC).

On October 8, 2000, an outbreak of an unusual febrile illness with occasional hemorrhage and significant mortality was reported to the Ministry of Health (MoH) in Kampala by the superintendent of St. Mary's Hospital in Lacor, and the District Director of Health Services in the Gulu District. A preliminary assessment conducted by MoH found additional cases in Gulu District and in Gulu Hospital, the regional referral hospital. On October 15, suspicion of Ebola hemorrhagic fever (EHF) was confirmed when the National Institute of Virology (NIV), Johannesburg, South Africa, identified Ebola virus infection among specimens from patients, including health-care workers at St. Mary's Hospital. This report describes surveillance and control activities related to the EHF outbreak and presents preliminary clinical and epidemiologic findings.
PMID: 11686289 [PubMed - indexed for MEDLINE]

2150. Wkly Epidemiol Rec. 2001 Feb 9;76(6):41-6.

Outbreak of Ebola haemorrhagic fever, Uganda, August 2000-January 2001.

[Article in English, French]

[No authors listed]

PMID: 11233580 [PubMed - indexed for MEDLINE]

2151. Biochem J. 2001 Feb 1;353(Pt 3):537-45.

Implication of the proprotein convertases furin, PC5 and PC7 in the cleavage of surface glycoproteins of Hong Kong, Ebola and respiratory syncytial viruses: a comparative analysis with fluorogenic peptides.

Basak A(1), Zhong M, Munzer JS, Chrétien M, Seidah NG.

Author information: (1)Laboratory of Molecular Medicine and Disease of Ageing Centre, Loeb Health Research Institute, Ottawa Civic Hospital, 725 Parkdale Avenue, Ottawa, Ontario, Canada K1Y 4K9. abasak@lri.ca

Fluorogenic peptides encompassing the processing sites of envelope glycoproteins of the infectious influenza A Hong Kong virus (HKV), Ebola virus (EBOV) and respiratory syncytial virus (RSV) were tested for cleavage by soluble recombinants of the proprotein convertases furin, PC5 and PC7. Kinetic studies with these intramolecularly quenched fluorogenic peptides revealed selective cleavages at the physiological dibasic sites. The HKV peptide is cleaved by both furin and PC5 with similar efficacy; in comparison, PC7 cleaves this substrate poorly. In contrast with the basic tetrapeptide insertion within the haemagglutinin sequence of HKV, two other dipeptide insertions revealed a poorer cleavage with a similar rank order of potency. These results demonstrate that the N-terminal RERR insertion to the wild-type avian RKKR downward arrow sequence is functionally significant, and suggest that the approx. 5-fold increase in cleavage efficacy contributes to the high infectivity of the H5N1 virus subtype. With regard to RSV peptide processing, PC7 is twice as effective as PC5 and furin. The EBOV peptide was processed with similar efficiency by the three enzymes. Our observations that all of these cleavages can be effectively inhibited by a plant andrographolide derivative at 250 microM or less might aid in the design of potent convertase inhibitors as alternative antiviral therapies.

PMCID: PMC1221599 PMID: 11171050 [PubMed - indexed for MEDLINE]

2152. Clin Infect Dis. 2001 Feb 1;32(3):446-56. Epub 2001 Jan 24.

Risks and prevention of nosocomial transmission of rare zoonotic diseases.

Weber DJ(1), Rutala WA.

Author information: (1)Division of Infectious Diseases, University of North Carolina at Chapel Hill, Chapel Hill, NC 27599-7030, USA. dweber@unch.unc.edu

Americans are increasingly exposed to exotic zoonotic diseases through travel, contact with exotic pets, occupational exposure, and leisure pursuits. Appropriate isolation precautions are required to prevent nosocomial transmission of rare zoonotic diseases for which person-to-person transmission has been documented. This minireview provides guidelines for the isolation of patients and management of staff exposed to the following infectious diseases with documented person-to-person transmission: Andes hantavirus disease, anthrax, B virus infection, hemorrhagic fevers (due to Ebola, Marburg, Lassa, Crimean-Congo hemorrhagic fever, Argentine hemorrhagic fever, and Bolivian hemorrhagic fever viruses), monkeypox, plague, Q fever, and rabies. Several of these infections may also be encountered as bioterrorism hazards (i.e., anthrax, hemorrhagic fever viruses, plague, and Q fever). Adherence to recommended isolation precautions will allow for proper patient care while protecting the health care workers who provide care to patients with known or suspected zoonotic infections capable of nosocomial transmission.

PMID: 11170953 [PubMed - indexed for MEDLINE]

2153. J Clin Microbiol. 2001 Feb;39(2):776-8.

Immunofluorescence method for detection of Ebola virus immunoglobulin g, using HeLa cells which express recombinant nucleoprotein.

Saijo M(1), Niikura M, Morikawa S, Kurane I.

Author information: (1)Special Pathogens Laboratory, Department of Virology 1, National Institute of Infectious Diseases, Gakuen 4-7-1, Musahimurayama, Tokyo 208-0011, Japan.

A novel recombinant baculovirus which expresses Ebola virus (EBO) nucleoprotein (NP) under the control of the cytomegalovirus immediate-early promoter was constructed. HeLa cells abortively infected with the baculovirus expressed EBO NP, and this was used as an immunofluorescent (IF) antigen to detect EBO immunoglobulin G (IgG) antibody. This IF method has high efficacy in detecting EBO IgG antibody in clinical specimens, indicating its usefulness in the diagnosis of EBO infections and seroepidemiological studies.

PMCID: PMC87819 PMID: 11158150 [PubMed - indexed for MEDLINE]

2154. J Virol. 2001 Feb;75(3):1576-80.

Ebola virus glycoprotein: proteolytic processing, acylation, cell tropism, and detection of neutralizing antibodies.

Ito H(1), Watanabe S, Takada A, Kawaoka Y.

Author information: (1)Department of Pathobiological Sciences, School of Veterinary Medicine, University of Wisconsin-Madison, Madison, Wisconsin 53706, USA.

Using the vesicular stomatitis virus (VSV) pseudotype system, we studied the functional properties of the Ebola virus glycoprotein (GP). Amino acid substitutions at the GP cleavage site, which reduce glycoprotein cleavability and viral infectivity in some viruses, did not appreciably change the infectivity of VSV pseudotyped with GP. Likewise, removal of two acylated cysteine residues in the transmembrane region of GP showed no discernible effects on infectivity. Although most filoviruses are believed to target endothelial cells and hepatocytes preferentially, the GP-carrying VSV showed greater affinity for epithelial cells than for either of these cell types, indicating that Ebola virus GP does not necessarily have strong tropism toward endothelial cells and hepatocytes. Finally, when it was used to screen for neutralizing antibodies against Ebola virus GP, the VSV pseudotype system allowed us to detect strain-specific

neutralizing activity that was inhibited by secretory GP (SGP). This finding provides evidence of shared neutralizing epitopes on GP and SGP molecules and indicates the potential of SGP to serve as a decoy for neutralizing antibodies.
PMCID: PMC114066 PMID: 11152533 [PubMed - indexed for MEDLINE]
2155. Nurs Times. 2001 Feb 1-7;97(5):14-5.
Ebola crisis.
Bleasedale M.
PMID: 11954170 [PubMed - indexed for MEDLINE]
2156. Wkly Epidemiol Rec. 2001 Jan 19;76(3):17-8.
Unverified rumours of viral haemorrhagic fever, Democratic Republic of the Congo.
[Article in English, French]
[No authors listed]
PMID: 11218694 [PubMed - indexed for MEDLINE]
2157. BMC Microbiol. 2001;1:1. Epub 2001 Feb 9.
The viral transmembrane superfamily: possible divergence of Arenavirus and Filovirus glycoproteins from a common RNA virus ancestor.
Gallaher WR(1), DiSimone C, Buchmeier MJ.

Author information: (1)Department of Microbiology, Immunology & Parasitology, Neuroscience Center of Excellence and Stanley S. Scott Cancer Center, Louisiana State University Medical Center, New Orleans, LA 70112-1393, USA. wgalla@lsuhsc.edu

BACKGROUND: Recent studies of viral entry proteins from influenza, measles, human immunodeficiency virus, type 1 (HIV-1), and Ebola virus have shown, first with molecular modeling, and then X-ray crystallographic or other biophysical studies, that these disparate viruses share a coiled-coil type of entry protein. RESULTS: Structural models of the transmembrane glycoproteins (GP-2) of the Arenaviruses, lymphochoriomeningitis virus (LCMV) and Lassa fever virus, are presented, based on consistent structural propensities despite variation in the amino acid sequence. The principal features of the model, a hydrophobic amino terminus, and two antiparallel helices separated by a glycosylated, antigenic apex, are common to a number of otherwise disparate families of enveloped RNA viruses. Within the first amphipathic helix, demonstrable by circular dichroism of a peptide fragment, there is a highly conserved heptad repeat pattern proposed to mediate multimerization by coiled-coil interactions. The amino terminal 18 amino acids are 28% identical and 50% highly similar to the corresponding region of Ebola, a member of the Filovirus family. Within the second, charged helix just prior to membrane insertion there is also high similarity over the central 18 amino acids in corresponding regions of Lassa and Ebola, which may be further related to the similar region of HIV-1 defining a potent antiviral peptide analogue. CONCLUSIONS: These findings indicate a common pattern of structure and function among viral transmembrane fusion proteins from a number of virus families. Such a pattern may define a viral transmembrane superfamily that evolved from a common precursor eons ago.
PMCID: PMC29097 PMID: 11208257 [PubMed - indexed for MEDLINE]
2158. Bull World Health Organ. 2001;79(3):267.
Role of the Red Cross movement in Uganda's Ebola outbreak.
Sandbladh H.
Comment on Bull World Health Organ. 2000;78(12):1476-7.
PMCID: PMC2566385 PMID: 11285677 [PubMed - indexed for MEDLINE]
2159. Bull World Health Organ. 2001;79(1):79. Epub 2003 Nov 5.
Experimental vaccine protects monkeys against Ebola virus.
Gottlieb S.
PMCID: PMC2566335 PMID: 11217674 [PubMed - indexed for MEDLINE]
2160. J Clin Microbiol. 2001 Jan;39(1):1-7.
Enzyme-linked immunosorbent assays for detection of antibodies to Ebola and Marburg viruses using recombinant nucleoproteins.
Saijo M(1), Niikura M, Morikawa S, Ksiazek TG, Meyer RF, Peters CJ, Kurane I.

Author information: (1)Special Pathogens Laboratory, Department of Virology 1, National Institute of Infectious Diseases, Gakuen 4-7-1, Musashimurayama, Tokyo 208-0011, Japan.

The full-length nucleoprotein (NP) of Ebola virus (EBO) was expressed as a His-tagged recombinant protein (His-EBO-NP) by a baculovirus system. Carboxy-terminal halves of NPs of EBO and Marburg virus (MBG) were expressed as glutathione S-transferase-tagged recombinant proteins in an Escherichia coli system. The antigenic regions on the NPs of EBO and MBG were determined by both Western blotting and enzyme-linked immunosorbent assay (ELISA) to be located on the C-terminal halves. The C-terminal 110 and 102 amino acids of the NPs of EBO and MBG, respectively, possess strong antigenicity. The full-length NP of EBO was strongly expressed in insect cells upon infection with the recombinant baculovirus, while expression of the full-length NP of MBG was weak. We developed an immunoglobulin G (IgG) ELISA using His-EBO-NP and the C-terminal halves of the NPs of EBO and MBG as antigens. We evaluated the IgG ELISA for the ability to detect IgG antibodies to EBO and MBG, using human sera collected from EBO and MBG patients. The IgG ELISA with the recombinant NPs showed high sensitivity and specificity in detecting EBO and MBG antibodies. The results indicate that ELISA systems prepared with the recombinant NPs of EBO and MBG are valuable tools for the diagnosis of EBO and MBG infections and for seroepidemiological field studies.
PMCID: PMC87670 PMID: 11136739 [PubMed - indexed for MEDLINE]
2161. Pharm Unserer Zeit. 2001;30(3):185-6.

[Hope for a vaccine against ebola virus].

[Article in German]

Holzgrabe U.

PMID: 11400662 [PubMed - indexed for MEDLINE]

2162. Qual Health Res. 2001 Jan;11(1):5-25.

The rhetorical construction of the predatorial virus: a Burkian analysis of nonfiction accounts of the Ebola virus.

Weldon RA(1).

Author information: (1)University of Louisville, Louisville, Kentucky, USA.

Over the past 5 years, a new subgenre of horror films, referred to as plague films, has turned our focus to the threat of a hemorrhagic viral pandemic, comparable to the Spanish Flu epidemic of 1916. Based on the Ebola viral outbreaks of 1976, various writers have presented their accounts under the guise of increasing interest and prevention strategies. Disregarding inappropriate health care practices as the cause of these epidemics, accountability is refocused onto the rhetorically constructed, predatory nature of the virus. By employing Burke's theory of dramatism and pentadic analysis, the author examines this rhetorical construction of Ebola as a predatorial virus and its implications for public perceptions of public health endeavors.

PMID: 11147163 [PubMed - indexed for MEDLINE]

2163. Trans Am Clin Climatol Assoc. 2001;112:79-84; discussion 86-8.

The Gordon Wilson Lecture: viruses and human disease.

Nabel GJ(1).

Author information: (1)Vaccine Research Center, National Institutes of Health, 40 Convent Drive, MSC-3005, Bethesda, MD 20892, USA. gnabel@mail.nih.gov

In many ways, Ebola virus infection provides a model for understanding the toxicity of viruses and their causal role in human disease. The highly aggressive course of Ebola virus infection provides a model for understanding the molecular mechanisms of viral cytotoxicity. In addition, the use of animal models and definition of immune correlates, which lead to protection, may provide lessons that are applicable to other viral infections. Perhaps the greatest challenge facing biomedical science today is the containment of the human immunodeficiency virus, the causative agent of AIDS. In many ways the critical obstacles to the development of a vaccine for HIV are similar to those observed with Ebola virus infection. Because the reservoir of infection is not known and human-to-human spread has been documented, vaccines may provide the best opportunity to contain and limit the spread of infection worldwide. Similar to Ebola virus, there are few convincing examples of immune resistance of HIV infection. In addition, it has been difficult to identify broadly neutralizing antibodies that can prevent infection in vitro or in vivo. In defining immune correlates, relevant animal models, and mechanisms of cytotoxicity, it is hoped that similar efforts may lead to effective vaccines for other infectious diseases. In this way, Ebola virus infection provides a useful paradigm for understanding the genetic determinants of viral disease and in facilitating the development of treatments and prevention of viral infections.

PMCID: PMC2194412 PMID: 11413785 [PubMed - indexed for MEDLINE]

2164. EMBO J. 2000 Dec 15;19(24):6732-41.

Membrane association induces a conformational change in the Ebola virus matrix protein.

Scianimanico S(1), Schoehn G, Timmins J, Ruigrok RH, Klenk HD, Weissenhorn W.

Author information: (1)European Molecular Biology Laboratory (EMBL) Grenoble Outstation, 6 rue Jules Horowitz, 38000 Grenoble, France.

The matrix protein VP40 from Ebola virus is targeted to the plasma membrane, where it is thought to induce assembly and budding of virions through its association with the lipid bilayer. Ebola virus VP40 is expressed as a monomeric molecule in solution, consisting of two loosely associated domains. Here we show that a C-terminal truncation of seven residues destabilizes the monomeric closed conformation and induces spontaneous hexamerization in solution, as indicated by chemical cross-linking and electron microscopy. Three-dimensional reconstruction of electron microscopy images shows ring-like structures consisting of the N-terminal domain along with evidence for flexibly attached C-terminal domains. In vitro destabilization of the monomer by urea treatment results in similar hexameric molecules in solution. In addition, we demonstrate that membrane association of wild-type VP40 also induces the conformational switch from monomeric to hexameric molecules that may form the building blocks for initiation of virus assembly and budding. Such a conformational change induced by bilayer targeting may be a common feature of many viral matrix proteins and its potential inhibition may result in new anti-viral therapies.

PMCID: PMC305896 PMID: 11118208 [PubMed - indexed for MEDLINE]

2165. Proc Natl Acad Sci U S A. 2000 Dec 5;97(25):13871-6.

A PPxY motif within the VP40 protein of Ebola virus interacts physically and functionally with a ubiquitin ligase: implications for filovirus budding.

Harty RN(1), Brown ME, Wang G, Huibregtse J, Hayes FP.

Author information: (1)Department of Pathobiology, School of Veterinary Medicine, University of Pennsylvania, 3800 Spruce Street, Philadelphia, PA 19104-6049, USA. rharty@vet.upenn.edu

VP40, the putative matrix protein of both Ebola and Marburg viruses, possesses a conserved proline-rich motif (PY motif) at its N terminus. We demonstrate that the VP40 protein can mediate its own release from mammalian cells, and that the PY motif is important for this self-exocytosis (budding) function. In addition, we used Western-ligand blotting to demonstrate that the PY motif of VP40 can mediate interactions with specific cellular proteins that have type I WW-domains, including the mammalian ubiquitin ligase, Nedd4. Single point mutations that disrupted the PY motif of VP40 abolished the PY/WW-domain interactions. Significantly, the full-length VP40 protein was shown to interact both physically and functionally with full-length Rsp5, a ubiquitin ligase of yeast and homolog of Nedd4. The VP40 protein was multiubiquitinated by Rsp5 in a PY-dependent manner in an in vitro ubiquitination assay. These data demonstrate that the VP40 protein of Ebola virus possesses a PY motif that is functionally similar to those described previously for Gag and M proteins of specific retroviruses and rhabdoviruses, respectively. Last, these studies imply that VP40 likely plays an important role in filovirus budding, and that budding of retroviruses, rhabdoviruses, and filoviruses may proceed via analogous mechanisms.

PMCID: PMC17668 PMID: 11095724 [PubMed - indexed for MEDLINE]

2166. Virology. 2000 Dec 5;278(1):20-6.

Downregulation of beta1 integrins by Ebola virus glycoprotein: implication for virus entry.

Takada A(1), Watanabe S, Ito H, Okazaki K, Kida H, Kawaoka Y.

Author information: (1)Laboratory of Microbiology, Graduate School of Veterinary Medicine, Sapporo, 060-0818, Japan.

Filoviruses, including Ebola virus, are cytotoxic. To investigate the role of the Ebola virus glycoprotein (GP) in this cytopathic effect, we transiently expressed the GP in human kidney 293T cells. Expression of wild-type GP, but not the secretory form of the molecule lacking a membrane anchor, induced rounding and detachment of the cells, as did a chimeric GP containing its ectodomain and influenza virus hemagglutinin transmembrane-cytoplasmic domain. These results indicate that the GP ectodomain and its anchorage to the membrane are required for GP-induced morphologic changes in host cells. Since cell rounding and detachment could be associated with reduced levels of cell adhesion molecules, we also studied the expression of integrins, which are major molecules for adhesion to extracellular matrices, and found that the beta1 integrin group is downregulated by the GP. This result was further extended by experiments in which anti-beta1 monoclonal antibodies or purified integrins inhibited the infectivity of vesicular stomatitis virus pseudotyped with the GP. We suggest that integrins, especially the beta1 group, might interact with the GP and perhaps be involved in Ebola virus entry into cells.

Copyright 2000 Academic Press.

PMID: 11112476 [PubMed - indexed for MEDLINE]

2167. Biosci Rep. 2000 Dec;20(6):597-612.

Virus membrane fusion proteins: biological machines that undergo a metamorphosis.

Dutch RE(1), Jardetzky TS, Lamb RA.

Author information: (1)Department of Biochemistry, University of Kentucky Medical Center, Lexington 40536, USA.

Fusion proteins from a group of widely disparate viruses, including the paramyxovirus F protein, the HIV and SIV gp160 proteins, the retroviral Env protein, the Ebola virus Gp, and the influenza virus haemagglutinin, share a number of common features. All contain multiple glycosylation sites, and must be trimeric and undergo proteolytic cleavage to be fusogenically active. Subsequent to proteolytic cleavage, the subunit containing the transmembrane domain in each case has an extremely hydrophobic region, termed the fusion peptide, or at near its newly generated N-terminus. In addition, all of these viral fusion proteins have 4-3 heptad repeat sequences near both the fusion peptide and the transmembrane domain. These regions have been demonstrated from a tight complex, in which the N-terminal heptad repeat forms a trimeric-coiled coil, with the C-terminal heptad repeat forming helical regions that buttress the coiled-coil in an anti-parallel manner. The significance of each of these structural elements in the processing and function of these viral fusion proteins is discussed.

PMID: 11426696 [PubMed - indexed for MEDLINE]

2168. Nat Med. 2000 Dec;6(12):1322-3.

Will we have and why do we need an Ebola vaccine?

Klenk HD.

PMID: 11100112 [PubMed - indexed for MEDLINE]

2169. Eur J Med Res. 2000 Nov 30;5(11):491-505.

Dermatological infectiology--Quo vadis? Symposium, Ruhr-University, September 29-30, 2000. Abstracts.

[No authors listed]

Infectious diseases remain a major cause of morbidity and mortality in the year 2000. 17 million deaths per year or roughly a third of all deaths are caused by infections. Infectious diseases also pose a serious economic threat. While many well-established pathogens have not been contained several new infectious agents have been discovered within the past 27 years which include rotavirus, legionella, HIV, ebola, campylobacter, helicobacter, nipah, HHV8, hepatitis C, and many others. Additionally many new pathogens have emerged as serious threats to the ever-growing number of immuno-compromised patients. Infectious etiologies have been found for many common diseases (certain leukemias, duodenal ulcers, etcetera). It is likely that infections are at least co-factors for many other diseases (transplant-associated atherosclerosis). Only specialized care and multi-disciplinary collaboration will enable us to cope with current problems and the inevitable emergence of new infectious diseases.

PMID: 11121370 [PubMed - indexed for MEDLINE]

2170. Nature. 2000 Nov 30;408(6812):605-9.

Development of a preventive vaccine for Ebola virus infection in primates.

Sullivan NJ(1), Sanchez A, Rollin PE, Yang ZY, Nabel GJ.

Author information: (1)Vaccine Research Center, National Institutes of Health, Bethesda, Maryland 20892, USA.

Comment in Nature. 2000 Nov 30;408(6812):527-8.

Outbreaks of haemorrhagic fever caused by the Ebola virus are associated with high mortality rates that are a distinguishing feature of this human pathogen. The highest lethality is associated with the Zaire subtype, one of four strains identified to date. Its rapid progression allows little opportunity to develop natural immunity, and there is currently no effective anti-viral therapy. Therefore, vaccination offers a promising intervention to prevent infection and limit spread. Here we describe a highly effective vaccine strategy for Ebola virus infection in non-human primates. A combination of DNA immunization and boosting with adenoviral vectors that encode viral proteins generated cellular and humoral immunity in cynomolgus macaques. Challenge with a lethal dose of the highly pathogenic, wild-type, 1976 Mayinga strain of Ebola Zaire virus resulted in uniform infection in controls, who progressed to a moribund state and death in less than one week. In contrast, all vaccinated animals were asymptomatic for more than six months, with no detectable virus after the initial challenge. These findings demonstrate that it is possible to develop a preventive vaccine against Ebola virus infection in primates.

PMID: 11117750 [PubMed - indexed for MEDLINE]

2171. Nature. 2000 Nov 30;408(6812):527-8.

Fighting the Ebola virus.

Burton DR, Parren PW.

Comment on Nature. 2000 Nov 30;408(6812):605-9.

PMID: 11117724 [PubMed - indexed for MEDLINE]

2172. Proc Natl Acad Sci U S A. 2000 Nov 21;97(24):13063-8.

A role for ubiquitin ligase recruitment in retrovirus release.

Strack B(1), Calistri A, Accola MA, Palu G, Gottlinger HG.

Author information: (1)Department of Cancer Immunology and AIDS, Dana-Farber Cancer Institute, Harvard Medical School, Boston, MA 02115, USA.

Comment in Proc Natl Acad Sci U S A. 2000 Nov 21;97(24):12945-7.

Retroviral Gag polyproteins have specific regions, commonly referred to as late assembly (L) domains, which are required for the efficient separation of assembled virions from the host cell. The L domain of HIV-1 is in the C-terminal p6(gag) domain and contains an essential P(T/S)AP core motif that is widely conserved among lentiviruses. In contrast, the L domains of oncoretroviruses such as Rous sarcoma virus (RSV) have a more N-terminal location and a PPxY core motif. In the present study, we used chimeric Gag constructs to probe for L domain activity, and observed that the unrelated L domains of RSV and HIV-1 both induced the appearance of Gag-ubiquitin conjugates in virus-like particles (VLP). Furthermore, a single-amino acid substitution that abolished the activity of the RSV L domain in VLP release also abrogated its ability to induce Gag ubiquitination. Particularly robust Gag ubiquitination and enhancement of VLP release were observed in the presence of the candidate L domain of Ebola virus, which contains overlapping P(T/S)AP and PPxY motifs. The release defect of a minimal Gag construct could also be corrected through the attachment of a peptide that serves as a physiological docking site for the ubiquitin ligase Nedd4. Furthermore, VLP formation by a full-length Gag polyprotein was sensitive to lactacystin, which depletes the levels of free ubiquitin through inhibition of the proteasome. Our findings suggest that the engagement of the ubiquitin conjugation machinery by L domains plays a crucial role in the release of a diverse group of enveloped viruses.

PMCID: PMC27178 PMID: 11087860 [PubMed - indexed for MEDLINE]

2173. Ugeskr Laeger. 2000 Nov 13;162(46):6269-70.

[Ebola fever].

[Article in Danish]

Pedersen C(1).

Author information: (1)Medicinsk afdeling C, Odense Universitetshospital.

PMID: 11107997 [PubMed - indexed for MEDLINE]

2174. Virology. 2000 Nov 10;277(1):147-55.

Molecular characterization of guinea pig-adapted variants of Ebola virus.

Volchkov VE(1), Chepurnov AA, Volchkova VA, Ternovoj VA, Klenk HD.

Author information: (1)Institut für Virologie, Philipps-Universität, Robert-Koch-Strasse 17, Marburg, 35037, Germany. Viktor.Volchkov@ens-lyon.fr

Serial passage of initially nonlethal Ebola virus (EBOV) in outbred guinea pigs resulted in the selection of variants with high pathogenicity. Nucleotide sequence analysis of the complete genome of the guinea pig-adapted variant 8mc revealed that it differed from wild-type virus by eight mutations. No mutations were identified in nontranscribed regions, including leader, trailer, and intragenic sequences. Among noncoding regions the only base change was found in the VP30 gene. Two silent base changes were found in the open reading frame (ORF) encoding NP protein. Nucleotide changes resulting in single-amino-acid exchanges were identified in both NP and L genes. Three other mutations found in VP24 caused amino acid substitutions, which are responsible for larger structural changes of this protein, as indicated by an alteration in electrophoretic mobility. A highly pathogenic EBOV variant K5 from another passaging series showed an amino acid substitution at nearly the same location in the VP24 gene, suggesting the importance of this protein in the adaptation process. In addition, sequence variability of the GP gene was found when plaque-purified clones of EBOV-8mc were analyzed. Three of five viral clones showed insertion of one uridine residue at the GP gene-editing site, which led to a significant change in the expression of virus glycoproteins. This observation suggests that the editing site is a hot spot for insertion and deletion of nucleotides, not only at the level of transcription but also of genome replication. Irrespective of the number of uridine residues at the editing site, all plaque-purified clones of EBOV variant 8mc resembled each other in their pathogenicity for guinea pigs, indicating either the absence or only supportive role of mutations in the GP gene on the adaptation process.

Copyright 2000 Academic Press.

PMID: 11062045 [PubMed - indexed for MEDLINE]

2175. Nurs Stand. 2000 Nov 8-14;15(8):20.

Under siege. An outbreak of the Ebola virus in Uganda has already taken its toll on nurses.

Hyde-Price C.

PMID: 11971462 [PubMed - indexed for MEDLINE]

2176. Proc Natl Acad Sci U S A. 2000 Nov 7;97(23):12411-2.

Emerging viral diseases.

Nichol ST(1), Arikawa J, Kawaoka Y.

Author information: (1)Special Pathogens Branch, Division of Viral and Rickettsial Diseases, Centers for Disease Control and Prevention, Atlanta, GA 30333, USA.

PMCID: PMC34064 PMID: 11035785 [PubMed - indexed for MEDLINE]

2177. Science. 2000 Nov 3;290(5493):923-5.

Emerging diseases. On the trail of Ebola and Marburg viruses.

Balter M.

PMID: 11184732 [PubMed - indexed for MEDLINE]

2178. J Virol. 2000 Nov;74(21):10194-201.

Functional importance of the coiled-coil of the Ebola virus glycoprotein.

Watanabe S(1), Takada A, Watanabe T, Ito H, Kida H, Kawaoka Y.

Author information: (1)Department of Pathobiological Sciences, School of Veterinary Medicine, University of Wisconsin-Madison, Madison, Wisconsin 53706, USA.
Ebola virus contains a single glycoprotein (GP) that is responsible for receptor binding and membrane fusion and is proteolytically cleaved into disulfide-linked GP1 and GP2 subunits. The GP2 subunit possesses a coiled-coil motif, which plays an important role in the oligomerization and fusion activity of other viral GPs. To determine the functional significance of the coiled-coil motif of GP2, we examined the effects of peptides corresponding to the coiled-coil motif of GP2 on the infectivity of a mutant vesicular stomatitis virus (lacking the receptor-binding/fusion protein) pseudotyped with the Ebola virus GP. A peptide corresponding to the C-terminal helix reduced the infectivity of the pseudotyped virus. We next introduced alanine substitutions into hydrophobic residues in the coiled-coil motif to identify residues important for GP function. None of the substitutions affected GP oligomerization, but some mutations, two in the N-terminal helix and all in the C-terminal helix, reduced the ability of GP to confer infectivity to the mutant vesicular stomatitis virus without affecting the transport of GP to the cell surface, its incorporation into virions, and the production of virus particles. These results indicate that the coiled-coil motif of GP2 plays an important role in facilitating the entry of Ebola virus into host cells and that peptides corresponding to this region could act as efficient antiviral agents.

PMCID: PMC102058 PMID: 11024148 [PubMed - indexed for MEDLINE]

2179. US News World Rep. 2000 Oct 30;129(17):39.

A killer virus pays a visit. Can Uganda contain the Ebola outbreak?

Lovgren S.

PMID: 11556383 [PubMed - indexed for MEDLINE]

2180. BMJ. 2000 Oct 28;321(7268):1037.

Ebola virus claims more lives in Uganda.

MacDonald R.

PMCID: PMC1118838 PMID: 11053156 [PubMed - indexed for MEDLINE]

2181. Nurs Times. 2000 Oct 26-Nov 1;96(43):12-3.

What is Ebola?

Gelbart M.

PMID: 11968675 [PubMed - indexed for MEDLINE]

2182. Proc Natl Acad Sci U S A. 2000 Oct 24;97(22):12289-94.

The Ebola virus VP35 protein functions as a type I IFN antagonist.

Basler CF(1), Wang X, Mühlberger E, Volchkov V, Paragas J, Klenk HD, García-Sastre A, Palese P.

Author information: (1)Department of Microbiology, Mount Sinai School of Medicine, One Gustave L. Levy Place, New York, NY 10029, USA.
An assay has been developed that allows the identification of molecules that function as type I IFN antagonists. Using this assay, we have identified an Ebola virus-encoded inhibitor of the type I IFN response, the Ebola virus VP35 protein. The assay relies on the properties of an influenza virus mutant, influenza delNS1 virus, which lacks the NS1 ORF and, therefore, does not produce the NS1 protein. When cells are infected with influenza delNS1 virus, large amounts of type I IFN are produced. As a consequence, influenza delNS1 virus replicates poorly. However, high-efficiency transient transfection of a plasmid encoding a protein that interferes with type I IFN-induced antiviral functions, such as the influenza A virus NS1 protein or the herpes simplex virus protein ICP34.5, rescues growth of influenza delNS1 virus. When plasmids expressing individual Ebola virus proteins were transfected into Madin Darby canine kidney cells, the Ebola virus VP35 protein enhanced influenza delNS1 virus growth more than 100-fold. VP35 subsequently was shown to block double-stranded RNA- and virus-mediated induction of an IFN-stimulated response element reporter gene and to block double-stranded RNA- and virus-mediated induction of the IFN-beta promoter. The Ebola virus VP35 therefore is likely to inhibit induction of type I IFN in Ebola virus-infected cells and may be an important determinant of Ebola virus virulence in vivo.

PMCID: PMC17334 PMID: 11027311 [PubMed - indexed for MEDLINE]

2183. Wkly Epidemiol Rec. 2000 Oct 20;75(42):337-8.

Ebola, Uganda.

[Article in English, French]
[No authors listed]
PMID: 11218329 [PubMed - indexed for MEDLINE]
2184. Clin Microbiol Rev. 2000 Oct;13(4):602-14.

Passive immunity in prevention and treatment of infectious diseases.

Keller MA(1), Stiehm ER.

Author information: (1)Department of Pediatrics, UCLA School of Medicine, Harbor-UCLA Medical Center, Torrance, California 90509-2910, USA. keller@humc.edu

Antibodies have been used for over a century in the prevention and treatment of infectious disease. They are used most commonly for the prevention of measles, hepatitis A, hepatitis B, tetanus, varicella, rabies, and vaccinia. Although their use in the treatment of bacterial infection has largely been supplanted by antibiotics, antibodies remain a critical component of the treatment of diptheria, tetanus, and botulism. High-dose intravenous immunoglobulin can be used to treat certain viral infections in immunocompromised patients (e.g., cytomegalovirus, parvovirus B19, and enterovirus infections). Antibodies may also be of value in toxic shock syndrome, Ebola virus, and refractory staphylococcal infections. Palivizumab, the first monoclonal antibody licensed (in 1998) for an infectious disease, can prevent respiratory syncytial virus infection in high-risk infants. The development and use of additional monoclonal antibodies to key epitopes of microbial pathogens may further define protective humoral responses and lead to new approaches for the prevention and treatment of infectious diseases.

PMCID: PMC88952 PMID: 11023960 [PubMed - indexed for MEDLINE]
2185. Comp Med. 2000 Oct;50(5):479-80.

Comments on the article "Marburg and Ebola virus infections in laboratory non-human primates: a literature review". Soren Schou and Axel Kornerup Hansen. Comparative Medicine, 2000. 50:108-123.

Weber H.

Comment on Comp Med. 2000 Apr;50(2):108-23.
PMID: 11099125 [PubMed - indexed for MEDLINE]
2186. J Virol. 2000 Oct;74(20):9738-41.

Critical role for the cysteines flanking the internal fusion peptide of avian sarcoma/leukosis virus envelope glycoprotein.

Delos SE(1), White JM.

Author information: (1)Department of Cell Biology, School of Medicine, University of Virginia Health System, Charlottesville, Virginia 22908, USA. sed7a@unix.virginia.edu

The transmembrane subunit (TM) of the envelope glycoprotein (Env) of the oncovirus avian sarcoma/leukosis virus (ASLV) contains an internal fusion peptide flanked by two cysteines (C9 and C45). These cysteines, as well as an analogous pair in the Ebola virus GP glycoprotein, are predicted to be joined by a disulfide bond. To examine the importance of these cysteines, we mutated C9 and C45 in the ASLV subtype A Env (EnvA), individually and together, to serine. All of the mutant EnvAs formed trimers that were composed of the proteolytically processed surface (SU) and TM subunits. All mutant EnvAs were incorporated into murine leukemia virus pseudotyped virions and bound receptor with wild-type affinity. Nonetheless, all mutant EnvAs were significantly impaired (approximately 1,000-fold) in their ability to support infectivity. They were also significantly impaired in their ability to mediate cell-cell fusion. Our data are consistent with a model in which the internal fusion peptide of ASLV-A EnvA exists as a loop that is stabilized by a disulfide bond at its base and in which this stabilized loop serves an important function during virus-cell fusion. The fusion peptide of the Ebola virus GP glycoprotein may conform to a similar structure.

PMCID: PMC112407 PMID: 11000247 [PubMed - indexed for MEDLINE]
2187. Vet Hum Toxicol. 2000 Oct;42(5):297-300.

The poison center role in biological and chemical terrorism.

Krenzelok EP(1), Allswede MP, Mrvos R.

Author information: (1)Pittsburgh Poison Center, Children's Hospital of Pittsburgh and School of Pharmacy and Medicine, University of Pittsburgh, PA 15213, USA.

Nuclear, biological and chemical (NBC) terrorism countermeasures are a major priority with municipalities, healthcare providers, and the federal government. Significant resources are being invested to enhance civilian domestic preparedness by conducting education at every response level in anticipation of a NBC terroristic incident. The key to a successful response, in addition to education, is integration of efforts as well as thorough communication and understanding the role that each agency would play in an actual or impending NBC incident. In anticipation of a NBC event, a regional counter-terrorism task force was established to identify resources, establish responsibilities and coordinate the response to NBC terrorism. Members of the task force included first responders, hazmat, law enforcement (local, regional, national), government officials, the health department, and the regional poison information center. Response protocols were developed and education was conducted, culminating in all members of the response task force becoming certified NBC instructors. The poison center participated actively in 3 incidents of suspected biologic and chemical terrorism: an alleged anthrax-contaminated letter sent to a women's health clinic; a possible sarin gas release in a high school: and a potential anthrax/ebola contamination incident at an international airport. All incidents were determined hoaxes. The regional response plan establishes the poison information center as a common repository for all cases in a biological or chemical incident. The poison center is one of several critical components of a regional counterterrorism response force. It can conduct active and passive toxicosurveillance and identify sentinel events. To be responsive, the poison center staff must be knowledgeable about biological and chemical agents. The development of basic protocols and a standardized staff education program is essential. The use of the RaPiD-T (R-recognition, P-protection, D-detection, T-triage/treatment) course can provide basic staff education for responding to this important but rare consultation to the poison center.

PMID: 11003124 [PubMed - indexed for MEDLINE]

2188. Lancet. 2000 Sep 30;356(9236):1173.

Hunting and logging linked to emerging infectious diseases.

Larkin M.

PMID: 11030306 [PubMed - indexed for MEDLINE]

2189. Ann Pathol. 2000 Sep;20(4):297.

[Emergence of new infectious disease: the anatomic pathologists's point of view].

[Article in French]

Loubière R.

Comment on Ann Pathol. 2000 Sep;20(4):323-42.

PMID: 11015645 [PubMed - indexed for MEDLINE]

2190. J Gen Virol. 2000 Sep;81(Pt 9):2155-9.

Differential induction of cellular detachment by envelope glycoproteins of Marburg and Ebola (Zaire) viruses.

Chan SY(1), Ma MC, Goldsmith MA.

Author information: (1)Gladstone Institute of Virology and Immunology, PO Box 419100, San Francisco, CA 94141-9100, USA.

Human infection by Marburg (MBG) or Ebola (EBO) virus is associated with fatal haemorrhagic fevers. While these filoviruses may both incite disease as a result of explosive virus replication, we hypothesized that expression of individual viral gene products, such as the envelope glycoprotein (GP), may directly alter target cells and contribute to pathogenesis. We found that expression of EBO GP in 293T cells caused significant levels of cellular detachment in the absence of cell death or virus replication. This detachment was induced most potently by membrane-bound EBO GP, rather than the shed glycoprotein products (sGP or GP1), and was largely attributable to a domain within the extracellular region of GP2. Furthermore, detachment was blocked by the Ser/Thr kinase inhibitor 2-aminopurine, suggesting the importance of a phosphorylation-dependent signalling cascade in inducing detachment. Since MBG GP did not induce similar cellular detachment, MBG and EBO GP interact with target cells by distinct processes to elicit cellular dysregulation.

PMID: 10950971 [PubMed - indexed for MEDLINE]

2191. Kansenshogaku Zasshi. 2000 Sep;74(9):687-93.

[Future direction of medical care system for patients with infectious disease and the new infectious diseases control law in Japan--centering around a category 1 hospital].

[Article in Japanese]

Takeda Y(1), Nomura T.

Author information: (1)Funabashi Public Health Center.

As of April 1, 1999, the new Infectious Diseases Control Law became effective in Japan. Under the new law, there are three types of category for medical care systems such as "Specified Infectious Disease Medical Hospital", "Category 1 Infectious Disease (Ebola virus hemorrhagic fever, Marburg disease, Lassa fever, Crimean-Congo hemorrhagic fever and plague) Designated Hospital" and "Category 2 Infectious Disease (Cholera, Sigellosis, Typhoid fever, Paratyphoid fever, Poliomyelitis and Diphtheria) Designated Hospital". In these categories, Category 1 Infectious Disease Designated Hospital should be designated by prefectural governments, one hospital per prefecture. Recently some papers indicated that (1) whether each government should arrange a category 1 hospital, (2) whether strict isolation with precautions against airborne spread including negative air pressure with anterior-room should be required, (3) plague is not a dangerous disease and the patient with plague is not required of Category 1 hospital but Category 2 hospital for medical care and infection control. The purpose of this article is, including a counterargument for these opinion, to summarize the point of view for the new medical care system under the new law and to search for the future medical care system in Japan. First of all, medical care for patients with infectious diseases should not be a special one but the extension of the general one. Second, we understand that one of the purposes for Category 1 hospital is the core hospital concerning the therapy, pre/post education and research for infectious diseases in each prefectures. Third, the constructive standard for Category 1 hospital should be a strict one including negative air pressure rooms with an anterior-room and an outside hall, and the air should not be recirculated. Under the big chance of enforcement of this new Infectious Diseases Control Law in Japan, we should try to restruct about medical care system for patients with infectious diseases in a long-range plan.

PMID: 11068360 [PubMed - indexed for MEDLINE]

2192. EMBO J. 2000 Aug 15;19(16):4228-36.

Crystal structure of the matrix protein VP40 from Ebola virus.

Dessen A(1), Volchkov V, Dolnik O, Klenk HD, Weissenhorn W.

Author information: (1)European Molecular Biology Laboratory Grenoble Outstation, 6 rue Jules Horowitz, 38000 Grenoble, France.

Ebola virus maturation occurs at the plasma membrane of infected cells and involves the clustering of the viral matrix protein VP40 at the assembly site as well as its interaction with the lipid bilayer. Here we report the X-ray crystal structure of VP40 from Ebola virus at 2.0 A resolution. The crystal structure reveals that Ebola virus VP40 is topologically distinct from all other known viral matrix proteins, consisting of two domains with unique folds, connected by a flexible linker. The C-terminal domain, which is absolutely required for membrane binding, contains large hydrophobic patches that may be involved in the

interaction with lipid bilayers. Likewise, a highly basic region is shared between the two domains. The crystal structure reveals how the molecule may be able to switch from a monomeric conformation to a hexameric form, as observed in vitro. Its implications for the assembly process are discussed.
PMCID: PMC302032 PMID: 10944105 [PubMed - indexed for MEDLINE]

2193. Vaccine. 2000 Aug 15;19(1):142-53.

Recombinant RNA replicons derived from attenuated Venezuelan equine encephalitis virus protect guinea pigs and mice from Ebola hemorrhagic fever virus.

Pushko P(1), Bray M, Ludwig GV, Parker M, Schmaljohn A, Sanchez A, Jahrling PB, Smith JF.

Author information: (1)Virology Division, US Army Medical Research Institute for Infectious Diseases, Fort Detrick, Frederick, MD 21702, USA.

RNA replicons derived from an attenuated strain of Venezuelan equine encephalitis virus (VEE), an alphavirus, were configured as candidate vaccines for Ebola hemorrhagic fever. The Ebola nucleoprotein (NP) or glycoprotein (GP) genes were introduced into the VEE RNA downstream from the VEE 26S promoter in place of the VEE structural protein genes. The resulting recombinant replicons, expressing the NP or GP genes, were packaged into VEE replicon particles (NP-VRP and GP-VRP, respectively) using a bipartite helper system that provided the VEE structural proteins in trans and prevented the regeneration of replication-competent VEE during packaging. The immunogenicity of NP-VRP and GP-VRP and their ability to protect against lethal Ebola infection were evaluated in BALB/c mice and in two strains of guinea pigs. The GP-VRP alone, or in combination with NP-VRP, protected both strains of guinea pigs and BALB/c mice, while immunization with NP-VRP alone protected BALB/c mice, but neither strain of guinea pig. Passive transfer of sera from VRP-immunized animals did not confer protection against lethal challenge. However, the complete protection achieved with active immunization with VRP, as well as the unique characteristics of the VEE replicon vector, warrant further testing of the safety and efficacy of NP-VRP and GP-VRP in primates as candidate vaccines against Ebola hemorrhagic fever.
PMID: 10924796 [PubMed - indexed for MEDLINE]

2194. Nat Med. 2000 Aug;6(8):886-9.

Identification of the Ebola virus glycoprotein as the main viral determinant of vascular cell cytotoxicity and injury.

Yang ZY(1), Duckers HJ, Sullivan NJ, Sanchez A, Nabel EG, Nabel GJ.

Author information: (1)Vaccine Research Center, National Institutes of Health, 40 Convent Drive, Bethesda, Maryland 20892-3005, USA.

Here we defined the main viral determinant of Ebola virus pathogenicity; synthesis of the virion glycoprotein (GP) of Ebola virus Zaire induced cytotoxic effects in human endothelial cells in vitro and in vivo. This effect mapped to a serine-threonine-rich, mucin-like domain of this type I transmembrane glycoprotein, one of seven gene products of the virus. Gene transfer of GP into explanted human or porcine blood vessels caused massive endothelial cell loss within 48 hours that led to a substantial increase in vascular permeability. Deletion of the mucin-like region of GP abolished these effects without affecting protein expression or function. GP derived from the Reston strain of virus, which causes disease in nonhuman primates but not in man, did not disrupt the vasculature of human blood vessels. In contrast, the Zaire GP induced endothelial cell disruption and cytotoxicity in both nonhuman primate and human blood vessels, and the mucin domain was required for this effect. These findings indicate that GP, through its mucin domain, is the viral determinant of Ebola pathogenicity and likely contributes to hemorrhage during infection.
PMID: 10932225 [PubMed - indexed for MEDLINE]

2195. Acta Trop. 2000 Jul 21;76(1):3-7.

Communicable disease surveillance with limited resources: the scope to link human and veterinary programmes.

Shears P(1).

Author information: (1)Centre for Tropical Medical Microbiology, Liverpool School of Tropical Medicine, UK. shears@liv.ac.uk

Zoonoses are an important cause of human disease in much of Africa, but limitations in current diagnosis and surveillance strategies restrict the effectiveness of control and prevention programmes. Outbreaks of disease, ranging from Ebola virus infection to Rift Valley Fever, that have occurred recently in Africa have demonstrated the need for improved disease surveillance and monitoring. Strategies are suggested for co-ordinating human and animal disease surveillance programmes, at the district and regional level, to make more effective use of limited resources.
PMID: 10913758 [PubMed - indexed for MEDLINE]

2196. Bull Soc Pathol Exot. 2000 Jul;93(3):172-5.

[Forest ecosystems and Ebola virus].

[Article in French]

Morvan JM(1), Nakouné E, Deubel V, Colyn M.

Author information: (1)Laboratoire des arbovirus, Institut Pasteur, Bangui, République Centrafricaine. morvan@intnet.cf

Despite data collected since the emergence of the Ebola virus in 1976, its natural transmission cycle and especially the nature of its reservoirs and means of transmission are still an enigma. This means that effective epidemiological surveillance and prevention are difficult to implement. The location of outbreak areas has suggested that the reservoir and the transmission cycle of the Ebola virus are closely linked to the rainforest ecosystem. The fact that outbreaks seldom occur suggests the presence of a rare animal reservoir having few contacts with man. Paradoxically, various serological investigations have shown a high prevalence in human beings, especially in forest areas of the Central African Republic (CAR), with no pathology associated. This would appear to suggest a circulation of both pathogenic and non-pathogenic strains as well as frequent contacts with man. The ecological changes resulting from human activity (agriculture and logging) account for the modification of the fauna (movement of rainforest fauna, introduction of savannah species) and could explain a multiplication of contacts. Likewise, it is interesting to note that the centre of outbreaks has always been in areas bordering on forests (ecotone foreset-

savannah in the Democratic Republic of Congo, savannah in Sudan). All these considerations have led us to establish a permanent "watch" in areas bordering on forests in the CAR, involving a multidisciplinary approach to the virological study (strain isolation, molecular biology) of the biodiversity of small terrestrial mammals. The results of a study conducted on 947 small mammals has shown for the first time the presence of the Ebola virus genome in two species of rodents and one species of shrew living in forest border areas. These animals must be considered as intermediary hosts and research should now focus on reservoirs in the ecosystem of forest border areas where contacts with man are likely to be more frequent.
PMID: 11030051 [PubMed - indexed for MEDLINE]
2197. Bull Soc Pathol Exot. 2000 Jul;93(3):156.

[Circulation of virus and interspecies contamination in wild animals].

[Article in French]

Osterhaus A(1).

Author information: (1)Université de Rotterdam, Pays-Bas.

Paradoxically, just when we have succeeded in eradicating and/or bringing under control the major viral infections (smallpox, poliomyelitis, measles) numerous viral infections are emerging in man and in animals. Changes in our social environment, technological and ecological equilibrium have facilitated this phenomenon. Furthermore, certain of these viruses have demonstrated an almost unlimited capacity to adapt genetically to environmental change. HIV has already infected 40 million individuals, but monkeypox, Ebola, simian herpes can cause epidemics with serious if not fatal outcomes. Haemorrhagic fever epidemics have resulted from human contact with Flavivirus infected rodents and insects. Paramyxoviruses and morbiliviruses can cause fatal outcomes in man and animals. And the three influenza epidemics having occurred in the 20th century all came from the type A avian reservoir. The often complex combinations of predisposing factors having facilitated the emergence of several epidemics merit further consideration.
PMID: 11030047 [PubMed - indexed for MEDLINE]
2198. J Health Hum Serv Adm. 2000 Summer;23(1):83-99.

International health and emerging infectious diseases.

Ebomoyi W(1), Ebomoyi JI.

Author information: (1)University of Northern Colorado, USA.

This article explored the role of international health in reducing the impact of infectious diseases by espousing the monumental application of global electronic communication and socioeconomic development initiatives. The interaction between the society and environmental changes have dramatic effects on the frequency of infectious diseases worldwide. Development of dams, human population expansion, migration patterns, urbanization and the invasion of hitherto virgin forests, and global warming enhance the proliferation of vectors of infectious diseases. Sustainable development and emphasis on primary prevention initiatives, coupled with the application of technology to improve farming, provision of safe water and electrification of rural communities, are significant steps in infectious disease control.
PMID: 11269207 [PubMed - indexed for MEDLINE]
2199. J Mol Biol. 2000 Jun 30;300(1):103-12.

Structural characterization and membrane binding properties of the matrix protein VP40 of Ebola virus.

Ruigrok RW(1), Schoehn G, Dessen A, Forest E, Volchkov V, Dolnik O, Klenk HD, Weissenhorn W.

Author information: (1)Grenoble Outstation, European Molecular Biology Laboratory (EMBL), 6 rue Jules Horowitz, Grenoble, 38000, France.

The matrix protein VP40 of Ebola virus is believed to play a central role in viral assembly as it targets the plasma membrane of infected cells and subsequently forms a tightly packed layer on the inner side of the viral envelope. Expression of VP40 in Escherichia coli and subsequent proteolysis yielded two structural variants differing by a C-terminal truncation 114 amino acid residues long. As indicated by chemical cross-linking studies and electron microscopy, the larger polypeptide was present in a monomeric form, whereas the truncated one formed hexamers. When analyzed for their in vitro binding properties, both constructs showed that only monomeric VP40 efficiently associated with membranes containing negatively charged lipids. Membrane association of truncated, hexameric VP40 was inefficient, indicating a membrane-recognition role for the C-terminal part. Based on these observations we propose that assembly of Ebola virus involves the formation of VP40 hexamers that is mediated by the N-terminal part of the polypeptide.
Copyright 2000 Academic Press.
PMID: 10864502 [PubMed - indexed for MEDLINE]
2200. Lancet. 2000 Jun 24;355(9222):2210-5.

Human asymptomatic Ebola infection and strong inflammatory response.

Leroy EM(1), Baize S, Volchkov VE, Fisher-Hoch SP, Georges-Courbot MC, Lansoud-Soukate J, Capron M, Debré P, McCormick JB, Georges AJ.

Author information: (1)Centre International de Recherches Médicales de Franceville, Gabon. leroy@cimf.sci.ga

Comment in Lancet. 2000 Jun 24;355(9222):2178-9.

BACKGROUND: Ebola virus is one of the most virulent pathogens, killing a very high proportion of patients within 5-7 days. Two outbreaks of fulminating haemorrhagic fever occurred in northern Gabon in 1996, with a 70% case-fatality rate. During both outbreaks we identified some individuals in direct contact with sick patients who never developed symptoms. We aimed to determine whether these individuals were indeed infected with Ebola virus, and how they maintained asymptomatic status. METHODS: Blood was collected from 24 close contacts of symptomatic patients. These asymptomatic individuals were sampled 2, 3, or 4 times during a 1-month period after the first exposure to symptomatic patients. Serum samples were analysed for the presence of Ebola antigens, virus-specific IgM and IgG (by ELISA and western blot), and different cytokines and chemokines. RNA was extracted from peripheral blood mononuclear cells, and reverse transcriptase-PCR assays were done to amplify RNA of Ebola virus. PCR products were then sequenced. FINDINGS: 11 of 24 asymptomatic individuals developed both IgM and IgG responses to Ebola antigens, indicating viral infection. Western-blot analysis showed that IgG responses were directed to nucleoprotein and viral protein of 40 kDa. The glycoprotein and viral protein of 24 kDa genes showed no nucleotide differences between symptomatic and asymptomatic individuals. Asymptomatic individuals had a strong inflammatory response characterised by high circulating concentrations of cytokines and chemokines. INTERPRETATION: This study showed that asymptomatic, replicative Ebola infection can and does occur in human beings. The lack of genetic differences between symptomatic and asymptomatic individuals suggest that asymptomatic Ebola infection did not result from viral mutations. Elucidation of the factors related to the genesis of the strong inflammatory response occurring early during the infectious process in these asymptomatic individuals could increase our understanding of the disease.

PMID: 10881895 [PubMed - indexed for MEDLINE]

2201. Lancet. 2000 Jun 24;355(9222):2178-9.

Symptomless infection with Ebola virus.

Baxter AG(1).

Author information: (1)Centenary Institute of Cancer Medicine and Cell Biology, Newtown NSW, Australia.

Comment on Lancet. 2000 Jun 24;355(9222):2210-5.

PMID: 10881884 [PubMed - indexed for MEDLINE]

2202. Acta Crystallogr D Biol Crystallogr. 2000 Jun;56(Pt 6):758-60.

Crystallization and preliminary X-ray analysis of the matrix protein from Ebola virus.

Dessen A(1), Forest E, Volchkov V, Dolnik O, Klenk HD, Weissenhorn W.

Author information: (1)European Molecular Biology Laboratory (EMBL), Grenoble, France.

The matrix protein from Ebola virus is a membrane-associated molecule that plays a role in viral budding. Despite its functional similarity to other viral matrix proteins, it displays no sequence similarity and hence may have a distinct fold. X-ray diffraction quality crystals of the Ebola VP40 matrix protein were grown by the hanging-drop vapour-diffusion method. The crystals belong to the monoclinic space group C2, with unit-cell parameters a = 64.4, b = 91.1, c = 47.9 A, beta = 96.3 degrees. A data set to 1.9 A resolution has been collected using synchrotron radiation. The unit cell contains one molecule of molecular weight 35 kDa per asymmetric unit, with a corresponding volume solvent content of 35%.

PMID: 10818356 [PubMed - indexed for MEDLINE]

2203. J Virol. 2000 May;74(10):4933-7.

Distinct mechanisms of entry by envelope glycoproteins of Marburg and Ebola (Zaire) viruses.

Chan SY(1), Speck RF, Ma MC, Goldsmith MA.

Author information: (1)Gladstone Institute of Virology and Immunology, San Francisco, California 94141-9100, USA.

Since the Marburg (MBG) and Ebola (EBO) viruses have sequence homology and cause similar diseases, we hypothesized that they associate with target cells by similar mechanisms. Pseudotype viruses prepared with a luciferase-containing human immunodeficiency virus type 1 backbone and packaged by the MBG virus or the Zaire subtype EBO virus glycoproteins (GP) mediated infection of a comparable wide range of mammalian cell types, and both were inhibited by ammonium chloride. In contrast, they exhibited differential sensitivities to treatment of target cells with tunicamycin, endoglycosidase H, or protease (pronase). Therefore, while they exhibit certain functional similarities, the MBG and EBO virus GP interact with target cells by distinct processes.

PMCID: PMC112022 PMID: 10775638 [PubMed - indexed for MEDLINE]

2204. Rinsho Byori. 2000 May;Suppl 112:15-20.

[Introduction to sterilization and disinfection of medical wastes contaminated with human virus].

[Article in Japanese]

Ichikawa S(1), Ohya H, Ito K.

Author information: (1)Kanagawa Prefectural College of Nursing and Medical Technology.

In this paper, we describe sterilization and disinfection of medical wastes contaminated with blood borne-virus, such as Ebola virus, Marburg virus, Crimean-Congo hemorrhagic fever virus, Lassa virus, Hepatitis B virus and Human immunodeficiency virus.

PMID: 10901040 [PubMed - indexed for MEDLINE]

2205. Trop Med Int Health. 2000 May;5(5):318-24.

Viewpoint: filovirus haemorrhagic fever outbreaks: much ado about nothing?

Borchert M(1), Boelaert M, Sleurs H, Muyembe-Tamfum JJ, Pirard P, Colebunders R, Van der Stuyft P, van der Groen G.

Author information: (1)Institute of Tropical Medicine, Antwerp, Belgium. mborchert@itg.be

The recent outbreak of Marburg haemorrhagic fever in the Democratic Republic of Congo has put the filovirus threat back on the international health agenda. This paper gives an overview of Marburg and Ebola outbreaks so far observed and puts them in a public health perspective. Damage on the local level has been devastating at times, but was marginal on the international level despite the considerable media attention these outbreaks received. The potential hazard of outbreaks, however, after export of filovirus from its natural environment into metropolitan areas, is argued to be considerable. Some avenues for future research and intervention are explored. Beyond the obvious need to find the reservoir and study the natural history, public health strategies for a more timely and efficient response are urgently needed.

PMID: 10886793 [PubMed - indexed for MEDLINE]

2206. Vopr Virusol. 2000 May-Jun;45(3):40-4.

[Monoclonal antibodies to Ebola virus: isolation, characteristics, and study of cross reactivity with Marburg virus].

[Article in Russian]

Kazachinskaia EI, Pereboev AV, Chepurnov AA, Belanov EF, Razumov IA.

Thirteen hybridoma strains producing monoclonal antibodies (Mabs) to Ebola virus were prepared by fusion of NS-0 mouse myeloma cells with splenocytes of BALB/c mice immunized with purified and inactivated Ebola virus (Mayinga strain). Mabs directed against viral proteins were selected and tested by ELISA. Protein specificity of 13 Mabs was determined by immunoblotting with SDS-PAGE proteins of Ebola virus. Of these, 11 hybridoma Mabs reacted with 116 kDa protein (NP) and 2 with Ebola virus VP35. Antigenic cross-reactivity between Ebola and Marburg viruses was examined in ELISA and immunoblotting with polyclonal and monoclonal antibodies. In ELISA, polyclonal antibodies of immune sera to Ebola or Marburg viruses reacted with heterologous filoviruses, and two anti-NP Ebola antibodies (Mabs 7E1 and 6G8) cross-reacted with both viruses. Target proteins for cross-reactivity, Ebola NP (116 kDa) and Marburg NP (96 kDa), and VP35 of both filoviruses were detected by immunoblotting with polyclonal and monoclonal antibodies (6G8) to Ebola virus.

PMID: 10867995 [PubMed - indexed for MEDLINE]

2207. Comp Med. 2000 Apr;50(2):108-23.

Marburg and Ebola virus infections in laboratory non-human primates: a literature review.

Schou S(1), Hansen AK.

Author information: (1)Department of Oral Surgery, School of Dentistry, Faculty of Health Sciences, University of Copenhagen and University Hospital (Rigshospitalet), Denmark.

Comment in Comp Med. 2000 Oct;50(5):479-80.

BACKGROUND AND PURPOSE: Several non-human primate species are used as laboratory animals for various types of studies. Although importation of monkeys may introduce different diseases, special attention has recently been drawn to Marburg and Ebola viruses. This review presented here discusses the potential risk of these viruses for persons working with non-human primates as laboratory animals by focusing on epidemiology, virology, symptoms, pathogenesis, natural reservoir, transmission, quarantine of non-human primates, therapy, and prevention. CONCLUSION: A total of 23 Marburg and Ebola virus outbreaks causing viral hemorrhagic fever has been reported among humans and monkeys since the first outbreak in Marburg, Germany in 1967. Most of the 1,100 human cases, with nearly 800 deaths, developed in Africa due mainly to direct and intimate contact with infected patients. Few human cases have developed after contact with non-human primates used for various scientific purposes. However, adequate quarantine should be applied to prevent human infections not only due to Marburg and Ebola viruses, but also to other infective agents. By following proper guidelines, the filovirus infection risk for people working with non-human primates during quarantine exists, but is minimal. There seems to be little risk for filovirus infections after an adequate quarantine period. Therefore, non-human primates can be used as laboratory animals, with little risk of filovirus infections, provided adequate precautions are taken.

PMID: 10857001 [PubMed - indexed for MEDLINE]

2208. J Med Virol. 2000 Apr;60(4):463-7.

Diagnosis of Ebola haemorrhagic fever by RT-PCR in an epidemic setting.

Leroy EM(1), Baize S, Lu CY, McCormick JB, Georges AJ, Georges-Courbot MC, Lansoud-Soukate J, Fisher-Hoch SP.

Author information: (1)Centre International de Recherches Médicales de Franceville, BP 769 Franceville, Gabon. leroy@cirmf.sci.ga

This study reports the first field evaluation of a new diagnostic technique for Ebola virus disease with sensitivity and specificity. Ebola virus causes rare but fulminating outbreaks in Equatorial Africa. Rapid differentiation from other infections is critical for timely implementation of public health measures. Patients usually die before developing antibodies, necessitating rapid virus detection. A reverse transcriptase-polymerase chain reaction (RT-PCR) assay was developed, implemented and evaluated at Centre International de Recherches Médicales de Franceville (CIRMF) in Gabon, to detect Ebola viral RNA in peripheral blood mononuclear cells (PBMC). Twenty-six laboratory-confirmed patients during and 5 after the acute phase of Ebola haemorrhagic fever, 15 healthy controls and 20 febrile patients not infected with Ebola virus were studied. RT-PCR results were compared with ELISA antigen capture, and Ebola specific IgM and IgG antibody detection. Ebola virus RNA was amplified from 26/26 specimens from the acute phase, 3/5 during recovery, 0/20 febrile patients and 1/15 negative controls. Sensitivity of RT-PCR in identifying acute infection and early convalescence compared with antigen or IgM detection was 100% and 91% respectively, and specificity compared with antigen detection and IgM assay combined was 97%. Antigen capture detected only 83% of those identified by PCR, and IgM only 67%. Ebola virus RNA was detected in all 13 fatalities, only 5 of whom had IgM and none IgG. RT-PCR detected Ebola RNA in PBMC one to three weeks after disappearance of symptoms when antigen was undetectable. RT-PCR was the most sensitive method and able to detect virus from early acute disease throughout early recovery.

Copyright 2000 Wiley-Liss, Inc.

PMID: 10686031 [PubMed - indexed for MEDLINE]

2209. Microbes Infect. 2000 Apr;2(5):489-95.

Emerging and reemerging infections in africa: the need for improved laboratory services and disease surveillance.

Shears P(1).

Author information: (1)Centre for Tropical Medical Microbiology, Liverpool School of Tropical Medicine, Pembroke Place, L3 5QA, Liverpool, UK.

Emerging and reemerging infections pose a serious public health threat to most countries of tropical Africa. In the past decade, epidemics of diseases including cholera, dysentery, meningitis, yellow fever and Ebola virus have resulted in significant morbidity and mortality. Improved laboratory services and disease surveillance systems are essential to monitor disease trends and to initiate public health action. The present situation of emerging and reemerging infections in Africa is described in this review, and strategies for improved disease surveillance and monitoring are discussed.

PMID: 10865194 [PubMed - indexed for MEDLINE]

2210. Rev Sci Tech. 2000 Apr;19(1):79-91.

Infections by viruses of the families Bunyaviridae and Filoviridae.

Zeller H(1), Bouloy M.

Author information: (1)Unité des arbovirus et virus des fièvres hémorragiques, Institut Pasteur, 25-28 rue du Docteur Roux, 75724 Paris, France.

Rift Valley fever is the most important bunyaviral disease of animals in Africa. The virus, transmitted by mosquitoes, causes abortions and mortality in young animals in addition to haemorrhagic fevers in humans. Although vaccines against this virus are available, the uses of these vaccines are limited because of deleterious effects or incomplete protection, justifying further studies to improve the existing vaccines or to develop others. Nairobi sheep disease is transmitted by ticks. The disease is endemic in East Africa and sporadic cases are reported in India and Sri Lanka. Other viruses transmitted by mosquitoes or midges are teratogenic in cattle or sheep, these include Akabane and related viruses in Asia, Australia and the Middle East, and Cache Valley in North America. The Marburg and Ebola viruses of the genus Filovirus are associated with epidemics in Central Africa with high fatality rates in humans; some outbreaks were related to contact with monkeys. Another subtype of Ebola virus was first described in a quarantine facility in the United States of America among cynomolgus monkeys (Macaca fascicularis) from the Philippines. The reservoir of these viruses remains unknown.

PMID: 11189728 [PubMed - indexed for MEDLINE]

2211. Rev Sci Tech. 2000 Apr;19(1):310-7.

Public health implications of emerging zoonoses.

Meslin FX(1), Stöhr K, Heymann D.

Author information: (1)Department of Communicable Disease Surveillance and Response, World Health Organization, 20 Avenue Appia, 1211 Geneva 27, Switzerland.

Many new, emerging and re-emerging diseases of humans are caused by pathogens which originate from animals or products of animal origin. A wide variety of animal species, both domestic and wild, act as reservoirs for these pathogens, which may be viruses, bacteria or parasites. Given the extensive distribution of the animal species affected, the effective surveillance, prevention and control of zoonotic diseases pose a significant challenge. The authors describe the direct and indirect implications for public health of emerging zoonoses. Direct implications are defined as the consequences for human health in terms of morbidity and mortality. Indirect implications are defined as the effect of the influence of emerging zoonotic disease on two groups of people, namely: health professionals and the general public. Professional assessment of the importance of these diseases influences public health practices and structures, the identification of themes for research and allocation of resources at both national and international levels. The perception of the general public regarding the risks involved considerably influences policy-making in the health field. Extensive outbreaks of zoonotic disease are not uncommon, especially as the disease is often not recognised as zoonotic at the outset and may spread undetected for some time. However, in many instances, the direct impact on health of these new, emerging or re-emerging zoonoses has been small compared to that of other infectious diseases affecting humans. To illustrate the tremendous indirect impact of emerging zoonotic diseases on public health policy and structures and on public perception of health risks, the authors provide a number of examples, including that of the Ebola virus, avian influenza, monkeypox and bovine spongiform encephalopathy. Recent epidemics of these diseases have served as a reminder of the existence of infectious diseases and of the capacity of these diseases to occur unexpectedly in new locations and animal species. The need for greater international co-operation, better local, regional and global networks for communicable disease surveillance and pandemic planning is also illustrated by these examples. These diseases have contributed to the definition of new paradigms, especially relating to food safety policies and more generally to the protection of public health. Finally, the examples described emphasise the importance of intersectorial collaboration for disease containment, and of independence of sectorial interests and transparency when managing certain health risks.

PMID: 11189723 [PubMed - indexed for MEDLINE]

2212. Circulation. 2000 Mar 14;101(10):E9020.

Antibodies that protect mice against ebola virus hold promise of vaccine and therapy for disease

SoRelle R.

PMID: 10715280 [PubMed - as supplied by publisher]

2213. Science. 2000 Mar 3;287(5458):1664-6.

Epitopes involved in antibody-mediated protection from Ebola virus.

Wilson JA(1), Hevey M, Bakken R, Guest S, Bray M, Schmaljohn AL, Hart MK.

Author information: (1)Virology Division, U.S. Army Medical Research Institute of Infectious Diseases, 1425 Porter Street, Fort Detrick, Frederick, MD 21702-5011, USA.

To determine the ability of antibodies to provide protection from Ebola viruses, monoclonal antibodies (mAbs) to the Ebola glycoprotein were generated and evaluated for efficacy. We identified several protective mAbs directed toward five unique epitopes on Ebola glycoprotein. One of the epitopes is conserved among all Ebola viruses that are known to be pathogenic for humans. Some protective mAbs were also effective therapeutically when administered to mice 2 days after exposure to lethal Ebola virus. The identification of protective mAbs has important implications for developing vaccines and therapies for Ebola virus.

PMID: 10698744 [PubMed - indexed for MEDLINE]

2214. J Intern Med. 2000 Mar;247(3):301-10.

Globalization, coca-colonization and the chronic disease epidemic: can the Doomsday scenario be averted?

Zimmet P(1).

Author information: (1)International Diabetes Institute, Melbourne, Australia.

There are at present approximately 110 million people with diabetes in the world but this number will reach over 220 million by the year 2010, the majority of them with type 2 diabetes. Thus there is an urgent need for strategies to prevent the emerging global epidemic of type 2 diabetes to be implemented. Tackling diabetes must be part of an integrated program that addresses lifestyle related disorders. The prevention and control of type 2 diabetes and the other major noncommunicable diseases (NCDs) can be cost- and health-effective through an integrated (i.e. horizontal) approach to noncommunicable diseases disease prevention and control. With the re-emergence of devastating communicable diseases including AIDS, the Ebola virus and tuberculosis, the pressure is on international and regional agencies to see that the noncommunicable disease epidemic is addressed. The international diabetes and public health communities need to adopt a more pragmatic view of the epidemic of type 2 diabetes and other noncommunicable diseases. The current situation is a symptom of globalization with respect to its social, cultural, economic and political significance. Type 2 diabetes will not be prevented by traditional medical approaches; what is required are major and dramatic changes in the socio-economic and cultural status of people in developing countries and the disadvantaged, minority groups in developed nations. The international diabetes and public health communities must lobby and mobilize politicians, other international agencies such as UNDP, UNICEF, and the World Bank as well as other international nongovernmental agencies dealing with the noncommunicable diseases to address the socio-economic, behavioural, nutritional and public health issues that have led to the type 2 diabetes and noncommunicable diseases epidemic. A multidisciplinary Task Force representing all parties which can contribute to a reversal of the underlying socio-economic causes of the problem is an urgent priority.

PMID: 10762445 [PubMed - indexed for MEDLINE]

2215. Antiviral Res. 2000 Feb;45(2):135-47.

Treatment of lethal Ebola virus infection in mice with a single dose of an S-adenosyl-L-homocysteine hydrolase inhibitor.

Bray M(1), Driscoll J, Huggins JW.

Author information: (1)Department of Viral Therapeutics, United States Army Medical Research Institute of Infectious Diseases, Fort Detrick, Frederick, MD 21702-5011, USA. bray@ncifcrf.gov

Ebola Zaire virus causes lethal hemorrhagic fever in humans, for which there is no effective treatment. A variety of adenosine analogues inhibit the replication of Ebola virus in vitro, probably by blocking the cellular enzyme, S-adenosyl-L-homocysteine hydrolase, thereby indirectly limiting methylation of the 5' cap of viral messenger RNA. We previously observed that adult, immunocompetent mice treated thrice daily for 9 days with 2.2-20 mg/kg of an adenosine analogue, carbocyclic 3-deazaadenosine, were protected against lethal Ebola virus challenge. We now report that a single inoculation of 80 mg/kg or less of the same substance, or of 1 mg/kg or less of another analogue, 3-deazaneplanocin A, provides equal or better protection, without causing acute toxicity. One dose of drug given on the first or second day after virus infection reduced peak viremia more than 1000-fold, compared with mock-treated controls, and resulted in survival of most or all animals. Therapy was less effective when administered on the day of challenge, or on the third day postinfection. Single or multiple doses of the same medications suppressed Ebola replication in severe combined immunodeficient mice, but even daily treatment for 15 consecutive days did not eliminate the infection.

PMID: 10809022 [PubMed - indexed for MEDLINE]

2216. Apoptosis. 2000 Feb;5(1):5-7.

Apoptosis in fatal Ebola infection. Does the virus toll the bell for immune system?

Baize S(1), Leroy EM, Mavoungou E, Fisher-Hoch SP.

Author information: (1)Centre International de Recherches Médicales de Franceville, Gabon, France. sbaize@cirmf.sci.ga

In fatal Ebola virus hemorrhagic fever massive intravascular apoptosis develops rapidly following infection and progressing relentlessly until death. While data suggest that T lymphocytes are mainly deleted by apoptosis in PBMC of human fatal cases, experimental Ebola infection in animal models have shown some evidence of destruction of lymphocytes in spleen and lymph nodes probably involving both T and B cells. Nevertheless, we are able to conclude from the accumulated evidence that early interactions between Ebola virus and the immune system, probably via macrophages, main targets for viral replication, lead to massive destruction of immune cells in fatal cases.

PMID: 11227491 [PubMed - indexed for MEDLINE]

2217. Immunol Lett. 2000 Feb 1;71(2):131-40.

Immune and pathophysiological processes in baboons experimentally infected with Ebola virus adapted to guinea pigs.

Ignatiev GM(1), Dadaeva AA, Luchko SV, Chepurnov AA.

Author information: (1)Institute of Molecular Biology, State Research Center of Virology and Biotechnology Vector, Koltsovo, Novosibirsk region, Russia.

The dynamics of pathophysiological and immunological parameters monitored in monkeys Papio hamadryas infected with the guinea pig-adapted Ebola virus strain demonstrated that this viral strain preserved its virulence for monkeys and caused the disease with characteristic features similar to those caused by non-adapted Ebola virus. However, certain previously unknown patterns have been observed: (1) prolongation of the febrile period by two days; (2) extended period was characterized by stability of serum biochemical parameters; (3) marked vacuolization of the neutrophil cytoplasm; (4) appearance of juvenile lymphocytes on day 3 and by the end of the disease; and (5) a considerable increase in the spontaneous mononuclear proliferation (along with a decrease in the mitogen-induced proliferation) during the terminal stage of infection. The severity of pathological coagulation was found to correlate with the activity of

serum cytokines IFN-alpha and TNF-alpha: their activities increased about 250- and 100-fold, respectively. There was significant alteration in the activity of natural killer cells, that dropped by the time of animal death.
PMID: 10714441 [PubMed - indexed for MEDLINE]
2218. Kansenshogaku Zasshi. 2000 Feb;74(2):87-95.

[Is MBSL-level ward needed for the treatment of viral hemorrhagic diseases and pest?].

[Article in Japanese]

Ebisawa I.

The recently revised Japanese Law on Infectious Diseases designates pest, Lassa, Marburg, Ebola and Crimean-Congo hemorrhagic diseases should be treated in an MBSL-level ward and that it should be constructed in each prefecture. However, pest can be treated with several antibiotics easily in an ordinary infectious disease ward. Lassa, Marburg and Ebola virus diseases are endemic in tropical Africa and only Lassa fever was imported into Japan in 1987. The probability of its importation to each prefecture is calculated on an assumption that a Lassa fever patient may be imported into Japan once in 10 years. Its incidence was calculated in comparison with the incidence of imported malaria from the African continent. Its probability P is calculated as follows. Corrected number of imported malaria patients from the African continent per year for each prefecture CN is divided by 445. 445 is the number of imported malaria patients from the African continent in ten years. Finally 445/CN is the number of years needed for each prefecture to import one case of Lassa fever. The results indicate that it takes 37 years for Metropolitan Tokyo where the largest number of malaria patients are imported annually. Other prefectures need more than 100 to 10,000 years, with an average of 1,017 years, for importation of one patient of Lassa fever. It is concluded that construction of an MBSL-level ward in each prefecture is unnecessary. The reports that the above mentioned viral hemorrhagic diseases can be treated safely in the ordinary infectious disease ward should be carefully reviewed.
PMID: 10740998 [PubMed - indexed for MEDLINE]
2219. Lab Invest. 2000 Feb;80(2):171-86.

Apoptosis induced in vitro and in vivo during infection by Ebola and Marburg viruses.

Geisbert TW(1), Hensley LE, Gibb TR, Steele KE, Jaax NK, Jahrling PB.

Author information: (1)Pathology Division, US Army Medical Research Institute of Infectious Diseases, Fort Detrick, Maryland 21702-5011, USA. tom.geisbert@amedd.army.mil

Induction of apoptosis has been documented during infection with a number of different viruses. In this study, we used transmission electron microscopy (TEM) and terminal deoxynucleotidyl transferase-mediated deoxyuridine triphosphate nick-end labeling to investigate the effects of Ebola and Marburg viruses on apoptosis of different cell populations during in vitro and in vivo infections. Tissues from 18 filovirus-infected nonhuman primates killed in extremis were evaluated. Apoptotic lymphocytes were seen in all tissues examined. Filoviral replication occurred in cells of the mononuclear phagocyte system and other well-documented cellular targets by TEM and immunohistochemistry, but there was no evidence of replication in lymphocytes. With the exception of intracytoplasmic viral inclusions, filovirus-infected cells were morphologically normal or necrotic, but did not exhibit ultrastructural changes characteristic of apoptosis. In lymph nodes, filoviral antigen was co-localized with apoptotic lymphocytes. Examination of cell populations in lymph nodes showed increased numbers of macrophages and concomitant depletion of CD8+ T cells and plasma cells in filovirus-infected animals. This depletion was particularly striking in animals infected with the Zaire subtype of Ebola virus. In addition, apoptosis was demonstrated in vitro in lymphocytes of filovirus-infected human peripheral blood mononuclear cells by TEM. These findings suggest that lymphopenia and lymphoid depletion associated with filoviral infections result from lymphocyte apoptosis induced by a number of factors that may include release of various chemical mediators from filovirus-infected or activated cells, damage to the fibroblastic reticular cell conduit system, and possibly stimulation by a viral protein.
PMID: 10701687 [PubMed - indexed for MEDLINE]
2220. J Immunol. 2000 Jan 15;164(2):953-8.

Ebola virus secretory glycoprotein (sGP) diminishes Fc gamma RIIIB-to-CR3 proximity on neutrophils.

Kindzelskii AL(1), Yang Z, Nabel GJ, Todd RF 3rd, Petty HR.

Author information: (1)Department of Biological Sciences, Wayne State University, Detroit, MI 48202, USA.

Previous studies have shown that Ebola virus' secretory glycoprotein (sGP) binds to Fc gamma RIIIB (CD16b) and inhibits L-selectin shedding. In this study, we test the hypothesis that sGP interferes with the physical linkage between CR3 and Fc gamma RIIIB. Neutrophils were stained with rhodamine-conjugated anti-CD16b mAb (which does not inhibit sGP binding) and fluorescein-conjugated anti-CR3 mAb reagents and then incubated in media with or without sGP. Physical proximity between fluorochrome-labeled CR3 and Fc gamma RIIIB on individual cells was measured by resonance energy transfer (RET) imaging, quantitative RET microfluorometry, and single-cell imaging spectrophotometry. Cells incubated with control supernatants displayed a significant RET signal, indicative of physical proximity (
PMID: 10623844 [PubMed - indexed for MEDLINE]
2221. Bull Soc Pathol Exot. 2000 Jan;93(5):340-7.

[Microbiological surveillance: viral hemorrhagic fever in Central African Republic: current serological data in man].

[Article in French]

Nakounné E(1), Selekon B, Morvan J.

Author information: (1)Laboratoire des fièvres hémorragiques virales, Centre OMS de référence pour les maladies émergentes, Institut Pasteur, BP 923, Bangui, République centrafricaine.

An investigation was conducted between 1994 and 1997 in forested areas of the Central African Republic (CAR) to determine the seroprevalence of IgG antibodies against several haemorrhagic fever viruses present in the region. Sera were obtained from 1762 individuals in two groups (Pygmy and Bantu located populations) living in 4 forested areas in the south of the country. Sera were tested for IgG antibodies against Ebola, Marburg, Rift Valley fever (RVF), Yellow fever (YF) and Hantaviruses by enzyme immunoassay (EIA), and against Lassa virus by immunofluorescent assay. The prevalence of IgG antibodies was 5.9% for Ebola, 2% for Marburg, 6.9% pour RVF, 6.5% for YF, 2% for Hantaan. No antibodies were detected against Lassa, Seoul, Puumala and Thottapalayam viruses. No IgM antibodies were detected against RVF and YF viruses. The distribution of antibodies appears to be related to tropical rain forest areas. This study indicates that several haemorrhagic fever viruses are endemic in forested areas of the CAR and could emerge due to environmental modification.
PMID: 11775321 [PubMed - indexed for MEDLINE]

2222. Bull World Health Organ. 2000;78(12):1476-7.

The Uganda Ebola outbreak--not all negative.

Maurice J.

Comment in Bull World Health Organ. 2001;79(3):267.

PMCID: PMC2560656 PMID: 11196502 [PubMed - indexed for MEDLINE]

2223. Crit Care Med. 2000 Jan;28(1):284-5.

An outbreak of Ebola virus: lessons for everyday activities in the intensive care unit.

Gradon J.

Comment on Crit Care Med. 2000 Jan;28(1):240-4.

PMID: 10667555 [PubMed - indexed for MEDLINE]

2224. Crit Care Med. 2000 Jan;28(1):240-4.

Unexpected Ebola virus in a tertiary setting: clinical and epidemiologic aspects.

Richards GA(1), Murphy S, Jobson R, Mer M, Zinman C, Taylor R, Swanepoel R, Duse A, Sharp G, De La Rey IC, Kassianides C.

Author information: (1)Department of Pulmonology and Critical Care, Johannesburg Hospital, and University of the Witwatersrand, South Africa.

Comment in Crit Care Med. 2000 Jan;28(1):284-5.

OBJECTIVES: To describe the clinical manifestations of viral hemorrhagic fever, and to increase clinicians' awareness and knowledge of these illnesses. DESIGN: Retrospective study of the clinical and laboratory data and management of two cases of Ebola virus infection with key epidemiologic data provided. SETTING: Two tertiary care hospitals. PATIENTS: Two adult patients, the index case and the source patient, both identified as having Ebola, one of whom originated in Gabon. INTERVENTIONS: One patient was admitted to the intensive care unit. The other was managed in a general ward. MEASUREMENT AND MAIN RESULTS: Clinical and laboratory data are reported. One patient, a healthcare worker who contracted this illness in the course of her work, died of refractory thrombocytopenia and an intracerebral bleed. The source patient survived. Despite a long period during which the diagnosis was obscure, none of the other 300 contacts contracted the illness. CONCLUSIONS: Identification of high-risk patients and use of universal blood and body fluid precautions will considerably decrease the risk of nosocomial spread of viral hemorrhagic fevers.
PMID: 10667531 [PubMed - indexed for MEDLINE]

2225. Immunol Res. 2000;21(2-3):265-78.

Antibodies in human infectious disease.

Parren PW(1), Poignard P, Ditzel HJ, Williamson RA, Burton DR.

Author information: (1)Department of Immunology, The Scripps Research Institute, La Jolla, CA 92037, USA.

Investigation of human antibody responses to viral pathogens at the molecular level is revealing novel aspects of the interplay of viruses with the humoral immune system. In viral infection, at least two types of human antibody responses exist: a response to mature envelope on virions that is neutralizing and a response to immature forms of envelope (viral debris) that is not. Many pathogens have, to varying degrees, evolved envelopes to minimize antibody responses against epitopes exposed on the virion. In this article, we review recent studies on human immunodeficiency virus type 1, Ebola virus, and respiratory syncytial virus. Prion diseases are diseases of protein conformation. We have generated a large panel of antibodies recognizing the cellular prion protein (PrP(c)), some of which also react with the abnormally folded infectious prion protein (PrP(Sc)). These antibodies are being used to gain insight into both the molecular events leading to the formation of infectious PrP and the physiologic role played by PrP in normal and prion-infected cells.
PMID: 10852127 [PubMed - indexed for MEDLINE]

2226. J Infect. 2000 Jan;40(1):16-20.

Ebola haemorrhagic fever--a review.

Colebunders R(1), Borchert M.

Author information: (1)Department of Clinical Sciences, Institute of Tropical Medicine, Antwerp, Belgium.

PMID: 10762106 [PubMed - indexed for MEDLINE]

2227. Med Trop (Mars). 2000;60(3):303-4.

[Ebola and Marburg virus: entomologic hypothesis to confirm].

[Article in French]

Darriet F.

PMID: 11258069 [PubMed - indexed for MEDLINE]

2228. Med Trop (Mars). 2000;60(2 Suppl):50.

[Ebola virus and virus reservoirs].

[Article in French]

Morvan JM(1).

Author information: (1)Institut Pasteur, Bangui, République Centrafricaine. morvan@intnet.cf

PMID: 11100460 [PubMed - indexed for MEDLINE]

2229. Microbes Infect. 2000 Jan;2(1):39-44.

Ebola and Marburg virus antibody prevalence in selected populations of the Central African Republic.

Gonzalez JP(1), Nakoune E, Slenczka W, Vidal P, Morvan JM.

Author information: (1)Institut Français de Recherche Scientifique pour le Développement en Coopération IRD-Orstom, Paris, France.

With the natural history of the filovirus family seemingly unknown, filovirus ecology in its natural environment remains a rudimentary field of research. In order to investigate the maintenance cycle of filovirus in Central Africa, a study was conducted within the rain forest of the Central African Republic. The epidemiological study determines the frequency and distribution of filovirus seroprevalence in a selected human population. Using an ELISA, serum samples from Pygmy and non-Pygmy populations were tested for Ebola-Zaire virus and Marburg (MBG) virus antibody. Filovirus antibody reacting sera were found in all zones investigated, and in all populations studied (Ebola virus IgG 5.3%; Marburg virus IgG 2.4%). Pygmies appeared to have a significantly higher seroprevalence (P < 0.03) against Ebola-Zaire virus (7.02%) than non-Pygmies (4.2%). MBG virus or related unknown filovirus strains also seem to be present in the western part of Central Africa. MBG virus antibodies were present in different Pygmy groups (ranging from 0.7 to 5.6%, mean 2.05%) and in several non-Pygmy populations (ranging from 0.0 to 3.9%, mean 3.4%) without an overall significant difference between the two groups (P = 0.14). The potentialities of nonpathogenic filovirus strains circulating in the Central African Republic are discussed.

PMID: 10717539 [PubMed - indexed for MEDLINE]

2230. Stem Cells. 2000;18(1):19-39.

Latest developments in gene transfer technology: achievements, perspectives, and controversies over therapeutic applications.

Romano G(1), Michell P, Pacilio C, Giordano A.

Author information: (1)Kimmel Cancer Institute, Jefferson Medical College, Thomas Jefferson University, Philadelphia, Pennsylvania 19107, USA. Gaetano.Romano@mail.tju.edu

Over the last decade, more than 300 phase I and phase II gene-based clinical trials have been conducted worldwide for the treatment of cancer and monogenic disorders. Lately, these trials have been extended to the treatment of AIDS and, to a lesser extent, cardiovascular diseases. There are 27 currently active gene therapy protocols for the treatment of HIV-I infection in the USA. Preclinical studies are currently in progress to evaluate the possibility of increasing the number of gene therapy clinical trials for cardiopathies, and of beginning new gene therapy programs for neurologic illnesses, autoimmuno diseases, allergies, regeneration of tissues, and to implement procedures of allogeneic tissues or cell transplantation. In addition, gene transfer technology has allowed for the development of innovative vaccine design, known as genetic immunization. This technique has already been applied in the AIDS vaccine programs in the USA. These programs aim to confer protective immunity against HIV-I transmission to individuals who are at risk of infection. Research programs have also been considered to develop therapeutic vaccines for patients with AIDS and generate either preventive or therapeutic vaccines against malaria, tuberculosis, hepatitis A, B and C viruses, influenza virus, La Crosse virus, and Ebola virus. The potential therapeutic applications of gene transfer technology are enormous. However, the effectiveness of gene therapy programs is still questioned. Furthermore, there is growing concern over the matter of safety of gene delivery and controversy has arisen over the proposal to begin in utero gene therapy clinical trials for the treatment of inherited genetic disorders. From this standpoint, despite the latest significant achievements reported in vector design, it is not possible to predict to what extent gene therapeutic interventions will be effective in patients, and in what time frame.

PMID: 10661569 [PubMed - indexed for MEDLINE]

2231. Virology. 1999 Dec 5;265(1):164-71.

Delta-peptide is the carboxy-terminal cleavage fragment of the nonstructural small glycoprotein sGP of Ebola virus.

Volchkova VA(1), Klenk HD, Volchkov VE.

Author information: (1)Institut für Virologie, Philipps-Universität Marburg, Marburg, 35011, Germany.

In the present study we have investigated processing and maturation of the nonstructural small glycoprotein (sGP) of Ebola virus. When sGP expressed from vaccinia virus vectors was analyzed by pulse-chase experiments using SDS-PAGE under reducing conditions, the mature form and two different precursors have been identified. First, the endoplasmic reticulum form sGP(er), full-length sGP with oligomannosidic N-glycans, was detected, sGP(er) was then replaced by the Golgi-specific precursor pre-sGP, full-length sGP containing complex N-glycans. This precursor was finally converted by proteolysis into mature sGP and a smaller cleavage fragment, Delta-peptide. Studies employing site-directed mutagenesis revealed that sGP was cleaved at a multibasic amino acid motif at positions 321 to 324 of the open reading frame. Cleavage was blocked by RVKR-chloromethyl ketone. Uncleaved pre-sGP forms a disulfide-linked homodimer and is secreted into the culture medium in the presence of the inhibitor as efficiently as proteolytically processed sGP. In vitro treatment of pre-sGP by purified recombinant furin resulted in efficient cleavage, confirming the importance of this proprotein convertase for the processing and maturation of sGP. Delta-peptide is also secreted into the culture medium and therefore represents a novel nonstructural expression product of the GP gene of Ebola virus. Both cleavage fragments contain sialic acid, but only Delta-peptide is highly O-glycosylated.

Copyright 1999 Academic Press.

PMID: 10603327 [PubMed - indexed for MEDLINE]
2232. J Med Virol. 1999 Dec;59(4):552-60.

Lassa and Mopeia virus replication in human monocytes/macrophages and in endothelial cells: different effects on IL-8 and TNF-alpha gene expression.

Lukashevich IS(1), Maryankova R, Vladyko AS, Nashkevich N, Koleda S, Djavani M, Horejsh D, Voitenok NN, Salvato MS.

Author information: (1)Department of Pathology, University of Wisconsin, Madison, Wisconsin, USA.

Cells of the mononuclear and endothelial lineages are targets for viruses which cause hemorrhagic fevers (HF) such as the filoviruses Marburg and Ebola, and the arenaviruses Lassa and Junin. A recent model of Marburg HF pathogenesis proposes that virus directly causes endothelial cell damage and macrophage release of TNF-alpha which increases the permeability of endothelial monolayers [Feldmann et al. , 1996]. We show that Lassa virus replicates in human monocytes/macrophages and endothelial cells without damaging them. Human endothelial cells (HUVEC) are highly susceptible to infection by both Lassa and Mopeia (a non-pathogenic Lassa-related arenavirus). Whereas monocytes must differentiate into macrophages before supporting even low level production of these viruses, the virus yields in the culture medium of infected HUVEC cells reach more than 7 log10 PFU/ml without cellular damage. In contrast to filovirus, Lassa virus replication in monocytes/macrophages fails to stimulate TNF-alpha gene expression and even down-regulates LPS-stimulated TNF-alpha mRNA synthesis. The expression of IL-8, a prototypic proinflammatory CXC chemokine, was also suppressed in Lassa virus infected monocytes/macrophages and HUVEC on both the protein and mRNA levels. This contrasts with Mopeia virus infection of HUVEC in which neither IL-8 mRNA nor protein are reduced. The cumulative down-regulation of TNF-alpha and IL-8 expression could explain the absence of inflammatory and effective immune responses in severe cases of Lassa HF.

PMCID: PMC2391009 PMID: 10534741 [PubMed - indexed for MEDLINE]
2233. Microbes Infect. 1999 Dec;1(14):1193-201.

Identification of Ebola virus sequences present as RNA or DNA in organs of terrestrial small mammals of the Central African Republic.

Morvan JM(1), Deubel V, Gounon P, Nakouné E, Barrière P, Murri S, Perpète O, Selekon B, Coudrier D, Gautier-Hion A, Colyn M, Volehkov V.

Author information: (1)Laboratoire des arbovirus et virus des fièvres hémorragiques, Institut Pasteur de Bangui Bangui, Central African Republic.

The life cycle of the Ebola (EBO) virus remains enigmatic. We tested for EBO virus in the organs of 242 small mammals captured during ecological studies in the Central African Republic. EBO virus glycoprotein or polymerase gene sequences were detected by reverse transcription PCR in RNA extracts of the organs of seven animals and by PCR in DNA extract of one animal. Neither live virus nor virus antigen was detected in any organ sample. Direct sequencing of amplicons identified the virus as being of the Zaire/Gabon subtype. Virus-like nucleocapsids were observed by electron microscopy in the cytoplasm of the spleen cells of one animal. The animals belonged to two genera of rodents (Muridae; Mus setulosus, Praomys sp1 and P. sp2) and one species of shrew (Soricidae; Sylvisorex ollula). These preliminary results provide evidence that common terrestrial small mammals living in peripheral forest areas have been in contact with the EBO virus and demonstrate the persistence of EBO virus RNA and DNA in the organs of the animals. Our findings should lead to better targeting of research into the life cycle of the EBO virus.

PMID: 10580275 [PubMed - indexed for MEDLINE]
2234. Mol Biol Cell. 1999 Dec;10(12):4191-200.

A discrete stage of baculovirus GP64-mediated membrane fusion.

Kingsley DH(1), Behbahani A, Rashtian A, Blissard GW, Zimmerberg J.

Author information: (1)Laboratory of Cellular and Molecular Biophysics, National Institute of Child Health and Human Development, National Institutes of Health, Bethesda, Maryland 20892-1855, USA.

Viral fusion protein trimers can play a critical role in limiting lipids in membrane fusion. Because the trimeric oligomer of many viral fusion proteins is often stabilized by hydrophobic 4-3 heptad repeats, higher-order oligomers might be stabilized by similar sequences. There is a hydrophobic 4-3 heptad repeat contiguous to a putative oligomerization domain of Autographa californica multicapsid nucleopolyhedrovirus envelope glycoprotein GP64. We performed mutagenesis and peptide inhibition studies to determine if this sequence might play a role in catalysis of membrane fusion. First, leucine-to-alanine mutants within and flanking the amino terminus of the hydrophobic 4-3 heptad repeat motif that oligomerize into trimers and traffic to insect Sf9 cell surfaces were identified. These mutants retained their wild-type conformation at neutral pH and changed conformation in acidic conditions, as judged by the reactivity of a conformationally sensitive mAb. These mutants, however, were defective for membrane fusion. Second, a peptide encoding the portion flanking the GP64 hydrophobic 4-3 heptad repeat was synthesized. Adding peptide led to inhibition of membrane fusion, which occurred only when the peptide was present during low pH application. The presence of peptide during low pH application did not prevent low pH-induced conformational changes, as determined by the loss of a conformationally sensitive epitope. In control experiments, a peptide of identical composition but different sequence, or a peptide encoding a portion of the Ebola GP heptad motif, had no effect on GP64-mediated fusion. Furthermore, when the hemagglutinin (X31 strain) fusion protein of influenza was functionally expressed in Sf9 cells, no effect on hemagglutinin-mediated fusion was observed, suggesting that the peptide does not exert nonspecific effects on other fusion proteins or cell membranes. Collectively, these studies suggest that the specific peptide sequences of GP64 that are adjacent to and include portions of the hydrophobic 4-3 heptad repeat play a dynamic role in membrane fusion at a stage that is downstream of the initiation of protein conformational changes but upstream of lipid mixing.

PMCID: PMC25752 PMID: 10588652 [PubMed - indexed for MEDLINE]
2235. Rinsho Biseibutshu Jinsoku Shindan Kenkyukai Shi. 1999 Dec;10(2):117-20.

[Topics of emerging, re-emerging infectious diseases].

[Article in Japanese]

Yamaguchi K(1).

Author information: (1)Dept. of Clinical Microbiology, Toho University School of Medicine.

PMID: 10866500 [PubMed - indexed for MEDLINE]

2236. Science. 1999 Oct 22;286(5440):654-5.

On the track of Ebola's hideout?

Hagmann M.

PMID: 10577212 [PubMed - indexed for MEDLINE]

2237. Science. 1999 Oct 15;286(5439):444-7.

Do-it-yourself gene watching.

Marshall E.

PMID: 10577207 [PubMed - indexed for MEDLINE]

2238. Air Med J. 1999 Oct-Dec;18(4):156-9.

Ebola and the filoviruses: reducing the threat by improving Third World medical care and education of aircrew members.

Gillen PB(1).

Author information: (1)Wright-Patterson Medical Center, Dayton, OH, USA.

PMID: 10622852 [PubMed - indexed for MEDLINE]

2239. J Virol. 1999 Oct;73(10):8907-12.

Mutational analysis of the putative fusion domain of Ebola virus glycoprotein.

Ito H(1), Watanabe S, Sanchez A, Whitt MA, Kawaoka Y.

Author information: (1)Department of Pathobiological Sciences, School of Veterinary Medicine, University of Wisconsin-Madison, Madison, Wisconsin 53706, USA. Ebola viruses contain a single glycoprotein (GP) spike, which functions as a receptor binding and membrane fusion protein. It contains a highly conserved hydrophobic region (amino acids 524 to 539) located 24 amino acids downstream of the N terminus of the Ebola virus GP2 subunit. Comparison of this region with the structural features of the transmembrane subunit of avian retroviral GPs suggests that the conserved Ebola virus hydrophobic region may, in fact, serve as the fusion peptide. To test this hypothesis directly, we introduced conservative (alanine) and nonconservative (arginine) amino acid substitutions at eight positions in this region of the GP2 molecule. The effects of these mutations were deduced from the ability of the Ebola virus GP to complement the infectivity of a vesicular stomatitis virus (VSV) lacking the receptor-binding G protein. Some mutations, such as Ile-to-Arg substitutions at positions 532 (I532R), F535R, G536A, and P537R, almost completely abolished the ability of the GP to support VSV infectivity without affecting the transport of GP to the cell surface and its incorporation into virions or the production of virus particles. Other mutations, such as G528R, L529A, L529R, I532A, and F535A, reduced the infectivity of the VSV-Ebola virus pseudotypes by at least one-half. These findings, together with previous reports of liposome association with a peptide corresponding to positions 524 to 539 in the GP molecule, offer compelling support for a fusion peptide role for the conserved hydrophobic region in the Ebola virus GP.

PMCID: PMC112919 PMID: 10482652 [PubMed - indexed for MEDLINE]

2240. Virology. 1999 Sep 15;262(1):114-28.

Ebola virus defective interfering particles and persistent infection.

Calain P(1), Monroe MC, Nichol ST.

Author information: (1)Division of Viral and Rickettsial Diseases, Centers for Disease Control and Prevention, Mailstop G14, 1600 Clifton Road, N.E., Atlanta, Georgia 30329-4018, USA. Ebola virus (Zaire subtype) is associated with high mortality disease outbreaks that commonly involve human to human transmission. Surviving patients can show evidence of prolonged virus persistence. The potential for Ebola virus to generate defective interfering (DI) particles and establish persistent infections in tissue culture was investigated. It was found that serial undiluted virus passages quickly resulted in production of an evolving population of virus minireplicons possessing both deletion and copyback type DI genome rearrangements. The tenth undiluted virus passage resulted in the establishment of virus persistently infected cell lines. Following one or two crises, these cells were stably maintained for several months with continuous shedding of infectious virus. An analysis of the estimated genome lengths of a selected set of the Ebola virus minireplicons and standard filoviruses revealed no obvious genome length rule, such as "the rule of six" found for the phylogenetically related Paramyxovirinae subfamily viruses. Minimal promoters for Ebola virus replication were found to be contained within 156 and 177 nucleotide regions of the genomic and antigenomic RNA 3' termini, respectively, based on the length of authentic termini retained in the naturally occurring minireplicons analyzed. In addition, using UV-irradiated preparations of virus released from persistently infected cells, it was demonstrated that Ebola virus DI particles could potentially be used as natural minireplicons to assay standard virus support functions.

PMID: 10489346 [PubMed - indexed for MEDLINE]

2241. Vopr Virusol. 1999 Sep-Oct;44(5):217-20.

[Effect of an infectios dose of the Ebola virus on survivability and immunologic indicators in guinea pigs].

[Article in Russian]

Dadaeva AA, Chepurnov AA, Sizikova LP, Chepurnova TS.

Analysis of the time course of immunological parameters in intact guinea pigs and animals immunized with inactivated Ebola virus (EV) inoculated with high and low doses of EV strain lethal for guinea pigs showed that high doses induced a higher resistance of the lymphocytic component of immunity than low doses, but activation of the neutrophil phagocytosis was far less expressed after high doses than after low ones. This indicates a qualitative effect of the infective dose of EV on the development of immunological reactions in animals, which modifies the ratio between the lymphocytic and neutrophilic components of immunity.
PMID: 10544449 [PubMed - indexed for MEDLINE]

2242. Vaccine. 1999 Aug 6;17(23-24):2991-8.

Cytotoxic T lymphocytes to Ebola Zaire virus are induced in mice by immunization with liposomes containing lipid A.

Rao M(1), Matyas GR, Grieder F, Anderson K, Jahrling PB, Alving CR.

Author information: (1)Department of Membrane Biochemistry, Walter Reed Army Institute of Research, Washington, DC 20307-5100, USA. dr._mangala_rao@wrsmtp-ccmail.army.mil

An eight amino acid sequence (TELRTFSI) present in the carboxy terminal end (aa 577-584) of membrane-anchored GP, the major structural protein of Ebola virus, was identified as an H-2k-specific murine cytotoxic T cell epitope. Cytotoxic T lymphocytes (CTLs) to this epitope were induced by immunizing B10.BR mice intravenously with either irradiated Ebola virus or with irradiated Ebola virus encapsulated in liposomes containing lipid A. The CTL response induced by irradiated Ebola virus could not be sustained after the second round of in vitro stimulation of immune splenocytes with the peptide, unless the irradiated virus was encapsulated in liposomes containing lipid A. The identification of an Ebola GP-specific CTL epitope and the requirement of liposomal lipid A for CTL memory recall responses could prove to be a promising approach for developing a vaccine against Ebola virus infection.
PMID: 10462234 [PubMed - indexed for MEDLINE]

2243. Dtsch Tierarztl Wochenschr. 1999 Aug;106(8):332-8.

[Emergence of "new" viral zoonoses].

[Article in German]

Greiser-Wilke I(1), Haas L.

Author information: (1)Institut für Virologie, Tierärztliche Hochschule Hannover.

In the last two to three decades a significant increase of viral zoonotic infections was observed. These zoonoses are not only newly (or previously unrecognized) emerging diseases, but also due to the reappearance of diseases thought to have been defeated (re-emerging diseases). "New" viral diseases can arise when viruses broaden their host-range (monkey poxvirus; equine morbillivirus), or can be a consequence of intrinsic properties of the virus itself, such as high mutation rates (influenza A virus). Most new or reemerging viral zoonoses are due to infections with hemorrhagic viruses. Many of them are transmitted by insects (arboviruses, e.g. yellow fever virus) or by rodents (e.g. Hanta viruses), others by contact with patients and nosocomial infections (e.g. Ebola virus). The emergence and increase of these diseases are a consequence of anthropogenic environmental changes, such as distortions of the ecological balance and changes in agriculture. In addition, the uncontrolled growth of the cities in tropical and subtropical regions without improvement of the public health measures and the increasing international animal trade and travel also favour the spread and recurrence of these diseases.
PMID: 10488638 [PubMed - indexed for MEDLINE]

2244. IUBMB Life. 1999 Aug;48(2):151-6.

Evolutionary conservation of the membrane fusion machine.

Poumbourios P(1), Center RJ, Wilson KA, Kemp BE, Kobe B.

Author information: (1)St. Vincent's Institute of Medical Research, Fitzroy, Victoria, Australia.

Recent structural studies of proteins mediating membrane fusion reveal intriguing similarities between diverse viral and mammalian systems. Particularly striking is the close similarity between the transmembrane envelope glycoproteins from the retrovirus HTLV-I and the filovirus Ebola. These similarities suggest similar mechanisms of membrane fusion. The model that fits most currently available data suggests fusion activation in viral systems is driven by a symmetrical conformational change triggered by an activation event such as receptor binding or a pH change. The mammalian vesicle fusion mediated by the SNARE protein complex most likely occurs by a similar mechanism but without symmetry constraints.
PMID: 10794590 [PubMed - indexed for MEDLINE]

2245. J Virol. 1999 Jul;73(7):6024-30.

Ebola virus can be effectively neutralized by antibody produced in natural human infection.

Maruyama T(1), Rodriguez LL, Jahrling PB, Sanchez A, Khan AS, Nichol ST, Peters CJ, Parren PW, Burton DR.

Author information: (1)Departments of Immunology and Molecular Biology, The Scripps Research Institute, La Jolla, California 92037, USA.

The activity of antibodies against filoviruses is poorly understood but has important consequences for vaccine design and passive prophylaxis. To investigate this activity, a panel of recombinant human monoclonal antibodies to Ebola virus antigens was isolated from phage display libraries constructed from RNA from donors who recovered from infection in the 1995 Ebola virus outbreak in Kikwit, Democratic Republic of Congo. Antibodies reactive with nucleoprotein (NP), envelope glycoprotein (GP), and secreted envelope glycoprotein (sGP) were characterized by immunofluorescence and radioimmunoprecipitation assays. Four antibodies reacting strongly with sGP and weakly with GP and two antibodies reacting with NP were not neutralizing. An antibody specific for GP neutralized Ebola virus to 50% at 0.4 microgram/ml as the recombinant Fab fragment and to 50% at 0.3 microgram/ml (90% at 2.6 microgram/ml) as the corresponding whole immunoglobulin G1 molecule. The studies indicate that neutralizing antibodies are produced in infection by Ebola virus although probably at a relatively low frequency. The neutralizing antibody may be useful in vaccine design and as a prophylactic agent against Ebola virus infection.
PMCID: PMC112663 PMID: 10364354 [PubMed - indexed for MEDLINE]

2246. Med Clin North Am. 1999 Jul;83(4):865-83, v.

Emerging infectious diseases and risk to the traveler.

Freedman DO(1), Woodall J.

Author information: (1)Department of Medicine, Microbiology, and Epidemiology and Public Health, University of Alabama at Birmingham, USA.

This article examines the relationship between travel and emerging infections. The authors begin with an overview of disease emergence and follow with a brief infection-by-infection examination of selected emerging pathogens of particular relevance to travelers and the medical care providers who counsel them. Emphasis is given to those agents that clearly have emerged as significant new or increased risk to travelers; or are of sufficiently new interest, even in the face of inadequate data in travelers, to be of potential immediate concern. The authors also discuss several novel pathogens, such as Ebola virus, that are clearly of insignificant or minimal risk to travelers, but are the subject of frequent questions from patients requesting pre-travel advice from medical providers.

PMID: 10453254 [PubMed - indexed for MEDLINE]

2247. Immunol Lett. 1999 Jun 1;68(2-3):257-61.

Suppressive effect of Ebola virus on T cell proliferation in vitro is provided by a 125-kDa GP viral protein.

Chepurnov AA(1), Tuzova MN, Ternovoy VA, Chernukhin IV.

Author information: (1)Laboratory of Extremely Dangerous Viral Infections, State Research Center of Virology and Biotechnology Vector, Koltsovo, Novosibirsk, Region, Russia. chepurnov@vector.nsk.su

Ebola virus (EV), an extremely infectious pathogen, causes severe hemorrhagic fever in humans and nonhuman primates. The disease pattern includes damage of parenchymal cells of vital organs in association with hemostatic and immune disorders. Vaccination with the inactivated virions does not provide an effective immune protection against the disease. The inadequate immune response may be directly caused by the virus, and, hence, it may presumably be crucial in the pathogenic process and prophylactic treatment of Ebola infection. The suggested immunosuppressive properties of EV were examined in this study. We have demonstrated that the whole heat-inactivated virions can dose-dependently suppress human lymphocyte mitogen-stimulated proliferation in vitro. In further analyses, we identified the viral protein responsible for the suppressive effect, and we showed that it was provided by a protein corresponding to a 125-kDa envelope glycoprotein (GP-125). The protein alone inhibited lymphocyte proliferation, whereas the other viral proteins were without significant effect on blastogenesis. To determine the immunosuppressive properties of different portions of GP-125, deletion mutants of GP were designed based on predicted localisation of antigen sites. They were expressed as recombinant proteins and studied in proliferation assays. We identified a 40-amino acid sequence at the N-terminus of GP-125 that exerted a suppressive effect on blastogenesis.

PMID: 10424429 [PubMed - indexed for MEDLINE]

2248. J Zoo Wildl Med. 1999 Jun;30(2):201-7.

Procedures utilized for primate import quarantine at the International Center for Gibbon Studies.

Mootnick AR(1), Ostrowski SR.

Author information: (1)International Center for Gibbon Studies, Santa Clarita, California 91380, USA.

The intent of the Foreign Quarantine requirements (42 CFR 71.53) for nonhuman primates (NHPs) is to prevent the importation of potentially serious infectious diseases that are not endemic to the United States. In 1990, prompted by an outbreak of Ebola (Reston) hemorrhagic fever at an (NHP) quarantine facility, the Centers for Disease Control and Prevention (CDC) initiated unannounced inspections of all NHP importers' quarantine facilities. During the inspections, the majority did not meet the required infection control and containment standards. Numerous discrepancies were identified in infection control and NHP quarantine protocols. Zoos should have knowledge of CDC requirements and recommendations for the importation of NHPs into the United States. Zoos planning to import NHPs should register with the CDC and have their NHP quarantine facility and protocols inspected and approved by CDC's Division of Quarantine. Specific areas addressed must include protocols for in-transit shipping and handling, transport to the quarantine facility, biocontainment procedures (transfer of NHPs from shipping containers to quarantine cages, entering/exiting the quarantine room, routine daily and emergency procedures, protective clothing, infection control, infectious waste disposal), occupational health, and employee training. Here, we provide information on the approved protocols used for import quarantine at a single registered importer facility specializing in importation of gibbons (Hylobatidae) for species conservation purposes. These procedures are site specific and are not intended to be applicable to the needs of all NHP import facilities.

PMID: 10484134 [PubMed - indexed for MEDLINE]

2249. J Theor Biol. 1999 May 21;198(2):173-81.

Are the fusion processes involved in birth, life and death of the cell depending on tilted insertion of peptides into membranes?

Peuvot J(1), Schanck A, Lins L, Brasseur R.

Author information: (1)Medical Affairs, UCB-Pharma, allée de la Recherche, 1070 Bruxelles, Belgium. Jacques.Peuvot@UCB-Group.com

Various peptide segments have been modeled as asymmetric amphipathic alpha-helices. Theoretical calculations have shown that they insert obliquely into model membranes. They have been named "tilted peptides". Molecular modeling results reported here also evidence the presence of tilted peptides in ADM-1 protein of Caenorhabditis elegans that may be involved in fusion events, in meltrin alpha, a protein implicated in myoblast fusion, in hemagglutinin of influenza virus, in the E2 glycoprotein of rubella virus, in the S protein of hepatitis B virus, in a subdomain of Ebola virus and in the malaria CS protein. Experimental results have indicated that tilted peptide fragments may be involved in cellular life events like sperm-egg fecondation, muscle development, protein translocation through signal sequences and cellular death caused by viral infection or parasite infestation. We speculate that membrane destabilization by these tilted peptides may be an important common step in life processes involving fusion phenomena.

PMID: 10339392 [PubMed - indexed for MEDLINE]
2250. Am J Trop Med Hyg. 1999 Apr;60(4):610-5.

Leptospirosis and Ebola virus infection in five gold-panning villages in northeastern Gabon.

Bertherat E(1), Renaut A, Nabias R, Dubreuil G, Georges-Courbot MC.

Author information: (1)Centre International de Recherches Médicales de Franceville, Gabon.

An exhaustive epidemiologic and serologic survey was carried out in five gold-panning villages situated in northeastern Gabon to estimate the degree of exposure of to leptospirosis and Ebola virus. The seroprevalence was 15.7% for leptospirosis and 10.2% for Ebola virus. Sixty years after the last seroepidemiologic survey of leptospirosis in Gabon, this study demonstrates the persistence of this infection among the endemic population and the need to consider it as a potential cause of hemorrhagic fever in Gabon. There was no significant statistical correlation between the serologic status of populations exposed to both infectious agents, indicating the lack of common risk factors for these diseases.
PMID: 10348236 [PubMed - indexed for MEDLINE]
2251. J Virol. 1999 Apr;73(4):3491-6.

Ebola virus selectively inhibits responses to interferons, but not to interleukin-1beta, in endothelial cells.

Harcourt BH(1), Sanchez A, Offermann MK.

Author information: (1)Program in Genetics and Molecular Biology, Department of Internal Medicine, Emory University, Atlanta, Georgia 30322, USA.

Ebola virus infection is highly lethal and leads to severe immunosuppression. In this study, we demonstrate that infection of human umbilical vein endothelial cells (HUVECs) with Ebola virus Zaire (EZ) suppressed basal expression of the major histocompatibility complex class I (MHC I) family of proteins and inhibited the induction of multiple genes by alpha interferon (IFN-alpha) and IFN-gamma, including those coding for MHC I proteins, 2'-5' oligoadenylate synthetase [2'-5'(A)N], and IFN regulatory factor 1 (IRF-1). Induction of interleukin-6 (IL-6) and ICAM-1 by IL-1beta was not suppressed by infection with EZ, suggesting that the inhibition of IFN signaling is specific. Gel shift analysis demonstrated that infection with EZ blocked the induction by IFNs of nuclear proteins that bind to IFN-stimulated response elements, gamma activation sequences, and IFN regulatory factor binding site (IRF-E). In contrast, infection with EZ did not block activation of the transcription factor NF-kappaB by IL-1beta. The events that lead to the blockage of IFN signaling may be critical for Ebola virus-induced immunosuppression and would play a role in the pathogenesis of Ebola virus infection.
PMCID: PMC104118 PMID: 10074208 [PubMed - indexed for MEDLINE]
2252. Nat Med. 1999 Apr;5(4):423-6.

Defective humoral responses and extensive intravascular apoptosis are associated with fatal outcome in Ebola virus-infected patients.

Baize S(1), Leroy EM, Georges-Courbot MC, Capron M, Lansoud-Soukate J, Debré P, Fisher-Hoch SP, McCormick JB, Georges AJ.

Author information: (1)Centre International de Recherches Médicales de Franceville, Gabon. sbaize@cirmf.sci.ga

Comment in Nat Med. 1999 Apr;5(4):373-4.

Ebola virus is very pathogenic in humans. It induces an acute hemorrhagic fever that leads to death in about 70% of patients. We compared the immune responses of patients who died from Ebola virus disease with those who survived during two large outbreaks in 1996 in Gabon. In survivors, early and increasing levels of IgG, directed mainly against the nucleoprotein and the 40-kDa viral protein, were followed by clearance of circulating viral antigen and activation of cytotoxic T cells, which was indicated by the upregulation of FasL, perforin, CD28 and gamma interferon mRNA in peripheral blood mononuclear cells. In contrast, fatal infection was characterized by impaired humoral responses, with absent specific IgG and barely detectable IgM. Early activation of T cells, indicated by mRNA patterns in peripheral blood mononuclear cells and considerable release of gamma interferon in plasma, was followed in the days preceding death by the disappearance of T cell-related mRNA (including CD3 and CD8). DNA fragmentation in blood leukocytes and release of 41/7 nuclear matrix protein in plasma indicated that massive intravascular apoptosis proceeded relentlessly during the last 5 days of life. Thus, events very early in Ebola virus infection determine the control of viral replication and recovery or catastrophic illness and death.
PMID: 10202932 [PubMed - indexed for MEDLINE]
2253. Nat Med. 1999 Apr;5(4):373-4.

Surviving Ebola virus infection.

Nabel GJ.

Comment on Nat Med. 1999 Apr;5(4):423-6.
PMID: 10202917 [PubMed - indexed for MEDLINE]
2254. Wkly Epidemiol Rec. 1999 Mar 26;74(12):89.

Ebola: the virus and the disease.

[Article in English, French]

[No authors listed]
PMID: 10207327 [PubMed - indexed for MEDLINE]
2255. Proc Natl Acad Sci U S A. 1999 Mar 16;96(6):2662-7.

Core structure of the envelope glycoprotein GP2 from Ebola virus at 1.9-A resolution.

Malashkevich VN(1), Schneider BJ, McNally ML, Milhollen MA, Pang JX, Kim PS.

Author information: (1)Howard Hughes Medical Institute, Whitehead Institute for Biomedical Research, Department of Biology, Massachusetts Institute of Technology, Nine Cambridge Center, Cambridge, MA 02142, USA.

Ebola virions contain a surface transmembrane glycoprotein (GP) that is responsible for binding to target cells and subsequent fusion of the viral and host-cell membranes. GP is expressed as a single-chain precursor that is posttranslationally processed into the disulfide-linked fragments GP1 and GP2. The GP2 subunit is thought to mediate membrane fusion. A soluble fragment of the GP2 ectodomain, lacking the fusion-peptide region and the transmembrane helix, folds into a stable, highly helical structure in aqueous solution. Limited proteolysis studies identify a stable core of the GP2 ectodomain. This 74-residue core, denoted Ebo-74, was crystallized, and its x-ray structure was determined at 1.9-A resolution. Ebo-74 forms a trimer in which a long, central three-stranded coiled coil is surrounded by shorter C-terminal helices that are packed in an antiparallel orientation into hydrophobic grooves on the surface of the coiled coil. Our results confirm the previously anticipated structural similarity between the Ebola GP2 ectodomain and the core of the transmembrane subunit from oncogenic retroviruses. The Ebo-74 structure likely represents the fusion-active conformation of the protein, and its overall architecture resembles several other viral membrane-fusion proteins, including those from HIV and influenza.
PMCID: PMC15825 PMID: 10077567 [PubMed - indexed for MEDLINE]

2256. Emerg Infect Dis. 1999 Mar-Apr;5(2):312-3.

Risk for Ebola virus infection in Côte d'Ivoire.

Kunii O, Formenty P, Diarra-Nama J, Nahounou N.

PMCID: PMC2640681 PMID: 10221898 [PubMed - indexed for MEDLINE]

2257. J Virol. 1999 Mar;73(3):2333-42.

Comparison of the transcription and replication strategies of marburg virus and Ebola virus by using artificial replication systems.

Mühlberger E(1), Weik M, Volchkov VE, Klenk HD, Becker S.

Author information: (1)Institut für Virologie der Philipps-Universität Marburg, 35037 Marburg, Germany.

The members of the family Filoviridae, Marburg virus (MBGV) and Ebola virus (EBOV), are very similar in terms of morphology, genome organization, and protein composition. To compare the replication and transcription strategies of both viruses, an artificial replication system based on the vaccinia virus T7 expression system was established for EBOV. Specific transcription and replication of an artificial monocistronic minireplicon was demonstrated by reporter gene expression and detection of the transcribed and replicated RNA species. As it was shown previously for MBGV, three of the four EBOV nucleocapsid proteins, NP, VP35, and L, were essential and sufficient for replication. In contrast to MBGV, EBOV-specific transcription was dependent on the presence of the fourth nucleocapsid protein, VP30. When EBOV VP30 was replaced by MBGV VP30, EBOV-specific transcription was observed but with lower efficiency. Exchange of NP, VP35, and L between the two replication systems did not lead to detectable reporter gene expression. It was further observed that neither MBGV nor EBOV were able to replicate the heterologous minigenomes. A chimeric minigenome, however, containing the EBOV leader and the MBGV trailer was encapsidated, replicated, transcribed, and packaged by both viruses.
PMCID: PMC104478 PMID: 9971816 [PubMed - indexed for MEDLINE]

2258. Bull Soc Pathol Exot. 1999 Feb;92(1):33-7.

[Intramuscular injections in Sub-saharan African children, apropos of a frequently misunderstood pathology: the complications related to intramuscular quinine injections].

[Article in French]

Barennes H(1).

Author information: (1)Unité de vaccinologie et de recherche opérationnelle, Centre Muraz, Bobo-Dioulasso, Burkina-Faso.

In West Africa, the incidence of poliomyelitis has decreased in the past years thanks to intensive immunization campaigns. Nowadays intramuscular injection is the main reason for paralysis of the legs in African children as well as attendance at Rehabilitation Centres. Intramuscular injection of quinine is the most frequently reported. Faced with the lack of sterile material, health workers do not rationalize the use of intramuscular injections. Although the use of the same needle has decreased, using the same syringe for many patients, with only a rapid washing between, is still commonplace Poor septic conditions and abuse of prescriptions also contribute to the transmission of severe diseases (hepatitis, malaria, syphilis, filariasis, Ebola virus, tetanus and HIV). Paralysis due to injection is often confused with poliomyelitis and health workers are often not aware of the sequelae of injection. It seems important to prevent risk related to intramuscular injection in Africa through educating health workers and the local population. Rationalization of practises, promotion of oral therapy and alternatives to intramuscular administration should be carried out. In this respect, the intrarectal administration of an injectable solution of diluted quinine--its efficiency and pharmacokinetic having been studied over the last ten years--offers interesting opportunities.
PMID: 10214519 [PubMed - indexed for MEDLINE]

2259. J Gen Virol. 1999 Feb;80 (Pt 2):355-62.

Characterization of the L gene and 5' trailer region of Ebola virus.

Volchkov VE(1), Volchkova VA, Chepurnov AA, Blinov VM, Dolnik O, Netesov SV, Feldmann H.

Author information: (1)Institut für Virologie, Philipps-Universität, Marburg, Germany. volchkov@mailer.uni-marburg.de

The nucleotide sequences of the L gene and 5' trailer region of Ebola virus strain Mayinga (subtype Zaire) have been determined, thus completing the sequence of the Ebola virus genome. The putative transcription start signal of the L gene was identical to the determined 5' terminus of the L mRNA (5' GAGGAAGAUUAA) and showed a high degree of similarity to the corresponding regions of other Ebola virus genes. The 3' end of the L mRNA terminated with 5' AUUAUAAAAAA, a sequence which is distinct from the proposed transcription termination signals of other genes. The 5' trailer sequence of the Ebola virus genomic RNA

consisted of 676 nt and revealed a self-complementary sequence at the extreme end which may play an important role in virus replication. The L gene contained a single ORF encoding a polypeptide of 2212 aa. The deduced amino acid sequence showed identities of about 73 and 44% to the L proteins of Ebola virus strain Maleo (subtype Sudan) and Marburg virus, respectively. Sequence comparison studies of the Ebola virus L proteins with several corresponding proteins of other non-segmented, negative-strand RNA viruses, including Marburg viruses, confirmed a close relationship between filoviruses and members of the Paramyxovirinae. The presence of several conserved linear domains commonly found within L proteins of other members of the order Mononegavirales identified this protein as the RNA-dependent RNA polymerase of Ebola virus.
PMID: 10073695 [PubMed - indexed for MEDLINE]
2260. J Infect Dis. 1999 Feb;179 Suppl 1:S287-8.

Gleanings from the harvest: suggestions for priority actions against Ebola virus epidemics.

Johnson KM(1).

Author information: (1)Department of Biology, University of New Mexico, Albuquerque, USA.
PMID: 9988198 [PubMed - indexed for MEDLINE]
2261. J Infect Dis. 1999 Feb;179 Suppl 1:S283-6.

Ebola hemorrhagic fever: lessons from Kikwit, Democratic Republic of the Congo.

Heymann DL(1), Barakamfitiye D, Szczeniowski M, Muyembe-Tamfum JJ, Bele O, Rodier G.

Author information: (1)Division of Emerging and Other Communicable Diseases, World Health Organization (WHO), Geneva, Switzerland. heymannd@who.ch
The outbreak of Ebola hemorrhagic fever in Kikwit, Democratic Republic of the Congo, clearly signaled an end to the days when physicians and researchers could work in relative obscurity on problems of international importance, and it provided many lessons to the international public health and scientific communities. In particular, the outbreak signaled a need for stronger infectious disease surveillance and control worldwide, for improved international preparedness to provide support when similar outbreaks occur, and for accommodating the needs of the press in providing valid information. A need for more broad-based international health regulations and electronic information systems within the World Health Organization also became evident, as did the realization that there are new and more diverse partners able to rapidly respond to international outbreaks. Finally, a need for continued and coordinated Ebola research was identified, especially as concerns development of simple and valid diagnostic tests, better patient management procedures, and identification of the natural reservoir.
PMID: 9988197 [PubMed - indexed for MEDLINE]
2262. J Infect Dis. 1999 Feb;179 Suppl 1:S281-2.

US policy for disease control among imported nonhuman primates.

DeMarcus TA(1), Tipple MA, Ostrowski SR.

Author information: (1)Division of Quarantine, National Center for Infectious Diseases, Centers for Disease Control and Prevention, Atlanta, Georgia 30333, USA.
In 1990, in response to the occurrence of Ebola virus (subsequently identified as subtype Reston) infection among cynomolgus monkeys imported from the Philippines, the United States implemented strict disease control measures for handling nonhuman primates during transit and quarantine and initiated importer facility compliance inspections. Disease control measures emphasized protection of workers from exposure, use of containment facilities and procedures, measures to prevent spread of infection among animals, and laboratory testing of animals that die or become ill during quarantine. From 1991-1995, no outbreaks of filovirus infection occurred, and only one other disease outbreak (caused by Mycobacterium species) was recognized. In April 1996, Ebola virus (subtype Reston) infection was identified in another group of cynomolgus monkeys imported from the Philippines. The disease control measures implemented since the first Ebola virus (subtype Reston) outbreak appeared to work well. Currently, the 27 registered importer facilities import approximately 8500 nonhuman primates annually, and mortality rates are
PMID: 9988196 [PubMed - indexed for MEDLINE]
2263. J Infect Dis. 1999 Feb;179 Suppl 1:S274-80.

Long-term disease surveillance in Bandundu region, Democratic Republic of the Congo: a model for early detection and prevention of Ebola hemorrhagic fever.

Lloyd ES(1), Zaki SR, Rollin PE, Tshioko K, Bwaka MA, Ksiazek TG, Calain P, Shieh WJ, Kondé MK, Verchueren E, Perry HN, Manguindula L, Kabwau J, Ndambi R, Peters CJ.

Author information: (1)Centers for Disease Control and Prevention, Atlanta, Georgia 30333, USA. pyr3@cdc.gov
After the large-scale outbreak of Ebola hemorrhagic fever (EHF) in Bandundu region, Democratic Republic of the Congo, a program was developed to help detect and prevent future outbreaks of EHF in the region. The long-term surveillance and prevention strategy is based on early recognition by physicians, immediate initiation of enhanced barrier-nursing practices, and the use of an immunohistochemical diagnostic test performed on formalin-fixed skin specimens of patients who die of suspected viral hemorrhagic fever. The program was implemented in September 1995 during a 4-day workshop with 28 local physicians representing 17 of 22 health zones in the region. Specimen collection kits were distributed to clinics in participating health zones, and a follow-up evaluation was conducted after 6 months. The use of a formalin-fixed skin specimen for laboratory confirmation of EHF can provide an appropriate method for EHF surveillance when linked with physician training, use of viral hemorrhagic fever isolation precautions, and follow-up investigation.
PMID: 9988195 [PubMed - indexed for MEDLINE]
2264. J Infect Dis. 1999 Feb;179 Suppl 1:S268-73.

Organization of patient care during the Ebola hemorrhagic fever epidemic in Kikwit, Democratic Republic of the Congo, 1995.

Guimard Y(1), Bwaka MA, Colebunders R, Calain P, Massamba M, De Roo A, Mupapa KD, Kibadi K, Kuvula KJ, Ndaberey DE, Katwiki KR, Mapanda BB, Nkuku OB, Fleerackers Y, Van den Enden E, Kipasa MA.

Author information: (1)Institute of Tropical Medicine, Antwerp, Belgium.

In contrast with procedures in previous Ebola outbreaks, patient care during the 1995 outbreak in Kikwit, Democratic Republic of the Congo, was centralized for a large number of patients. On 4 May, before the diagnosis of Ebola hemorrhagic fever (EHF) was confirmed by the Centers for Disease Control and Prevention, an isolation ward was created at Kikwit General Hospital. On 11 May, an international scientific and technical committee established as a priority the improvement of hygienic conditions in the hospital and the protection of health care workers and family members; to this end, protective equipment was distributed and barrier-nursing techniques were implemented. For patients living far from Kikwit, home care was organized. Initially, hospitalized patients were given only oral treatments; however, toward the end of the epidemic, infusions and better nutritional support were given, and 8 patients received blood from convalescent EHF patients. Only 1 of the transfusion patients died (12.5%). It is expected that with improved medical care, the case fatality rate of EHF could be reduced.

PMID: 9988194 [PubMed - indexed for MEDLINE]

2265. J Infect Dis. 1999 Feb;179 Suppl 1:S263-7.

Interventions to control virus transmission during an outbreak of Ebola hemorrhagic fever: experience from Kikwit, Democratic Republic of the Congo, 1995

Kerstiëns B(1), Matthys F.

Author information: (1)Médecins sans Frontières, Brussels, Belgium. bkerstie@jhsph.edu

On 6 May 1995, the Médecins sans Frontières (MSF) coordinator in Kinshasa, Democratic Republic of the Congo (DRC), received a request for assistance for what was believed to be a concurrent outbreak of bacillary dysentery and viral hemorrhagic fever (suspected Ebola hemorrhagic fever [EHF]) in the town of Kikwit, DRC. On 11 May, the MSF intervention team assessed Kikwit General Hospital. This initial assessment revealed a nonfunctional isolation ward for suspected EHF cases; a lack of water and electricity; no waste disposal system; and no protective gear for medical staff. The priorities set by MSF were to establish a functional isolation ward to deal with EHF and to distribute protective supplies to individuals who were involved with patient care. Before the intervention, 67 health workers contracted EHF; after the initiation of control measures, just 3 cases were reported among health staff and none among Red Cross volunteers involved in body burial.

PMID: 9988193 [PubMed - indexed for MEDLINE]

2266. J Infect Dis. 1999 Feb;179 Suppl 1:S259-62.

Ebola outbreak in Kikwit, Democratic Republic of the Congo: discovery and control measures.

Muyembe-Tamfum JJ(1), Kipasa M, Kiyungu C, Colebunders R.

Author information: (1)Kinshasa University, Democratic Republic of the Congo.

The Ebola epidemic in Kikwit, Democratic Republic of the Congo, was recognized because of a nosocomial outbreak in Kikwit General Hospital. Initially, a diagnosis of shigella infection was suspected because many patients presented with bloody diarrhea. On 4 May 1995, blood samples from 14 acutely ill patients were sent to the Centers for Disease Control and Prevention (Atlanta), and on 9 May, a diagnosis of Ebola hemorrhagic fever was confirmed. The major disease control measures that were undertaken were the isolation of patients in a quarantine ward at Kikwit General Hospital, the distribution of protective equipment to health care workers and family members caring for Ebola patients, the use of barrier nursing techniques, the distribution of health education material, active and passive case finding, and the burying of the deceased in plastic bags by a trained team of Red Cross volunteers who wore gloves and protective clothing.

PMID: 9988192 [PubMed - indexed for MEDLINE]

2267. J Infect Dis. 1999 Feb;179 Suppl 1:S248-58.

A mouse model for evaluation of prophylaxis and therapy of Ebola hemorrhagic fever.

Bray M(1), Davis K, Geisbert T, Schmaljohn C, Huggins J.

Author information: (1)Division of Virology, US Army Medical Research Institute of Infectious Diseases, Fort Detrick, Frederick, Maryland 21702-5011, USA. bray@ncifcrf.gov

The Zaire subtype of Ebola virus (EBO-Z) is lethal for newborn mice, but adult mice are resistant to the virus, which prevents their use as an animal model of lethal Ebola infection. We serially passed EBO-Z virus in progressively older suckling mice, eventually obtaining a plaque-purified virus that was lethal for mature, immunocompetent BALB/c and C57BL/6 inbred and ICR (CD-1) outbred mice. Pathologic changes in the liver and spleen of infected mice resembled those in EBO-Z-infected primates. Virus titers in these tissues reached $10(9)$ pfu/g. The LD50 of mouse-adapted EBO-Z virus inoculated into the peritoneal cavity was approximately 1 virion. Mice were resistant to large doses of the same virus inoculated subcutaneously, intradermally, or intramuscularly. Mice injected peripherally with mouse-adapted or intraperitoneally with non-adapted EBO-Z virus resisted subsequent challenge with mouse-adapted virus.

PMID: 9988191 [PubMed - indexed for MEDLINE]

2268. J Infect Dis. 1999 Feb;179 Suppl 1:S240-7.

Antiviral drug therapy of filovirus infections: S-adenosylhomocysteine hydrolase inhibitors inhibit Ebola virus in vitro and in a lethal mouse model.

Huggins J(1), Zhang ZX, Bray M.

Author information: (1)Virology Division, US Army Medical Research Institute of Infectious Diseases, Fort Detrick, Frederick, Maryland 21702-5011, USA. huggins@ncifcrf.gov

Ebola (subtype Zaire) viral replication was inhibited in vitro by a series of nine nucleoside analogue inhibitors of S-adenosylhomocysteine hydrolase, an important target for antiviral drug development. Adult BALB/c mice lethally infected with mouse-adapted Ebola virus die 5-7 days after infection. Treatment initiated on day 0 or 1 resulted in dose-dependent protection, with mortality completely prevented at doses > or =0.7 mg/kg every 8 h. There was significant protection (90%) when treatment was begun on day 2, at which time, the liver had an average titer of $3 \times 10(5)$ pfu/g virus and the spleen had $2 \times 10(6)$ pfu/g. Treatment with 2.2 mg/kg initiated on day 3, when the liver had an average titer of $2 \times 10(7)$ pfu/g virus and the spleen had $2 \times 10(8)$ pfu/g, resulted in 40% survival. As reported here, Carbocyclic 3-deazaadenosine is the first compound demonstrated to cure animals from this otherwise lethal Ebola virus infection.

PMID: 9988190 [PubMed - indexed for MEDLINE]

2269. J Infect Dis. 1999 Feb;179 Suppl 1:S235-9.

Recombinant human monoclonal antibodies to Ebola virus.

Maruyama T(1), Parren PW, Sanchez A, Rensink I, Rodriguez LL, Khan AS, Peters CJ, Burton DR.

Author information: (1)Department of Immunology, The Scripps Research Institute, La Jolla, California 92037, USA.

Human Fab (IgG1kappa) phage display libraries were constructed from bone marrow RNA from 2 donors who recovered from infection with Ebola (EBO) virus during the 1995 outbreak in Kikwit, Democratic Republic of the Congo. The libraries were initially panned against a radiation-inactivated EBO virus-infected Vero cell lysate, but only weak binders were identified. In contrast, panning against secreted EBO glycoprotein (SGP) resulted in Fabs showing very strong reactivity with SGP in ELISA. These Fabs also reacted with a virion membrane preparation. The Fabs were strongly positive in IFAs with cells infected with EBO (subtype Zaire) virus but negative with uninfected cells, with a characteristic punctate staining pattern in the cytoplasm. The Fabs showed weak or no reactivity with the virus cell lysate although donor serum did react. The Fabs are now being characterized in structural and functional terms. Major interest will focus on the ability of antibodies to neutralize EBO virus and, later, to protect animals against infection.

PMID: 9988189 [PubMed - indexed for MEDLINE]

2270. J Infect Dis. 1999 Feb;179 Suppl 1:S224-34.

Evaluation of immune globulin and recombinant interferon-alpha2b for treatment of experimental Ebola virus infections.

Jahrling PB(1), Geisbert TW, Geisbert JB, Swearengen JR, Bray M, Jaax NK, Huggins JW, LeDuc JW, Peters CJ.

Author information: (1)United States Army Research Institute of Infectious Diseases, Fort Detrick, Frederick, Maryland 21702-5011, USA. PBJ@Detrick.Army.Mil

A passive immunization strategy for treating Ebola virus infections was evaluated using BALB/ c mice, strain 13 guinea pigs, and cynomolgus monkeys. Guinea pigs were completely protected by injection of hyperimmune equine IgG when treatment was initiated early but not after viremia had developed. In contrast, mice were incompletely protected even when treatment was initiated on day 0, the day of virus inoculation. In monkeys treated with one dose of IgG on day 0, onset of illness and viremia was delayed, but all treated animals died. A second dose of IgG on day 5 had no additional beneficial effect. Pretreatment of monkeys delayed onset of viremia and delayed death several additional days. Interferon-alpha2b ($2 \times 10(7)$ IU/kg/day) had a similar effect in monkeys, delaying viremia and death by only several days. Effective treatment of Ebola infections may require a combination of drugs that inhibit viral replication in monocyte/macrophage-like cells while reversing the pathologic effects (e.g., coagulopathy) consequent to this replication.

PMID: 9988188 [PubMed - indexed for MEDLINE]

2271. J Infect Dis. 1999 Feb;179 Suppl 1:S218-23.

Preparation and use of hyperimmune serum for prophylaxis and therapy of Ebola virus infections.

Kudoyarova-Zubavichene NM(1), Sergeyev NN, Chepurnov AA, Netesov SV.

Author information: (1)State Research Center of Virology and Biotechnology Vector, Koltsovo, Russia.

To obtain hyperimmune serum appropriate for the treatment of filovirus infection, methods were developed to immunize nonsusceptible animals with live Ebola (EBO) virus preparations. Immune plasma with high ELISA and neutralization-specific antibody titers was obtained by multiple immunization of sheep and goats with preparations of live EBO virus. Goat immunoglobulin was prepared by Cohn's method and tested on guinea pigs, using an EBO virus strain that is highly pathogenic for guinea pigs. Prophylaxis with these immunoglobulins within 48 h after infection was effective in challenge experiments, with a log10 prophylaxis index as high as 1.92+/-0.52. Other studies have shown that equine anti-EBO virus immunoglobulins worked well in baboons. The goat immunoglobulins were also tested in preclinical trials on laboratory animals; after being positively evaluated, they were administered to volunteers in clinical trials for biologic safety and reactivity, and they were administered to researchers suspected of becoming infected with EBO during their experimental work. These immunoglobulins may be useful for the emergency treatment of persons accidentally infected with EBO.

PMID: 9988187 [PubMed - indexed for MEDLINE]

2272. J Infect Dis. 1999 Feb;179 Suppl 1:S203-17.

Pathogenesis of experimental Ebola virus infection in guinea pigs.

Connolly BM(1), Steele KE, Davis KJ, Geisbert TW, Kell WM, Jaax NK, Jahrling PB.

Author information: (1)Virology Division, United States Army Medical Research Institute of Infectious Diseases, Fort Detrick, Frederick, Maryland 21702-5011, USA.

The subtype Zaire of Ebola (EBO) virus (Mayinga strain) was adapted to produce lethal infections in guinea pigs. In many ways, the disease was similar to EBO infections in nonhuman primates and humans. The guinea pig model was used to investigate the pathologic events in EBO infection that lead to death. Analytical methods included immunohistochemistry, in situ hybridization, and electron microscopy. Cells of the mononuclear phagocyte system, primarily macrophages, were identified as the early and sustained targets of EBO virus. During later stages of infection, interstitial fibroblasts in various tissues were infected, and there was evidence of endothelial cell infection and fibrin deposition. The distribution of lesions, hematologic profiles, and increases in serum biochemical enzymes associated with EBO virus infection in guinea pigs was similar to reported findings in experimentally infected nonhuman primates and naturally infected humans.

PMID: 9988186 [PubMed - indexed for MEDLINE]

2273. J Infect Dis. 1999 Feb;179 Suppl 1:S199-202.

An analysis of features of pathogenesis in two animal models of Ebola virus infection.

Ryabchikova EI(1), Kolesnikova LV, Luchko SV.

Author information: (1)State Research Center of Virology and Biotechnology Vector, Research Institute of Molecular Biology, Koltsovo, Russia. elena@vector.nsk.su

Virus reproduction and the time course of changes in liver and kidney functions and in the blood clotting system were studied in the visceral organs of green monkeys and baboons infected with Ebola virus (subtype Zaire). It was shown that monocytes and macrophages were the first cells to be infected with the virus, followed by hepatocytes, adrenocorticocytes, fibroblasts, and endotheliocytes. The early and late pathologic changes in the monkey organs are described. Biochemical data on changes in blood clotting and liver and kidney functions in the course of the infection are presented. The responses of blood clotting and vascular permeability were species specific: Fibrin deposited in blood vessels in green monkeys, while hemorrhages developed in baboons. The results show that species-specific features of monkeys must be taken into account when choosing an experimental model for studying Ebola virus infection.

PMID: 9988185 [PubMed - indexed for MEDLINE]

2274. J Infect Dis. 1999 Feb;179 Suppl 1:S192-8.

ELISA for the detection of antibodies to Ebola viruses.

Ksiazek TG(1), West CP, Rollin PE, Jahrling PB, Peters CJ.

Author information: (1)Disease Assessment Division, US Army Medical Research Institute of Infectious Disease, Fort Detrick, Frederick, Maryland, USA.

EIAs for IgG and IgM antibodies directed against Ebola (EBO) viral antigens have been developed and evaluated using sera of animals and humans surviving infection with EBO viruses. The IgM capture assay detected anti-EBO (subtype Reston) antibodies in the sera of 5 of 5 experimentally infected animals at the time they succumbed to lethal infections. IgM antibodies were also detected in the serum of a human who was infected with EBO (subtype Reston) during a postmortem examination of an infected monkey. The antibody was detectable as early as day 6 after infection in experimentally infected animals and persisted for 400 days in 3 animals who survived infection, and it persisted for approximately 10 years after infection in the sera of 2 humans. Although these data are limited by the number of sera available for verification, the IgM assay seems to have great promise as a diagnostic tool. Furthermore the long-term persistence of the IgG antibodies measured by this test strongly suggests that the ELISA will be useful in field investigations of EBO virus.

PMID: 9988184 [PubMed - indexed for MEDLINE]

2275. J Infect Dis. 1999 Feb;179 Suppl 1:S188-91.

Markedly elevated levels of interferon (IFN)-gamma, IFN-alpha, interleukin (IL)-2, IL-10, and tumor necrosis factor-alpha associated with fatal Ebola virus infection.

Villinger F(1), Rollin PE, Brar SS, Chikkala NF, Winter J, Sundstrom JB, Zaki SR, Swanepoel R, Ansari AA, Peters CJ.

Author information: (1)Department of Pathology and Laboratory Medicine, School of Medicine, Emory University, Atlanta, Georgia 30322, USA. fvillin@emory.edu

The role of immune mechanisms in the pathogenesis of Ebola hemorrhagic fever (EHF) remains to be elucidated. In this report, the serum cytokine levels of patients who died of EHF were compared with those of patients who recovered and those of control patients. A marked elevation of interferon (IFN)-gamma levels (>100 pg/mL) was observed in sequential serum samples from all fatal EHF cases compared with patients who recovered or controls. Markedly elevated serum levels of interleukin (IL)-2, IL-10, tumor necrosis factor (TNF)-alpha, and IFN-alpha were also noted in fatal EHF cases; however, they had a greater degree of variability. No differences were noted in serum levels of IL-4 and IL-6. mRNA quantitation from blood clots of the same patients showed relatively elevated levels of TNF-alpha and IFN-alpha in samples from EHF patients. Taken together, these results suggest that a high degree of immune activation accompanies and potentially contributes to a fatal outcome in EHF patients.

PMID: 9988183 [PubMed - indexed for MEDLINE]

2276. J Infect Dis. 1999 Feb;179 Suppl 1:S177-87.

Clinical virology of Ebola hemorrhagic fever (EHF): virus, virus antigen, and IgG and IgM antibody findings among EHF patients in Kikwit, Democratic Republic of the Congo, 1995.

Ksiazek TG(1), Rollin PE, Williams AJ, Bressler DS, Martin ML, Swanepoel R, Burt FJ, Leman PA, Khan AS, Rowe AK, Mukunu R, Sanchez A, Peters CJ.

Author information: (1)Special Pathogens Branch, Division of Viral and Rickettsial Diseases, National Center for Infectious Diseases, Centers for Disease Control and Prevention, Atlanta, Georgia 30333, USA.

Ebola hemorrhagic fever (EHF) patients treated at Kikwit General Hospital during the 1995 outbreak were tested for viral antigen, IgG and IgM antibody, and infectious virus. Viral antigen could be detected in virtually all patients during the acute phase of illness, while antibody was not always detectable before death. Virus was also isolated from patients during the course of their febrile illness, but attempts to quantify virus in Vero E6 cells by standard plaque assay were often unsuccessful. IgG and IgM antibody appeared at approximately the same time after disease onset (8-10 days), but IgM persisted for a much shorter period among the surviving convalescent patients. IgG antibody was detectable in surviving patients through about 2 years after onset, the latest time that samples were obtained. Detection of Ebola virus antigens or virus isolation appears to be the most reliable means of diagnosis for patients with suspected acute EHF, since patients with this often-fatal disease (80% mortality) may not develop detectable antibodies before death.

PMID: 9988182 [PubMed - indexed for MEDLINE]

2277. J Infect Dis. 1999 Feb;179 Suppl 1:S170-6.

Persistence and genetic stability of Ebola virus during the outbreak in Kikwit, Democratic Republic of the Congo, 1995.

Rodriguez LL(1), De Roo A, Guimard Y, Trappier SG, Sanchez A, Bressler D, Williams AJ, Rowe AK, Bertolli J, Khan AS, Ksiazek TG, Peters CJ, Nichol ST.

Author information: (1)Special Pathogens Branch, Division of Viral and Rickettsial Diseases, National Center for Infectious Diseases, Centers for Disease Control and Prevention, Atlanta, Georgia 30329-4018, USA.

Ebola virus persistence was examined in body fluids from 12 convalescent patients by virus isolation and reverse transcription-polymerase chain reaction (RT-PCR) during the 1995 Ebola hemorrhagic fever outbreak in Kikwit, Democratic Republic of the Congo. Virus RNA could be detected for up to 33 days in vaginal, rectal, and conjunctival swabs of 1 patient and up to 101 days in the seminal fluid of 4 patients. Infectious virus was detected in 1 seminal fluid sample obtained 82 days after disease onset. Sequence analysis of an RT-PCR fragment of the most variable region of the glycoprotein gene amplified from 9 patients revealed no nucleotide changes. The patient samples were selected so that they would include some from a suspected line of transmission with at least three human-to-human passages, some from 5 survivors and 4 deceased patients, and 2 from patients who provided multiple samples through convalescence. There was no evidence of different virus variants cocirculating during the outbreak or of genetic variation accumulating during human-to-human passage or during prolonged persistence in individual patients.

PMID: 9988181 [PubMed - indexed for MEDLINE]

2278. J Infect Dis. 1999 Feb;179 Suppl 1:S164-9.

Detection and molecular characterization of Ebola viruses causing disease in human and nonhuman primates.

Sanchez A(1), Ksiazek TG, Rollin PE, Miranda ME, Trappier SG, Khan AS, Peters CJ, Nichol ST.

Author information: (1)Special Pathogens Branch, Division of Viral and Rickettsial Diseases, National Center for Infectious Diseases, Centers for Disease Control and Prevention, Atlanta, Georgia 30333, USA. ans1@cdc.gov

Ebola (EBO) viruses were detected in specimens obtained during the hemorrhagic fever outbreak among humans in Kikwit, Democratic Republic of the Congo (DRC), in 1995 (subtype Zaire) and during an outbreak of disease in cynomolgus macaques in Alice, Texas, and the Philippines in 1996 (subtype Reston). Reverse transcriptase-polymerase chain reaction assays were developed and proven effective for detecting viral RNA in body fluids and tissues of infected individuals. Little change was seen in the nucleotide or deduced amino acid sequences of the glycoprotein (GP) of these EBO virus subtypes compared with those of their original representatives (i.e., the 1976 Yambuku, DRC, EBO isolate [subtype Zaire] and the 1989 Philippines and Reston, Virginia, isolates [subtype Reston]). The nonstructural secreted GP (SGP), the primary product of the GP gene, was more highly conserved than the structural GP, indicating different functional roles or evolutionary constraints for these proteins. Significant amounts of SGP were detected in acutely infected humans.

PMID: 9988180 [PubMed - indexed for MEDLINE]

2279. J Infect Dis. 1999 Feb;179 Suppl 1:S155-63.

Search for the Ebola virus reservoir in Kikwit, Democratic Republic of the Congo: reflections on a vertebrate collection.

Leirs H(1), Mills JN, Krebs JW, Childs JE, Akaibe D, Woollen N, Ludwig G, Peters CJ, Ksiazek TG.

Author information: (1)Danish Pest Infestation Laboratory, Lyngby. h.leirs@ssl.dk

A 3-month ecologic investigation was done to identify the reservoir of Ebola virus following the 1995 outbreak in Kikwit, Democratic Republic of the Congo. Efforts focused on the fields where the putative primary case had worked but included other habitats near Kikwit. Samples were collected from 3066 vertebrates and tested for the presence of antibodies to Ebola (subtype Zaire) virus: All tests were negative, and attempts to isolate Ebola virus were unsuccessful. The investigation was hampered by a lack of information beyond the daily activities of the primary case, a lack of information on Ebola virus ecology, which precluded the detailed study of select groups of animals, and sample-size limitations for rare species. The epidemiology of Ebola hemorrhagic fever suggests that humans have only intermittent contact with the virus, which complicates selection of target species. Further study of the epidemiology of human outbreaks to further define the environmental contact of primary cases would be of great value.

PMID: 9988179 [PubMed - indexed for MEDLINE]

2280. J Infect Dis. 1999 Feb;179 Suppl 1:S148-54.

Field investigations of an outbreak of Ebola hemorrhagic fever, Kikwit, Democratic Republic of the Congo, 1995: arthropod studies.

Reiter P(1), Turell M, Coleman R, Miller B, Maupin G, Liz J, Kuehne A, Barth J, Geisbert J, Dohm D, Glick J, Pecor J, Robbins R, Jahrling P, Peters C, Ksiazek T.

Author information: (1)Dengue Branch, Centers for Disease Control and Prevention, San Juan, Puerto Rico 00921-3200, USA. iprl@cdc.gov

During the final weeks of a 6-month epidemic of Ebola hemorrhagic fever in Kikwit, Democratic Republic of the Congo, an extensive collection of arthropods was made in an attempt to learn more of the natural history of the disease. A reconstruction of the activities of the likely primary case, a 42-year-old man who lived in the city, indicated that he probably acquired his infection in a partly forested area 15 km from his home. Collections were made throughout this area, along the route he followed from the city, and at various sites in the city itself. No Ebola virus was isolated, but a description of the collections and the ecotopes involved is given for comparison with future studies of other outbreaks.

PMID: 9988178 [PubMed - indexed for MEDLINE]

2281. J Infect Dis. 1999 Feb;179 Suppl 1:S139-47.

A search for Ebola virus in animals in the Democratic Republic of the Congo and Cameroon: ecologic, virologic, and serologic surveys, 1979-1980. Ebola Virus Study Teams.

Breman JG(1), Johnson KM, van der Groen G, Robbins CB, Szczeniowski MV, Ruti K, Webb PA, Meier F, Heymann DL.

Author information: (1)Smallpox Eradication Unit, World Health Organization, Geneva, Switzerland. jbreman@nih.gov

More than 30 years after the first outbreak of Marburg virus disease in Germany and Yugoslavia and 20 years after Ebola hemorrhagic fever first occurred in central Africa, the natural history of filoviruses remains unknown. In 1979 and 1980, animals in the Democratic Republic of the Congo and Cameroon were collected during the dry season near the site of the 1976 Ebola hemorrhagic fever epidemic. The study objectives were to identify local animals and search for evidence of Ebola virus in their tissues. A total of 1664 animals representing 117 species was collected, including >400 bats and 500 rodents. Vero and CV-1 cells and IFA and RIA were used for virus and antibody detection, respectively. No evidence of Ebola virus infection was found. This study was limited in time and animal collections and excluded insects and plants. Long-term, prospective, multidisciplinary comparative studies will yield more information than will repeat short forays on the ecology of filoviruses.
PMID: 9988177 [PubMed - indexed for MEDLINE]

2282. J Infect Dis. 1999 Feb;179 Suppl 1:S127-38.

Ecology of Marburg and Ebola viruses: speculations and directions for future research.

Monath TP(1).

Author information: (1)Research and Medical Affairs, OraVax, Inc., Cambridge Massachusetts 02139, USA. tmonath@oravax.com

Marburg and virulent Ebola viruses are maintained in hosts that are rare and have little contact with humans or do not readily transmit virus. Bats (particularly solitary microchiropteran species) are leading contenders as reservoir hosts. Virus transfer to humans occurs by contact with the primary reservoir or via an intermediate animal that acquired infection from the reservoir and is, in turn, hunted by humans. An interesting possibility is that filoviruses may be arthropod or plant viruses, with non-blood-feeding arthropods transmitting the virus to intermediate hosts or humans during oral ingestion or envenomation. Paradoxically, in Africa, Ebola virus disease has high lethality and high seroprevalence as determined by the IFA test. If the seroreactivity is confirmed by more specific tests, then the Ebola virus serogroup in Africa probably contains an antigenically cross-reactive, enzootic, nonpathogenic agent(s). Such viruses may have separate life cycles or may give rise to virulent strains by mutation.
PMID: 9988176 [PubMed - indexed for MEDLINE]

2283. J Infect Dis. 1999 Feb;179 Suppl 1:S120-6.

Ebola virus outbreak among wild chimpanzees living in a rain forest of Côte d'Ivoire.

Formenty P(1), Boesch C, Wyers M, Steiner C, Donati F, Dind F, Walker F, Le Guenno B.

Author information: (1)World Health Organization (WHO) Taï Forest Project, and Centre Suisse de recherches scientifiques, Abidjan, Côte d'Ivoire. formenty@globeaccess.net

An outbreak of Ebola in nature is described for the first time. During a few weeks in November 1994, approximately 25% of 43 members of a wild chimpanzee community disappeared or were found dead in the Taï National Park, Côte d'Ivoire. A retrospective cohort study was done on the chimpanzee community. Laboratory procedures included histology, immunohistochemistry, bacteriology, and serology. Ebola-specific immunohistochemical staining was positive for autopsy tissue sections from 1 chimpanzee. Demographic, epidemiologic, and ecologic investigations were compatible with a point-source epidemic. Contact activities associated with a case (e.g., touching dead bodies or grooming) did not constitute significant risk factors, whereas consumption of meat did. The relative risk of meat consumption was 5.2 (95% confidence interval, 1.3-21.1). A similar outbreak occurred in November 1992 among the same community. A high mortality rate among apes tends to indicate that they are not the reservoir for the disease causing the illness. These points will have to be investigated by additional studies.
PMID: 9988175 [PubMed - indexed for MEDLINE]

2284. J Infect Dis. 1999 Feb;179 Suppl 1:S115-9.

Epidemiology of Ebola (subtype Reston) virus in the Philippines, 1996.

Miranda ME(1), Ksiazek TG, Retuya TJ, Khan AS, Sanchez A, Fulhorst CF, Rollin PE, Calaor AB, Manalo DL, Roces MC, Dayrit MM, Peters CJ.

Author information: (1)Research Institute for Tropical Medicine, and Field Epidemiology Training Program, Department of Health, Manila, Philippines.

Ebola (subtype Reston [EBO-R]) virus infection was detected in macaques imported into the United States from the Philippines in March 1996. Studies were initiated in the Philippines to identify the source of the virus among monkey-breeding and export facilities, to establish surveillance and testing, and to assess the risk and significance of EBO-R infections in humans who work in these facilities. Over a 5-month period, acutely infected animals were found at only one facility, as determined using Ebola antigen detection. Three of 1732 monkeys and 1 of 246 animal handlers tested had detectable antibodies; all were from the same facility, which was the source of infected monkeys imported to the United States. Virus transmission, which was facilitated by poor infection-control practices, continued for several months in one facility and was stopped only when the facility was depopulated. None of the 246 employees of the facilities or 4 contacts of previously antibody-positive individuals reported an Ebola-like illness. This investigation suggests that human EBO-R infection is rare.
PMID: 9988174 [PubMed - indexed for MEDLINE]

2285. J Infect Dis. 1999 Feb;179 Suppl 1:S108-14.

Ebola (subtype Reston) virus among quarantined nonhuman primates recently imported from the Philippines to the United States.

Rollin PE(1), Williams RJ, Bressler DS, Pearson S, Cottingham M, Pucak G, Sanchez A, Trappier SG, Peters RL, Greer PW, Zaki S, Demarcus T, Hendricks K, Kelley M, Simpson D, Geisbert TW, Jahrling PB, Peters CJ, Ksiazek TG.

Author information: (1)Special Pathogens Branch and Molecular Pathology and Ultrastructure Activity, Division of Viral and Rickettsial Diseases, National Center for Infectious Diseases, Centers for Disease Control and Prevention, Atlanta, Georgia 30333, USA. PYR3@CDC.GOV

In April 1996, laboratory testing of imported nonhuman primates (as mandated by quarantine regulations) identified 2 cynomolgus macaques (Macaca fascicularis) infected with Ebola (subtype Reston) virus in a US-registered quarantine facility. The animals were part of a shipment of 100 nonhuman primates recently imported from the Philippines. Two additional infected animals, who were thought to be in the incubation phase, were identified among the remaining 48 animals in the affected quarantine room. The other 50 macaques, who had been held in a separate isolation room, remained asymptomatic, and none of these animals seroconverted during an extended quarantine period. Due to the rigorous routine safety precautions, the facility personnel had no unprotected exposures and remained asymptomatic, and no one seroconverted. The mandatory quarantine and laboratory testing requirements, put in place after the original Reston outbreak in 1989-1990, were effective for detecting and containing Ebola virus infection in newly imported nonhuman primates and minimizing potential human transmission.

PMID: 9988173 [PubMed - indexed for MEDLINE]

2286. J Infect Dis. 1999 Feb;179 Suppl 1:S102-7.

Prevalence of IgG antibodies to Ebola virus in individuals during an Ebola outbreak, Democratic Republic of the Congo, 1995.

Busico KM(1), Marshall KL, Ksiazek TG, Roels TH, Fleerackers Y, Feldmann H, Khan AS, Peters CJ.

Author information: (1)Special Pathogens Branch, Division of Viral and Rickettsial Diseases, National Center for Infectious Diseases, Centers for Disease Control and Prevention, Atlanta, Georgia 30333, USA.

During the 1995 outbreak of Ebola (EBO) hemorrhagic fever in Kikwit, Democratic Republic of Congo, two surveys using a new ELISA for EBO (subtype Zaire) virus antigen were conducted to assess the prevalence of EBO IgG antibodies among residents of Kikwit and the surrounding area. The first study determined the proportion of antibody-positive individuals who were self-identified forest and city workers from the Kikwit area. Serum samples from 9 (2.2%) of 414 workers had IgG EBO antibodies. The second study determined the proportion of EBO antibody-positive individuals who lived in villages surrounding Kikwit. The prevalence of IgG EBO antibodies in this population was 9.3% (15|161). The difference in the overall prevalence of EBO antibodies may indicate that villagers have a greater chance of exposure to EBO virus compared with those living in and in close proximity to cities.

PMID: 9988172 [PubMed - indexed for MEDLINE]

2287. J Infect Dis. 1999 Feb;179 Suppl 1:S98-101.

Serologic survey among hospital and health center workers during the Ebola hemorrhagic fever outbreak in Kikwit, Democratic Republic of the Congo, 1995.

Tomori O(1), Bertolli J, Rollin PE, Fleerackers Y, Guimard Y, De Roo A, Feldmann H, Burt F, Swanepoel R, Killian S, Khan AS, Tshioko K, Bwaka M, Ndambe R, Peters CJ, Ksiazek TG.

Author information: (1)World Health Organization, Harare, Zimbabwe.

From May to July 1995, a serologic and interview survey was conducted to describe Ebola hemorrhagic fever (EHF) among personnel working in 5 hospitals and 26 health care centers in and around Kikwit, Democratic Republic of the Congo. Job-specific attack rates estimated for Kikwit General Hospital, the epicenter of the EHF epidemic, were 31% for physicians, 11% for technicians/room attendants, 10% for nurses, and 4% for other workers. Among 402 workers who did not meet the EHF case definition, 12 had borderline positive antibody test results; subsequent specimens from 4 of these tested negative. Although an old infection with persistent Ebola antibody production or a recent atypical or asymptomatic infection cannot be ruled out, if they occur at all, they appear to be rare. This survey demonstrated that opportunities for transmission of Ebola virus to personnel in health facilities existed in Kikwit because blood and body fluid precautions were not being universally followed.

PMID: 9988171 [PubMed - indexed for MEDLINE]

2288. J Infect Dis. 1999 Feb;179 Suppl 1:S92-7.

Ebola hemorrhagic fever, Kikwit, Democratic Republic of the Congo, 1995: risk factors for patients without a reported exposure.

Roels TH(1), Bloom AS, Buffington J, Muhungu GL, Mac Kenzie WR, Khan AS, Ndambi R, Noah DL, Rolka HR, Peters CJ, Ksiazek TG.

Author information: (1)Epidemic Intelligence Service, Division of Applied Public Health Training, National Center for Chronic Disease Prevention and Health Promotion, Centers for Disease Control and Prevention, Atlanta, Georgia, USA. tbr6@cdc.gov

In 1995, 316 people became ill with Ebola hemorrhagic fever (EHF) in Kikwit, Democratic Republic of the Congo. The exposure source was not reported for 55 patients (17%) at the start of this investigation, and it remained unknown for 12 patients after extensive epidemiologic evaluation. Both admission to a hospital and visiting a person with fever and bleeding were risk factors associated with infection. Nineteen patients appeared to have been exposed while visiting someone with suspected EHF, although they did not provide care. Fourteen of the 19 reported touching the patient with suspected EHF; 5 reported that they had no physical contact. Although close contact while caring for an infected person was probably the major route of transmission in this and previous EHF outbreaks, the virus may have been transmitted by touch, droplet, airborne particle, or fomite; thus, expansion of the use of barrier techniques to include casual contacts might prevent or mitigate future epidemics.

PMID: 9988170 [PubMed - indexed for MEDLINE]

2289. J Infect Dis. 1999 Feb;179 Suppl 1:S87-91.

Transmission of Ebola hemorrhagic fever: a study of risk factors in family members, Kikwit, Democratic Republic of the Congo, 1995. Commission de Lutte contre les Epidémies à Kikwit.

Dowell SF(1), Mukunu R, Ksiazek TG, Khan AS, Rollin PE, Peters CJ.

Author information: (1)Division of Viral and Rickettsial Diseases, Centers for Disease Control and Prevention, Atlanta, Georgia 30333, USA. SFD2@cdc.gov

The surviving members of 27 households in which someone had been infected with Ebola virus were interviewed in order to define the modes of transmission of Ebola hemorrhagic fever (EHF). Of 173 household contacts of the primary cases, 28 (16%) developed EHF. All secondary cases had direct physical contact with the ill person (rate ratio [RR], undefined; P < .001), and among those with direct contact, exposure to body fluids conferred additional risk (RR, 3.6; 95%

confidence interval [CI], 1.9-6.8). After adjusting for direct contact and exposure to body fluids, adult family members, those who touched the cadaver, and those who were exposed during the late hospital phase were at additional risk. None of the 78 household members who had no physical contact with the case during the clinical illness were infected (upper 95% CI, 4%). EHF is transmitted principally by direct physical contact with an ill person or their body fluids during the later stages of illness.

PMID: 9988169 [PubMed - indexed for MEDLINE]

2290. J Infect Dis. 1999 Feb;179 Suppl 1:S76-86.

The reemergence of Ebola hemorrhagic fever, Democratic Republic of the Congo, 1995. Commission de Lutte contre les Epidémies à Kikwit.

Khan AS(1), Tshioko FK, Heymann DL, Le Guenno B, Nabeth P, Kerstiëns B, Fleerackers Y, Kilmarx PH, Rodier GR, Nkuku O, Rollin PE, Sanchez A, Zaki SR, Swanepoel R, Tomori O, Nichol ST, Peters CJ, Muyembe-Tamfum JJ, Ksiazek TG.

Author information: (1)Special Pathogens Branch and Infectious Disease Pathology Activity, Division of Viral and Rickettsial Diseases, National Center for Infectious Diseases, and Epidemiology Program Office, Centers for Disease Control and Prevention,

In May 1995, an international team characterized and contained an outbreak of Ebola hemorrhagic fever (EHF) in Kikwit, Democratic Republic of the Congo. Active surveillance was instituted using several methods, including house-to-house search, review of hospital and dispensary logs, interview of health care personnel, retrospective contact tracing, and direct follow-up of suspect cases. In the field, a clinical case was defined as fever and hemorrhagic signs, fever plus contact with a case-patient, or fever plus at least 3 of 10 symptoms. A total of 315 cases of EHF, with an 81% case fatality, were identified, excluding 10 clinical cases with negative laboratory results. The earliest documented case-patient had onset on 6 January, and the last case-patient died on 16 July. Eighty cases (25%) occurred among health care workers. Two individuals may have been the source of infection for >50 cases. The outbreak was terminated by the initiation of barrier-nursing techniques, health education efforts, and rapid identification of cases.

PMID: 9988168 [PubMed - indexed for MEDLINE]

2291. J Infect Dis. 1999 Feb;179 Suppl 1:S65-75.

Ebola hemorrhagic fever outbreaks in Gabon, 1994-1997: epidemiologic and health control issues.

Georges AJ(1), Leroy EM, Renaut AA, Benissan CT, Nabias RJ, Ngoc MT, Obiang PI, Lepage JP, Bertherat EJ, Bénoni DD, Wickings EJ, Amblard JP, Lansoud-Soukate JM, Milleliri JM, Baize S, Georges-Courbot MC.

Author information: (1)Centre International de Recherches Médicales de Franceville, Gabon. ajgeorges@wanadoo.fr

From the end of 1994 to the beginning of 1995, 49 patients with hemorrhagic symptoms were hospitalized in the Makokou General Hospital in northeastern Gabon. Yellow fever (YF) virus was first diagnosed in serum by use of polymerase chain reaction followed by blotting, and a vaccination campaign was immediately instituted. The epidemic, known as the fall 1994 epidemic, ended 6 weeks later. However, some aspects of this epidemic were atypical of YF infection, so a retrospective check for other etiologic agents was undertaken. Ebola (EBO) virus was found to be present concomitantly with YF virus in the epidemic. Two other epidemics (spring and fall 1996) occurred in the same province. GP and L genes of EBO virus isolates from all three epidemics were partially sequenced, which showed a difference of

PMID: 9988167 [PubMed - indexed for MEDLINE]

2292. J Infect Dis. 1999 Feb;179 Suppl 1:S60-4.

Ebola between outbreaks: intensified Ebola hemorrhagic fever surveillance in the Democratic Republic of the Congo, 1981-1985.

Jezek Z(1), Szczeniowski MY, Muyembe-Tamfum JJ, McCormick JB, Heymann DL.

Author information: (1)World Health Organization, Geneva, Switzerland.

Surveillance for Ebola hemorrhagic fever was conducted in the Democratic Republic of the Congo from 1981 to 1985 to estimate the incidence of human infection. Persons who met the criteria of one of three different case definitions were clinically evaluated, and blood was obtained for antibody confirmation by IFA. Contacts of each case and 4 age- and sex-matched controls were also clinically examined and tested for immunofluorescent antibody. Twenty-one cases of Ebola infection (persons with an antibody titer of > or = 1:64, or lower if they fit the clinical case definition) were identified, with a maximum 1-year incidence of 9 and a case fatality rate of 43%. Cases occurred throughout the year, but most (48%) occurred early in the rainy season. Fifteen percent of contacts had antibody titers > or =1:64 to Ebola virus, compared with 1% of controls (P < .0001). Results suggest that Ebola virus periodically emerges from nature to infect humans, that person-to-person transmission is relatively limited, and that amplification to large epidemics is unusual.

PMID: 9988166 [PubMed - indexed for MEDLINE]

2293. J Infect Dis. 1999 Feb;179 Suppl 1:S54-9.

Histopathological and immunohistochemical studies of lesions associated with Ebola virus in a naturally infected chimpanzee.

Wyers M(1), Formenty P, Cherel Y, Guigand L, Fernandez B, Boesch C, Le Guenno B.

Author information: (1)Laboratoire d'histopathologie animale, Ecole nationale vétérinaire, Nantes, France. wyers@vet-nantes.fr

Lesions caused by the Côte d'Ivoire subtype of Ebola virus in a naturally infected young chimpanzee were characterized by histopathological and immunohistochemical methods. The predominant lesions consisted of multifocal necrosis in the liver and diffuse fibrinoid necrosis in the red pulp of the spleen. In these sites, macrophages contained large eosinophilic intracytoplasmic inclusion bodies. Immunohistochemical staining indicated that macrophages were a major site of viral replication. The absence of bronchiolar and pulmonary lesions and the paucity of antigen-containing macrophages in the lung suggested that aerosol transmission by this animal was unlikely. There were necrotic foci and antigen-containing macrophages in intestinal lymph nodes, in association with lesions caused by intestinal parasites, suggesting the possibility of virus entry through the digestive tract.

PMID: 9988165 [PubMed - indexed for MEDLINE]

498

2294. J Infect Dis. 1999 Feb;179 Suppl 1:S48-53.

Human infection due to Ebola virus, subtype Côte d'Ivoire: clinical and biologic presentation.

Formenty P(1), Hatz C, Le Guenno B, Stoll A, Rogenmoser P, Widmer A.

Author information: (1)World Health Organization and Polyclinique Internationale Sainte Anne-Marie, Abidjan, Côte d'Ivoire. formenty@globeaccess.net

In November 1994 after 15 years of epidemiologic silence, Ebola virus reemerged in Africa and, for the first time, in West Africa. In Côte d'Ivoire, a 34-year-old female ethologist was infected while conducting a necropsy on a wild chimpanzee. Eight days later, the patient developed a syndrome that did not respond to antimalarial drugs and was characterized by high fever, headache, chills, myalgia, and cough. The patient had abdominal pain, diarrhea, vomiting, and a macular rash, and was repatriated to Switzerland. The patient suffered from prostration and weight loss but recovered without sequelae. Laboratory findings included aspartate aminotransferase and alanine aminotransferase activity highly elevated, thrombocytopenia, lymphopenia, and, subsequently, neutrophilia. A new subtype of Ebola was isolated from the patient's blood on days 4 and 8. No serologic conversion was detected among contact persons in Côte d'Ivoire (n = 22) or Switzerland (n = 52), suggesting that infection-control precautions were satisfactory.

PMID: 9988164 [PubMed - indexed for MEDLINE]

2295. J Infect Dis. 1999 Feb;179 Suppl 1:S36-47.

A novel immunohistochemical assay for the detection of Ebola virus in skin: implications for diagnosis, spread, and surveillance of Ebola hemorrhagic fever. Commission de Lutte contre les Epidémies à Kikwit.

Zaki SR(1), Shieh WJ, Greer PW, Goldsmith CS, Ferebee T, Katshitshi J, Tshioko FK, Bwaka MA, Swanepoel R, Calain P, Khan AS, Lloyd E, Rollin PE, Ksiazek TG, Peters CJ.

Author information: (1)Division of Viral and Rickettsial Diseases, National Center for Infectious Diseases, Centers for Disease Control and Prevention, Atlanta, Georgia 30333, USA. sxzl@cdc.gov

Laboratory diagnosis of Ebola hemorrhagic fever (EHF) is currently performed by virus isolation and serology and can be done only in a few high-containment laboratories worldwide. In 1995, during the EHF outbreak in the Democratic Republic of Congo, the possibility of using immunohistochemistry (IHC) testing of formalin-fixed postmortem skin specimens was investigated as an alternative diagnostic method for EHF. Fourteen of 19 cases of suspected EHF met the surveillance definition for EHF and were positive by IHC. IHC, serologic, and virus isolation results were concordant for all EHF and non-EHF cases. IHC and electron microscopic examination showed that endothelial cells, mononuclear phagocytes, and hepatocytes are main targets of infection, and IHC showed an association of cellular damage with viral infection. The finding of abundant viral antigens and particles in the skin of EHF patients suggests an epidemiologic role for contact transmission. IHC testing of formalin-fixed skin specimens is a safe, sensitive, and specific method for laboratory diagnosis of EHF and should be useful for EHF surveillance and prevention.

PMID: 9988163 [PubMed - indexed for MEDLINE]

2296. J Infect Dis. 1999 Feb;179 Suppl 1:S28-35.

Clinical, virologic, and immunologic follow-up of convalescent Ebola hemorrhagic fever patients and their household contacts, Kikwit, Democratic Republic of the Congo. Commission de Lutte contre les Epidémies à Kikwit.

Rowe AK(1), Bertolli J, Khan AS, Mukunu R, Muyembe-Tamfum JJ, Bressler D, Williams AJ, Peters CJ, Rodriguez L, Feldmann H, Nichol ST, Rollin PE, Ksiazek TG.

Author information: (1)Epidemiology Program Office and Special Pathogens Branch, Division of Viral and Rickettsial Diseases, National Center for Infectious Diseases, Centers for Disease Control and Prevention, Atlanta, Georgia 30341, USA.

A cohort of convalescent Ebola hemorrhagic fever (EHF) patients and their household contacts (HHCs) were studied prospectively to determine if convalescent body fluids contain Ebola virus and if secondary transmission occurs during convalescence. Twenty-nine EHF convalescents and 152 HHCs were monitored for up to 21 months. Blood specimens were obtained and symptom information was collected from convalescents and their HHCs; other body fluid specimens were also obtained from convalescents. Arthralgias and myalgia were reported significantly more often by convalescents than HHCs. Evidence of Ebola virus was detected by reverse transcription-polymerase chain reaction in semen specimens up to 91 days after disease onset; however, these and all other non-blood body fluids tested negative by virus isolation. Among 81 initially antibody negative HHCs, none became antibody positive. Blood specimens of 5 HHCs not identified as EHF patients were initially antibody positive. No direct evidence of convalescent-to-HHC transmission of EHF was found, although the semen of convalescents may be infectious. The existence of initially antibody-positive HHCs suggests that mild cases of Ebola virus infection occurred and that the full extent of the EHF epidemic was probably underestimated.

PMID: 9988162 [PubMed - indexed for MEDLINE]

2297. J Infect Dis. 1999 Feb;179 Suppl 1:S24-7.

Ebola hemorrhagic fever, Democratic Republic of the Congo, 1995: determinants of survival.

Sadek RF(1), Khan AS, Stevens G, Peters CJ, Ksiazek TG.

Author information: (1)Special Pathogens Branch, Centers for Disease Control and Prevention, USA. RFSADEK@MKG.COM

In May 1995, an international team characterized and contained an outbreak of Ebola hemorrhagic fever in Kikwit, Democratic Republic of the Congo. This study reports the descriptive features of this outbreak along with a statistical analysis of the outbreak data. Proportional hazards analysis was used to examine the effect of age, phase of the outbreak, and sex on the risk of death, and a conditional probability analysis was used to examine the effectiveness of whole blood transfusion from convalescent patients on survival. Two hundred fifty case-patients (80.7%) died. The main predictor of survival in the proportional hazards model was age. No statistical evidence of a survival benefit of transfusion of blood from convalescent patients was evident after adjusting for age, sex, and the days since onset of symptoms (P = .1713).

PMID: 9988161 [PubMed - indexed for MEDLINE]
2298. J Infect Dis. 1999 Feb;179 Suppl 1:S18-23.

Treatment of Ebola hemorrhagic fever with blood transfusions from convalescent patients. International Scientific and Technical Committee.

Mupapa K(1), Massamba M, Kibadi K, Kuvula K, Bwaka A, Kipasa M, Colebunders R, Muyembe-Tamfum JJ.

Author information: (1)Kinshasa University, Ministry of Public Health, Democratic Republic of the Congo.

Between 6 and 22 June 1995, 8 patients in Kikwit, Democratic Republic of the Congo, who met the case definition used in Kikwit for Ebola (EBO) hemorrhagic fever, were transfused with blood donated by 5 convalescent patients. The donated blood contained IgG EBO antibodies but no EBO antigen. EBO antigens were detected in all the transfusion recipients just before transfusion. The 8 transfused patients had clinical symptoms similar to those of other EBO patients seen during the epidemic. All were seriously ill with severe asthenia, 4 presented with hemorrhagic manifestations, and 2 became comatose as their disease progressed. Only 1 transfused patient (12.5%) died; this number is significantly lower than the overall case fatality rate (80%) for the EBO epidemic in Kikwit and than the rates for other EBO epidemics. The reason for this low fatality rate remains to be explained. The transfused patients did receive better care than those in the initial phase of the epidemic. Plans should be made to prepare for a more thorough evaluation of passive immune therapy during a new EBO outbreak.

PMID: 9988160 [PubMed - indexed for MEDLINE]
2299. J Infect Dis. 1999 Feb;179 Suppl 1:S15-7.

Isolated case of Ebola hemorrhagic fever with mucormycosis complications, Kinshasa, Democratic Republic of the Congo.

Kalongi Y(1), Mwanza K, Tshisuaka M, Lusiama N, Ntando E, Kanzake L, Shieh WJ, Zaki SR, Lloyd ES, Ksiazek TG, Rollin PE.

Author information: (1)Médecine Interne, Clinique Bondeko, Kinshasa-Limete, Democratic Republic of the Congo.

A patient with undiagnosed Ebola (EBO) hemorrhagic fever (EHF) was transferred from Kikwit to a private clinic in Kinshasa, Democratic Republic of the Congo. A diagnosis of EHF was suspected on clinical grounds and was confirmed by detection of EBO virus-specific IgM and IgG in serum of the patient. During the course of the disease, although she had no known predisposing factors, the patient developed a periorbital mucormycosis abscess on eyelid tissue that was biopsied during surgical drainage; the abscess was histologically confirmed. Presence of EBO antigen was also detected by specific immunohistochemistry on the biopsied tissue. The patient survived the EBO infection but had severe sequelae associated with the mucormycosis. Standard barrier-nursing precautions were taken upon admission and upgraded when EHF was suspected; there was no secondary transmission of the disease.

PMID: 9988159 [PubMed - indexed for MEDLINE]
2300. J Infect Dis. 1999 Feb;179 Suppl 1:S13-4.

Late ophthalmologic manifestations in survivors of the 1995 Ebola virus epidemic in Kikwit, Democratic Republic of the Congo.

Kibadi K(1), Mupapa K, Kuvula K, Massamba M, Ndaberey D, Muyembe-Tamfum JJ, Bwaka MA, De Roo A, Colebunders R.

Author information: (1)Kikwit General Hospital, Democratic Republic of the Congo.

Three (15%) of 20 survivors of the 1995 Ebola outbreak in the Democratic Republic of the Congo enrolled in a follow-up study and 1 other survivor developed ocular manifestations after being asymptomatic for 1 month. Patients complained of ocular pain, photophobia, hyperlacrimation, and loss of visual acuity. Ocular examination revealed uveitis in all 4 patients. All patients improved with a topical treatment of 1% atropine and steroids.

PMID: 9988158 [PubMed - indexed for MEDLINE]
2301. J Infect Dis. 1999 Feb;179 Suppl 1:S11-2.

Ebola hemorrhagic fever and pregnancy.

Mupapa K(1), Mukundu W, Bwaka MA, Kipasa M, De Roo A, Kuvula K, Kibadi K, Massamba M, Ndaberey D, Colebunders R, Muyembe-Tamfum JJ.

Author information: (1)Department of Microbiology, University of Kinshasa, and Ministry of Public Health, Democratic Republic of the Congo.

Fifteen (14%) of 105 women with Ebola hemorrhagic fever hospitalized in the isolation unit of the Kikwit General Hospital (Democratic Republic of the Congo) were pregnant. In 10 women (66%) the pregnancy ended with an abortion. In 3 of them, a curettage was performed, and all 3 received a blood transfusion from an apparently healthy person. One woman was prematurely delivered of a stillbirth. Four pregnant women died during the third trimester of their pregnancy. All women presented with severe bleeding. Only 1 survived; she had a curettage because of an incomplete abortion after 8 months of amenorrhea. The mortality among pregnant women with Ebola hemorrhagic fever (95.5%) was slightly but not significantly higher than the overall mortality observed during the Ebola epidemic in Kikwit (77%; 245/316 infected persons).

PMID: 9988157 [PubMed - indexed for MEDLINE]
2302. J Infect Dis. 1999 Feb;179 Suppl 1:S8-10.

Epidemiologic and clinical aspects of the Ebola virus epidemic in Mosango, Democratic Republic of the Congo, 1995.

Ndambi R(1), Akamituna P, Bonnet MJ, Tukadila AM, Muyembe-Tamfum JJ, Colebunders R.

Author information: (1)Mosango General Hospital, Democratic Republic of the Congo.

Twenty-three Ebola hemorrhagic fever (EHF) cases (15 males, 8 females) were identified in Mosango, Democratic Republic of the Congo; 18 (78%) of them died. Eight of the patients came from Kikwit General Hospital and were hospitalized at Mosango General Hospital, 10 acquired their infection at the Mosango hospital and were treated there, and 5 acquired their infection through contact with a hospitalized patient but were never hospitalized themselves. For most of the EHF cases, it was clear that they had been in contact with blood or body fluids of another EHF patient. The Ebola outbreak in Mosango remained relatively small, probably because hygienic conditions in this hospital were relatively good at the time of the outbreak and because as soon as the epidemic was recognized, barrier nursing techniques were used.

PMID: 9988156 [PubMed - indexed for MEDLINE]

2303. J Infect Dis. 1999 Feb;179 Suppl 1:S1-7.

Ebola hemorrhagic fever in Kikwit, Democratic Republic of the Congo: clinical observations in 103 patients.

Bwaka MA(1), Bonnet MJ, Calain P, Colebunders R, De Roo A, Guimard Y, Katwiki KR, Kibadi K, Kipasa MA, Kuvula KJ, Mapanda BB, Massamba M, Mupapa KD, Muyembe-Tamfum JJ, Ndaberey E, Peters CJ, Rollin PE, Van den Enden E, Van den Enden E.

Author information: (1)Hôpital Général de Référence de Kikwit, Diocèse de Kikwit, and 5ème Région Militaire, Democratic Republic of the Congo.

During the 1995 outbreak of Ebola hemorrhagic fever in the Democratic Republic of the Congo, a series of 103 cases (one-third of the total number of cases) had clinical symptoms and signs accurately recorded by medical workers, mainly in the setting of the urban hospital in Kikwit. Clinical diagnosis was confirmed retrospectively in cases for which serum samples were available (n = 63, 61% of the cases). The disease began unspecifically with fever, asthenia, diarrhea, headaches, myalgia, arthralgia, vomiting, and abdominal pain. Early inconsistent signs and symptoms included conjunctival injection, sore throat, and rash. Overall, bleeding signs were observed in

PMID: 9988155 [PubMed - indexed for MEDLINE]

2304. J Infect Dis. 1999 Feb;179 Suppl 1:ix-xvi.

An introduction to Ebola: the virus and the disease.

Peters CJ(1), LeDuc JW.

Author information: (1)National Center for Infectious Diseases, Centers for Disease Control and Prevention, Atlanta, Georgia 30333, USA.

PMID: 9988154 [PubMed - indexed for MEDLINE]

2305. J Virol. 1999 Feb;73(2):1419-26.

Endoproteolytic processing of the ebola virus envelope glycoprotein: cleavage is not required for function.

Wool-Lewis RJ(1), Bates P.

Author information: (1)Department of Microbiology, University of Pennsylvania School of Medicine, Philadelphia, Pennsylvania 19104-6076, USA.

Proteolytic processing is required for the activation of numerous viral glycoproteins. Here we show that the envelope glycoprotein from the Zaire strain of Ebola virus (Ebo-GP) is proteolytically processed into two subunits, GP1 and GP2, that are likely covalently associated through a disulfide linkage. Murine leukemia virions pseudotyped with Ebo-GP contain almost exclusively processed glycoprotein, indicating that this is the mature form of Ebo-GP. Mutational analysis identified a dibasic motif, reminiscent of furin-like protease processing sites, as the Ebo-GP cleavage site. However, analysis of Ebo-GP processing in LoVo cells that lack the proprotein convertase furin demonstrated that furin is not required for processing of Ebo-GP. In sharp contrast to other viral systems, we found that an uncleaved mutant of Ebo-GP was able to mediate infection of various cell lines as efficiently as the wild-type, proteolytically cleaved glycoprotein, indicating that cleavage is not required for the activation of Ebo-GP despite the conservation of a dibasic cleavage site in all filoviral envelope glycoproteins.

PMCID: PMC103966 PMID: 9882347 [PubMed - indexed for MEDLINE]

2306. Adv Pediatr Infect Dis. 1999;14:1-27.

Emerging viral infections.

Khabbaz RF(1).

Author information: (1)Division of Viral and Rickettsial Diseases, Centers for Disease Control and Prevention, Atlanta, Georgia, USA.

PMID: 10079847 [PubMed - indexed for MEDLINE]

2307. Arch Virol Suppl. 1999;15:159-69.

The glycoproteins of Marburg and Ebola virus and their potential roles in pathogenesis.

Feldmann H(1), Volchkov VE, Volchkova VA, Klenk HD.

Author information: (1)Institut für Virologie, Philipps-Universität Marburg, Germany.

Filoviruses cause systemic infections that can lead to severe hemorrhagic fever in human and non-human primates. The primary target of the virus appears to be the mononuclear phagocytic system. As the virus spreads through the organism, the spectrum of target cells increases to include endothelial cells, fibroblasts, hepatocytes, and many other cells. There is evidence that the filovirus glycoprotein plays an important role in cell tropism, spread of infection, and pathogenicity. Biosynthesis of the glycoprotein forming the spikes on the virion surface involves cleavage by the host cell protease furin into two disulfide linked subunits GP1 and GP2. GP1 is also shed in soluble form from infected cells. Different strains of Ebola virus show variations in the cleavability of the glycoprotein, that may account for differences in pathogenicity, as has been observed with influenza viruses and paramyxoviruses. Expression of the spike glycoprotein of Ebola virus, but not of Marburg virus, requires transcriptional editing. Unedited GP mRNA yields the nonstructural glycoprotein sGP, which is secreted extensively from infected cells. Whether the soluble glycoproteins GP1 and sGP interfere with the humoral immune response and other defense mechanisms remains to be determined.

PMID: 10470276 [PubMed - indexed for MEDLINE]

2308. Biull Eksp Biol Med. 1999 Jan;127(1):81-5.

[Effects of repeated administration of Ebola virus preparations on dynamics of immunologic parameters].

[Article in Russian]

Chepurnov AA, Dadaeva AA, Sizikova LP.

PMID: 10190013 [PubMed - indexed for MEDLINE]

2309. Br Homeopath J. 1999 Jan;88(1):24-7.

Sicarius (six-eyed crab spider): a homeopathic treatment for Ebola haemorrhagic fever and disseminated intravascular coagulation?

Richardson-Boedler C.

PMID: 10228601 [PubMed - indexed for MEDLINE]

2310. Br J Biomed Sci. 1999;56(4):280-4.

Ebola virus.

Streether LA(1).

Author information: (1)Virology Department, Grampian University Hospitals NHS Trust, Aberdeen Royal Infirmary, Foresterhill, Scotland, UK.

Ebola virus was first identified as a filovirus in 1976, following epidemics of severe haemorrhagic fever in sub-Saharan Africa. Further outbreaks have occurred since, but, despite extensive and continued investigations, the natural reservoir for the virus remains unknown. The mortality rate is high and there is no cure for Ebola virus infection. Molecular technology is proving useful in extending our knowledge of the virus. Identification of the host reservoir, control and prevention of further outbreaks, rapid diagnosis of infection, and vaccine development remain areas of continued interest in the fight against this biosafety level-four pathogen.

PMID: 10795373 [PubMed - indexed for MEDLINE]

2311. Bull World Health Organ. 1999;77(10):789-800.

Unsafe injections in the developing world and transmission of bloodborne pathogens: a review.

Simonsen L(1), Kane A, Lloyd J, Zaffran M, Kane M.

Author information: (1)World Health Organization, Geneva, Switzerland.

Unsafe injections are suspected to occur routinely in developing countries. We carried out a literature review to quantify the prevalence of unsafe injections and to assess the disease burden of bloodborne infections attributable to this practice. Quantitative information on injection use and unsafe injections (defined as the reuse of syringe or needle between patients without sterilization) was obtained by reviewing the published literature and unpublished WHO reports. The transmissibility of hepatitis B and C viruses and human immunodeficiency virus (HIV) was estimated using data from studies of needle-stick injuries. Finally, all epidemiological studies that linked unsafe injections and bloodborne infections were evaluated to assess the attributable burden of bloodborne infections. It was estimated that each person in the developing world receives 1.5 injections per year on average. However, institutionalized children, and children and adults who are ill or hospitalized, including those infected with HIV, are often exposed to 10-100 times as many injections. An average of 95% of all injections are therapeutic, the majority of which were judged to be unnecessary. At least 50% of injections were unsafe in 14 of 19 countries (representing five developing world regions) for which data were available. Eighteen studies reported a convincing link between unsafe injections and the transmission of hepatitis B and C, HIV, Ebola and Lassa virus infections and malaria. Five studies attributed 20-80% of all new hepatitis B infections to unsafe injections, while three implicated unsafe injections as a major mode of transmission of hepatitis C. In conclusion, unsafe injections occur routinely in most developing world regions, implying a significant potential for the transmission of any bloodborne pathogen. Unsafe injections currently account for a significant proportion of all new hepatitis B and C infections. This situation needs to be addressed immediately, as a political and policy issue, with responsibilities clearly defined at the global, country and community levels.

PIP: Unsafe injections and the consequent transmission of bloodborne pathogens are suspected to occur routinely in the developing world. This paper presents a review of the literature to determine the prevalence of unsafe injection practices and assess the disease burden of bloodborne infections. Quantitative data on injection usage and unsafe injection practices, such as the reuse of unsterilized syringe or needles between patients, is obtained by reviewing published articles and unpublished reports of the WHO. In addition, the transmissibility of hepatitis B and C viruses and HIV was determined using information from studies of needle-stick injuries. All epidemiological researches that associate injections with bloodborne diseases were examined to assess the attributable burden of bloodborne infections. It was estimated that each person in developing countries receives an average of 1.5 injections per annum. However, institutionalized children, children and adults who are sick or confined in hospitals, often receive 10-100 times as many injections. Of these injections, 95% are therapeutic, a majority of which are unnecessary. At least 50% of injections in 14 of 19 countries were unsafe. Furthermore, 18 studies present convincing evidence on the association of unsafe injection practices and the transmission of bloodborne viruses such as hepatitis B and C, Ebola, Lassa virus infections and malaria. Such practices account for a significant number of hepatitis B and C infections. PMCID: PMC2557743 PMID: 10593026 [PubMed - indexed for MEDLINE]

2312. Curr Top Microbiol Immunol. 1999;235:77-84.

Ebola virus outbreaks in the Ivory Coast and Liberia, 1994-1995.

Le Guenno B(1), Formenty P, Boesch C.

Author information: (1)WHO Collaborating Center for Arboviruses and Haemorrhagic Fevers, Institut Pasteur, Paris, France.

PMID: 9893379 [PubMed - indexed for MEDLINE]

2313. Curr Top Microbiol Immunol. 1999;235:35-47.

Processing of the Ebola virus glycoprotein.

Volchkov VE(1).

Author information: (1)Institut für Virologie, Philipps-Universität Marburg, Germany.

PMID: 9893377 [PubMed - indexed for MEDLINE]

2314. Med Trop (Mars). 1999;59(4):411.

[A case of Ebola virus hemorrhagic fever in Libreville (Gabon), fatal after evacuation to South Africa].

[Article in French]

Okome-Nkoumou M, Kombila M.

PMID: 10816757 [PubMed - indexed for MEDLINE]

2315. Mol Membr Biol. 1999 Jan-Mar;16(1):3-9.

Structural basis for membrane fusion by enveloped viruses.

Weissenhorn W(1), Dessen A, Calder LJ, Harrison SC, Skehel JJ, Wiley DC.

Author information: (1)Laboratory of Molecular Medicine, Children's Hospital, Boston, MA 02215, USA. weissen@embl-grenoble.fr

Enveloped viruses such as HIV-1, influenza virus, and Ebola virus express a surface glycoprotein that mediates both cell attachment and fusion of viral and cellular membranes. The membrane fusion process leads to the release of viral proteins and the RNA genome into the host cell, initiating an infectious cycle. This review focuses on the HIV-1 gp41 membrane fusion protein and discusses the structural similarities of viral membrane fusion proteins from diverse families such as Retroviridae (HIV-1), Orthomyxoviridae (influenza virus), and Filoviridae (Ebola virus). Their structural organization suggests that they have all evolved to use a similar strategy to promote fusion of viral and cellular membranes. This observation led to the proposal of a general model for viral membrane fusion, which will be discussed in detail.

PMID: 10332732 [PubMed - indexed for MEDLINE]

2316. Naturwissenschaften. 1999 Jan;86(1):8-17.

Characteristics of Filoviridae: Marburg and Ebola viruses.

Beer B(1), Kurth R, Bukreyev A.

Author information: (1)Paul-Ehrlich-Institute, Langen, Germany.

Filoviruses are enveloped, nonsegmented negative-stranded RNA viruses. The two species, Marburg and Ebola virus, are serologically, biochemically, and genetically distinct. Marburg virus was first isolated during an outbreak in Europe in 1967, and Ebola virus emerged in 1976 as the causative agent of two simultaneous outbreaks in southern Sudan and northern Zaire. Although the main route of infection is known to be person-to-person transmission by intimate contact, the natural reservoir for filoviruses still remains a mystery.

PMID: 10024977 [PubMed - indexed for MEDLINE]

2317. Prehosp Disaster Med. 1999 Jan-Mar;14(1):18-26.

KAMEDO--a Swedish Disaster Medicine Study organization.

Kulling PE(1), Lorin H.

Author information: (1)Emergency and Disaster Planning Division, Socialstyrelsen/The National Board of Health and Welfare, Stockholm, Sweden.

Kamedo is a Swedish Disaster Medicine study organization that sends observers to disaster areas anywhere in the world to study recent events, collect useful information, and identify problems relative to the practice of Disaster Medicine. The results of these investigations are published in the KAMEDO Reports, and the English versions will be published in Prehospital and Disaster Medicine. Three of the recent reports follow: 1) KAMEDO Report 69: Ebolus Virus Epidemic in Zaire, 1995; 2) KAMEDO Report 70: The German Rescue and Emergency Organizations: a) Industrial Chemical Fire, Memmingen, Germany 23 January 1997; b) Fire at the Düsseldorf Airport, 01 April 1996; and c) Bus Accident on the Autobahn in Rosenheim, Germany; and 3) Terrorist Attack with Sarin, 20 March 1995. In addition, a catalog listing all of the KAMEDO Reports available in English is provided.

PMID: 10537595 [PubMed - indexed for MEDLINE]

2318. Ryoikibetsu Shokogun Shirizu. 1999;(23 Pt 1):85-9.

[Ebola hemorrhagic fever and Marburg virus disease: their virological and clinical aspects].

[Article in Japanese]

Hirabayashi Y(1).

Author information: (1)Clinical Research Laboratory, International Medical Center of Japan.

PMID: 10088344 [PubMed - indexed for MEDLINE]

2319. Virology. 1998 Dec 5;252(1):179-88.

Ebola virus inhibits induction of genes by double-stranded RNA in endothelial cells.

Harcourt BH(1), Sanchez A, Offermann MK.

Author information: (1)Winship Cancer Center, Emory University, Atlanta, Georgia 30322, USA.

Fatal cases of filoviral infection are accompanied by a marked immunosuppression. Endothelial cells play a vital role in the host immune response through the expression of several immunomodulatory genes in addition to the expression of the antiviral genes, 2',5'-oligoadenylate synthetase [2'-5'(A)N], and the double-stranded RNA (dsRNA)-activated protein kinase (PKR). dsRNA, an intermediate generated during viral replication and gene transcription of many viruses, leads to the induction of immunomodulatory genes in endothelial cells. In this report, we show that induction of the major histocompatibility complex class I family of genes, 2'-5'(A)N, interleukin-6 (IL-6), PKR, interferon (IFN)-regulatory factor-1, and intercellular adhesion molecule-1 (ICAM-1) by dsRNA in human umbilical vein endothelial cells is suppressed by infection with the filovirus Ebola-Zaire (EZ). In contrast, induction of IL-6 and ICAM-1 by IL-1 is intact in EZ-infected cells. Gel shift analysis demonstrates that dsRNA-induced protein binding to IFN-responsive elements is strongly suppressed by EZ-IFN, whereas NF-kappa B activation by dsRNA remains intact. We previously reported that IFN signaling is suppressed by EZ infection, and these data strongly suggest that elements shared between IFN and dsRNA signaling are being inhibited by EZ. Inhibition of IFN and dsRNA responsiveness could play a role in the immunosuppression seen in EZ infections and would play a role in the pathogenesis of disease caused by EZ.

PMID: 9875327 [PubMed - indexed for MEDLINE]

2320. Braz J Infect Dis. 1998 Dec;2(6):265-268.

Epidemiology of the Ebola Virus: Facts and Hypotheses.

Portela Câmara F(1).

Author information: (1)Department of Virology, Institute of Microbiology Federal University of Rio de Janeiro.

Marburg and Ebola viruses are emerging pathogens recognized since 1967, and in 1976, when they were first identified. These viruses are the only members of the Filoviridae family. They cause severe, frequently fatal, hemorrhagic fever. Each genus includes some serotypes with the distinctive characteristics to cause high mortality rate during outbreaks. The Ebola-Zaire subtype is the most lethal variant. The epidemiology of human pathogenic filovirus is reviewed in this paper considering the most relevant facts. Primary human cases arise probably through close contact with infected primates. This point may be the key to preventing the introduction of these viruses in human populations. Once introduced in humans, the infection may spread through close contact with infected individuals or their body fluids, particularly in hospital environments. A main feature of filovirus outbreaks is the occurrence of cycles of secondary infection.

PMID: 11103018 [PubMed - as supplied by publisher]

2321. Russ J Immunol. 1998 Dec;3(3-4):263-265.

The Effect of Inactivated Ebola Virus on Immune and Hemopoietic Cell Activity.

Tuzova MN(1), Khaldoyanidi SK, Gaidul KV, Kozlov VA, Chepurnov AA.

Author information: (1)Institute of Clinical Immunology Russian Academy of Medical Scienses, Siberian Branch, Novosibirsk, Russia.

PMID: 12687104 [PubMed - as supplied by publisher]

2322. Clin Excell Nurse Pract. 1998 Nov;2(6):343-51.

Historical analysis of the Ebola virus: prospective implications for primary care nursing today.

Amundsen SB(1).

Author information: (1)Simmons College, Boston, Massachusetts, USA. MBUW62A@prodigy.com

Ebola continues to attract worldwide attention as a highly lethal virus of unknown origin that leaves victims bleeding to death and has no known vaccine or cure. The purpose of this historical research was to review and analyze the primary and secondary sources available on Ebola for use by primary care nurses in the event of future outbreaks. A rich resource of history has been well documented by some of the original physicians, virologists, and members of international teams, but nothing was found to be documented by nurses during these outbreaks. Multiple themes emerged including the origins of the viral strains of Ebola, transmission factors, epidemiology, virology, nonhuman and genetic research, treatment, and clinical implications. This research will provide primary care nurses with historical information about Ebola to help in future treatment options and algorithm development.

PMID: 12596837 [PubMed - indexed for MEDLINE]

2323. J Gen Virol. 1998 Nov;79 (Pt 11):2565-72.

Recombinant Ebola virus nucleoprotein and glycoprotein (Gabon 94 strain) provide new tools for the detection of human infections.

Prehaud C(1), Hellebrand E, Coudrier D, Volchkov VE, Volchkova VA, Feldmann H, Le Guenno B, Bouloy M.

Author information: (1)Unité des Arbovirus et virus des Fièvres Hémorragiques, Institut Pasteur, Paris, France.

After cloning and sequencing the glycoprotein (GP) gene of one of the Gabonese strains of Ebola virus isolated during the 1994-1996 outbreak, it was shown that the circulating virus was of the Zaire subtype. This was confirmed in this study by cloning and sequencing the nucleoprotein (NP) gene of this strain. These two structural proteins were also expressed as recombinant proteins and used in ELISA tests. NP was expressed as a His-tagged fusion protein in Escherichia coli and was purified on resins charged with nickel ions. GP was expressed by means of recombinant baculoviruses in Spodoptera frugiperda cells. Both recombinant proteins reacted positively in ELISAs for the detection of IgG antibodies in convalescent human sera from Gabon and Zaire. The difference in the relative titres of anti-NP and -GP antibodies was variable, depending on the sera. In addition, the recombinant NP reacted with heterologous sera from Côte d'Ivoire and was used successfully to detect IgM antibodies by mu-capture ELISA in sera from Gabonese patients.

PMID: 9820131 [PubMed - indexed for MEDLINE]

2324. Mol Cell. 1998 Nov;2(5):605-16.

Crystal structure of the Ebola virus membrane fusion subunit, GP2, from the envelope glycoprotein ectodomain.

Weissenhorn W(1), Carfí A, Lee KH, Skehel JJ, Wiley DC.

Author information: (1)Laboratory of Molecular Medicine, Howard Hughes Medical Institute, Children's Hospital, Boston, Massachusetts 02115, USA.

We have determined the structure of GP2 from the Ebola virus membrane fusion glycoprotein by X-ray crystallography. The molecule contains a central triple-stranded coiled coil followed by a disulfide-bonded loop homologous to an immunosuppressive sequence in retroviral glycoproteins, which reverses the chain direction and connects to an alpha helix packed antiparallel to the core helices. The structure suggests that fusion peptides near the N termini form disulfide-bonded loops at one end of the molecule and that the C-terminal membrane anchors are at the same end. In this conformation, GP2 could both bridge two membranes and facilitate their apposition to initiate membrane fusion. We also find a heptad irregularity like that in low-pH-induced influenza HA2 and a solvent ion trapped in a coiled coil like that in retroviral TMs.

PMID: 9844633 [PubMed - indexed for MEDLINE]

2325. Rinsho Byori. 1998 Nov;Suppl 108:105-10.

[Laboratory diagnosis of viral infections. 8. Viral hemorrhagic fever].

[Article in Japanese]

Morikawa S.

PMID: 9921238 [PubMed - indexed for MEDLINE]

2326. Todays Surg Nurse. 1998 Nov-Dec;20(6):3-6.

Biological warfare: what happens if we are attacked?

Ball K.

PMID: 9875006 [PubMed - indexed for MEDLINE]

2327. Trop Med Int Health. 1998 Nov;3(11):883-5.

Survey among survivors of the 1995 Ebola epidemic in Kikwit, Democratic Republic of Congo: their feelings and experiences.

De Roo A(1), Ado B, Rose B, Guimard Y, Fonck K, Colebunders R.

Author information: (1)Institute of Tropical Medicine, Antwerp, Belgium.

This study describes experiences of the survivors of the 1995 Ebola epidemic in Kikwit, Democratic Republic of Congo. Most of the survivors in our sample had cared for a sick family member before becoming ill themselves, and most had never heard of Ebola before they developed symptoms and therefore did not suspect that they were infected by the virus. Fear, denial and shame were their principal initial feelings. After release from hospital, survivors were abandoned by family or friends more often than they had expected. Belief in god was an important aid to all of them. Their most negative experiences were witnessing other people dying in the isolation ward of the Kikwit General Hospital, and the reluctance of hospital personnel to treat them. During Ebola outbreaks more attention should be given to the psychosocial implications of such an epidemic. Information campaigns should include antidiscrimination messages and more psychosocial support should be given to patients and their families.

PMID: 9855400 [PubMed - indexed for MEDLINE]

2328. Virology. 1998 Oct 25;250(2):408-14.

The nonstructural small glycoprotein sGP of Ebola virus is secreted as an antiparallel-orientated homodimer.

Volchkova VA(1), Feldmann H, Klenk HD, Volchkov VE.

Author information: (1)Institut für Virologie, Philipps-Universität, Robert-Koch-Strasse 17, Marburg, D-35037, Germany. volchkov@mailer.uni-marburg.de

The nonstructural small glycoprotein sGP, which unlike the transmembrane GP is synthesized from primary nonedited mRNA species, is secreted from infected cells as a disulfide-linked homodimer. Site-directed mutagenesis of all cysteine residues revealed that dimerization is due to an intermolecular disulfide linkage between cysteine residues at positions 53 and 306. Formic acid hydrolysis of sGP demonstrated that sGP dimers consist of monomers in antiparallel orientation. Another editing product of the GP gene of Ebola virus (ssGP), which shares 295 amino-terminal amino acid residues with sGP, is secreted from cells in a monomeric form due to the lack of the carboxyl-terminal part (present in sGP), including cysteine at position 306.

Copyright 1998 Academic Press.

PMID: 9792851 [PubMed - indexed for MEDLINE]

2329. Curr Opin Neurol. 1998 Oct;11(5):539-44.

Tropical myeloneuropathies revisited.

Román G(1).

Author information: (1)Department of Internal Medicine, University of Texas, San Antonio, USA. roman@uthsesa.edu

An interesting neurological syndrome, characterized by recurrent optic neuritis, cervical myelopathy from syringomyelia, paraparesis, amenorrhea-galactorrhea, and other endocrine problems, has been described among young black women in the French West Indies. The etiology remains unknown, but possible links with Devic's disease, acute disseminated encephalomyelitis, and neurotoxicity from quinolines in Annona muricata teas have been postulated. The largest epidemic of neuropathy in this century occurred in Cuba in 1991-1994. Clinical features and etiologic studies are reviewed. Its primary cause was nutritional. A similar epidemic was recently described in Tanzania. A number of infectious neuropathies and myopathies are reviewed, including leprosy, tuberculosis, hemorrhagic fevers (Ebola and Marburg filoviruses, Lassa, Argentinean and Bolivian arenaviruses), the human retrovirus human T-cell lymphotropic virus type I, Lyme disease and postimmunization neuropathies. The tropics continue to contribute interesting and important clinical conditions that may illuminate the etiopathiogenesis of other common disorders.

PMID: 9848004 [PubMed - indexed for MEDLINE]

2330. J Infect Dis. 1998 Sep;178(3):651-61.

A mouse model for evaluation of prophylaxis and therapy of Ebola hemorrhagic fever.

Bray M(1), Davis K, Geisbert T, Schmaljohn C, Huggins J.

Author information: (1)Division of Virology, US Army Medical Research Institute of Infectious Diseases, Fort Detrick, Frederick, Maryland 21702-5011, USA. bray@ncifcrf.gov

Erratum in J Infect Dis 1998 Nov;178(5):1553.

The Zaire subtype of Ebola virus (EBO-Z) is lethal for newborn mice, but adult mice are resistant to the virus, which prevents their use as an animal model of lethal Ebola infection. We serially passed EBO-Z virus in progressively older suckling mice, eventually obtaining a plaque-purified virus that was lethal for mature, immunocompetent BALB/c and C57BL/6 inbred and ICR (CD-1) outbred mice. Pathologic changes in the liver and spleen of infected mice resembled those in EBO-Z-infected primates. Virus titers in these tissues reached 10(9) pfu/g. The LD50 of mouse-adapted EBO-Z virus inoculated into the peritoneal cavity was approximately 1 virion. Mice were resistant to large doses of the same virus inoculated subcutaneously, intradermally, or intramuscularly. Mice injected peripherally with mouse-adapted or intraperitoneally with non-adapted EBO-Z virus resisted subsequent challenge with mouse-adapted virus.

PMID: 9728532 [PubMed - indexed for MEDLINE]

2331. J Urban Health. 1998 Sep;75(3):471-9.

Emerging and resurgent pathogens in New York City.

Hamburg M(1).

Author information: (1)Department of Health and Human Services, Washington, DC 20201, USA.

PMID: 9762644 [PubMed - indexed for MEDLINE]

2332. Acta Clin Belg. 1998 Aug;53(4):245-50.

Import infectious diseases in Belgium.

Van Gompel A, Van den Ende J.

PMID: 9795443 [PubMed - indexed for MEDLINE]

2333. Clin Infect Dis. 1998 Aug;27(2):404-6.

Marburg and Ebola hemorrhagic fevers: does the primary course of infection depend on the accessibility of organ-specific macrophages?

Schnittler HJ(1), Feldmann H.

Author information: (1)Institute of Physiology, Westfälische-Wilhelms-Universität, Münster, Germany.

PMID: 9709901 [PubMed - indexed for MEDLINE]

2334. J Virol. 1998 Aug;72(8):6442-7.

Biochemical analysis of the secreted and virion glycoproteins of Ebola virus.

Sanchez A(1), Yang ZY, Xu L, Nabel GJ, Crews T, Peters CJ.

Author information: (1)Special Pathogens Branch, Division of Viral and Rickettsial Diseases, National Center for Infectious Diseases, Centers for Disease Control and Prevention, Atlanta, Georgia 30333, USA. ansl@cdc.gov

The glycoproteins expressed by a Zaire species of Ebola virus were analyzed for cleavage, oligomerization, and other structural properties to better define their functions. The 50- to 70-kDa secreted and 150-kDa virion/structural glycoproteins (SGP and GP, respectively), which share the 295 N-terminal residues, are cleaved near the N terminus by signalase. A second cleavage event, occurring in GP at a multibasic site (RRTRR downward arrow) that is likely mediated by furin, results in two glycoproteins (GP1 and GP2) linked by disulfide bonding. This furin cleavage site is present in the same position in the GPs of all Ebola viruses (R[R/K]X[R/K]R downward arrow), and one is predicted for Marburg viruses (R[R/K]KR downward arrow), although in a different location. Based on the results of cross-linking studies, we were able to determine that Ebola virion peplomers are composed of trimers of GP1-GP2 heterodimers and that aspects of their structure are similar to those of retroviruses, paramyxoviruses, and influenza viruses. We also determined that SGP is secreted from infected cells almost exclusively in the form of a homodimer that is joined by disulfide bonding.

PMCID: PMC109803 PMID: 9658086 [PubMed - indexed for MEDLINE]

2335. Emerg Infect Dis. 1998 Jul-Sep;4(3):508-10.

Unrecognized Ebola hemorrhagic fever at Mosango Hospital during the 1995 epidemic in Kikwit, Democratic Republic of the Congo.

Bonnet MJ, Akamituna P, Mazaya A.

PMCID: PMC2640276 PMID: 9716990 [PubMed - indexed for MEDLINE]

2336. Euro Surveill. 1998 Jul;3(7):80.

Establishing a European network for the diagnosis of.

Niedrig M, Niklasson B, Lloyd G, Schmitz H, LeGuenno B.

The epidemics in recent years of Ebola haemorrhagic fever in Zaire and Gabon acted as a reminder that dangerous infections can be imported very quickly into Europe. Meetings on emerging and re-emerging pathogens organised by the World Health Organization

PMID: 12631763 [PubMed - as supplied by publisher]

2337. Rinsho Byori. 1998 Jul;46(7):651-5.

[Viral hemorrhagic fever--Ebola hemorrhagic fever, Marburg disease and Lassa fever].

[Article in Japanese]

Hotta H(1).

Author information: (1)Department of Microbiology, Kobe University School of Medicine.

Viral hemorrhagic fevers include Ebola hemorrhagic fever, Marburg disease and Lassa fever. The etiologic agents of the diseases, Ebola virus, Marburg virus and Lassa virus, respectively, are categorized as viruses with biosafety level 4, because of their high mortality, high transmissibility and the lack of effective vaccines and therapeutic measures. Ebola and Marburg viruses are members of the Filoviridae family and easily distinguishable from viruses of other families by the characteristic morphology of the virion. The natural reservoir(s) of Ebola and Marburg viruses remain unknown. On the other hand, Lassa virus is a member of the Arenaviridae family and its natural reservoir is a kind of rodent of the Mastomys species, which are asymptomtically infected with the virus and continue to excrete the virus throughout their lifetime. Ebola, Marburg and Lassa viruses exist almost exclusively in Africa, with a minor fraction of Ebola virus being present in southeast Asia and possibly other tropical areas. However, these viruses can be imported to any part of the world industrialized countries.

When attending patients with viral hemorrhagic fevers, "barrier nursing" using face shields (or goggles), masks, rubber gloves, etc., is recommended to avoid direct contact with blood and other body fluids of the patients.

PMID: 9721531 [PubMed - indexed for MEDLINE]

2338. Trans R Soc Trop Med Hyg. 1998 Jul-Aug;92(4):469.

Pathophysiology of Ebola haemorrhagic fever.

Clark IA, Awburn MM, Cowden WB.

Comment on Trans R Soc Trop Med Hyg. 1998 Jan-Feb;92(1):1-2.

PMID: 9850413 [PubMed - indexed for MEDLINE]

2339. Trends Microbiol. 1998 Jul;6(7):258-9.

Pathogenesis of Ebola virus infection: recent insights.

Takada A(1), Kawaoka Y.

Author information: (1)Dept of Disease Control, Graduate School of Veterinary Medicine, Hokkaido University, Sapporo, Japan.

PMID: 9717212 [PubMed - indexed for MEDLINE]

2340. Vopr Virusol. 1998 Jul-Aug;43(4):163-9.

[Dynamics of immunologic indicators in guinea pigs upon administering various preparations of the Ebola virus].

[Article in Russian]

Dadaeva AA, Sizikova LP, Zhukov VA, Chepurnov AA.

Immunological and hematological values are analyzed in guinea pigs infected with Ebola virus (EV) strain weakly pathogenic for these animals, inactivated EV, and EV strain adapted to guinea pigs and causing a lethal infection in them. The disease induced by lethal EV differed from that induced by other EV strains. Blastic wave in lymphoid organs in the absence of antibodies to EV detected by enzyme immunoassay, elimination of circulating immune complexes, and appearance of eosinophils in the blood of guinea pigs infected with lethal EV suggest the formation of aggressive immune complexes actively precipitating in tissues and contributing to the development of pathological process typical of Ebola infection.

PMID: 9791881 [PubMed - indexed for MEDLINE]

2341. Nurs Spectr (Wash D C). 1998 Jun 29;8(13):8, 24.

Biological warfare: would you recognize an attack?

Sabatini M.

PMID: 10562136 [PubMed - indexed for MEDLINE]

2342. Virology. 1998 Jun 20;246(1):134-44.

DNA vaccines expressing either the GP or NP genes of Ebola virus protect mice from lethal challenge.

Vanderzanden L(1), Bray M, Fuller D, Roberts T, Custer D, Spik K, Jahrling P, Huggins J, Schmaljohn A, Schmaljohn C.

Author information: (1)Virology Division, United States Army Medical Research Institute of Infectious Diseases, Ft. Detrick, Maryland 21702-5011, USA.

DNA vaccines expressing the envelope glycoprotein (GP) or nucleocapsid protein (NP) genes of Ebola virus were evaluated in adult, immunocompetent mice. The vaccines were delivered into the skin by particle bombardment of DNA-coated gold beads with the Powderject-XR gene gun. Both vaccines elicited antibody responses as measured by ELISA and elicited cytotoxic T cell responses as measured by chromium release assays. From one to four vaccinations with 0.5 microgram of the GP DNA vaccine resulted in a dose-dependent protection from Ebola virus challenge. Maximal protection (78% survival) was achieved after four vaccinations. Mice were completely protected with a priming dose of 0.5 microgram of GP DNA followed by three or four subsequent vaccinations with 1.5 micrograms of DNA. Partial protection could be observed for at least 9 months after three immunizations with 0.5 microgram of the GP DNA vaccine. Comparing the GP and NP vaccines indicated that approximately the same level of protection could be achieved with either vaccine.

PMID: 9657001 [PubMed - indexed for MEDLINE]

2343. Soc Sci Med. 1998 Jun;46(12):1637-53.

The refugee crisis in Africa and implications for health and disease: a political ecology approach.

Kalipeni E(1), Oppong J.

Author information: (1)Department of Geography, University of Illinois at Urbana-Champaign, Urbana 61801, USA.

Political violence in civil war and ethnic conflicts has generated millions of refugees across the African continent with unbelievable pictures of suffering and unnecessary death. Using a political ecology framework, this paper examines the geographies of exile and refugee movements and the associated implications for re-emerging and newly emerging infectious diseases in great detail. It examines how the political ecologic circumstances underlying the refugee crisis influences health services delivery and the problems of disease and health in refugee camps. It has four main themes, namely, an examination of the geography of the refugee crisis: the disruption of health services due to political ecologic forces that produce refugees; the breeding of disease in refugee camps due to the prevailing desperation and destitution; and the creation of an optimal environment for emergence and spread of disease due to the chaotic nature of war and violence that produces refugees. We argue in this paper that there is great potential of something more virulent than cholera and Ebola emerging and taking a big toll before being identified and controlled. We conclude by noting that once such a disease is out in the public rapid diffusion despite political boundaries is likely, a fact that has a direct bearing on global health. The extensive evidence presented in this paper of the overriding role of political factors in the refugee health problem calls for political reform and peace accords, engagement and empowerment of Pan-African organizations, foreign policy changes by Western governments and greater vigilance of non-governmental organizations (NGOs) in the allocation and distribution of relief aid.

PMID: 9672401 [PubMed - indexed for MEDLINE]

2344. Proc Natl Acad Sci U S A. 1998 May 26;95(11):6032-6.

The central structural feature of the membrane fusion protein subunit from the Ebola virus glycoprotein is a long triple-stranded coiled coil.

Weissenhorn W(1), Calder LJ, Wharton SA, Skehel JJ, Wiley DC.

Author information: (1)Laboratory of Molecular Medicine, Howard Hughes Medical Institute, The Children's Hospital, 320 Longwood Avenue Boston, MA 02215, USA.

The ectodomain of the Ebola virus Gp2 glycoprotein was solubilized with a trimeric, isoleucine zipper derived from GCN4 (pIIGCN4) in place of the hydrophobic fusion peptide at the N terminus. This chimeric molecule forms a trimeric, highly alpha-helical, and very thermostable molecule, as determined by chemical crosslinking and circular dichroism. Electron microscopy indicates that Gp2 folds into a rod-like structure like influenza HA2 and HIV-1 gp41, providing further evidence that viral fusion proteins from diverse families such as Orthomyxoviridae (Influenza), Retroviridae (HIV-1), and Filoviridae (Ebola) share common structural features, and suggesting a common membrane fusion mechanism.

PMCID: PMC27580 PMID: 9600912 [PubMed - indexed for MEDLINE]

2345. Virology. 1998 May 25;245(1):110-9.

Release of viral glycoproteins during Ebola virus infection.

Volchkov VE(1), Volchkova VA, Slenczka W, Klenk HD, Feldmann H.

Author information: (1)Institut für Virologie, Philipps-Universität Marburg, Germany. Volchkov@mailer.uni-marburg.de

Maturation and release of the Ebola virus glycoprotein GP were studied in cells infected with either Ebola or recombinant vaccinia viruses. Significant amounts of GP were found in the culture medium in nonvirion forms. The major form represented the large subunit GP1 that was shed after release of its disulfide linkage to the smaller transmembrane subunit GP2. The minor form were intact GP1,2 complexes incorporated into virosomes. Vector-expressed GP formed spikes morphologically indistinguishable from spikes on virus particles, indicating that spike assembly is independent of other viral proteins. Analysis of a truncation mutant revealed an early and almost complete release of GP1,2 molecules, showing that membrane anchoring is mediated by the carboxy-terminal hydrophobic domain of GP2. We have also compared wild-type virus which requires transcriptional editing for synthesis of full-length GP with a variant that does not depend on editing. Both viruses released comparable amounts of GP1, but the variant expressed only minute amounts of the small, soluble GP which is the expression product of nonedited mRNA species of the GP gene. The abundant shedding of soluble GP1 may play an important role in the immunopathology of Ebola hemorrhagic fever in experimentally and naturally infected hosts.

PMID: 9614872 [PubMed - indexed for MEDLINE]

2346. Proc Natl Acad Sci U S A. 1998 May 12;95(10):5762-7.

Processing of the Ebola virus glycoprotein by the proprotein convertase furin.

Volchkov VE(1), Feldmann H, Volchkova VA, Klenk HD.

Author information: (1)Institut für Virologie, Philipps-Universität Marburg, 35011 Marburg, Germany. volchkov@mailer.uni-marburg.de

In the present study, we have investigated processing and maturation of the envelope glycoprotein (GP) of Ebola virus. When GP expressed from vaccinia virus vectors was analyzed by pulse-chase experiments, the mature form and two different precursors were identified. First, the endoplasmic reticulum form preGPer, full-length GP with oligomannosidic N-glycans, was detected. preGPer (110 kDa) was replaced by the Golgi-specific form preGP (160 kDa), full-length GP containing mature carbohydrates. preGP was finally converted by proteolysis into mature GP1,2, which consisted of two disulfide-linked cleavage products, the amino-terminal 140-kDa fragment GP1, and the carboxyl-terminal 26-kDa fragment GP2. GP1,2 was also identified in Ebola virions. Studies employing site-directed mutagenesis revealed that GP was cleaved at a multibasic amino acid motif located at positions 497 to 501 of the ORF. Cleavage was blocked by a peptidyl chloromethylketone containing such a motif. GP is cleaved by the proprotein convertase furin. This was indicated by the observation that cleavage did not occur when GP was expressed in furin-defective LoVo cells but that it was restored in these cells by vector-expressed furin. The Reston subtype, which differs from all other Ebola viruses by its low human pathogenicity, has a reduced cleavability due to a mutation at the cleavage site. As a result of these observations, it should now be considered that proteolytic processing of GP may be an important determinant for the pathogenicity of Ebola virus.

PMCID: PMC20453 PMID: 9576958 [PubMed - indexed for MEDLINE]

2347. J Virol. 1998 Apr;72(4):3155-60.

Characterization of Ebola virus entry by using pseudotyped viruses: identification of receptor-deficient cell lines.

Wool-Lewis RJ(1), Bates P.

Author information: (1)Department of Microbiology, University of Pennsylvania School of Medicine, Philadelphia 19104-6076, USA.

Studies analyzing Ebola virus replication have been severely hampered by the extreme pathogenicity of this virus. To permit analysis of the host range and function of the Ebola virus glycoprotein (Ebo-GP), we have developed a system for pseudotyping these glycoproteins into murine leukemia virus (MLV). This pseudotyped virus, MLV(Ebola), can be readily concentrated to titers which exceed 5 x 10(6) infectious units/ml and is effectively neutralized by antibodies specific for Ebo-GP. Analysis of MLV(Ebola) infection revealed that the host range conferred by Ebo-GP is very broad, extending to cells of a variety of species. Notably, all lymphoid cell lines tested were completely resistant to infection; we speculate that this is due to the absence of a cellular receptor for Ebo-GP on B and T cells. The generation of high-titer MLV(Ebola) pseudotypes will be useful for the analysis of immune responses to Ebola virus infection, development of neutralizing antibodies, analysis of glycoprotein function, and isolation of the cellular receptor(s) for the Ebola virus.

PMCID: PMC109772 PMID: 9525641 [PubMed - indexed for MEDLINE]

2348. Lit Med. 1998 Spring;17(1):149-74.

Ebola goes pop: the filovirus from literature into film.

Semmler IA(1).

Author information: (1)State University of New York at Albany, USA.

PMID: 9604849 [PubMed - indexed for MEDLINE]

2349. Nat Med. 1998 Apr;4(4):388-9.

Two strings to the bow of Ebola virus.

Klenk HD, Volchkov VE, Feldmann H.

PMID: 9546777 [PubMed - indexed for MEDLINE]

2350. J Virol. 1998 Mar;72(3):1775-81.

Phosphatidylinositol-dependent membrane fusion induced by a putative fusogenic sequence of Ebola virus.

Ruiz-Argüello MB(1), Goñi FM, Pereira FB, Nieva JL.

Author information: (1)Grupo de Biomembranas (Unidad Asociada al CSIC), Departamento de Bioquímica, Universidad del País Vasco, Bilbao, Spain.

The membrane-interacting abilities of three sequences representing the putative fusogenic subdomain of the Ebola virus transmembrane protein have been investigated. In the presence of calcium, the sequence EBO(GE) (GAAIGLAWIPYFGPAAE) efficiently fused unilamellar vesicles composed of phosphatidylcholine, phosphatidylethanolamine, cholesterol, and phosphatidylinositol (molar ratio, 2:1:1:0.5), a mixture that roughly resembles the lipid composition of the hepatocyte plasma membrane. Analysis of the lipid dependence of the process demonstrated that the fusion activity of EBO(GE) was promoted by phosphatidylinositol but not by other acidic phospholipids. In comparison, EBO(EA) (EGAAIGLAWIPYFGPAA) and EBO(EE) (EGAAIGLAWIPYFGPAAE) sequences, which are similar to EBO(GE) except that they bear the negatively charged glutamate residue at the N terminus and at both the N and C termini, respectively, induced fusion to a lesser extent. As revealed by binding experiments, the glutamate residue at the N terminus severely impaired peptide-vesicle interaction. In addition, the fusion-competent EBO(GE) sequence did not associate significantly with vesicles lacking phosphatidylinositol. Tryptophan fluorescence quenching by vesicles containing brominated phospholipids indicated that the EBO(GE) peptide penetrated to the acyl chain level only when the membranes contained phosphatidylinositol. We conclude that binding and further penetration of the Ebola virus putative fusion peptide into membranes might be governed by the nature of the N-terminal residue and by the presence of phosphatidylinositol in the target membrane. Moreover, since insertion of such a peptide leads to membrane destabilization and fusion, the present data would be compatible with the involvement of this sequence in Ebola virus fusion.

PMCID: PMC109466 PMID: 9499027 [PubMed - indexed for MEDLINE]

2351. Ned Tijdschr Geneeskd. 1998 Feb 28;142(9):448-51.

[Viral hemorrhagic fever].

[Article in Dutch]

Kager PA(1).

Author information: (1)Academisch Medisch Centrum, afd. Inwendige Geneeskunde, Tropische Geneeskunde en Aids, Amsterdam.

Viral haemorrhagic fevers, such as Lassa fever and yellow fever, cause tens of thousands of deaths annually outside the Netherlands. The viruses are mostly transmitted by mosquitoes, ticks or via excreta of rodents. Important to travellers are yellow fever, dengue and Lassa and Ebola fever. For yellow fever there is an efficacious vaccine. Dengue is frequently observed in travellers; prevention consists in avoiding mosquito bites, the treatment is symptomatic. Lassa and Ebola fever are extremely rare among travellers; a management protocol can be obtained from the Netherlands Ministry of Health, Welfare and Sports. Diagnostics of a patient from the tropics with fever and haemorrhagic diathesis should be aimed at treatable disorders such as malaria, typhoid fever, rickettsiosis or bacterial sepsis, because the probability of such a disease is much higher than that of Lassa or Ebola fever.

PMID: 9562757 [PubMed - indexed for MEDLINE]

2352. Science. 1998 Feb 13;279(5353):983-4.

A method in Ebola's madness.

Wickelgren I.

Comment on Science. 1998 Feb 13;279(5353):1034-7.

PMID: 9490485 [PubMed - indexed for MEDLINE]

2353. Science. 1998 Feb 13;279(5353):1034-7.

Distinct cellular interactions of secreted and transmembrane Ebola virus glycoproteins.

Yang Z(1), Delgado R, Xu L, Todd RF, Nabel EG, Sanchez A, Nabel GJ.

Author information: (1)Howard Hughes Medical Institute and Department of Internal Medicine, University of Michigan, Ann Arbor, MI 48109, USA.

Comment in Science. 1998 Feb 13;279(5353):983-4. Science. 1998 Oct 30;282(5390):843.

The mechanisms by which Ebola virus evades detection and infects cells to cause hemorrhagic fever have not been defined, though its glycoprotein, synthesized in either a secreted or transmembrane form, is likely involved. Here the secreted glycoprotein was found to interact with neutrophils through CD16b, the neutrophil-specific form of the Fc gamma receptor III, whereas the transmembrane glycoprotein was found to interact with endothelial cells but not neutrophils. A murine retroviral vector pseudotyped with the transmembrane glycoprotein preferentially infected endothelial cells. Thus, the secreted glycoprotein inhibits early neutrophil activation, which likely affects the host response to infection, whereas binding of the transmembrane glycoprotein to endothelial cells may contribute to the hemorrhagic symptoms of this disease.

PMID: 9461435 [PubMed - indexed for MEDLINE]

2354. Virology. 1998 Jan 5;240(1):138-46.

Variation in the glycoprotein and VP35 genes of Marburg virus strains.

Sanchez A(1), Trappier SG, Ströher U, Nichol ST, Bowen MD, Feldmann H.

Author information: (1)Special Pathogens Branch, National Center for Infectious Diseases, Centers for Disease Control and Prevention, Atlanta, Georgia, USA. ans1@cdc.gov

Marburg virus, the prototype of the family Filoviridae, differs genetically, serologically, and morphologically from Ebola viruses. To better define the genetic variation within the species, VP35 and glycoprotein (GP) genes of representative human isolates from four known episodes of Marburg virus hemorrhagic fever were analyzed. The percentage nucleotide differences in the GP gene coding regions of Marburg viruses (0.1-21%) was nearly equal to the percentage amino acid changes (0-23%), while the percentage nucleotide differences in VP35 coding regions (0.3-20.9%) were higher than the percentage amino acid changes (0.9-6.1%), indicating a greater number of nonsynonymous changes occurring in the GP gene. The higher variation in the GP gene and the corresponding protein, especially those changes in the variable middle region of the GP, suggests that the variability may be the result of responses to natural host pressures. Analysis of the GP gene open reading frame shows a nonrandom distribution of nonsynonymous mutations that may indicate positive Darwinian selection is operating within the variable region. A heptad repeat region and an adjoining predicted fusion peptide are found in the C-terminal third of Marburg virus GPs, as has been previously shown for Ebola virus, and are similar to those found in transmembrane glycoproteins of retroviruses, paramyxoviruses, coronaviruses, and influenza viruses. Comparative analyses showed that there are two lineages within the Marburg virus species of filoviruses. The most recent isolate from Kenya (1987) represents a separate genetic lineage within the Marburg virus species (21-23% amino acid difference). However, this lineage likely does not represent a separate Marburg subtype, as the extent of divergence is less than that separating Ebola virus subtypes.

PMID: 9448698 [PubMed - indexed for MEDLINE]

2355. Emerg Infect Dis. 1998 Jan-Mar;4(1):134.

Ebola/Athens revisited.

Olson PE, Benenson AS, Genovese EN.

PMCID: PMC2627670 PMID: 9452412 [PubMed - indexed for MEDLINE]

2356. Med Trop (Mars). 1998;58(2):177-86.

[Ebola virus: what the practitioner needs to know].

[Article in French]

Georges AJ(1), Baize S, Leroy EM, Georges-Courbot MC.

Author information: (1)Unité de Biologie des Rétrovirus et Pathogènes Viraux Spéciaux, Centre International de Recherche Médicale de Franceville (CIRMF), Franceville, Gabon. ajgeorges@wanadoo.fr

The Ebola virus is an RNA virus of Filoviridae family. The earliest documented fatal epidemic of Ebola hemorrhagic occurred in 1976. There are four genetically different subtypes of Ebola virus. The virus remains in the blood for several weeks, can maintain its infectivity for several weeks at 20 degrees C outside the body, and survives for several weeks in corpses. Isolation of Ebola virus requires level 4 laboratory security conditions. Specimens are obtained by culturing mammal cells. Identification is achieved using reference serums. Serologic diagnosis is made using mainly ELISA technique for immunocapture of IgM or EBO Ag. The natural reservoir for Ebola virus is unknown. One possibility is that each isolated strain has a different reservoir. In recorded outbreaks, the index case has often had a history of contact with non-human primates. However since these animals are also highly sensitive to the virus, they cannot be considered as reservoirs but only as intermediate hosts. Transmission requires close contact such as occurs in association with health care, local customs, or funeral rites. In humans, infection causes hemorrhagic fever that progresses to diarrhea within 5 to 10 days. Recovery is observed in only 25% of cases. During outbreaks containment depends on implementation of simple precautions including isolation of suspected cases, appropriate protective clothing, disinfection with hypochlorite solutions, and proper waste disposal.

PMID: 9791600 [PubMed - indexed for MEDLINE]

2357. Nat Med. 1998 Jan;4(1):37-42.

Immunization for Ebola virus infection.

Xu L(1), Sanchez A, Yang Z, Zaki SR, Nabel EG, Nichol ST, Nabel GJ.

Author information: (1)Department of Biological Chemistry, University of Michigan Medical Center, Ann Arbor 48109-0650, USA.

Comment in Nat Med. 1998 Jan;4(1):16-7.

Infection by Ebola virus causes rapidly progressive, often fatal, symptoms of fever, hemorrhage and hypotension. Previous attempts to elicit protective immunity for this disease have not met with success. We report here that protection against the lethal effects of Ebola virus can be achieved in an animal model by immunizing with plasmids encoding viral proteins. We analyzed immune responses to the viral nucleoprotein (NP) and the secreted or transmembrane forms of the glycoprotein (sGP or GP) and their ability to protect against infection in a guinea pig infection model analogous to the human disease. Protection was achieved and correlated with antibody titer and antigen-specific T-cell responses to sGP or GP. Immunity to Ebola virus can therefore be developed through genetic vaccination and may facilitate efforts to limit the spread of this disease.

PMID: 9427604 [PubMed - indexed for MEDLINE]

2358. Nat Med. 1998 Jan;4(1):16-7.

Ebola takes a punch.

Folks T.

Comment on Nat Med. 1998 Jan;4(1):37-42.

PMID: 9427596 [PubMed - indexed for MEDLINE]

2359. Trans R Soc Trop Med Hyg. 1998 Jan-Feb;92(1):1-2.

Ebola haemorrhagic fever.

Rollin PE(1), Ksiazek TG.

Author information: (1)Division of Viral and Rickettsial Diseases, National Center for Infectious Diseases, Centers for Disease Control and Prevention, Atlanta, GA 30333, USA. pyr3@cdc.gov

Comment in Trans R Soc Trop Med Hyg. 1998 Jul-Aug;92(4):469.

PMID: 9692135 [PubMed - indexed for MEDLINE]

2360. Ultrastruct Pathol. 1998 Jan-Feb;22(1):3-17.

Marburg hemorrhagic fever: report of a case studied by immunohistochemistry and electron microscopy.

Geisbert TW(1), Jaax NK.

Author information: (1)Pathology Division, United States Medical Research Institute of Infectious Diseases, Fort Detrick, MD 21702-5011, USA. Tom_Geisbert@DETRICK.ARMY.MIL

The histologic and ultrastructural findings in a fatal human case of Marburg hemorrhagic fever are reported. Marburg virus was isolated from fluids and tissues and was identified in tissues by immunohistochemistry and electron and immunoelectron microscopy. The distribution of viral antigen by light level immunohistochemistry correlated with histologic lesions and also with the ultrastructural localization of virions. The tissue distribution and lesions of Marburg virus in this patient were consistent with the disease described in other human Marburg infections. Immunocytochemistry and ultrastructural examination revealed several previously unreported findings. A striking predilection for viral infection of the pancreatic islet cells was noted. In other tissues, macrophages were the primary cellular target for Marburg virus infection, with hepatocytes, adrenal cortical and medullary cells, and fibroblast-like cells also serving as important sites of viral replication. This case demonstrates the value of transmission electron microscopy as a tool for assisting in the definitive diagnosis of Marburg or Ebola hemorrhagic fever, as well as providing insight into the pathogenesis of these agents.

PMID: 9491211 [PubMed - indexed for MEDLINE]

2361. Vestn Ross Akad Med Nauk. 1998;(4):24-9.

[Developing methods of specific heterologic immunoglobulins preparation for urgent prevention of Ebola fever and study of their properties].

[Article in Russian]

Cherpunov AA, Kudoiarova-Zubavichene NM, Dedkova LM, Sergeev NN, Netesov SV.

Methods for preventing and treating Ebola virus hemorrhagic fever are not still available despite the fact that this virus have been studied for 20 years. Methods of immunization of the animals (sheep, goats) non-susceptible to Ebola virus with live virus preparations were developed to obtain the hyperimmune anti-Ebola virus sera required to have highly immune antivirus gamma-globulins. These methods made it possible to obtain the immune sera having high virus-neutralizing antibodies. Caprine immunoglobulins were obtained from sera by fractionation of immune sera by Kohn's method. The neutralization indices of the immunoglobulins obtained were at least Ig. When administered in the first hours of infection, the protective effect of these preparations was shown on guinea pigs infected with LD50 of the strain pathogenic to the animals. Preclinical trials of these immunoglobulins on laboratory animals and clinical trials on volunteers were performed. The preparation was used as a preventive agent when accidents took place at the laboratory working with Ebola virus. The similar preparation from equine sera having high neutralizing and protective properties was elaborated at the Virological Center, Microbiological Institute, Russian Ministry of Defense. Its prophylactic efficiency was also shown in infected gamadrias.

PMID: 9633237 [PubMed - indexed for MEDLINE]

2362. Vestn Ross Akad Med Nauk. 1998;(3):51-5.

[Microscopic study of species specific features of hemostatic impairment in Ebola virus infected monkeys].

[Article in Russian]

Riabchikova EI, Kolesnikova LV, Rassadkin IuN.

Pathological changes were studied in the blood vessels of baboons, green, rhesus, and cynomolgus monkeys at the end-stage Ebola (Zaire) infection. Marked microvascular lesions (capillary stasis, blood engorgement, thrombosis with blood cells, neutrophil accumulation, endothelial edema) were found in all the monkeys. These changes clearly indicate impaired organ blood supply. Multiple hemorrhages were formed by diapedesis without vascular wall destruction. Fibrin deposition and thrombi were features of hemostatic impairment in green and rhesus monkeys. Fibrin deposition and hemorrhages were not found in the cynomolgus monkeys. The possible mechanisms responsible for end-stage shock in Ebola virus-infection associated with microcirculatory disorders.

PMID: 9608279 [PubMed - indexed for MEDLINE]

2363. Proc Natl Acad Sci U S A. 1997 Dec 23;94(26):14764-9.

A system for functional analysis of Ebola virus glycoprotein.

Takada A(1), Robison C, Goto H, Sanchez A, Murti KG, Whitt MA, Kawaoka Y.

Author information: (1)Department of Virology and Molecular Biology, St. Jude Children's Research Hospital, 332 North Lauderdale, P.O. Box 318, Memphis, TN 38101, USA.

Ebola virus causes hemorrhagic fever in humans and nonhuman primates, resulting in mortality rates of up to 90%. Studies of this virus have been hampered by its extraordinary pathogenicity, which requires biosafety level 4 containment. To circumvent this problem, we developed a novel complementation system

for functional analysis of Ebola virus glycoproteins. It relies on a recombinant vesicular stomatitis virus (VSV) that contains the green fluorescent protein gene instead of the receptor-binding G protein gene (VSVDeltaG*). Herein we show that Ebola Reston virus glycoprotein (ResGP) is efficiently incorporated into VSV particles. This recombinant VSV with integrated ResGP (VSVDeltaG*-ResGP) infected primate cells more efficiently than any of the other mammalian or avian cells examined, in a manner consistent with the host range tropism of Ebola virus, whereas VSVDeltaG* complemented with VSV G protein (VSVDeltaG*-G) efficiently infected the majority of the cells tested. We also tested the utility of this system for investigating the cellular receptors for Ebola virus. Chemical modification of cells to alter their surface proteins markedly reduced their susceptibility to VSVDeltaG*-ResGP but not to VSVDeltaG*-G. These findings suggest that cell surface glycoproteins with N-linked oligosaccharide chains contribute to the entry of Ebola viruses, presumably acting as a specific receptor and/or cofactor for virus entry. Thus, our VSV system should be useful for investigating the functions of glycoproteins from highly pathogenic viruses or those incapable of being cultured in vitro.
PMCID: PMC25111 PMID: 9405687 [PubMed - indexed for MEDLINE]
2364. Dev Sante. 1997 Dec;(132):2.

[Infections always present at the dawn of the 21st century].

[Article in French]

Reinert P.

PIP: Despite the many scientific achievements realized in recent years, infectious diseases still remain the main cause of premature mortality worldwide. It is also growing increasingly difficult to fight infections. Tuberculosis and malaria are making a comeback, cholera and yellow fever are making new inroads into countries where they¿ve never been before, other diseases are developing resistance to antibiotics and have in some cases become incurable, and new diseases such as Ebola-induced hemorrhagic fever and Hantavirus pneumonia are being observed. These infections and resulting diseases are having major adverse impacts upon both human health and countries¿ economic development. However, hygienic measures can largely prevent the transmission of infectious agents leading to such diseases. Obstacles to prevention include widespread poverty and human misery, population growth, war-related population migrations, and economic crises in some countries, which render their healthcare systems ineffective. Regarding such problems, the World Health Organization¿s three priorities are to continue with efforts already in place to eradicate a number of diseases, to attack longstanding diseases like tuberculosis and malaria, and to engage in an international coalition against infectious diseases. PMID: 12322621 [PubMed - indexed for MEDLINE]
2365. Rev Med Virol. 1997 Dec;7(4):239-246.

Threat to Humans from Virus Infections of Non-human Primates.

Brown DW(1).

Author information: (1)Enteric and Respiratory Virus Laboratory Central Public Health Laboratory, 61 Colindale Avenue, London NW9 5HT, UK.
Several hundred distinct non human primate species are recognised, and they are likely to harbour a similar range of viruses to humans. Simians such as cynomolgus and rhesus macaques, African green monkeys, and marmosets are widely used for biomedical research, but despite this extensive close contact very few simian viruses have been shown to pose a threat of infection or illness to humans. Herpesvirus Simiae is the best recognised zoonotic hazard of simians. It is an alphaherpes virus of Asiatic macaques, which causes a mild or subclinical primary infection followed by latency in its natural host. It can be acquired by humans following a bite and causes an ascending meningoencephalitis. Less than 40 human cases have been described and the mortality rate in untreated human infections is 70%. The infection is treatable with acyclovir and extensive guidelines for managing simians and potential exposures have been developed. Ebola virus and Marburg virus have caused epizootics in cynomolgus macaques and vervet monkeys respectively, which have resulted in human infection and fatalities. However, non human primates are unlikely to be their natural host. More recently simian immunodeficiency virus and simian foamy virus have infected researchers, but infection has not been linked to illness. Simian viruses also pose a direct threat to humans through the use of primary monkey tissue cultures in laboratory work and vaccine manufacture, indeed a significant exposure of the human population occurred when cells contaminated with SV40 a polyomavirus of rhesus monkeys were used for polio vaccine production. New medical interventions such as xenotransplantation using primate organs pose a potential risk which requires careful assessment. Copyright 1997 by John Wiley & Sons Ltd.
PMID: 10398488 [PubMed - as supplied by publisher]
2366. Nihon Naika Gakkai Zasshi. 1997 Nov 10;86(11):2016-22.

[Emerging infectious diseases--Ebola hemorrhagic fever].

[Article in Japanese]

Kurata T.

PMID: 9480303 [PubMed - indexed for MEDLINE]
2367. J R Soc Med. 1997 Nov;90(11):622-4.

The enigmatic haemorrhagic fevers.

Suresh V(1).

Author information: (1)General Hospital, Tata Tea Limited, Munnar, India.
PMCID: PMC1296673 PMID: 9496275 [PubMed - indexed for MEDLINE]
2368. Clin Microbiol Rev. 1997 Oct;10(4):650-73.

A week in the life of a travel clinic.

Blair DC(1).

Author information: (1)Infectious Disease Division, State University of New York--Health Science Center, Syracuse 13210, USA. blaird@mailbox.hscsyr.edu

International travel has increased enormously in recent years. With the greater movement of people have come increased encounters with a wide variety of diseases: malaria, dengue, cholera, typhoid fever, Ebola virus, and many more. The need for greater scope, consistency, and knowledgeability in pretravel health care to meet these challenges has been met by the emergence of the discipline of travel medicine. Travelers are well advised to become informed of the risks they face and to take steps to minimize those risks. After reviewing a traveler's medical history and a detailed itinerary, a travel medicine practitioner can offer expert advice on behavioral modifications, immunizations, and chemoprophylaxis regimens which will increase the traveler's margin of safety. The issues most frequently addressed in a travel clinic include treatment of traveler's diarrhea, malaria chemoprophylaxis, and immunizations, for hepatitis A, typhoid fever, tetanus/diphtheria, influenza, pneumococcus, hepatitis B, polio, meningococcus, measles, mumps, rubella, varicella, and rabies. Pretravel consultation must consider the age and underlying health problems of the traveler, the nature of the trip (wilderness, jungle, rural, urban, resort, or cruise), the duration of travel, and the latest available information on the site in terms of disease outbreaks, terrorism, and natural calamities.
PMCID: PMC172939 PMID: 9336667 [PubMed - indexed for MEDLINE]
2369. J Infect Dis. 1997 Oct;176(4):1058-63.

International Colloquium on Ebola Virus Research: summary report.

Breman JG(1), van der Groen G, Peters CJ, Heymann DL.

Author information: (1)Fogarty International Center, National Institutes of Health, Bethesda, Maryland 20892, USA.

PMID: 9333167 [PubMed - indexed for MEDLINE]
2370. Lakartidningen. 1997 Oct 1;94(40):3489-91.

[Care of a patient with a rare and highly contagious virus disease. An emergency situation resulted in good preparedness].

[Article in Swedish]

Frydén A(1).

Author information: (1)Infektionskliniken, Universitetssjukhuset i Linköping.

Ever since the eradication of smallpox, Sweden has been poorly furnished with emergency facilities for the care of patients with serious, very infectious diseases. National interest in creating such facilities was aroused by epidemics of haemorrhagic disease (first and foremost due to Ebola virus during the present decade), at the same time as the first Scandinavian case of haemorrhagic fever associated with a risk of person-to-person infection occurred in Linköping. A special laboratory which has been set up at the Centre for Disease Control, in Stockholm, and University Hospital, Linköping, in collaboration with the Board of Health and Welfare, has introduced a high-security infectious disease unit for the care of such patients, with separate ventilation and waste-water treatment systems. The unit is also equipped to provide intensive care, and a laboratory can be rapidly set up and fully operative within 12-24 hours. Most important of all, personnel are available who are trained both for laboratory work and the care of such patients, and used to working as a team and familiar with the special protective equipment. If a patient can not be transported to the special unit, a team is available to travel to the hospital where the patient has been admitted, to give instruction and help to set up infection control routines and even supply protective equipment.
PMID: 9411086 [PubMed - indexed for MEDLINE]
2371. Afr Health. 1997 Sep;19(6):10-1.

Infection control in Africa. Nosocomial infection.

Pearse J.

PIP: This article discusses infection prevention and control in Africa and describes an available manual for infection control. The effectiveness of prevention and control efforts is dependent on health care services and the prevalence of disease. Funding for health care, the perceived economic impact of infection control, and trained administrators determine the availability of health services and the spread of disease. The challenge is to provide cleanliness, aseptic techniques in patient care, and protection for the health worker. If the hospital infection rate is as high as 15% of admissions and each case requires an additional 7 days of hospitalization, the estimated costs nationally could exceed US $110 million. Africa has a massive infectious disease burden, in addition to HIV and tuberculosis. The spread of Ebola fever shows how out-of-control infections can become. Most African countries are unequipped with infrastructure to handle surveillance of the new resistant bacterial strains resulting from indiscriminate use of antibiotics. In Zimbabwe, infection and prevention control was proved possible and cost effective. Education was provided at the village level in basic hygiene, home nursing, construction of fly-proof pit toilets, and a safe water supply. Training of trainers expanded the process of education. The "Infection Control Manual" provides the manager with the principles and background knowledge for prevention and control of infections. The Infection Control Association of Southern Africa is a useful source of information, standards, and support base. PMID: 12321236 [PubMed - indexed for MEDLINE]
2372. J Infect Dis. 1997 Sep;176(3):549-59.

Summary of antibody workshop: The Role of Humoral Immunity in the Treatment and Prevention of Emerging and Extant Infectious Diseases.

Krause RM(1), Dimmock NJ, Morens DM.

Author information: (1)Fogarty International Center, National Institutes of Health, Bethesda, Maryland 20892, USA.

In the era before antibiotics, human diseases were commonly treated with immune animal and human sera, often with life-saving results. With the advent of emerging infectious diseases, many of which cannot be adequately treated or prevented, attempts to develop antibody treatments have taken on new importance. The role of humoral immunity in treatment and prevention was the focus of discussion at a 1996 workshop. The cellular and molecular mechanisms of neutralization were examined in detail. It was noted that success in passive immunity has frequently been the key element in devising a successful strategy to develop a vaccine for active immunization. The workshop concluded on a cautious note of optimism that antibody-based treatment and prevention for diseases such as human immunodeficiency virus infection, Ebola fever, and others of clinical and public health importance deserve further development and clinical trial.

PMID: 9291299 [PubMed - indexed for MEDLINE]

2373. Vopr Virusol. 1997 Sep-Oct;42(5):226-9.

[Study of the treatment-prophylactic effect of immunomodulators in experimental infections, caused by Marburg, Ebola, and Venezuelan equine encephalitis viruses].

[Article in Russian]

Sergeev AN, Ryzhikov AB, Bulychev LE, Evtin NK, P'iankov OV, P'iankova OG, Slezkina EI, Kotliarov LA, Petrishchenko VA, Pliasunov IV.

Therapeutic and prophylactic effects of immunomodifiers ridostin, reaferon, and polyribonate used alone and in various combinations were assessed in experiments on guinea pigs infected with Venezuelan equine encephalomyelitis (VEE) (strain Trinidad), Marburg (strain Popp), and Ebola (M/C-8 variant of Zaire strain) viruses at doses 5 to 20 respiratory LD50 through the respiratory airways. Urgent prophylactic simultaneous intramuscular and intranasal administration of ridostin protected the animals infected with Marburg virus (p = 0.1) and prolonged their life span by 2.4 days (p = 0.15). In Ebola infection a combination of ridostin and reaferon appreciably prolonged the mean life span: by 2.9 days (p = 0.04). In VEE ridostin alone or in combination with reaferone appreciably increased the share of survivors; ridostin with reaferon and polyribonate notably prolonged the mean life span of infected animals. None of these drugs or combinations produced an appreciable therapeutic effect in any of the studied infections.

PMID: 9424849 [PubMed - indexed for MEDLINE]

2374. JAMA. 1997 Aug 6;278(5):438-9.

The agents of biological warfare.

Vogel P(1), Fritz DL, Kuehl K, Davis KJ, Geisbert T.

Author information: (1)Pathology Division, US Army Military Research Institute for Infectious Disease (USAMRIID), Fort Detrick, MD 21702-5011, USA.

PMID: 9244340 [PubMed - indexed for MEDLINE]

2375. Arch Pathol Lab Med. 1997 Aug;121(8):805-19.

Pathology of experimental Ebola virus infection in African green monkeys. Involvement of fibroblastic reticular cells.

Davis KJ(1), Anderson AO, Geisbert TW, Steele KE, Geisbert JB, Vogel P, Connolly BM, Huggins JW, Jahrling PB, Jaax NK.

Author information: (1)Pathology Division, USAMRIID, Ft Detrick, MD 21702-5011, USA.

BACKGROUND: Ebola virus has been responsible for explosive lethal outbreaks of hemorrhagic fever in both humans and nonhuman primates. Previous studies showed a predilection of Ebola virus for cells of the mononuclear phagocyte system and endothelial cells. OBJECTIVE: To examine the distribution of lesions and Ebola virus antigen in the tissues of six adult male African green monkeys (Cercopithecus aethiops) that died 6 to 7 days after intraperitoneal inoculation of Ebola-Zaire (Mayinga) virus. METHODS: Tissues were examined histologically, immunohistochemically, and ultrastructurally. RESULTS: A major novel finding of this study was that fibroblastic reticular cells were immunohistochemically and ultrastructurally identified as targets of Ebola virus infection. CONCLUSIONS: The role of Ebola virus-infected fibroblastic reticular cells in the pathogenesis of Ebola hemorrhagic fever warrants further investigation. This is especially important because of recent observations indicating that fibroblastic reticular cells, along with the reticular fibers they produce, maximize the efficiency of the immune response.

PMID: 9278608 [PubMed - indexed for MEDLINE]

2376. Arch Pathol Lab Med. 1997 Aug;121(8):776-84.

Emerging and reemerging infections. Progress and challenges in the subspecialty of infectious disease pathology.

Schwartz DA(1).

Author information: (1)Department of Pathology, Emory University School of Medicine, Atlanta, Ga, USA.

Emerging and reemerging infections are attracting greater attention from the public health and medical communities. Pathologists and other physicians are increasingly aware of the importance of the subspecialty of infectious disease pathology as a tool for diagnosis, surveillance, and research of emerging infections. In this communication, we describe the role that infectious disease pathologists have played during the last 2 years in broadening our understanding of selected emerging infections, including such examples as new variant Creutzfeldt-Jakob disease and bovine spongiform encephalopathy, leptospirosis, microsporidiosis, Ebola hemorrhagic fever, and cyclosporiasis. The significance of providing pathology services, especially the autopsy, to patients with potentially hazardous communicable diseases is discussed with the supposition that it is unethical to exclude or withhold health care from a patient based on his or her underlying disease or on risk factors for acquiring a disease. The increasing occurrence of infectious diseases imported into the United States and other nations, including human immunodeficiency virus-I group O, dengue fever, tuberculosis, malaria, diphtheria and cholera in immigrants and travelers, and Ebola virus in nonhuman primates, emphasizes the necessity for pathologists of having competence with infectious disease pathology. It is critical that new generations of pathologists not only be trained in the subspecialty of infectious disease pathology, but that they also be willing participants in the diagnosis and investigation of infectious diseases. The lack of training programs for infectious disease pathologists, as well as the deficiency in infectious disease pathology support for ongoing and future epidemiologic investigations and research, has led to the broadening of pathology services and initiation of a dedicated section of Infectious Disease Pathology at one of the nation's premier public health institutions, the Centers for Disease Control and Prevention in Atlanta, Ga. Together with preexisting groups of medical and veterinary infectious disease pathologists at universities, the Armed Forces Institute of Pathology, the US Army Medical Research Institute of Infectious Diseases, and the National Institutes of Health, this new program will significantly strengthen the capability of the United States to respond to future challenges of emerging and reemerging infections, both in this country and abroad.

PMID: 9278604 [PubMed - indexed for MEDLINE]
2377. FEMS Immunol Med Microbiol. 1997 Aug;18(4):281-9.

Ebola and hantaviruses.

Peters CJ(1).

Author information: (1)Division of Viral and Rickettsial Diseases, National Center for Infectious Diseases, Centers for Disease Control and Prevention, Atlanta, GA 30333, USA. cjp1@ciddvdl.em.cdc.gov
PMID: 9348164 [PubMed - indexed for MEDLINE]
2378. Mol Biol Evol. 1997 Aug;14(8):800-6.

The origin and evolution of Ebola and Marburg viruses.

Suzuki Y(1), Gojobori T.

Author information: (1)Center for Information Biology, National Institute of Genetics, Mishima, Japan.
Molecular evolutionary analyses for Ebola and Marburg viruses were conducted with the aim of elucidating evolutionary features of these viruses. In particular, the rate of nonsynonymous substitutions for the glycoprotein gene of Ebola virus was estimated to be, on the average, $3.6 \times 10(-5)$ per site per year. Marburg virus was also suggested to be evolving at a similar rate. Those rates were a hundred times slower than those of retroviruses and human influenza A virus, but were of the same order of magnitude as that of the hepatitis B virus. When these rates were applied to the degree of sequence divergence, the divergence time between Ebola and Marburg viruses was estimated to be more than several thousand years ago. Moreover, most of the nucleotide substitutions were transitions and synonymous for Marburg virus. This suggests that purifying selection has operated on Marburg virus during evolution.
PMID: 9254917 [PubMed - indexed for MEDLINE]
2379. Rinsho Byori. 1997 Aug;45(8):751-6.

[Viral haemorrhagic fever].

[Article in Japanese]
Masuda G(1).
Author information: (1)Department of Infectious Diseases, Tokyo Metropolitan Komagome Hospital.
Viral haemorrhagic fever denotes various kinds of febrile illness caused by certain viruses which often presents with bleeding tendency and occasionally shock. Out of these, the four maladies, Lassa fever, Ebola haemorrhagic fever, Marburg haemorrhagic fever and Crimean-Congo haemorrhagic fever which are endemically present in Africa or eastern Europe, are known to be such diseases with high man-to-man communicability. These four haemorrhagic fevers are, therefore, designated as special conditions requiring isolation during the period when the infected patients are shedding the viruses, not only in Japan but also in many other countries. We have so far only one such case of Lassa fever who returned to Japan from Sierra Leone in 1987. Some haemorrhagic fevers including dengue (haemorrhagic) fever and hantavirus infections (e.g. haemorrhagic fever with renal syndrome) are not known to be man-to-man transmissible and requiring no isolation. We have a number of dengue and dengue haemorrhagic fevers here in Japan today among imported febrile cases from tropical or subtropical countries. Every physician should take viral haemorrhagic fevers into consideration as one of the possibilities in diagnosing patients returning from overseas travel.
PMID: 9283226 [PubMed - indexed for MEDLINE]
2380. Bol Asoc Med P R. 1997 Jul-Sep;89(7-9):127-33.

The investigation of emerging and re-emerging viral diseases: a paradign.

Ríos Olivares E(1).

Author information: (1)Department of Microbiology and Immunology, Universidad Central del Caribe School of Medicine, Bayamón, Puerto Rico 00960-6032.
Emerging virus infections are defined as previously nonthreatening viruses that can decimate new populations by finding fresh hosts and vectors--often with the help of humans who introduce new species into virgen environment, Several etiologic agents of these diseases, some of the interacting factors that contribute to their development and the role of molecular medicine in their understanding is discussed.
PMID: 9419931 [PubMed - indexed for MEDLINE]
2381. Popul Bull. 1997 Jul;52(2):1-52.

Infectious diseases -- new and ancient threats to world health.

Olshansky SJ, Carnes B, Rogers RG, Smith L.
PIP: Infectious and parasitic diseases remain a leading cause of death and disability in developing countries and are re-emerging as a serious health problem in developed countries. Outbreaks of Ebola, dengue hemorrhagic fever, cholera, and bubonic plague have occurred in low-income countries and multidrug-resistant organisms have surfaced throughout the world. Since 1973, over 28 new disease-causing microbes have been identified. This issue of Population Bulletin analyzes the impact of factors such as population growth, urbanization, migration, poverty, travel, agricultural practices, climate changes, natural disasters, and medical technology on the resurgence of infectious and parasitic diseases as well as the influence of diseases such as AIDS on population dynamics and socioeconomic development. Most of these diseases could be prevented, cured, or eradicated with known public health measures. National governments can help reduce poverty, step up immunization programs, and lessen the chances of introducing new diseases. Nongovernmental organizations can disseminate preventive knowledge and monitor disease outbreaks. The medical profession can strengthen infection control precautions and institute surveillance of the use of antibiotics and other antimicrobial agents. Since the geographic isolation that used to contain disease outbreaks has been replaced by permeable international borders, the campaign against infectious and parasitic diseases must be global. PMID: 12292663 [PubMed - indexed for MEDLINE]

2382. Vopr Virusol. 1997 Jul-Aug;42(4):189-91.

[Methods for controlling colonization of air and laboratory surfaces by pathogens of certain especially dangerous viral infections].

[Article in Russian]

Chepurnov AA, P'iankov OV, Chepurnova TS, Makhova NV, Bakulina LF, Tiunnikov GI.

Regular check-ups of the laboratory environment (air and working surfaces) for contamination with the objects of investigations are obligatory for laboratories working with viruses causing grave diseases, such as Ebola, Marburg, and Machupo fevers and Venezuelan equine encephalomyelitis. Methods for indication and identification of these agents have been developed and experimentally tried.

PMID: 9304303 [PubMed - indexed for MEDLINE]

2383. Vopr Virusol. 1997 Jul-Aug;42(4):171-5.

[Change in biochemical and hemostatic indicators in guinea pigs upon administering Ebola virus preparations].

[Article in Russian]

Chepurnov AA, Dadaeva AA, Zhukov VA, Sizikov LP, Merzlikin NV.

The biochemical and hemostatic parameters were compared in guinea pigs after inoculation of Ebola virus strains lethal and nonlethal for them and of inactivated antigen of this virus. The time course of the main hemostatic and biochemical parameters in animals challenged with the lethal strain of Ebola virus differed much from that in other groups. This permits us to hypothesize that modification of the virus in the course of adaptation to the host results in the appearance of properties boosting the enzymatic processes and, hence, in depletion and failure of antioxidant and hemostatic defence, which aggravates the pathological process.

PMID: 9304298 [PubMed - indexed for MEDLINE]

2384. Virology. 1997 May 26;232(1):139-44.

Emergence of subtype Zaire Ebola virus in Gabon.

Volchkov V(1), Volchkova V, Eckel C, Klenk HD, Bouloy M, LeGuenno B, Feldmann H.

Author information: (1)Institut für Virologie, Philipps-Universität, Marburg, Germany.

Gabon has recently been struck three times by Ebola hemorrhagic fever. The first isolate originating from the 1994 outbreak has been subjected to molecular characterization of its GP and VP24 genes. Sequence analysis demonstrates that the agent, Gabon-94 virus, belongs to subtype Zaire of Ebola virus. The isolate is closely related to the Kikwit-95 isolate, and both viruses seem to have evolved from a progenitor virus different from that of the Zaire-76 isolates. The relatively close relationship of all subtype Zaire viruses isolated at different geographical locations and up to 20 years apart suggests an extreme conservation in the yet unknown natural reservoir of Ebola viruses. The level of genetic variability in the human host might be different as indicated by the comparison of isolates from a single outbreak (Mayinga-76 and Eckron-76), but needs further investigation on clinical material of patients by PCR since both isolates have different levels of passages in tissue culture.

PMID: 9185597 [PubMed - indexed for MEDLINE]

2385. Vopr Virusol. 1997 May-Jun;42(3):140-3.

[Changes in certain indicators of hemostasis in rabbits upon administration of Ebola virus preparations].

[Article in Russian]

Chepurnov AA, Dadaeva AA, Sizikova LP, Pisanko VA.

Changes in some parameters of hemostasis in rabbits insusceptible to Ebola virus (EV) in various periods after reinoculations with live and inactivated virus are described. Challenge with both control protein and live and inactivated EV leads to imbalance in the hemostasis system, which is compensated for in the course of follow-up and does not result in clinically manifest disorders of blood clotting. However, the mechanisms of development of the hemostasis imbalance caused by the control protein and virus preparations were different. In the former case no fibrinogen degradation products were detected in the blood serum, whereas in the latter they appeared in the serum after each reinoculation of the virus. This indicates a peculiar effect of EV on hemostasis.

PMID: 9297348 [PubMed - indexed for MEDLINE]

2386. Vopr Virusol. 1997 May-Jun;42(3):115-20.

[Immunobiological properties of vp24 protein of Ebola virus expressed by recombinant vaccinia virus].

[Article in Russian]

Chepurnov AA, Ternovoĭ VA, Dadaeva AA, Dmitriev IP, Sizikova LP, Volchkov VE, Kudoiarova NM, Rudzevich TN, Netesov SV.

Immunological and biochemical parameters were studied in guinea pigs immunized with recombinant vaccinia virus containing full-sized gene of Ebola virus vp24 protein and then infected with virulent strain of Ebola virus. The majority of the studied parameters changed similarly in guinea pigs immunized with recombinant vaccinia virus and control guinea pigs inoculated with vaccinia virus both before and after challenge with Ebola virus. However, in animals immunized with recombinant vaccinia virus producing vp24 some biochemical parameters, the mean life span after challenge with Ebola virus, the level of antibodies to the virus, and the phagocytic activity of neutrophils indicated the development of immunological processes other than in controls, namely, the development of immune response to vp24. Although these processes did not eventually lead to the survival of animals, they prolonged the mean life span and resulted in the production of anti-Ebola antibodies, though the level thereof was low. These data demonstrate that recombinant vaccines against Ebola fever are a promising trend of research.

PMID: 9297340 [PubMed - indexed for MEDLINE]

2387. Emerg Infect Dis. 1997 Apr-Jun;3(2):223-8.

Global aspects of emerging and potential zoonoses: a WHO perspective.

Meslin FX(1).

Author information: (1)Division of Emerging and Other Communicable Diseases--Surveillance and Control, World Health Organization, Geneva, Switzerland. Many new human pathogens that have emerged or reemerged worldwide originated from animals or from products of animal origin. Many animal species as well as categories of agents have been involved in the emergence of diseases. Wild (e.g., bats, rodents) as well as draught animals (e.g., horses) and food animals (e.g., poultry, cattle) were implicated in the epidemiologic cycles of these diseases. Many of the agents responsible for new infections and diseases in humans were viruses (e.g., hantaviruses, lyssaviruses, and morbilliviruses), but bacteria, especially enteritic bacteria (e.g., Salmonellae and Escherichia coli) and parasites (e.g., Cryptosporidium) of animal origin, were also involved in major food and waterborne outbreaks. The public health relevance of some of these agents (e.g., new lyssaviruses and morbilliviruses) is not yet fully assessed. In addition the zoonotic nature of some other human diseases, such as Ebola and the new variant form of Creutzfeldt-Jakob disease, is suspected but not yet demonstrated. Finally, the possible future use of xenografts may lead, if precautions are not taken, to the emergence of new diseases called xenozoonoses.

PMCID: PMC2627609 PMID: 9204308 [PubMed - indexed for MEDLINE]

2388. Ghana Off News Bull. 1997 Apr 1-30;2(7):3.

UN Sec-Gen on World Health Day.

[No authors listed]

PIP: In a speech on April 7, 1997, World Health Day, UN Secretary-General Kofi Annan stated that the globalization of trade, changes in ecology and climate, and mass movements of people are some factors which contribute to the spread of infectious diseases. As such, Mr. Annan called for international solidarity to combat such diseases. He believes that uncontrolled urbanization in many countries forces people to live in unhygienic and overcrowded conditions. In keeping with the day's theme of emerging infectious diseases, the Secretary-General noted that emerging and re-emerging infectious diseases have become a global public health concern during the 1990s. New diseases such as Ebola and HIV/AIDS have emerged, while old diseases once thought to be under control have re-emerged. Considerable progress has, however, been made in controlling some very deadly diseases through the global efforts of the World Health Organization, international organizations, and nongovernmental organizations. PMID: 12321711 [PubMed - indexed for MEDLINE]

2389. Zhonghua Liu Xing Bing Xue Za Zhi. 1997 Apr;18(2):102-5.

[Study of the reasons for spread of communicable diseases].

[Article in Chinese]

Wei CY.

PMID: 9812510 [PubMed - indexed for MEDLINE]

2390. Health Millions. 1997 Mar-Apr;23(2):19.

Emerging infectious disease: global response, global alert.

Nakajima H.

PIP: Despite spectacular progress in the eradication of infectious diseases, malaria and tuberculosis are making a comeback in many parts of the world. After years of decline, plague, diphtheria, dengue, meningococcal meningitis, yellow fever, and cholera have reappeared as public health threats. In the last 20 years [before 1997] more than 30 new and highly infectious diseases have been identified, including Ebola-type hemorrhagic fever, HIV/AIDs, and hepatitis C. Antibiotic resistance has also emerged during this period, and fewer new antibiotics are being produced because of high development costs and licensing. Drugs no longer offer protection or cure for many infectious diseases, and consequently more people need hospitalization with higher treatment costs. The causes of the appearance of new diseases and the resurgence of old ones include the rapid increase in international travel, the growth of mega-cities with high population densities, inadequate safe water and sanitation, food-borne diseases by the globalization of trade, and human penetration into remote animal and insect habitats. Meanwhile, resources for public health are being reduced, with the result that either the appearance of new diseases or resistance to drugs go unnoticed. A recent example is the human immunodeficiency virus, which went unrecognized until a large number of people got infected. For this very reason the 1997 World Health Day featured the theme of emerging infectious diseases and global response. Such forums are held to help countries rebuild the foundations of disease surveillance and control, while the public and private sectors may be encouraged to develop better techniques for surveillance to confront a common global threat. PMID: 12348002 [PubMed - indexed for MEDLINE]

2391. Lancet. 1997 Mar 1;349(9052):621.

Konzo and Ebola in Bandundu region of Zaire.

Banea M, Tylleskär T, Rosling H.

PMID: 9057741 [PubMed - indexed for MEDLINE]

2392. Sante. 1997 Mar-Apr;7(2):81-7.

[Virus transmission in the tropical environment, the socio-ecology of primates and the balance of ecosystems].

[Article in French]

Galat G(1), Galat-Luong A.

Author information: (1)Laboratoire de primatologie, ORSTOM, Dakar, Sénégal. We studied the contribution of non human primates to the transmission of yellow fever and HIV in the wild. We demonstrate the consequences of the modification of ecosystems on the emergence of new viral diseases and the reappearance of diseases believed to be eradicated. In the primary forest, the natural yellow fever cycle is limited to monkeys and mosquitoes living high in the canopy. Transmission to man is an anomaly, requiring the circumstances

found in the forest and savanna contact zones, where man has changed the forest to a mosaic and decimated the simian population, favoring contact between mosquitoes and man. In these contact zones, the amaril virus circulates in episodic cycles. During each episode, most of the local monkeys are infected, and thereby acquire immunity. Yellow fever can only reappear subsequently when a sufficiently large new generation of non-immune young monkeys is available. Monkeys do not become ill when infected, presumably as a result of typical host-parasite cross selection having led to the development of a balance between the parasite and its host. AIDS is a transmissible viral disease which appeared recently. Various African non-human primates are hosts to SIV, a retrovirus closely related to HIV which causes AIDS in man. SIV-infected African monkeys do not develop AIDS. However, when used to infect species from other continents (for example Asian macaco monkeys) SIV can cause AIDS. Does pathogenicity appear during transmission of the virus from one primate host to another, and is this the case for human AIDS? Experimental inoculations, the demonstration of SIVagm in other species, the mosaic structure of the genome (implying cross species recombinations), and the high probability of cross-species transmission of the viruses in the wild all favor this idea. Possibly counterbalancing the pessimism about the development of an HIVI vaccine in the near future, the non-human SIV models holds out some hope. The emergence of new diseases, such as Ebola, or diseases from other niches, and the reappearance of diseases believed to be eradicated, are frequent when man modifies the ecosystem, the structure and balance of which he does not control, and when he puts into contact species which have never met before.
PMID: 9273125 [PubMed - indexed for MEDLINE]

2393. Vopr Virusol. 1997 Mar-Apr;42(2):91-2.

[Effect of inactivated Ebola virus on colony forming activity of human hematopoietic stem cells].

[Article in Russian]

Chepurnov AA, Tiunnikov GI, Chernukhin IV.

The effect of Ebola virus antigen on the growth of hemopoietic precursors was studied. Incubation of mononuclear cells with the viral antigen led to a dose-dependent decrease of erythroid colony formation but did not alter the growth of the granulocyto-macrophagal precursors. Hence, Ebola virus antigen is capable of directly affecting the hemopoietic activity of precursors in man by inhibiting the growth of erythroid colonies.
PMID: 9182409 [PubMed - indexed for MEDLINE]

2394. Vopr Virusol. 1997 Mar-Apr;42(2):66-70.

[False-positive reactions in laboratory diagnosis of Lassa, Marburg, and Ebola viral hemorrhagic fevers and AIDS].

[Article in Russian]

Vladyko AS, Zaĭtseva VN, Trofimov NM, Shkolina TV, Scheslenok EP, Boshchenko IuA, Petkevich AS.

Sera of normal subjects and AIDS patients living in Minsk and Odessa were tested for antibodies to hazardous viral infections Lassa, Marburg, and Ebola. Four to 16% of examinees were seropositive to Ebola virus, 0.8 to 2.3% to Lassa, and up to 0.8% to Marburg virus. Common B-epitopes were found in viruses belonging to different families: Lassa, Ebola, and HIV. Antibodies specific to these viruses antigens were found in the reference sera to influenza A and B, respiratory syncytial virus, and adenovirus. Sera of convalescents after malaria and of AIDS patients contained antibodies to Lassa virus.
PMID: 9182402 [PubMed - indexed for MEDLINE]

2395. Vopr Virusol. 1997 Mar-Apr;42(2):56-9.

[Study of the phagocytic ability of blood polymorphonuclear leukocytes from rabbits and guinea pigs upon administering Ebola virus].

[Article in Russian]

Dadaveva AA, Sizikova LP, Bakulina LF, Chepurnov AA.

Study of the phagocytic activity of polymorphonuclear leukocytes (PMNL) of rabbits resistant to Ebola virus and guinea pigs susceptible to it, repeatedly challenged with live or inactivated Ebola virus in accordance with the immunization protocols, showed a much higher phagocytic activity in animals resistant to the virus than in those susceptible to it. Such behavior of PMNL in guinea pigs may be explained by the absence of the necessary cytokine background activating the neutrophils.
PMID: 9182399 [PubMed - indexed for MEDLINE]

2396. Biull Eksp Biol Med. 1997 Feb;123(2):205-8.

[Ultrastructural stereological analysis of monkey lungs during experimental Ebola fever].

[Article in Russian]

Kolesnikova LV, Riabchikova EI, Rassadkin IuN, Grazhdantseva AA.
PMID: 9280497 [PubMed - indexed for MEDLINE]

2397. Zhonghua Liu Xing Bing Xue Za Zhi. 1997 Feb;18(1):47-9.

[Surveillance and control of some emerging zoonoses].

[Article in Chinese]

Yu ES.
PMID: 9812483 [PubMed - indexed for MEDLINE]

2398. Lancet. 1997 Jan 18;349(9046):181-2.

Identification of the Ebola virus in Gabon in 1994.

Amblard J, Obiang P, Edzang S, Prehaud C, Bouloy M, Guenno BL.
PMID: 9111553 [PubMed - indexed for MEDLINE]

2399. Lancet. 1997 Jan 18;349(9046):181.

Isolation and partial molecular characterisation of a strain of Ebola virus during a recent epidemic of viral haemorrhagic fever in Gabon.

Georges-Courbot MC, Lu CY, Lansoud-Soukate J, Leroy E, Baize S.

PMID: 9111552 [PubMed - indexed for MEDLINE]

2400. Wkly Epidemiol Rec. 1997 Jan 3-10;72(1-2):7-8.

Ebola haemorrhagic fever. A summary of the outbreak in Gabon.

[Article in English, French]

[No authors listed]

PMID: 9002779 [PubMed - indexed for MEDLINE]

2401. Afr J Health Sci. 1997 Jan-Mar;4(1):1.

The Eighteenth African Health Sciences Congress: dissemination of research results for utilisation.

Koech DK(1).

Author information: (1)African Forum for Health Sciences.

The African Health Sciences Congress for 1997 will be held in Cape Town, South Africa, from 14 to 18 April. This congress has been an annual event where scientists from across the world meet to present research results and to discuss meaningful approaches to solving some of the world's pressing health problems. The congress which is under the aegis of the African Forum for Health Sciences (AFHES), focusses special attention on ways of finding solutions for problems that afflict the African. The AFHES aims to accentuate, through these meetings, practical approaches that can be used by African governments to tackle health-related matters in order to improve the socio-economic status of the people on the African continent. The common health-related matters that one would be expected to be covered at such a congress are the six major tropical diseases identified by the World Health Organisation (WHO), namely malaria, filariasis, schistosomiasis, leishmaniasis, trypanosomiasis and leprosy. But now, there are other health-related problems on the continent that must be dealt with in order to ensure quality of life. Among them are the new and re-emerging diseases like the haemorrhagic fevers (Ebola and Marbug) and yellowfever, the sexually-transmitted diseases including HIV/AIDS, acute respiratory infections and reproductive health. Then there are the less often mentioned health-related problems currently afflicting the African continent that are not given so much attention as the others. These include sanitation, famine and drought, and malnutrition which arise from political upheavals leading to refugees. The consequences of these socio-economic difficulties further exacerbate the prevalence of the existing tropical and other diseases. Scientists working in Africa should play leading roles in tackling the many health problems that afflict the peoples of Africa. They are well placed to collect direct information on these health issues and to provide practical and meaningful strategies for their solution. The WHO Africa Region has taken a meaningful step towards finding mechanisms of eliminating female mutilation in Africa, and this is highlighted in the Newsdesk pages of this issue of the Journal. This, it is hoped, will be achieved through the use of the African traditional foundation and wisdom. Similarly, the African traditional culture of health should provide the basis for utilising the wisdom of the traditional healers and traditional midwives for dealing with primary health care matters on the African continent. The Journal congratulates all the scientists working in Africa, be they Africans or non-Africans, and those outside Africa, who work tirelessly to solve problems that will pave the way for an acceptable quality of life for the world's peoples. It is earnestly hoped that the scientists in Cape Town during the 18th African Health Sciences Congress will deliberate, discuss and dedicate themselves to solving Africa's pressing health problems. The Journal also acknowledges with gratitude, the organisers of this congress, namely the South African Medical Research Council, the Kenya Medical Research Institute and the Epidemiological Society of Southern Africa (ESSA), which, under the auspices of the African Forum for Health Sciences, have made it possible to hold the Congress in cape Town this year.

PMID: 17583970 [PubMed]

2402. Arch Virol Suppl. 1997;13:191-9.

Haemorrhagic fevers and ecological perturbations.

Le Guenno B(1).

Author information: (1)WHO Collaborating Center for Arboviruses and Hemorrhagic Fever Viruses, Institut Pasteur, Paris, France.

Hemorrhagic fever is a clinical and imprecise definition for several different diseases. Their main common point is to be zoonoses. These diseases are due to several viruses which belong to different families. The Flaviviridae have been known for the longest time. They include the Amaril virus that causes yellow fever and is transported by mosquitoes. Viruses that have come to light more recently belong to three other families: Arenaviridae, Bunyaviridae, and Filoviridae. They are transmitted by rodents (hantaviruses and arenaviruses) or from unknown reservoirs (Ebola Marburg). The primary cause of most outbreaks of hemorrhagic fever viruses is ecological disruption resulting from human activities. The expansion of the world population perturbs ecosystems that were stable a few decades ago and facilitates contacts with animals carrying viruses pathogenic to humans. Another dangerous human activity is the development of hospitals with poor medical hygiene. Lassa, Crimean-Congo or Ebola outbreaks are mainly nosocomial. There are also natural environmental changes: the emergence of Sin Nombre in the U.S. resulted from heavier than usual rain and snow during spring 1993 in the Four Corners. Biological industries also present risks. In 1967, collection of organs from monkeys allowed the discovery in Marburg of a new family of viruses, the Filoviridae. Hemorrhagic fever viruses are cause for worry, and the avenues to reduce their toll are still limited.

PMID: 9413538 [PubMed - indexed for MEDLINE]

2403. Biol Trace Elem Res. 1997 Jan;56(1):93-106.

Computational genomic analysis of hemorrhagic fever viruses. Viral selenoproteins as a potential factor in pathogenesis.

Ramanathan CS(1), Taylor EW.

Author information: (1)Computational Center for Molecular Structure and Design, University of Georgia, Athens 30601-2352, USA. wtaylor@rx.uga.edu

A number of distinct viruses are known as hemorrhagic fever viruses based on a shared ability to induce hemorrhage by poorly understood mechanisms, typically involving the formation of blood clots ("disseminated intravascular coagulation"). It is well documented that selenium plays a significant role in the regulation of blood clotting via its effects on the thromboxane/prostacyclin ratio, and effects on the complement system. Selenium has an anticlotting effect, whereas selenium deficiency has a proclotting or thrombotic effect. It is also well documented that extreme dietary selenium deficiency, which is almost never seen in humans, has been associated with hemorrhagic effects in animals. Thus, the possibility that viral selenoprotein synthesis might contribute to hemorrhagic symptoms merits further consideration. Computational genomic analysis of certain hemorrhagic fever viruses reveals the presence of potential protein coding regions (PPCRs) containing large numbers of in-frame UGA codons, particularly in the -1 reading frame. In some cases, these clusterings of UGA codons are very unlikely to have arisen by chance, suggesting that these UGAs may have some function other than being a stop codon, such as encoding selenocysteine. For this to be possible, a downstream selenocysteine insertion element (SECIS) is required. Ebola Zaire, the most notorious hemorrhagic fever virus, has a PCR with 17 UGA codons, and several potential SECIS elements can be identified in the viral genome. One potential viral selenoprotein may contain up to 16 selenium atoms per molecule. Biosynthesis of this protein could impose an unprecedented selenium demand on the host, potentially, leading to severe lipid peroxidation and cell membrane destruction, and contributing to hemorrhagic symptoms. Alternatively, even in the absence of programmed selenoprotein synthesis, it is possible that random slippage errors would lead to increased encounters with UGA codons in overlapping reading frames, and thus potentially to nonspecific depletion of SeC in the host.
PMID: 9152513 [PubMed - indexed for MEDLINE]

2404. Emerg Infect Dis. 1997 Jan-Mar;3(1):59-62.

Isolation and phylogenetic characterization of Ebola viruses causing different outbreaks in Gabon.

Georges-Courbot MC(1), Sanchez A, Lu CY, Baize S, Leroy E, Lansout-Soukate J, Tévi-Bénissan C, Georges AJ, Trappier SG, Zaki SR, Swanepoel R, Leman PA, Rollin PE, Peters CJ, Nichol ST, Ksiazek TG.

Author information: (1)Centre International de Recherches Médicales, Franceville, Gabon.

Three outbreaks of Ebola hemorrhagic fever have recently occurred in Gabon. Virus has been isolated from clinical materials from all three outbreaks, and nucleotide sequence analysis of the glycoprotein gene of the isolates and virus present in clinical samples has been carried out. These data indicate that each of the three outbreaks should be considered an independent emergence of a different Ebola virus of the Zaire subtype. As in earlier Ebola virus outbreaks, no genetic variability was detected between virus samples taken during an individual outbreak.
PMCID: PMC2627600 PMID: 9126445 [PubMed - indexed for MEDLINE]

2405. Prehosp Disaster Med. 1997 Jan-Mar;12(1):30-5.

The role of EMS systems in public health emergencies.

McIntosh BA(1), Hinds P, Giordano LM.

Author information: (1)Department of Emergency Medicine, Maimonides Medical Center, Brooklyn, New York 11219, USA.

INTRODUCTION: Until now, the public health response to the threat of an epidemic has involved coordination of efforts between federal agencies, local health departments, and individual hospitals, with no defined role for prehospital emergency medical services (EMS) providers. METHODS: Representatives from the local health department, hospital consortium, and prehospital EMS providers developed an interim plan for dealing with an epidemic alert. The plan allowed for the prehospital use of appropriate isolation procedures, prophylaxis of personnel, and predesignation of receiving hospitals for patients suspected of having infection. Additionally, a dual notification system utilizing an EMS physician and a representative from the Office of Infectious Diseases from the hospital group was implemented to ensure that all potential cases were captured. Initially, the plan was employed only for those cases arising from the Centers for Disease Control and Prevention (CDC)/Public Health Service (PHS) quarantine unit at the airport, but its use later was expanded to include all potential cases within the 9-1-1 system. RESULTS: In the two test situations in which it was employed, the plan incorporating the prehospital EMS sector worked well and extended the surveillance net further into the community. During the Pneumonic Plague alert, EMS responded to the quarantine facilities at the airport five times and transported two patients to isolation facilities. Two additional patients were identified and transported to isolation facilities from calls within the 9-1-1 system. In all four isolated cases, Pneumonic Plague was ruled out. During the Ebola alert, no potential cases were identified. CONCLUSIONS: The incorporation of the prehospital sector into an already existing framework for public health emergencies (i.e., epidemics), enhances the reach of the public safety surveillance net and ensure that proper isolation is continued from identification of a possible case to arrive at a definitive treatment facility.
PMID: 10166372 [PubMed - indexed for MEDLINE]

2406. Vopr Virusol. 1997 Jan-Feb;42(1):31-4.

[Developing principles for emergency prevention and treatment of Ebola fever].

[Article in Russian]

Markin VA, Mikhaĭlov VV, Krasnianskiĭ VP, Borisevich IV, Firsova IV.

The authors validate the efficiency of pathogenetic approach to the development of urgent measures for the prevention and therapy of Ebola fever. The virus circulating in the body is to be blocked as soon as possible and the impaired functions and systems repaired. Therapy of Ebola fever should be based on the earliest possible and sufficiently prolonged administration of specific immunoglobulins in combination with pathogenetic drugs.
PMID: 9103042 [PubMed - indexed for MEDLINE]

2407. Ann Intern Med. 1996 Dec 1;125(11):917-28.

Occupationally acquired infections in health care workers. Part II.

Sepkowitz KA(1).

Author information: (1)Infectious Disease Service, Memorial Sloan-Kettering Cancer Center, New York, NY 10021, USA.

Erratum in Ann Intern Med 1997 Apr 1;126(7):588.

BACKGROUND: Health care workers are at occupational risk for a vast array of infections that cause substantial illness and occasional deaths. Despite this, few studies have examined the incidence, prevalence, or exposure-associated rates of infection or have considered infection-specific interventions recommended to maintain worker safety. OBJECTIVE: To characterize the type and frequency of infections, the recommended interventions, and the costs of protecting health care workers. Part II of this two-part review focuses on infections caused by bloodborne organisms, organisms spread through the oral-fecal route, and organisms spread through direct contact. It also reviews established interventions for controlling transmission. DATA SOURCES: A MEDLINE search and examination of infectious disease and infection control journals. DATA SELECTION: All English-language articles and meeting abstracts published from January 1983 to February 1996 related to occupationally acquired infections among health care workers were reviewed. Outbreak- and non-outbreak-associated incidence and prevalence rates were derived, as were costs to prevent, control, and treat infections in health care workers. DATA SYNTHESIS: Occupational transmission to health care workers was identified for numerous diseases, including infections caused by bloodborne organisms (human immunodeficiency virus, hepatitis B virus, hepatitis C virus, Ebola virus), organisms spread through the oral-fecal route (salmonella, hepatitis A virus), and organisms spread through direct contact (herpes simplex virus, Sarcoptes scabiei). Most outbreak-associated attack rates range from 15% to 40%. Occupational transmission is usually associated with violation of one or more of three basic principles of infection control: handwashing, vaccination of health care workers, and prompt placement of infectious patients into appropriate isolation. CONCLUSIONS: The risk for occupationally acquired infections is an unavoidable part of daily patient care. Occupationally acquired infections cause substantial illness and occasional death among health care workers. Further studies are needed to enhance compliance with established infection control approaches. As health care is being reformed, the risk for and costs of occupationally acquired infection must be considered.

PMID: 8967673 [PubMed - indexed for MEDLINE]

2408. Clin Immunol Immunopathol. 1996 Dec;81(3):303-6.

A novel hypothesis to explain the hemorrhagic and connective tissue manifestations of Ebola virus infection.

Tilson MD(1), Ozsvath KJ, Hirose H, Xia S, Lahita R.

Author information: (1)St. Luke's/Roosevelt Hospital Center, Columbia University, New York 10027, USA.

The hemorrhagic and connective tissue complications of infection with Ebola virus are poorly understood. While searching for homologies and motifs of the aortic aneurysm-associated autoantigenic protein 40 kDa (AAAP-40), we have noted some short sequences (possibly shared epitopes) that occur in the envelope glycoprotein (40 kDa) of the Ebola virus. As a first step toward determining whether molecular mimicry of human matrix proteins by the Ebola virus protein might explain some of the severe connective tissue manifestations of infection, we have tested whether immunoglobulin (IgG) purified from the sera of patients with abdominal aortic aneurysm (AAA) are immunoreactive with the 40-kDa protein of the Ebola virus. Immunoblots of soluble Ebola proteins (strain Mayinga/Zaire) were probed with IgG's purified from the sera of eight patients with AAA and two healthy young control volunteers. The proteins were also probed with IgG extracted from the walls of two surgical aneurysm specimens. Serum IgG from eight consecutively studied AAA patients was immunoreactive with an Ebola virus protein of 40 kDa, consistent with the envelope glycoprotein. IgG's extracted from the walls of two AAAs were also reactive. The control sera were not reactive. In addition to the Ebola sequences in AAAP-40, an Ebola sequence also occurs in the microfibril-associated glycoprotein-4 (MAGP-4), which is distributed ubiquitously throughout connective tissue with elastin. We hypothesize that the catastrophic hemorrhagic and connective tissue complications of Ebola virus infection may be the result of these shared epitopes.

PMID: 8938109 [PubMed - indexed for MEDLINE]

2409. Infect Dis Clin North Am. 1996 Dec;10(4):917-37.

Perspectives in fatal epidemics.

Butler JC(1), Kilmarx PH, Jernigan DB, Ostroff SM.

Author information: (1)National Center for Infectious Diseases, Centers for Disease Control and Prevention, Atlanta, Georgia, USA.

This article discusses four epidemics of fatal infectious diseases: a 1993 cluster of deaths among previously healthy persons in the southwestern United States that led to the identification of a new clinical syndrome, hantavirus pulmonary syndrome; the first epidemic of Ebola hemorrhagic fever identified in nearly two decades occurring in 1995 in Zaire, which resulted in 317 cases with a mortality rate of 77%; an outbreak of Legionnaires' disease among cruise ship passengers in 1994; and a 1989 cluster of illnesses among nonhuman primates in Reston, Virginia leading to the identification of a new strain of Ebola virus. In each outbreak, the public health emergency was recognized and reported by alert clinicians, and the control of disease was facilitated through rapid, coordinated responses involving multiple agencies. Such collaboration between clinical and public health entities and among various agencies will be increasingly needed as surveillance and diagnostic capabilities for emerging and reemerging infectious diseases are enhanced around the world.

PMID: 8958175 [PubMed - indexed for MEDLINE]

2410. Sci Am. 1996 Dec;275(6):60-5.

The specter of biological weapons.

Cole LA.

PMID: 8923762 [PubMed - indexed for MEDLINE]

2411. BMJ. 1996 Nov 30;313(7069):1351.

Fears over Ebola spread as nurse dies.

Sidley P.

PMID: 8956694 [PubMed - indexed for MEDLINE]

2412. Lancet. 1996 Nov 23;348(9039):1427-30.

In the heart of darkness: sleeping sickness in Zaire.

Ekwanzala M(1), Pépin J, Khonde N, Molisho S, Bruneel H, De Wals P.

Author information: (1)Bureau Central de la Trypanosomiase, Kinshasa, Zaire.

Comment in Lancet. 1997 Feb 8;349(9049):438.

PIP: Human African trypanosomiasis (HAT) control programs existed during the colonial era in the Belgian Congo. HAT cases peaked in 1930 at 33,562. They declined gradually to about 1000 cases in 1959. The civil war that erupted after Zaire's independence in 1960 crippled the public health system. During 1960-1967, no active case finding was conducted and notification of HAT cases fell greatly. Mismanagement and corruption maintained a severe social and economic crisis after the civil war. At the end of the 1980s, the number of new HAT cases began to increase from the relatively stable numbers of 4000-6000 during 1969-1981 to almost 10,000. Socioeconomic conditions deteriorated quickly in the 1990s. The withdrawal of foreign aid in 1991 devastated many governmental health facilities that had been dependent on these funds. In much of Zaire, Catholic and Protestant missions were the only health care providers. The breakdown of the health system contributed to epidemics of Ebola fever, dysentery, the plague, and cholera. The specialized mobile teams providing trypanocidal drugs to HAT patients could no longer operate, resulting in drug shortages and thousands of deaths. The teams were somewhat remobilized during 1993-1994, when some foreign aid was again available. A return to neglected areas in 1994 found the HAT prevalence to be 15.4/1000 in the Equator region. In Kimbanzi, Bandundu region, it was 718/1000 among 241 persons examined. Had the teams not arrived when they did, the entire village of Kimbanzi could have disappeared within 1-2 years. The high prevalence rates in neglected areas were the highest rates recorded this century. The neglect brought about an increase in the number of infectious people, an increase in transmission, and a higher cost and toxicity of treatment due to an increase in late-stage HAT cases. The estimated true total incidence of HAT in Zaire in 1994 was about 34,400 new cases. The number of HAT deaths in 1994 was probably at least 80 times higher than that of Ebola deaths in 1995. Proper HAT control methods need to be fully funded and implemented to control this curable disease. PMID: 8937285 [PubMed - indexed for MEDLINE]

2413. Ann Intern Med. 1996 Nov 15;125(10):844-51.

Are all diseases infectious?

Lorber B(1).

Author information: (1)Section of Infectious Diseases, Temple University Hospital, Philadelphia, PA 19140, USA.

The complex interactions between microorganisms and human hosts include the well-known, traditional infectious diseases and the symbiotic relation we have with our normal flora. The media have brought to the public's attention many newly described infectious diseases, such as Ebola virus hemorrhagic fever, that were not part of common medical parlance a decade ago. While flooding us with interesting and often dramatic reports of so-called emerging infectious diseases, the media have largely ignored a more fundamental change in our appreciation of human-microorganism interactions: the discovery that transmissible agents may play important roles in diseases not suspected of being infectious in origin. A well-known example is ulcer disease; other examples include neurodegenerative disease, inflammatory disease, and cancer. These fascinating instances of host-pathogen interaction open new prospects for the prevention of disease through immunization.

PMID: 8928993 [PubMed - indexed for MEDLINE]

2414. Nurs Times. 1996 Nov 6-12;92(45):20-1.

Bug busters.

Cole A.

PMID: 9000967 [PubMed - indexed for MEDLINE]

2415. Afr J Health Sci. 1996 Nov;3(4):141-8.

Hemorrhagic fevers: few clues after 25 years.

Petit PL(1), Johnson BK, Hermans J, Tukei PM.

Author information: (1)Department of Microbiology, Schieland Hospital, Burg. Knappertlaan 25, 3116 BA Schiedam, The Netherlands.

There is a high prevalence of Ebola antibodies found in the Kenya population, related to geographical area and season, although the clinical disease was never found and the virus was not isolated. A field study was carried out in 7 hospitals in western Kenya, 1986 -1987 (including surveillance studies in suspect areas), to intensify collection and transport of samples, testing facilities, patient observation with record keeping and follow-up. This study involved 1109 admitted patients with fever and/or bleeding, 155 contacts of haemorrahagic fever antibody (Hfab) patients, and 916 people in suspect areas. Respectively 160,44 and 80 persons were found Hfab positive mainly to Ebola, using an indirect immunofluorescent assay. From 676 viral cultures no virus was isolated. A relationship between antibody titres and ecological factors, social habitat, age, sex or season was not found. The non-specificity of IF testing was demonstrated by: 1) the disagreement between the results of two reference laboratories; 2) the unpredictability of the titre conversation course; and 3) by proving a significant cross-reactivity with Borrelia burgdorferii antibodies, Plasmodium falcparum antibodies and Salmonella typhi antibodies. Renewed testing in 1995 of 90 positive sera (with low titres) showed 19 sera to be positive by Elisa (2 in Zaire, 1 in Sudan, 9 in Reston and 7 in Cote d'Ivoire) from which 4 were confirmed by IFI 2 in Reston and 2 in Cote d'Ivoire. These findings are more proof that non-human virulent strains of Filoviridae, especially Ebola virus, are around in Kenya.

PMID: 17451318 [PubMed]

2416. Glob Issues. 1996 Nov;1(17):6-9.

Here to stay. An interview with Dr. David Satcher, Director, U.S. Centers for Disease Control and Prevention.

Stilkind J.

PIP: This paper presents an interview with Dr. David Satcher of the US Centers for Disease Control and Prevention (CDC) on the issue of infectious and chronic diseases. The problem of new and reemerging infectious diseases around the world, particularly in developing countries, is discussed. While drug resistant malaria and sporadic outbreaks of Ebola in Africa have alarmed health programs, AIDS is the major emerging infectious disease throughout the world. Microorganisms have a way of surviving: they mutate, they adapt, and they emerge. The CDC¿s major partner in the global response to emerging infections is WHO. The CDC has learned lessons from its experience with AIDS and Ebola virus events. A system of domestic surveillance and global prevention should be developed. Poverty, hunger and malnutrition may contribute to the rise of chronic diseases in developing countries. The introduction of richer diets higher in cholesterol in combination with a sedentary lifestyle also will also lead to more chronic diseases among people in developing countries. In the future, smoking will have a greater impact on mortality than will any other factor in these countries. Infectious diseases are much less predictable. Drug resistant microorganisms and urbanization counterbalance the development of vaccines. The U.S. health care system wrongly prioritizes tertiary care while spending only 1% of its health budget on the prevention of diseases. Dr. Satcher would like to see the implementation of programs dealing with human behavior, sanitation, immunization and health education as preventive measures. PMID: 12349258 [PubMed - indexed for MEDLINE]

2417. Glob Issues. 1996 Nov;1(17):31-4.

The threat of emerging infections.

[No authors listed]

PIP: A variety of newly discovered pathogens and new forms of older infectious agents threaten to reemerge. Typical symptoms of acute infection are fever, headache, malaise, vomiting, and diarrhea. Some of the better-known emerging viral infections include dengue, filoviruses (Ebola, Marburg), hantaviruses, hepatitis B, hepatitis C, HIV, influenza, lassa fever, measles, rift valley fever, rotavirus, and yellow fever. Emerging bacterial infections include cholera, Escherichia coli O157:H7, legionnaires disease (Legionella), lyme disease, streptococcus infections (group A), tuberculosis, and typhoid. Emerging parasitic infections include cryptosporidium and other waterborne pathogens and malaria. The causes of many diseases are still shrouded in mystery; thus, treatments and cures for them are as yet unknown. PMID: 12349257 [PubMed - indexed for MEDLINE]

2418. Glob Issues. 1996 Nov;1(17):20-6.

The return of infectious disease.

Garrett L.

PIP: This article presents the history of efforts to control the spread of infectious disease from the post-antibiotic era to 1995. Since World War II, public health strategy has focused on the eradication of microbes using powerful medical weaponry. The goal was to push humanity through a ¿health transition,¿ leaving the age of infectious disease permanently behind. But recent developments have shown that this grandiose optimism was premature. As people move across international borders, unwanted microbial hitch-hikers tag along, as happened in the case of Ebola. In large cities, sex industries arise and multiple-partner sex becomes more common, prompting rapid increases in sexually transmitted disease. Moreover, the practice of sharing syringes is a ready vehicle for the transmission of microbes while unhygienic health facilities become centers for the dissemination of disease rather than its control. Black market access to antimicrobials has led to overuse or outright misuse of the drugs and the emergence of resistant bacteria and parasites. Consequently, old organisms, aided by mankind's misuse of disinfectants and drugs, may take on new and more lethal forms. Even when allegations of biological warfare are not flying, it is often difficult to obtain accurate information about outbreaks of disease, particularly in countries dependent on foreign investment or tourism or both. Unfortunately, only 6 laboratories in the world meet security and safety standards that would make them suitable sites for research on the world's deadliest microbes. National security warrants bolder steps involving focusing not only on microbes directly dangerous to humans, but also on those that could pose major threats to crops or livestock. Unfortunately, economic crises have led to budget cuts, particularly in health care, at all levels of government in the US. PMID: 12349255 [PubMed - indexed for MEDLINE]

2419. Glob Issues. 1996 Nov;1(17):10-3.

New drugs, new vaccines, new diseases. An interview with Dr. Anthony Fauci, Director of the National Institute of Allergy and Infectious Diseases (NIAID).

Fuller J.

PIP: This document presents an interview with Dr. Anthony Fauci on the development of a new generation of vaccines to prevent and possibly eradicate a legion of deadly diseases ranging from tuberculosis to AIDS. Infections that have caused major devastations in the world today include tuberculosis, malaria, schistosomiasis, filariasis, pneumococcal pneumonia, influenza, AIDS, and Ebola. Agencies should be making sure that the basic research base in microbiology, immunology, antimicrobials, and vaccinology is at the very highest level. The integration of research efforts between countries depends on collaboration between the investigators of home countries with foreign investigators. Among new developments in vaccinology are an acellular pertussis vaccine for pertussis/whooping cough (an extremely contagious disease that causes death), DNA immunization (a new technique applicable to all types of diseases), and transgenic plants for immunization against hepatitis, pertussis, and polio. As of now, AIDS in Western countries has declined, while in Africa and Asia its spread has accelerated. Combination therapy for AIDS has had a profound impact on the level of the virus in the body; however, the treatment is still vague. The good news with regard to AIDS is that education is having an impact; this is exemplified by the situation in Thailand, where the government together with nongovernmental organizations and the military has begun a crash education campaign regarding prostitutes and the use of condoms. Progress is being made in the search for better vaccine candidates. AIDS-like epidemics involving new diseases are bound to emerge at some future point, though, given the long-term historical trend. PMID: 12349252 [PubMed - indexed for MEDLINE]

2420. Wkly Epidemiol Rec. 1996 Oct 18;71(42):320.

Ebola haemorrhagic fever.

[Article in English, French]

[No authors listed]

PMID: 8937257 [PubMed - indexed for MEDLINE]

2421. Proc Natl Acad Sci U S A. 1996 Oct 15;93(21):11354-8.

Negative-strand RNA viruses: genetic engineering and applications.

Palese P(1), Zheng H, Engelhardt OG, Pleschka S, García-Sastre A.

Author information: (1)Department of Microbiology, Mount Sinai School of Medicine, New York, NY 10029, USA. ppalese@smtplink.mssm.edu

The negative-strand RNA viruses are a broad group of animal viruses that comprise several important human pathogens, including influenza, measles, mumps, rabies, respiratory syncytial, Ebola, and hantaviruses. The development of new strategies to genetically manipulate the genomes of negative-strand RNA viruses has provided us with new tools to study the structure-function relationships of the viral components and their contributions to the pathogenicity of these viruses. It is also now possible to envision rational approaches--based on genetic engineering techniques--to design live attenuated vaccines against some of these viral agents. In addition, the use of different negative-strand RNA viruses as vectors to efficiently express foreign polypeptides has also become feasible, and these novel vectors have potential applications in disease prevention as well as in gene therapy.

PMCID: PMC38061 PMID: 8876139 [PubMed - indexed for MEDLINE]

2422. Emerg Infect Dis. 1996 Oct-Dec;2(4):321-5.

Experimental inoculation of plants and animals with Ebola virus.

Swanepoel R(1), Leman PA, Burt FJ, Zachariades NA, Braack LE, Ksiazek TG, Rollin PE, Zaki SR, Peters CJ.

Author information: (1)National Institute for Virology, Sandringham, South Africa.

Thirty-three varieties of 24 species of plants and 19 species of vertebrates and invertebrates were experimentally inoculated with Ebola Zaire virus. Fruit and insectivorous bats supported replication and circulation of high titers of virus without necessarily becoming ill; deaths occurred only among bats that had not adapted to the diet fed in the laboratory.

PMCID: PMC2639914 PMID: 8969248 [PubMed - indexed for MEDLINE]

2423. Emerg Infect Dis. 1996 Oct-Dec;2(4):259-69.

Social inequalities and emerging infectious diseases.

Farmer P(1).

Author information: (1)Harvard Medical School, Department of Social Medicine, Boston, MA 02115, USA. pefarmer@bics.bwh.harvard.edu

Although many who study emerging infections subscribe to social-production-of-disease theories, few have examined the contribution of social inequalities to disease emergence. Yet such inequalities have powerfully sculpted not only the distribution of infectious diseases, but also the course of disease in those affected. Outbreaks of Ebola, AIDS, and tuberculosis suggest that models of disease emergence need to be dynamic, systemic, and critical. Such models--which strive to incorporate change and complexity, and are global yet alive to local variation--are critical of facile claims of causality, particularly those that scant the pathogenic roles of social inequalities. Critical perspectives on emerging infections ask how large-scale social forces influence unequally positioned individuals in increasingly interconnected populations; a critical epistemology of emerging infectious diseases asks what features of disease emergence are obscured by dominant analytic frameworks. Research questions stemming from such a reexamination of disease emergence would demand close collaboration between basic scientists, clinicians, and the social scientists and epidemiologists who adopt such perspectives.

PMCID: PMC2639930 PMID: 8969243 [PubMed - indexed for MEDLINE]

2424. Health Facil Manage. 1996 Oct;9(10):68, 70, 72 passim.

Innovative new equipment lowers risks of needlesticks.

Garvin M(1).

Author information: (1)University of Iowa Hospitals and Clinics, Iowa City, USA.

PMID: 10160386 [PubMed - indexed for MEDLINE]

2425. Virology. 1996 Sep 15;223(2):376-80.

Termini of all mRNA species of Marburg virus: sequence and secondary structure.

Mühlberger E(1), Trommer S, Funke C, Volchkov V, Klenk HD, Becker S.

Author information: (1)Institut für Virologie, Philipps-Universität Marburg, Germany. muehlber@mailer.uni-marburg.de

The 3' and 5' ends of Marburg virus (MBG)-specific mRNA species have been determined using reverse transcription-PCR, rapid amplification of cDNA ends, or the reverse ligation-mediated PCR procedure after removal of cap structures with tobacco acid pyrophosphatase. The polyadenylation sites of all MBG-specific mRNAs were strictly conserved and corresponded to the predicted transcriptional stop signals of genomic RNA. Determination of the 5' ends of the mRNA species showed that mRNA synthesis started precisely at the first nucleotide of a highly conserved transcriptional start site. The 5' ends of the mRNA species can build a stable secondary structure with the conserved nucleotides always located in the stem region of a hairpin. Nucleotide substitutions in the conserved 5' regions are accompanied by compensatory mutations of the complementary nucleotide thus leading to a conservation of the secondary structures. Compensatory mutations were also found when 5' ends of mRNA of MBG strain Musoke were compared with MBG strain Popp or the closely related Ebola virus, indicating that the secondary structures will be conserved even if the sequence is altered.

PMID: 8806574 [PubMed - indexed for MEDLINE]

2426. Med Clin (Barc). 1996 Sep 7;107(7):255-6.

[Ebola virus infection].

[Article in Spanish]

Roca B, Simón E.

PMID: 8975095 [PubMed - indexed for MEDLINE]

2427. J Travel Med. 1996 Sep 1;3(3):192-193.

Malaria Prophylaxis During an Ebola Outbreak: A Difficult Choice.

Colebunders R(1).

Author information: (1)Institute of Tropical Medicine, Antwerp, Belgium.

PMID: 9815453 [PubMed - as supplied by publisher]

2428. Pediatr Ann. 1996 Sep;25(9):511-7.

Emerging and newly identified viral infections.

DeVincenzo JP(1).

Author information: (1)Division of Infectious Diseases, University of Tennessee, Memphis, USA.

PMID: 8880884 [PubMed - indexed for MEDLINE]

2429. Prof Nurse. 1996 Sep;11(12):798-9.

Ebola fever.

Payling KJ.

Ebola fever is a serious, life-threatening disease found in areas of Africa, South America and Asia. This update examines transmission, symptoms, diagnosis and nursing management.

PMID: 9137050 [PubMed - indexed for MEDLINE]

2430. Vopr Virusol. 1996 Sep-Oct;41(5):232-4.

[Development of the immunoenzyme test-system for detection of Ebola virus antigen].

[Article in Russian]

Borisevich IV, Mikhaĭlov VV, Potryvaeva NV, Malinkin IuN, Kirillov AP, Krasnianskiĭ VP, Markov VI, Makhlaĭ AA, Lebedinskaia EV.

An enzyme immunoassay system has been developed for the detection of Ebola virus antigen. It permits a highly accurate and sensitive rapid detection of the antigen. Optimal dilutions of specific immunoglobulin (1:500, corresponding to protein concentration of 50 micrograms/ml) and conjugate were found. The resolving capacity of the new test system is $1.9 \times 10(-7)$ g protein.

PMID: 8967072 [PubMed - indexed for MEDLINE]

2431. Nature. 1996 Aug 29;382(6594):744.

Ebola bar creates monkey shortage.

Nathan R.

PMID: 8752264 [PubMed - indexed for MEDLINE]

2432. Am Fam Physician. 1996 Jul;54(1):66, 68.

Public health policies for HIV/AIDS prevention.

Handsfield HH.

Comment on Am Fam Physician. 1995 Nov 1;52(6):1682.

PMID: 8677854 [PubMed - indexed for MEDLINE]

2433. Am J Trop Med Hyg. 1996 Jul;55(1):89-90.

Short report: lack of virus replication in arthropods after intrathoracic inoculation of Ebola Reston virus.

Turell MJ(1), Bressler DS, Rossi CA.

Author information: (1)U.S. Army Medical Research Institute of Infectious Diseases, Fort Detrick, Frederick, Maryland 21702-5011, USA.

To evaluate the potential for arthropods to serve as reservoir hosts of Ebola virus, three mosquito species, Aedes albopictus, Aedes taeniorhynchus, and Culex pipiens, and a soft tick, Ornithodoros sonrai, were inoculated with 102.5 plaque-forming units of Ebola Reston virus. After incubation at 22 degrees C for 11 days, at least six specimens of each species were triturated and examined for evidence of viral replication by enzyme-linked immunosorbent assay and plaque assay. There was no evidence of viral replication in any of the arthropods tested. Because intrathoracic inoculation bypasses various barriers to viral infection, the lack of replication of Ebola Reston virus in these inoculated arthropods indicates that these mosquito species and soft ticks probably are not involved as natural reservoirs of Ebola virus.

PMID: 8702028 [PubMed - indexed for MEDLINE]

2434. Bol Asoc Med P R. 1996 Jul-Sep;88(7-9):69-72.

[Ebola: "a fatal syndrome"].

[Article in Spanish]

Martínez GA(1), Ramírez Ronda CH.

Author information: (1)Departamento de Medicina Interna Hospital de Veteranos (III), Escuela de Medicina UPR, San Juan, P.R. 00927-5800.

No other clinical entity has attached more attention now-a-day than those precipitated by the infection with a Hemorrhagic Fever Virus. Potentially caused by Arena, Bunya, Flavi, and Filoviradae, only the latter has had such a major impact throughout the world. Two major genuses have been recognized since they become evident for the first time in 1967, the single-species Marburg, and the 3-species-Ebola (E. zaire, sudan and reston). With the exception of the 2 outbreaks of E. reston (Washington, USA 1989-1993), all of them have taken place in Africa, where the virus is still hiding among the wild-life of the Tropical Rain Forest. Currently (in April 1995) the reemergence of Ebola virus has once more proven its fatality, leaving around 170 deaths in Zaire, 250 miles from its capital, Kinshasa. There is worldwide alert, sponsored by the CDC in Atlanta, the World Health Organization and the authorities in Zaire regarding its potential spreading to naive regions, in and out of Africa. The characteristic clinical picture of a viral hemorrhagic fever has no match. After a 2-21 days incubation period a viral-like illness develops. As days go by, symptoms worsen, and by the 7th day, a severe and diffuse bleeding tendency ensues. The individual's death is the most likely outcome in the great majority of cases. As a lethal virus, without an available treatment and a possible airborne-route of transmission, Ebola virus will always be considered a persistent threat to the global health.
PMID: 9004731 [PubMed - indexed for MEDLINE]
2435. JAMA. 1996 Jun 19;275(23):1816-7.

Infectious diseases.

Stoeckle MY(1), Douglas RG Jr.
Author information: (1)Cornell University Medical College, New York, NY, USA.
PMID: 8642726 [PubMed - indexed for MEDLINE]
2436. Cell. 1996 May 17;85(4):477-8.

Similar structural models of the transmembrane proteins of Ebola and avian sarcoma viruses.

Gallaher WR.
PMID: 8653783 [PubMed - indexed for MEDLINE]
2437. Am Fam Physician. 1996 May 15;53(7):2283-4.

HIV, Ebola virus and public health measures.

Clarke P.
Comment on Am Fam Physician. 1995 Nov 1;52(6):1682.
PMID: 8638503 [PubMed - indexed for MEDLINE]
2438. MLO Med Lab Obs. 1996 May;28(5):40-6, 48-51; quiz 53-4.

New and emerging pathogens, Part 4. New and emerging viral diseases--the ultimate parasites.

Fratz GR(1), Wolf BC, Pizzuti WB, Brown JW.
Author information: (1)New Jersey State Department of Health, Division of Public Health and Environmental Laboratories, Trenton, USA.
PMID: 10157594 [PubMed - indexed for MEDLINE]
2439. Mt Sinai J Med. 1996 May-Sep;63(3-4):159-66.

The emergence of "emerging diseases": a lesson in holistic epidemiology.

Kilbourne ED(1).
Author information: (1)Department of Microbiology and Immunology, New York Medical College, Valhalla 10595, USA.
The term "emerging diseases" is a loosely defined category of entities comprising resurgent or recurrent old diseases (usually caused by "new" or mutated previously known agents), diseases truly new to man, but caused by preexisting ("old") zoonotic agents, and syndromes newly defined by the discovery of new agents through advances in biotechnology. Identification and solution of these problems depends, first, on recognition of their differences, and then upon tailoring appropriate strategies for their control. Thus, new influenza viruses appear each year to challenge immunity to their antecedents, but evoke the unchanged and centuries old symptom complex of influenza. Tuberculosis, is resurgent because of mycobacterial mutation to antibiotic resistance, immunosuppression by AIDS, and laxity in public health surveillance. Parvovirus B19 and herpesvirus 6 were revealed as cryptic infectors of white blood cells in studies of hepatitis B and AIDS, but since have been shown to be important causes of childhood rashes, aplastic anemia, and neurologic disease. The encroachment of human habitation on wilderness perimeters (ecosystem change) has increased contact with vectors of zoonotic viruses and bacteria, as evidenced by Lyme disease, Ebola virus infection, and the hemorrhagic fevers. The term "holistic epidemiology" embraces all these problems, from the molecular to the macroenvironmental level. Humans, parasites, and their environment will continue their ancient, fluctuating, dynamic relationship in the future, and new diseases will continue to emerge.
PMID: 8692162 [PubMed - indexed for MEDLINE]
2440. Nat Struct Biol. 1996 May;3(5):465-9.

Retrovirus envelope domain at 1.7 angstrom resolution.

Fass D(1), Harrison SC, Kim PS.
Author information: (1)Howard Hughes Medical Institute, Cambridge, Massachusetts, 02142, USA.
We report the crystal structure of an extraviral segment of a retrovirus envelope protein, the Moloney murine leukemia virus (MoMuLV) transmembrane (TM) subunit. This segment, which comprises a region of the MoMuLV TM protein analogous to that contained within the X-ray crystal structure of low-pH converted influenza hemagglutinin, contains a trimeric coiled coil, with a hydrophobic cluster at its base and a strand that packs in an antiparallel orientation against the

coiled coil. This structure gives the first high-resolution insight into the retrovirus surface and serves as a model for a wide range of viral fusion proteins; key residues in this structure are conserved among C- and D-type retroviruses and the filovirus ebola.

PMID: 8612078 [PubMed - indexed for MEDLINE]

2441. Postgrad Med. 1996 May;99(5):75-6, 78.

Ebola virus disease. Recognizing the face of a rare killer.

Sodhi A(1).

Author information: (1)University of Southern California-Los Angeles County Medical Center 90033, USA. asodhi@hsc.usc.edu

Because of international travel and immigration, US physicians should be aware of the signs and symptoms of Ebola virus disease. It should be suspected in any recent traveler who presents with manifestations of viral hemorrhagic fever and in laboratory workers exposed to animals from endemic areas who show symptoms. Infected persons should be given supportive care to help them survive the acute phase of infection. Fortunately, adequate preventive measures are already in place in US hospitals and laboratories because of the prevalence of AIDS and hepatitis. However, aid should be provided to the World Health Organization and developing countries such as Zaire to support further research into the epidemiology and natural history of the virus, which may help prevent future deadly epidemics.

PMID: 8650097 [PubMed - indexed for MEDLINE]

2442. MMWR Morb Mortal Wkly Rep. 1996 Apr 19;45(15):314-6.

Ebola-Reston virus infection among quarantined nonhuman primates--Texas, 1996.

Centers for Disease Control and Prevention (CDC).

PMID: 8602131 [PubMed - indexed for MEDLINE]

2443. Proc Natl Acad Sci U S A. 1996 Apr 16;93(8):3602-7.

The virion glycoproteins of Ebola viruses are encoded in two reading frames and are expressed through transcriptional editing.

Sanchez A(1), Trappier SG, Mahy BW, Peters CJ, Nichol ST.

Author information: (1)Division of Viral and Ricketsial Diseases, National Center for Infectious Diseases, Centers for Disease Control and Prevention, Atlanta, GA 30333, USA.

In late 1994 and early 1995, Ebola (EBO) virus dramatically reemerged in Africa, causing human disease in the Ivory Coast and Zaire. Analysis of the entire glycoprotein genes of these viruses and those of other EBO virus subtypes has shown that the virion glycoprotein (130 kDa) is encoded in two reading frames, which are linked by transcriptional editing. This editing results in the addition of an extra nontemplated adenosine within a run of seven adenosines near the middle of the coding region. The primary gene product is a smaller (50-70 kDa), nonstructural, secreted glycoprotein, which is produced in large amounts and has an unknown function. Phylogenetic analysis indicates that EBO virus subtypes are genetically diverse and that the recent Ivory Coast isolate represents a new (fourth) subtype of EBO virus. In contrast, the EBO virus isolate from the 1995 outbreak in Kikwit, Zaire, is virtually identical to the virus that caused a similar epidemic in Yambuku, Zaire, almost 20 years earlier. This genetic stability may indicate that EBO viruses have coevolved with their natural reservoirs and do not change appreciably in the wild.

PMCID: PMC39657 PMID: 8622982 [PubMed - indexed for MEDLINE]

2444. Hosp Pract (1995). 1996 Apr 15;31(4):85-91, 96-101, 104 passim.

Patterns and predictability in emerging infections.

Morse SS(1).

Author information: (1)Rockefeller University, New York, N.Y., USA.

Many seemingly novel infections have a long history as zoonoses, and perhaps in sporadic human hosts; they gain access to new host populations through ecologic changes and human activity. identification of patterns in the emergence of such illnesses--ranging from influenza and Lyme disease to Ebola fever and AIDS--suggests that worldwide surveillance may be more feasible than once thought.

PMID: 8609193 [PubMed - indexed for MEDLINE]

2445. Br Dent J. 1996 Apr 6;180(7):264-6.

Ebola virus infection: an overview.

Samaranayake LP(1), Peiris JS, Scully C.

Author information: (1)Faculty of Dentistry, University of Hong Kong.

The current outbreak of the Ebola virus infection in Africa has yet again proven that highly dangerous diseases that are transmitted via the blood-borne route may be endemic in some parts of the world and may emerge as sporadic outbreaks causing worldwide concern. Health care professionals are at the forefront of combatting these diseases and treating infected individuals. Though dental professionals are unlikely to be directly involved in the management of such acute infections, with very high mortality rates, they may encounter patients seeking dental treatment who are either from, or who have recently toured the endemic disease areas. This overview, therefore, is a thumb nail sketch of the Ebola virus infection and its implications for dentistry.

PMID: 8935292 [PubMed - indexed for MEDLINE]

2446. Emerg Infect Dis. 1996 Apr-Jun;2(2):155-6.

The Thucydides syndrome: Ebola déjà vu? (or Ebola reemergent?)

Olson PE, Hames CS, Benenson AS, Genovese EN.

PMCID: PMC2639821 PMID: 8964060 [PubMed - indexed for MEDLINE]

2447. Lancet. 1996 Mar 9;347(9002):691.

Research on Ebola virus.

Kelly MJ.

Comment on Lancet. 1995 Dec 23-30;346(8991-8992):1669-71.

PMID: 8596404 [PubMed - indexed for MEDLINE]

2448. Commun Dis Rep CDR Wkly. 1996 Mar 1;6(9):75, 78.

Outbreak of Ebola haemorrhagic fever in Gabon.

[No authors listed]

PMID: 8839188 [PubMed - indexed for MEDLINE]

2449. Mol Med Today. 1996 Mar;2(3):120-8.

The role of molecular techniques in the understanding of emerging infections.

Sable CA(1), Mandell GL.

Author information: (1)Merck Research Labs BL3-3, Blue Bell, PA 19422, USA.

Emerging infections are defined as infections that are newly identified or recognized, or those whose incidence in humans has significantly increased over the past 20 years. The interaction of several factors contributes to the emergence of infectious disease, including changes in human behavior, technological advances, economic development, increased international travel, microbial adaptation and lapses in public health measures. Biomedical research has allowed us to identify and classify previously uncultured pathogens, characterize microbial virulence factors, create new diagnostic tests and develop vaccines. Here, we highlight a few emerging infections and illustrate the role that molecular medicine has played in furthering our understanding of these diseases.

PMID: 8796869 [PubMed - indexed for MEDLINE]

2450. Oncol Rep. 1996 Mar;3(2):339-50.

Comparative virology and AIDS (review).

Kodama M(1), Kodama T.

Author information: (1)NATL CANC CTR,RES INST,DIV BIOPHYS,TOKYO 104,JAPAN.

The scientific debate between pros and cons of the HIV criminal theory of AIDS still remains unsettled. The purpose of this review is to promote resolution of the problem by extracting a common principle of the host-virus relation using data resources for each of 4 viruses as follows: a) polyoma virus, b) Marek's disease virus, c) Ebola virus, d) Korean hemorrhagic fever virus. Conclusions drawn from this study are given as follows: i) Environment emerged as the cardinal factor to modify the process of virus infection in all of the 4 viruses studied. Above all, an accelerating effect of environmental stress on the progression of virus infection was noted in vivo in the majority of viral diseases. ii) Evidence is available to indicate that a healthy cell (or a healthy individual) may harbor virus genes of multiple species without manifesting any pathologic sign. iii) Evidence also suggests that the biological property as well as morphological structure of a virus may vary in reponse to a change of the bioenvironment. On the basis of the above information, we propose to renounce 2 assumptions of classical infection model: a) the hereditarily determined virulence of a microorganism (including virus) be the sole determinant of infection to the effect that its invasion into the host should automatically complete the programmed course of infection; b) virus, a quasi-living creature, should reserve its behavioral independence irrespective of a change of the bioenvironment. The new infection model was constructed on the basis of the selfish gene concept that had been invented by Richard Dawkins to explain the altruistic behavior of an individual. That is, the fate of an exogenous or endogenous virus is under the dual control of the host genome (selfish gene) and the outer environment. The progression of virus infection is conditioned by a crosstalk between them. The selfish gene may use virus (a lifeless substance) as a magic bullet to induce a designated host response. In that sense, virus is not allowed to retain behavioral independence in the practice of its task. The above new model of virus infection was tested for its validity in the recent data of AIDS epidemiology.

PMID: 21594370 [PubMed]

2451. Pediatr Infect Dis J. 1996 Mar;15(3):189-91.

Ebola hemorrhagic fever: why were children spared?

Dowell SF(1).

Author information: (1)Division of Bacterial and Mycotic Diseases, Centers for Disease Control and Prevention, Atlanta, GA 30333, USA. SFD2@ciddbdl.em.cdc.gov

PMID: 8852904 [PubMed - indexed for MEDLINE]

2452. Arch Pathol Lab Med. 1996 Feb;120(2):140-55.

Lethal experimental infection of rhesus monkeys with Ebola-Zaire (Mayinga) virus by the oral and conjunctival route of exposure.

Jaax NK(1), Davis KJ, Geisbert TJ, Vogel P, Jaax GP, Topper M, Jahrling PB.

Author information: (1)Pathology Division, Unites States Army Medical Research Institute of Infectious Diseases, Fort Detrick, MD 21702-5011, USA.

OBJECTIVE: The source of infection or mode of transmission of Ebola virus to human index cases of Ebola fever has not been established. Field observations in outbreaks of Ebola fever indicate that secondary transmission of Ebola virus is linked to improper needle hygiene, direct contact with infected tissue or fluid samples, and close contact with infected patients. While it is presumed that the virus infects through either breaks in the skin or contact with mucous membranes, the only two routes of exposure that have been experimentally validated are parenteral inoculation and aerosol inhalation. Epidemiologic evidence suggests that aerosol exposure is not an important means of virus transmission in natural outbreaks of human Ebola fever; this study was designed to verify that Ebola virus could be effectively transmitted by oral or conjunctival exposure in nonhuman primates. MATERIALS AND METHODS: Adult rhesus monkeys

(Macaca mulatta) were exposed to Ebola-Zaire (Mayinga) virus orally (N=4), conjunctivally (N=4), or by intramuscular inoculation (N=1, virus-positive control). RESULTS: Four of four monkeys exposed by the conjunctival route, three of four monkeys exposed by the oral route, and the intramuscularly inoculated positive control monkey (one of one) were successfully infected with Ebola-Zaire (Mayinga). Seven monkeys died of Ebola fever between days 7 and 8 postexposure. One monkey was given aggressive supportive therapy and a platelet transfusion; it lived until day 12 postexposure. CONCLUSIONS: Findings in this study experimentally confirm that Ebola virus can be effectively transmitted via the oral or conjunctival route of exposure in nonhuman primates.
PMID: 8712894 [PubMed - indexed for MEDLINE]

2453. J Med Virol. 1996 Feb;48(2):141-6.

Evaluation of arthropod-borne viruses and other infectious disease pathogens as the causes of febrile illnesses in the Khartoum Province of Sudan.

McCarthy MC(1), Haberberger RL, Salib AW, Soliman BA, El-Tigani A, Khalid IO, Watts DM.

Author information: (1)U.S. Naval Medical Research Unit No 3, Cairo, Egypt.

The relative importance of arthropod-borne and other disease pathogens as the cause of an outbreak of febrile illnesses was assessed during August 1988, following severe flooding in Khartoum, Sudan. A total of 200 patients with acute febrile illness and 100 afebrile controls were enrolled in the study during October and November 1988; at the Omdurman Military Hospital, Khartoum, Sudan. Sera were tested for IgM and IgG antibodies to six arthropod-borne viruses by an enzyme-linked immunoabsorbent assay, and for similar antibodies to Lassa fever, Crimean-Congo hemorrhagic fever, and Ebola and Marburg viruses by an indirect fluorescence assay. Thick and thin blood smears were examined microscopically for malaria parasites, and fecal and blood specimens were tested for bacteria by standard culture methods. Among the acute and convalescent sera collected from 67 febrile patients, five cases were caused by sandfly fever Sicilian (SFS), six by sandfly fever Naples (SFN), and 12 by unidentified phleboviruses. Of 233 remaining unpaired, acute-phase sera collected from cases and controls, 49 (21%) had IgM antibodies to SFS or SFN, RVF, West Nile (WN), and Chikungunya (CHIK) viruses. Forty-three (22%) of 192 febrile cases and two of the 100 afebrile controls were positive for Plasmodium falciparum, and bacterial enteropathogens were associated with 25 (13%) cases and four controls. These data indicated that phleboviruses and to a lesser extent, WN, P. falciparum, and enterobacterial pathogens were causes of acute febrile illnesses following the 1988 flood in Khartoum, Sudan.
PMID: 8835346 [PubMed - indexed for MEDLINE]

2454. Med J Aust. 1996 Jan 15;164(2):79-83.

Viral haemorrhagic fevers: current status, future threats.

Speed BR(1), Gerrard MP, Kennett ML, Catton MG, Harvey BM.

Author information: (1)Fairfield Hospital, VIC.

In developing countries, the major outbreaks of viral haemorrhagic fevers such as Marburg, Ebola and Lassa fever viruses have been nosocomially spread. The high mortality and absence of specific treatment have had a devastating effect. Epidemics of this highly contagious disease remain a constant threat to Australia and, as a result, carefully planned laboratory and public health strategies and clinical infection control measures have been instituted for the management of suspected cases.
PMID: 8569577 [PubMed - indexed for MEDLINE]

2455. Filoviruses.

Feldmann H, Klenk HD. In: Baron S, editor. Medical Microbiology. 4th edition. Galveston (TX): University of Texas Medical Branch at Galveston; 1996. Chapter 72.

Filoviruses were first discovered in 1967 as the causative agents of a hemorrhagic fever outbreak among laboratory workers in Europe. These workers had been exposed to tissues and blood from African green monkeys (Cercopithecus aethiops) imported from Uganda and infected with Marburg virus. Since then, sporadic cases of Marburg hemorrhagic fever in man have occurred in Kenya and Zimbabwe (Table 72-1). Ebola hemorrhagic fever was first reported from northern Zaire and southern Sudan in 1976 when two distinct subtypes were isolated during simultaneous epidemics. Ebola Sudan reemerged in 1979 at the same location, causing a smaller epidemic of viral hemorrhagic fever. The third subtype (Reston) was isolated from cynomolgus monkeys (Macaca fascicularis) imported from the Philippines into the United States in 1989 and into Italy in 1992. Another distinct Ebola virus emerged on the Ivory Coast in 1994. The virus was isolated from a nonfatal case, in which a worker was infected during the autopsy of a wild chimpanzee. Recently Ebola reemerged in southwestern Zaire in the city of Kikwit and the surrounding villages in Bandundu Province. The isolated virus was closely related to the 1976 Zairian isolate, and the outbreak in these regions resembled the previous Ebola hemorrhagic fever epidemics (Table 72-1).
PMID: 21413301 [PubMed]

2456. Adv Pediatr Infect Dis. 1996;12:21-53.

Viral hemorrhagic fevers.

Lacy MD(1), Smego RA.

Author information: (1)Section of infectious Diseases, Robert C. Byrd Health Sciences Center, West Virginia University, Morgantown, USA.
PMID: 9033974 [PubMed - indexed for MEDLINE]

2457. Adv Virus Res. 1996;47:1-52.

Marburg and Ebola viruses.

Feldmann H(1), Klenk HD.

Author information: (1)Institute of Virology, Philipps University, Marburg, Germany.
PMID: 8895830 [PubMed - indexed for MEDLINE]

2458. Am J Med Sci. 1996 Jan;311(1):55-9.

Lessons learned from the hantaviruses and other hemorrhagic fever viruses.

Butler JC(1), Peters CJ.

Author information: (1)Centers for Disease Control and Prevention, Atlanta, Georgia 30333, USA.

In recent years, numerous previously known infections pathogens and their associated diseases have been recognized. Among these newly identified agents are the viruses that cause the hemorrhagic fevers, including Sin Nombre virus, the etiologic agent of the 1993 outbreak of hantavirus pulmonary syndrome in the American Southwest. Epidemiologic and laboratory investigations of the hemorrhagic fevers and their etiologic agents provide lessons that may be used collectively as a paradigm of the nature of emerging and re-emerging infectious diseases.

PMID: 8571987 [PubMed - indexed for MEDLINE]

2459. Arch Virol. 1996;141(5):909-21.

Ebola virus infection in guinea pigs: presumable role of granulomatous inflammation in pathogenesis.

Ryabchikova E(1), Kolesnikova L, Smolina M, Tkachev V, Pereboeva L, Baranova S, Grazhdantseva A, Rassadkin Y.

Author information: (1)State Research Center of Virology and Biotechnology "Vector" Research Institute of Molecular Biology, Koltsovo, Novosibirsk Region, Russia.

An approach combining virology with light and electron microscopy was used to study the organs of guinea pigs during nine serial passages of Ebola virus, strain Zaire. It was observed that the wild type of Ebola virus causes severe granulomatous inflammation in the liver and reproduces in the cells of the mononuclear phagocyte system (MPS). Based on morphological characterization, two types of virus-cell interactions were demonstrated. The obtained data evidenced for heterogeneity of the population of wild type of Ebola virus. The virus accumulated in the liver of the infected animals, and the lesions became more pronounced with passage. Degenerative changes appeared, and their severity was increased with passage in the other organs as well. The set of target cells diversified and, as a result, not only the MPS cells, but also hepatocytes, spongiocytes, endotheliocytes and fibroblasts became involved in the reproduction of Ebola virus. The possible role of granulomatous inflammation in the development of the adaptive mechanism of Ebola virus to guinea pigs is discussed.

PMID: 8678836 [PubMed - indexed for MEDLINE]

2460. Arch Virol Suppl. 1996;11:77-100.

Emerging and reemerging of filoviruses.

Feldmann H(1), Slenczka W, Klenk HD.

Author information: (1)Institute of Virology, Philipps-University, Marburg, Federal Republic of Germany.

Filoviruses are causative agents of a hemorrhagic fever in man with mortalities ranging from 22 to 88%. They are enveloped, nonsegmented negative-stranded RNA viruses and are separated into two types, Marburg and Ebola, which can be serologically, biochemically and genetically distinguished. In general, there is little genetic variability among viruses belonging to the Marburg type. The Ebola type, however, is subdivided into at least three distinct subtypes. Marburg virus was first isolated during an outbreak in Europe in 1967. Ebola virus emerged in 1976 as the causative agent of two simultaneous outbreaks in southern Sudan and northern Zaire. The reemergence of Ebola, subtype Zaire, in Kikwit 1995 caused a worldwide sensation, since it struck after a sensibilization on the danger of Ebola virus disease. Person-to-person transmission by intimate contact is the main route of infection, but transmission by droplets and small aerosols among infected individuals is discussed. The natural reservoir for filoviruses remains a mystery. Filoviruses are prime examples for emerging pathogens. Factors that may be involved in emergence are international commerce and travel, limited experience in diagnosis and case management, import of nonhuman primates, and the potential of filoviruses for rapid evolution.

PMID: 8800808 [PubMed - indexed for MEDLINE]

2461. Arch Virol Suppl. 1996;11:135-40.

Passive immunization of Ebola virus-infected cynomolgus monkeys with immunoglobulin from hyperimmune horses.

Jahrling PB(1), Geisbert J, Swearengen JR, Jaax GP, Lewis T, Huggins JW, Schmidt JJ, LeDuc JW, Peters CJ.

Author information: (1)United States Army Research Institute of Infectious Diseases, Fort Detrick, Frederick, Maryland 21702-5011, USA.

A commercially available immunoglobulin G (IgG) from horses, hyperimmunized to Ebola virus, was evaluated for its ability to protect cynomolgus monkeys against disease following i.m. inoculation with 1 000 PFU Ebola virus (Zaire '95 strain). Six monkeys were treated immediately after infection by i.m. infection of 6.0 ml IgG; these animals developed passive ELISA titers of 1:160 to 1:320 to Ebola, two days afer inoculation. However, the beneficial effects of IgG treatment were limited to a delay in onset of viremia and clinical signs, in comparison with untreated controls. The six IgG recipients had no detectable viremia day 5, in contrast with three virus infected controls whose viremias exceeded 7.0 log10 PFU/ml that day. The controls died on days 6, 6, and 7, while two IgG recipients died day 7 and the remaining 4 died day 8, all with high viremias. These results document that passively acquired antibody can have a beneficial effect in reducing the viral burden in Ebola-infected primates; however, effective treatment of human patients may require antibodies with higher specific activities and more favorable pharmacokinetic properties than the presently available equine IgG.

PMID: 8800795 [PubMed - indexed for MEDLINE]

2462. Arch Virol Suppl. 1996;11:115-34.

Experimental infection of cynomolgus macaques with Ebola-Reston filoviruses from the 1989-1990 U.S. epizootic.

Jahrling PB(1), Geisbert TW, Jaax NK, Hanes MA, Ksiazek TG, Peters CJ.

Author information: (1)United States Army Research Institute of Infectious Diseases, Fort Detrick, Frederick, Maryland 21702-5011, USA.

This study describes the pathogenesis of the Ebola-Reston (EBO-R) subtype of Ebola virus for experimentally infected cynomolgus monkeys. The disease course of EBO-R in macaques was very similar to human disease and to experimental diseases in macaques following EBO-Zaire and EBO-Sudan infections. Cynomolgus monkeys infected with EBO-R in this experiment developed anorexia, occasional nasal discharge, and splenomegaly, petechial facial hemorrhages and severe subcutaneous hemorrhages in venipuncture sites, similar to human Ebola fever. Five of the six EBO-R infected monkeys died, 8 to 14 days after inoculation. One survived and developed high titered neutralizing antibodies specific for EBO-R. The five acutely ill monkeys shed infectious virus in various bodily secretions. Further, abundant virus was visualized in alveolar interstitial cells and free in the alveoli suggesting the potential for generating infectious aerosols. Thus, taking precautions against aerosol exposures to filovirus infected primates, including humans, seems prudent. This experiment demonstrated that EBO-R was lethal for macaques and was capable of initiating and sustaining the monkey epizootic. Further investigation of this animal model should facilitate development of effective immunization, treatment, and control strategies for Ebola hemorrhagic fever.
PMID: 8800793 [PubMed - indexed for MEDLINE]

2463. Arch Virol Suppl. 1996;11:101-14.
Characterization of a new Marburg virus isolated from a 1987 fatal case in Kenya.
Johnson ED(1), Johnson BK, Silverstein D, Tukei P, Geisbert TW, Sanchez AN, Jahrling PB.

Author information: (1)United States Army Medical Research Institute of Infectious Diseases, Fort Detrick, Frederick, Maryland 21702-5011, USA.
In 1987, an isolated case of fatal Marburg disease was recognized during routine clinical haemorrhagic fever virus surveillance conducted in Kenya. This report describes the isolation and partial characterization of the new Marburg virus (strain Ravn) isolated from this case. The Ravn isolate was indistinguishable from reference Marburg virus strains by cross-neutralization testing. Virus particles and aggregates of Marburg nucleocapsid matrix in Ravn-infected vero cells, were visualized by immunoelectron microscopic techniques, and also in tissues obtained from the patient and from inoculated monkeys. The cell culture isolate produced a haemorrhagic disease typical of Marburg virus infection when inoculated into rhesus monkeys. Disease was characterized by the sudden appearance of fever and anorexia within 4 to 7 days, and death by day 11. Comparison of nucleotide sequences for portions of the glycoprotein genes of Marburg-Ravn were compared with Marburg reference strains Musoki (MUS) and Popp (POP). Nucleotide identity in this alignment between RAV and MUS is 72.3%, RAV and POP is 71%, and MUS and POP is 91.7%. Amino acid identity between RAV and MUS is 72%, RAV and POP is 67%, and MUS and POP is 93%. These data suggest that Ravn is another subtype of Marburg virus, analogous to the emerging picture of a spectrum of Ebola geographic isolates and subtypes.
PMID: 8800792 [PubMed - indexed for MEDLINE]

2464. Asepsis. 1996;18(4):20-2.
Ground zero: Ebola.
Dowell S.
PMID: 9271926 [PubMed - indexed for MEDLINE]

2465. East Afr Med J. 1996 Jan;73(1):27-31.
Threat of Marburg and Ebola viral haemorrhagic fevers in Africa.
Tukei PM(1).
Author information: (1)Virus Research Centre, Kenya Medical Research Institute, Nairobi, Kenya.
Marburg and Ebola viruses are members of the filovirus family that can be regarded as recently emerged. These viruses have caused sporadic outbreaks of fatal haemorrhagic disease in Africa, Europe and recently in the USA. The case fatality rates rank among the highest ranging from 33-80%. The mode of transmission of these viruses are clearly through close contact with blood and body fluids. Disease outbreaks have been amplified in hospital situations with poor blood precautions. In villages disease has been amplified through contamination with blood and fluids during nursing the sick and burial rituals. The source of the viruses has eluded discovery and new theories regarding the nature of these viruses are being entertained. The threat of new outbreaks in Africa is real since serological evidence of the presence of the virus has been documented in Kenya, Sudan, Zaire, Zimbabwe, Gabon, Cote-d'Ivoire and Gabon.
PMID: 8625857 [PubMed - indexed for MEDLINE]

2466. S Afr Med J. 1996 Jan;86(1):19-20.
Ebola questions still unanswered.
van der Linde I.
PMID: 8685773 [PubMed - indexed for MEDLINE]

2467. Virus Genes. 1996;13(3):189-201.
Computer simulations of proteolysis of Marburg and Ebola-Zaire filovirus coded proteins to generate nonapeptides with motifs of known HLA class I haplotypes and detection of antigenic domains in the viral glycoproteins.
Becker Y(1).
Author information: (1)Department of Molecular Virology, Faculty of Medicine, Hebrew University of Jerusalem, Israel.
The primary amino acid sequences of the proteins coded by Marburg and Ebola-Zaire filoviruses were studied by computer programs to search for putative proteolytic cleavages which yield nonapeptides with motifs of binding to known HLA class I haplotypes. The computer analyses predicted that numerous nonapeptides with motifs to bind HLA class I A68 and A2 haplotypes were detected. A few nonapeptides with motifs HLA class I A24, B8, B27 and B35 were predicted in Marburg virus proteins. A similar finding is reported for Ebola-Zaire viral proteins (the viral polymerase was not studied). The search for antigenic domains that may induce the humoral immune response in the viral glycoproteins was based on computer analyses of the physical properties and antigenicity predictions of amino acids in certain domains of the primary amino acid sequences. Twelve putative antigenic domains were detected in Marburg virus

glycoprotein and 11 putative antigenic domains in Ebola-Zaire virus glycoprotein. Despite the marked differences in the primary amino acid sequences in the putative antigenic domains of the two viral glycoproteins, 8 antigenic domains were found to have similar locations in the viral glycoproteins of the two viruses. Each pair of antigenic domains resemble each other in the physical properties of the amino acids that are different. These computer analyses may provide an approach to developing synthetic peptides capable of induction of both the cellular and humoral responses to protect against infection with Marburg or Ebola viruses.

PMID: 9035363 [PubMed - indexed for MEDLINE]

2468. West J Med. 1996 Jan;164(1):36-8.

Emerging infections--Ebola and other filoviruses.

Peters CJ(1).

Author information: (1)Viral Pathogens Branch, Centers for Disease Control and Prevention, Atlanta, GA 30333, USA.

PMCID: PMC1303291 PMID: 8779200 [PubMed - indexed for MEDLINE]

2469. Lancet. 1995 Dec 23-30;346(8991-8992):1669-71.

Transmission of Ebola virus (Zaire strain) to uninfected control monkeys in a biocontainment laboratory.

Jaax N(1), Jahrling P, Geisbert T, Geisbert J, Steele K, McKee K, Nagley D, Johnson E, Jaax G, Peters C.

Author information: (1)United States Army Medical Research Institute of Infectious Diseases, Frederick, Maryland 21702-5011, USA.

Comment in Lancet. 1996 Mar 9;347(9002):691.

Secondary transmission of Ebola virus infection in humans is known to be caused by direct contact with infected patients or body fluids. We report transmission of Ebola virus (Zaire strain) to two of three control rhesus monkeys (Macaca mulatta) that did not have direct contact with experimentally inoculated monkeys held in the same room. The two control monkeys died from Ebola virus infections at 10 and 11 days after the last experimentally inoculated monkey had died. The most likely route of infection of the control monkeys was aerosol, oral or conjunctival exposure to virus-laden droplets secreted or excreted from the experimentally inoculated monkeys. These observations suggest approaches to the study of routes of transmission to and among humans.

PMID: 8551825 [PubMed - indexed for MEDLINE]

2470. Virology. 1995 Dec 20;214(2):421-30.

GP mRNA of Ebola virus is edited by the Ebola virus polymerase and by T7 and vaccinia virus polymerases.

Volchkov VE(1), Becker S, Volchkova VA, Ternovoj VA, Kotov AN, Netesov SV, Klenk HD.

Author information: (1)State Research Centre of Virology and Biotechnology Vector, Institute of Molecular Biology, Koltsovo, Novosibirsk Region, Russia.

The glycoprotein gene of Ebola virus contains a translational stop codon in the middle, thus preventing synthesis of full-length glycoprotein. Twenty percent of the mRNA isolated from Ebola virus-infected cells was shown to be edited, containing one additional nontemplate A in a stretch of seven consecutive A residues. Only the edited mRNA species encoded full-length glycoprotein, whereas the exact copies of the viral template coded for a smaller secreted glycoprotein. Expression of the glycoprotein by an in vitro transcription/translation system, by the vaccinia virus/T7 polymerase system, and by recombinant vaccinia virus revealed that full-length glycoprotein was synthesized not only when the edited glycoprotein gene (8A's) was used as a template for T7 and vaccinia virus polymerases, but also when the nonedited (genomic) glycoprotein gene was used. Analysis of mRNA produced by T7 and vaccinia virus polymerase from the 7A's construct revealed that 1-5% contained alterations at the same site that was also edited by the Ebola virus polymerase. Our data indicate that the editing site in the Ebola virus glycoprotein gene is recognized not only by Ebola virus polymerase but also by DNA-dependent RNA polymerases of different origin.

PMID: 8553543 [PubMed - indexed for MEDLINE]

2471. Rev Infirm. 1995 Dec;(19):8-12.

[Nightmare in Zaire...from a medical and a humane viewpoint].

[Article in French]

Chlous P.

PMID: 8850830 [PubMed - indexed for MEDLINE]

2472. Virus Res. 1995 Dec;39(2-3):129-50.

Differentiation of filoviruses by electron microscopy.

Geisbert TW(1), Jahrling PB.

Author information: (1)Pathology Division, United States Army Medical Research Institute of Infectious Diseases, Fort Detrick, MD 21702-5011, USA.

Cultured monolayers of MA-104, Vero 76, SW-13, and DBS-FRhL-2 cells were infected with Marburg (MBG), Ebola-Sudan (EBO-S), Ebola-Zaire (EBO-Z), and Ebola-Reston (EBO-R) viruses (Filoviridae, Filovirus) and examined by electron microscopy to provide ultrastructural details of morphology and morphogenesis of these potential human pathogens. Replication of each filovirus was seen in all cell systems employed. Filoviral particles appeared to enter host cells by endocytosis. Filoviruses showed a similar progression of morphogenic events, from the appearance of nascent intracytoplasmic viral inclusions to formation of mature virions budded through plasma membranes, regardless of serotype or host cell. However, ultrastructural differences were demonstrated between MBG and other filoviruses. MBG virions recovered from culture fluids were uniformly shorter in mean unit length than EBO-S, EBO-Z, or EBO-R particles. Examination of filovirus-infected cells revealed that intermediate MBG inclusions were morphologically distinct from EBO-S, EBO-Z, and EBO-R inclusions. No structural difference of viral inclusion material was observed among EBO-S, EBO-Z, and EBO-R. Immunoelectron microscopy showed that the filoviral matrix protein (VP40) and nucleoprotein (NP) accumulated in EBO-Z inclusions, and were closely associated during viral morphogenesis. These details facilitate the efficient and definitive diagnosis of filoviral infections by electron microscopy.

PMID: 8837880 [PubMed - indexed for MEDLINE]

2473. Am Fam Physician. 1995 Nov 1;52(6):1682.

Ebola virus and HIV: a contrast in public health measures.

Felmar E.

Comment in Am Fam Physician. 1996 Jul;54(1):66, 68. Am Fam Physician. 1996 May 15;53(7):2283-4.

PMID: 7484678 [PubMed - indexed for MEDLINE]

2474. Vopr Virusol. 1995 Nov-Dec;40(6):270-3.

[Development and study of the properties of immunoglobulin against Ebola fever].

[Article in Russian]

Borisevich IV, Mikhaĭlov VV, Krasnianskiĭ VP, Gradoboev VN, Lebedinskaia EV, Potryvaeva NV, Timan'kova GD.

Immunoglobulin to Ebola fever has been for the first time prepared from hyperimmune equine blood sera by alcohol fractionation after Cohn. Preclinical study of the physicochemical and immunobiological properties of immunoglobulin showed that it protects up to 100% Papio hamadryas infected intramuscularly at doses of 110 to 29 LD50 Ebola virus. Scheme for the use of Ebola immunoglobulin has been experimentally validated.

PMID: 8686265 [PubMed - indexed for MEDLINE]

2475. Vopr Virusol. 1995 Nov-Dec;40(6):257-60.

[Attempts to develop a vaccine against Ebola fever].

[Article in Russian]

Chupurnov AA, Chernukhin IV, Ternovoĭ VA, Kudoiarova NM, Makhova NM, Azaev MSh, Smolina MP.

Data on the immunopathogenesis of Ebola fever in laboratory animals are presented and the efficacy of some methods of vaccine prophylaxis discussed. Antiviral immunity induced in guinea pigs by injection of inactivated viral agents did not protect them from infection, whereas injections of a nonlethal strain of the virus in ascending doses led to the formation of immunity preventing the development of disease upon inoculation with a lethal strain in high doses. The role of some viral peptides in the development of immune response is shown and variants of recombinant constructions for the prevention of Ebola fever are offered.

PMID: 8686261 [PubMed - indexed for MEDLINE]

2476. Lab Anim Sci. 1995 Oct;45(5):523-5.

Detection of Ebola-Reston (Filoviridae) virus antibody by dot-immunobinding assay.

Kalter SS(1), Heberling RL, Barry JD, Tian PY.

Author information: (1)Virus Reference Laboratory, Inc., San Antonio, TX 78229, USA.

Thirty human and nonhuman primate sera tested at the Centers for Disease Control by enzyme-linked immunosorbent assay (ELISA), immunofluorescent antibody assay (IFA), and Western blotting were retested at the Virus Reference Laboratory, Inc. by the dot-immunobinding assay (DIA). The Ebola-Reston strain of virus received from the Centers for Disease Control was prepared into a suitable DIA antigen as described for other antigens. All six Western blotting-positive sera were also positive by DIA, as were the five ELISA-positive sera. Testing by IFA, the original test of choice, indicated an additional four seropositives, all negative by the other test systems. Of 288 randomly selected macaque sera, 19 were also found to be Ebola-Reston virus-positive by DIA.

PMID: 8569150 [PubMed - indexed for MEDLINE]

2477. Can Commun Dis Rep. 1995 Sep 30;21(18):164, 167.

The Ebola fever epidemic officially declared over in Zaire.

[Article in English, French]

[No authors listed]

PMID: 8547920 [PubMed - indexed for MEDLINE]

2478. Biull Eksp Biol Med. 1995 Sep;120(9):302-4.

[Experimental study of Ebola hemorrhagic fever in baboon models].

[Article in Russian]

Luchko SV, Dadaeva AA, Ustinova EN, Sizikova LP, Riabchikova EI, Sandakhchiev LS.

PMID: 8593345 [PubMed - indexed for MEDLINE]

2479. Int Nurs Rev. 1995 Sep-Oct;42(5):139-40.

Combating Ebola: model of international collaboration.

[No authors listed]

PMID: 8575871 [PubMed - indexed for MEDLINE]

2480. Sci Am. 1995 Sep;273(3):34-6.

Hide-and-seek. Ebola--and the funds to study it--eludes researchers.

Leutwyler K.

PMID: 7652534 [PubMed - indexed for MEDLINE]

2481. Wkly Epidemiol Rec. 1995 Aug 25;70(34):241-2.

Ebola haemorrhagic fever.

[Article in English, French]

[No authors listed]

PMID: 7547206 [PubMed - indexed for MEDLINE]

2482. JAMA. 1995 Aug 2;274(5):374-5.

From the Centers for Disease Control and Prevention. Update: management of patients with suspected viral hemorrhagic fever--United States.

[No authors listed]

PMID: 7616624 [PubMed - indexed for MEDLINE]

2483. JAMA. 1995 Aug 2;274(5):373-4.

From the Centers for Disease Control and Prevention. Update: outbreak of Ebola viral hemorrhagic fever--Zaire, 1995.

[No authors listed]

PMID: 7616623 [PubMed - indexed for MEDLINE]

2484. Cent Afr J Med. 1995 Aug;41(8):264.

AIDS, Ebola and other new epidemics: theme of European Conference on Tropical Medicine in Hamburg.

Papendorf J.

PMID: 7585919 [PubMed - indexed for MEDLINE]

2485. Int J Exp Pathol. 1995 Aug;76(4):227-36.

Lethal experimental infections of rhesus monkeys by aerosolized Ebola virus.

Johnson E(1), Jaax N, White J, Jahrling P.

Author information: (1)US Army Medical Research Institute of Infectious Diseases, Frederick, Maryland 21702-5011, USA.

The potential of aerogenic infection by Ebola virus was established by using a head-only exposure aerosol system. Virus-containing droplets of 0.8-1.2 microns were generated and administered into the respiratory tract of rhesus monkeys via inhalation. Inhalation of viral doses as low as 400 plaque-forming units of virus caused a rapidly fatal disease in 4-5 days. The illness was clinically identical to that reported for parenteral virus inoculation, except for the occurrence of subcutaneous and venipuncture site bleeding and serosanguineous nasal discharge. Immunocytochemistry revealed cell-associated Ebola virus antigens present in airway epithelium, alveolar pneumocytes, and macrophages in the lung and pulmonary lymph nodes; extracellular antigen was present on mucosal surfaces of the nose, oropharynx and airways. Aggregates of characteristic filamentous virus were present within type I pneumocytes, macrophages, and air spaces of the lung by electron microscopy. Demonstration of fatal aerosol transmission of this virus in monkeys reinforces the importance of taking appropriate precautions to prevent its potential aerosol transmission to humans.

PMCID: PMC1997182 PMID: 7547435 [PubMed - indexed for MEDLINE]

2486. Int J Exp Pathol. 1995 Aug;76(4):225-6.

Ebola virus transmission.

Irving WL.

PMCID: PMC1997188 PMID: 7547434 [PubMed - indexed for MEDLINE]

2487. Ann Saudi Med. 1995 Jul;15(4):311-2.

Ebola virus update.

Al-Hajjar S(1).

Author information: (1)Consultant, Pediatric Infectious Diseases and Virology, Department of Pediatrics and Pathology, Laboratory Medicine, King Faisal Specialist Hospital and Research Centre, Riyadh, Saudi Arabia.

PMID: 17590596 [PubMed]

2488. Emerg Infect Dis. 1995 Jul-Sep;1(3):96-7.

Reemergence of Ebola virus in Africa.

Sanchez A, Ksiazek TG, Rollin PE, Peters CJ, Nichol ST, Khan AS, Mahy BW.

PMCID: PMC2626881 PMID: 8903173 [PubMed - indexed for MEDLINE]

2489. Epidemiol Bull. 1995 Jul;16(2):16.

Outbreak of Ebola hemorrhagic fever--Zaire, 1995.

[No authors listed]

PMID: 7646952 [PubMed - indexed for MEDLINE]

2490. S D J Med. 1995 Jul;48(7):207-8.

VRE--a more immediate threat than Ebola.

Barlow JF.

Comment in S D J Med. 1995 Sep;48(9):299.

PMID: 7660100 [PubMed - indexed for MEDLINE]

2491. MMWR Morb Mortal Wkly Rep. 1995 Jun 30;44(25):475-9.

Update: management of patients with suspected viral hemorrhagic fever--United States.

Centers for Disease Control and Prevention (CDC).

In 1988, CDC published guidelines for managing patients with suspected viral hemorrhagic fever (VHF) (1). Pending a comprehensive review of the 1988 guidelines, this notice provides interim recommendations that update the 1988 guidelines for healthcare settings in the United States. This update applies to four viruses that cause syndromes of VHF: Lassa, Marburg, Ebola, and Congo-Crimean hemorrhagic fever viruses; although the risk and/or mode of nosocomial transmission differs for each of these viruses, the limited data do not permit clear distinctions.

PMID: 7783731 [PubMed - indexed for MEDLINE]

2492. MMWR Morb Mortal Wkly Rep. 1995 Jun 30;44(25):468-9, 475.

Update: outbreak of Ebola viral hemorrhagic fever--Zaire, 1995.

Centers for Disease Control and Prevention (CDC).

As of June 25, public health authorities have identified 296 persons with viral hemorrhagic fever (VHF) attributable to documented or suspected Ebola virus infection in an outbreak in the city of Kikwit and the surrounding Bandundu region of Zaire (1,2); 79% of the cases have been fatal, and 90 (32%) of 283 cases in persons for whom occupation was known occurred in health-care workers. This report summarizes characteristics of persons with VHF from an initial description of cases and preliminary findings of an assessment of risk factors for transmission.

PMID: 7783730 [PubMed - indexed for MEDLINE]

2493. Can Commun Dis Rep. 1995 Jun 15;21(11):103-4.

Ebola hemorrhagic fever. A brief description.

[Article in English, French]

[No authors listed]

PMID: 7647744 [PubMed - indexed for MEDLINE]

2494. Harefuah. 1995 Jun 15;128(12):772-6.

[Ebola disease].

[Article in Hebrew]

Aizenstein O, Paz I, Vazina A, Michaeli D.

PMID: 7557687 [PubMed - indexed for MEDLINE]

2495. JAMA. 1995 Jun 14;273(22):1748.

From the Centers for Disease Control and Prevention. Update: outbreak of Ebola viral hemorrhagic fever--Zaire, 1995.

[No authors listed]

PMID: 7769766 [PubMed - indexed for MEDLINE]

2496. JAMA. 1995 Jun 14;273(22):1747-8.

From the Centers for Disease Control and Prevention. Outbreak of Ebola viral hemorrhagic fever--Zaire, 1995.

[No authors listed]

PMID: 7769765 [PubMed - indexed for MEDLINE]

2497. Fortschr Med. 1995 Jun 10;113(16):43-5.

[Ebola virus and hemorrhagic fever--still a mysterious disease. Pathogens are endemic in tropical Africa--humans and monkeys are apparently only secondary hosts].

[Article in German]

Burkhardt U(1), Blessing J.

Author information: (1)Institut für medizinische und mikrobiologische Diagnostik, Singen/Hohentwiel.

PMID: 7635379 [PubMed - indexed for MEDLINE]

2498. Lancet. 1995 Jun 3;345(8962):1448.

Ebola haemorrhagic fever in Kikwit, Zaire. International Scientific and Technical Committee and WHO Collaborating Centre for Haemorrhagic Fevers.

Muyembe T, Kipasa M.

PMID: 7760645 [PubMed - indexed for MEDLINE]

2499. Wkly Epidemiol Rec. 1995 Jun 2;70(22):158.

Ebola haemorrhagic fever.

[Article in English, French]

[No authors listed]

PMID: 7619683 [PubMed - indexed for MEDLINE]

2500. Am J Infect Control. 1995 Jun;23(3):214.

Ebola again.

[No authors listed]

PMID: 7677271 [PubMed - indexed for MEDLINE]

2501. Rev Med Liege. 1995 Jun;50(6):241-3.

[Ebola virus disease, a tropical hemorrhagic fever].

[Article in French]

Piérard GE(1).

Author information: (1)Service de Dermatopathologie, CHU du Sart Tilman.

PMID: 7618000 [PubMed - indexed for MEDLINE]

2502. Nurs Times. 1995 May 31-Jun 6;91(22):18.

Infectious terror.

Lee F.

PMID: 7603847 [PubMed - indexed for MEDLINE]

2503. BMJ. 1995 May 27;310(6991):1353.

Ebola threat eases.

Dyer O.

PMID: 7787528 [PubMed - indexed for MEDLINE]

2504. BMJ. 1995 May 27;310(6991):1344-5.

Ebola virus.

Bennett D, Brown D.

PMCID: PMC2549737 PMID: 7787519 [PubMed - indexed for MEDLINE]

2505. MMWR Morb Mortal Wkly Rep. 1995 May 26;44(20):399.

Update: outbreak of Ebola viral hemorrhagic fever--Zaire, 1995.

Centers for Disease Control and Prevention (CDC).

PMID: 7746265 [PubMed - indexed for MEDLINE]

2506. Wkly Epidemiol Rec. 1995 May 26;70(21):149-51.

Ebola haemorrhagic fever.

[Article in English, French]

[No authors listed]

PMID: 7619681 [PubMed - indexed for MEDLINE]

2507. Lancet. 1995 May 20;345(8960):1271-4.

Isolation and partial characterisation of a new strain of Ebola virus.

Le Guenno B(1), Formenty P, Wyers M, Gounon P, Walker F, Boesch C.

Author information: (1)WHO Collaborating Center for Arboviruses and Haemorragic Fevers, Institut Pasteur, Paris, France.

Erratum in Lancet. 2006 Mar 11;367(9513):816. Formenty, P [corrected to Formenty, P].

Comment in Lancet. 1995 May 20;345(8960):1252-3. Lancet. 1995 Jul 29;346(8970):322.

We have isolated a new strain of Ebola virus from a non-fatal human case infected during the autopsy of a wild chimpanzee in the Côte-d'Ivoire. The wild troop to which this animal belonged has been decimated by outbreaks of haemorrhagic syndromes. This is the first time that a human infection has been connected to naturally-infected monkeys in Africa. Data from the long-term survey of this troop of chimpanzees could answer questions about the natural reservoir of the Ebola virus.

PMID: 7746057 [PubMed - indexed for MEDLINE]

2508. Lancet. 1995 May 20;345(8960):1252-3.

The filovirus enigma.

Simpson DI(1).

Author information: (1)Department of Microbiology and Immunobiology, Queen's University of Belfast, UK.

Comment on Lancet. 1995 May 20;345(8960):1271-4.

PMID: 7746050 [PubMed - indexed for MEDLINE]

2509. Commun Dis Rep CDR Wkly. 1995 May 19;5(20):93.

Viral haemorrhagic fever in Zaire: update.

[No authors listed]

PMID: 7613589 [PubMed - indexed for MEDLINE]

2510. MMWR Morb Mortal Wkly Rep. 1995 May 19;44(19):381-2.

Outbreak of Ebola viral hemorrhagic fever--Zaire, 1995.

Centers for Disease Control and Prevention (CDC).

On May 6, 1995, CDC was notified by health authorities and the U.S. Embassy in Zaire of an outbreak of viral hemorrhagic fever (VHF)-like illness in Kikwit, Zaire (1995 population: 400,000), a city located 240 miles east of Kinshasa. The World Health Organization and CDC were invited by the Government of Zaire to participate in an investigation of the outbreak. This report summarizes preliminary findings from this ongoing investigation.

PMID: 7739512 [PubMed - indexed for MEDLINE]

2511. Science. 1995 May 19;268(5213):974-5.

Chimpanzee outbreak heats up search for Ebola origin.

Morell V.

PMID: 7754392 [PubMed - indexed for MEDLINE]

2512. Wkly Epidemiol Rec. 1995 May 19;70(20):147-8.

Ebola haemorrhagic fever.

[Article in English, French]

[No authors listed]

Erratum in Wkly Epidemiol Rec. 2004 May 14;79(2):200.

PMID: 7786718 [PubMed - indexed for MEDLINE]

2513. Commun Dis Rep CDR Wkly. 1995 May 12;5(19):89.

Viral haemorrhagic fever: outbreak in Zaire.

[No authors listed]

PMID: 7787924 [PubMed - indexed for MEDLINE]

2514. Antibiot Khimioter. 1995 May;40(5):24-7.

[The efficacy of the emergency prophylactic and therapeutic actions of immunomodulators in experimental filovirus infections].

[Article in Russian]

Sergeev AN, Lub MIu, P'iankova OG, Kotliarov LA.

The study of the preventive and therapeutic action of some immunomodulators (ridostin, reaferon and polyribonate) used alone and in combinations was conducted on laboratory animals infected aerogenically by Marburg or Ebola virus. It was found that special preventive intranasal and intramuscular administration of ridostin provided protection of the animals infected by Marburg virus (p = 0.1) and an increase in their mean lifespan by 2.4 days (p = 0.15). In the Ebola infection combined administration of ridostin and reaferon caused an essential increase in the mean lifespan of the animals by 2.9 days (p = 0.04). None of the tested drugs had any significant positive effect when used in various combinations according to the treatment schemes in Marburg and Ebola infections in guinea pigs.

PMID: 8534175 [PubMed - indexed for MEDLINE]

2515. Sante. 1995 May-Jun;5(3):145-6.

[Ebola, a tranquil river in the heart of Africa].

[Article in French]

Gonzalez JP.

PMID: 7640895 [PubMed - indexed for MEDLINE]

2516. Sante. 1995 May-Jun;5(3):143-4.

[Ebola 1995: history repeats itself].

[Article in French]

Camprasse MA.

PMID: 7640894 [PubMed - indexed for MEDLINE]

2517. Vopr Virusol. 1995 May-Jun;40(3):138-40.

[Preparation of hyperimmune horse serum against Ebola virus].

[Article in Russian]

Krasnianskiĭ BP, Mikhaĭlov VV, Borisevich IV, Gradoboev VN, Evseev AA, Pshenichnov VA.

Immunization of horses with Ebola virus resulted in production of specific virus-neutralizing antibodies with their maximal level attained on days 28 to 42 postimmunization. Repeated cycles of immunization lead to increase of antibodies titer to 1:4096.

PMID: 7676681 [PubMed - indexed for MEDLINE]

2518. Vopr Virusol. 1995 May-Jun;40(3):113-5.

[Experimental Ebola fever in Macaca mulatta].

[Article in Russian]

P'iankov OV, Sergeev AN, P'iankova OG, Chepurnov AA.

Aerogenic infection of M. rhesus with Ebola virus causes in them a disease similar in the principal clinical and virological parameters a grave form of Ebola fever in humans, as it is described in literature. Rapid development of symptoms of total intoxication in the presence of fever, hemorrhagic diathesis, and high viremia are indicative of the infection severity in monkeys.

PMID: 7676671 [PubMed - indexed for MEDLINE]

2519. Biochem Mol Biol Int. 1995 Mar;35(3):605-13.

Complete nucleotide sequences of Marburg virus genes 5 and 6 encoding VP30 and VP24 proteins.

Bukreyev AA(1), Belanov EF, Blinov VM, Netesov SV.

Author information: (1)State Research Center of Virology and Biotechnology Vector, Institute of Molecular Biology, Koltsovo, Novosibirsk Region, Russia. Nucleotide sequences of the genes 5 and 6 of the Marburg virus, Popp strain, were determined. ORFs encoding polypeptides VP30 (281 a.a., MW 32,640) and VP24 (253 a.a., MW 28,621) were found. The putative transcription start and stop signals for viral RNA-dependent RNA polymerase were revealed for both genes. Overlapping of genes 5 and 6 was shown. The deduced amino acid sequences of VP30 and VP24 proteins displayed significant homology with the analogous proteins of another filovirus, the Ebola virus (33% and 37%, respectively). The VP24 appeared to have a hydrophobic amino acid composition; content of hydrophobic amino acids was 40.7%. Model of VP24 location in the virion was suggested.
PMID: 7773195 [PubMed - indexed for MEDLINE]

2520. Vopr Virusol. 1995 Mar-Apr;40(2):74-6.

[The effect of some physical and chemical factors on inactivation of the Ebola virus].

[Article in Russian]

Chepurnov AA, Chuev IuP, P'iankov OV, Efimova IV.

Ebola virus was found to survive multiple freezing and thawing, stable at storage, and poorly inactivated by UV irradiation. At the same time, common disinfectants reliably inactivate this virus.
PMID: 7762236 [PubMed - indexed for MEDLINE]

2521. Duodecim. 1995;111(14):1277-9.

[Ebola virus epidemic].

[Article in Finnish]

Vapalahti O, Vaheri A.
PMID: 9244676 [PubMed - indexed for MEDLINE]

2522. Med Trop (Mars). 1995;55(2):133-4.

[Ebola virus and yellow fever: lessons to learn from the epidemics].

[Article in French]

Baudon D.
PMID: 7564992 [PubMed - indexed for MEDLINE]

2523. Virus Genes. 1995;11(2-3):191-5.

Retrovirus and filovirus "immunosuppressive motif" and the evolution of virus pathogenicity in HIV-1, HIV-2, and Ebola viruses.

Becker Y(1).

Author information: (1)Department of Molecular Virology, Faculty of Medicine, Hebrew University of Jerusalem, Israel.

The "immunosuppressive motif" was found to be present in the glycoproteins of retroviruses and filoviruses. This sequence is also conserved in the pathogenic lentiviruses, HIV-1 and SIV, and is absent from HIV-2 gp41 and from an apathogenic simian retrovirus. The present analysis deals with the possible involvement of the "immunosupressessive motif" in the pathogenicity of retroviruses and filoviruses, and the reasons for the conservation of this motif. The ancestral gene from which the "immunosuppressive motif" originated is not known.
PMID: 8828145 [PubMed - indexed for MEDLINE]

2524. Vopr Virusol. 1995 Jan-Feb;40(1):31-5.

[Development and application of an immunoenzyme test system for diagnosing Ebola fever].

[Article in Russian]

Merzlikin NV, Chepurnov AA, Istomina NN, Ofitserov VI, Vorob'eva MS.

Enzyme immunoassay (EIA) test systems for the detection of antigens of and antibodies to Ebola virus were developed and tried. The test system for the detection of Ebola virus antigens based on direct solid-phase EIA detects viral antigens in culture fluid of infected Vero cells, in the blood sera, and in homogenates of infected tissues. Use of this test system allows detection of at least 10 ng of viral proteins or 5.0 x 10(3) to 1.0 x 10(4) PFU/ml in infectious material. The test system is prepared on the basis of protein A - horseradish peroxidase conjugate. It is universal for the testing of animal and human sera and is characterized by high resolution and reproducibility of results. It allows detection of antibodies to Ebola virus starting from days 8-9 of infection. A higher sensitivity of direct solid-phase EIA in comparison with complement fixation or indirect immunofluorescence tests is demonstrated.
PMID: 7740786 [PubMed - indexed for MEDLINE]

2525. Lancet. 1994 Dec 17;344(8938):1693-4.

Renewed UN drive against AIDS.

McGregor A.

PIP: After a 1-day meeting of agency directors on December 12 in New York, UN Secretary-General Boutros Boutros-Ghali announced the appointment of Dr. Peter Piot as director of a renewed UN program against human immunodeficiency virus (HIV) and acquired immunodeficiency syndrome (AIDS), provisionally entitled "UN Joint and Co-sponsored Programme on AIDS." The 6 UN agencies already involved (UNICEF, UNDP, UNESCO, UN Population Fund, the World Bank, and WHO) will be more tightly coordinated; the World Health Organization (WHO) will remain in charge. Dr. Piot, a 45-year-old Belgian physician and co-discoverer of the Ebola virus (1976), assisted and effectively succeeds Dr. Michael Merson, the director of the World Health Organizations's global program on AIDS. While professor of microbiology at the Institute of Tropical Medicine in Antwerp, Dr. Piot launched a series of collaborative projects in Africa, including "Project SIDA" in Kinshasa in 1984. The new program will not be fully operational until 1996. The World Bank is expected to provide additional money. Dr.

Merson's predecessor, Dr. Jonathan Mann (now director of the International Center at the Harvard School Of Public Health) expressed hopefulness about the new leadership and concern that what has been learned about AIDS in the last decade will be applied in the new program. A transition team has been working on a provisional program blueprint that provides for a resident coordinator and the full integration of local staff in each country. Additional emphasis will be given to education. An estimated 17 million people are infected with HIV, 3 million more since June of last year. 20-40 million are expected to be infected by 1999. PMID: 7996968 [PubMed - indexed for MEDLINE]

2526. Vopr Virusol. 1994 Nov-Dec;39(6):286-8.

[Preparation of rabbit antiserum to Ebola virus].

[Article in Russian]

Chepurnov AA, Merzlikin NV, Chepurnova TS, Vorob'eva MS.

Humoral immunity of rabbits insusceptible to Ebola virus infection were studied after challenge with infectious Ebola virus and inactivated antigen of this virus. Administration of Ebola virus antigen induced the production of specific antibodies in proportion with the antigen dose injected.

PMID: 7716928 [PubMed - indexed for MEDLINE]

2527. Vopr Virusol. 1994 Nov-Dec;39(6):254-7.

[Isolation of purified Ebola virus].

[Article in Russian]

Chepurov AA, Merzlikin NV, Rabchikova EI, Chepurnova TS, Volchkov VE, Istomina NN, Kuz'min VA, Vorob'eva MS.

Purified concentrates of Ebola virus were prepared by two methods, adsorption on polyethylenglycol-600 followed by ultracentrifugation in sucrose density gradient and ultrafiltration. The ultrafiltration method permits preparation of concentrated Ebola virus with better preserved virion structure and infective activity than the traditional method.

PMID: 7716917 [PubMed - indexed for MEDLINE]

2528. Vopr Virusol. 1994 Sep-Oct;39(5):229-32.

[Composition and immunochemical properties of goat immunoglobulins against the Ebola virus].

[Article in Russian]

Dedkova LM, Kudoiarova NM, Chepurpov AA, Ofitserov VI.

Serum samples containing Ebola Virus neutralizing antibodies were prepared by prolonged immunization of goats with 10% liver homogenate from guinea pigs infected with Ebola virus. Differences in IgG fractions of normal and hyperimmune caprine blood sera were detected. Analytical chromatography on Polysil SA and immunodiffusion showed the presence of three IgG-containing fractions in hyperimmune sera. Immunochemical properties of these fractions were studied by solid-phase enzyme immunoassay and neutralization test. Antibodies to viral antigens were referred to IgG2 and IgG1a, and virus neutralizing properties were found mainly in IgG2 antibodies. Immunoglobulins were isolated from hyperimmune serum by alcohol sedimentation. The principal IgG fraction was found to contain much lower levels of antibodies to guinea pig liver antigens than intact serum, but at the same time it was characterized by a higher neutralization index.

PMID: 7716910 [PubMed - indexed for MEDLINE]

2529. AIDS. 1994 May;8(5):705-6.

The laboratory, epidemiology, nosocomial infection and HIV.

Heymann DL, Piot P.

PMID: 8060553 [PubMed - indexed for MEDLINE]

2530. Virology. 1994 Mar;199(2):469-73.

Characterization of filoviruses based on differences in structure and antigenicity of the virion glycoprotein.

Feldmann H(1), Nichol ST, Klenk HD, Peters CJ, Sanchez A.

Author information: (1)Special Pathogens Branch, Centers for Disease Control and Prevention, Atlanta, Georgia 30333.

Eight different filovirus isolates, representing major episodes of filovirus hemorrhagic disease, were propagated for structural and antigenetic analyses of their glycoprotein (GP). Carbohydrate analysis revealed that N- and O-glycosylation are features of filovirus GPs. Oligosaccharide side chains differed in their sialylation pattern and seemed to be cell line-dependent. Marburg virus (MBG) isolates are clearly distinguished from Ebola (EBO) and Reston viruses by a lack of terminal sialic acids when propagated in E6 and MA-104 cells. It was also determined that GP-specific antisera failed to show any cross-reactivity between MBG isolates and other filoviruses. These data, together with prior findings, indicate that the genus Filovirus can be divided into a MBG group and EBO group.

PMID: 8122375 [PubMed - indexed for MEDLINE]

2531. Vopr Virusol. 1994 Mar-Apr;39(2):91-2.

[The isolation of hyperimmune horse serum to the Ebola virus].

[Article in Russian]

Krasnianskiĭ VP, Mikhaĭlov VV, Borisevich IV, Gradoboev VN, Evseev AA, Pshenichnov VA.

Immunization of horses with Ebola virus resulted in the production of specific virus-neutralizing antibody with maximum titres at 28-42 days. Repeated cycles of immunization led to a rise in antibody titres to 1:4096.

PMID: 8017064 [PubMed - indexed for MEDLINE]

2532. Vopr Virusol. 1994 Mar-Apr;39(2):82-4.

[The evaluation in hamadryas baboons of the possibility for the specific prevention of Ebola fever].

[Article in Russian]

Mikhaĭlov VV, Borisevich IV, Chernikova NK, Potryvaeva NV, Krasnianskiĭ VP.

The protective role of virus-neutralizing antibody was demonstrated in Ebola virus-infected animals (Papio hamadryas) used in experiments on the development of passive humoral immunity by using specific immunoglobulin. Two immunizations of the monkeys with purified concentrated Ebola virus antigen with complete Freund adjuvant was shown to confirm intensive immunity to subsequent challenge protecting 80% of the immunized animals. It is concluded that effective preparations may be developed for specific prophylaxis of Ebola fever.

PMID: 8017061 [PubMed - indexed for MEDLINE]

2533. Antiviral Res. 1993 Sep;22(1):45-75.

Molecular approaches for the treatment of hemorrhagic fever virus infections.

Andrei G(1), De Clercq E.

Author information: (1)Rega Institute for Medical Research, Katholieke Universiteit Leuven, Belgium.

Viruses causing hemorrhagic fevers in man belong to the following virus groups: togavirus (Chikungunya), flavivirus (dengue, yellow fever, Kyasanur Forest disease, Omsk hemorrhagic fever), arenavirus (Argentinian hemorrhagic fever, Bolivian hemorrhagic fever, Lassa fever), filovirus (Ebola, Marburg), phlebovirus (Rift Valley fever), nairovirus (Crimian-Congo hemorrhagic fever) and hantavirus (hemorrhagic fever with renal syndrome, nephropathic epidemia). Hemorrhagic fever virus infections can be approached by different therapeutic strategies: (i) vaccination; (ii) administration of high-titered antibodies; and (iii) treatment with antiviral drugs. Depending on the molecular target of their interaction, antiviral agents could be classified as follows: IMP dehydrogenase inhibitors (i.e., ribavirin and its derivatives); OMP decarboxylase inhibitors (i.e., pyrazofurin); CTP synthetase inhibitors (i.e., cyclopentylcytosine and cyclopentenylcytosine); SAH hydrolase inhibitors (i.e., neplanocin A); polyanionic substances (i.e., sulfated polymers); interferon and immunomodulators.

PMID: 8250543 [PubMed - indexed for MEDLINE]

2534. Trans R Soc Trop Med Hyg. 1993 Sep-Oct;87(5):536-8.

Filovirus activity among selected ethnic groups inhabiting the tropical forest of equatorial Africa.

Johnson ED(1), Gonzalez JP, Georges A.

Author information: (1)United States Army Medical Research Institute of Infectious Diseases, Frederick, Maryland.

Seroepidemiological surveys were conducted to determine the frequency and distribution of filovirus activity among selected ethnic groups inhabiting the tropical forests of the Central African Republic. 427 serum specimens were collected from hunter-gatherers and subsistence farmers living in forest environs in the Lobaye District south of the river Lobaye and west of the river Oubangui. Striking serological evidence for filovirus activity was found in both populations. Ebola virus appears to be the most active filovirus; 17.6% (75/427) of the Lobaye survey population were seropositive for Ebola virus reactive antibody while 1.2% (5/427) were seroreactive with Marburg viral antigens. Ethnic background appeared to be an important risk factor influencing filovirus exposure in the forest communities. The filovirus antibody prevalence among 21-40 years old male Aka Pygmy hunter-gatherers was significantly (P = 0.03) 3 times higher (37.5%) than that in similarly aged male Monzombo and Mbati subsistence farmers (13.2%). Continued epidemiological investigations are needed to define ethnic-related events influencing human filovirus activity in the Congo basin of equatorial Africa.

PMID: 8266403 [PubMed - indexed for MEDLINE]

2535. Trans R Soc Trop Med Hyg. 1993 Sep-Oct;87(5):530-5.

Haemorrhagic fever virus activity in equatorial Africa: distribution and prevalence of filovirus reactive antibody in the Central African Republic.

Johnson ED(1), Gonzalez JP, Georges A.

Author information: (1)United States Army Medical Research Institute of Infectious Diseases, Frederick, Maryland.

Seroepidemiological surveys were conducted to determine the frequency and distribution of haemorrhagic fever virus (HFV) activity in the Central African Republic. Human serum specimens (4295) were collected from 5 ecologically distinct zones. Serological evidence of HFV activity was found in all the zones. The filovirus antibody prevalence (24.4%, 1051/4295) was greater than the combined prevalence for Lassa virus, Rift Valley fever virus and Crimean-Congo HFV antibody (1.1%, 45/4295; P < 0.01). Evidence of filovirus activity was found in all zones: 21.3% (914/4295) of the population were seropositive for Ebola virus antibody while only 3.2% (137/4295) were seroreactive with Marburg viral antigens. Age and sex were important host-related factors influencing filovirus activity, particularly in dry grassland and moist forest communities. These communities shared many factors, but differences, such as agricultural practices and ethnic backgrounds, may also affect the risk of infection. Filovirus infections appear to occur without apparent disease. Continued investigations are needed to evaluate the true pathogenicity of the African filoviruses and the likelihood that unidentified serologically cross-reacting and non-pathogenic members of the filovirus family are active in equatorial Africa.

PMID: 8266402 [PubMed - indexed for MEDLINE]

2536. Virus Res. 1993 Sep;29(3):215-40.

Sequence analysis of the Ebola virus genome: organization, genetic elements, and comparison with the genome of Marburg virus.

Sanchez A(1), Kiley MP, Holloway BP, Auperin DD.

Author information: (1)Division of Viral and Rickettsial Diseases, Centers for Disease Control and Prevention, Atlanta, GA 30333.

Sequence analysis of the second through the sixth genes of the Ebola virus (EBO) genome indicates that it is organized similarly to rhabdoviruses and paramyxoviruses and is virtually the same as Marburg virus (MBG). In vitro translation experiments and predicted amino acid sequence comparisons showed that the order of the EBO genes is: 3'-NP-VP35-VP40-GP-VP30-VP24-L. The transcriptional start and stop (polyadenylation) signals are conserved and all

contain the sequence 3'-UAAUU. Three base intergenic sequences are present between the NP and VP35 genes (3'-GAU) and VP40 and GP genes (3'-AGC), and a large intergenic sequence of 142 bases separates the VP30 and VP24 genes. Novel gene overlaps were found between the VP35 and VP40, the GP and VP30, and the VP24 and L genes. Overlaps are 20 or 18 bases in length and are limited to the conserved sequences determined for the transcriptional signals. Stem-and-loop structures were identified in the putative (+) leader RNA and at the 5' end of each mRNA. Hybridization studies showed that a small second mRNA is transcribed from the glycoprotein gene, and is produced by termination of transcription at an atypical polyadenylation signal located in the middle of the coding region. The predicted amino acid sequence of the glycoprotein contains an N-terminal signal peptide sequence, a hydrophobic anchor sequence, and 17 potential N-linked glycosylation sites. Alignment of predicted amino acid sequences showed that the structural proteins of EBO and MBG contain large regions of homology despite the absence of serologic cross-reactivity.
PMID: 8237108 [PubMed - indexed for MEDLINE]

2537. Vopr Virusol. 1993 Jul-Aug;38(4):179-82.

[The ultrastructural changes in guinea pig organs during the serial passage of the Ebola virus].

[Article in Russian]

Pereboeva LA, Tkachev VK, Kolesnikova LV, Krendeleva LIa, Riabchikova EI, Smolina MP.

Morphological study of internal organs of guinea pigs inoculated with Ebola virus at 2-8 passages was carried out. In the course of these passages the number of infected cells and virus particles in the organs was shown to increase, and the destructive changes in organs became more pronounced. In the 1st-3rd passages Ebola virus replication was observed in macrophagal cells only but beginning from the 4th passage of virus reproduction was found also in hepatocytes, spongiocytes, and fibroblasts.
PMID: 8236945 [PubMed - indexed for MEDLINE]

2538. Vopr Virusol. 1993 Jul-Aug;38(4):176-9.

[The morphological changes in Ebola infection in guinea pigs].

[Article in Russian]

Riabchikova EI, Baranova SG, Tkachev VK, Grazhdantseva AA.

Ebola virus reproduction and morphological lesions were investigated in infected guinea pigs by electron microscopy. The liver was found to be the main target organ, whereas in other internal organs the pathological changes were insignificant. Ebola virus reproduction was demonstrated only in cells of the mononuclear phagocyte system.
PMID: 8236944 [PubMed - indexed for MEDLINE]

2539. FEBS Lett. 1993 May 24;323(1-2):183-7.

The GP-protein of Marburg virus contains the region similar to the 'immunosuppressive domain' of oncogenic retrovirus P15E proteins.

Bukreyev A(1), Volchkov VE, Blinov VM, Netesov SV.

Author information: (1)NPO VECTOR, Institute of Molecular Biology, Koltsovo, Novosibirsk Region, Russian Federation.

cDNA was synthesized and cloned on the template of the genomic RNA of Marburg virus (strain Popp). Recombinant plasmids with specific cDNA inserts were selected and sequenced. The length of the open reading frame encoding the GP-protein is 681 amino acids. GP-protein is proposed to be an integral membrane protein. Computer-assisted comparison of the deduced amino acid sequence with those of different viruses revealed significant homology with the GP-protein of Ebola virus and with the 'immunosuppressive domain' of the P15E envelope proteins of some oncogenic retroviruses.
PMID: 8495737 [PubMed - indexed for MEDLINE]

2540. FEBS Lett. 1993 May 3;322(1):41-6.

The VP35 and VP40 proteins of filoviruses. Homology between Marburg and Ebola viruses.

Bukreyev AA(1), Volchkov VE, Blinov VM, Netesov SV.

Author information: (1)Institute of Molecular Biology, Koltsovo, Novosibirsk Region, Russian Federation.

The fragments of genomic RNA sequences of Marburg (MBG) and Ebola (EBO) viruses are reported. These fragments were found to encode the VP35 and VP40 proteins. The canonic sequences were revealed before and after each open reading frame. It is suggested that these sequences are mRNA extremities and at the same time the regulatory elements for mRNA transcription. Homology between the MBG and EBO proteins was discovered.
PMID: 8482365 [PubMed - indexed for MEDLINE]

2541. Zh Mikrobiol Epidemiol Immunobiol. 1993 May-Jun;(3):99-105.

[Ebola hemorrhagic fever].

[Article in Russian]

Titenko AM.
PMID: 8067102 [PubMed - indexed for MEDLINE]

2542. J Clin Invest. 1993 Apr;91(4):1301-9.

Replication of Marburg virus in human endothelial cells. A possible mechanism for the development of viral hemorrhagic disease.

Schnittler HJ(1), Mahner F, Drenckhahn D, Klenk HD, Feldmann H.

Author information: (1)Institut für Virologie, Philipps-Universität Marburg, Germany.

Marburg and Ebola virus, members of the family Filoviridae, cause a severe hemorrhagic disease in humans and primates. The disease is characterized as a pantropic virus infection often resulting in a fulminating shock associated with hemorrhage, and death. All known histological and pathophysiological parameters of the disease are not sufficient to explain the devastating symptoms. Previous studies suggested a nonspecific destruction of the endothelium as a possible mechanism. Concerning the important regulatory functions of the endothelium (blood pressure, anti-thrombogenicity, homeostasis), we examined Marburg virus replication in primary cultures of human endothelial cells and organ cultures of human umbilical cord veins. We show here that Marburg virus replicates in endothelial cells almost as well as in monkey kidney cells commonly used for virus propagation. Our data support the concept that the destruction of endothelial cells resulting from Marburg virus replication is a possible mechanism responsible for the hemorrhagic disease and the shock syndrome typical of this infection.

PMCID: PMC288099 PMID: 8473483 [PubMed - indexed for MEDLINE]

2543. J Virol. 1993 Mar;67(3):1203-10.

Marburg virus gene 4 encodes the virion membrane protein, a type I transmembrane glycoprotein.

Will C(1), Mühlberger E, Linder D, Slenczka W, Klenk HD, Feldmann H.

Author information: (1)Institut für Virologie, Philipps-Universität, Marburg, Germany.

Gene 4 of Marburg virus, strain Musoke, was subjected to nucleotide sequence analysis. It is 2,844 nucleotides long and extends from genome position 5821 to position 8665 (EMBL Data Library, emnew: MVREPCYC [accession no. Z12132]). The gene is flanked by transcriptional signal sequences (start signal, 3'-UACUUCUUGUAAUU-5'; termination signal, 3'-UAAUUCUUUUU-5') which are conserved in all Marburg virus genes. The major open reading frame encodes a polypeptide of 681 amino acids (M(r), 74,797). After in vitro transcription and translation, as well as expression in Escherichia coli, this protein was identified by its immunoreactivity with specific antisera as the unglycosylated form of the viral membrane glycoprotein (GP). The GP is characterized by the following four different domains: (i) a hydrophobic signal peptide at the amino terminus (1 to 18), (ii) a predominantly hydrophilic external domain (19 to 643), (iii) a hydrophobic transmembrane anchor (644 to 673), and (iv) a small hydrophilic cytoplasmic tail at the carboxy terminus (674 to 681). Amino acid analysis indicated that the signal peptide is removed from the mature GP. The GP therefore has the structural features of a type I transmembrane glycoprotein. The external domain of the protein has 19 N-glycosylation sites and several clusters of hydroxyamino acids and proline residues that are likely to be the attachment sites for about 30 O-glycosidic carbohydrate chains. The region extending from positions 585 to 610 shows significant homology to a domain observed in the envelope proteins of several retroviruses and Ebola virus that has been suspected to be responsible for immunosuppressive properties of these viruses. A second open reading frame of gene 4 has the coding capacity for an unidentified polypeptide 112 amino acids long.

PMCID: PMC237485 PMID: 8437211 [PubMed - indexed for MEDLINE]

2544. Trans R Soc Trop Med Hyg. 1993 Mar-Apr;87(2):162.

The yellow fever epidemic in Ethiopia, 1961-1962: retrospective serological evidence for concomitant Ebola or Ebola-like virus infection.

Tignor GH(1), Casals J, Shope RE.

Author information: (1)Yale University School of Medicine, Department of Epidemiology and Public Health, New Haven, CT 06510.

PMID: 8337716 [PubMed - indexed for MEDLINE]

2545. Vopr Virusol. 1993 Mar-Apr;38(2):54-8.

[Research with the Marburg, Lassa and Ebola viruses].

[Article in Russian]

Pshenichnov VA, Makhlaĭ AA, Mikhaĭlov VV.

PMID: 8059520 [PubMed - indexed for MEDLINE]

2546. Arch Virol. 1993;133(3-4):423-36.

Ebola protein analyses for the determination of genetic organization.

Elliott LH(1), Sanchez A, Holloway BP, Kiley MP, McCormick JB.

Author information: (1)Division of Viral and Rickettsial Diseases, Centers for Disease Control and Prevention, Atlanta, Georgia.

Amino-acid sequencing of the purified major nucleoprotein (NP), VP35 and VP40 from purified Ebola virus proved that they are the protein products of the first three genes, and that the open reading frame (ORF) of the NP begins at nucleotide 470. Because of the many unusual features of the ORFs of Ebola virus, we thought that our conclusions should be substantiated. Comparisons of in vitro-translation products to purified viral proteins were used to demonstrate conclusively that the NP, VP35 and VP40 were the protein products of genes one, two, and three, respectively. Studies using antibodies to synthetic peptides matching the N- and C-termini of the deduced sequences from these genes confirmed these conclusions and that the ORF for the NP begins at nucleotide 470. Subsequent studies confirmed that VP30 is encoded by the fifth gene.

PMID: 8257297 [PubMed - indexed for MEDLINE]

2547. Arch Virol Suppl. 1993;7:81-100.

Molecular biology and evolution of filoviruses.

Feldmann H(1), Klenk HD, Sanchez A.

Author information: (1)Institut für Virologie, Philipps-Universität, Marburg, Federal Republic of Germany.

The family Filoviridae contains extremely pathogenic human viruses causing a fulminating, febrile hemorrhagic disease. Filoviruses are enveloped, filamentous particles with a nonsegmented negative-strand RNA genome showing the gene arrangement 3'-NP-VP35-VP40-GP-VP30-VP24-L-5'. Genes are flanked by highly conserved transcriptional signals and are generally separated by variable intergenic regions. They are transcribed into monocistronic polyadenylated messenger RNAs which contain relatively long 5' and 3' untranslated regions. Seven structural proteins are encoded by the genome of which four form the helical nucleocapsid (NP-VP35-VP30-L), two are membrane-associated (VP40-VP24), and one is a transmembrane glycoprotein (GP). Comparison of filovirus genomes with those of other nonsegmented negative-strand RNA viruses suggest comparable mechanisms of transcription and replication and a common evolutionary lineage for all these viruses. Sequence analyses of single genes, however, showed that filoviruses are more closely related to paramyxoviruses, particularly human respiratory syncytial virus. These data support the concept of the taxonomic order Mononegavirales for all nonsegmented negative-strand RNA viruses and the classification of Marburg virus, Ebola virus, and Reston virus in the family Filoviridae, separate from the families Paramyxoviridae and Rhabdoviridae.

PMID: 8219816 [PubMed - indexed for MEDLINE]

2548. Vopr Virusol. 1993 Jan-Feb;38(1):17-8.

[A comparative evaluation of an immunoenzyme analytical method using a fluorogenic or chromogenic substrate in determining the Marburg virus antigen].

[Article in Russian]

Kutuzov VA, Mikhaĭlov VV, Kruglova SE, Kutuzov VV, Kirillov AP, Krasnianskiĭ VP, Pshenichnov VA, Lebedinskaia EV.

A comparative evaluation of the developed variants of indirect solid-phase enzyme immunoassay using fluorogenic and chromogenic substrates for the determination of Marburg virus antigen was carried out. The resolving capacity of this method was 3.8 x 10(-9) g of protein for the former and 3.1 x 10(-8) g of protein for the latter substrate. Cross titrations demonstrated the lack of common antigens with Ebola virus.

PMID: 8073738 [PubMed - indexed for MEDLINE]

2549. J Infect Dis. 1992 Oct;166(4):753-63.

Pathogenic potential of filoviruses: role of geographic origin of primate host and virus strain.

Fisher-Hoch SP(1), Brammer TL, Trappier SG, Hutwagner LC, Farrar BB, Ruo SL, Brown BG, Hermann LM, Perez-Oronoz GI, Goldsmith CS, et al.

Author information: (1)Special Pathogens Branch, Research Animal Section, Centers for Disease Control, Atlanta, Georgia.

African filoviruses have caused outbreaks of fulminating hemorrhagic fever among humans. In 1989, related filoviruses were isolated from cynomolgus monkeys imported into the United States from the Philippines. The pathogenic potential of these new filoviruses was compared in 16 Asian monkeys (Macaca fascicularis-cynomolgus) and 16 African monkeys (Cercopithecus aethiops-African green) using African filoviruses from Zaire (Ebola virus) and Sudan or Asian filoviruses (Reston and Pennsylvania). African filovirus infections resulted in earlier death (P = .005), had a shorter duration of disease and median incubation period (3-4 vs. 7 days), and had earlier peak viremia (5-7 vs. 7-9 days). African green monkeys showed significantly higher survival than cynomolgus monkeys (P less than .01), and some were asymptomatic as have been humans accidentally infected with Asian filovirus. Rechallenge experiments showed that protection in survivors of filovirus infections against fatal challenge with Ebola (Zaire) virus is unpredictable. The minimal clinical disease observed in humans infected with the Reston strain is consistent with host- and virus-dependent pathogenicity.

PMID: 1527410 [PubMed - indexed for MEDLINE]

2550. Lancet. 1992 Aug 22;340(8817):451-3.

Filovirus clearance in non-human primates.

Fisher-Hoch SP(1), Perez-Oronoz GI, Jackson EL, Hermann LM, Brown BG.

Author information: (1)Special Pathogens Branch, Centers for Disease Control, Atlanta, Georgia 30333.

There has been concern in the USA and Europe about filovirus outbreaks in recently imported monkeys, and possible transmission to human beings. Healthy monkeys have been found to have low-titre immunofluorescence antibody (IFA) to Asian filoviruses (Reston and Pennsylvania viruses) as well as to the African filoviruses that caused fulminating human outbreaks in the 1970s (Ebola [Zaire] and Sudan viruses). We have assessed whether such monkeys are a risk to man. We studied 42 non-human primates; 31 were experimentally infected with African and Asian filoviruses, 6 were infected during a documented Reston filovirus outbreak, and 5 had serological evidence suggestive of recent filovirus infection. During the first 15 days after infection, virus could be routinely recovered from serum or biopsy or necropsy tissue, and Asian filovirus RNA could be detected by polymerase chain reaction. 20 to 600 days after challenge, filovirus could no longer be recovered nor viral RNA detected in 141 serum, liver, spleen, or kidney specimens. Animals surviving filovirus infection develop high-titre, cross-reacting filovirus-specific antibody 14 to 21 days after infection, and this coincides with virus clearance. Healthy monkeys with low-titre filovirus antibody may be regarded as uninfected.

PMID: 1354784 [PubMed - indexed for MEDLINE]

2551. FEBS Lett. 1992 Jul 6;305(3):181-4.

The envelope glycoprotein of Ebola virus contains an immunosuppressive-like domain similar to oncogenic retroviruses.

Volchkov VE(1), Blinov VM, Netesov SV.

Author information: (1)Institute of Molecular Biology, Novosibirsk Region, Russia.

Genomic RNA of a Zaire strain of Ebola virus was cloned, and cDNA inserts specific for the glycoprotein gene were isolated and sequenced. The determined sequence has only one open reading frame encoding 318 amino acids and is part of ORF-4 on the plus RNA strand. The putative transcriptional stop site (3' AAUUCUUUUU 5') and the transcriptional start site (3' AACUACUUCUAAUU..5') were identified. Computer-assisted comparison of the amino acid sequence of the C-terminal part of protein encoded by ORF-4 of Ebola virus with sequences of the proteins present in the SWISSPROT and EMBL banks revealed significant homology with the 'immunosuppressive domain' of the p15E envelope proteins of various oncogenic retroviruses. The possible role of such a homology is discussed.

PMID: 1299611 [PubMed - indexed for MEDLINE]

2552. Am J Trop Med Hyg. 1992 Jun;46(6):664-71.

Outbreak of fatal illness among captive macaques in the Philippines caused by an Ebola-related filovirus.

Hayes CG(1), Burans JP, Ksiazek TG, Del Rosario RA, Miranda ME, Manaloto CR, Barrientos AB, Robles CG, Dayrit MM, Peters CJ.

Author information: (1)U.S. Naval Medical Research Unit No. 2, Manila, Philippines.

Following the detection of an Ebola-like virus in cynomolgus macaques recently imported into the United States from The Philippines, studies were initiated to document transmission at export facilities located in the latter country. At one export facility, 52.8% of 161 monkeys that died over a 2.5-month period were shown to be infected with this virus using an enzyme-linked immunosorbent assay to detect antigen in liver homogenates. A case fatality rate of 82.4% was documented for the infected monkeys. The initial anti-viral antibody prevalence among the captive macaques at this facility was 25.9% (indirect fluorescent antibody titer greater than or equal to 1:16). Followup documented infection of 24.4% of initially seronegative animals and 8.7% of initially seropositive monkeys. Being held in a gang cage versus a single cage was found to be a significant risk factor for subsequent virus infection, and the presence of IFA antibody was shown to predict protection. This study documents unequivocally for the first time the presence of an Ebola-related filovirus in Asia.

PMID: 1621890 [PubMed - indexed for MEDLINE]

2553. J Clin Microbiol. 1992 Apr;30(4):947-50.

Enzyme immunosorbent assay for Ebola virus antigens in tissues of infected primates.

Ksiazek TG(1), Rollin PE, Jahrling PB, Johnson E, Dalgard DW, Peters CJ.

Author information: (1)Disease Assessment Division, U.S. Army Medical Research Institute of Infectious Diseases, Frederick, Maryland 21702-5011.

A sandwich enzyme immunosorbent assay (EIA) using a mixture of mouse monoclonal antibodies for antigen capture and polyclonal hyperimmune rabbit anti-Ebola virus serum for antigen detection was developed and evaluated on the tissues of monkeys naturally or experimentally infected with strains of Ebola viruses. When compared with virus isolation, the antigen detection EIA was both sensitive and specific: 44 of 45 (97.7%) liver homogenates and 38 of 41 (92.7%) spleen homogenates that were culture positive and tested by both techniques were positive for viral antigen, while 85 of 87 (97.7%) culture-negative liver homogenates and 66 of 66 culture-negative spleen homogenates were found to be antigen negative. The assay, initially developed to detect antigens of prototype African strains of Ebola virus, reliably detected related strains of Ebola virus found during two recent outbreaks of Ebola virus infection among imported, quarantined Macaca fascicularis monkeys in the United States. The assay allows economical and rapid testing of large numbers of tissue specimens. Antigen was found in homogenates of spleen and liver and in serum.

PMCID: PMC265191 PMID: 1572982 [PubMed - indexed for MEDLINE]

2554. Lab Anim Sci. 1992 Apr;42(2):152-7.

Combined simian hemorrhagic fever and Ebola virus infection in cynomolgus monkeys.

Dalgard DW(1), Hardy RJ, Pearson SL, Pucak GJ, Quander RV, Zack PM, Peters CJ, Jahrling PB.

Author information: (1)Hazelton Washington, Vienna, VA.

Simian hemorrhagic fever (SHF) virus and a new strain of Ebola virus were isolated concurrently in recently imported cynomolgus monkeys (Macaca fascicularis) being maintained in a quarantine facility. Ebola virus had never been isolated in the U.S. previously and was presumed to be highly pathogenic for humans. A chronology of events including measures taken to address the public health concerns is presented. The clinicopathologic features of the disease were abrupt anorexia, splenomegaly, marked elevations of lactate dehydrogenase, alanine aminotransferase, and aspartate aminotransferase, with less prominent elevations of blood urea nitrogen, creatinine, and other serum chemistry parameters. Histologically, fibrin deposition, hemorrhage, and necrosis of lymphoid cells and reticular mononuclear phagocytes were present in the spleens of SHF and of Ebola virus-infected animals. Intravascular fibrin thrombi and hemorrhage were also present in the renal medulla and multifocally in the gastrointestinal tract. Necrosis of lymphoid and epithelial cells was occasionally noted in the gastrointestinal tract. The histopathologic findings considered specific for Ebola virus infection include hepatocellular necrosis, necrosis of the zona glomerulosa of the adrenal cortex, and interstitial pneumonia, all of which were generally associated with the presence of 1 to 4 mu intracytoplasmic amphophilic inclusion bodies. The disease spread within rooms despite discontinuation of all direct contact with animals, and droplet or aerosol transmission was suspected. Antibody to Ebola virus developed in animal handlers but no clinical disease was noted, suggesting a less virulent strain of virus.(ABSTRACT TRUNCATED AT 250 WORDS)

PMID: 1318446 [PubMed - indexed for MEDLINE]

2555. Vopr Virusol. 1992 Mar-Apr;37(2):110-3.

[Ebola virus reproduction in cell cultures].

[Article in Russian]

Titenko AM, Novozhilov SS, Andaev EI, Borisova TI, Kulikova EV.

Ebola-Zaire virus production in Vero and BGM cells was studied. The CPE developed in both cell cultures. The cell monolayer destruction by 80-90% was seen at a low multiplicity of infection in 7-8 days after virus inoculation. An overlay composition was developed for virus titration using plaque assay. The plaque production was shown to be directly proportional to the virus dose. The curve of Ebola virus production in Vero cell culture fluid was determined. At a multiplicity of infection of 0.01 PFU/cell, the maximum virus titer of 10(6.4) PFU/ml was reached in 7 days postinfection. Specific antisera were generated by inoculation of guinea pigs. Indirect immunofluorescent assay was used for testing of virus-specific antigen and antibody.

PMID: 1279896 [PubMed - indexed for MEDLINE]

2556. J Comp Pathol. 1992 Feb;106(2):137-52.

Association of Ebola-related Reston virus particles and antigen with tissue lesions of monkeys imported to the United States.

Geisbert TW(1), Jahrling PB, Hanes MA, Zack PM.

Author information: (1)Disease Assessment Division, U.S. Army Medical Research Institute of Infectious Diseases, Fort Detrick, Frederick, Maryland 21702-5011. During 1989-1990, an epizootic involving a filovirus closely related to Ebola virus occurred in a Reston, Virginia, primate-holding facility. Tissues were collected from cynomolgus monkeys and examined by electron microscopy and immunohistochemistry for Ebola-related viral antigen. Viral replication was extensive in fixed tissue macrophages, interstitial fibroblasts of many organs, circulating macrophages and monocytes, and was observed less frequently in vascular endothelial cells, hepatocytes, adrenal cortical cells and renal tubular epithelium. Viral replication was observed infrequently in epithelial cells lining ducts or mucous membranes, intestinal epithelial cells, eosinophils and plasma cells. Replication of Reston virus in lymphocytes was never observed, in contrast to reports of lymphocytes of monkeys experimentally infected with the Ebola-Zaire virus. Free filoviral particles were seen in pulmonary alveoli and renal tubular lumina, which correlates with epidemiological evidence of droplet and fomite transmission. Viral infection of interstitial fibroblasts and macrophages caused multisystemic disruptive lesions involving connective tissue. Focal necrosis in organs where viral replication was minimal may have been secondary to ischaemia caused by fibrin deposition and occasional platelet-fibrin thrombi. Immunoelectron microscopy on sections of liver, differentiated viral tubular inclusion masses and precursor material from non-viral tubuloreticular inclusions. Immunohistochemistry showed that the distribution of viral antigen in affected tissue correlated well with ultrastructural localization of virions.

PMID: 1597531 [PubMed - indexed for MEDLINE]

2557. J Gen Virol. 1992 Feb;73 (Pt 2):347-57.

Sequence analysis of the Marburg virus nucleoprotein gene: comparison to Ebola virus and other non-segmented negative-strand RNA viruses.

Sanchez A(1), Kiley MP, Klenk HD, Feldmann H.

Author information: (1)Department of Biology, Georgia State University, Atlanta 30302-4010.

The first 3000 nucleotides from the 3' end of the Marburg virus (MBG) genome were determined from cDNA clones produced from genomic RNA and mRNA. Identified in the sequence was a short putative leader sequence at the extreme 3' end, followed by the complete nucleoprotein (NP) gene. The 5' end of the NP mRNA was determined as was the polyadenylation site for the NP gene. The transcriptional start (3' UUCUUCUUAUAAUU..) and termination (3' ..UAAUUCUUUUU) signals of the MBG NP gene are very similar to those seen with Ebola virus (EBO). In comparison to other non-segmented negative-strand RNA viruses, filovirus transcriptional signals are most similar to members of the Paramyxovirus and Morbillivirus genera. In vitro translation of a run-off transcript containing the entire MBG NP coding region produced an authentic NP. Sequence comparisons of the 3' end of the MBG and EBO genomes revealed weak nucleotide sequence similarity, but the predicted sequence of the first 400 amino acids of these viruses showed a high degree. This homology is encoded in divergent nucleotide sequences through different codon usages and substitutions of similar amino acids. A small region in the middle of the MBG and EBO NP sequences was found to contain a significant amino acid homology with NPs of paramyxoviruses and to a lesser extent with rhabdoviruses. Specific sites of conserved sequence are contained in hydrophobic domains and may have a common function. Alignments of the entire NP amino acid sequences of these viruses also suggest that filoviruses are more closely related to paramyxoviruses than to rhabdoviruses.

PMID: 1538192 [PubMed - indexed for MEDLINE]

2558. Dev Biol Stand. 1992;76:267-74.

Filovirus contamination of cell cultures.

Peters CJ(1), Jahrling PB, Ksiazek TG, Johnson ED, Lupton HW.

Author information: (1)Disease Assessment Division, U.S. Army Medical Research Institute of Infectious Diseases, Fort Detrick, Frederick, MD 21701-5011.

The filoviruses Marburg and Ebola comprise a newly recognized family of viruses. The first filovirus to be isolated was Marburg virus in 1967. This virus was imported in shipments of African green monkeys from Uganda and infected several cell-culture technicians, with serious illness resulting. The rarity of Marburg and Ebola virus transmission, decreasing use of imported African monkeys, and quarantine efforts have presumably been responsible for the lack of additional episodes until 1989, when a new filovirus related to Ebola was isolated from quarantined monkeys in Reston, Virginia. This virus was imported on multiple occasions from a Philippine supplier of cynomolgus macaques as a consequence of an epidemic of acute infections in the foreign holding facility. While quarantine procedures prevented the use of any of these animals in research and the three human infections that occurred were asymptomatic, this episode emphasizes that these little understood viruses have considerable potential for mischief. The finding of antibodies reacting with Ebola viruses in many biomedically important Old World primates, including colonized monkeys in the U.S., emphasizes the need for more research to understand the specificity of the antibodies, spectrum of filovirus strains in nature, potential hosts, and true distribution of the family. The filoviruses grow well in primary and established cell strains and cell lines, and cytopathogenic effects may be absent or require several days to be manifest, leading to the possibility of occult contamination. The known viruses are readily detected by polyclonal and monoclonal antibody staining of cells and by electron microscopy; nucleic acid probes exist to develop more sensitive techniques if warranted.

PMID: 1478345 [PubMed - indexed for MEDLINE]

2559. Med Microbiol Immunol. 1992;181(1):43-55.

Evidence for occurrence of filovirus antibodies in humans and imported monkeys: do subclinical filovirus infections occur worldwide?

Becker S(1), Feldmann H, Will C, Slenczka W.

Author information: (1)Institut für Virologie, Philipps-Universität, Marburg, Federal Republic of Germany.

In the present serological study 120 monkey sera from different species originating from the Philippines, China, Uganda and undetermined sources and several groups of human sera comprising a total of 1288 specimens from people living in Germany were examined for the presence of antibodies directed against filoviruses (Marburg virus, strain Musoke/Ebola virus, subtype Zaire, strain Mayinga/Reston virus). Sera were screened using a filovirus-specific enzyme-linked immunosorbent assay (ELISA). ELISA-positive sera were then confirmed by the indirect immunofluorescence technique, Western blot technique, and a

blocking assay, and declared positive when at least one confirmation test was reactive. Altogether 43.3% of the monkey sera and 6.9% of the human sera reacted positively with at least one of the three different filovirus antigens. The blocking assays show that antibodies, detected in the sera, are directed to specific filovirus antigens and not caused by antigenic cross-reactivity with hitherto unknown agents. Data presented in this report suggest that subclinical filovirus infections may also occur in humans and in subhuman primates. They further suggest that filoviruses are not restricted to the African continent.
PMID: 1579085 [PubMed - indexed for MEDLINE]

2560. World Health Stat Q. 1992;45(2-3):200-7.

Surveillance and control of emerging zoonoses.

Meslin FX(1).

Author information: (1)Division of Communicable Diseases, World Health Organization, Geneva.

Emerging zoonoses are defined as zoonotic diseases caused either by apparently new agents, or by previously known microorganisms, appearing in places or in species in which the disease was previously unknown. New animal diseases with an unknown host spectrum are also included in this definition. Natural animal reservoirs represent a more frequent source of new agents of human disease than the sudden appearance of a completely new agent. Factors explaining the emergence of a zoonotic or potentially zoonotic disease are usually complex, involving mechanisms at the molecular level, such as genetic drift and shift, and modification of the immunological status of individuals and populations. Social and ecological conditions influencing population growth and movement, food habits, the environment and many other factors may play a more important role than changes at the molecular level. Diseases associated with changing farming practices, trade and consumer habits. Bacterial enteric diseases due to Salmonella enteritidis and Echerichia coli 0:157 are examples of diseases associated with changing farming practices and consumer habits. The increasing trade in live animals for animal production and research led to the introduction of the New World screwworm to the Libyan Arab Jamahiriya in 1989 and an Ebola-like virus in monkeys in quarantine facilities in the United States of America. The development of the epidemics of bovine spongiform encephalopathy (BSE) in the United Kingdom is due to multiple factors including the increasing use of ruminant proteins as feed for animals. Diseases associated with changing environmental conditions which influence reservoirs, vectors and/or victim species population parameters.(ABSTRACT TRUNCATED AT 250 WORDS)
PMID: 1462655 [PubMed - indexed for MEDLINE]

2561. MMWR Morb Mortal Wkly Rep. 1991 Oct 11;40(40):684-5, 691.

Update: nonhuman primate importation.

Centers for Disease Control (CDC).

Beginning in November 1989, a number of cynomolgus monkeys (Macaca fascicularis) imported into the United States were found to have been infected with a previously unrecognized Ebola-like filovirus. This report summarizes findings of surveillance and serologic testing of nonhuman primates imported under special permits from June 1990 through September 1991.
PMID: 1656185 [PubMed - indexed for MEDLINE]

2562. J Clin Pathol. 1991 Jun;44(6):521-2.

Rapid identification of Ebola virus and related filoviruses in fluid specimens using indirect immunoelectron microscopy.

Geisbert TW(1), Rhoderick JB, Jahrling PB.

Author information: (1)Disease Assessment Division, US Army Medical Research Institute of Infectious Diseases, Fort Detrick, Frederick, Maryland 21702-5011. Recent filoviral outbreaks in animal primates have raised public awareness of the potential for filoviruses to become a public health concern; methods that efficiently identify these viruses are therefore of high priority. An indirect immunoelectron microscopy method, which uses homologous guinea pig polyclonal antiserum, successfully identified Ebola-related (Reston) virus particles in serum and tissue culture fluid specimens with infectivity titres of 300 plaque forming units (pfu) per ml or more. The sensitivity of this procedure is sufficient to show virus in most acute phase sera, and is equal to that of the antigen capture enzyme linked immunosorbent assay (ELISA). The immunoelectron microscopy fluid technique can differentiate among antigenically distinct filoviruses in less than three hours. It should be valuable in the rapid diagnosis of potential filoviral infections.
PMCID: PMC496840 PMID: 2066435 [PubMed - indexed for MEDLINE]

2563. J Gen Virol. 1991 Mar;72 (Pt 3):677-85.

Sequence of the major nucleocapsid protein gene of pneumonia virus of mice: sequence comparisons suggest structural homology between nucleocapsid proteins of pneumoviruses, paramyxoviruses, rhabdoviruses and filoviruses.

Barr J(1), Chambers P, Pringle CR, Easton AJ.

Author information: (1)Department of Biological Sciences, University of Warwick, Coventry, U.K.

The complete nucleotide sequence of gene 3 of pneumonia virus of mice has been determined, and the 5' end of the mRNA mapped using a modification of the polymerase chain reaction technique. The gene contains a single open reading frame, beginning with a 5'-proximal AUG initiation codon, encoding a polypeptide with a predicted Mr of 43141. Expression of the gene 3 protein in Escherichia coli and in vitro showed that it reacted with virus-specific antiserum and comigrated with the major nucleocapsid (N) polypeptide. The predicted amino acid sequence has extensive identity with that of the N protein of human respiratory syncytial virus. Comparisons with the amino acid sequences of N proteins of other paramyxoviruses, vesicular stomatitis virus and Ebola virus suggest that these proteins may have retained much of the same structure. These regions of conserved structure would most likely have the common functions of RNA binding and protein/protein interactions in the virus nucleocapsid.
PMID: 1848602 [PubMed - indexed for MEDLINE]

2564. Lancet. 1991 Feb 16;337(8738):425-6.

Seroepidemiological study of filovirus related to Ebola in the Philippines.

Miranda ME, White ME, Dayrit MM, Hayes CG, Ksiazek TG, Burans JP.

PMID: 1671441 [PubMed - indexed for MEDLINE]

2565. Dev Biol Stand. 1991;75:183-9.

Virus zoonoses and their potential for contamination of cell cultures.

Mahy BW(1), Dykewicz C, Fisher-Hoch S, Ostroff S, Tipple M, Sanchez A.

Author information: (1)Division of Viral and Rickettsial Diseases, Centers for Disease Control, Atlanta, GA 30333.

Silent virus infections of laboratory animals present a human health hazard, from direct exposure and from contamination of biological products for human use. Here we report two recent examples. In 1989, an outbreak of lymphocytic choriomeningitis virus (LCMV) infections was recognized among workers at a cancer research center after an animal caretaker developed viral meningitis. Investigation revealed that multiple tumor cell lines at the facility were infected with LCMV, as were research animals injected with these cell lines. Of 82 workers tested, eight (10%) were found to have been infected. The infected workers were more likely than other animal handlers to report handling athymic (nude) mice (p less than .0.007). The number of nude mice used in this facilty had increased five-fold in the previous year, possibly explaining the timing of the outbreak. This is the first reported LCMV outbreak since 1975, and the first to implicate nude mice as a source of human LCMV infections. In November 1989 and January 1990, infections caused by two distinct Ebola-like filoviruses were discovered in non-human primates at quarantine facilities in Virginia and Pennsylvania. Although 22 persons were considered to have high- or medium-risk exposures for Ebola infection, no Ebola-compatible illnesses occurred. One of the medium-risk persons had Ebola IgG antibodies confirmed by IFA and Western blot. Rigorous use of barrier precautions may have limited exposure and infection with these filoviruses. In February 1990, new groups of filovirus-infected monkeys were identified in Virginia and in Texas. Seroconversion occurred in four animal handlers, including one to very high titer, but again no illness was observed.(ABSTRACT TRUNCATED AT 250 WORDS)

PMID: 1794619 [PubMed - indexed for MEDLINE]

2566. Lancet. 1990 Dec 22-29;336(8730):1591.

Detection of Ebola-like viruses by immunofluorescence.

Rollin PE, Ksiazek TG, Jahrling PB, Haines M, Peters CJ.

PMID: 1979412 [PubMed - indexed for MEDLINE]

2567. Science. 1990 Oct 26;250(4980):502.

Not enough monkey business.

Palca J.

PMID: 2237402 [PubMed - indexed for MEDLINE]

2568. Science. 1990 Oct 26;250(4980):492.

Filovirus infection in newly imported monkeys.

Roper WL.

Comment on Science. 1990 Jun 1;248(4959):1071-3.

PMID: 2237399 [PubMed - indexed for MEDLINE]

2569. J Clin Pathol. 1990 Oct;43(10):813-6.

Use of immunoelectron microscopy to show Ebola virus during the 1989 United States epizootic.

Geisbert TW(1), Jahrling PB.

Author information: (1)Disease Assessment Division, United States Army Medical Research Institute of Infectious Diseases, Fort Detrick, Frederick, Maryland 21701-5011.

A filovirus, serologically related to Ebola virus, was detected by post-embedment immunoelectron microscopical examination of MA-104 cells. These had been infected by inoculation with serum samples obtained during the 1989 epizootic in cynomolgus monkeys (Macaca fascicularis), imported from the Philippines and maintained at Reston, Virginia, USA, a primate holding facility. The immunoelectron microscopy method, when used in conjunction with standard transmission electron microscopy (TEM) of infected cells, provided consistent results and was simple to perform in this epizootic. It is concluded that immunoelectron microscopy is potentially useful in the direct immunological diagnosis of Ebola and related filoviral infections (such as Marburg) in clinical samples obtained from those with acute infection.

PMCID: PMC502829 PMID: 2229429 [PubMed - indexed for MEDLINE]

2570. MMWR Morb Mortal Wkly Rep. 1990 Jun 22;39(24):404-5.

Update: filovirus infection associated with contact with nonhuman primates or their tissues.

Centers for Disease Control (CDC).

PMID: 2112686 [PubMed - indexed for MEDLINE]

2571. Rev Prat. 1990 Jun 21;40(18):1656-9.

[The other types of viral hepatitis].

[Article in French]

Miguet JP(1), Coaquette A, Bresson-Hadni S, Lab M.

Author information: (1)Service d'hépatologie, CHU Jean-Minjoz, Besançon.

Hepatitis due to viruses other than A, B, C, D, E are numerous but uncommon in adults. Among the group of Herpesviridae (HSV, CMV, EBV, VZV), clinical hepatitis is usually suggestive of disseminated viral infection. Fulminant hepatitis occasionally observed in immunocompromised hosts are due to HSV, and VZV, but exceptionally to EBV. Many new techniques using specific monoclonal antibodies permit an accurate and fast diagnosis. Three drugs (vidarabine, acyclovir, ribavirine) have been shown to be efficient in the treatment of severe forms of the disease. Hepatitis due to exotic viruses (Amaril, Ebola, Lassa) are exceptional in France, but require specific prophylactic measures.
PMID: 2164704 [PubMed - indexed for MEDLINE]

2572. Science. 1990 Jun 1;248(4959):1071-3.

Import rules threaten research on primates.

Palca J.

Comment in Science. 1990 Oct 26;250(4980):492.

PMID: 2160732 [PubMed - indexed for MEDLINE]

2573. MMWR Morb Mortal Wkly Rep. 1990 May 4;39(17):296-7.

Update: evidence of filovirus infection in an animal caretaker in a research/service facility.

Centers for Disease Control (CDC).

PMID: 2109176 [PubMed - indexed for MEDLINE]

2574. MMWR Morb Mortal Wkly Rep. 1990 Apr 27;39(16):266-7; 273.

Update: filovirus infections among persons with occupational exposure to nonhuman primates.

Centers for Disease Control (CDC).

PMID: 2109172 [PubMed - indexed for MEDLINE]

2575. MMWR Morb Mortal Wkly Rep. 1990 Apr 6;39(13):221.

Update: filovirus infection in animal handlers.

Centers for Disease Control (CDC).

PMID: 2107388 [PubMed - indexed for MEDLINE]

2576. Science. 1990 Mar 30;247(4950):1538.

Imported monkey puzzle.

Sun M.

Comment in Science. 1990 Jun 22;248(4962):1473.

PMID: 2321012 [PubMed - indexed for MEDLINE]

2577. Nature. 1990 Mar 29;344(6265):369.

US shuts down monkey trade.

Anderson GC.

PMID: 2320102 [PubMed - indexed for MEDLINE]

2578. Nature. 1990 Mar 22;344(6264):280.

Monkey imports may be curtailed in US.

Anderson GC.

PMID: 2314464 [PubMed - indexed for MEDLINE]

2579. Lancet. 1990 Mar 3;335(8688):502-5.

Preliminary report: isolation of Ebola virus from monkeys imported to USA.

Jahrling PB(1), Geisbert TW, Dalgard DW, Johnson ED, Ksiazek TG, Hall WC, Peters CJ.

Author information: (1)Disease Assessment Division, US Army Medical Research Institute of Infectious Disease, Fort Detrick, Frederick, MD 21701.

An epizootic caused by an Ebola-related filovirus and by simian haemorrhagic fever virus began among cynomolgus monkeys in a US quarantine facility after introduction of monkeys from the Philippines. This incident, the first in which a filovirus has been isolated from non-human primates without deliberate infection, raises the possibility that cynomolgus monkeys could be a reservoir of Ebola virus infection.

PMID: 1968529 [PubMed - indexed for MEDLINE]

2580. Wkly Epidemiol Rec. 1990 Feb 16;65(7):45-7.

Ebola virus.

[Article in English, French]

[No authors listed]

PMID: 2167118 [PubMed - indexed for MEDLINE]

2581. Can Dis Wkly Rep. 1990 Jan 27;16(4):17-8.

Ebola virus infection in imported primates--United States.

[Article in English, French]

[No authors listed]

In late November 1989, Ebola virus was isolated from cynomolgus monkeys (Macaca fascicularis) imported into the United States from the Philippines via Amsterdam and New York. During quarantine in a primate facility in Virginia, numerous macaques died, some with findings consistent with simian hemorrhagic fever (SHF). The US Army Medical Research Institute of Infectious Diseases tested 10 animals and, from 3, isolated SHF from tissues and serum; however, 5 other animals of the 10 tested were positive for Ebola virus. Monkeys from a later shipment quarantined in a second room also had unusually high mortality and were tested by a rapid antigen detection enzyme-linked immunosorbent assay. Ebola viral antigen was detected in serum and/or tissues from 7 of these monkeys. Primary liver material from animals in both rooms exhibited particles with typical filovirus morphology by electron microscopy and Ebola virus antigen by immunohistochemistry.

PMID: 2302743 [PubMed - indexed for MEDLINE]

2582. MMWR Morb Mortal Wkly Rep. 1990 Jan 19;39(2):22-4, 29-30.

Update: Ebola-related filovirus infection in nonhuman primates and interim guidelines for handling nonhuman primates during transit and quarantine.

Centers for Disease Control (CDC).

PMID: 2104655 [PubMed - indexed for MEDLINE]

2583. Science. 1990 Jan 19;247(4940):279-80.

Emerging viruses, emerging threat.

Culliton BJ.

PMID: 2153314 [PubMed - indexed for MEDLINE]

2584. J Med Primatol. 1990;19(6):519-35.

Primate viral diseases in perspective.

Kalter SS(1), Heberling RL.

Author information: (1)Virus Reference Laboratory, WHO Collaborating Center, for Reference and Research in Simian Viruses, San Antonio, TX.

The recent occurrence of fatal Herpesvirus simiae (B virus) infection in human subjects has again focused the attention of primatologists on this virus. B virus, however, is only one of a number of viral diseases that plays a role in primate colony management. This report is to emphasize to the primatologist a number of viruses other than H. simiae, with high morbidity and mortality rates, of importance for health management of nonhuman primate animal colonies. This concept is supported by the recent occurrence in colonies of nonhuman primates of simian hemorrhagic fever virus, SA8, herpesvirus, respiratory syncytial virus, encephalomyocarditis virus, Ebola virus, and simian immunodeficiency viruses.

PMID: 2174083 [PubMed - indexed for MEDLINE]

2585. MMWR Morb Mortal Wkly Rep. 1989 Dec 8;38(48):831-2, 837-8.

Ebola virus infection in imported primates--Virginia, 1989.

Centers for Disease Control (CDC).

PMID: 2511410 [PubMed - indexed for MEDLINE]

2586. Trans R Soc Trop Med Hyg. 1989 Nov-Dec;83(6):851-4.

Arbovirus infections and viral haemorrhagic fevers in Uganda: a serological survey in Karamoja district, 1984.

Rodhain F(1), Gonzalez JP, Mercier E, Helynck B, Larouze B, Hannoun C.

Author information: (1)Unité d'Ecologie des Systèmes Vectoriels, Institut Pasteur, Paris, France.

Sera collected in May 1984 from 132 adult residents of Karamoja district, Uganda, were examined by haemagglutination inhibition tests for antibodies against selected arboviruses, namely Chikungunya and Semliki Forest alphaviruses (Togaviridae); dengue type 2, Wesselsbron, West Nile, yellow fever and Zika flaviviruses (Flaviviridae); Bunyamwera, Ilesha and Tahyna bunyaviruses (Bunyaviridae); and Sicilian sandfly fever phlebovirus (Bunyaviridae); and by immunofluorescence tests against certain haemorrhagic fever viruses, Lassa fever arenavirus (Arenaviridae), Ebola-Sudan, Ebola-Zaïre and Marburg filoviruses (Filoviridae), Crimean-Congo haemorrhagic fever nairovirus and Rift Valley fever phlebovirus (Bunyaviridae). Antibodies against Chikungunya virus were the most prevalent (47%), followed by flavivirus antibodies (16%), which were probably due mainly to West Nile virus. No evidence of yellow fever or dengue virus circulation was observed. A few individuals had antibodies against Crimean-Congo haemorrhagic fever, Lassa, Ebola and Marburg viruses, suggesting that these viruses all circulate in the area.

PMID: 2559514 [PubMed - indexed for MEDLINE]

2587. Res Virol. 1989 Jul-Aug;140(4):319-31.

Antibody prevalence against haemorrhagic fever viruses in randomized representative Central African populations.

Gonzalez JP(1), Josse R, Johnson ED, Merlin M, Georges AJ, Abandja J, Danyod M, Delaporte E, Dupont A, Ghogomu A, et al.

Author information: (1)Institut Français de Recherche Scientifique, Développement en Coopération, Bangui.

Between 1985 and 1987, 5,070 randomly selected persons living in 6 central African countries (Cameroon, Central African Republic, Chad, Congo, Equatorial Guinea and Gabon) were checked for serological evidence of haemorrhagic fever. Rural and urban areas were studied, including ecoclimatic zones ranging from dry savana to tropical rain forest. Virus-reactive antibodies were found with all antigens tested, and the global prevalence of positive sera was distributed as follows: Crimean-Congo haemorrhagic fever virus, 0.22%; Rift Valley fever virus, 0.18%; Ebola virus, 12.40%; Marburg virus, 0.39%; Lassa virus, 0.06%; and Hantaan virus, 6.15%. A significant variation in antibody prevalence was observed within the study regions. Association between the viruses was not observed.

PMID: 2505350 [PubMed - indexed for MEDLINE]

2588. Rev Infect Dis. 1989 May-Jun;11 Suppl 4:S790-3.

Firsthand clinical observations of hemorrhagic manifestations in Ebola hemorrhagic fever in Zaire.

Sureau PH(1).

Author information: (1)Viral Hemorrhagic Diseases Laboratory, Institut Pasteur, Paris, France.

About 5 weeks after the beginning of the outbreak of Ebola virus fever in Yambuku, Zaire, several acute cases of the disease were observed. All of those affected had the following common signs and symptoms: sudden onset of high fever, with chills, headache, myalgia, anorexia, nausea, abdominal pain, sore throat, expressionless face, and profound prostration. In some cases, on around the fifth day of the acute phase, the appearance of an exanthematous rash on the trunk announced the hemorrhagic manifestations: hemorrhagic conjunctivitis, bleeding ulcerations in the mouth and on the lips, gingival bleeding, hematemesis, and melena; epistaxis, ear bleeding, hematuria, and postpartum hemorrhages were also reported. All these hemorrhagic cases had a fatal outcome within about a week. The hemorrhagic manifestations were less severe in the cases that occurred by the end of the outbreak than in the first reported cases. Hemorrhagic manifestations were less frequent and less severe, or even absent, in the nonfatal cases (convalescents, serologically confirmed). No biologic investigation of the hemostatic impairment could be performed under the emergency conditions of this field study.

PMID: 2749110 [PubMed - indexed for MEDLINE]

2589. Rev Infect Dis. 1989 May-Jun;11 Suppl 4:S750-61.

Prospects for treatment of viral hemorrhagic fevers with ribavirin, a broad-spectrum antiviral drug.

Huggins JW(1).

Author information: (1)Department of Antiviral Studies, U.S. Army Medical Research Institute of Infectious Diseases, Frederick, Maryland 21701-5011.

Ribavirin, a broad-spectrum antiviral drug, is active against hemorrhagic fever viruses (with the exception of Ebola virus) in cell culture systems. In model infections with arenaviruses in guinea pigs and monkeys, ribavirin has demonstrated both prophylactic and therapeutic efficacy. In therapeutic studies it has not prevented late-onset neurologic disease. In human cases of Lassa fever, it significantly reduces mortality when administered before day 7 of illness to persons at high risk. In rodents and monkeys infected with Rift Valley fever virus, ribavirin therapy resulted in reduced mortality; prophylactic administration to volunteers infected with sandfly fever virus, Sicilian strain, prevented development of illness. Ribavirin increased the number of survivors and the mean time to death in suckling mice infected with Crimean-Congo hemorrhagic fever virus and in suckling mice infected with Hantaan virus. In the People's Republic of China, ribavirin significantly reduced mortality in patients with hemorrhagic fever with renal syndrome. Ribavirin has not been effective in animal models of filoviral and flaviviral infections. The only important adverse effect of ribavirin in humans is manageable, reversible anemia.

PMID: 2546248 [PubMed - indexed for MEDLINE]

2590. Rev Infect Dis. 1989 May-Jun;11 Suppl 4:S730-5.

Epidemiology of hemorrhagic fever viruses.

LeDuc JW(1).

Author information: (1)Disease Assessment Division, U.S. Army Medical Research Institute of Infectious Diseases, Frederick, Maryland 21701-5001.

Twelve distinct viruses associated with hemorrhagic fever in humans are classified among four families: Arenaviridae, which includes Lassa, Junin, and Machupo viruses; Bunyaviridae, which includes Rift Valley fever, Crimean-Congo hemorrhagic fever, and Hantaan viruses; Filoviridae, which includes Marburg and Ebola viruses; and Flaviviridae, which includes yellow fever, dengue, Kyasanur Forest disease, and Omsk viruses. Most hemorrhagic fever viruses are zoonoses, with the possible exception of the four dengue viruses, which may continually circulate among humans. Hemorrhagic fever viruses are found in both temperate and tropical habitats and generally infect both sexes and all ages, although the age and sex of those infected are frequently influenced by the possibility of occupational exposure. Transmission to humans is frequently by bite of an infected tick or mosquito or via aerosol from infected rodent hosts. Aerosol and nosocomial transmission are especially important with Lassa, Junin, Machupo, Crimean-Congo hemorrhagic fever, Marburg, and Ebola viruses. Seasonality of hemorrhagic fever among humans is influenced for the most part by the dynamics of infected arthropod or vertebrate hosts. Mammals, especially rodents, appear to be important natural hosts for many hemorrhagic fever viruses. The transmission cycle for each hemorrhagic fever virus is distinct and is dependent upon the characteristics of the primary vector species and the possibility for its contact with humans.

PMID: 2546247 [PubMed - indexed for MEDLINE]

2591. Trans R Soc Trop Med Hyg. 1989 May-Jun;83(3):407-9.

Antibodies to haemorrhagic fever viruses in Madagascar populations.

Mathiot CC(1), Fontenille D, Georges AJ, Coulanges P.

Author information: (1)Institut Pasteur, Bangui, Central African Republic.

Sera of 381 adult people from 5 areas in Madagascar were tested by the indirect immunofluorescence method for antibodies against Congo-Crimean haemorrhagic fever and Rift Valley fever viruses (Bunyaviridae), Ebola (strains Zaire and Sudan) and Marburg viruses (Filoviridae), and Lassa virus (Arenaviridae). The highest prevalence rate was that of Ebola virus (4.5%). As no haemorrhagic syndrome has been found associated with this virus, the possible presence of a less pathogenic, antigenically related, strain is discussed. The prevalences of Congo-Crimean haemorrhagic fever and Rift Valley viruses were very low, despite previous viral isolations from potential vectors. No serum reacted against Lassa or Marburg antigens. The results are analysed in the light of the geographical and bioecological characteristics of Madagascar, which is a true 'microcontinent' very different from the African mainland.

PMID: 2515626 [PubMed - indexed for MEDLINE]

2592. Virology. 1989 May;170(1):81-91.

The nucleoprotein gene of Ebola virus: cloning, sequencing, and in vitro expression.

Sanchez A(1), Kiley MP, Holloway BP, McCormick JB, Auperin DD.

Author information: (1)Division of Viral Diseases, Centers for Disease Control, Atlanta, Georgia 30333

Genomic and messenger RNAs of a Zaire strain of Ebola virus were cloned, and inserts specific for the nucleoprotein gene were isolated and sequenced. The nucleoprotein gene is located proximal to the 3' end of the genome and is preceeded by a putative leader sequence. The gene begins with the transcriptional start site sequence 3'-UACUCCUUCUAAUU..., and ends with the polyadenylation site sequence 3'-... UAAUUCUUUUUU. The predicted coding region is 2217 bases in length and encodes a protein that contains 739 amino acids, with a calculated molecular weight of 83.3 kDa. The protein has an approximate net charge of -30 and can be divided into a hydrophobic N-terminal half and a hydrophilic and highly acidic C-terminal half. An in vitro transcript, generated from plasmid DNA containing the entire coding region, directs the synthesis of authentic nucleoprotein in a rabbit reticulocyte lysate system. The genomic organization and transcriptional signals of Ebola are similar to those of other nonsegmented, negative-strand RNA viruses, but nucleic acid or amino acid sequence comparisons indicate a lack of similarity.

PMID: 2718390 [PubMed - indexed for MEDLINE]

2593. Johns Hopkins Mag. 1989 Feb;41(1):10-1.

A syringe that self-destructs.

Newman A.

PIP: The reuse of unsterilized syringes is spreading AIDS, hepatitis B and the African Ebola-Marburg virus. In the US 25% of the AIDS cases are related to intravenous drug abuse. In developing countries syringe reuse is related to poor health care delivery systems. In these countries syringes are used over 5 times before sterilization; in some countries the syringes are distributed by people who sell injections of vitamins and antibiotics. In 1986 Halsey challenged the medical community to design a syringe that would not transmit these diseases, and shortly thereafter a separate challenge was issued by the World Health Organization. The requirements of this syringe are its self destruction after use, little requiring retraining of medical personal, and no more than 1 cent to the cost, and be simple to make. These challenges brought 70 various syringe entries and all but 3 were eliminated. The Hopkins syringe is similar to a regular syringe except it has a polymer insert that seals up after one use. When water flows around the polymer insert it swells and closes off the passageway preventing any liquid from flowing in or out of the syringe. Another syringe seals up in 2.5 minutes which allows the health worker time to draw and inject a patient before the syringe destructs. By using hydrogels that are already approved for use in contact lenses and food substances, the safety has been tested. Companies looking at production costs estimate that the polymer insert will add only 1/4 of a cent to the cost of a syringe. PMID: 12282933 [PubMed - indexed for MEDLINE]

2594. Dev Biol Stand. 1989;70:173-9.

Adventitious viral agents in biological products.

Minor P(1).

Author information: (1)National Institute for Biological Standards and Control, South Mimms, Potters Bar, Herts.

The objectives of tests for extraneous agents will be discussed in the light of quality requirements for biological products published over the last twenty years, current developments of novel production methods and products, and past and current virological findings.

PMID: 2547677 [PubMed - indexed for MEDLINE]

2595. J Gen Virol. 1988 Aug;69 (Pt 8):1957-67.

Physicochemical properties of Marburg virus: evidence for three distinct virus strains and their relationship to Ebola virus.

Kiley MP(1), Cox NJ, Elliott LH, Sanchez A, DeFries R, Buchmeier MJ, Richman DD, McCormick JB.

Author information: (1)Division of Viral Diseases, Centers for Disease Control, Atlanta, Georgia 30333

The physicochemical and antigenic properties of three groups of Marburg (MBG) virus isolates, separated temporally and geographically, were compared to each other and to another member of the same family, Ebola (EBO) virus. Each MBG isolate contained seven virion proteins, one of which was a glycosylated surface protein. Peptide mapping of glycoproteins, nucleoproteins (NP) and viral structural protein (VP40) demonstrated extensive sequence conservation in the proteins of viruses isolated over a 13-year period, but homology was not evident in VP24. Some homology between the NPs of MBG and EBO was observed. A close antigenic relationship between MBG strains was found by radioimmunoassay but no evidence was found of antigenic cross-reactivity with EBO viruses. MBG virion proteins are produced from virus-specific monocistronic mRNA species. Five of the seven viral proteins were produced by in vitro translation of these RNAs. MBG virions contained one RNA species with an Mr of 4.2 x 10(6) and virions had a density of 1.14 g/ml in potassium tartrate. Virus isolates from different outbreaks had distinct T1 oligonucleotide maps, but had approximately 95% homology in base sequence. No two geographically distinct virus pairs were more closely related to each other than to a third virus isolate. MBG viruses are thus similar to EBO viruses in morphology and other physicochemical properties and are very similar to each other in RNA and protein composition. Each of the three geographically and temporally distinct MBG virus outbreaks appears to have been due to a genetically distinguishable, but antigenically closely related virus strain. In addition, these studies confirm the belief that MBG and EBO viruses are members of the new virus family, the Filoviridae.

PMID: 3404120 [PubMed - indexed for MEDLINE]

2596. Am J Trop Med Hyg. 1988 Mar;38(2):407-10.

Viral hemorrhagic fever antibodies in Nigerian populations.

Tomori O(1), Fabiyi A, Sorungbe A, Smith A, McCormick JB.

Author information: (1)Department of Virology, College of Medicine, University of Ibadan, Nigeria.

Using the immunofluorescence test, a serosurvey for antibodies to five viral agents associated with hemorrhagic febrile infections was conducted with 1,677 human sera from different parts of Nigeria. Three hundred fifty-seven (21.3%) were positive for Lassa virus antibody, while antibodies to Rift Valley fever virus were detected in 42 (2.5%) of the sera. Testing for Rift Valley fever virus antibody was confirmed by plaque reduction neutralization test. Antibodies to Ebola and Marburg viruses were detected in 30 and 29 sera, respectively. Of the 357 Lassa virus antibody-positive sera, 297 (83.2%) were positive for Lassa only. In contrast, sera positive for Marburg were positive in combination with Lassa, Ebola, or Rift Valley fever viruses. Antibodies to Lassa and Rift Valley fever viruses were found in all locations in Nigeria, whereas Ebola and Marburg antibodies were found mainly in the northern savanna zones of Benue and Gongola, but not in the rain forest area of Ondo.

PMID: 3128130 [PubMed - indexed for MEDLINE]

2597. MMWR Morb Mortal Wkly Rep. 1988 Feb 26;37 Suppl 3:1-16.

Management of patients with suspected viral hemorrhagic fever.

Centers for Disease Control (CDC).

PMID: 3126390 [PubMed - indexed for MEDLINE]

2598. Bull Soc Pathol Exot Filiales. 1988;81(4):679-82.

[Serological study of the virus responsible for hemorrhagic fever in an urban population of Cameroon].

[Article in French]

Paix MA(1), Poveda JD, Malvy D, Bailly C, Merlin M, Fleury HJ.

Author information: (1)Laboratoire de Virologie, Université de Bordeaux II, France.

A sero-epidemiological study of Hemorrhagic Fever Viruses in a urban population of Cameroon. The authors report the results of a sero-epidemiological survey undertaken in a urban population of Cameroon and concerning Congo, Rift (RVF), Lassa, Ebola, Marburg and Yellow Fever Viruses. On 375 human sera tested, 1.06% show antibodies against RVF virus and 1.87% are positive for anti-Ebola antibodies thus yielding evidence that these two viruses are present in this area of Cameroon. 33.75% have antibodies against Yellow Fever Virus as determined with an Hemagglutination-inhibition test. This quite high percentage, in spite of the weak specificity of the method for this virus, could raise the problem of the opportunity of a vaccination campaign. No antibody to Marburg, Lassa or Congo viruses is detected.

PMID: 3064937 [PubMed - indexed for MEDLINE]

2599. Trans R Soc Trop Med Hyg. 1988;82(5):761-6.

A study of viral and rickettsial exposure and causes of fever in Juba, southern Sudan.

Woodruff PW(1), Morrill JC, Burans JP, Hyams KC, Woody JN.

Author information: (1)US Naval Medical Research Unit No. 3, Cairo, Egypt.

Patients presenting at the Juba Teaching Hospital, either with fever of undetermined origin or with a clinical cause of fever, gave evidence of exposure to a wide range of viral and rickettsial agents. Serological tests showed high antibody levels to flaviviruses (56.9%) and alphaviruses (29.2%), with lesser levels of bunyamweraviruses (3.8%), Rift Valley fever (2.3%), and sandfly fever (0.75%). Flavivirus exposure was significantly associated with clinical evidence of liver disease; repeated exposure to flaviviruses was particularly prevalent in those with poor sanitation and who had received previous injections. A significant focus of Ebola and Marburg exposure in Juba has been identified. Clinical evidence of liver disease was evident in 37% of patients studied, and 24.6% were HBsAg positive. The first 2 HIV-positive individuals from the southern Sudan are reported, including one with clinical AIDS. A high prevalence of positive antibodies to Rickettsia typhi in the population indicated that murine typhus was common locally. This study indicates the need for further public health measures in the southern Sudan to control the spread of these infections.

PMID: 2855284 [PubMed - indexed for MEDLINE]

2600. Southeast Asian J Trop Med Public Health. 1987 Sep;18(3):390-1.

Pathophysiology of shock and haemorrhage in viral haemorrhagic fevers.

Fisher-Hoch S(1).

Author information: (1)Special Pathogens Branch, Centers for Disease Control, Atlanta, Ga 30333.

PMID: 3433168 [PubMed - indexed for MEDLINE]

2601. Baillieres Clin Gastroenterol. 1987 Apr;1(2):211-30.

Viral diseases involving the liver.

Tandon BN, Acharya SK.

Even though HAV, HBV and HNANB viruses are responsible for most of the viral hepatitis cases, many other viruses have been reported to cause hepatic injury. These viruses may involve the liver, either as part of a systemic illness (e.g. EBV, CMV, HSV) or as the primary target organ (e.g. yellow fever virus, Lassa fever virus, Ebola virus). Clinically overt hepatocellular dysfunction is rare in such viral infections. Biochemical disturbance of hepatic functions shown, for example, by rises in AST and ALT, is a frequent event and indicates hepatic damage. Morphological changes of the liver include varying degrees of hepatic necrosis with a paucity of inflammatory activities. Intranuclear or cytoplasmic inclusion bodies may be characteristic findings in these diseases. Laboratory diagnosis depends upon serology and liver histology. Treatment is still largely supportive in most of these diseases, although recent trials of antiviral agents show promise against some viruses. Chronic sequelae, such as cirrhosis or hepatocellular cancer, are not encountered. More work is needed to elucidate the pathogenesis of hepatic injury in these illnesses.

PMID: 2822180 [PubMed - indexed for MEDLINE]

2602. Virology. 1987 Apr;157(2):414-20.

Identification and analysis of Ebola virus messenger RNA.

Sanchez A, Kiley MP.

Six messenger RNA species of Ebola virus were identified in infected Vero E6 cells. Virion RNA hybridizes to each of the mRNAs, confirming that Ebola virus possesses a negative-stranded RNA genome. The mRNAs are monocristronic transcripts, are synthesized in the presence of actinomycin D, and are polyadenylated. In vitro translation of mRNA preparations results in the synthesis of five authentic viral proteins and a putative unglycosylated form of the glycoprotein, demonstrated by immunoprecipitation with virus-specific antisera and SDS-PAGE. No mRNA species was detected for the polymerase (L protein) gene.

PMID: 2881398 [PubMed - indexed for MEDLINE]

2603. Bull Soc Pathol Exot Filiales. 1987;80(1):51-61.

[Current serologic data on viral hemorrhagic fevers in the Central African Republic].

[Article in French]

Meunier DM, Johnson ED, Gonzalez JP, Georges-Courbot MC, Madelon MC, Georges AJ.

During the years 1984-1985, 1,528 serum samples were taken through out the CAR. Of these sera, 319 (20.8%) contained anti-Filoviridae antibodies (Ebola, Marburg). This figure is higher than those found in Cameroon, Sudan, Gabon and Zaïre. Three zones of the country are particularly exposed, the North-East where the population is in the contact with Sudan Ebola, the South-East where it is in contact with Zaïre Ebola, and the South-West where it is in contact with Sudan Ebola. The authors believe that there could exist either a Central African Ebola strain or an Ebola-Like less pathogenic virus which is responsible for cross reactions. Results concerning Rift Valley Fever virus, Congo virus and Lassa virus seem less interesting. However RVF and Congo strains were isolated.

PMID: 3607998 [PubMed - indexed for MEDLINE]

2604. Bull Soc Pathol Exot Filiales. 1987;80(4):607-12.

[Clinico-epidemiologic and laboratory research on hemorrhagic fevers in Guinea].

[Article in French]

Boiro I(1), Lomonossov NN, Sotsinski VA, Constantinov OK, Tkachenko EA, Inapogui AP, Balde C.

Author information: (1)Université de Conakry, République de Guinée.

In 1982-1983, were reported the cases of haemorrhagic fevers among populations living in the Madina-Ula district of Guinea. Clinico-epidemiological and serological studies (experimental studies) reveal into presumption of Ebola and Lassa fever viruses significance in the etiology of the disease outbreaks. Antibodies to Ebola virus were recognized in 19% from total number of sweating reconvalescent patients with the same clinical features, in order to 8% in healthy local populations. Antibodies to Lassa virus were detected in 3 cases, in 4 cases was revealed Lassa virus antigen in small rodents.

PMID: 3440310 [PubMed - indexed for MEDLINE]

2605. Bull Soc Pathol Exot Filiales. 1987;80(1):68-73.

[Hemorrhagic fever viruses. Principal epidemiologic aspects].

[Article in French]

Fleury HJ.

PMID: 3038354 [PubMed - indexed for MEDLINE]

2606. J Infect. 1986 Sep;13(2):103-6.

Viral haemorrhagic fevers.

Emond RT.

PMID: 3760594 [PubMed - indexed for MEDLINE]

2607. Trop Geogr Med. 1986 Sep;38(3):209-14.

Hemorrhagic fever virus infections in an isolated rainforest area of central Liberia. Limitations of the indirect immunofluorescence slide test for antibody screening in Africa.

Van der Waals FW, Pomeroy KL, Goudsmit J, Asher DM, Gajdusek DC.

Serum samples from 119 healthy individuals and 106 epilepsy patients inhabiting Grand Bassa County, Liberia, were tested for antibodies to hemorrhagic fever viruses (HFV) by indirect immunofluorescence. E6 Vero cells infected with Lassa fever virus (LAS), Rift Valley Fever virus (RVF), Congo Hemorrhagic Fever virus (CON), Marburg virus (MBG) and the Ebola (EBO) virus strains Mayinga (May) and Boniface (Bon) were used as antigen. To obtain reproducible and specific test results sera had to be absorbed extensively with uninfected E6 Vero cells, tested for reactivity to both virus infected and uninfected E6 Vero cells and read blindly by two independent observers. Antibodies to EBO were shown to be highly prevalent (13.4%) in the population of this rainforest area, while prevalences of antibodies to LAS (1.3%), RVF (0.4%) and MBG (1.3%) were much lower. No correlation between past HFV infection and post-encephalitic epilepsy or other reported febrile illnesses could be established.

PMID: 3092415 [PubMed - indexed for MEDLINE]

2608. Blut. 1986 Aug;53(2):115-7.

No evidence of LAV infection in the Republic of Liberia, West Africa, in the year 1973

Neppert J, Göhring S, Schneider W, Wernet P.

Sera collected 13 years ago from 592 residents of the Republic of Liberia have been tested for antibodies to LAV polypeptides. 7 sera were positive by ELISA using two commercially available test kits whereas immunoblotting did not confirm antibodies specific for LAV.

PIP: Liberian sera collected in 1973 from 592 residents of agricultural and iron ore mining companies were tested for LAV (HTLV-III), now known as HIV, by ELISA and western blotting, and no positives were found. The ELISA tests were kits from ELAVIA, Institute Pasteur, France, and VIRAMED, Electro Nucleonics, USA, and the immunoblot method was that of Towbin et al. The subjects included 430 men and non-pregnant women who had no positive findings, and 162 pregnant women at parturition, of whom 7 had positive ELISAs but negative confirmatory western blots. This population had high rates of onchocerciasis, hepatitis B, nematodes, Schistosomas, Marburg virus and Ebola virus. PMID: 3015288 [PubMed - indexed for MEDLINE]

2609. Lancet. 1986 May 17;1(8490):1160.

Seasonal variation in antibodies against Ebola virus in Kenyan fever patients.

Johnson BK, Wambui C, Ocheng D, Gichogo A, Oogo S, Libondo D, Gitau LG, Tukei PM, Johnson ED.

PMID: 2871413 [PubMed - indexed for MEDLINE]

2610. Virology. 1986 Mar;149(2):251-4.

Conservation of the 3' terminal nucleotide sequences of Ebola and Marburg virus.

Kiley MP, Wilusz J, McCormick JB, Keene JD.

The 3' RNA base sequences of several Marburg (MBG) and Ebola (EBO) virus isolates have been determined. A comparison of these 3' terminal noncoding sequences with those of other negative strand RNA viruses suggests a unique phylogenic niche for Marburg and Ebola viruses. The translation initiation site and 35 N-terminal amino acids of the 3' proximal coding gene of a Zaire strain of Ebola virus was predicted. In addition, putative leader RNA sequences preceding the first gene are discussed in terms of possible regulatory functions.

PMID: 3946083 [PubMed - indexed for MEDLINE]

2611. Vopr Virusol. 1986 Mar-Apr;31(2):186-90.

[Indirect immunoenzyme method for the laboratory diagnosis of Lassa and Ebola hemorrhagic fevers].

[Article in Russian]

Ivanov AP, Tkachenko EA, van der Groen G, Butenko AM, Konstantinov OK.

Conditions for performing solid-phase indirect enzyme-immunoassay (SPEIA) for the detection of Lassa and Ebola virus antigens and antibodies to them using horseradish peroxidase-labeled antispecific globulins were developed. The method is highly sensitive, specific, and reproducible. By this method, antigens of Lassa and Ebola viruses could be detected in tissue culture fluid of the infected cell cultures and in animal organ suspensions. Detection of antibodies to Lassa and Ebola viruses in human convalescent sera and in normal donors by means of SPEIA opens possibilities for its use in large-scale diagnostic and seroepidemiological surveys.

PMID: 3524001 [PubMed - indexed for MEDLINE]

2612. Leuk Res. 1986;10(2):167-77.

In-vitro infection of chronic lymphocytic leukemia cells by Epstein-Barr virus (EBV).

Tatsumi E, Harada S, Bechtold T, Lipscomb H, Davis J, Kuszynski C, Volsky DJ, Han T, Armitage J, Purtilo DT.

We sought to determine the potential of infecting lymphoid cells from patients with chronic leukemia (CLL) with Epstein-Barr virus (EBV) by testing for EBV receptors (EBVR) by flow cytometry, assessing for infectability of these cells by culturing with B95-8-derived virus, and staining for EB nuclear-associated antigens (EBNA) at various times post-infection. EBVR were present on 54-91% of lymphoid cells in seven cases of CLL and on 46% of prolymphocytic leukemia cells. Dynamic changes regarding EBNA positivity, morphology, and viability occurred post-infection with the virus. On day 2 only a few EBNA-positive lymphoblasts were observed. On days 11-21 positivity increased from 2 to 34% of cells. Simultaneously, the viable cell number declined to approximately 1/10th of original number. A significant proportion of the EBNA-positive cells corresponded to the original CLL cells. In 3 of 7 cases of CLL a Pan T-cell phenotype was demonstrated by Leu-1 monoclonal antibody testing. The infected cells did not react with two monoclonal antibodies, EBV-CS 1 and 4, which react with B-cell lymphoblastoid cell lines (B-LCL). Moreover, the B-LCL derived at 1-2 months post-infection of CLL cells did not express the Leu-1 antigen, but expressed EBV-CS 1 or 4 defined antigens. In the prolymphocytic leukemia, 64% of the cells showed EBNA positivity on day 7 and giant cells with huge round or multiple nuclei appeared which were EBNA-positive. CLL and prolymphocytic leukemia cells can be infected as demonstrated by EBNA-positivity. This infection does not lead to immediate transformation, but evokes lymphoblast and multinucleated giant cell production prior to the death of cells.

PMID: 3512923 [PubMed - indexed for MEDLINE]

2613. J Infect Dis. 1985 Nov;152(5):887-94.

Pathophysiology of shock and hemorrhage in a fulminating viral infection (Ebola).

Fisher-Hoch SP, Platt GS, Neild GH, Southee T, Baskerville A, Raymond RT, Lloyd G, Simpson DI.

Eleven rhesus monkeys were monitored intensively during experimental infection with Ebola virus. Prominent neutrophilia with left shift and lymphopenia were the earliest abnormalities and were statistically significant by day 4 (P less than .02 and P less than .01, respectively). By day 4 falls in platelet counts were not statistically significant, whereas in vitro platelet aggregation was markedly depressed, progressing rapidly to complete failure by the time of maximum illness. Intraplatelet protein studies suggested this event was the result of in vivo activation and degranulation. Coagulation cascade defects were mainly in the intrinsic system and were surprisingly mild, with no evidence of selective consumption or production deficit of factor VII or VIII. When the possibility of indirectly mediated damage to endothelium possibly by a nonspecific immune response was examined, weight loss was less severe in drug-treated monkeys, and all had detectable plasma prostacyclin metabolites, but there was no improvement in survival.

PMID: 4045253 [PubMed - indexed for MEDLINE]

2614. J Pathol. 1985 Nov;147(3):199-209.

Ultrastructural pathology of experimental Ebola haemorrhagic fever virus infection.

Baskerville A, Fisher-Hoch SP, Neild GH, Dowsett AB.

The organs of monkeys infected with Ebola haemorrhagic fever were examined by light and electron microscopy during the acute stage of the disease. The virus caused focal coagulative necrosis in the liver, spleen, kidney, lung and testis and widespread mild vascular damage. In the brain there was intense congestion, with erythrocyte 'sludging', but no inflammatory reaction. There was significant injury to the microvasculature in all organs. Virus replicated in endothelial cytoplasm causing focal necrosis, separation of tight junctions and detachment from basement membranes. These changes were associated with oedema and haemorrhage, but though contributing to the hypovolaemic shock were not sufficiently extensive to account for the severity of vascular collapse. Renal involvement was also clinically important. Some renal cellular injury was caused by direct virus invasion of glomerular endothelium and tubular epithelium, but much tubular damage was probably due to ischaemia resulting from thrombosis in the peritubular capillaries. The virus also replicated in lymphocytes and monocytes and in interstitial cells of the testis. Since particles were not found in seminiferous epithelium, the degeneration of spermatogonia and spermatocytes was probably secondary to ischaemia.

PMID: 4067737 [PubMed - indexed for MEDLINE]

2615. Virology. 1985 Nov;147(1):169-76.

Descriptive analysis of Ebola virus proteins.

Elliott LH, Kiley MP, McCormick JB.

The virion proteins of two strains of Ebola virus were compared by SDS-polyacrylamide gel electrophoresis (PAGE) and radioimmunoprecipitation (RIP). Seven virion proteins were described; an L (180K), GP (125K), NP (104K), VP40 (40K), VP35 (35K), VP30 (30K), and VP24 (24K). The RNP complex of the virus contained the L, the NP, and VP30, with VP35 in loose association with them. The GP was the major spike protein, with VP40 and VP24 making up the remaining protein content of the multilayered envelope.

PMID: 4060597 [PubMed - indexed for MEDLINE]

2616. Vopr Virusol. 1985 Sep-Oct;30(5):624-6.

[Method for the simultaneous detection of immunofluorescing antibodies to the causative agents of different hemorrhagic fevers].

[Article in Russian]

Lukashevich IS, van der Groen G.

PMID: 3907144 [PubMed - indexed for MEDLINE]

2617. J Clin Microbiol. 1984 Sep;20(3):486-9.

Physicochemical inactivation of Lassa, Ebola, and Marburg viruses and effect on clinical laboratory analyses.

Mitchell SW, McCormick JB.

Clinical specimens from patients infected with Lassa, Ebola, or Marburg virus may present a serious biohazard to laboratory workers. We have examined the effects of heat, alteration of pH, and gamma radiation on these viruses in human blood and on the electrolytes, enzymes, and coagulation factors measured in laboratory tests that are important in the care of an infected patient. Heating serum at 60 degrees C for 1 h reduced high titers of these viruses to noninfectious levels without altering the serum levels of glucose, blood urea nitrogen, and electrolytes. Dilution of blood in 3% acetic acid, diluent for a leukocyte count, inactivated all of these viruses. All of the methods tested for viral inactivation markedly altered certain serum proteins, making these methods unsuitable for samples that are to be tested for certain enzyme levels and coagulation factors.

PMCID: PMC271356 PMID: 6490832 [PubMed - indexed for MEDLINE]

2618. Antiviral Res. 1984 Aug;4(4):169-85.

Viral haemorrhagic fevers: properties and prospects for treatment and prevention.

Howard CR.

PMID: 6091539 [PubMed - indexed for MEDLINE]

2619. Radiography. 1984 Jan;50(589):11-3.

Radiography in a secure isolation unit.

Walters A, Pilkington DB.

PMID: 6538049 [PubMed - indexed for MEDLINE]

2620. Lancet. 1983 Nov 5;2(8359):1055-8.

Haematological and biochemical monitoring of Ebola infection in rhesus monkeys: implications for patient management.

Fisher-Hoch SP, Platt GS, Lloyd G, Simpson DI, Neild GH, Barrett AJ.

Patients with severe viral infections such as Lassa or Ebola may be denied adequate laboratory investigations because of justifiable fears among laboratory staff. This study in monkeys was designed to provide comprehensive haematological and biochemical monitoring in a contained environment during all stages of Ebola infection. Marked neutrophilia, depletion of lymphocytes, and early failure of platelet aggregation preceded a consumption coagulopathy with a microangiopathic haemolytic anaemia, thrombocytopenia, and failure of prostacyclin production by vascular endothelium. Liver dysfunction was moderate but in conjunction with the dehydration and hypoalbuminaemia could be expected to precipitate renal failure and shock. It seems reasonable to anticipate successful patient support with a patient management isolator and treatment with platelet transfusions, fresh frozen plasma, and possibly prostacyclin when haemostasis is defective during this otherwise self-limiting illness.

PMID: 6138602 [PubMed - indexed for MEDLINE]

2621. Am J Trop Med Hyg. 1983 Nov;32(6):1465-6.

Ebola virus infection in man: a serological and epidemiological survey in the Cameroons.

Bouree P, Bergmann JF.

The presence of antibodies to Ebola virus among 1,517 apparently healthy persons in five regions of the Cameroons was tested using indirect immunofluorescence. A positive rate of 9.7% was found, confirming that the virus circulates in the absence of clinical cases. Highest rates were found among Pygmies, young adults, and rain forest farmers.

PMID: 6650749 [PubMed - indexed for MEDLINE]

2622. East Afr Med J. 1983 Oct;60(10):718-22.

A probable case of Ebola virus haemorrhagic fever in Kenya.

Teepe RG, Johnson BK, Ocheng D, Gichogo A, Langatt A, Ngindu A, Kiley M, Johnson KM, McCormick JB.

PMID: 6671431 [PubMed - indexed for MEDLINE]

2623. J Clin Microbiol. 1983 Aug;18(2):416-9.

Development of an immunofluorescence focus assay for Ebola virus.

Truant AL, Regnery RL, Kiley MP.

A 48-h indirect immunofluorescence focus assay for the quantitation of Ebola virus was developed, utilizing HeLa-229 cell monolayers. The dose dependency and the sensitivity of this assay as compared with conventional assays are reported. This indirect immunofluorescence focus assay can be used as a rapid, quantitative test for the detection of Ebola virus, an agent from Africa known to cause hemorrhagic fever.

PMCID: PMC270815 PMID: 6352735 [PubMed - indexed for MEDLINE]

2624. Lancet. 1983 Mar 19;1(8325):654.

Modifications to indirect immunofluorescence tests on Lassa, Marburg, and Ebola material.

van der Groen G, Kurata T, Mets C.

PMID: 6131336 [PubMed - indexed for MEDLINE]

2625. Trop Geogr Med. 1983 Mar;35(1):43-7.

Viral haemorrhagic fever surveillance in Kenya, 1980-1981.

Johnson BK, Ocheng D, Gitau LG, Gichogo A, Tukei PM, Ngindu A, Langatt A, Smith DH, Johnson KM, Kiley MP, Swanepoel R, Isaacson M.

Following two cases of Marburg virus disease in Kenya in 1980, viral haemorrhagic fever surveillance was undertaken in western Kenya. Over a 21-month period investigations, including virus isolation attempts, patient and contact serology, visits to areas where suspected cases occurred, interviewing family members and neighbours of suspected cases and following up any additional illnesses in these areas, were carried out. During the study two cases were found that were likely to have been Ebola haemorrhagic fever based on rising antibody titres or positive serology in contacts. Diagnoses of hepatitis A, hepatitis B, malaria, bacterial septicaemia or other causes were arrived at in 24 cases. No diagnosis could be made in 26 instances. 741 human sera were tested for antibodies against Marburg, Ebola, Congo haemorrhagic fever, Rift Valley fever or Lassa fever viruses by indirect fluorescence. Eight sera were positive for Ebola virus antibodies, all of which were from suspected cases or contacts of suspected cases. Two sera were antibody positive to Congo virus and one had antibodies against Rift Valley fever virus. No Marburg or Lassa virus antibodies were detected.

PMID: 6684336 [PubMed - indexed for MEDLINE]

2626. J Infect Dis. 1983 Feb;147(2):276-81.

Comparative analysis of the structural polypeptides of Ebola viruses from Sudan and Zaire.

Buchmeier MJ, DeFries RU, McCormick JB, Kiley MP.

Polypeptide structural analyses were performed by tryptic peptide mapping to assess the relationship between isolates of Ebola virus obtained in Sudan and Zaire. The results of these analyses indicate (1) that the Sudan and Zaire isolates are unique viral agents, (2) that multiple isolates within each group bear close resemblance to one another, (3) that suggestive evidence exists of conservation of homologous structure in the VP-2 (virion protein no. 2) nucleocapsid proteins of these viruses, and (4) that protein differences between the two Ebola virus subtypes appear to reside in the VP-1 and VP-3 virion polypeptides.

PMID: 6827145 [PubMed - indexed for MEDLINE]

2627. J Infect Dis. 1983 Feb;147(2):272-5.

Evidence for two subtypes of Ebola virus based on oligonucleotide mapping of RNA.

Cox NJ, McCormick JB, Johnson KM, Kiley MP.

Ebola viruses isolated during outbreaks of acute hemorrhagic fever in Africa from 1976 to 1979 were examined by T1 oligonucleotide mapping of virion RNA. Two Ebola virus subtypes distinguishable by their oligonucleotide patterns were involved in the outbreaks of the disease during this three-year period. The first type was isolated in Zaire in 1976 and again in 1977; the second type caused outbreaks in Sudan in 1976 and again in 1979. Oligonucleotide patterns of the two groups of Ebola viruses (Zaire and Sudan) were remarkably similar within the group but differed between groups by approximately 60 oligonucleotides. We can conclude from this study (1) that the outbreaks of hemorrhagic fever which occurred concurrently in 1976 in Zaire and Sudan were caused by viruses that are

genetically distinct; (2) that compared with other RNA viruses there was an unusually high genetic stability among viruses within Zaire and Sudan over two- and three-year periods, respectively; and (3) that the two genetic subtypes probably evolved from a common ancestor since they share common oligonucleotides.
PMID: 6827144 [PubMed - indexed for MEDLINE]

2628. J Infect Dis. 1983 Feb;147(2):268-71.

Antigenic analysis of strains of Ebola virus: identification of two Ebola virus serotypes.

Richman DD, Cleveland PH, McCormick JB, Johnson KM.

A sensitive radioimmunoassay has been adapted for Ebola virus antigens and antibodies to them. It uses 125I-labeled staphylococcal protein A and a specially designed filter manifold. The assay is applicable to the sera of humans and to a wide range of animal sera. Virus isolates from two discrete outbreaks of Ebola hemorrhagic fever that occurred in 1976 were shown by this assay to be antigenically distinct. This lack of identity was further confirmed by cross-absorbing antisera to each isolate with antigens of the heterologous virus strain. The advantages of this assay include the use of noninfectious antigens, the requirement for only small quantities of serum, the capability of screening large numbers of sera, the speed of execution, and the objectivity of end point determination.
PMID: 6827143 [PubMed - indexed for MEDLINE]

2629. J Infect Dis. 1983 Feb;147(2):264-7.

Biologic differences between strains of Ebola virus from Zaire and Sudan.

McCormick JB, Bauer SP, Elliott LH, Webb PA, Johnson KM.
PMID: 6827142 [PubMed - indexed for MEDLINE]

2630. Ann N Y Acad Sci. 1983;420:192-207.

Detection of viral antigens in formalin-fixed specimens by enzyme treatment.

Kurata T, Hondo R, Sato S, Oda A, Aoyama Y, McCormick JB.

Enzyme treatment (protease or trypsin) was applied to formalin-fixed paraffin-embedded materials and virus-infected cultured cells to detect viral antigens by immunofluorescence. The viral antigens were demonstrated in several organs of autopsy or biopsy cases of which diagnoses had been established by immunofluorescence or virus isolation using frozen materials, or suspected on the basis of serology and/or histopathological findings. These included herpes simplex, varicella-zoster, cytomegalo, subacute sclerosing panencephalitis, progressive multifocal leukoencephalopathy, Japanese B encephalitis, measles, acute hemorrhagic conjunctivitis, Lassa and Korean hemorrhagic fever. Antigen could be recovered also in virus-infected cells (herpes simplex, measles, Lassa, Ebola, Marburg, Rift Valley, Congo and Korean Hemorrhagic fever) by enzyme treatment after periods of formalin fixation of four weeks and storage of three months. In herpes simplex virus-infected mouse brain, antigen was detected after fixation for three months in formalin.
PMID: 6326644 [PubMed - indexed for MEDLINE]

2631. Bull World Health Organ. 1983;61(6):997-1003.

Ebola virus disease in southern Sudan: hospital dissemination and intrafamilial spread.

Baron RC, McCormick JB, Zubeir OA.

Between 31 July and 6 October 1979, 34 cases of Ebola virus disease (22 of which were fatal) occurred among five families in a rural district of southern Sudan; the disease was introduced into four of the families from a local hospital. Chains of secondary spread within the family units, accounting for 29 cases resulted from direct physical contact with an infected person. Among all persons with such contact in the family setting, those who provided nursing care had a 5.1-fold increased risk of infection, emphasizing the importance of intimate contact in the spread of this disease. The absence of illness among persons who were exposed to cases in confined spaces, but without physical contact, confirmed previous impressions that there is no risk of airborne transmission. While the ecology of Ebola virus is unknown, the presence of anti-Ebola antibodies in the sera of 18% of persons who were unassociated with the outbreak suggests that the region is an endemic focus of Ebola virus activity.
PMCID: PMC2536233 PMID: 6370486 [PubMed - indexed for MEDLINE]

2632. Trans R Soc Trop Med Hyg. 1983;77(5):731-3.

Antibodies against haemorrhagic fever viruses in Kenya populations.

Johnson BK, Ocheng D, Gichogo A, Okiro M, Libondo D, Tukei PM, Ho M, Mugambi M, Timms GL, French M.

Human sera from Lodwar (77 sera), Nzoia (841 sera), Masinga (251 sera), Laisamis (174 sera) and the Malindi/Kilifi area (556 sera) in Kenya were tested by indirect immunofluorescence for antibodies against Marburg, Ebola (Zaire and Sudan strains), Congo haemorrhagic fever, Rift Valley fever and Lassa viruses. Antibodies against Ebola virus, particularly the Zaire strain, were detected in all regions and were, over-all, more abundant than antibodies against the other antigens. Ebola and Marburg antibody prevalence rates were highest in the samples from Lodwar and Laisamis, both semi-desert areas. Antibodies against Rift Valley fever virus were also highest in the Lodwar sample followed by Malindi/Kilifi and Laisamis. Congo haemorrhagic fever virus antibodies were rare and no antibodies against Lassa virus were detected in the 1899 sera tested.
PMID: 6419422 [PubMed - indexed for MEDLINE]

2633. Verh K Acad Geneeskd Belg. 1983;45(1-2):201-25.

[The epidemic of hemorrhagic fever in Zaire (August-November 1976) and its implications].

[Article in Dutch]
Pattyn SR.
PMID: 6613302 [PubMed - indexed for MEDLINE]

2634. Verh K Acad Geneeskd Belg. 1983;45(1-2):31-200.

[Epidemic hemorrhagic fevers].

[Article in Dutch]

Janssens PG, Pattyn SR.

PMID: 6310907 [PubMed - indexed for MEDLINE]

2635. J Clin Microbiol. 1982 Oct;16(4):704-8.

Inactivation of Lassa, Marburg, and Ebola viruses by gamma irradiation.

Elliott LH, McCormick JB, Johnson KM.

Because of the cumbersome conditions experienced in a maximum containment laboratory, methods for inactivating highly pathogenic viruses were investigated. The infectivity of Lassa, Marburg, and Ebola viruses was inactivated without altering the immunological activity after radiation with Co60 gamma rays. At 4 degrees C, Lassa virus was the most difficult to inactivate with a rate of 5.3 X 10(-6) log 50% tissue culture infective dose per rad of CO60 radiation, as compared with 6.8 X 10(-6) log 50% tissue culture infective dose per rad for Ebola virus and 8.4 X 10(-6) log 50% tissue culture infective dose per rad for Marburg virus. Experimental inactivation curves, as well as curves giving the total radiation needed to inactivate a given concentration of any of the three viruses, are presented. We found this method of inactivation to be superior to UV light or beta-propiolactone inactivation and now routinely use it for preparation of material for protein-chemistry studies or for preparation of immunological reagents.

PMCID: PMC272450 PMID: 7153317 [PubMed - indexed for MEDLINE]

2636. J Infect Dis. 1982 Oct;146(4):483-6.

Antibody to Ebola virus in guinea pigs: Tandala, Zaire.

Stansfield SK, Scribner CL, Kaminski RM, Cairns T, McCormick JB, Johnson KM.

A case-control study was conducted to investigate the findings of antibody to Ebola virus in the serum of a guinea pig from Tandala, Zaire. Case households, defined by the possession of one or more guinea pigs, were compared to neighboring households without guinea pigs. Seven (5.1%) of 138 samples of human sera and 36 (26%) of 138 samples of guinea pig sera had antibody to Ebola virus. There was no clustering of seropositivity among humans or guinea pigs within households, nor was there any association between the ownership of guinea pigs and seropositivity among household members. These data suggest sporadic subclinical infection of guinea pigs and humans without a dominant role for person-to-person or guinea pig-to-guinea pig transmission.

PMID: 6750007 [PubMed - indexed for MEDLINE]

2637. Lancet. 1982 Jul 17;2(8290):155.

Inactivating Lassa and Marburg/Ebola viruses.

Pereira MS.

PMID: 6123862 [PubMed - indexed for MEDLINE]

2638. Lancet. 1982 Apr 10;1(8276):816-20.

Marburg-virus disease in Kenya.

Smith DH, Johnson BK, Isaacson M, Swanapoel R, Johnson KM, Killey M, Bagshawe A, Siongok T, Keruga WK.

PMID: 6122054 [PubMed - indexed for MEDLINE]

2639. Ann Soc Belg Med Trop. 1982 Mar;62(1):49-54.

Use of betapropionolactone inactivated Ebola, Marburg and Lassa intracellular antigens in immunofluorescent antibody assay.

Van der Groen G, Elliot LH.

PMID: 7049096 [PubMed - indexed for MEDLINE]

2640. Ann Soc Belg Med Trop. 1982 Mar;62(1):67-8.

Lack of cross reactivity of rhabdovirus antibodies with Marburg and Ebola antigens in the indirect immunofluorescent antibody test.

Van der Groen G, Elliot LH.

PMID: 6179483 [PubMed - indexed for MEDLINE]

2641. Sem Hop. 1982 Feb 18;58(7):427-34.

[Diagnosis of fever in a patient returning from black Africa (author's transl)].

[Article in French]

Chagnon A.

The diagnostic problems which arise when fever occurs in a patient returning from black Africa are more and more frequently encountered because of the multiplication of rapid connections with this continent. Analysis of the main etiologies leads the author to review most of the specifically tropical diseases. However, cosmopolitan diseases should not be underrated. The author emphasizes the high incidence of pernicious malaria, liver amebiasis, and typho-paratyphoid fevers, along with the necessity of keeping in mind the new viral diseases (Lassa, Marburg, Ebola).

PMID: 6280318 [PubMed - indexed for MEDLINE]

2642. Intervirology. 1982;18(1-2):24-32.

Filoviridae: a taxonomic home for Marburg and Ebola viruses?

Kiley MP, Bowen ET, Eddy GA, Isaäcson M, Johnson KM, McCormick JB, Murphy FA, Pattyn SR, Peters D, Prozesky OW, Regnery RL, Simpson DI, Slenczka W, Sureau P, van der Groen G, Webb PA, Wulff H.

PMID: 7118520 [PubMed - indexed for MEDLINE]

2643. Prog Liver Dis. 1982;7:495-515.

Viral hemorrhagic fevers with hepatic involvement: pathologic aspects with clinical correlations.

Ishak KG, Walker DH, Coetzer JA, Gardner JJ, Gorelkin L.

PMID: 6125993 [PubMed - indexed for MEDLINE]

2644. Trans R Soc Trop Med Hyg. 1982;76(6):719-20.

Haemorrhagic fever in Gabon. I. Incidence of Lassa, Ebola and Marburg viruses in Haut-Ogooué.

Ivanoff B, Duquesnoy P, Languillat G, Saluzzo JF, Georges A, Gonzalez JP, McCormick J.

A serological enquiry aimed at determining the incidence of infection with Lassa, Ebola and Marburg viruses was conducted on the human population of the region of Haut-Ogooué (Gabon) and on primates. The results, obtained by the indirect immunofluorescence technique, showed that more than 6% of the human population had had contact with Ebola virus but no antibodies against Marburg or Lassa viruses were found. Most sera reacted to an Ebola antigen from a Zairian strain, but showed little or no reaction to an antigen from a Sudanese strain.

PMID: 7164137 [PubMed - indexed for MEDLINE]

2645. Trans R Soc Trop Med Hyg. 1982;76(3):307-10.

Marburg, Ebola and Rift Valley Fever virus antibodies in East African primates.

Johnson BK, Gitau LG, Gichogo A, Tukei PM, Else JG, Suleman MA, Kimani R, Sayer PD.

Sera from 464 primates held at four institutes in Kenya were tested by indirect immunofluorescence for the presence of antibodies against Marburg, Ebola, Congo haemorrhagic fever, Rift Valley fever and Lassa viruses. Four of 136 vervet monkeys were positive for Marburg virus antibodies and three of 184 baboons had antibodies against Ebola virus. One baboon was positive for Marburg virus antibodies. Two vervet monkeys, three baboons and one grivet monkey (of 56 tested) had antibodies against Rift Valley fever virus. No Congo or Lassa virus antibodies were detected. A sample of 88 sera of more arboreal primates (Sykes, blue and colobus monkeys) were negative against all five antigens, as were sera from 58 staff members of the institutes who worked with or near the animals.

PMID: 6810518 [PubMed - indexed for MEDLINE]

2646. Trans R Soc Trop Med Hyg. 1982;76(6):803-5.

Viral haemorrhagic fever antibodies in Zimbabwe schoolchildren.

Blackburn NK, Searle L, Taylor P.

PMID: 6761909 [PubMed - indexed for MEDLINE]

2647. S Afr Med J. 1981 Nov 7;60(19):751-3.

Marburg virus disease. The diagnosis and management of suspected cases.

Andrijich VB.

Marburg virus disease is an African disease of unknown epidemiology. The infection is pantropic and highly contagious. Haemorrhage and other features cause serious morbidity and high mortality, and early diagnosis is essential. Viral haemorrhagic fever is diagnosed clinically and confirmed by coagulation studies. Electron microscopy and serology are necessary for the identification of the virus, as Lassa and Ebola viruses (among other organisms) give similar symptoms, and Ebola virus is morphologically indistinguishable from Marburg virus. Treatment is essentially supportive. Patients and contacts must be isolated and monitored, and extreme precautions must be taken by hospital and laboratory staff to prevent their own infection.

PMID: 7029731 [PubMed - indexed for MEDLINE]

2648. J Clin Microbiol. 1981 Nov;14(5):527-9.

Preparation of polyvalent viral immunofluorescent intracellular antigens and use in human serosurveys.

Johnson KM, Elliott LH, Heymann DL.

A method is described for preparation of polyvalent antigens for use in rapid screening for immunofluorescent antibodies to Lassa, Marburg, and Ebola viruses. The technique uses mixtures of specifically infected Vero cells placed on Teflon-templated microscopy slides. It was found to be as sensitive as the use of monovalent antigens for detection and quantitation of antibodies to these highly hazardous human pathogens.

PMCID: PMC273981 PMID: 7031084 [PubMed - indexed for MEDLINE]

2649. J Virol Methods. 1981 Sep;3(2):61-9.

A comparison of indirect immunofluorescence and electron microscopy for the diagnosis of some haemorrhagic viruses in cell cultures.

El Mekki AA, van der Groen G.

Yellow fever, dengue (types 1, 2 and 4), Chikungunya, Rift Valley fever, Ebola, Marburg, and Lassa viruses were inoculated into susceptible cell cultures and daily investigated by indirect immunofluorescence (IFA) and electron microscopy (EM) with a view to achieve an early detection-identification of these agents. Compared to the other cell lines tested (Vero, BHK-21 and Aedes albopictus), CV-1 cells were found to be more sensitive. Viral antigens were detected by IFA from a few hours post inoculation (CHIK and RVF) to a maximum of 3 days (YF and EBO). For most of the viruses studied, the cytopathic effect (CPE) commenced 2-3 days after the detection of viral antigens. Virus particles were detected by EM only in the case of EBO, MBG and LAS, before any CPE was observed in cell cultures.

PMID: 7024293 [PubMed - indexed for MEDLINE]

2650. Lancet. 1981 Jun 27;1(8235):1420-1.

Marburg and Ebola virus antibodies in Kenyan primates.

Johnson BK, Gitau LG, Gichogo A, Tukei PM, Else JG, Suleman MA, Kimani R.
PMID: 6113374 [PubMed - indexed for MEDLINE]

2651. J Infect Dis. 1981 May;143(5):749-51.

Ecology of ebola virus: a first clue?

Johnson KM, Scribner CL, McCormick JB.
PMID: 7017023 [PubMed - indexed for MEDLINE]

2652. J Clin Microbiol. 1981 Apr;13(4):791-3.

Plaque assay for Ebola virus.

Moe JB, Lambert RD, Lupton HW.

A plaque assay for Ebola virus is reported. The procedure has real potential for future research, although it is less sensitive than indirect fluorescent-antibody and mouse inoculation tests.

PMCID: PMC273881 PMID: 7014628 [PubMed - indexed for MEDLINE]

2653. Med Trop (Mars). 1981 Mar-Apr;41(2):191-9.

[Marburg, Lassa and Ebola viral hemorrhagic fevers (author's transl)].

[Article in French]

Ardouin C, Chevalier JM, Algayres JP.

For each of these three fevers recently described, the authors report the history of their identification. The features of the three viruses, and the clinical aspects of the diseases they induce, are also indicated. The laboratory diagnosis is described. Practical indications are given for the transportation of the specimens to the only three high security laboratories in the world. The laboratory diagnosis is described. Some cautions are indicated handling and treating patients. It must be envisaged also to organize a four degrees quarantine cautions; compulsory for necropsies, burials, and occasionally for long distant transportations of patients are indicated.

PMID: 7242302 [PubMed - indexed for MEDLINE]

2654. J Infect Dis. 1981 Feb;143(2):291.

Inactivation of Ebola virus with 60Co irradiation.

Lupton HW.
PMID: 7217722 [PubMed - indexed for MEDLINE]

2655. Infect Control. 1981 Jan-Feb;2(1):38-49.

Nosocomial viral infections: III. Guidelines for prevention and control of exanthematous viruses, gastroenteritis viruses, picornaviruses, and uncommonly seen viruses.

Valenti WM, Hruska JF, Menegus MA, Freeburn MJ.

This communication is the third in a four-part series on nosocomial viral infections from the Strong Memorial Hospital. This third article discusses guidelines for prevention and control of exanthematous viruses, gastroenteritis, viruses, adenoviruses and the picornaviruses other than rhinoviruses. Several uncommonly seen viruses, such as the virus of Creutzfeldt-Jakob disease and Marburg, Ebola, and Lassa fever viruses, also are reviewed briefly.

PMID: 6260699 [PubMed - indexed for MEDLINE]

2656. Verh Dtsch Ges Pathol. 1981;65:100-2.

[Light microscopy study of Ebola virus hepatitis in guinea pigs].

[Article in German]

Korb G, Slenczka W.
PMID: 7347447 [PubMed - indexed for MEDLINE]

2657. Lancet. 1980 Dec 13;2(8207):1294-5.

Inactivated vaccine for Ebola virus efficacious in guineapig model.

Lupton HW, Lambert RD, Bumgardner DL, Moe JB, Eddy GA.
PMID: 6108462 [PubMed - indexed for MEDLINE]

2658. Tropenmed Parasitol. 1980 Dec;31(4):389-98.

Clinical observations in 42 patients with Lassa fever.

Knobloch J, McCormick JB, Webb PA, Dietrich M, Schumacher HH, Dennis E.

Under continuous observation of several months, 42 patients from the eastern province of Sierra Leone, Liberia (Lofa County), and neighbouring Guinea were identified as Lassa fever cases by indirect immunofluorescent antibody technique, indicating that the disease is endemic in these areas. The clinical course varied from mild disease to severe illness with haemorrhagic disorders. The fatality rate was 14%. The occurrence of only two possible secondary cases suggests that person-to-person spread of the disease is unimportant epidemiologically. There was a wide range of patients' ages, tribes, and occupations, including a 2 months old baby and a white US citizen. Clinical, laboratory, and histopathological investigations demonstrated the panorganotropism of Lassa virus. Haematological tests in few selected haemorrhagic cases with Lassa fever did not support coagulation disorders or thrombocytopenia as causing the bleeding tendency. The histopathologic changes bear resemblance to those observed in Argentinian and Bolivian haemorrhagic fever, both being caused by viruses of the Arena group. However, Lassa virus hepatitis may be differentiated from liver lesions occurring in yellow fever, Marburg virus disease, and Ebola (Maridi) haemorrhagic fever.

PMID: 7233535 [PubMed - indexed for MEDLINE]

2659. J Virol. 1980 Nov;36(2):465-9.

Virion nucleic acid of Ebola virus.

Regnery RL, Johnson KM, Kiley MP.

The virion nucleic acid of Ebola virus consists of a single-stranded RNA with a molecular weight of approximately 4.0 x 10(6). The virion RNA did not bind to oligodeoxythymidylic acid-cellulose under conditions known to bind RNAs rich in polyadenylic acid and was not infectious under conditions which yielded infectious RNA from Sindbis virus, suggesting that Ebola virus virion nucleic acid is a negative-stranded RNA.

PMCID: PMC353663 PMID: 7431486 [PubMed - indexed for MEDLINE]

2660. J Infect Dis. 1980 Sep;142(3):372-6.

Ebola hemorrhagic fever: Tandala, Zaire, 1977-1978.

Heymann DL, Weisfeld JS, Webb PA, Johnson KM, Cairns T, Berquist H.

Ebola virus was recovered from a nine-year-old girl who died of acute hemorrhagic fever in June 1977 at Tandala Hospital in northwestern Zaire, in the first reported recognized case of this disease since the discovery epidemics of 1976 in Zaire and Sudan. Investigations undertaken in the Tandala region revealed that two previous clinical infections with Ebola virus had occurred in 1972 and that about 7% of the residents had immunofluorescent antibodies to the virus. Females younger than 30 years of age had a higher prevalence of antibodies than males of comparable age, but above the age of 30 years there was no sex difference. No other clues to the still-mysterious natural reservoir of Ebola virus were uncovered.

PMID: 7441008 [PubMed - indexed for MEDLINE]

2661. Br Med J. 1980 Aug 9;281(6237):427-30.

Changing patterns of communicable disease in England and Wales. Part i--Newly recognised diseases.

Galbraith NS, Forbes P, Mayon-White RT.

PMCID: PMC1713331 PMID: 7000261 [PubMed - indexed for MEDLINE]

2662. J Gen Virol. 1980 Aug;49(2):333-41.

Ebola virus: identification of virion structural proteins.

Kiley MP, Regnery RL, Johnson KM.

Polyacrylamide gel electrophoresis of purified Ebola virus revealed the presence of four major virion structural proteins which we have designated VP1, VP2, VP3 and VP4. Vesicular stomatitis virus (VSV) proteins were used as mol. wt. markers, and the virion proteins were found to have mol. wt. of 125000 (VP1), 104000 (VP2), 40000 (VP3) and 26000 (VP4). VP1 was labelled with glucosamine and is probably a glycoprotein. The density of the Ebola virion was approx. 1.14g/ml in potassium tartrate. Virus nucleocapsids with a density of 1.32g/ml in caesium chloride were released when virions were treated with detergents. Proteins VP2 and VP3 were consistently associated with released nucleocapsids and are probably the major structural nucleocapsid proteins analogous to the N protein of VSV. Protein VP4 was reduced or absent in released nucleocapsids and is probably analogous to the membrane (M) protein of VSV and similar viruses. The glycoprotein (VP1) is larger than the glycoprotein of any known negative-strand RNA virus and is not labelled well with 35S-methionine. VP1 is solubilized by detergent treatment, suggesting that it is a component of the virion spikes and analogous to the G protein of VSV. Our results, in conjunction with analysis of Ebola virion RNA (Regnery et al. 1980), strongly suggest that the virus is a negative-strand RNA virus and, along with marburg virus, may constitute a new taxon within this group.

PMID: 7441205 [PubMed - indexed for MEDLINE]

2663. Bull Soc Pathol Exot Filiales. 1980 May-Jun;73(3):238-41.

[Preliminary note on the presence of antibodies to Ebola virus in the human population in the eastern part of the Central African Republic].

[Article in French]

Saluzzo JF, Gonzalez JP, Hervé JP, Georges AJ, Johnson KM.

The authors reported a preliminary serological survey on Ebola virus infection in Central African Republic. They have tested 499 sera samples by using indirect immunofluorescent technique. The positivity with Ebola antigen was 3,4% (17 cases). It has been found a high antibody titre (greater than or equal to 1/64) with 3 sera, which reflects a possible recent contact with Ebola virus.

PMID: 7014009 [PubMed - indexed for MEDLINE]

2664. R Soc Health J. 1980 Apr;100(2):52-6.

Exotic infectious diseases: Marburg/Ebola/haemorrhagic fevers.

Simpson DI.

PMID: 6770413 [PubMed - indexed for MEDLINE]

2665. Med Klin. 1980 Feb 15;75(4):135-42.

[Developments and trends in virology].

[Article in German]

Siegert R.

PMID: 6154883 [PubMed - indexed for MEDLINE]

2666. Nihon Rinsho. 1980 Feb 10;38(2):308-14.

[Ebola haemorrhagic fever: epidemiology, symptomatology, management and prognosis].

[Article in Japanese]

Imagawa Y.

PMID: 7392222 [PubMed - indexed for MEDLINE]

2667. Nihon Rinsho. 1980 Feb 10;38(2):289-94.

[Pathogenic microbiology of international communicable diseases].

[Article in Japanese]

Oya A.

PMID: 6771443 [PubMed - indexed for MEDLINE]

2668. Br J Hosp Med. 1980 Feb;23(2):191, 193-4.

The nasty viruses--Lassa, Marburg, and Ebola.

Simpson DI.

PMID: 6768412 [PubMed - indexed for MEDLINE]

2669. J Med Virol. 1980;6(2):129-38.

A comparative study of strains of Ebola virus isolated from southern Sudan and northern Zaire in 1976.

Bowen ET, Platt GS, Lloyd G, Raymond RT, Simpson DI.

During the 1976 Ebola virus outbreak in Sudan, the investigations team gained the impression that fewer haemorrhagic manifestations and few fatalities occurred during the later stages of the epidemic after the virus had undergone several generations in man. This impression was also noted in guinea pigs experimentally infected with Sudanese and Zairean strains of Ebola virus. The virulence of the Sudanese isolates was less intense than isolates emanating from Zaire. Similar findings were seen in monkeys; a Zairean isolated produced fatal infections, whereas monkeys inoculated with a Sudan strain generally recovered. Two monkeys, which had recovered from Sudanese strain infections and had developed high levels of antibody detectable by immunofluorescence, were challenged with the Zairean strain. Both developed viraemias and died. The mechanisms of this "failed protection" are discussed.

PMID: 6165800 [PubMed - indexed for MEDLINE]

2670. Mikrobiyol Bul. 1980 Jan;14(1):65-73.

[A new viral infectious disease: Ebola haemorrhagic fever (author's transl)].

[Article in Turkish]

Tuncer A.

All references about a new viral infection, which was seen in Sudan and Zaire at 1976 called "Ebola Haemorrhagic Fever" with high fever, diarrhoea, vomiting and great systemic haemorrhagic manifestations were reviewed. We discussed the history, etiology, epidemiology, source of infections, mode of transmission, period of communicability, clinical and laboratory findings and control measures of the disease. Some comments were made about what could be done, if a new disease of unknown etiology is seen in any part of our country.

PMID: 7453587 [PubMed - indexed for MEDLINE]

2671. Yale J Biol Med. 1980 Jan-Feb;53(1):109-15.

Exotic viral diseases.

Dowdle WR.

Marburg virus disease, Lassa fever, monkeypox, and Ebola virus diseases of humans have all been recognized since 1967. These are examples of some of the exotic virus diseases which through importation may present a potential public health problem in the United States. Some of these viruses are also highly hazardous to laboratory and medical personnel. This paper is a review of the general characteristics, the epidemiology, and laboratory diagnosis of the exotic viruses which have been described during the last 25 years.

PMCID: PMC2595835 PMID: 6246685 [PubMed - indexed for MEDLINE]

2672. Med Trop (Mars). 1979 Nov-Dec;39(6):675-84.

[Ebola virus three years later (author's transl)].

[Article in French]

Courtois D.

Sporadic cases and data from serologic surveys give evidence that Ebola virus is still active in Northern Zaïre after the first outbreak in 1976. It is also active in Southern Sudan where it is, from August 1979, responsible of a new epidemic focus. In addition, serological surveys demonstrate that its dispersion area comprises several other african countries. Physicians practising in central Africa must be aware of this fact. Serological test is necessary to confirm the diagnosis. This confirmation is necessary to obtain convalescent patient plasma, the only specific treatment. The clinical, epidemiological and virological aspects of Ebola virus disease are reviewed as well as precautionary measures to be taken by medical and nursing staff to avoid infection.

PMID: 119124 [PubMed - indexed for MEDLINE]

2673. Fortschr Med. 1979 Sep 6;97(33):1387-90.

[African hemorrhagic fever as a new problem in medicine].

[Article in German]

Stille W.
PMID: 573738 [PubMed - indexed for MEDLINE]
2674. Pol Tyg Lek. 1979 Jul 23;34(30):1203-5.

[African hemorrhagic fever caused by Ebola virus].

[Article in Polish]
Kornaszewski W, Muyembe T, Kintoki V.
PMID: 503930 [PubMed - indexed for MEDLINE]
2675. Ann Intern Med. 1979 Jul;91(1):117-9.

Ebola virus and hemorrhagic fever: Andromeda strain or localized pathogen?

Johnson KM.
PMID: 111590 [PubMed - indexed for MEDLINE]
2676. Ann Soc Belg Med Trop. 1979 Mar;59(1):87-92.

Measurement of antibodies to Ebola virus in human sera from N. W.-Zaire.

Van der Groen G, Pattyn SR.
PMID: 395911 [PubMed - indexed for MEDLINE]
2677. Public Health. 1979 Mar;93(2):67-75.

44 contacts of Ebola virus infection--Salisbury.

Williams EH.
PMID: 432398 [PubMed - indexed for MEDLINE]
2678. Can Med Assoc J. 1979 Jan 20;120(2):146-55.

Lassa fever, Marburg and Ebola virus diseases and other exotic diseases: is there a risk to Canada?

Clayton AJ.
There are seven exotic diseases of concern; three of these, the most unpredictable and least understood, are Lassa fever, Marburg virus disease and Ebola virus disease. In this article the epidemiologic aspects of these diseases are discussed, with particular emphasis on exportation from their indigenous areas in Africa and on the occurrence of secondary cases. Any of these conditions could be brought into Canada either by aeromedical evacuation or inadvertently. Between 1972 and 1978 there were seven occasions when Canada could have been involved with handling cases of Lassa fever. The Government of Canada has purchased several containment bed and transit isolators. These units, with filtered air under negative pressure, accommodate infectious patients being transported and cared for without contaminating medical attendants or the environment.
PMCID: PMC1818857 PMID: 570088 [PubMed - indexed for MEDLINE]
2679. Dakar Med. 1979;24(1):56-9.

[Virological and clinical notes on recent viral epidemics in Zaïre].

[Article in French]
Wone I, de Lauture H.
PMID: 574073 [PubMed - indexed for MEDLINE]
2680. Dakar Med. 1979;24(1):51-5.

[Marburg, Ebole and Lassa virus infections].

[Article in French]
Denis F, Robin Y.
PMID: 574072 [PubMed - indexed for MEDLINE]
2681. J Med Virol. 1979;4(3):239-40.

Ebola virus virulence for newborn mice.

van der Groen G, Jacob W, Pattyn SR.
PMID: 536744 [PubMed - indexed for MEDLINE]
2682. J Med Virol. 1979;4(3):213-25.

Ebola and Marburg viruses: II. Thier development within Vero cells and the extra-cellular formation of branched and torus forms.

Ellis DS, Stamford S, Tvoey DG, Lloyd G, Bowen ET, Platt GS, Way H, Simpson DI.
The development of Marburg virus and the Sudanese and Zaire strains of Ebola virus in Vero cells as visualized by electron microscopy is described. Despite differences in timing, all three strains appear to pass through identical stages of development. Initially there is a large increase in nucleolus material, and viral precursor material arranges itself in spirals and then into tubes. The cells fill with core material, which passes to the plasmalemma, which often proliferates. Each virion passes through the plasmalemma, acquiring a coat of host material. The formation of torus forms is discussed; the branched appearance that is often seen is believed to be an aberrant form. The reasons for this view are put forward.
PMID: 119829 [PubMed - indexed for MEDLINE]
2683. J Med Virol. 1979;4(3):201-11.

Ebola and Marburg viruses: I. Some ultrastructural differences between strains when grown in Vero cells.

Ellis DS, Stamford S, Lloyd G, Bowen ET, Platt GS, Way H, Simpson DI.

A strain of Marburg virus and two strains of Ebola virus grown in Vero cells were compared by electron microscopy. The outer coat of the Marburg virion appeared to be more resistant to erosion by negative staining techniques than that of the Epbola strains. Marburg virus commonly produced "torus" forms and short filaments; the Zaire strain of Ebola produced extensive branched forms and very long filaments; the Sudan strain of Ebola produced shorter, less branched structures but very many aberrant forms. The mechanism for the production of these aberrant forms is described.

PMID: 94087 [PubMed - indexed for MEDLINE]

2684. Ter Arkh. 1979;51(11):119-23.

[New African hemorrhagic fevers].

[Article in Russian]

Pokrovskiĭ VV.

PMID: 392795 [PubMed - indexed for MEDLINE]

2685. Br J Exp Pathol. 1978 Dec;59(6):584-93.

Ebola virus: a comparison, at ultrastructural level, of the behaviour of the Sudan and Zaire strains in monkeys.

Ellis DS, Bowen ET, Simpson DI, Stamford S.

Histopathological and electron microscopical examination of human liver specimens collected during the Ebola haemorrhagic fever outbreaks in Zaire and Sudan indicated that Zairean strains of the virus produced more extensive lesions. Experimental infection of rhesus monkeys wiht Zairean and Sudanese strains of Ebola virus produced similar changes to those found in man. In Zairean strain infections large numbers of virus particles were found in the liver, lung and spleen accompanied by extensive necrosis in the spleen. In Sudan strain infections particles were found only in the liver and in greatly reduced numbers. The main distinction lay in the high proportion of aberrant particles found with the Sudanese strain. The possibility of these being defective particles is discussed.

PMCID: PMC2041404 PMID: 106868 [PubMed - indexed for MEDLINE]

2686. Nouv Presse Med. 1978 Oct 7;7(34):3007-12.

[Lassa, Marbourg and Ebola viruses: new features of African tropical pathology. II. Epidemiology. Public health problems (author's transl)].

[Article in French]

Brès P.

Lassa, Marbourg and Ebola viruses are characterised by their endemo-epidemicity in tropical Africa, by their potential of inter-human transmission, by their gravity (30 to 50% mortality in cases admitted to hospital) and by the difficulty of their aetiological diagnosis. This results in a public health problem for countries in non-endemic regions receiving travellers coming from Africa. This problem is related to the risk of importation of cases, a risk which should not be exaggerated but nor should it be underestimated. Appropriate measures may be suggested in the light of assessment of the risk: organisation of specialised hospital facilities, laboratory and coordination service.

PMID: 364408 [PubMed - indexed for MEDLINE]

2687. Nouv Presse Med. 1978 Sep 30;7(33):2921-6.

[Recent Lassa, Marbourg and Ebola viruses in African tropical viruses. I. Semiology--physiopathology--diagnosis--treatment (author's transl)].

[Article in French]

Brès P.

Three new viruses have been identified in Africa during the present decade. They may cause sporadic cases or limited outbreaks, and they are probably endemic in areas which are still ill-defined. Severe forms of infection lead to the haemorrhagic syndrome or to hypovolemic shock, the physiopathology of which is being studied. The case-fatality ratio of severe cases is between 30 and 85 per cent. Nosocomial outbreaks have been observed, but they can be avoided if appropriate barrier nursing measures are carried out for the treatment of patients or adequate protection measures for sampling and examination of laboratory specimens. As such cases may be transferred outside the endemic zone, this implies that countries receiving travellers from Africa should have hospitals with specialized units for strict isolation and treatment of these patients.

PMID: 569288 [PubMed - indexed for MEDLINE]

2688. Dtsch Med Wochenschr. 1978 Jul 21;103(29):1176-81.

[Marburg, Lassa and Ebola virus as cause of hemorrhagic fever].

[Article in German]

Siegert R.

PMID: 352653 [PubMed - indexed for MEDLINE]

2689. Bol Oficina Sanit Panam. 1978 Jul;85(1):54-72.

[Infections by Marburg and Ebola viruses: guide for their diagnosis, treatment and control].

[Article in Spanish]

Simpson DI.

PMID: 150845 [PubMed - indexed for MEDLINE]

2690. J Pathol. 1978 Jul;125(3):131-8.

The pathology of experimental Ebola virus infection in monkeys.

Baskerville A, Bowen ET, Platt GS, McArdell LB, Simpson DI.

Six rhesus and two vervet monkeys were infected intraperitoneally with Ebola virus. They developed an acute haemorrhagic fever with skin rash 4 days later and died 6--12 days after infection. Histopathological lesions of acute necrosis were present in the liver, spleen, lymph nodes, lungs and testes. The presence of fibrin thrombi in several organs was suggestive of the occurrence of disseminated intravascular coagulation during the infection.

PMID: 102747 [PubMed - indexed for MEDLINE]

2691. J Clin Pathol. 1978 Mar;31(3):201-8.

Ultrastructure of Ebola virus particles in human liver.

Ellis DS, Simpson IH, Francis DP, Knobloch J, Bowen ET, Lolik P, Deng IM.

Electron microscopy of tissues from two necropsies carried out in the Sudan on patients with Ebola virus infection identified virus particles in lung and spleen, but the main concentrations of Ebola particles were seen in liver sections. Viral precursor proteins and cores were found in functional liver cells, often aligned in membrane-bound aggregations. Complete virions, usually found only extracellularly, were mainly seen as long tubular forms, some without cores. Many tubular forms had 'enlarged heads' or 'spores' and some branched and torus forms were identified. The size and structure of the Ebola virus forms appear to be virtually indistinguishable from those of Marburg virus.

PMCID: PMC1145228 PMID: 641193 [PubMed - indexed for MEDLINE]

2692. J Infect Dis. 1978 Mar;137(3):298-308.

Isolation of the etiologic agent of Korean Hemorrhagic fever.

Lee HW, Lee PW, Johnson KM.

Lung tissues from 73 rodents (Apodemus agrarius coreae) gave specific immunofluorescent reactions when they reacted with sera from patients convalescing from Korean hemorrhagic fever. Similar staaining was observed in the lungs of A. agrarius inoculated with acute-phase sera obtained from two patients with this disease. The unidentified agent was successfully propagated in adult A. agrarius through eight passages representing a cumulative dilution of greater than 10(-17). Experimentally inoculated rodents developed specific fluorescent antigen in the lung, kidney, liver, parotid glands, and bladder. Organs, especially lungs, were positive beginning 10 days and continuing through 69 days after inoculation. The agent could not be cultivated in several types of cell cultures nor in laboratory animals. No fluorescence was observed when infected A. agrarius lung tissues were reacted with antisera to Marburg virus, Ebola virus, and serval arenaviruses. Diagnostic increases in immunofluorescent antibodies occurred in 113 of 116 severe and 11 of 34 milder cases of clinically suspected Korean hemorrhagic fever. Antibodies were present during the first week of symptoms, reached a peak at the end of the second week, and persisted for up to 14 years. Convalescent-phase sera from four persons suffering a similar disease in the Soviet Union were also positive for antibodies.

PMID: 24670 [PubMed - indexed for MEDLINE]

2693. Can Med Assoc J. 1978 Feb 18;118(4):347-8, 350.

Lassa, Marburg and Ebola: newly described African fevers.

Seah SK.

PMCID: PMC1817968 PMID: 564739 [PubMed - indexed for MEDLINE]

2694. Bull World Health Organ. 1978;56(6):819-32.

Viral haemorrhagic fevers of man.

Simpson DI.

This article reviews the current state of knowledge on the viral haemorrhagic fevers that infect man, namely smallpox, chikungunya fever, dengue fever, Rift Valley fever, yellow fever, Crimean haemorrhagic fever, Kyasanur Forest disease, Omsk haemorrhagic fever, Argentinian haemorrhagic fever (Junin virus), Bolivian haemorrhagic fever (Machupo virus), Lassa fever, haemorrhagic fever with renal syndrome, and Marburg and Ebola virus diseases.

PMCID: PMC2395691 PMID: 310725 [PubMed - indexed for MEDLINE]

2695. Bull World Health Organ. 1978;56(2):271-93.

Ebola haemorrhagic fever in Zaire, 1976.

[No authors listed]

Between 1 September and 24 October 1976, 318 cases of acute viral haemorrhagic fever occurred in northern Zaire. The outbreak was centred in the Bumba Zone of the Equateur Region and most of the cases were recorded within a radius of 70 km of Yambuku, although a few patients sought medical attention in Bumba, Abumombazi, and the capital city of Kinshasa, where individual secondary and tertiary cases occurred. There were 280 deaths, and only 38 serologically confirmed survivors.The index case in this outbreak had onset of symptoms on 1 September 1976, five days after receiving an injection of chloroquine for presumptive malaria at the outpatient clinic at Yambuku Mission Hospital (YMH). He had a clinical remission of his malaria symptoms. Within one week several other persons who had received injections at YMH also suffered from Ebola haemorrhagic fever, and almost all subsequent cases had either received injections at the hospital or had had close contact with another case. Most of these occurred during the first four weeks of the epidemic, after which time the hospital was closed, 11 of the 17 staff members having died of the disease. All ages and both sexes were affected, but women 15-29 years of age had the highest incidence of disease, a phenomenon strongly related to attendance at prenatal and outpatient clinics at the hospital where they received injections. The overall secondary attack rate was about 5%, although it ranged to 20% among close relatives such as spouses, parent or child, and brother or sister.Active surveillance disclosed that cases occurred in 55 of some 550 villages which were examined house-by-house. The disease was hitherto unknown to the people of the affected region. Intensive search for cases in the area of north-eastern Zaire between the Bumba Zone and the Sudan frontier near Nzara and Maridi failed to detect definite evidence of a link between an epidemic of the disease in that country and the outbreak near Bumba. Nevertheless it was established that people can and do make the trip between Nzara and Bumba in not more than four days; thus it was regarded as quite possible that an infected person had travelled from Sudan to Yambuku and transferred the virus to a needle of the hospital while receiving an injection at the outpatient clinic.Both the incubation period, and the duration of the clinical disease averaged about one week. After 3-4 days of non-specific symptoms and signs, patients typically experienced progressively severe sore throat, developed a maculopapular rash, had intractable abdominal pain, and began to bleed from multiple sites, principally the gastrointestinal tract. Although laboratory determinations were limited and not conclusive, it was concluded that pathogenesis of the disease included non-icteric hepatitis and possibly acute pancreatitis as well as disseminated intravascular coagulation.This syndrome was caused by a virus morphologically similar to Marburg virus, but immunologically distinct. It was named Ebola virus. The agent was isolated from the blood of 8 of 10 suspected cases using Vero cell cultures. Titrations of serial specimens obtained from one patient disclosed persistent viraemia of 10(6.5)-10(4.5) infectious units from the third day of illness until death on the eighth day. Ebola virus particles were found in formalin-

PMCID: PMC2395567 PMID: 307456 [PubMed - indexed for MEDLINE]

2696. Bull World Health Organ. 1978;56(2):247-70.

Ebola haemorrhagic fever in Sudan, 1976. Report of a WHO/International Study Team.

[No authors listed]

A large outbreak of haemorrhagic fever (subsequently named Ebola haemorrhagic fever) occurred in southern Sudan between June and November 1976. There was a total of 284 cases; 67 in the source town of Nzara, 213 in Maridi, 3 in Tembura, and 1 in Juba. The outbreak in Nzara appears to have originated in the workers of a cotton factory. The disease in Maridi was amplified by transmission in a large, active hospital. Transmission of the disease required close contact with an acute case and was usually associated with the act of nursing a patient. The incubation period was between 7 and 14 days. Although the link was not well established, it appears that Nzara could have been the source of infection for a similar outbreak in the Bumba Zone of Zaire.In this outbreak Ebola haemorrhagic fever was a unique clinical disease with a high mortality rate (53% overall) and a prolonged recovery period in those who survived. Beginning with an influenza-like syndrome, including fever, headache, and joint and muscle pains, the disease soon caused diarrhoea (81%), vomiting (59%), chest pain (83%), pain and dryness of the throat (63%), and rash (52%). Haemorrhagic manifestations were common (71%), being present in half of the recovered cases and in almost all the fatal cases.Two post mortems were carried out on patients in November 1976. The histopathological findings resembled those of an acute viral infection and although the features were characteristic they were not exclusively diagnostic. They closely resembled the features described in Marburg virus infection, with focal eosinophilic necrosis in the liver and destruction of lymphocytes and their replacement by plasma cells. One case had evidence of renal tubular necrosis.Two strains of Ebola virus were isolated from acute phase sera collected from acutely ill patients in Maridi hospital during the investigation in November 1976. Antibodies to Ebola virus were detected by immunofluorescence in 42 of 48 patients in Maridi who had been diagnosed clinically, but in only 6 of 31 patients in Nzara. The possibility of the indirect immunofluorescent test not being sufficiently sensitive is discussed.Of Maridi case contacts, in hospital and in the local community, 19% had antibodies. Very few of them gave any history of illness, indicating that Ebola virus can cause mild or even subclinical infections. Of the cloth room workers in the Nzara cotton factory, 37% appeared to have been infected, suggesting that the factory may have been the prime source of infection.

PMCID: PMC2395561 PMID: 307455 [PubMed - indexed for MEDLINE]

2697. Bull World Health Organ. 1978;56(2):245.

[The epidemic of Ebola haemorrhagic fever in Sudan and Zaire, 1976: introductory note].

Brès P.

PMCID: PMC2395566 PMID: 307454 [PubMed - indexed for MEDLINE]

2698. Trans R Soc Trop Med Hyg. 1978;72(2):188-91.

Ebola haemorrhagic fever: experimental infection of monkeys.

Bowen ET, Platt GS, Simpson DI, McArdell LB, Raymond RT.

Experimental infection of rhesus and vervet monkeys with Ebola virus produced a uniformly fatal illness. The course of the disease resembled that found in man with weight loss, anorexia, fever, haemorrhages and skin rash being frequently seen. Viraemia was obvious within two days of infection and persisted until death which occurred between days five and eight. Virus was found in high concentrations in several organs but particularly in the liver, spleen, and lungs.

PMID: 418537 [PubMed - indexed for MEDLINE]

2699. Disasters. 1977 Dec;1(4):309-14. doi: 10.1111/j.1467-7717.1977.tb00049.x.

Haemorrhagic Fever in Africa due to marburg-ebola viruses.

Draper CC(1).

Author information: (1)London School of Hygiene and Tropical Medicine.

PMID: 20958370 [PubMed]

2700. Br Med J. 1977 Aug 27;2(6086):559-61.

Negative-pressure plastic isolator for patients with dangerous infections.

Trexler PC, Emond RT, Evans B.

A negative-pressure plastic isolator is effective for dealing with patients suffering from dangerous infections. So far it has been used to treat seven patients suspected of having infections due to Lassa, Marburg, or Ebola viruses. One patient spent 32 days in the isolator. The isolator was proved comfortable and acceptable to patients, and it gives the nursing and medical attendants a high degree of protection. All routine nursing and medical procedures can be carried out with minimal interference by the physical barrier, though it is not practicable to undertake artificial respiration or haemodialysis.

PMCID: PMC1631473 PMID: 890419 [PubMed - indexed for MEDLINE]
2701. Br Med J. 1977 Aug 27;2(6086):541-4.

A case of Ebola virus infection.

Emond RT, Evans B, Bowen ET, Lloyd G.

In November 1976 an investigator at the Microbiological Research Establishment accidentally inoculated himself while processing material from patients in Africa who had been suffering from a haemorrhagic fever of unknown cause. He developed an illness closely resembling Marburg disease, and a virus was isolated from his blood that resembled Marburg virus but was distinct serologically. The course of the illness was mild and may have been modified by treatment with human interferon and convalescent serum. Convalescence was protracted; there was evidence of bone-marrow depression and virus was excreted in low titre for some weeks. Recovery was complete. Infection was contained by barrier-nursing techniques using a negative-pressure plastic isolator and infection did not spread to attendant staff or to the community.

PMCID: PMC1631428 PMID: 890413 [PubMed - indexed for MEDLINE]
2702. Br Med J. 1977 Aug 27;2(6086):539-40.

Ebola virus infectons.

[No authors listed]
PMCID: PMC1631468 PMID: 890411 [PubMed - indexed for MEDLINE]
2703. Lancet. 1977 Mar 12;1(8011):581-2.

After Marburg, Ebola.

[No authors listed]
PMID: 65668 [PubMed - indexed for MEDLINE]